KU-522-908

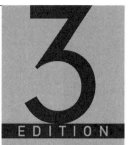

3
EDITION

The Handbook of Health Behavior Change

Sally A. Shumaker, PhD, is a tenured Professor in Public Health Sciences —Social Sciences and Health Policy, Senior Associate Dean for Research, and Co-Director of the Translational Science Institute. She received her PhD in Social Psychology from the University of Michigan and completed postdoctoral training in environmental and health psychology from the University of California, at Irvine and Los Angeles, respectively. Dr. Shumaker's research is by nature interdisciplinary and translational, and she has worked with scientists from throughout the world representing a range of health, basic, and social/behavioral science disciplines. In addition to her senior leadership roles, she has an active research portfolio and is the recipient of a number of grants and contracts from the NIH, Foundations and Industry. Dr. Shumaker has written more than 200 journal articles, books, and chapters in the areas of cognitive aging and dementia, disability, HRQL, adherence, and psychosocial factors in disease progression. She holds Fellow status in several professional organizations and is the former president and current secretary-treasurer of an international public policy association. Dr. Shumaker has received national awards in mentoring, behavioral health science, research, and leadership training.

Judith K. Ockene, PhD, MEd, MA, is a tenured Professor of Medicine and Chief of the Division of Preventive and Behavioral Medicine in the Department of Medicine at the University of Massachusetts Medical School (UMMS). She holds the Barbara Helen Smith Chair in Preventive and Behavioral Medicine and is Interim Vice Provost for Faculty Affairs at UMMS. Dr. Ockene is the recipient of numerous NIH grants funding research in the prevention of illness and disability and the promotion of health and quality of life for individuals and communities. Much of her research now focuses on women's health affecting morbidity, mortality, and quality of life in older women. Dr. Ockene teaches medical and public health students, residents in training, community physicians, and a variety of other health care providers how to help patients make lifestyle changes for the prevention and control of disease and adaptation to illness. Dr. Ockene's work is at the intersection of clinical medicine and public health. She has more than 150 publications in preventive and behavioral medicine.

Kristin A. Riekert, PhD, is an Assistant Professor of Medicine in the Division of Pulmonary and Critical Care Medicine, Department of Medicine at The Johns Hopkins University and Co-Director of the Johns Hopkins Adherence Research Center (JHARC). The JHARC serves as a national advisory center on the assessment of adherence in clinical trials and conducts ongoing studies of adherence assessment and promotion. Dr. Riekert received her PhD in Clinical Psychology from Case Western Reserve University where she specialized in pediatric psychology. She completed postdoctoral training in health psychology at The Johns Hopkins University. Dr. Riekert is the Principal Investigator or Co-Principal Investigator of several NH and foundation sponsored intervention trials focused on improving adherence and health outcomes in cystic fibrosis and asthma. Dr. Riekert's primary areas of research interest are: psychosocial predictors of adherence in pediatric chronic illness, measurement of adherence, development of culturally and developmentally appropriate interventions to improve adherence, developmental aspects of transitioning responsibility for health behaviors and care, patient-reported outcome methodology, health care disparities, and doctor-patient communication.

The Handbook of Health Behavior Change

3 EDITION

Sally A. Shumaker, PhD

Judith K. Ockene, PhD, MEd, MA

Kristin A. Riekert, PhD

Editors

SPRINGER PUBLISHING COMPANY

New York

Copyright © 2009 Springer Publishing Company, LLC

All rights reserved.

No part of this publication may be reproduced, stored in a retrieval system, or transmitted in any form or by any means, electronic, mechanical, photocopying, recording, or otherwise, without the prior permission of Springer Publishing Company, LLC.

Springer Publishing Company, LLC
11 West 42nd Street
New York, NY 10036
www.springerpub.com

Acquisitions Editor: Sheri W. Sussman
Production Editor: Julia Rosen
Cover design: Joanne E. Honigman
Composition: Apex CoVantage

   09 10 11 12/5 4 3 2

Library of Congress Cataloging-in-Publication Data

The handbook of health behavior change / Sally A. Shumaker, Judith K. Ockene, Kristin A. Riekert, editors.–3rd ed.
     p. ; cm.
   Includes bibliographical references and index.
   ISBN 978-0-8261-1545-4 (alk. paper)
  1. Health behavior.   2. Health attitudes.   3. Self-care, Health.   4. Behavior modification.   I. Shumaker, Sally A.   II. Ockene, Judith K.   III. Riekert, Kristin A.
     [DNLM: 1. Health Promotion.   2. Behavior Therapy.   3. Health Behavior.
4. Patient Compliance.   WA 590 H2356 2008]
   RA776.9.H36   2008
   613–dc22   2008024564

Printed in the United States of America by Hamilton Printing Company.

The author and the publisher of this Work have made every effort to use sources believed to be reliable to provide information that is accurate and compatible with the standards generally accepted at the time of publication. The author and publisher shall not be liable for any special, consequential, or exemplary damages resulting, in whole or in part, from the readers' use of, or reliance on, the information contained in this book.

The publisher has no responsibility for the persistence or accuracy of URLs for external or third-party Internet Web sites referred to in this publication and does not guarantee that any content on such Web sites is, or will remain, accurate or appropriate.

This book is dedicated to all of the people who work hard to maintain a healthy lifestyle in the midst of multiple personal, social and cultural challenges—and to all the health care professionals who work hard to help their patients succeed in meeting the challenges of healthy living.

Contents

Tables and Figures

Section V

Section VI

Chapter 34

Chapter 35

Section VII

Chapter 36

Contributors

David B. Abrams, PhD
Office of the Director
National Institutes of Health
Bethesda, MD

Barbara E. Ainsworth, PhD, MPH
Department of Exercise and Wellness
Arizona State University
Mesa, AZ

David G. Altman, PhD
Center for Creative Leadership
Greensboro, NC

Bettina M. Beech, DrPH
Division of Internal Medicine and Public
  Health
Vanderbilt University School of
  Medicine
Nashville, TN

Ronny A. Bell, PhD, MS
Department of Epidemiology and
  Prevention
Division of Public Health Sciences
Maya Angelou Research Center on
  Minority Health
Wake Forest University School of
  Medicine
Winston-Salem, NC

Beth C. Bock, PhD
Department of Psychiatry and Human
  Behavior
Centers for Behavioral and Preventive
  Medicine
Brown Medical School and
  The Miriam Hospital
Providence, RI

Jamie S. Bodenlos, PhD
Division of Preventive and Behavioral
  Medicine
Department of Medicine
University of Massachusetts Medical
  School
Worcester, MA

Uli Boehmer, PhD
Social and Behavioral Sciences
  Department
School of Public Health
Boston University
Boston, MA

Viktor E. Bovbjerg, MPH, PhD
Department of Public Health Sciences
University of Virginia School of Medicine
Charlottesville, VA

Deborah J. Bowen, PhD
Social and Behavioral Sciences Department
School of Public Health
Boston University
Boston, MA

Suzanne B. Cashman, ScD
Department of Family Medicine and
  Community Health
University of Massachusetts Medical
  School
Worcester, MA

David Cella, PhD
Center on Outcomes, Research, and
  Education
Evanston Northwestern Healthcare
  and Northwestern University Feinberg
  School of Medicine
Evanston, IL

Margaret A. Chesney, PhD
National Center for Complementary and
   Alternative Medicine
National Institutes of Health
Bethesda, MD

Joseph T. Ciccolo, PhD
Department of Psychiatry and Human
   Behavior
Centers for Behavioral and Preventive
   Medicine
Brown Medical School and
   The Miriam Hospital
Providence, RI

Noreen M. Clark, PhD
Center for Managing Chronic Disease
University of Michigan
Ann Arbor, MI

**Emmanuelle Clerisme-Beaty, MD,
MHS**
Division of Pulmonary and Critical
   Care Medicine
The Johns Hopkins University
Baltimore, MD

Laura H. Coker, PhD
Department of Social Sciences and
   Health Policy
Division of Public Health Sciences
Wake Forest University School of Medicine
Winston-Salem, NC

Mark R. Conaway, PhD
Division of Biostatistics and
   Epidemiology
Department of Public Health
University of Virginia Health Systems
Charlottesville, VA

Susan J. Curry, PhD
Institute for Health Research and Policy
University of Illinois at Chicago
Chicago, IL

Susan M. Czajkowski, PhD
Clinical Applications and Prevention Branch
Division of Prevention and Population
   Sciences
National Heart, Lung, and Blood Institute
National Institutes of Health
Bethesda, MD

Michael A. Dawes, MD
Neurobehavioral Research Laboratory
   and Clinic
University of Texas Health Science
   Center at San Antonio
San Antonio, TX

Judith DePue, EdD, MPH
Centers for Behavioral and Preventive
   Medicine
The Miriam Hospital/Brown Medical
   School
Providence, RI

M. Robin DiMatteo, PhD
Department of Psychology
University of California,
   Riverside
Riverside, CA

Katherine Dodd, MPH
Division of Geriatric Medicine
University of Massachusetts Medical
   School and
The Meyers Primary Care
   Institute
Worcester, MA

Donald M. Dougherty, PhD
Neurobehavioral Research Laboratory
   and Clinic
University of Texas Health Science
   Center at San Antonio
San Antonio, TX

Elizabeth Dugan, PhD
Division of Geriatric Medicine
University of Massachusetts Medical
   School and
The Meyers Primary Care
   Institute
Worcester, MA

**Jacqueline Dunbar-Jacob, PhD, RN,
FAAN**
School of Nursing
Pittsburgh, PA

Shellie Ellis, MA
Translational Science Institute
Wake Forest University School of
   Medicine
Winston-Salem, NC

Beth M. Ewy, MPH, CHES
Center for Tobacco Treatment Research
  and Training
Division of Preventive and Behavioral
  Medicine
University of Massachusetts Medical
  School
Worcester, MA

Ramesh Farzanfar, PhD
Medical Information Systems Unit
Boston University Medical Center
Boston, MA

Marian L. Fitzgibbon, PhD
Institute for Health Research
  and Policy
University of Illinois at Chicago
Chicago, IL

Laurie G. Forlano, DO, MPH
Department of Family Medicine and
  Community Health
University of Massachusetts
Worcester, MA

**Patricia D. Franklin, MD,
MPH, MBA**
Department of Orthopedics and Physical
  Rehabilitation
University of Massachusetts Medical
  Center
Worcester, MA

Elizabeth Galik, PhD, CRNP
University of Maryland School
  of Nursing
Baltimore, MD

Leigh A. Gemmell, PhD
VA Pittsburgh Healthcare System
Pittsburgh, PA

William H. George, PhD
Department of Psychology
University of Washington
Seattle, WA

Michael G. Goldstein, MD
Clinical Education and Research
Institute for Healthcare
  Communication
New Haven, CT

Neil E. Grunberg, PhD
Department of Medical and Clinical
  Psychology
Uniformed Services University of the
  Health Sciences
University of the Health Sciences
Bethesda, MD

Kelly B. Haskard, PhD
Department of Psychology
Texas State University
San Marcos, TX

Laura L. Hayman, PhD
Nursing College of Nursing and Health
  Sciences
University of Massachusetts-Boston
Boston, MA

Christian S. Hendershot, MS
Department of Psychology
University of Washington
Seattle, WA

**Kenneth C. Hergenrather, PhD,
MSEd, MRC**
Department of Counseling Human and
  Organizational Studies
Graduate School of Education and
  Human Development
The George Washington University
Washington, D.C.

Christina K. Holub, MPH
Department of Health Behavior and
  Health Education
University of North Carolina at Chapel
  Hill
Chapel Hill, NC

Christy R. Houle, MPH
Center for Managing Chronic Disease
University of Michigan
Ann Arbor, MI

Carolyn E. Ievers-Landis, PhD
Division of Behavioral Pediatrics and
  Psychology
Rainbow Babies and Children's
  Hospital
Case Western Reserve University School
  of Medicine
Cleveland, OH

Kathleen Insel, RN, PhD
Division of Nursing Practice
University of Arizona
Tucson, AZ

Christine Jackson, PhD
Public Health and Environment
RTI International
Research Triangle Park, NC

Sharon A. Jackson, PhD
Northrop Grumman
Division of Heart Disease and Stroke
    Prevention
National Center for Chronic Disease
    Prevention and Health Promotion
Centers for Disease Control and Prevention
Atlanta, GA

Sara Johnson, PhD
Pro-Change Behavior Systems, Inc.
West Kingston, RI

Denise G. Jolicoeur, MPH, CHES
Division of Preventive and Behavioral
    Medicine
University of Massachusetts Medical School
Worcester, MA

Jon Kabat-Zinn, PhD
Department of Medicine (Emeritus)
Center for Mindfulness in Medicine,
    Health Care, and Society
University of Massachusetts Medical School
Worcester, MA

Robert M. Kaplan, PhD
Department of Health Services
UCLA School of Public Health
Los Angeles, CA

Alessandra N. Kazura, MD
Center for Tobacco Independence
    Maine Health
Portland, ME

Nancy M. P. King, JD
Department of Social Sciences and
    Health Policy
Wake Forest University School of
    Medicine
Winston-Salem, NC

Teresa K. King, PhD
Department of Psychology
Bridgewater State College
Bridgewater, MA

Laura Cousino Klein, PhD
Department of Biobehavioral Health
Pennsylvania State University
University Park, PA

Claire A. Lane, PhD
Cardiff University
Nursing, Health and Social Care
    Research Center
Cardiff, UK

Patricia Lee, MA
University of Alabama at Birmingham
School of Public Health
Birmingham, AL

Kismet A. Loftin-Bell, MALS, MSL
Department of Epidemiology and
    Prevention
Wake Forest University School of
    Medicine
Winston-Salem, NC

Bess H. Marcus, PhD
Department of Community Health and
    Psychiatry and Human Behavior
Brown University
Providence, RI

G. Alan Marlatt, PhD
Department of Psychology
University of Washington
Seattle, WA

Barbara S. McCann, PhD
Department of Psychiatry and Behavioral
    Sciences
University of Washington School of
    Medicine
Seattle, WA

Kathleen Michael, PhD, CCRN
Baltimore Veterans Administration
    Medical Center Geriatrics Research
Education and Clinical Center
University of Maryland School
    of Nursing
Baltimore, MD

Michael E. Miller, PhD
Department of Biostatistical Sciences
Wake Forest University School of
  Medicine
Winston-Salem, NC

David L. Mount, PsyD, MA
Department of Internal Medicine
Maya Angelou Research Center on
  Minority Health
Hypertension and Vascular Research
  Center
Wake Forest University School of
  Medicine
Winston-Salem, NC

Carolyn L. Murdaugh, RN, PhD, FAAN
Professor and Associate Dean for
  Research
University of Arizona
Tucson, AZ

Eun Shim Nahm, PhD, RN
University of Maryland School
  of Nursing
Baltimore, MD

Michelle J. Naughton, PhD
Department of Social Sciences and
  Health Policy
Wake Forest University School of
  Medicine
Winston-Salem, NC

Sylvain Nouvion, PhD
Department of Psychiatry and Behavioral
  Medicine
Wake Forest University School of
  Medicine
Winston-Salem, NC

Michiko Otsuki, PhD
Department of Psychology
University of South Florida,
  St. Petersburg
St. Petersburg, FL

Lori Pbert, PhD
Division of Preventive and Behavioral
  Medicine
University of Massachusetts Medical
  School
Worcester, MA

Amy H. Peterman, PhD
Department of Psychology
University of North Carolina at Charlotte
Charlotte, NC

James O. Prochaska, PhD
Cancer Prevention Research Center
University of Rhode Island
Kingston, RI

Janice M. Prochaska, PhD
Pro-Change Behavior Systems, Inc.
West Kingston, RI

Judith J. Prochaska, PhD, MPH
Department of Psychiatry
University of California, San Francisco
San Francisco, CA

Cynthia S. Rand, PhD
Department of Medicine
The Johns Hopkins University
Baltimore, MD

Michael A. Rapoff, PhD
Department of Pediatrics
University of Kansas Medical Center
Kansas City, KS

W. Jack Rejeski, PhD
Department of Health and Exercise Science
Wake Forest University
Winston-Salem, NC

Barbara Resnick, PhD, CRNP, FAAN, FAANP
Ziporkin Gershowitz Chair in
  Gerontological Nursing
University of Maryland School
  of Nursing
Baltimore, MD

Scott D. Rhodes, PhD, MPH
Department of Social Sciences and
  Health Policy
Wake Forest University School
  of Medicine
Winston-Salem, NC

Stephen Rollnick, PhD
Department of General Practice
Cardiff University
Centre for Health Sciences Research
Cardiff, UK

Milagros C. Rosal, PhD
Division of Preventive and Behavioral
  Medicine
Department of Medicine
University of Massachusetts Medical School
Worcester, MA

Paul G. Salmon, PhD
Department of Psychological and Brain
  Sciences
University of Louisville
Louisville, KY

Saki F. Santorelli, EdD, MA
Center for Mindfulness in Medicine,
  Health Care, and Society
Division of Preventive and Behavioral
  Medicine
Department of Medicine
University of Massachusetts Medical School
Worcester, MA

Elizabeth A. Schlenk, PhD, RN
School of Nursing
Pittsburgh, PA

Margaret Schneider, PhD
Department of Planning, Policy, and Design
School of Social Ecology
University of California
Irvine, CA

Sandra E. Sephton, PhD
Department of Psychological and Brain
  Sciences and James Graham Brown
  Cancer Center
University of Louisville
Louisville, KY

Marianne Shaughnessy, PhD
Baltimore Veterans Administration
  Medical Center Geriatrics Research
Education and Clinical Center
University of Maryland School of Nursing
Baltimore, MD

Ashley W. Smith, PhD, MPH
Outcomes Research Branch, Applied
  Research Program
Division of Cancer Control and
  Population Sciences
National Cancer Institute
National Institutes of Health
Bethesda, MD

Ralph L. Smith, PhD
Department of Pediatrics
University of Kansas Medical Center
Kansas City, KS

Daniel Stokols, PhD
Department of Planning, Policy, and
  Design
Department of Psychology and Social
  Behavior
School of Social Ecology
University of California
Irvine, CA

Deborah D. Thompson, PhD
USDA/ARS Children's Nutrition
  Research Center
Department of Pediatrics
Baylor College of Medicine
Houston, TX

David Victorson, PhD
Center on Outcomes, Research and
  Education
Evanston Northwestern Healthcare and
  Northwestern University Feinberg
  School of Medicine
Evanston, IL

Dori Whitehead, PhD
Department of Psychiatry and Human
  Behavior
Centers for Behavioral and Preventive
  Medicine
Brown Medical School and The Miriam
  Hospital
Providence, RI

Melicia C. Whitt-Glover, PhD
Department of Epidemiology and
  Prevention
Division of Public Health Sciences
Maya Angelou Research Center on
  Minority Health
Wake Forest University School of Medicine
Winston-Salem, NC

Sara Wilcox, PhD
Department of Exercise Science
Arnold School of Public Health
University of South Carolina
Columbia, SC

Aimee M. Wilkin, MD, MPH
Department of Internal Medicine
Wake Forest University School of Medicine
Winston-Salem, NC

Summer L. Williams, MA
Department of Psychology
University of California,
   Riverside
Riverside, CA

Dawn Witherspoon, MA
Department of Psychology
Case Western University
Cleveland, OH

Richard Wooldredge, MA
Northwest Care
   Consortium
Winston-Salem, NC

Preface

The first edition of this book was published in 1988, growing out of a recognition in medicine and public health that many acute and chronic diseases can be prevented or at least have their impact lessened by increased attention to the adoption and maintenance of behaviors for optimal health. This recognition evolved from the many epidemiologic investigations demonstrating the existence of a strong relationship among the onset, progression, and exacerbation of diseases and alteration of lifestyles, such as smoking cessation, developing healthy eating habits, taking medications as prescribed, increasing physical activity, and practicing safe sex. There was also increased awareness that for the adoption of healthy behaviors to occur and be sustained there were not only demands and responsibilities placed on the individual at risk. There were also demands placed on the health care system and its providers; on other channels within the community such as schools, worksites, and churches; and on the social and political context in which change occurs. That first edition included 24 chapters covering theory, lifestyle interventions, obstacles to change and adherence, population-specific issues, and what we then termed "the broader context."

More than 20 years later, a comparison of this third edition to the original provides a vivid view of just how much this field has grown and, to a lesser degree, how many challenges remain the same. There is no question that research on behavior change and adherence has become more central to clinical research and care—no longer a peripheral or add-on element but recognized as an essential part of the health and well-being of the public. Further, there is an increased recognition of just how complex the issue of behavior change and maintenance is, and how embedded this issue is in the entire fabric of a society—going far beyond the ability of a single individual to change his or her approach to preventive care and treatment. And yet people and their health professionals continue to struggle with achieving optimal lifestyles and adhering to the medical regimens and health behaviors that will minimize diseases and their impact. This book provides an updated and substantially expanded view of the theoretical and empirical literature on the factors that influence the adoption of healthy behaviors and the individual, interpersonal, social, and cultural factors that can inhibit or promote behavior change. In keeping with the evolution of this field, we have added a number of new chapters to fully reflect this important area of health research and care.

Chapters 1–9 in Section I of the book provide a review of past and current theoretical models of health behavior change, disease prevention, disease management, and relapse prevention. In addition, models of the maintenance of new behaviors are considered. Reviews are provided of some of the more current techniques used to enhance adherence are provided—such as motivational interviewing and shared decision-making.

Chapters 10–15, Section II, focus on a range of some of the more critical areas of health behaviors—providing updated reviews and the complexities of these specific lifestyle interventions among diverse patient populations. Health behaviors considered include tobacco use, diet, physical activity, safer sexual practices, and stress reduction. Recognizing that healthy lifestyles most often encompass multiple behaviors and are best considered within the context of their interdependence, the final chapter tackles the complexities of multiple risk behavior change.

In the earlier two editions of this book, measurement issues were addressed within other chapters or as a single chapter within a section as there was limited information on this topic at that time. As a further demonstration of the growth of this field, the current edition dedicates a full section to measurement. Chapters 16–19 in Section III review adherence assessment in both clinical care and research, assessing physical activity and substance abuse reliably, and some of the statistical issues addressed when measuring and analyzing adherence behavior in the research setting.

In Section IV, chapters 20–24 address the factors that predict or serve as obstacles to lifestyle change and adherence. Authors consider individual patient characteristics, biological and psychosocial factors, the social context, and the unique challenges associated in trying to change physician practices in clinical settings to be more congruent with best practices as they relate to health behavior recommendations. With the growing recognition of the multiple levels of influences—from intrapersonal to societal and policy—in determining behavior, all of the authors in this section ground their presentations in this broader and, admittedly, more complex view of behavior change and maintenance.

Chapters 25–29 in Section V consider the unique and similar issues associated with maintained behavior change within specific populations. Populations considered include: the young, the elderly, adults with cognitive impairments, and adolescents with chronic diseases. In addition, the final chapter addresses the complicated interrelationships among health disparities, minority status, and heath behavior change.

Medical regimen adherence is a major problem in clinical care and research. In Section VI (chapters 30–35), authors discuss the challenges associated with adhering to the often complicated health regimens faced by people with chronic diseases. These include patients with chronic obstructive pulmonary disease (COPD), diabetes, cancer, and HIV. In addition, chapter 34 looks at adherence issues among patients with multiple chronic diseases, while chapter 35 considers the role of cognition in adherence behavior among patients with type 2 diabetes.

In the final section of the book (chapters 36–40), authors consider the issues of behavior change and adherence within a broader context. The first chapter addresses the subtle interaction between placebo effects and adherence and the implications of this interaction for any behavior change believed by an individual to be health enhancing. In the second chapter, authors consider the value of social determinants of health coupled with community-based participatory research in realizing the full potential of achieving lasting lifestyle changes. The role of ethics is explored as it relates to the issue of adherence and how it is framed—particularly with respect to the clinical versus research setting. The final two chapters of the book ask two very different but critical issues that, in some ways, bring us back to the beginning: Does adherence matter? And, have we really learned anything in our years of research on this topic?

In total, this book represents an updated and thorough examination of the factors that influence people's choices to change their behaviors in order to enhance their health, and the intrapersonal, interpersonal, sociocultural, and policy factors that can both positively and negatively affect the choices made and one's ability to achieve a desired behavior. This book is particularly valuable at the graduate student level in the fields of public or population health, health psychology, health communications, and medical sociology and anthropology. In addition, advanced-level undergraduate students in or population health-related courses within the social sciences will find this of value. The content of this book will also be informative to clinical investigators, behavioral and social scientists, and practitioners who grapple with the issues confronting individuals who must make well-informed decisions regarding their health-related behaviors, change many difficult health habits, and adopt new behaviors.

Acknowledgments

The editors kindly acknowledge the following individuals who contributed to making this new edition possible:

Sonya Ashburn, Assistant to the Editors, *The Handbook of Health Behavior Change* (3rd ed.)

The following people provided content expertise in reviewing chapters in *The Handbook of Health Behavior Change* (3rd ed.):

Michiko Otsuki, PhD

Stephenie Lemon, PhD

Sherry Pagoto, PhD

Roger Luckmann, PhD

Milagros Rosal, PhD

Jacki Hecht, RN, MSN

Gbenga Ogedegbe, MD, MPH, MS

Jamie Bodenlos, PhD

Karen Potvin Klein, MA, ELS (Wake Forest University School of Medicine) provided proofreading and editorial assistance.

Health Behavior
Change and
Maintenance:
Theory and
Techniques

Section
1

Judith K. Ockene
Editor

Chapters in Section I provide a detailed review of a wide variety of theories of behavior change addressing cognitive, interpersonal, social, and cultural factors that are proposed to have an effect on an individual's behavior and change of those behaviors. Section I also includes chapters that address specific strategies that help facilitate behavior change.

Theories attempt to explain cause-effect relationships and help to provide a basis for understanding and predicting behavior, behavior change, and maintenance; for developing interventions to achieve changes in health-risk behaviors; and for evaluating the outcomes of the interventions. No single theory is all-encompassing.

The first chapter in Section I, by Curry and Fitzgibbon, provides "Theories of Prevention" that the authors posit is needed to close the "gap between what we can achieve and what we do achieve for disease prevention." The second chapter, by Clark and Houle, "Theoretical Models and Strategies for Improving Disease Management by Patients," reviews several models and theories that have been used to address adherence in self-management of health and disease. Other chapters present the transtheoretical model of behavior change, multilevel theories of behavior change, and models of provider-patient interaction and shared decision-making. Chapters addressing techniques for health behavior change and maintenance also are included. The techniques include intervention for relapse prevention and maintenance, motivational interviewing, and e-health strategies to support adherence. There also is a chapter on the influence of culture on behavior.

Even though there are many theories and models available, there is still much we have not been able to explain or prove about why and how people make changes in health-risk behaviors and, just as importantly, maintain those changes. To fill in the black box of behavior change, we must be able to move outside the box. Theories can be used to guide us but should not constrain our creativity. We must be open to integrating, expanding, and testing our theories in order to expand our base of knowledge and to using what we learn from practice to alter our theories.

Theories of Prevention

1

Susan J. Curry and
Marian L. Fitzgibbon

At the beginning of the 20th century, the three leading causes of death were pneumonia/influenza, tuberculosis, and gastritis. These three diseases accounted for more than a third of all deaths at the time (Brownson & Bright, 2004). Advances in microbiology formed the foundation for infectious disease prevention during the first half of the 20th century. Following Koch's work in the late 1800s on the anthrax bacillus showing how bacteria could cause disease, numerous pathogenic organisms were discovered, and the germ theory of prevention emerged as a driving force in medicine and public health (Bullough & Rosen, 1992). Some prevention efforts were derived from advances in the biomedical sciences after the discovery that antibodies from infected organisms could be used to inoculate healthy individuals against pathogen-borne diseases. By identifying environmental sources of exposure to disease-causing bacteria, the germ theory of prevention also spurred wide-scale investments in the public health infrastructure to create healthier environments (e.g., clean water, better sanitation, improved nutrition).

The success of interventions derived from the germ theory of prevention were evident by the mid-20th century. By 1951, death rates from infectious diseases had fallen dramatically, and increases in life expectancy also were evident. In 1900, average life expectancy at birth was 46 years for males and 48 years for females. By 1950, life expectancy had increased to 66 and 71 years, respectively (National Center for Health Statistics, 2006).

Currently, heart disease, cancer, and stroke are the leading causes of death, and they account for approximately two-thirds of all deaths (Brownson & Bright, 2004; Brownson, Remington, & Davis, 1998). The shift from infectious to chronic diseases as major causes of premature morbidity and mortality necessitated a shift in theories of prevention. Chronic diseases, in contrast to infectious diseases, are characterized by a noncontagious origin, a long period of illness or disability, a prolonged latency period between exposure to the risk factors and negative health outcome, and multiple risk-factor etiology (McKenna, Taylor, Marks, & Koplan, 1998).

Three tenets of this chapter are that (1) a significant proportion of premature morbidity and mortality from chronic disease is preventable; (2) there is a substantial gap between what we can achieve and what we do achieve for disease prevention; and (3) closing this gap may be facilitated by a simple and clearly articulated "health behavior theory of prevention."

What do we mean by a health behavior theory of prevention? Let's start with what we mean by theory. First, there is nothing magical or mystical about theory. It is simply a statement about causal relationships. The validity of these causal relationships may or may not be *conclusively* proven (Deutsch & Krause, 1965). Theories of prevention, therefore, are statements about causal relationships between exposures or risk factors and disease incidence (primary prevention) and progression (secondary prevention). Given our focus on health behavior, we can narrow this definition further by defining a health behavior theory of prevention as statements about causal relationships between health behaviors and disease incidence and progression.

Prevention theory enhances our work as scientists and practitioners in many ways. Theory helps us build the science of prevention by directing our hypotheses and research questions and informs the selection of appropriate populations to study. Ultimately, theories of prevention determine intervention approaches including individual treatments, models of health care delivery, public health practice, and health policy.

In the years following World War II, epidemiologists began to focus on the etiology of chronic diseases, particularly lung cancer and coronary heart disease (CHD) (Susser, 1985; White, 1990). The epidemiological evidence for an association between cigarette smoking and lung cancer initially received the most attention as a behavioral risk factor, because it posed a challenge to a large and powerful industry that was then perceived to be invulnerable (Glantz, Slade, Bero, Hanauer, & Barnes, 1996; Kluger, 1996). Early studies that suggested this association encountered numerous objections. The objections resulted, in part, from the fact that the conclusions were based on statistical correlations from observational studies, which could never in themselves prove causation, and the fact that cigarette smoking as a single behavior was linked to a large number of chronic disease outcomes (Berkson, 1958; Doll, 1999). However, strong and consistent evidence for the association continued to emerge from laboratory studies and autopsy reports, as well as from observational studies. In 1957, a national scientific study group concluded that there was a causal relationship between smoking and cancer (Study Group on Smoking and Health, 1957). However, the tobacco industry and some scientists continued to argue that none of the studies had actually demonstrated a causal relationship. Their response contributed inadvertently to an overdue expansion in methodological rigor in the fields of statistics and epidemiology and a related increase in our understanding of how epidemiologic research can support laboratory studies and clinical research (Cornfield et al., 1959). Ultimately, there was consensus that this groundbreaking research had demonstrated that tobacco use, particularly cigarette smoking, causes or contributes to a number of chronic diseases (Parascandola, 2004; Talley, Kushner, & Sterk, 2004; White, 1990).

These first epidemiologic studies conducted in the 1940s and 1950s led an advisory committee to the U.S. Surgeon General to conclude that cigarette smoking was a cause of lung and laryngeal cancer and the primary cause of chronic bronchitis (Surgeon General, 1964). This information ultimately culminated in the Surgeon General's Report on smoking and health and led to a number of advances, including increased research into the development of chronic disease and tobacco use, evaluation of prevention and cessation programs, campaigns to reduce or prevent smoking, and the dissemination of this information to the public (Brownson & Bright, 2004).

On a related but somewhat different pathway, researchers began to think in terms of "risk factors" for the development of coronary heart disease, with the idea that certain behaviors moderated the probability of disease. For example, in the 1940s, the Framingham Heart Study was launched as a major, prospective epidemiological study to determine the major risk factors for heart disease. The study identified six major risk factors, including hypertension, elevated blood lipids, cigarette smoking, sedentary lifestyle, obesity, and diabetes (Bullough & Rosen, 1992). The concept of "risk factors" forced researchers to think of chronic disease as the outcome of multiple factors and required a strategic change in thinking about chronic diseases and their complications as being preventable rather than inevitable (Brownson & Bright, 2004). In other words, a reduction in chronic disease could best be achieved by altering factors that place a person at increased risk. Burgeoning research in this area has led to a better understanding of the tremendous influence that certain behaviors can exert upon health.

By 1979 the Surgeon General's Report on Health Promotion and Disease Prevention noted that an analysis of the 10 leading causes of death in the United States in 1976 indicated that as much as half of mortality was due to unhealthy behavior or lifestyle (U.S. Department of Health Education and Welfare, 1979). The health behavior theory of disease prevention had emerged.

Disease Prevention Through Health Behavior Change

In 1993, McGinnis and Foege published an analysis of the actual causes of death in the United States (McGinnis & Foege, 1993). They showed that tobacco use, unhealthy diet and activity patterns, and alcohol use are the top three actual causes of death in the United States. Together these health behaviors account for nearly 40% of all deaths. Extrapolating from their data, each hour, we can conclude that as many as 85 Americans die prematurely due to tobacco use, poor nutrition, and inactivity.

In addition to the devastating human costs, the health care costs associated with treating chronic diseases are staggering. The combined total of private, public, and personal dollars spent on health care in the United States is almost $2 trillion dollars per year, which amounts to more than 15% of our gross domestic product (GDP) (Heffler et al., 2005). No other industrialized nation spends more than 10% of its GDP on health care. Fries and colleagues estimated that preventable illnesses were responsible for 70% of all medical care spending, and health insurance claims are higher for individuals with at least one behavioral risk factor than for individuals with no behavioral risk factors (Fries et al., 1993; Millman & Robertson Inc., 1995). Unfortunately, spending all of this money does not lead to better health outcomes. The United States ranks behind 44 other countries in life expectancy and 41 countries in infant mortality (Central Intelligence Agency, 2007). In a recent study, out of 13 countries studied, the United States ranked 12th when compared on 16 health indicators (Starfield, 2000).

Disease prevention is not new, and links between behavior and prevention have been articulated for thousands of years. For example, traditional Chinese medicine's (TCM) focus on prevention dates back more than 2,500 years and recommends eating healthful foods, engaging in physical labor, and doing breathing exercises (Selin, 2003). More than 2,000 years ago, Hippocrates (c. 460–377 B.C.) taught that "If we could give every individual the right amount of nourishment and exercise, not too little and not too much, we would have found the safest way to health." The following sections focus on the evidence for three behavioral risk factors for a number of chronic diseases: tobacco use, unhealthy diets, and physical inactivity.

The Top Three Behavioral Risk Factors

Tobacco Use

Tobacco use remains the leading cause of preventable morbidity and mortality in the United States and is responsible for more than 30% of all cancer deaths (American Cancer Society, 2005). For the most part, smoking prevalence has declined, but recently there has been a troubling leveling off. Currently, approximately 21% of the adult population, or 45 million adults, smoke cigarettes (American Cancer Society, 2007). Even with the dramatic decline in prevalence from 60% before World War I, tobacco-related diseases still contribute to approximately 440,000 premature deaths each year (American Cancer Society, 2007). Current smokers have 20 times the rate of lung cancer of those who have never smoked (U.S. Public Health Service, Office of the Surgeon General, 1989) The risk of lung cancer among cigarette smokers increases with the duration of smoking, as well as with the number of cigarettes smoked per day (Doll & Peto, 1978). In a model developed by Doll and Peto, duration of smoking increased the probability of disease more than the number of cigarettes smoked per day (Doll

& Peto, 1978). Therefore, individuals who initiate smoking at a young age have a greater likelihood of developing lung cancer than those who started later (U.S. Department of Health and Human Services, 1988). This strongly suggests that approaches that delay the age of onset of smoking in a population or prevent smoking altogether could have a substantial impact on the incidence of lung cancer by shortening the average duration of smoking. That said, numerous studies have also shown that cigarette smokers can derive benefit by quitting at any age (U.S. Public Health Service, Office of the Surgeon General, 1989). And it is clear that the likelihood of developing lung cancer is lower among people who quit smoking than among those who continue to smoke (U.S. Department of Health and Human Services, 1990).

Diet and Nutrition

In addition to smoking, it is now widely understood that unhealthful diets and physical inactivity play a significant role in the causation and progression of chronic disease, although the numbers attributable to these causes vary (Centers for Disease Control & National Center for Chronic Disease Prevention and Health Promotion, 2003). The concentrated focus on changes in nutrition and physical activity as avenues to promote heath is relatively recent. Until the 1970s and the hearings held by the U.S. Senate Select Committee on Nutrition and Human Needs, the focus of nutrition policy had been on undernutrition, rather than chronic disease prevention (Brownson, Remington, & Davis, 1998). Since the controversial dietary goals for the United States were published in 1977, numerous scientific papers have supported the relationship between a typical U.S. diet and chronic diseases such as heart disease, cancer, diabetes, and stroke (U.S. Senate Select Committee on Nutrition and Human Needs, 1977) These efforts have contributed to improvements in the dietary habits of Americans.

Overall, a diet that includes a large variety of fruits, vegetables, and whole grains has been strongly associated with reductions in coronary heart disease, stroke, and type 2 diabetes (Michels, 2005). However, the results of studies attempting to isolate nutritional factors related to cancer prevention have been less compelling (McCullough & Giovannucci, 2004). This may be because specific nutrients do not exert a protective effect in isolation. Protective effects may also depend on dose, timing, and duration of exposure or nutrient status (Kushi et al., 2006). On the other hand, diets low in fat and high in fruits, vegetables, and whole grains are consistent with energy balance and may contribute to a lower body weight (Rolls, Ello-Martin, & Tohill, 2004). An unhealthful diet, overall, appears to be an independent risk factor for certain chronic diseases but also plays a crucial role in its effect on chronic disease through the influence on the development and maintenance of obesity by altering energy balance (Centers for Disease Control & National Center for Chronic Disease Prevention and Health Promotion, 2003).

Physical Activity and Energy Expenditure

Energy expenditure, while also an independent risk factor for certain chronic diseases, is also an important component of energy balance (Hill & Wyatt, 2005). Unfortunately, it is estimated that only 38.5% of adults in the United States meet the national guidelines for physical activity (Simpson et al., 2003). A recent study found that physically inactive women had a rate of all-cause mortality that was 52% higher than that of physically active women; their risk of cardiovascular mortality was doubled, and their risk of cancer-related mortality was 29% higher (Hu et al., 2004).

When energy intake is balanced with energy expenditure, body weight remains constant. Thus, overweight and obesity can occur when energy intake is greater than energy expenditure for a sustained period of time (Hill & Wyatt, 2005). However, there are gaps in our knowledge about the health risks of obesity, and deaths attributable to obesity are difficult to calculate for a variety of reasons. Body mass index (BMI) is influenced by energy intake and energy expenditure levels, which may affect health in ways independent of or mediated by BMI. Estimates of the number of deaths attributable to obesity have ranged from 112,000 (Flegal, Graubard, Williamson, & Gail, 2005) to 280,000 (Allison, Fontaine, Manson, Stevens, & Van Itallie, 1999) to 400,000 (Mokdad, Marks, Stroup, & Gerberding, 2004; Mokdad, Marks, Stroup, & Gerberding, 2005). These disparate findings in obesity-attributable deaths underscore the need to develop more sophisticated approaches that could lead to more consistent estimations. Nonetheless, despite the varying estimations, there is no doubt that a decrease in unhealthful dietary and sedentary behavior patterns could translate into a lowering of the elevated risk of morbidity and mortality associated with obesity.

Excess body weight is an independent risk factor for cardiovascular disease, as well as a contributor to other risk factors such as hypertension and type 2 diabetes (Eckel, 1997). Moreover, in 2002, a working group at the International Agency for Research on Cancer concluded that there was convincing evidence that being overweight (body mass index [BMI] $\geq$ 25 kg/m^2) or obese (BMI $\geq$ 30 kg/m^2) is associated with risk of cancers of the endometrium, colon, and kidney (Calle, Rodriguez, Walker-Thurmond, & Thun, 2003). Recent data also suggest that successful weight loss and the avoidance of adult weight gain could translate into significant reductions in breast cancer rates (Harvie et al., 2005). Calle and colleagues estimated that 90,000 deaths due to cancer could be prevented annually if individuals could achieve and maintain a BMI of 25 kg/m^2 (Calle et al., 2003).

While there is widespread debate as to how individuals can best achieve energy balance, it is clear that the balance between energy intake and energy expenditure through physical activity is a critical component in the maintenance of a healthy body weight (Hill & Wyatt, 2005). The consistency of the energy balance message, along with similar messages from the American Heart Association (Mosca et al., 2004; Pearson et al., 2002; Williams et al., 2002), the National Cholesterol Education Program Adult Treatment Panel (Expert Panel on Detection Evaluation and Treatment of High Blood Cholesterol in Adults, 2001), and the American Academy of Pediatrics (Krebs, Jacobson, & the American Academy of Pediatrics Committee on Nutrition, 2003) underscores the incontrovertible evidence that the burden of illness today due to chronic disease is, in part, preventable (McGinnis & Foege, 1993).

National Prevention Priorities

Because a considerable number of early deaths among Americans could be prevented through modification of behavioral risk factors, there needs to be a commitment, combined with a comprehensive plan, to make the changes possible (McGinnis & Foege, 1993). Decisions about smoking, level of activity, and dietary intake are fundamentally and intrinsically linked to individual, cultural, environmental, and commercial factors (Ammerman et al., 2003). Therefore, messages related to preventive health care need to address these root causes of chronic disease in a format that can enhance motivation and promote and monitor effective action (Ammerman et al., 2003; McGinnis & Foege, 2004). Efforts to set health objectives that can be monitored are a recent phenomenon. A 1978 paper published by the Institute of Medicine (IOM) was the first to establish objectives for public health (Nightingale, Cureton, Kalmar, & Trudeau, 1978). The work of the IOM in this area led to the 1979 *Surgeon General's Report on Health Promotion and Disease Prevention* (U.S. Department of Health Education and Welfare Public Health Service, 1979) and culminated in 1990 in the publication of *Healthy People 2000*, which contained 22 priority areas and 319 health objectives to be achieved by the year 2000 (U.S. Department of Health and Human Services, Public Health Service, 1990). Many of the objectives of *Healthy People 2000* were achieved (U.S. Department of Health and Human Services, 2000). However, phenomena such as increasing overweight and obesity rates, as well as an increase in the incidence of diabetes, ultimately led to a set of objectives that focused more specifically on lifestyle behavior change (U.S. Department of Health and Human Services, 2000).

Currently, the U.S. Public Health Service has established two primary health goals for the year 2010: (1) to increase quality and years of health life; and (2) to eliminate health disparities among Americans. In an effort to achieve these goals, the U.S. Public Health Service has published 467 health objectives divided into 26 specific areas (U.S. Department of Health and Human Services, 2000). The core of the objectives for *Healthy People 2010* is based on the scientific evidence documenting the relationship between behavioral risk factors and the development of chronic disease. In fact, 5 of the 10 leading indicators for the health of the nation are health behaviors. The objectives for these behaviors are quite ambitious and include reducing the prevalence of smoking among adults by 50%, doubling the percentage of adults who engage in regular physical activity, and reducing the proportion of overweight and obese children by at least 50% and the proportion of such adults by 35%.

While there is considerable debate regarding the effectiveness of setting ambitious and, some believe, unachievable goals, there is little doubt that modification of behavioral risk factors will make the largest contribution to reductions in morbidity and mortality from the major diseases. For example, Byers and colleagues estimated achievable reductions in cancer incidence and mortality rates between 1990 and 2010 (Byers et al., 1999). Overall, 47% of the achievable reductions in cancer incidence and 51% of the achievable reductions in cancer mortality came from reductions in tobacco use. A similar analysis for coronary mortality conducted in the United Kingdom indicates that 44% of achievable reductions would come from reductions in tobacco use (Critchley & Capewell, 2003).

Indeed, over the past few decades, there have been substantial improvements in chronic disease morbidity and mortality rates (Strong, Mathers, Leeder, & Beaglehole, 2005). For example, deaths from cardiovascular disease have been reduced significantly (Minino, Heron, & Smith, 2006), and cancer mortality also has declined (Minino et al., 2006). While the reasons for this improvement are multifaceted, health behavior changes have contributed to the decline, particularly adherence to recommendations involving diet, physical activity, and abstinence from smoking.

In summary, the underlying science is available to support the health behavior theory of prevention. Over the past several decades, our knowledge of the causes of chronic disease, including effective intervention techniques, has increased exponentially. However, we continue to face challenges in translating preventive health knowledge into improved health (Glasgow, Lichtenstein, & Marcus, 2003). A more rapid translation of scientific results could significantly reduce the burden of chronic disease, as well as the health disparities in chronic disease that exist for many underserved segments of our population (Kumanyika & Morssink, 2006).

From Theory to Action

High-Risk and Population-Based Prevention Strategies

The previous section highlights evidence for two basic tenets of a health behavior theory of prevention: reductions in the prevalence of health risk behaviors are associated with reductions in premature morbidity and mortality (e.g., declines in smoking prevalence and decreases in lung cancer and cardiovascular disease), and increases in the prevalence of health risk behaviors are associated with increases in premature morbidity and mortality (e.g., increased weight from unhealthful diets and lack of physical activity and increases in the incidence of type 2 diabetes). Unfortunately, science and practice are not inextricably linked. A fundamental challenge for the health behavior theory of prevention is moving from theory to action, which involves pull-through from research to practice. In this section we consider two types of prevention strategies—high-risk and population-based approaches.

In his seminal book, *The Strategy of Preventive Medicine,* Geoffrey Rose introduces the high-risk approach to prevention in the context of "the prevention paradox," which he defines as "a preventive measure that brings large benefits to the community offers little to each participating individual" (Rose, 1992). One way to deal with this paradox is to adopt a high-risk strategy that focuses on identifying individuals or groups of individuals known to be at high risk for disease and concentrates prevention and intervention efforts on reversing or reducing their risk level. Individuals with no or mildly elevated risk are essentially left alone. Examples of high-risk strategies for behavioral risk-factor modification include tobacco cessation interventions targeted at smokers with genetic markers of susceptibility to lung cancer (e.g., Bize, Burnand, Mueller, & Cornuz, 2005), diet and physical activity interventions targeted to nondiabetic individuals with elevated blood glucose and body mass indices greater than 25 (e.g., Diabetes Prevention Research Group, 2002), and interventions to increase compliance with mammography screening targeted at women with a family history of breast cancer (e.g., Curry, Taplin, Barlow, Anderman, & McBride, 1993). Appealing aspects of a high-risk approach to prevention include its practicability, appropriateness, cost-effectiveness, and potentially high benefit-to-risk ratio. Wilson and Jungner elaborated these advantages 40 years ago and noted that targeting interventions to clearly identified high-risk individuals can be easily integrated into the current organization and culture of health care, provides a cost-effective use of resources, provides interventions that are appropriate to the individual, and avoids "interference" with those who are not at special risk (Wilson & Jungner, 1968). Moreover, because all interventions bring some costs and possible adverse effects, the benefit-to-risk ratio for prevention interventions is likely to be higher in populations where the potential benefits are greatest.

The prospective advantages of a high-risk prevention strategy are tempered by several potential limitations. Wilson and Junger raise concerns that if prevention becomes "medicalized," there may be negative effects on individuals who are "labeled" and that high-risk strategies focus primarily on individuals and so can fail to address key contextual determinants of risk factors and/or diseases. As a result, the high-risk approach can "isolate" high-risk individuals by asking them to adopt behaviors that have minimal social and environmental supports. Most important is their observation, echoed by many others, that the high-risk approach is limited by imprecise prediction; most risk, including behavioral risk, is probabilistic, not deterministic. This means that some (even many) "high-risk" individuals will stay well and that some low-risk individuals will get sick. Rose aptly summarizes the implications of imprecise risk as a fundamental axiom of preventive medicine: "A large number of people exposed to a small risk may generate many more cases than a small number exposed to a high risk." He further notes that in the context of this axiom a high-risk prevention strategy would be addressing only the margins of the problem (Rose, 1992).

The information in Table 1.1 helps to illustrate this axiom and the potential limitations of a high-risk prevention strategy. These are data for men aged 40 to 59 years who were screened for risk factors related to myocardial infarction (MI), as well as for the presence of early disease. The second column of the table indicates that among all men in this group, 15% were found to have elevated risk factors and 2% were found to have elevated risk factors plus early disease. Thus, 85% of the population would be considered risk-free. The third column shows the percentage of men who had an MI in the 5 years following screening. Among those with elevated risk factors and early disease, nearly one-quarter,

1.1 5-Year Myocardial Infarction (MI) Risk and Risk Factors

Screening Result	% of men	% with MI	% of all MIs in this group
All men	100	4	100
Elevated risk factors	15	7	32
Elevated risk factors + early disease	2	22	12

Note. From *The Strategy of Preventive Medicine*, by G. Rose, 1992, p. 50. New York: Oxford University Press. Copyright 1999 by Oxford University Press. Reprinted with permission.

22%, of them had an MI, whereas 7% of those with only elevated risk factors had an MI. Across the entire population of men, there was a 4% incidence of MI. The last column of the table shows the percentage of all MIs that are accounted for by those in the elevated-risk categories; 32% of all MIs occurred among men with elevated risk factors, and 12% occurred among those with elevated risk factors and early disease.

Thus, the majority of MIs (~68%) occurred in men with no known risk factors. These data lead to two important observations. First, even among men with elevated risk factors, the majority did not have MIs (93% and 78%, respectively). Second, a high-risk prevention approach, even if 100% successful, would prevent only one-third of all future MIs.

As the name implies, a population-based approach to prevention targets all individuals, regardless of risk status, with the goal of shifting the entire risk factor distribution in a positive direction. In many ways, the strengths and limitations of a population-based prevention strategy are the mirror image of those outlined for the high-risk approach. On the plus side, population-based prevention takes a less "medical-model" approach and includes social, organizational, environmental, and policy strategies that change the context and social norms for individual change. Conversely, a population-based strategy may be less cost-effective; since resources are allocated for a much broader spectrum of the population, it may fail to leverage the resources and influence of the health care system, and, by exposing more individuals to interventions with potential adverse effects, may have a smaller overall benefit-to-risk ratio (cf. Jeffery, 1989; Lichtenstein & Glasgow, 1992). In essence, a population-based prevention strategy brings us to a fundamental question derived from the prevention paradox: will moderate and achievable change in the population as a whole lead to reductions in the prevalence and negative consequences of disease?

With regard to behavioral risk factors, Rose points out that this question can be addressed by observing the correlation between the population average and the prevalence of deviance (Rose & Day, 1990). Population averages can be calculated without the "outliers" to reduce the influence of extreme values (which determine the prevalence of deviance) on the observed associations. Using data from a large, longitudinal cohort study, Rose reports correlations between the prevalence of high blood pressure and population averages of salt intake, weight, and alcohol intake that range from .64 to .78. Extrapolating further, he calculates the expected reduction in the prevalence of risk factors associated with changes in the population average. For example, Rose calculated a 25% reduction in the prevalence of obesity with an average loss of 1 kg (2.25 lbs) in the population and a 25% drop in the prevalence of heavy drinking if the average intake of all drinkers fell by 10% (Rose, 1992, p. 65). These data lend support to population-based approaches to behavioral risk factor modification that aim for modest changes across a broad spectrum of individuals.

Of course, high-risk and population-based approaches are not mutually exclusive. Optimal health outcomes through behavioral risk-factor modification are more likely to be achieved by the two approaches combined. Moreover, as definitions of risk and disease are modified to encompass larger proportions of the general population, the distinction may become increasingly blurred. The trend toward defining "pre-disease" (e.g., prehypertension, prediabetes) as well as toward lowering diagnostic thresholds (e.g., hypercholesterolemia, type 2 diabetes, overweight, and obesity) results in a decrease in the proportion of the population defined as "well" (Kaplan, 2005). One estimate is that lower thresholds for hypercholesterolemia, hypertension, type 2 diabetes, and overweight would result in fully 75% of the entire U.S. adult population qualifying for a chronic disease diagnosis (Kaplan, Ganiats, & Frosch, 2004). Given the common pathway of health behaviors as important for both the prevention and the management of chronic disease, we can see that the population and high-risk approaches may very well converge.

Health Behavior Theory of Prevention and Emerging Paradigms of Disease Prevention

Thought leaders in health psychology point to the need for health psychologists to "look beyond current concepts and methods in prevention science" to achieve the considerable potential of health psychology, which includes health behavior theory (Smith, Orleans, & Jenkins, 2004). Dr. Elias Zerhouni, Director of the National Institutes of Health, presents a vision for the future of NIH in the context of the "4 Ps" of medicine that "will be more predictive, personalized, preemptive, and participatory" (Zerhouni, 2006; Zerhouni, 2007). Dr. Zerhouni describes a transformation of the health care process in which there is a "continuous participation of individuals, communities, and healthcare institutions as early as possible in the natural cycle of a disease process." By identifying biomarkers (e.g., genetic variants, molecular changes, individual-level measures of environmental exposures) that are predictive of later development of serious disease, the vision is for biological "preemption" of disease before it occurs. Notably absent in this vision is any explicit attention to prevention beyond the level of individual biology (Glasgow, Fisher, Haire-Joshu, & Goldstein, 2007).

What we can see in this vision is a merging of the population and high-risk approaches to prevention. In essence, all individuals become "high risk" as they are monitored throughout the life cycle for "predisease," and the indicators of predisease will largely be at the molecular level. However, behavior will still play a large role in the translation and adoption of biomedical advances, particularly as associations between molecular markers of disease and known environmental factors are articulated. Moreover, the predictive, personalized, and preemptive vision raises a number of key questions that an expanded health behavior model of prevention can address (cf. McBride, 2005). At what point in the life span should intensive screening for biomarkers of disease begin? What are the criteria for determining the value of a biomarker in formulating a prevention strategy at the individual level? Important considerations include issues of sensitivity and specificity of a biomarker in predicting future disease, the potential for detecting "pseudodisease" (i.e., markers of disease that do not affect overall life expectancy and quality of life; Black & Welch, 1997), and the availability of proven preventive interventions and their risk-benefit profiles (cf. Mahadevia, Kamanger, & Samet, 2003). How can we communicate complex biomedical information to individuals with average to low health literacy? What are the psychological consequences of looking for markers of predisease and of finding "false positive" indications? Will individuals avoid the health care system for fear of being labeled "at risk" and losing health coverage, employment opportunities, and so on? Will more precise feedback on the risk of serious disease result in meaningful reductions in behavioral risk factors? Will this expanded medical model of disease prevention overload the medical system logistically and financially?

None of these are new questions; they are critical issues for effective translation from theory practice. It is notable that even with our rich scientific evidence that behavioral risk factors contribute substantially to premature morbidity and mortality, that improvements in rates of heart disease and cancer are inextricably linked to reductions in tobacco use, and that the increased prevalence of type 2 diabetes is associated with increased rates of overweight and obesity, the biomedical community has not embraced the health behavior theory of disease prevention. There is a wide translational gap between what we as a society can do and what we actually do to address behavioral risk factors (Curry, 2004). Our health behavior research is often "chasing the bus" of new knowledge, for example, trying to understand why individuals fail to obtain recommended screening tests or how to better achieve successful behavior change. Accelerated translation of findings from these emerging prevention paradigms will occur only if the theory, science, practice, and policy related to a health behavior theory of prevention are an integral part of the transdisciplinary collaboration for actualizing this new vision.

References

Allison, D. B., Fontaine, K. R., Manson, J. E., Stevens, J., & Van Itallie, T. B. (1999). Annual deaths attributable to obesity in the United States. *Journal of the American Medical Association, 282,* 1530–1580.

American Cancer Society. (2005). *Cancer facts and figures, 2005.* Atlanta: American Cancer Society.

American Cancer Society. (2007). *Cancer facts & figures, 2007.* Atlanta: American Cancer Society.

Ammerman, A., Corbie-Smith, G., St. George, D. M., Washington, C., Weathers, B., & Jackson-Christian, B. (2003). Research expectations among African American church leaders in the PRAISE! project: A randomized trial guided by community-based participatory research. *American Journal of Public Health, 93,* 1720–1727.

Berkson, J. (1958). Smoking and lung cancer: Some observations on two recent reports. *Journal of the American Statistical Association, 53,* 28–38.

Bize, R., Burnand, B., Mueller, Y., & Cornuz, J. (2005). Biomedical risk assessment as an aid for smoking cessation. *Cochrane Database of Systematic Reviews, 4,* CD004705.

Black, W. C., & Welch, H. G. (1997). Screening for disease. *American Journal of Roentgenol, 168* (January), 3–11.

Brownson, R. C., & Bright, F. S. (2004). Chronic disease control in public health practice: Looking back and moving forward. *Public Health Reports, 119,* 230–238.

Brownson, R. C., Remington, P. L., & Davis, J. R. (Eds.). (1998). *Chronic disease epidemiology and control* (2nd ed.). Washington, DC: American Public Health Association.

Bullough, B., & Rosen, G. (1992). *Preventive medicine in the United States: 1900–1990: Trends and interpretations.* Canton, MA: Watson Publishing International.

Byers, T., Mouchawar, J., Marks, J., Cady, B., Lins, N., Swanson, G. M., et al. (1999). The American Cancer Society challenge goals. How far can cancer rates decline in the U.S. by the year 2015? *Cancer, 5,* 715–727.

Calle, E. E., Rodriguez, C., Walker-Thurmond, K., & Thun, M. J. (2003). Overweight, obesity, and mortality from cancer in a prospectively studied cohort of U.S. adults. *New England Journal of Medicine, 348,* 1625–1638.

Centers for Disease Control & National Center for Chronic Disease Prevention and Health Promotion. (2003). Physical activity and good nutrition: Essential elements to prevent chronic diseases and obesity 2003. *Nutrition in Clinical Care, 6,* 135–138.

Central Intelligence Agency. (2007). *The world factbook*. Retrieved April 20, 2007, from https://www.cia.gov/cia/publications/factbook/index.html

Cornfield, J., Haenszel, W., Hammond, W., Lilienfeld, E., Shimkin, A., & Synder, E. (1959). Smoking and lung cancer: Recent evidence and a discussion of some questions. *Journal of the National Cancer Institute, 22,* 173–201.

Critchley, J. A., & Capewell, S. (2003). Substantial potential for reductions in coronary heart disease mortality in the U.K. through changes in risk factor levels. *Journal of Epidemiology and Community Health, 57*(4), 243–247.

Curry, S. J. (2004). Toward a public policy agenda for addressing multiple health risk behaviors in primary care. *American Journal of Preventive Medicine, 27*(2 Suppl), 106–108.

Curry, S., Taplin, S., Barlow, W., Anderman, C., & McBride, C. (1993) A randomized trial of the impact of risk assessment and feedback on participation in mammography screening. *Preventive Medicine, 22*(3), 350–360.

Deutsch, M., & Krause, R. M. (1965). *Theories in social psychology*. New York: Basic Books.

Diabetes Prevention Research Group. (2002). Reduction in the incidence of type 2 diabetes with lifestyle intervention or metformin. *New England Journal of Medicine, 346*(6), 393–403.

Doll, R. (1999). Tobacco: A medical history. *Journal of Urban Health, 76,* 289–313.

Doll, R., & Peto, R. (1978). Cigarette smoking and bronchial carcinoma: Dose and time relationships among regular smokers and lifelong non-smokers. *Journal of Epidemiology & Community Health, 32,* 303–313.

Eckel, R. H. (1997). Obesity and heart disease: A statement for healthcare professionals from the Nutrition Committee, American Heart Association. *Circulation, 96,* 3248–3250.

Expert Panel on Detection Evaluation and Treatment of High Blood Cholesterol in Adults. (2001). Executive Summary of the Third Report of the National Cholesterol Education Program (NCEP) Expert Panel on Detection, Evaluation, and Treatment of High Blood Cholesterol in Adults (Adult Treatment Panel III). *Journal of the American Medical Association, 285,* 2486–2497.

Flegal, K. M., Graubard, B. I., Williamson, D. F., & Gail, M. H. (2005). Excess deaths associated with underweight, overweight, and obesity. *Journal of the American Medical Association, 293,* 1861–1867.

Fries, J. F., Koop, C. E., Beadle, C. E., Cooper, P. P., England, M. J., Greaves, R. F., et al. (1993). Reducing health care costs by reducing the need and demand for medical services. The Health Project Consortium. *New England Journal of Medicine, 329,* 321–325.

Glantz, S. A., Slade, J., Bero, L., Hanauer, P., & Barnes, D. (1996). *The cigarette papers*. Berkeley: University of California Press.

Glasgow, R. E., Fisher, E. B., Haire-Joshu, D., & Goldstein, M. G. (2008). NIH science agenda: A public health perspective. *American Journal of Public Health, 97,* 1936–1938.

Glasgow, R. E., Lichtenstein, E., & Marcus, A. C. (2003). Why don't we see more translation of health promotion research to practice? Rethinking the efficacy-to-effectiveness transition. *American Journal of Public Health, 93,* 1261–1267.

Harvie, M., Howell, A., Vierkant, R. A., Kumar, N., Cerhan, J. R., Kelemen, L. E., et al. (2005). Association of gain and loss of weight before and after menopause with risk of postmenopausal breast cancer in the Iowa women's health study. *Cancer Epidemiology Biomarkers and Prevention, 14,* 656–661.

Heffler, S., Smith, S., Keehan, S., Borger, C., Clemens, M. K., & Truffer, C. (2005). U.S. health spending projections for 2004–2014. *Health Affairs* (January–June), Suppl. Web Exclusives: W5-74–W5-85.

Hill, J. O., & Wyatt, H. R. (2005). Role of physical activity in preventing and treating obesity. *Journal of Applied Physiology, 99,* 765–770.

Hu, F. B., Willett, W. C., Li, T., Stampfer, M. J., Colditz, G. A., & Manson, E. (2004). Adiposity as compared with physical activity in predicting mortality among women. *New England Journal of Medicine, 351,* 2694–2703.

Jeffery, R. W. (1989). Risk behaviors and health: Contrasting individual and population perspectives. *American Psychologist, 44*(9), 1194–1202.

Kaplan, R. M. (2005). Screening for cancer: Are resources being used wisely? *Recent Results in Cancer Research, 166,* 315–334.

Kaplan, R. M., Ganiats, T. G., & Frosch, D. L. (2004). Diagnostic and treatment decisions in U.S. healthcare. *Journal of Health Psychology, 9*(1), 29–40.

Kluger, R. (1996). *Ashes to ashes, America's hundred-year cigarette war, the public health and the unabashed triumph of Philip Morris.* New York: Vintage Books.

Krebs, N. F., Jacobson, M. S., & the American Academy of Pediatrics Committee on Nutrition. (2003). Prevention of pediatric overweight and obesity. *Pediatrics, 112,* 424–430.

Kumanyika, S. K., & Morssink, C. B. (2006). Bridging domains in efforts to reduce disparities in health and health care. *Health Education & Behavior, 33,* 440–458.

Kushi, L. H., Byers, T., Doyle, C., Bandera, E. V., McCullough, M., McTiernan, A., et al. (2006). American Cancer Society 2006 Nutrition and Physical Activity Guidelines Advisory Committee. American Cancer Society Guidelines on Nutrition and Physical Activity for cancer prevention: Reducing the risk of cancer with healthy food choices and physical activity. *CA: A Cancer Journal for Clinicians, 56,* 254–281.

Lichtenstein, E., & Glasgow, R. E. (1992). Smoking cessation: What have we learned over the past decade? *Journal of Consulting and Clinical Psychology, 60*(4), 518–527.

Mahadevia, P. J., Kamangar, F., & Samet, J. (2003). Background paper for chapter 7, Adopting new technology in the face of uncertain science: The case of screening for lung cancer. In S. J. Curry, T. Byers, & M. Hewitt (Eds.), *Fulfilling the potential for cancer prevention and early detection.* Washington, DC: National Academies Press.

McBride, C. M. (2005). Blazing a trail: A public health research agenda in genomics and chronic disease. *Prevention of Chronic Disease.* Retrieved April 16, 2007, from http://www.cdc.gov/pcd/issues/2005/apr/05_008.htm

McCullough, M. L., & Giovannucci, E. L. (2004). Diet and cancer prevention. *Oncogene, 23,* 6349–6364.

McGinnis, J. M., & Foege, W. H. (1993). Actual causes of death in the United States [see comments]. *Journal of the American Medical Association, 270,* 2207–2212.

McGinnis, J. M., & Foege, W. H. (2004). The immediate vs. the important. *Journal of the American Medical Association, 291,* 1263–1264.

McKenna, M. T., Taylor, W. R., Marks, J. S., & Koplan, J. P. (1998). Current issues and challenges in chronic disease control. In R. C. Brownson, P. L. Remington, & J. R. Davis (Eds.), *Chronic disease epidemiology and control* (2nd ed., pp. 1–26). Washington, DC: American Public Health Association.

Michels, K. B. (2005). The role of nutrition in cancer development and prevention. *International Journal of Cancer, 114,* 163–165.

Millman & Robertson Inc. (1995). *Health risks and their impact on medical costs.* Minneapolis, MN: Millman & Robertson Inc.

Minino, A. M., Heron, M. P., & Smith, B. L. (2006). Deaths: Preliminary data for 2004. *National Vital Statistics Reports, 54,* 1–49.

Mokdad, A. H., Marks, J. S., Stroup, D. F., & Gerberding, J. L. (2004). Actual causes of death in the United States, 2000. *Journal of the American Medical Association, 291,* 1238–1245.

Mokdad, A. H., Marks, J. S., Stroup, D. F., & Geberding, J. L. (2005). Correction: Actual causes of death in the United States, 2002. *Journal of the American Medical Association, 293*(3), 293–294.

Mosca, L., Appel, L. J., Benjamin, E. J., Berra, K., Chandra-Strobos, N., Fabunmi, R. P., et al. (2004). Evidence-based guidelines for cardiovascular disease prevention in women. *Circulation, 109,* 672–693.

National Center for Health Statistics. (2006). *Health, United States, 2006 with chartbook on trends in the health of Americans.* Hyattsville, MD: National Center for Health Statistics.

Nightingale, E. O., Cureton, M., Kalmar, V., & Trudeau, M. B. (1978). *Perspectives on health promotion and disease prevention in the United States.* Washington DC: National Academy of Sciences (staff paper).

Parascandola, M. (2004). Two approaches to etiology: The debate over smoking and lung cancer in the 1950s. *Endeavour, 28,* 81–86.

Pearson, T. A., Blair, S. N., Daniels, S. R., Eckel, R. H., Fair, J. M., Fortmann, S. P., et al. (2002). AHA guidelines for primary prevention of cardiovascular disease and stroke: 2002 update: Consensus panel guide to comprehensive risk reduction for adult patients without coronary or other atherosclerotic vascular diseases. American Heart Association Science Advisory and Coordinating Committee. *Circulation, 106,* 388–391.

Public Health Service. (1964). *Smoking and health: Report of the advisory committee to the Surgeon General of the Public Health Service.* Washington, DC: Public Health Service (DHEW publication no. PHS 64–1103).

Rolls, B. J., Ello-Martin, J. A., & Tohill, B. C. (2004). What can intervention studies tell us about the relationship between fruit and vegetable consumption and weight management? *Nutrition Reviews, 62,* 1–17.

Rose, G. (1992). *The strategy of preventive medicine.* New York: Oxford University Press.

Rose, G., & Day, S. (1990). The population mean predicts the number of deviant individuals. *British Medical Journal, 301,* 1031–1034.

Selin, H. (Ed.). (2003). *Medicine across cultures: History and practice of medicines in non-Western cultures.* Dordrecht: Kluwer Academic Publishers.

Simpson, M. E., Serdula, M., Galuska, D. A., Gillespie, C., Donehoo, R., Macera, C., et al. (2003). Walking trends among U.S. adults: The Behavioral Risk Factor Surveillance System, 1987–2000. *American Journal of Preventive Medicine, 25,* 95–100.

Smith, T. W., Orleans, C. T., & Jenkins, C. D. (2004). Prevention and health promotion: Decades of progress, new challenges, and an emerging agenda. *Health Psychology, 23*(2), 126–131.

Starfield, B. (2000). Is U.S. health really the best in the world? [Editorial] *Journal of the American Medical Association, 284*(4), 483–485.

Strong, K., Mathers, C., Leeder, S., & Beaglehole, R. (2005). Preventing chronic diseases: How many lives can we save? *Lancet, 366,* 1578–1582.

Study Group on Smoking and Health. (1957). Smoking and health. *Science, 125,* 1129–1133.

Surgeon General. (1964). *Smoking and health. Report of the Advisory Committee to the Surgeon General of the Public Health Service.* Retrieved March 9, 2007, from http://profiles.nlm.nih.gov/NN/B/C/X/B/

Susser, M. (1985). Epidemiology in the United States after World War II: The evolution of technique. *Epidemiologic Reviews, 7,* 147–177.

Talley, C., Kushner, H. I., & Sterk, C. E. (2004). Lung cancer, chronic disease epidemiology, and medicine, 1948–1964. *Journal of the History of Medicine & Allied Sciences, 59,* 329–374.

U.S. Department of Health and Human Services. (1988). *The health consequences of smoking: Nicotine addiction: A report of the Surgeon General, 1988.* Retrieved March 9, 2007, from http://profiles.nlm.nih.gov/NN/B/B/Z/D/

U.S. Department of Health and Human Services. (1990). *The health benefits of smoking cessation: A report of the Surgeon General.* Retrieved March 9, 2007, from http://profiles.nlm.nih.gov/NN/B/C/T/

U.S. Department of Health and Human Services. (2000). *Healthy People 2010.* Washington, DC: Author.

U.S. Department of Health and Human Services, Public Health Service. (1990). *Healthy People 2000* (No. DHHS Publication No. PHS 91-50212). Washington, DC: Author.

U.S. Department of Health, Education, and Welfare, Public Health Service. (1979). *Healthy People: The Surgeon General's report on health promotion and disease prevention.* Retrieved March 9, 2007, from http://profiles.nlm.nih.gov/NN/B/B/G/K/_nnbbgk.pdf

U.S. Public Health Service, Office of the Surgeon General. (1989). *Reducing the health consequences of smoking: 25 years of progress: a report of the Surgeon General.* Retrieved March 9, 2007, from http://profiles.nlm.nih.gov/NN/B/B/X/S/

U.S. Senate Select Committee on Nutrition and Human Needs. (1977). *Dietary goals for the United States.*

White, C. (1990). Research on smoking and lung cancer: A landmark in the history of chronic disease epidemiology. *Yale Journal of Biology and Medicine, 63,* 29–46.

Williams, C. L., Hayman, L. L., Daniels, S. R., Robinson, T. N., Steinberger, J., Paridon, S., et al. (2002). Cardiovascular health in childhood: A statement for health professionals from the Committee on Atherosclerosis, Hypertension, and Obesity in the Young (AHOY) of the Council on Cardiovascular Disease in the Young, American Heart Association. *Circulation, 106,* 143–160.

Wilson, J. M. G., & Jungner, G. (1968). The principles and practice of screening for disease. *WHO Public Health Papers 34.* Geneva: World Health Organization.

Zerhouni, E. A. (2006). NIH in the post-doubling era: Realities and strategies. *Science, 314*(5802), 1088–1090.

Zerhouni, E. A. (2007). *FY2008 Director's Budget Request Statement, March 6, 2007.* U.S. Department of Health & Human Services, National Institutes of Health. Retrieved April 13, 2007, from http://www.nih.gov/about/director/budgetrequest/fy2008directors budgetrequest.htm

Theoretical Models and Strategies for Improving Disease Management by Patients

2

Noreen M. Clark and
Christy R. Houle

It is apparent that the ultimate success of efficacious preventive and curative regimens is dependent upon individuals' willingness to undertake and maintain the required behaviors. Unfortunately, data indicate that poor adherence to professional advice often occurs wherever some form of discretionary action or self-administration is involved. Scheduled appointments for treatment are missed about 35% of the time, and significant numbers of patients do not take prescribed medications in accordance with instructions (DiMatteo, 2004). Adherence to recommended changes for lifestyle behaviors is disappointing. For instance, smoking cessation programs are considered to be unusually effective if 20% of the participants have stopped smoking for at least 1 year

This chapter is revised and expanded by the authors. It is based on
original work by Dr. Marshall H. Becker and is dedicated to his memory.

(U.S. Department of Health and Human Services [USDHHS], 2000); fewer than one-half of adults engage in recommended levels of physical activity (Sapkota, Bowles, Ham, & Kohl, 2005); and large percentages drop out of weight-control programs (Dansinger, Tatsioni, Wong, Chung, & Balk, 2007).

Given the extensive documentation of suboptimal public participation in screening, immunization, and other preventive health efforts, as well as low levels of individual adherence to prescribed medical therapies (cf. Kimmel et al., 2007; Osterberg & Blaschke, 2005; Sackett & Snow, 1979) it is not surprising that behavioral scientists devote extensive conceptual and empirical effort toward the explanation and prediction of individuals' health-related decisions. In the past three decades, discussions of the concept of compliance or adherence to use of medicines as prescribed by clinicians have been expanded to include a wider range of activities patients must undertake to manage their health problems more effectively. Therefore, this chapter reviews theoretical and conceptual frameworks that have been used to address adherence in self-management of health and disease. Given the need to increase the impact of effective preventive and curative therapies population-wide, a challenge for the future is to evolve models that integrate community-wide and individual-level health behavior change. To this end, this chapter also includes a discussion of decision making and action through community coalitions as a means to address the systems, policies, and other large-scale measures necessary to ensure that significant numbers of people have the access and assistance required to prevent and control disease. Important approaches and techniques have been identified that help health professionals to ameliorate problems in adherence and effective patient management of disease, but these are not covered in this chapter since they are covered in chapter 6 in this book.

Models of Adherence and Disease Management

The reasons individuals voluntarily elect to engage in health-directed activities were categorized years ago (Kasl & Cobb, 1966) into three major classes:

1. To prevent illness or to detect it at an asymptomatic stage ("health behavior");
2. In the presence of symptoms, to obtain diagnosis and to discover suitable treatment ("illness behavior"); and
3. In the presence of defined illness, to undertake/receive treatment aimed at restoration of health or at halting disease progression ("sick-role behavior").

More recently, the first category (health behavior) has been discussed as "health promotion and preventive behavior" (Glanz, Rimer, & Lewis, 2002). Illness and sick-role behavior are often referred to as "disease management" by patients (Clark, Gong, & Kaciroti, 2001; Lorig et al., 1999).

Health Belief Model

The Health Belief Model (HBM) was developed in the early 1950s by a group of social psychologists at the U.S. Public Health Service (Rosenstock, 1974) in an attempt to understand "the widespread failure of people to accept disease preventives or screening tests for the early detection of asymptomatic disease" (p. 328); it was later applied to patients' responses to symptoms (Kirscht, 1974) and to following prescribed medical regimens (Becker, 1974).

The basic components of the HBM are derived from a well-established body of psychological and behavioral theory whose various models hypothesize that behavior depends mainly upon two variables: (1) the value placed by an individual on a particular goal, and (2) the individual's estimate of the likelihood that a given action will achieve that goal (Maiman & Becker, 1974). When these variables were conceptualized in the context of health-related behavior, the correspondences were (1) the desire to avoid illness (or, if ill, to get well), and (2) the belief that a specific health action will prevent (or ameliorate) illness (i.e., the individual's estimate of the threat of illness and of the likelihood of being able, through personal action, to reduce that threat).

The HBM consists of the following dimensions (Figure 2.1).

Perceived susceptibility, or one's subjective perception of the risk of contracting a condition; *perceived severity,* or feelings concerning the seriousness of contracting an illness (or of leaving it untreated) (while low perceptions of seriousness might provide insufficient motivation for behavior, very high perceived severity might inhibit action); *perceived benefits,* or beliefs regarding the effectiveness of the various actions available to reduce disease threat; *perceived barriers,* or the potential negative aspects of a particular health action that may act as impediments to undertaking the recommended behavior; and *cues to action,* or stimuli to trigger the decision-making process.

In the HBM context, it is understood that diverse demographic, personal, structural, and social factors are capable of influencing health behaviors.

2.1

The Health Belief Model.

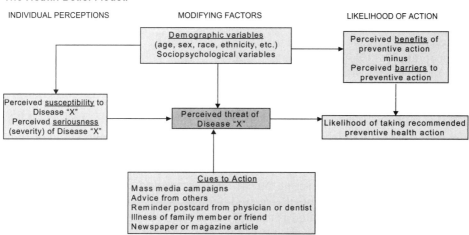

Note. From "A New Approach to Explaining Sick-Role Behavior in Low-income Populations," by M. H. Becker, R. H. Drachman, & J. P. Kirscht, 1974, *American Journal of Public Health, 64,* p. 206. Copyright 1974 by the American Public Health Association. Reprinted with permission from the American Public Health Association.

However, these variables are believed to work through their effects on the individual's health motivations and subjective perceptions, rather than functioning as direct causes of health action (Becker et al., 1977).

The HBM has received extensive research attention (cf. Menon, Champion, Monahan, Daggy, Hui, & Skinner, 2007; Silk et al., 2006). A large body of evidence has accumulated in support of the HBM's ability to account for individuals' undertaking preventive health actions, seeking diagnoses, and following prescribed medical advice (i.e., adhering to regimens), although the variance in difference it accounts for has not always been great. In the mid-1980s, a critical review summarized findings from 46 HBM-related investigations (18 prospective, 28 retrospective) and provided considerable empirical support for the model (Janz & Becker, 1984). Of all the HBM dimensions, "perceived barriers" proved the strongest predictor across all studies and behaviors. A systematic review of studies in the early 1990s found the model inconsistent in predictive power for a number of behaviors (Harrison, Mullen, & Green, 1992).

While the frequency of application has declined in recent years, the Health Belief Model continues to be widely used in published studies and program descriptions. In more current research, the model has been shown to be associated with a range of preventive behaviors, for example, cancer screening (Janz, Wren, Schottenfeld, & Guire, 2003); condom use (Hounton, Carabin, & Henderson, 2005); vaccination (de Wit, Vet, Schutten, & van Steenbergen, 2005); malaria chemoprophylaxis (Farquharson, Noble, Barker, & Beherns, 2004); and dental behavior (Barker, 1994; Pine et al., 2000). Constructs from the HBM have also predicted disease management for heart disease (George & Shalansky, 2007), diabetes (Pinto, Lively, Siganga, Holiday-Goodman, & Kamm, 2006), and HIV disease (Barclay et al., 2007; Catt, Stygall, & Catalan, 1995).

Investigators have examined the HBM constructs in combination with constructs from other theoretical models, such as Social Cognitive Theory. Specifically, self-efficacy, that is, the confidence people have in their ability to undertake given behaviors, has been explored in combination with HBM constructs by numerous researchers. Clark and colleagues (1988) added self-efficacy to dimensions of the HBM and found that the variance explained in the management of asthma by school-age children did not increase significantly. Adih and Alexander (1999), however, found self-efficacy along with constructs from the HBM was a significant predictor of condom use among youth. Although never explicitly incorporated into the original model, self-efficacy may prove to be a useful addition to the model when the focus is on long-term behavior change (Janz, Champion, & Strecher, 2002).

Despite the body of findings relating HBM dimensions to health actions, the HBM is a psychosocial model; as such, it is limited to accounting for as much of the variance in individuals' health-related behaviors as can be explained by their attitudes and beliefs. It is clear that other forces influence health actions as well; for example: (1) some behaviors (e.g., cigarette smoking, tooth brushing) have a substantial habitual component, obviating any ongoing psychosocial decision-making process; (2) many health-related behaviors are undertaken for what are ostensibly non-health-related reasons (e.g., dieting to appear more attractive); and (3) economic or environmental factors may prevent the individual from undertaking a preferred course of action (e.g., a worker in a hazardous environment; a resident in a city with high levels of air pollution). The model is based on the premises that "health" is a highly valued concern or goal for most individuals and that "cues to action" are widely prevalent; where these conditions are not satisfied, the model may not be useful in, or relevant to, predicting behavior.

Theory of Reasoned Action and the Theory of Planned Behavior

In the approach taken by Ajzen and Fishbein (1980), intention to perform a behavior is the central determinant of that behavior. More specifically, the Theory of Reasoned Action (TRA) focused on intention as predicted by the individual's attitude toward the behavior (i.e., the person's beliefs that the behavior leads to certain outcomes and the value attached to those outcomes) and the subjective norm associated with the behavior (i.e., the person's beliefs that certain individuals or groups think that she should or should not undertake the behavior, weighted by the person's desire to comply with their wishes). The relative influence of attitude and subjective norms on intention is dependent on the behavioral goal. For some behaviors, the attitudinal component will be the major determinant of intention, while for others, more external factors apply; the more the individual believes that significant others are in favor of his behavioral attempt, the stronger will be his intention to try. As with the HBM, sociodemographic factors operate only through their influences on the determinants of behavioral intention. This model also emphasizes normative influences that might affect intention for any reason, health-related or otherwise, thus adding a strong cultural component to the prediction of behavior.

The TRA has been effectively applied to explain and predict a variety of health behaviors, including preventive oral health behavior (Syrjala, Niskanen, & Knuuttila, 2002); breast-feeding (Swanson, Power, Kaur, Carter, & Shepherd, 2006); sun protection (Steen, Peay, & Owen, 1998); and condom use (Albarracin, Johnson, Fishbein, & Muellerleile, 2001).

The Theory of Planned Behavior (TPB) is an extension of Ajzen and Fishbein's Theory of Reasoned Action and considers both volitional and non-volitional behaviors. This model proposes that intention is not the exclusive determinant of behavior where an individual's control over the behavior is imperfect. Ajzen and colleagues (Ajzen, 1991; Ajzen & Driver, 1991) added the dimension of perceived behavioral control to the TRA as an additional predictor of intention, reflecting the notion that factors outside an individual's control can affect both intention and behavior. Control includes both personal and external factors that influence the behavior, such as having a workable plan, skills, social support, knowledge, time, money, willpower, and opportunity. Consistent with the TRA, intention to try to perform the behavior is the immediate determinant of an attempt to perform the behavior in the Theory of Planned Behavior. Intention is seen as a function of individuals' attitudes toward trying and their subjective norms.

In summary, the Theory of Planned Behavior states that individuals will try to perform a behavior if they believe that the benefits of success are outweighed by the benefits of failure and if they feel that significant others (with whom they want to comply) believe they should attempt to perform the behavior. Successful performance of the behavior will be the end result if individuals have sufficient control over internal and external factors that influence such performance. The Theory of Planned Behavior is posited as more appropriate when the probability of success and actual control over performance of a behavior are less than perfect.

A meta-analytic review of the 185 studies published through 1997 that examined the theory found that the TPB accounted for 27% of the variance in behavior and 39% of the variance in intention, although the study was not limited to health behavior (Armitage & Conner, 2001). In recent years, the TPB has proven increasingly useful in predicting both intention and actual health behavior. Constructs from the model have predicted intentions related to cancer screening (Steele & Porche, 2005), bicycle helmet use (O'Callaghan & Nausbaum, 2006), and fruit consumption (Brug, de Vet, de Noorijer, & Verplanken, 2006). Elements from the TPB have also predicted actual behavior, including sexual risk behaviors (Koniak-Griffin & Stein, 2006), safe-lifting behavior (Johnson & Hall, 2005), and physical activity (Armitage, 2005). In summary, it is evident from the multitude of studies applying the model that the TPB provides a useful framework for conceptualizing factors that determine a wide range of health behaviors.

Health Decision Model

Proposed as a "third generation model of patient behavior that focused more specifically on health decisions" (Eraker, Kirscht, & Becker, 1984, p. 260), the Health Decision Model attempted to combine decision analysis, behavioral decision theory, and health beliefs to yield a unifying model of health decisions and resultant behavior. The model was the first to include contributions from the "patient preferences" literature (Eraker & Politser, 1982), and interest continues to build around health care decision making conducted in a manner that incorporates these preferences (Institute of Medicine [IOM], 2003). Decision analysis provides quantitative means for patients to communicate their preferences about critical trade-offs between benefits and risk—and, at times, between quantity and quality of life (Hunink, 2001; Weinstein & Fineberg, 1980). Behavioral decision theory extends this quantitative emphasis by identifying a number of general inferential rules that patients use to reduce difficult mental tasks to simpler ones (Eraker & Sox, Jr., 1981).

Eraker and colleagues (1985) have observed that the relationships among health beliefs, decision analysis, and behavioral decision theory were demonstrated in a study on patient preferences as related to variations in the way information is presented to patients. For example, McNeil, Pauker, Sox, and Tversky (1982) examined the results of surgery and radiation treatment for lung cancer and found that preferences for alternative therapies shifted when the outcomes were framed in terms of probability of living or the probability of dying. The investigation also found that people relied more on preexisting beliefs regarding the treatments than on statistical data presented to them. These preexisting beliefs may help to explain why some patients, based on decision-analysis criteria, are treated in a manner not reflecting their underlying preferences.

The Health Decision Model also recognizes the importance of other factors affecting health decisions and behavior, such as knowledge, experience, and social and demographic variables. The bidirectional arrows and feedback loops reflect the notion that adherence behavior can change health beliefs. The model also includes concepts related to the efficacy of the prescribed regimen, motivational variables involving the person's assessment of the importance of good health, and "cues to action" that refer specifically to the patient-physician interaction (Eraker, Becker, Strecher, & Kirscht, 1985).

Self-Regulation Model

Leventhal and colleagues (1980, 1998) view self-regulation as a solution to dealing with the basic problem of locus of control in adherence theory. The fundamental notion is that:

> *The individual functions as a feedback system. He or she establishes behavioral goals, generates plans and responses to reach these goals, and establishes criteria for monitoring the effects of his/her responses on movement toward or away from the goal. This information is then used to alter coping techniques, set new criteria for evaluating response outputs and revise goals. The individual is, therefore, an information processing system that regulates his/her relationship to the environment. (1980, p. 34)*

Leventhal, Leventhal, and Contrada (1998) posit that:

> *(1) People are active problem solvers, they see and define their worlds, select and elaborate coping procedures to manage threats, and change the way they represent problems when they obtain disconfirming feedback; (2) Problem-solving processes occur in context; and (3) The energy expended or motivation to enhance health and to prevent and cure disease is directed to what is perceived to be the most immediate and urgent threat and is limited by resources and a satisfaction rule. (p. 718)*

The analogy provided is one of the person as scientist—formulating hypotheses about physiology and the effects of illness and creating a mental picture of ability to take actions to prevent or cure illness.

Leventhal's self-regulation model contains components that depict a process that an individual goes through: (1) extracting information from the environment; (2) generating a representation of the illness danger to oneself; and (3) planning and acting, which involves imagining response alternatives to deal with the problem and emotions it generates, then taking selected actions to achieve specific effects. Here the feedback loop is achieved by the last step: (4) monitoring or appraising how one's coping reactions affected the environmental problem and oneself.

In a self-regulation model, patients' adherence to a regimen is thought to be influenced by their perceptions and evaluations of the presence or absence of health threats, for example, symptoms. Using the model, Halm, Mora, and Leventhal (2006) have shown that individuals who conceptualized asthma as an acute, episodic illness were significantly more likely than individuals who did not see it as an acute episodic illness to report lower rates of adherence to inhaled corticosteroids at three separate time periods and after controlling for factors thought to affect medication adherence. Similarly, Brewer, Chapman, Brownlee, and Leventhal (2002) have demonstrated relationships between LDL cholesterol control and the degree to which patients' mental models of disease were similar to those of experts (i.e., physician-like).

In a study of 366 men and women using a clinic of a University Hospital, Cameron, Leventhal, and Leventhal (1995) found that care seeking was a function of the characteristics of the symptoms patients identified as distinctive signs of illness and not of the level of life stresses they experience. Also, this model relies to a fair degree on Bandura's formulations regarding reciprocal determinism and self-regulation, and both this work and Bandura's (1986) Social Cognitive Theory arise from a common theoretical heritage that strongly suggests the importance of the approach to understanding adherence behaviors.

Social Cognitive Theory

Bandura's (1986, 1997, 2004) discussion of social learning attempts to explain and predict behavior using several key concepts: incentives, outcome expectations, and efficacy expectations. Bandura (1977) outlined the roles of these concepts in a paradigm of a person engaging in a behavior that will have a consequent outcome; here, behavior change and maintenance are a function of (1) expectations about the outcomes that will result from engaging in behavior, and (2) expectations about one's ability to engage in or execute the behavior. Thus, "outcome expectations" consist of beliefs about whether given behaviors will lead to given outcomes, whereas "efficacy expectations" consist of beliefs about how capable one is of performing the behavior that leads to those outcomes. The two have been shown to be linked in predicting, for example, exercise behavior (Hallam & Petosa, 2004) and self-management of diabetes (Ianotti et al., 2006). It should be emphasized that both outcome and efficacy expectations reflect a person's beliefs about capabilities and the connections between behavior and outcome. Thus, it is these perceptions, and not necessarily "true" capabilities, that influence behavior. In addition, it is important to understand that the concept of self-efficacy relates to beliefs about one's capacity to perform specific behaviors in particular situations (Marks, Allegrante, & Lorig, 2005); self-efficacy does not refer to a personality characteristic or to a global trait that operates independent of contextual factors (Bandura, 1986, 1997). This means that individuals' efficacy expectations will vary greatly depending on the particular task and context that confronts them.

Bandura (1997) argued that perceived self-efficacy influences all aspects of behavior, including the acquisition of new behaviors (e.g., a sexually active young adult learning how to use a particular contraceptive device), inhibition of existing behaviors (e.g., decreasing or stopping cigarette smoking), and disinhibition of behaviors (e.g., resuming sexual activity after a myocardial infarction). Self-efficacy also affects people's choices on behaviors settings, the amount of effort they will expend on a task, and the length of time they will persist in the face of obstacles. Finally, self-efficacy affects people's emotional reactions, such as anxiety and distress and thought patterns. Thus, individuals with low self-efficacy about a particular task may ruminate about their personal deficiencies, rather than thinking about accomplishing or attending to the task at hand; this, in turn, impedes successful performance of the task.

Efficacy expectations are learned from four major sources (Bandura, 1977, 1986, 1997). The first, termed "performance accomplishments," refers to learning through personal experience in which one has achieved mastery over a difficult or previously feared task and thereby enjoys an increase in self-efficacy. Performance accomplishments attained through personal experience are the most potent source of efficacy expectations.

The second source is "vicarious experience," which includes learning that occurs through observation of events or other people. These events or people are referred to as "models" when they display a set of behaviors or stimulus array that illustrates a certain principle, rule, or response. In order for modeling to affect an observer's self-efficacy positively, however, it is important that the model can be viewed as having overcome difficulties through determined effort rather than with ease and that the model be similar to the observer with regard to other characteristics (e.g., age, gender). "Verbal persuasion" constitutes the third source of efficacy expectations. This method is quite familiar to all health workers who have exhorted patients to persevere in their efforts to change behavior. Finally, one's "physiological state" provides information that can influence efficacy expectations. Bandura noted that because high physiological arousal usually impairs performance, people are more likely to expect failure when they are very tense and viscerally agitated. For example, people who experience extremely sweaty palms, a racing heartbeat, and trembling knees prior to giving a talk find that their self-efficacy plummets; to someone just beginning an exercise program, fatigue and mild aches and pains may be mistakenly interpreted as a sign of physical inefficacy.

Individuals' sense of self-efficacy has been shown to predict asthma outcomes (Mancuso, Rincon, McCulloch, & Charlson, 2001); HIV risk behavior among low-income women (Sikkema et al., 1995); exercise behavior among arthritis patients (Gyurcsik, Estabrooks, & Frahm-Templar, 2003); disease management of older women with heart disease (Clark & Dodge, 1999); and glycosylated hemogoblin (HbA1c) levels among young adults with diabetes (Johnston-Brooks, Lewis, & Garg, 2002), among other outcomes.

A Model of Disease Self-Management

Drawing from Social Cognitive Theory and especially the construct of self-regulation, Clark (1997), Clark and Gong (2000), Clark, Gong, and Kaciroti (2001), and Clark and colleagues (1988) have proposed a framework for conceptualizing disease management by patients with acute or chronic conditions. In the refined version of this model (see Figure 2.2), self-regulation is viewed as a means by which patients determine what is effective and what isn't, given their specific goals. They make these determinations influenced by their social context and according to the resources they have available. The model is based on three assumptions. First, several factors predispose one to manage a disease. Second, patient management is the conscious use of strategies to manipulate situations to reduce the impact of disease on daily life. One learns which strategies do or do not work through processes of self-regulation. Third, a person is motivated

2.2

The continuous and reciprocal nature of self-regulation processes in disease prevention and management.

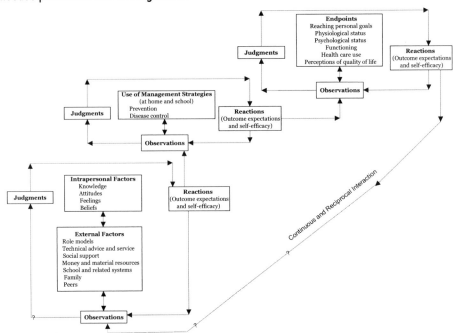

Note. Based on the model from "A Model of Self-Regulation for Control of Chronic Disease" by N. M. Clark, M. Gong & N. Kaciroti, 2001, *Health Education & Behavior,* 28, pp. 769–782. Copyright.

to be self-regulating by a desired goal or end point. The more salient the goal, the more self-regulating a person will try to be. The model is also predicated on the idea that the processes that make up self-regulation are continuous and reciprocal. Information, behavior, understanding, feelings, and conclusions generated from any one element of self-regulation as defined in the model (i.e., observation, judging, reacting) continually influence the other elements.

The model posits that, when taking a disease management action, people are influenced by internal factors, that is, information and beliefs concerning the specific problem. The action is also influenced by what they believe to be the benefits of engaging in the behavior to reach their personal goals and their beliefs that the benefits outweigh the costs. The extent to which people hold the requisite knowledge and beliefs to support an action depends, in part, on a range of external factors. These include interpersonal relationships through which emotional and instrumental (social) support is given and received. Almost certainly involved is technical advice from a clinician who provides therapeutic recommendations. Availability of money and other resources (e.g., the price of medicine and the ability to get to a pharmacy) also influence behavior. It also must be noted that while knowledge, attitudes, and feelings are the basis for action, these can also change as a result of behavior (Bandura, 1986).

Management strategies comprise the individual's means to keep the disease and its effects under control (Clark, Gong, & Kaciroti, 2001). These strategies may be effective or ineffective and may be consistent with clinicians' recommendations or not. Strategies evolve from people's observations, judgments, and reactions given the aforementioned internal and external factors. Others can influence the strategy chosen, but, in the end, individual personal goals, combined internal and external resources, and degree of self-regulation will dictate which management strategy will be derived and further employed. An example is a child who wants to play full-court basketball who believes he is susceptible to respiratory problems, thinks medicines will help and so uses them preventively, works out a procedure for taking a breather when active, seeks moral support from friends and coaches, and uses other strategies that enable him to reach his personal goal. The child learns which strategies are effective through self-regulation. Self-regulation may be particularly important in diseases where there is no sure-fire formula that an individual can use to control symptoms or deal with crucial interpersonal relationships. In these illnesses, patients (and families) must exercise a high level of decision making in the absence of health professionals. The self-regulatory processes in which they engage entail observing situations where the disease contributes to problems in reaching their goals; judging what types of actions might ameliorate the situation; using management strategies, that is, trying out new behaviors; and drawing conclusions or reacting to the effects of the behavior. Two important reactions are that the behavior resulted in the desired effect and that one can effectively carry out the behavior, that is, self-efficacy (as defined by Bandura, 1997, 2004). Using strategies to prevent symptoms, to manage them effectively, and to manage the interpersonal relationships needed to control the effects of the disease should lead to important outcomes.

The motivating factor in taking disease management action is a personal goal. Goals are highly idiosyncratic. When an educator or clinician (or any other person attempting to assist with disease management) has a goal that is different from that of the individual, the opportunity for successful goal attainment is attenuated. Usually, the clinician has a clinical goal, but this end point is not likely to be as important to the patient as her personal goal. When an educator or clinician focus on achieving the patient's personal goal, the chances are greater that the therapeutic regimen will appeal to the interests of the patient and that she will implement it.

This model was developed in an effort to delineate the discrete elements of self-regulation (observation, judgment, reaction). The assumption of the model presented here is that enabling people to be the best managers of their disease requires helping them to improve their self-regulation skills and modifying external factors so that these influences enhance the patient's ability to be self-regulating. Elements of the model have been shown to be predictive of disease self-management outcomes (cf. Cabana et al., 2006; Clark, Evans, Zimmerman, Levison, & Mellins, 1994; Clark, Gong, & Kaciroti, 2001).

Behavior Modification

Finally, an approach to understanding and influencing adherence behaviors that is substantially different from the cognitive themes emphasized in the previously described models and frameworks is represented by behavior modification. This approach emphasizes the roles played by habit and skill in attempts to modify undesirable personal (or "lifestyle") behaviors and brings to bear a wide variety of techniques (e.g., contingency contracting, self-monitoring, counterconditioning, covert sensitization, relaxation, environmental engineering) (Miltenberger, 2007). It is not reasonable to suggest a single "model" for behavior modification, although the concepts of behavioral consequences and stimulus control are fairly common elements of them. The general plan that this approach frequently follows is this: identify the problem and describe it in behavioral terms; select a target behavior that is measurable; identify the antecedents and consequences of the behavior; set behavioral objectives; devise and implement a behavior-change program; and evaluate the program. Since cognitive and behavioral models and approaches both have much to offer, it seems reasonable to assume that our best bets for effective interventions will be strategies that combine elements of both.

A Community Decision-Making and Action Model

Given the need to have a broader impact on population health and to reach large numbers of people, an important question is whether there are decision-making models for community-wide health behavior change? The challenge of public health, especially given advances in life sciences that will enable the most refined tailoring of medical therapies to an individual's biological profile, is developing interventions that can be highly specific to individuals but at the same time reach across populations. A health provider can help individual patients and families, but, to effect large-scale change, there must be effective systems, policies, and practices in place that extend assistance to all patients. Communities are finding it increasingly effective to work collectively to bring about policy and system change to prevent and control health problems by developing partnerships and collaborations. Community coalitions are one example (see, e.g., Clark, Malveaux, & Friedman, 2006).

Coalitions as a means to improve health status are widely evident in public health for a range of conditions, and there is an extensive literature regarding coalitions as vehicles for amassing community resources, influence, and energy in pursuit of a health goal (Clark et al., 2006). The key feature of such efforts is collaboration (Alexander et al., 2003), that is, the willingness of stakeholders in a problem to work together cooperatively toward its solution.

Coalition does not refer to the type of stakeholders engaged in collaboration. Rather, the term depicts a way of working. The type of coalition most discussed currently in the literature and, indeed, most often promoted in the field of public health is that which aims to give voice to constituencies not often at the table when the health problems affecting them and their families are considered. By employing this term, Butterfoss, Goodman, and Wandersman (1993) wished to describe a type of coalition that is representative of a given, defined community whose membership reflects all segments of that community's population, not just one sector or type of stakeholder. Reflected in the term is the idea that much of the know-how for resolving problems rests with those who experience them most directly and that they and their experience must be acknowledged in decisions about solutions. These stakeholders can be individuals with the problem or representatives of community-based organizations that understand the problem in its most compelling form. Implicitly, *community coalition* appears to mean that the given coalition (a) serves a defined community (usually having a common location or experience) recognized by those within it as a community, (b) is purposeful and has a time-specific duration, (c) exists to serve the broader community, (d) is viewed by community residents as representing and serving them, (e) reflects the diversity evident in the community, (f) addresses the problem(s) systematically and comprehensively, and (g) builds community independence and capacity. In bringing about change, coalitions must attend to how they function as a collective of members, as well as how they use strategies to achieve their change goals (Butterfoss, Kelly, & Taylor-Fishwick, 2005).

A comprehensive review conducted by Roussos and Fawcett (2000) identified a number of studies that provide population-wide outcomes where improvements appeared to be attributable to the efforts of a coalition. Examples include declines in lead poisoning in New York City (Freudenberg & Golub, 1987), reduction of infant mortality in Boston (Plough & Olafson, 1994), and improvements in the physical fitness of older adults (Hooker & Cirill, 2006).

A model referred to as the Allies model (Clark et al., 2006) for functioning of coalitions is presented in Figure 2.3. It holds still for an instant the dynamic movement of many factors that are thought to contribute to changed policies, enhanced systems, and improved practices of individuals thought to enable

2.3

Allies coalition model.

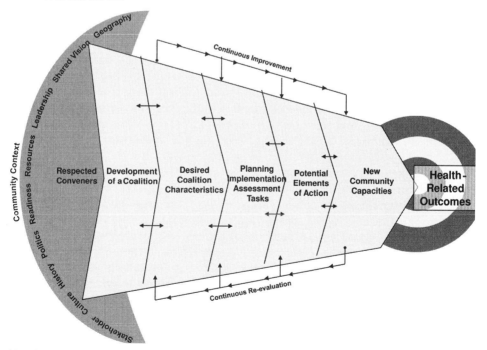

Note. From "Community Coalitions to Control Chronic Disease Allies Against Asthma as a Model and Case Study," by N. M. Clark, L. J. Doctor, A. R. Friedman, L. L. Lachance, C. R. Houle, X. Geng, et al., 2006, *Health Promotion Practice, 7*(2 suppl.), pp. 145–225. Copyright 2006 by Sage Publications. Reprinted with permission.

communities to reach health goals. However, it is important to acknowledge that it is only in the figure that the elements are static. Each factor influences every other one continually and over time within the turbulent field that constitutes any community. Nonetheless, it is likely that, at given moments over the life of a community coalition, it is possible to get very rough measures of these factors.

A pervasive factor for any coalition is the collective characteristics of the community where it strives to do work. A set of community characteristics provides a backdrop for the coalition's efforts and can either support or inhibit its success. It is, therefore, important for coalitions to pay attention to these characteristics, particularly during the formative stage.

Another important asset is the respected convener(s). Is there a respected person or agency seen by the community as important to resolving the problem and at the same time not closely associated with perspectives, factions, or authorities that are not trusted?

There is a need for ongoing internal leadership. Members must have an adequate understanding of the magnitude and importance of the problem the coalition is addressing. An infrastructure for functioning must be developed and maintained. Credibility in the wider community and participation that is diverse and representative of the entire community must be engendered. Stakeholders' commitment to the mission must be elicited and maintained. Trust levels must be sufficient to enable real collaboration, and mutual benefit must be recognized. Communication must be adequate and benefits for participation clear. Expert assistance must be available and used as needed.

When optimal structures and internal procedures are in place and a coalition reflects the organizational characteristics of success, it effectively moves toward its goals. Careful planning that draws on the collective wisdom, experience, and skills of the stakeholding members is necessary. Strategies to translate the plan into action and taking the indicated actions are required.

A coalition's characteristics reflect the intrapersonal characteristics described in self-regulation models. An additional similarity between the Allies coalition model and the previously discussed self-regulation model of disease self-management is evident. The elements of self-regulation—observation, judgment, trial behavior, and reaction—are clearly part of the Allies model as they are carried out community-wide. For example, ongoing evaluation and continuous feedback about the extent or level of the characteristics of a coalition is crucial to effective stakeholder engagement and commitment, and ongoing evaluation and continuous feedback are necessary to continually refine and modify plans and strategies the coalition has implemented or as it puts new ones into place.

Through these "self-regulating" features, a coalition structures itself and takes effective action. Action can take the form of coordination and integration of community services, establishment of exemplar programs or services, leadership in advocacy, or policy formation. Coalition action has been documented to include coordinating and providing systemic services for children with asthma and their families in seven communities around the United States, as well as providing families in the community with the skills they need to manage respiratory disease, and training health providers to both practice at the standard of care and support family self-management efforts (Clark et al., 2006). These were achievements institutionalized through policy changes that ensured adequate provision of quality care and directed resources for asthma control. More comprehensive studies are needed to illuminate the connection between aspects of coalition functioning and changes in community-wide behavior, health care systems, and health-related conditions.

Summary

This chapter has summarized and depicted the major elements of a number of well-known and widely employed psychological, behavioral, and sociological models of health-related decision making and action and has summarized some of the major strategies advanced in the empirical literature for increasing adherence and self-management. While further theoretical conceptualization and empirical investigation regarding behavioral determinants of (and strategies for influencing) patient health status are certainly still needed, the variables identified and suggestions offered in this chapter provide the foundation for programs that can be implemented by health care providers and public health planners wishing to improve levels of patient cooperation and ability to use health-related recommendations.

References

Adih, W. K., & Alexander, C. S. (1999). Determinants of condom use to prevent HIV infection among youth in Ghana. *The Journal of Adolescent Health, 24*(1), 63–72.

Ajzen, I. (1991). The theory of planned behavior. *Organizational Behavior and Human Decision Processes, 50,* 179–211.

Ajzen, I., & Driver, B. L. (1991). Prediction of leisure participation from behavioral, normative, and control beliefs: An application of the theory of planned behavior. *Leisure Sciences, 13,* 184–204.

Ajzen, I., & Fishbein, M. (1980). *Understanding attitudes and predicting social behavior.* Englewood Cliffs, NJ: Prentice-Hall.

Albarracin, D., Johnson, B. T., Fishbein, M., & Muellerleile, P. A. (2001). Theories of reasoned action and planned behavior as models of condom use: A meta-analysis. *Psychological Bulletin, 127*(1), 142–161.

Alexander, J. A., Weiner, B. J., Metzger, M. E., Shortell, S. M., Bazzoli, G. J., Hasnain-Wynia, R., et al. (2003). Sustainability of collaborative capacity in community health partnerships. *Medical Care Research and Review, 60*(4 Suppl.), 130–160.

Armitage, C. J. (2005). Can the theory of planned behavior predict the maintenance of physical activity? *Health Psychology, 24*(3), 235–245.

Armitage, C. J., & Conner, M. (2001). Efficacy of the theory of planned behaviour: A meta-analytic review. *The British Journal of Social Psychology, 40*(Pt. 4), 471–499.

Bandura, A. (1977). Self-efficacy: Toward a unifying theory of behavioral change. *Psychological Review, 84*(2), 191–215.

Bandura, A. (1986). *Social learning theory.* Englewood Cliffs, NJ: Prentice-Hall.

Bandura, A. (1997). *Self-efficacy: The exercise of control.* New York: W. H. Freeman.

Bandura, A. (2004). Health promotion by social cognitive means. *Health Education & Behavior, 31*(2), 143–164.

Barclay, T. R., Hinkin, C. H., Castellon, S. A., Mason, K. I., Reinhard, M. J., Marion, S. D., et al. (2007). Age-associated predictors of medication adherence in HIV-positive adults: Health beliefs, self-efficacy, and neurocognitive status. *Health Psychology, 26*(1), 40–49.

Barker, T. (1994). Role of health beliefs in patient compliance with preventive dental advice. *Community Dentistry and Oral Epidemiology, 22*(5 Pt. 1), 327–330.

Becker, M. H. (1974). The health belief model and sick role behavior. *Health Education Monographs, 2,* 409–419.

Becker, M. H., Drachman, R. H., & Kirscht, J. P. (1974). A new approach to explaining sick role behavior in low-income populations. American Journal of Public Health, 64.

Becker, M. H., Haefner, D. P., Kasl, S. V., Kirscht, J. P., Maiman, L. A., & Rosenstock, I. M. (1977). Selected psychosocial models and correlates of individual health-related behaviors. Medical Care, 15(5 Suppl.), 27–46.

Brewer, N. T., Chapman, G. B., Brownlee, S., & Leventhal, E. A. (2002). Cholesterol control, medication adherence and illness cognition. British Journal of Health Psychology, 7(Part 4), 433–447.

Brug, J., de Vet, E., de Nooijer, J., & Verplanken, B. (2006). Predicting fruit consumption: Cognitions, intention, and habits. Journal of Nutrition Education and Behavior, 38(2), 73–81.

Butterfoss, F. D., Goodman, R. M., & Wandersman, A. (1993). Community coalitions for prevention and health promotion. Health Education Research, 8(3), 315–330.

Butterfoss, F. D., Kelly, C., & Taylor-Fishwick, J. (2005). Health planning that magnifies the community's voice: Allies Against Asthma. Health Education & Behavior, 32(1), 113–128.

Cabana, M. D., Slish, K. K., Evans, D., Mellins, R. B., Brown, R. W., Lin, X., et al. (2006). Impact of physician asthma care education on patient outcomes. Pediatrics, 117(6), 2149–2157.

Cameron, L., Leventhal, E. A., & Leventhal, H. (1995). Seeking medical care in response to symptoms and life stress. Psychosomatic Medicine, 57(1), 37–47.

Catt, S., Stygall, J., & Catalan, J. (1995). Acceptance of zidovudine (AZT) in early HIV disease: The role of health beliefs. AIDS Care, 7(2), 229–225.

Clark, N. M. (1997). Self-regulation of heart disease and hypertension. In D. S. Gochman (Ed.), Handbook of health behavior research (pp. 149–168). New York: Plenum.

Clark, N. M., Doctor, L. J., Friedman, A. R., Lachance, L. L., Houle, C. R., Geng, X., et al. (2006). Community coalitions to control chronic disease: Allies Against Asthma as a model and case study. Health Promotion Practice, 7(2 Suppl), 14S–22S.

Clark, N. M., & Dodge, J. A. (1999). Exploring self-efficacy as a predictor of disease management. Health Education & Behavior, 26(1), 72–89.

Clark, N. M., Evans, D., Zimmerman, B. J., Levison, M. J., & Mellins, R. B. (1994). Patient and family management of asthma: Theory-based techniques for the clinician. The Journal of Asthma, 31(6), 427–435.

Clark, N. M., & Gong, M. (2000). Management of chronic disease by practitioners and patients: Are we teaching the wrong things? BMJ (Clinical research ed.), 320(7234), 572–575.

Clark, N. M., Gong, M., & Kaciroti, N. (2001). A model of self-regulation for control of chronic disease. Health Education & Behavior, 28(6), 769–782.

Clark, N. M., Malveaux, F., & Friedman, A. R. (2006). An introduction to Allies Against Asthma and this special issue. Health Promotion Practice, 7(2 Suppl), 8S-12S.

Clark, N. M., Rosenstock, I., Hassan, H., Evans, D., Feldman, C., & Mellins, R. (1988). The effect of health beliefs and feelings of self-efficacy on self-management behavior of children with a chronic disease. Patient Counseling and Education, 11, 131–139.

Dansinger, M. L., Tatsioni, A., Wong, J. B., Chung, M., & Balk, E. M. (2007). Meta-analysis: The effect of dietary counseling for weight loss. Annals of Internal Medicine, 147(1), 41–50.

de Wit, J. B., Vet, R., Schutten, M., & van Steenbergen, J. (2005). Social-cognitive determinants of vaccination behavior against hepatitis B: An assessment among men who have sex with men. Preventive Medicine, 40(6), 795–802.

DiMatteo, M. R. (2004). Variations in patients' adherence to medical recommendations: A quantitative review of 50 years of research. Medical Care, 42(3), 200–209.

Eraker, S. A., Becker, M. H., Strecher, V. J., & Kirscht, J. P. (1985). Smoking behavior, cessation techniques, and the health decision model. The American Journal of Medicine, 78(5), 817–825.

Eraker, S. A., Kirscht, J. P., & Becker, M. H. (1984). Understanding and improving patient compliance. Annals of Internal Medicine, 100(2), 258–268.

Eraker, S. A., & Politser, P. (1982). How decisions are reached: Physician and patient. Annals of Internal Medicine, 97(2), 262–268.

Eraker, S. A., & Sox, H. C., Jr. (1981). Assessment of patients' preferences for therapeutic outcomes. Medical Decision Making, 1(1), 29–39.

Farquharson, L., Noble, L. M., Barker, C., & Behrens, R. H. (2004). Health beliefs and communication in the travel clinic consultation as predictors of adherence to malaria chemoprophylaxis. British Journal of Health Psychology, 9(Pt. 2), 201–217.

Freudenberg, N., & Golub, M. (1987). Health education, public policy and disease prevention: A case history of the New York City coalition to end lead poisoning. *Health Education Quarterly, 14*(4), 387–401.

George, J., & Shalansky, S. J. (2007). Predictors of refill non-adherence in patients with heart failure. *British Journal of Clinical Pharmacology, 63*(4), 488–493.

Glanz, K., Rimer, B. K., & Lewis, F. M. (2002). The scope of health behavior and health education. In K. Glanz, B. K. Rimer, & F. M. Lewis (Eds.), *Health behavior and health education: Theory, research, and practice* (3rd ed., pp. 3–21). San Francisco: Jossey-Bass.

Gyurcsik, N. C., Estabrooks, P. A., & Frahm-Templar, M. J. (2003). Exercise-related goals and self-efficacy as correlates of aquatic exercise in individuals with arthritis. *Arthritis and Rheumatism, 49*(3), 306–313.

Hallam, J. S., & Petosa, R. (2004). The long-term impact of a four-session work-site intervention on selected social cognitive theory variables linked to adult exercise adherence. *Health Education & Behavior, 31*(1), 88–100.

Halm, E. A., Mora, P., & Leventhal, H. (2006). No symptoms, no asthma: The acute episodic disease belief is associated with poor self-management among inner-city adults with persistent asthma. *Chest, 129*(3), 573–580.

Harrison, J. A., Mullen, P. D., & Green, L. W. (1992). A meta-analysis of studies of the Health Belief Model with adults. *Health Education Research, 7*(1), 107–116.

Hooker, S. P., & Cirill, L. A. (2006). Evaluation of community coalitions' ability to create safe, effective exercise classes for older adults. *Evaluation and Program Planning, 29* (3), 242–250.

Hounton, S. H., Carabin, H., & Henderson, N. J. (2005). Towards an understanding of barriers to condom use in rural Benin using the health belief model: A cross sectional survey. *BMC Public Health, 5,* 8.

Hunink, M. G. (2001). In search of tools to aid logical thinking and communicating about medical decision making. *Medical Decision Making, 21*(4), 267–277.

Institute of Medicine. (2003). *Crossing the quality chasm: A new health system for the 21st century.* Washington, DC: National Academy Press.

Janz, N. K., & Becker, M. H. (1984). The health belief model: A decade later. *Health Education Quarterly, 11*(1), 1–47.

Janz, N. K., Champion, V. L., & Strecher, V. J. (2002). The health belief model. In K. Glanz, B. K. Rimer, & F. M. Lewis (Eds.), *Health behavior and health education: Theory, research, and practice* (3rd ed., pp. 45–66). San Francisco: Jossey-Bass.

Janz, N. K., Wren, P. A., Schottenfeld, D., & Guire, K. E. (2003). Colorectal cancer screening attitudes and behavior: A population-based study. *Preventive Medicine, 37*(6 Pt. 1), 627–634.

Johnson, S. E., & Hall, A. (2005). The prediction of safe lifting behavior: An application of the theory of planned behavior. *Journal of Safety Research, 36*(1), 63–73.

Johnston-Brooks, C. H., Lewis, M. A., & Garg, S. (2002). Self-efficacy impacts self-care and HbA1c in young adults with type I diabetes. *Psychosomatic Medicine, 64*(1), 43–51.

Kasl, S. V., & Cobb, S. (1966). Health behavior, illness behavior, and sick-role behavior. II. Sick-role behavior. *Archives of Environmental Health, 12*(4), 531–541.

Kimmel, S. E., Chen, Z., Price, M., Parker, C. S., Metlay, J. P., Christie, J. D., et al. (2007). The influence of patient adherence on anticoagulation control with warfarin: Results from the international normalized ratio adherence and genetics (IN-RANGE) study. *Archives of Internal Medicine, 167*(3), 229–235.

Kirscht, J. P. (1974). The health belief model and illness behavior. *Health Education Monographs, 2,* 387–408.

Koniak-Griffin, D., & Stein, J. A. (2006). Predictors of sexual risk behaviors among adolescent mothers in a human immunodeficiency virus prevention program. *The Journal of Adolescent Health, 38*(3), 297.e1–297.ell.

Leventhal, H., Leventhal, E. A., & Contrada, L. (1998). Self-regulation, health, and behavior: A perceptual-cognitive approach. *Psychology and Health, 13*(4), 717–733.

Leventhal, H., Meyer, D., & Gutmann, M. (1980). The role of theory in the study of compliance to high blood pressure regimens. In R. B. Haynes, M. E. Mattson, & T. O. Engebretson, Jr. (Eds.), *Patient compliance to prescribed antihypertensive medication regimens: A report to the National Heart, Lung, and Blood Institute* (NIH Publication No. 81-2102; pp. 1–58). Washington, DC: U.S. Department of Health and Human Services.

Lorig, K. R., Sobel, D. S., Stewart, A. L., Brown, B. W., Jr., Bandura, A., Ritter, P., et al. (1999). Evidence suggesting that a chronic disease self-management program can improve health status while reducing hospitalization: A randomized trial. *Medical Care, 37*(1), 5–14.

Maiman, L. A., & Becker, M. H. (1974). The health belief model: Origins and correlates in psychological theory. *Health Education Monographs, 2,* 336–353.

Mancuso, C. A., Rincon, M., McCulloch, C. E., & Charlson, M. E. (2001). Self-efficacy, depressive symptoms, and patients' expectations predict outcomes in asthma. *Medical Care, 39*(12), 1326–1338.

Marks, R., Allegrante, J. P., & Lorig, K. (2005). A review and synthesis of research evidence for self-efficacy-enhancing interventions for reducing chronic disability: Implications for health education practice (part I). *Health Promotion Practice, 6*(1), 37–43.

McNeil, B. J., Pauker, S. G., Sox, H. C., Jr., & Tversky, A. (1982). On the elicitation of preferences for alternative therapies. *New England Journal of Medicine, 306*(21), 1259–1262.

Menon, U., Champion, V., Monahan, P. O., Daggy, J., Hui, S., & Skinner, C. S. (2007). Health belief model variables as predictors of progression in stage of mammography adoption. *American Journal of Health Promotion, 21*(4), 255–261.

Miltenberger, R. G. (2007). *Behavior modification: Principles and procedures* (4th ed.). Belmont, MA: Wadsworth.

O'Callaghan, F. V., & Nausbaum, S. (2006). Predicting bicycle helmet wearing intentions and behavior among adolescents. *Journal of Safety Research, 37*(5), 425–431.

Osterberg, L., & Blaschke, T. (2005). Adherence to medication. *New England Journal of Medicine, 353*(5), 487–497.

Pine, C. M., McGoldrick, P. M., Burnside, G., Curnow, M. M., Chesters, R. K., Nicholson, J., et al. (2000). An intervention programme to establish regular toothbrushing: Understanding parents' beliefs and motivating children. *International Dental Journal,* 312–323.

Pinto, S. L., Lively, B. T., Siganga, W., Holiday-Goodman, M., & Kamm, G. (2006). Using the health belief model to test factors affecting patient retention in diabetes-related pharmaceutical care services. *Research in Social & Administrative Pharmacy, 2*(1), 38–58.

Plough, A., & Olafson, F. (1994). Implementing the Boston Healthy Start initiative: A case study of community empowerment and public health. *Health Education Quarterly, 21*(2), 221–234.

Rosenstock, I. M. (1974). Historical origins of the health belief model. *Health Education Monographs, 2,* 328–335.

Roussos, S. T., & Fawcett, S. B. (2000). A review of collaborative partnerships as a strategy for improving community health. *Annual Review of Public Health, 21,* 369–402.

Sackett, D. L., & Snow, J. C. (1979). The magnitude of compliance and noncompliance. In R. B. Haynes, D. W. Taylor, & D. L. Sackett (Eds.), *Compliance in health care* (pp. 11–22). Baltimore, MD: Johns Hopkins University Press.

Sapkota, S., Bowles, H. R., Ham, S. A., & Kohl, H. W. (2005). Adult participation in recommended levels of physical activity—United States, 2001 and 2003. *Morbidity and Mortality Weekly Report, 54*(47), 1208–1212.

Sikkema, K. J., Koob, J. J., Cargill, V. C., Kelly, J. A., Desiderato, L. L., Roffman, R. A., et al. (1995). Levels and predictors of HIV risk behavior among women in low-income public housing developments. *Public Health Reports, 110*(6), 707–713.

Silk, K., Bigsby, E., Volkman, J., Kingsley, C., Atkin, C., Ferrara, M., et al. (2006). Formative research on adolescent and adult perceptions of risk factors for breast cancer. *Social Science & Medicine, 63*(12), 3124–3136.

Steele, S. K., & Porche, D. J. (2005). Testing the theory of planned behavior to predict mammography intention. *Nursing Research, 54*(5), 332–338.

Steen, D. M., Peay, M. Y., & Owen, N. (1998). Predicting Australian adolescents' intentions to minimize sun exposure. *Psychology and Health, 13,* 111–119.

Swanson, V., Power, K., Kaur, B., Carter, H., & Shepherd, K. (2006). The impact of knowledge and social influences on adolescents' breast-feeding beliefs and intentions. *Public Health Nutrition, 9*(3), 297–305.

Syrjala, A. M., Niskanen, M. C., & Knuuttila, M. L. (2002). The theory of reasoned action in describing tooth brushing, dental caries and diabetes adherence among diabetic patients. *Journal of Clinical Periodontology, 29*(5), 427–432.

U.S. Department of Health and Human Services. (2000). *Reducing tobacco use: A report of the Surgeon General.* Atlanta: U.S. Department of Health and Human Services, Centers for Disease Control and Prevention, National Center for Chronic Disease Prevention and Health Promotion, Office on Smoking and Health.

Weinstein, M. C., & Fineberg, H. V. (1980). *Clinical decision analysis.* Philadelphia: W. B. Saunders.Becker, M. H., Drachman, R. H., & Kirscht, J. P. (1974). A new approach to explaining sick role behavior in low-income populations. American Journal of Public Health, 64.

Culture and Health-Related Behavior

3

Milagros C. Rosal
and Jamie S.
Bodenlos

Culture, defined as *what is learned, shared, transmitted intergenerationally, and reflected in a group's values, beliefs, norms, behaviors, communication, and social roles,* can affect health-related behaviors both directly and indirectly (Kreuter & Haughton, 2006). In clinical settings, health care providers are responsible for delivering evidence-based care that meets their patients' needs for maintaining health, preventing and managing chronic disease, and decreasing human suffering. Given the increasing diversity of the American population, clinical trials must provide evidence of efficacy and effectiveness of health-enhancing interventions in diverse samples and populations. Evaluating the generalizability of research findings across diverse groups (Office of Minority Health & U.S. Department of Health and Human Services, 2007) is an important stepping stone to decrease health disparities.

Current literature on culture and health, and particularly health behaviors, is very limited. However, interest in culture is growing due to numerous findings that ethnic minority patients are less likely to receive, or have differential outcomes from, preventive, diagnostic, medical, or surgical interventions, even after adjusting for severity of illness, access to care, and poverty (Ang, Ibrahim, Burant, Siminoff, & Kwoh, 2002; Escarce, Epstein, Colby, & Schwartz, 1993; Ford & Cooper, 1995; Hannan et al., 1999; Keppel, 2007; Lee, Gehlbach, Hosmer, Reti, & Baker, 1997; Shi, 1999; Smedley, Stith, & Nelson, 2003; Suarez-Almazor et al., 2005). An understanding of an individual's or a group's cultural context is essential for targeting health behavior change and decreasing health disparities, an important public health issue. Although there has been a movement in many disciplines to increase cultural competence, many researchers and clinicians still do not assess or understand culture appropriately.

In this chapter, we approach the topic of culture from an empirical and a theoretical perspective and discuss the importance of conducting theory-based research to enhance our understanding of cultural influences on behavior. The first section of this chapter is a review of commonly used culture-related concepts and definitions. The second section presents empirical evidence of the influence of culture on screening and preventive behaviors, illness and symptom perception, and disease management behaviors. The third section summarizes some of the most frequently cited theoretical models of behavior, which can be useful in accounting for the effect of culture on behavior. Last, we conclude with implications of culture for health care and for clinical and population research.

Culture-Related Definitions

Cultural Influence

Cultural influence refers to the degree to which the values, beliefs, norms, and traditions common to a particular group affect or sway the behavior of the individual members of the group. Culture can influence behavior through its influence on values and beliefs and traditional roles and social customs and its impact on what people see as acceptable, appropriate, and desirable behavior. These values, beliefs, and roles ultimately guide how someone acts (Haviland, 1999).

Cultural Change

There is a certain degree of permanency in cultures. However, cultures are not static. Changes in culture can occur to various degrees and at varying rates. Aspects of a culture may change and affect other aspects of that culture; for example, changes in politics often affect economics. Likewise, the learning of a new language (an important cultural symbol) by a group can bring on the adoption of other behaviors (e.g., greater engagement in the health care system) among members of that group. Cultural changes such as changes in beliefs and behaviors also can occur as a result of "lived experiences," that is, experiences that people (or groups of people) go through as they live their lives (Garro, 2000). At the individual level, these can include but are not limited to acquisition of education or migration to a new country, county, or region. Recent examples at the group level include disasters that affect regions (Hurricane Katrina's effect on the Gulf Coast or the effect of 911 on New York City and the United States).

Society and Subcultures

Society is defined as a group of people who have a common homeland, are dependent on one another for survival, and share a common culture often referred to as "mainstream" culture (Haviland, 1999). However, no member of a society experiences the same exact culture; culture shared by members of a society is not uniform, and multiple subcultures coexist within a single society. An example of one aspect of the mainstream American culture (or society) that affects Americans from all subcultures is the high number of fast-food chains. Many researchers believe that the high accessibility of calorie-dense food has contributed enormously to the obesity epidemic.

Individuals can belong to many different cultures and subcultures (Haviland, 1999). A subculture is defined as a group within a society that functions by its own distinctive standards of behavior, while at the same time sharing some standards in common with the general culture (Haviland, 1999). For example, although members of a society may share a common homeland and language (e.g., English in the United States), multiple subcultures exist and are represented by age (e.g., senior citizen), gender, religion, sexuality, occupation, social class, and regional (e.g., northeast) groups, among other factors. Although race and ethnicity are often considered proxies for culture, they exhibit great subgroup variation. For example, regional and socioeconomic differences between groups may be more important in determining behavior and some health disparities than racial or ethnic differences (Coughlin et al., 2006; Foster, 2006; McGory, Zingmond, Sekeris, Bastani, & Ko, 2006; Parikh-Patel, Bates, & Campleman, 2006); likewise, significant differences among Hispanic groups exist, organized by country of origin (birthplace) and socioeconomic status (Caban & Walker, 2006).

Culture Transmission

Transmission of culture is the process by which specific aspects of a culture (i.e., language, beliefs, rituals, appropriate behavior) are passed down from one generation to the next. Multiple factors affect the transmission of culture, including the family, peers, schools, work groups, geography, politics, and societal forces such as the media. Transmission of a culture begins soon after a child is born, through enculturation and socialization (Berry, Poortinga, Segall, & Dasen, 1992). Early in a child's life, the most important role models and transmitters of culture are the child's parents and siblings, who shape the child's behavior. As the child ages and begins to spend more time outside the home, other influences become important. These include rewards experienced for adherence to cultural standards in the form of "social acceptance," which can become especially important during adolescence. Transmission of culture also occurs via the media. This has a powerful effect shaping the views and attitudes of individuals in and across societies in the world (Wilson, Gutierrez, & Chao, 2003).

Acculturation

Transmission of a new culture can also occur later in life (as an adult) and after one has already become rooted in a different culture. This usually results when an individual changes geographic location and has to adapt to new cultural sanctions. Acculturation is the degree to which cultural elements of a mainstream culture are adopted by another group (e.g., a migrant group). Individuals may have varying levels of acculturation to a mainstream culture. Degree of acculturation has been measured by a combination of factors, including language spoken at home, years in the United States, citizenship status, and place of birth, as well as along various psychosocial measurements. The impact of acculturation on health has been studied particularly among Hispanics and Asian Americans, and an association between level of acculturation and health and health behaviors has been shown (Borrayo & Guarnaccia, 2000; Elder et al., 1991; Goel et al., 2003; Gonzalez, Haan, & Hinton, 2001; Lara, Gamboa, Kahramanian, Morales, & Bautista, 2005). It is likely that, as the United States continues to increase in diversity, acculturation will be an important variable to examine in health care settings and research.

Ethnocentrism

Transmission of culture from one generation to the next depends, to some extent, on how individuals feel about their culture. Ethnocentrism is the belief that one's own culture is superior to all others. This belief is adaptive for transmission of a culture or preserving key aspects of a particular culture. However, ethnocentrism can also become a barrier when one needs to understand or gain information about another culture. This is relevant to developing health promotion or disease management interventions that meet the needs of individuals of a particular culture. In order to gain an unbiased view of someone else's culture and thus understand individuals in their own cultural terms, researchers and health care providers must be able to see their own cultural biases and suspend judgment on culture-related practices of targeted individuals or groups. This process is referred to as cultural relativism (Haviland, 1999).

Cultural Competence

Cultural competence is having the capacity to function effectively as an individual or an organization within the context of the cultural beliefs, behaviors, and needs presented by a particular group or community (U.S. Department of Health and Human Services & Office of Minority Health, 2001). It requires (1) awareness of one's own cultural values and biases, (2) knowledge of others' views and perspectives, and (3) the skills to design and effectively deliver culturally appropriate interventions (Harris-Davis & Haughton, 2000).

Cultural Sensitivity

Cultural sensitivity refers to the extent to which ethnic and cultural aspects of a target population, as well as relevant historical, political, environmental, and social forces, are incorporated in the design, delivery, and evaluation of targeted interventions, materials, and programs (Resnicow, Baranowski, Ahluwalia, & Braithwaite, 1999). There are two types of cultural sensitivity: surface structure and deep structure. Surface-structure strategies involve matching behavioral interventions to characteristics of a target population. For example, an intervention for promoting physical activity among African American women based on surface structure may include materials that show pictures of African American women walking or lifting weights, with no attention to values and beliefs of the population of interest. Deep-structure strategies, on the other hand, target beliefs and values and incorporate messages to the population of interest that are in line with their beliefs and values as a culture (Resnicow et al., 1999). For instance, some within the African American community believe that the government is somehow facilitating the spread of HIV among members of their community (Bogart & Thorburn, 2005). Thus, a deep-structure culturally sensitive intervention would need to directly address this belief.

Empirical Evidence of Cultural Influences on Health-Related Behaviors

In this section, we review empirical evidence suggesting that elements of culture influence health behaviors and, ultimately, can have an impact on health disparities. There is much evidence to suggest that, even when the effects of socioeconomic status (SES) factors are accounted for, numerous racial and ethnic differences still exist in health outcomes and behaviors (Smedley et al., 2003). We review this evidence as it pertains to definitions of disease and disorders and to a variety of health-related behaviors, including use of health screenings, disease prevention and disease management, and treatment behaviors.

Culture and Health Screening Behavior

Health screenings are an important component of preventive care, yet adherence to health screening guidelines is suboptimal among certain groups and contribute to health disparities (Ata et al., 2006; Boltri, Okosun, Davis-Smith, & Vogel, 2005; Finney, Tumiel-Berhalter, Fox, & Jaen, 2006; Neal, Magwood, Jenkins, & Hossler, 2006).

An example of how cultural beliefs influence screening behaviors can be observed among Asian Americans. Asian Americans are the only racial group in the United States to experience cancer as the leading cause of death (Centers for Disease Control, 2004b; Fried, Prager, MacKay, & Xia, 2003). Rates of both breast and cervical cancer screening are very low among this population (Kagawa-Singer & Pourat, 2000). In fact, the proportion of Asian American women who receive mammograms and who adhere to cancer screening guidelines is the lowest among any of the racial or ethnic groups (MacLean, 2004). The cancer burden that affects this group might be significantly reduced by increasing earlier detection. Attitudes and beliefs of Asian American women have been found to be related to cancer screening rates. For instance, cultural traditions such as Buddhism, Taoism, and Confucianism, which focus on acceptance of the natural order of life (Allinson, 1989; Graham, 1990), lead Asians to view disease and illness as a part of the life cycle and as something out of their control, which is likely to influence engagement in screening behaviors (Kwok & Sullivan, 2006). In the Chinese culture, for instance, people often explain life events, including health and illness, in terms of luck, fortune, or fate (Allinson, 1989). These culturally influenced perceptions are likely to influence Asian individuals' perceptions of health screenings.

Culture and Preventive Behavior

The current medical literature provides ample evidence that several prevalent and costly diseases can be prevented, or their onset delayed, through interventions (e.g., lifestyle, medications) that decrease disease risk factors (Davidson & Toth, 2004; Ferdinand, 2005; Khan et al., 2006; Knowler et al., 2002; Turnbull, 2003). Thus, behavioral adherence to preventive interventions may be key to prolonging health and quality of life.

Empirical evidence of the influence of culture on prevention can be observed in the area of HIV prevention. In the United States, the African American community is disproportionally affected by HIV/AIDS, with a higher incidence of new AIDS cases and a death rate from AIDS seven times that of Whites (Centers for Disease Control and Prevention, 2001, 2002). This is despite the significant advances that have been made in the treatment of HIV/AIDS, in particular the availability of Highly Active Anti-Retroviral Treatment (HAART). Cultural factors may partially explain these disparities. Evidence exists that several minority groups (i.e., African Americans and Hispanics) (Bogart & Bird, 2003; Bogart & Thorburn, 2005; Herek & Capitanio, 1994; Klonoff & Landrine, 1999; Ross, Essien, & Torres, 2006) hold common conspiracy beliefs about HIV, including the belief that HIV is created by the government and planted in Black communities, that a cure is being withheld from the poor, that people who take new medications are guinea pigs for the government, that a lot of information about AIDS is being withheld from the public, and that medicines that are used to treat HIV actually cause AIDS (Bogart & Bird, 2003; Bogart & Thorburn, 2005; Herek & Capitanio, 1994; Herek & Glunt, 1991; Klonoff & Landrine, 1999). These conspiracy beliefs have been associated with negative attitudes toward condoms and inconsistent condom use in African American populations, thus minimizing the effect of HIV prevention interventions.

Although the examples described here illustrate ways in which culture can negatively impact adherence to prescribed health behaviors, there also is evidence of positive cultural influences on preventive behaviors. Evidence exists that Hispanics have lower rates of smoking than most other racial and ethnic groups with the exception of Asian Americans (Centers for Disease Control and Prevention, 2005a). Among Hispanics who do currently smoke, reports suggest that they smoke fewer cigarettes per day (Haynes, Harvey, Montes, Nickens, & Cohen, 1990; Marcus & Crane, 1985; Perez-Stable, Marin, & Marin, 1994), have lower average serum cotinine levels, and have lower nicotine addiction (Palinkas et al., 1993; Perez-Stable, Marin, Marin, & Benowitz, 1992; Winkleby, Schooler, Kraemer, Lin, & Fortmann, 1995). The Hispanic culture may in part explain differential prevalence rates of smoking. For example, Hispanics were more likely to cite family and interpersonal relationships as important reasons to quit smoking, suggesting that the interdependence (traditionally emphasized over independence) and the importance of the family (*familialismo*) that are characteristic of the Hispanic culture may, at least partly, explain the fact that Hispanics have lower smoking rates than do Whites. Likewise, lack of family approval has been shown to keep many young Hispanics from initiating smoking (Foraker, Patten, Lopez, Croghan, & Thomas, 2005). The wish to avoid or minimize interpersonal conflict (*simpatia*), another traditional trait of Hispanic cultures, may be another motivator in a Hispanic person's decisions not to start smoking (Perez-Stable, Marin, & Posner, 1998).

Culture, Illness Perception, and Disease Management

Individuals from different cultures may have different experiences or interpretations of bodily symptoms, what constitutes a disease, and what interventions and treatments are acceptable (Betancourt, 2006; Surbone, 2006; Waite, 2006; Ward, 2007). Interventions to treat or manage diseases, especially chronic diseases, require that a patient follow a set of behavioral prescriptions, including taking the appropriate medications in the prescribed dosage and schedule, undergoing diagnostic tests, adhering to lifestyle changes, and scheduling and attending medical visits, among other behaviors. In this section, we summarize empirical evidence that support the impact of cultural factors on illness perception and diagnosis, treatment-seeking behaviors, treatment choice, and adherence.

Perceptual differences potentially affect what individuals from different cultures do and what interventions they are willing to adhere to in the face of specific bodily symptoms or health conditions. These differences pose difficulty for health care providers who may not be aware of diverse cultural definitions of illness. Culture-bound syndromes are a clear example of this issue. The Diagnostic and Statistical Manual of Mental Disorders of the American Psychiatric Association (DSM-IV) defined these as "recurrent, locality-specific patterns of aberrant behavior and troubling experience that may or may not be linked to a particular DSM-IV diagnostic category" (American Psychiatric Association, 1994, p. 844). Many of these patterns are indigenously considered to be "illnesses," or at least afflictions, and most have local names. One example of a culture-bound syndrome is susto, which is present in Latin American or Hispanic populations. Susto is usually associated with a broad array of symptoms, including nervousness, anorexia, insomnia, listlessness, despondency, involuntary muscle tics, and diarrhea. The causes of susto are thought to be fright that results in a loss of soul from the body and can result from natural or supernatural events. For instance, susto may occur after one is in a near-accident or an actual accident or after one has witnessed a supernatural phenomenon such as a ghost. The symptoms associated with susto are often misinterpreted by health care providers, and the most frequent diagnosis that is given in the United States for these symptoms is tuberculosis (Rubel, O'Nell, & Collado-Ardon, 1984).

Symptom reporting and coping among various cultural groups may affect providers' response to patients and the interventions and treatments prescribed. For example, a review of cross-cultural studies (Calvillo & Flaskerud, 1991) concluded that White Americans of northern European origin react to pain stoically and withdraw if pain intensifies. This response to pain has become the cultural norm in the United States and is the behavior that providers expect and value.

Treatment preferences for common medical conditions also are influenced by the patient's culture. An example of this is the considerable influence of ethnicity on whether one chooses knee replacement as the treatment for knee osteoarthritis. Joint replacements, the number one most common procedure among hospital discharges in the United States, are elective procedures that provide substantial benefits in pain relief and quality of life (Callahan, Drake, Heck, & Dittus, 1995). However, despite these benefits, Hispanic and African Americans patients are half as likely as Whites to undergo surgery, even after controlling for income and access to care (Ibrahim, Siminoff, Burant, & Kwoh, 2002a, 2002b). African American patients in particular are the least likely to consider surgery, despite reporting more severe symptoms, even when significant physician counseling has been provided (Ibrahim et al., 2002a, 2002b). Willingness to undergo surgery is related to beliefs about the efficacy of the procedure, expectations of postsurgical pain and functional difficulties, and whether one knows individuals in one's close social environment who has undergone the procedure (Ibrahim et al., 2002a, 2002b; Suarez-Almazor et al., 2005). Also, perception of prayer as helpful in coping with arthritis has been associated with willingness to undergo surgery among African Americans (Ang et al., 2002).

Another example of the impact of culture on disease management is the use of pharmacotherapy for depression in Hispanic and African American populations. Depression is a highly prevalent condition, affecting 20% of Americans at some point in their lives (Gotlib & Hammen, 2002), and the burden of depression is especially high among the poor and minorities (Cooper et al., 2003; Falcon & Tucker, 2000; Lagomasino et al., 2005; Miller et al., 2004; Miranda & Cooper, 2004). Although African Americans and Hispanics may be less likely to receive appropriate treatment for depression than Whites (Miranda & Cooper, 2004; Simpson, Krishnan, Kunik, & Ruiz, 2007), even when primary-care providers recommend depression treatment, African American and Hispanic patients are much less likely to accept antidepressant treatment than their White counterparts (Miranda & Cooper, 2004) and are less likely to adhere to antidepressant therapy once they begin treatment (Diaz, Woods, & Rosenheck, 2005).

Hispanics consider antidepressant medication a less acceptable treatment than do Whites (whose rates of antidepressant use tripled between 1988–1994 and 1999–2000) (Centers for Disease Control, 2004a). As explained by Kleinman's model (Kleinman, Eisenberg, & Good, 1978), the physician and the patient are operating under two different explanations of the symptoms. Health care providers of Western medicine who prescribe antidepressant medications for treatment of depressive symptoms operate under the belief system that depression is a disease. Patients, on the other hand, may be operating under a different set of beliefs regarding the reason for their symptoms. For example, findings from qualitative research suggest that both cultural beliefs, including spiritual and religious attitudes, and stigma may explain the lack of acceptability of, and low adherence to, treatment with antidepressant medication in these populations (Cooper-Patrick et al., 1997). These cultural differences are likely to lead to noncompliance, strained patient-provider relations, and untreated symptoms. Kleinman's model is one way to view and explain the disparities in mental health treatment, especially in the case of taking antidepressant medications, among individuals with different cultural views on medicine (Kleinman et al., 1978).

Theoretical Frameworks That Account for Cultural Influences on Behavior

As stated earlier, empirical evidence suggests an important role of culture on the health behavior of individuals. In this section, we review theoretical frameworks that help explain the specific mechanisms by which culture influences behavior. This review is limited to commonly cited theories in the fields of preventive and behavioral medicine. Traditionally, theories have emphasized intraindividual factors as they affect health behaviors. Several well-known theories emphasize the role of cognition on human behavior: the *Folk Model* (otherwise known as Cultural Model) (Shore, 1996), *Prototype Theory* (Rosch, Mervis, Gray, Johnson, & Bayes-Braem, 1976), and the *Health Belief Model* (Becker, 1974; Janz & Becker, 1984). Others, such as *Social Cognitive* (Bandura, 1986) and *Operant* (Skinner, 1953, 1969, 1983) theories, emphasize an interaction between the individual and the environment. Recently, there has been greater recognition of the need to expand current theoretical frameworks and models to include the immediate and more distant environments in our understanding of human behavior (Matson-Koffman, Brownstein, Neiner, & Greaney, 2005). An example of this is the *Ecological Model* (Stokols, 1992, 1996). These theories and models are briefly reviewed in this section.

The Folk Model

The Folk Model proposes that behavior is influenced by "cultural models," thought of as loose, interpretative frameworks or cognitive categories used by people to understand the world and human behavior. These are taught through other members of a group, both overtly and unconsciously. These models are not fixed but malleable through the individual's personal experiences, which can either reinforce existing models or challenge these models (Shore, 1996). The Folk Model (Holy & Stuchlik, 1981; Shore, 1996) can be useful in explaining phenomena such as the low rates of mammogram screening among Asian Americans described earlier. It may be that specific beliefs associated with the Asian culture, including the belief that illness and disease are part of the life cycle over which they have little control, affect their health prevention behavior. Chinese people often explain health and illness in terms of luck, fortune, or fate (Allinson, 1989), and these beliefs result from generations of learning (the Folk Model) from other members of the culture, either overtly through verbal statements regarding health or health behaviors or through watching how people deal with illness, treatment, diagnoses, and the health care system. The Folk Model can also explain individual differences in behavior among Asian women. Personal experiences (i.e., interactions with a coworker who was diagnosed with early-stage breast cancer through mammography) can modify these folk models and thus influence that individual's behavior.

Prototype Theory

Prototype Theory proposes that, given the complexity of the stimuli in our world, individuals develop categorization systems in order to understand the environment and to deal with the overwhelming stimuli in it (Rosch et al., 1976). Individuals then base their judgments and decisions regarding a behavior, person, or object on the similarity between its features and the prototype (Cantor & Mischel, 1979). The types of prototypes that one has are likely to differ depending on one's culture. For instance, an individual's prototype of a high-socioeconomic-status (SES) middle-aged White female is likely to differ depending on (1) who the individual is and what that individual has learned through his own culture about high-SES White females, and (2) what the individual's personal experience has been like with high-SES White females. A young African American male from a low-SES background is likely to have a different prototype of high-SES White females than a woman from this "prototypical group." This prototype model has been used to explain stereotypes (Hilton & von Hippel, 1996). A stereotype is a generalization about a group of people in which identical characteristics are assigned to virtually all members of the group, regardless of actual variations among group members (i.e., characteristics of a culture are overgeneralized to all individuals of that culture). Overgeneralization of a negative characteristic is known as prejudice (Berry et al., 1992). Another type of prototype consists of "exemplary" examples for different categories (Lakoff, 1982). For instance, in discussing exercise with a patient, exemplary examples that may come to a clinician's mind at first are jogging or weight lifting. Examples of exercise that may not come to mind at first are yoga, Pilates, or marital arts. Prototype theory can be useful in understanding biases that affect perceptions and behaviors of patients and providers alike.

The Health Belief Model

The Health Belief Model (HBM) (Becker, 1974; Janz & Becker, 1984) is discussed in depth in chapter 2. Briefly, it provides a cognitive theoretical framework for understanding mediators of health-related behavior. The HBM is a value-expectancy theory that emphasizes that behaviors are mediated by thoughts and "expectations" regarding the behavior. Specifically, the model suggests that an individual's health behavior is affected by that person's desire to avoid illness or to get well (value) and the individual's belief that a specific health action available to him or her will prevent or improve illness (expectation). Accordingly, people will take action to prevent, screen for, or control their disease-health conditions if they believe that they are susceptible to disease (perceived susceptibility), that the disease will have serious consequences (perceived severity), that there are benefits to engaging in the behavior (perceived benefits), and that there are few barriers that prevent this behavior (perceived barriers). Thus, an individual will weigh her perceived susceptibility and the severity of the disease against the benefits and barriers to making the necessary changes. More recently, the concept of self-efficacy, or one's confidence in one's ability to take action, has been included in the model (Rosenstock, Strecher, & Becker, 1988). This model can be useful in our understanding of the influence of culturally based beliefs on health-related behaviors described earlier.

Social Cognitive Theory (SCT)

Social Cognitive Theory is one of the most commonly used theoretical frameworks in behavioral science (Bandura, 1986). SCT is discussed in depth in chapter 2. It posits that human behavior is the result of a triadic, dynamic, and reciprocal interaction among personal factors, behavior, and the environment, mediated by cognitive processes. The constructs of self-efficacy (belief in one's capacity to successfully perform a particular behavior) and outcome expectations (anticipated result of performing a specific behavior) are used to explain initiation of behavior as well as the persistence of the behavior over time and in the face of challenges (Bandura, 1997). An individual's standards (learned from experiences with the environment) and social sanctions have a role in behavioral self-regulation. Behavior that is consistent with the prevailing social norms is approved and rewarded by members of the society, whereas behaviors that violate these norms are punished. Individuals behave in ways that bring self-satisfaction and refrain from behaving in ways that are inconsistent with their own set of standards (Bandura, 1997). This model has had great applicability in understanding of individual behavior and has potential for use in understanding of culturally based group behavior. For instance, the low rates of breast cancer screening among Asians and African Americans (described earlier) can be explained by weak outcome expectations regarding screening mammograms. Likewise, cultural beliefs leading to lack of trust in the health care system among African Americans can affect the beliefs that they will adhere to a prescribed medication regimen (self-efficacy) and that taking a prescribed medication (e.g., antihypertensives) will reduce their risk of stroke (outcome expectation). Also, an important feature of Social Cognitive Theory, and relevant to the study of culture and cultural transmission and acculturation, is the role of modeling. Observation of others' behavior and the consequences of those behaviors plays a role in the transfer of culture among individuals by communicating which behaviors will be rewarded and which will be punished and in what contexts (Iversen & Lattal, 1991).

Operant Theory

Operant Theory, another well-known psychological paradigm for understanding behavior, is relevant to culture and has been applied to acculturation (Landrine & Klonoff, 2004). It proposes that behavioral antecedents and consequences regulate behavior (Glenn, Ellis, & Greenspoon, 1992; Skinner, 1969, 1983). The same general principles of discriminative stimuli, reinforcers, and punishers used to explain individual behavior in accordance with Operant Theory are applied to understand the behavior of groups and entire cultures. Antecedents (also referred to as discriminative stimuli) are features of the context or environment that signal whether and what contingencies will follow a behavior, whereas consequences are events that occur contingent upon the behavior of interest and that either increase (through reinforcement) or decrease (through punishment) the probability that that behavior will reoccur (Skinner, 1953, 1969, 1983). Culture determines what events become antecedents or discriminative stimulus for the occurrence of a particular behavior. For example, it is hypothesized that antecedent factors play a role in increased drinking among acculturated Hispanic women. A combination of social acceptance (in the United States) of relatively high amounts of alcohol consumption by women and a variety of environmental cues for drinking (including media that target women) lead to higher rates of drinking among highly acculturated Hispanic women, even when they differ on country of origin (Puerto Rican, Cuban, and Mexican) than among Hispanic women who are less assimilated (Black & Markides, 1993; Lara et al., 2005; Marks, Garcia, & Solis, 1990). With regard to consequences or contingencies, the culturally dominant values of the individual culture affect, at least partly, the reinforcing or punishing value of a contingency. Contingencies that explain how behavior at the population level is shaped (relevant to cultural transmission) are known as meta-contingencies or cultural contingencies (Skinner, 1969).

Ecological Models

Ecological models focus on the interactions of people with their physical and sociocultural environments and the impact that these transactions have on the individual's behavior (see chapter 5 for an in-depth discussion of this model). The Social Ecological Model of health behavior include the impact of culture on behavior (Stokols, 1992, 1996). This model makes four assumptions: (1) health is influenced by multiple aspects of physical and social environments, (2) environments are multidimensional, (3) human-environment interactions can be described at varying levels of organization, and (4) there is feedback across the different levels of environments and aggregates of individuals. These multilevel models can be used to understand phenomena such as neighborhood effects on behavior, where variables such as media ads that target specific groups can be studied as they affect the health behavior of those groups. Health behavior interventions based on the ecological model target the multiple levels (i.e., interpersonal, sociocultural, and environmental) of influences on health behavior.

Other Considerations and Concluding Remarks

In this chapter we have provided an overview of frequently used culture-related terminology; reviewed empirical evidence of cultural characteristics of ethnic and racial groups in the United States that may have an impact on health behaviors; and reviewed frequently used theoretical frameworks that account for the impact of culture on health behavior and adherence. Up to this point, we have discussed primarily the influence of culture on the individual behavior from the patients' perspective. However, the culture of the provider in the context of developing and delivering interventions to culturally diverse populations is also of great importance.

Increasing cultural competence and developing culturally sensitive interventions among health care providers have the potential to improve health outcomes of ethnically and culturally diverse individuals (Brach & Fraser, 2000). Culturally based beliefs, attitudes, and behaviors of health care providers are likely to influence and be influenced by cultural diversity, as well. Empirical evidence exists that providers' cultural biases have the potential to adversely affect patients. For instance, there is a greater delay in providing HIV treatment to African Americans and Hispanics than to Whites (Turner et al., 2000). Patients who are racially concordant with their physician are more likely to receive HIV treatment than are African American patients whose provider is White (King, Wong, Shapiro, Landon, & Cunningham, 2004). Stereotypical perceptions of patient adherence may account for this differential treatment; providers' beliefs regarding poor adherence to Highly Active Anti-retroviral Treatment (HAART) among African Americans and other populations may influence their provision of prescriptions of HIV medications to these populations (Bogart, Catz, Kelly, & Benotsch, 2001; Bogart, Kelly, Catz, & Sosman, 2000; Wong et al., 2004). Thus, at a minimum, it is important to know the limits of one's cultural competencies and abilities and how personally held prototypes of certain groups impact our own behavior (Harris-Davis & Haughton, 2000).

It makes intuitive sense that awareness of ethnocentric tendencies and cultural differences may enhance the effectiveness of interventions in culturally diverse populations. However, although much has been written about the importance of cultural sensitivity in the design and implementation of health-promoting interventions, less is known about efficacious strategies to enhance cultural competency and sensitivity among clinicians and researchers working with diverse cultural groups (Beagan, 2003; Godkin & Savageau, 2001). As reviewed earlier, strategies to increase the cultural sensitivity of interventions have been proposed. However, the efficacy of these strategies has not been scientifically studied.

We remind the reader at this juncture of the multitude of cultures and subcultures that coexist in many societies, especially in the United States population. We chose to review ethnic- and race-specific cultural differences that affect health as there is overwhelming evidence that minority Americans have greater prevalence and poorer health outcomes than do White Americans from preventable and treatable conditions, including cardiovascular disease and stroke (Centers for Disease Control and Prevention, 2005b), type 2 diabetes mellitus (Cowie et al., 2006; Lanting, Joung, Mackenbach, Lamberts, & Bootsma, 2005; Mainous et al., 2006), asthma (Centers for Disease Control, 2004a; Gold & Wright, 2005; Smith, Hatcher-Ross, Wertheimer, & Kahn, 2005), HIV/AIDS (Cargill & Stone, 2005; "Racial/ethnic disparities in diagnoses of HIV/AIDS—33 states, 2001–2004," 2006) and obesity (Ogden et al., 2006; Zhang & Wang, 2004). However, significant heterogeneity exists among ethnic and racial groups, and failure to recognize and appreciate the differences within ethnic groups can lead to inappropriate conclusions. For example, when analyses of racial and ethnic data are conducted, "White" is commonly used as the referent (majority) to which all other minority groups are compared (Kumanyika & Morssink, 2006), despite the fact that there is much diversity in the ancestry and biological characteristics of the White group (Bhopal & Donaldson, 1998), as well as in their cultural traditions, belief systems, and behaviors, including health behaviors. Similar issues also exist with the ethnic label "Hispanic" or "Latino," given the great diversity among individuals classified as Hispanic or Latino. Likewise, overt and subtle cultural differences exist among many other groups in society, including groups formed according to age, gender, sexual orientation, profession, and many other classifications. Often, our need to categorize information may minimize important differences among individuals within a particular category.

As the United States continues to become increasingly diverse, a greater emphasis on addressing the health care needs of diverse populations will be critical. This will require awareness of diversity issues and a comprehensive theoretical and empirical understanding of how specific cultural factors within diverse groups influence health behaviors and, ultimately, how to utilize limited health care resources to improve the health of our culturally diverse population. Much of our understanding of culture and its influences on behavior is atheoretical and retrospective. Future research should include the use of well-studied program planning, implementation, and evaluation models. Among these are the PRECEDE-PROCEED framework (Gielen & McDonald, 2002), which was developed in order to enable program planners and their communities to work together (Green & Kreuter, 1999) and is able to account for cultural influences that impact on program success. The PEN-3 Model (Airhihenbuwa, 1995) also can be considered, as this model is unique in its emphasis on the role of culture on health behavior. New models may be needed that facilitate our understanding of culture. It also will be important to explore models from other disciplines (such as sociology and anthropology) to address the varied culturally based needs of target groups. Although economic concerns favor capitalizing on similarities among cultures, it is unclear that a single universal model to approach cultural influences will have the impact desired.

Cultural awareness, competence, and sensitivity are likely to facilitate the influence of health care providers and researchers alike. Understanding culture will enhance patient-provider communication and potentially the effectiveness of the provider in facilitating behavior change in the patient. For researchers, cultural understanding is likely to enhance the ability to develop interventions compatible with the cultural needs and traditions of diverse populations and to test those interventions with culturally diverse groups. For example, understanding the function of behaviors of interest within a culture (such as social function of specific food-related patterns) can facilitate the understanding of factors that maintain those behaviors; capitalizing on elements of cultures that support adherence to desirable health behaviors (such as the importance of the family) can work in favor of cultural compatibility of interventions; and studying cultural factors relevant to specific groups can assist in the choice of variables, methodologies, and measurements (Rosal, Carbone, & Goins, 2003). Finally, researchers' cultural competence will be crucial to recruiting representative culturally diverse individuals into research studies and retaining these individuals until study completion so that conclusive statements can be made about the generalizability of the interventions.

References

Airhihenbuwa, C. O. (1995). Developing culturally appropriate health programs. In *Health and culture: Beyond the Western paradigm* (pp. 25–43). Thousand Oaks, CA: Sage.

Allinson, R. E. (1989). *Understanding the Chinese mind.* Hong Kong: Oxford University Press.

American Psychiatric Association. (1994). *Diagnostic and statistical manual of mental disorders* (4th ed.). Washington, DC: Author.

Ang, D. C., Ibrahim, S. A., Burant, C. J., Siminoff, L. A., & Kwoh, C. K. (2002). Ethnic differences in the perception of prayer and consideration of joint arthroplasty. *Medical Care, 40*(6), 471–476.

Ata, A., Elzey, J. D., Insaf, T. Z., Grau, A. M., Stain, S. C., & Ahmed, N. U. (2006). Colorectal cancer prevention: Adherence patterns and correlates of tests done for screening purposes within United States populations. *Cancer Detection and Prevention, 30*(2), 134–143.

Bandura, A. (1986). *Social foundation of thought and action: A social cognitive theory.* Englewood Cliffs, NJ: Prentice-Hall.

Bandura, A. (1997). *Self-efficacy: The exercise of control.* New York: W. H. Freeman.

Beagan, B. L. (2003). Teaching social and cultural awareness to medical students: "It's all very nice to talk about it in theory, but ultimately it makes no difference." *Academic Medicine, 78*(6), 605–614.

Becker, M. H. (1974). The health belief model and personal health behavior. *Health Education Monographs, 2,* 324–473.

Berry, J. W., Poortinga, Y. H., Segall, M. H., & Dasen, P. R. (1992). *Cross-cultural psychology: Research and applications.* New York: Cambridge University Press.

Betancourt, J. R. (2006). Cultural competency: Providing quality care to diverse populations. *Consultant Pharmacist, 21*(12), 988–995.

Bhopal, R., & Donaldson, L. (1998). White, European, Western, Caucasian, or what? Inappropriate labeling in research on race, ethnicity, and health. *American Journal of Public Health, 88*(9), 1303–1307.

Black, S. A., & Markides, K. S. (1993). Acculturation and alcohol consumption in Puerto Rican, Cuban-American, and Mexican-American women in the United States. *American Journal of Public Health, 83*(6), 890–893.

Bogart, L. M., & Bird, S. T. (2003). Exploring the relationship of conspiracy beliefs about HIV/AIDS to sexual behaviors and attitudes among African-American adults. *Journal of the National Medical Association, 95*(11), 1057–1065.

Bogart, L. M., Catz, S. L., Kelly, J. A., & Benotsch, E. G. (2001). Factors influencing physicians' judgments of adherence and treatment decisions for patients with HIV disease. *Medical Decision Making, 21*(1), 28–36.

Bogart, L. M., Kelly, J. A., Catz, S. L., & Sosman, J. M. (2000). Impact of medical and nonmedical factors on physician decision making for HIV/AIDS antiretroviral treatment. *Journal of Acquired Immune Deficiency Syndromes, 23*(5), 396–404.

Bogart, L. M., & Thorburn, S. (2005). Are HIV/AIDS conspiracy beliefs a barrier to HIV prevention among African Americans? *Journal of Acquired Immune Deficiency Syndromes, 38*(2), 213–218.

Boltri, J. M., Okosun, I. S., Davis-Smith, M., & Vogel, R. L. (2005). Hemoglobin A1c levels in diagnosed and undiagnosed Black, Hispanic, and White persons with diabetes: Results from NHANES 1999–2000. *Ethnicity & Disease, 15*(4), 562–567.

Borrayo, E. A., & Guarnaccia, C. A. (2000). Differences in Mexican-born and U.S.-born women of Mexican descent regarding factors related to breast cancer screening behaviors. *Health Care for Women International, 21*(7), 599–613.

Brach, C., & Fraser, I. (2000). Can cultural competency reduce racial and ethnic health disparities? A review and conceptual model. *Medical Care Research and Review, 57*(Suppl. 1), 181–217.

Caban, A., & Walker, E. A. (2006). A systematic review of research on culturally relevant issues for Hispanics with diabetes. *Diabetes Educator, 32*(4), 584–595.

Callahan, C. M., Drake, B. G., Heck, D. A., & Dittus, R. S. (1995). Patient outcomes following unicompartmental or bicompartmental knee arthroplasty. A meta-analysis. *Journal of Arthroplasty, 10*(2), 141–150.

Calvillo, E. R., & Flaskerud, J. H. (1991). Review of literature on culture and pain of adults with focus on Mexican-Americans. *Journal of Transcultural Nursing, 2*(2), 16–23.

Cantor, N., & Mischel, W. (1979). Prototypes in person perception. In L. Berkowitz (Ed.), *Advances in experimental social psychology* (Vol. 12, pp. 3–52). New York: Academic Press.

Cargill, V. A., & Stone, V. E. (2005). HIV/AIDS: A minority health issue. *Medicine Clinics of North America, 89*(4), 895–912.

Centers for Disease Control. (2004a, April 2). *Fact sheet: Racial/ethnic health disparities.* Retrieved April 24, 2007, from http://www.cdc.gov/od/oc/media/pressrel/fs040402.htm

Centers for Disease Control. (2004b). *Leading causes of death: Females—United States, 2003.* Retrieved March 3, 2007, from www.cdc.gov/wome/lcod.htm

Centers for Disease Control and Prevention. (2001). *HIV/AIDS surveillance report.* Retrieved April 2, 2007, from www.cdc.gov/omh/AMH/AMH.htm

Centers for Disease Control and Prevention. (2002). *HIV/AIDS surveillance supplemental report: Deaths among persons with AIDS through December 2000.* Retrieved April 3, 2007, from www.cdc.gov/omh/AMH/AMH.htm

Centers for Disease Control and Prevention. (2005a). Cigarette smoking among adults—United States, 2004. *MMWR Morbid Mortality Weekly Report, 54*(44), 1121–1124.

Centers for Disease Control and Prevention. (2005b). Health disparities experienced by Black or African Americans—United States. *MMWR Morbid Mortality Weekly Report, 54*(1), 1–3.

Cooper, L. A., Gonzales, J. J., Gallo, J. J., Rost, K. M., Meredith, L. S., Rubenstein, L. V., et al. (2003). The acceptability of treatment for depression among African-American, Hispanic, and White primary care patients. *Medical Care, 41*(4), 479–489.

Cooper-Patrick, L., Powe, N. R., Jenckes, M. W., Gonzales, J. J., Levine, D. M., & Ford, D. E. (1997). Identification of patient attitudes and preferences regarding treatment of depression. *Journal of General Internal Medicine, 12*(7), 431–438.

Coughlin, S. S., Richards, T. B., Thompson, T., Miller, B. A., VanEenwyk, J., Goodman, M. T., et al. (2006). Rural/nonrural differences in colorectal cancer incidence in the United States, 1998–2001. *Cancer, 107*(5 Suppl.), 1181–1188.

Cowie, C. C., Rust, K. F., Byrd-Holt, D. D., Eberhardt, M. S., Flegal, K. M., Engelgau, M. M., et al. (2006). Prevalence of diabetes and impaired fasting glucose in adults in the U.S. population: National Health and Nutrition Examination Survey 1999–2002. *Diabetes Care, 29*(6), 1263–1268.

Davidson, M. H., & Toth, P. P. (2004). Comparative effects of lipid-lowering therapies. *Progress in Cardiovascular Diseases, 47*(2), 73–104.

Diaz, E., Woods, S. W., & Rosenheck, R. A. (2005). Effects of ethnicity on psychotropic medications adherence. *Community Mental Health Journal, 41*(5), 521–537.

Elder, J. P., Castro, F. G., de Moor, C., Mayer, J., Candelaria, J. I., Campbell, N., et al. (1991). Differences in cancer-risk-related behaviors in Latino and Anglo adults. *Preventive Medicine, 20*(6), 751–763.

Escarce, J. J., Epstein, K. R., Colby, D. C., & Schwartz, J. S. (1993). Racial differences in the elderly's use of medical procedures and diagnostic tests. *American Journal of Public Health, 83*(7), 948–954.

Falcon, L. M., & Tucker, K. L. (2000). Prevalence and correlates of depressive symptoms among Hispanic elders in Massachusetts. *Journals of Gerontology, Series B, Psychological Sciences and Social Sciences, 55*(2), S108–116.

Ferdinand, K. C. (2005). Primary prevention trials: Lessons learned about treating high-risk patients with dyslipidemia without known cardiovascular disease. *Current Medical Research and Opinion, 21*(7), 1091–1097.

Finney, M. F., Tumiel-Berhalter, L. M., Fox, C., & Jaen, C. R. (2006). Breast and cervical cancer screening for Puerto Ricans, African Americans, and non-Hispanic Whites attending inner-city family practice centers. *Ethnicity and Disease, 16*(4), 994–1000.

Foraker, R. E., Patten, C. A., Lopez, K. N., Croghan, I. T., & Thomas, J. L. (2005). Beliefs and attitudes regarding smoking among young adult Latinos: A pilot study. *Preventive Medicine, 41*(1), 126–133.

Ford, E. S., & Cooper, R. S. (1995). Racial/ethnic differences in health care utilization of cardiovascular procedures: A review of the evidence. *Health Services Research, 30*(1 Pt 2), 237–252.

Foster, M. W. (2006). Analyzing the use of race and ethnicity in biomedical research from a local community perspective. *Journal of Law, Medicine & Ethics, Fall,* 508–512.

Fried, V. M., Prager, K., MacKay, A. P., & Xia, H. (2003). *Chartbook on trends in the health of Americans. Health, United States, 2003.* Hyattsville, MD: National Center for Health Statistics.

Garro, L. C. (2000). Remembering what one knows and the construction of the past: A comparison of cultural consensus theory and cultural schema theory. *Ethos, 3,* 275–319.

Gielen, A. C., & McDonald, E. M. (2002). Using the precede-proceed planning model to apply health behavior theories. In K. Glanz, B. K. Rimer, & F. M. Lewis (Eds.), *Health behavior and health education: Theory, research, and practice* (3rd ed., pp. 409–436). San Francisco: Jossey-Bass.

Glenn, S. S., Ellis, J., & Greenspoon, J. (1992). On the revolutionary nature of the operant as a unit of behavioral selection. *American Psychologist, 47*(11), 1329–1336.

Godkin, M. A., & Savageau, J. A. (2001). The effect of a global multiculturalism track on cultural competence of preclinical medical students. *Family Medicine, 33*(3), 178–186.

Goel, M. S., Wee, C. C., McCarthy, E. P., Davis, R. B., Ngo-Metzger, Q., & Phillips, R. S. (2003). Racial and ethnic disparities in cancer screening: The importance of foreign birth as a barrier to care. *Journal of General Internal Medicine, 18*(12), 1028–1035.

Gold, D. R., & Wright, R. (2005). Population disparities in asthma. *Annual Review of Public Health, 26,* 89–113.

Gonzalez, H. M., Haan, M. N., & Hinton, L. (2001). Acculturation and the prevalence of depression in older Mexican Americans: Baseline results of the Sacramento Area Latino Study on Aging. *Journal of the American Geriatrics Society, 49*(7), 948–953.

Gotlib, I. H., & Hammen, C. L. (Eds.). (2002). *Handbook of depression.* New York: Guilford Press.

Graham, A. C. (1990). *Studies in Chinese philosophy and philosophical literature.* Albany: SUNY Press.

Green, L. W., & Kreuter, M. (1999). *Health promotion planning: An educational and ecological approach* (3rd ed.). Mountain View, CA: Mayfield.

Hannan, E. L., van Ryn, M., Burke, J., Stone, D., Kumar, D., Arani, D., et al. (1999). Access to coronary artery bypass surgery by race/ethnicity and gender among patients who are appropriate for surgery. *Medical Care, 37*(1), 68–77.

Harris-Davis, E., & Haughton, B. (2000). Model for multicultural nutrition counseling competencies. *Journal of the American Dietetic Association, 100*(10), 1178–1185.

Haviland, W. A. (1999). *Cultural anthropology* (9th ed.). Fort Worth, TX: Harcourt Brace College Publishers.

Haynes, S. G., Harvey, C., Montes, H., Nickens, H., & Cohen, B. H. (1990). Patterns of cigarette smoking among Hispanics in the United States: Results from HHANES 1982–84. *American Journal of Public Health, 80 Suppl,* 47–53.

Herek, G. M., & Capitanio, J. P. (1994). Conspiracies, contagion, and compassion: Trust and public reactions to AIDS. *AIDS Education and Prevention, 6*(4), 365–375.

Herek, G. M., & Glunt, E. K. (1991). AIDS-related attitudes in the United States: A preliminary conceptualization. *Journal of Sex Research, 28,* 99–123.

Hilton, J. L., & von Hippel, W. (1996). Stereotypes. *Annual Reviews of Psychology, 47,* 237–271.

Holy, L., & Stuchlik, M. (Eds.). (1981). *The structure of folk models.* London: Academic Press.

Ibrahim, S. A., Siminoff, L. A., Burant, C. J., & Kwoh, C. K. (2002a). Differences in expectations of outcome mediate African American/White patient differences in "willingness" to consider joint replacement. *Arthritis & Rheumatism, 46*(9), 2429–2435.

Ibrahim, S. A., Siminoff, L. A., Burant, C. J., & Kwoh, C. K. (2002b). Understanding ethnic differences in the utilization of joint replacement for osteoarthritis: The role of patient-level factors. *Medical Care, 40*(1 Suppl.), I44–51.

Iversen, I. H., & Lattal, K. A. (Eds.). (1991). *Experimental analysis of behavior, Part 1 and Part 2.* Amsterdam: Elsevier.

Janz, N. K., & Becker, M. H. (1984). The health belief model: A decade later. *Health Education Quarterly, 11,* 1–47.

Kagawa-Singer, M., & Pourat, N. (2000). Asian American and Pacific Islander breast and cervical carcinoma screening rates and Healthy People 2000 objectives. *Cancer, 89*(3), 696–705.

Keppel, K. G. (2007). Ten largest racial and ethnic health disparities in the United States based on Healthy People 2010 objectives. *American Journal of Epidemiology, 166*(1), 97–103.

Khan, N. A., McAlister, F. A., Rabkin, S. W., Padwal, R., Feldman, R. D., Campbell, N. R., et al. (2006). The 2006 Canadian Hypertension Education Program recommendations for the management of hypertension: Part II—Therapy. *Canadian Journal of Cardiology, 22*(7), 583–593.

King, W. D., Wong, M. D., Shapiro, M. F., Landon, B. E., & Cunningham, W. E. (2004). Does racial concordance between HIV-positive patients and their physicians affect the time to receipt of protease inhibitors? *Journal of General Internal Medicine, 19*(11), 1146–1153.

Kleinman, A., Eisenberg, L., & Good, B. (1978). Culture, illness, and care: Clinical lessons from anthropologic and cross-cultural research. *Annals of Internal Medicine, 88*(2), 251–258.

Klonoff, E. A., & Landrine, H. (1999). Do Blacks believe that HIV/AIDS is a government conspiracy against them? *Preventive Medicine, 28*(5), 451–457.

Knowler, W. C., Barrett-Connor, E., Fowler, S. E., Hamman, R. F., Lachin, J. M., Walker, E. A., et al. (2002). Reduction in the incidence of type 2 diabetes with lifestyle intervention or metformin. *New England Journal of Medicine, 346*(6), 393–403.

Kreuter, M. W., & Haughton, L. T. (2006). Integrating culture into health information for African American women. *American Behavioral Scientist, 49*(6), 794–811.

Kumanyika, S. K., & Morssink, C. B. (2006). Bridging domains in efforts to reduce disparities in health and health care. *Health Education & Behavior, 33*(4), 440–458.

Kwok, C., & Sullivan, G. (2006). Chinese-Australian women's beliefs about cancer: Implications for health promotion. *Cancer Nursing, 29*(5), E14–21.

Lagomasino, I. T., Dwight-Johnson, M., Miranda, J., Zhang, L., Liao, D., Duan, N., et al. (2005). Disparities in depression treatment for Latinos and site of care. *Psychiatric Services, 56*(12), 1517–1523.

Lakoff, G. (1982). *Categories and cognitive models' series A, No. 96.* Trier: Linguistic Agency University Trier.

Landrine, H., & Klonoff, E. A. (2004). Culture change and ethnic-minority health behavior: An operant theory of acculturation. *Journal of Behavioral Medicine, 27*(6), 527–555.

Lanting, L. C., Joung, I. M., Mackenbach, J. P., Lamberts, S. W., & Bootsma, A. H. (2005). Ethnic differences in mortality, end-stage complications, and quality of care among diabetic patients: A review. *Diabetes Care, 28*(9), 2280–2288.

Lara, M., Gamboa, C., Kahramanian, M. I., Morales, L. S., & Bautista, D. E. (2005). Acculturation and Latino health in the United States: A review of the literature and its sociopolitical context. *Annual Review of Public Health, 26,* 367–397.

Lee, A. J., Gehlbach, S., Hosmer, Reti, M., & Baker, C. S. (1997). Medicare treatment differences for Blacks and Whites. *Medical Care, 35*(12), 1173–1189.

MacLean, J. (2004). *Breast cancer in California: A closer look.* Oakland: Breast Cancer Research Program, University of California.

Mainous, A. G., III, Baker, R., Koopman, R. J., Saxena, S., Diaz, V. A., Everett, C. J., et al. (2006). Impact of the population at risk of diabetes on projections of diabetes burden in the United States: An epidemic on the way. *Diabetologia, 50*(5), 934–940.

Marcus, A., & Crane, L. (1985). Smoking behavior among U.S. Latinos: An emerging challenge for public health. *American Journal of Public Health, 75,* 169–172.

Marks, G., Garcia, M., & Solis, J. M. (1990). Health risk behaviors of Hispanics in the United States: Findings from HHANES, 1982–84. *American Journal of Public Health, 80 Suppl,* 20–26.

Matson-Koffman, D. M., Brownstein, J. N., Neiner, J. A., & Greaney, M. L. (2005). A site-specific literature review of policy and environmental interventions that promote physical activity and nutrition for cardiovascular health: What works? *American Journal of Health Promotion, 19*(3), 167–193.

McGory, M. L., Zingmond, D. S., Sekeris, E., Bastani, R., & Ko, C. Y. (2006). A patient's race/ethnicity does not explain the underuse of appropriate adjuvant therapy in colorectal cancer. *Diseases of the Colon and Rectum, 49*(3), 319–329.

Miller, D. K., Malmstrom, T. K., Joshi, S., Andresen, E. M., Morley, J. E., & Wolinsky, F. D. (2004). Clinically relevant levels of depressive symptoms in community-dwelling middle-aged African Americans. *Journal of the American Geriatric Society, 52*(5), 741–748.

Miranda, J., & Cooper, L. A. (2004). Disparities in care for depression among primary care patients. *Journal of General Internal Medicine, 19*(2), 120–126.

Neal, D., Magwood, G., Jenkins, C., & Hossler, C. L. (2006). Racial disparity in the diagnosis of obesity among people with diabetes. *Journal of Health Care for the Poor and Underserved, 17*(2 Suppl), 106–115.

Office of Minority Health, & U.S. Department of Health and Human Services. (2007, May 7). *Federal health leaders unveil new programs to recruit minorities into clinical trials.* Retrieved May 7, 2007, from http://www.omhrc.gov/templates/content.aspx?ID = 5046&1v1ID = 40

Ogden, C. L., Carroll, M. D., Curtin, L. R., McDowell, M. A., Tabak, C. J., & Flegal, K. M. (2006). Prevalence of overweight and obesity in the United States, 1999–2004. *Journal of the American Medical Association, 295*(13), 1549–1555.

Palinkas, L. A., Pierce, J., Rosbrook, B. P., Pickwell, S., Johnson, M., & Bal, D. G. (1993). Cigarette smoking behavior and beliefs of Hispanics in California. *American Journal of Preventive Medicine, 9*(6), 331–337.

Parikh-Patel, A., Bates, J. H., & Campleman, S. (2006). Colorectal cancer stage at diagnosis by socioeconomic and urban/rural status in California, 1988–2000. *Cancer, 107*(5 Suppl.), 1189–1195.

Perez-Stable, E. J., Marin, G., & Marin, B. V. (1994). Behavioral risk factors: A comparison of Latinos and non-Latino Whites in San Francisco. *American Journal of Public Health, 84*(6), 971–976.

Perez-Stable, E. J., Marin, G., Marin, B. V., & Benowitz, N. L. (1992). Misclassification of smoking status by self-reported cigarette consumption. *American Review of Respiratory Disease, 145*(1), 53–57.

Perez-Stable, E. J., Marin, G., & Posner, S. F. (1998). Ethnic comparison of attitudes and beliefs about cigarette smoking. *Journal of General Internal Medicine, 13*(3), 167–174.

Racial/ethnic disparities in diagnoses of HIV/AIDS—33 states, 2001–2004. (2006). *Morbid Mortality Weekly Report, 55*(5), 121–125.

Resnicow, K., Baranowski, T., Ahluwalia, J. S., & Braithwaite, R. L. (1999). Cultural sensitivity in public health: Defined and demystified. *Ethnicity and Disease, 9*(1), 10–21.

Rosal, M. C., Carbone, E. T., & Goins, K. V. (2003). Use of cognitive interviewing to adapt measurement instruments for low-literate Hispanics. *Diabetes Education, 29*(6), 1006–1017.

Rosch, E., Mervis, B., Gray, W. D., Johnson, D. M., & Bayes-Braem, P. (1976). Basic objects in natural categories. *Cognitive Psychology, 8,* 382–439.

Rosenstock, I. M., Strecher, V. J., & Becker, M. H. (1988). Social learning theory and the Health Belief Model. *Health Education Quarterly, 15*(2), 175–183.

Ross, M. W., Essien, E. J., & Torres, I. (2006). Conspiracy beliefs about the origin of HIV/AIDS in four racial/ethnic groups. *Journal of Acquired Immune Deficiency Syndromes, 41*(3), 342–344.

Rubel, A. J., O'Nell, C. W., & Collado-Ardon, R. (1984). *Susto: A folk illness.* Berkeley: University of California Press.

Shi, L. (1999). Experience of primary care by racial and ethnic groups in the United States. *Medical Care, 37*(10), 1068–1077.

Shore, B. (1996). *Culture in mind: Cognition, culture, and the problem of meaning.* Oxford: Oxford University Press.

Simpson, S. M., Krishnan, L. L., Kunik, M. E., & Ruiz, P. (2007). Racial disparities in diagnosis and treatment of depression: A literature review. *Psychiatric Quarterly, 78*(1), 3–14.

Skinner, B. F. (1953). *Science and human behavior.* New York: Free Press.

Skinner, B. F. (1969). *Contingencies of reinforcement.* Englewood Cliffs, NJ: Prentice-Hall.

Skinner, B. F. (1983). *A matter of consequences.* New York: Knopf.

Smedley, B. D., Stith, A. Y., & Nelson, A. R. (Eds.). (2003). *Unequal treatment: Confronting racial and ethnic disparities in health care.* Washington, DC: National Academies Press.

Smith, L. A., Hatcher-Ross, J. L., Wertheimer, R., & Kahn, R. S. (2005). Rethinking race/ethnicity, income, and childhood asthma: Racial/ethnic disparities concentrated among the very poor. *Public Health Reports, 120*(2), 109–116.

Stokols, D. (1992). Establishing and maintaining healthy environments: Toward a social ecology of health promotion. *American Psychologist, 47,* 6–22.

Stokols, D. (1996). Translating social ecological theory into guidelines for community health promotion. *American Journal of Health Promotion, 10*(4), 282–298.

Suarez-Almazor, M. E., Souchek, J., Kelly, P. A., O'Malley, K., Byrne, M., Richardson, M., et al. (2005). Ethnic variation in knee replacement: patient preferences or uninformed disparity? *Archives of Internal Medicine, 165*(10), 1117–1124.

Surbone, A. (2006). Cultural aspects of communication in cancer care. *Recent Results in Cancer Research, 168,* 91–104.

Turnbull, F. (2003). Effects of different blood-pressure-lowering regimens on major cardiovascular events: Results of prospectively-designed overviews of randomised trials. *Lancet, 362*(9395), 1527–1535.

Turner, B. J., Cunningham, W. E., Duan, N., Andersen, R. M., Shapiro, M. F., Bozzette, S. A., et al. (2000). Delayed medical care after diagnosis in a U.S. national probability sample of persons infected with human immunodeficiency virus. *Archives of Internal Medicine, 160*(17), 2614–2622.

U.S. Department of Health and Human Services & Office of Minority Health. (2001). *National standards for culturally and linguistically appropriate services in health care: Final report.* Hyattsville, MD: Author.

Waite, R. L. (2006). Variations in the experiences and expressions of depression among ethnic minorities. *Journal of National Black Nurses Association, 17*(1), 29–35.

Ward, E. C. (2007). Examining differential treatment effects for depression in racial and ethnic minority women: A qualitative systematic review. *Journal of the National Medical Association, 99*(3), 265–274.

Wilson, C. C., Gutierrez, F., & Chao, L. M. (2003). *Racism, sexism and the media: The rise of class communication in multicultural America* (3rd ed.). Thousand Oaks, CA: Sage.

Winkleby, M. A., Schooler, C., Kraemer, H. C., Lin, J., & Fortmann, S. P. (1995). Hispanic versus White smoking patterns by sex and level of education. *American Journal of Epidemiology, 142*(4), 410–418.

Wong, M. D., Cunningham, W. E., Shapiro, M. F., Andersen, R. M., Cleary, P. D., Duan, N., et al. (2004). Disparities in HIV treatment and physician attitudes about delaying protease inhibitors for nonadherent patients. *Journal of General Internal Medicine, 19*(4), 366–374.

Zhang, Q., & Wang, Y. (2004). Socioeconomic inequality of obesity in the United States: Do gender, age, and ethnicity matter? *Social Science & Medicine, 58*(6), 1171–1180.

The Transtheoretical Model of Behavior Change

4

James O. Prochaska,
Sara Johnson, and
Patricia Lee

The Transtheoretical Model (TTM) is an integrative framework for understanding how individuals and populations progress toward adopting and maintaining health behavior change for optimal health. The Transtheoretical Model uses stages of change to integrate processes and principles of change from across major theories of intervention, hence the name "Transtheoretical." This model emerged from a comparative analysis of leading theories of psychotherapy and behavior change. The search was for a systematic integration of a field that had fragmented into more than 300 theories of psychotherapy (Prochaska, 1979). The comparative analysis identified only 10 processes of change, such as consciousness raising from the Freudian tradition, contingency management from the Skinnerian tradition, and helping relationships from the Rogerian tradition.

In an empirical analysis that compared self-changers to smokers in professional treatments, we assessed how frequently each group used each of the 10 processes (Prochaska & DiClemente, 1983). Our research participants kept saying that they used different processes at different times in their struggles with smoking. These naive subjects were teaching us about a phenomenon that was not included in any of the multitude of therapy theories. They were revealing to us that behavior change unfolds through a series of stages (Prochaska & DiClemente, 1983).

From the initial studies of smoking, the stage model rapidly expanded in scope to include investigations of and applications to a broad range of health and mental health behaviors. These include alcohol and substance abuse, anxiety and panic disorders, stress and depression, partner violence and bullying, delinquency, eating disorders and obesity, high-fat diets, exercise, HIV/AIDS, use of mammography screening, medication compliance, unplanned pregnancy, pregnancy and smoking, radon testing, sedentary lifestyles, sun exposure, and the practice of preventive medicine. Over time, these studies have expanded, validated, applied, and challenged the core constructs of the Transtheoretical Model.

Core Constructs

The Transtheoretical Model has concentrated on six stages of change; 10 processes of change; the pros and cons of changing; self-efficacy; and temptation as core constructs. The Transtheoretical Model is also based on critical assumptions about the nature of behavior change and interventions that can best facilitate such change. Each core construct has been subjected to a wide variety of studies across a broad range of behaviors and populations. These core constructs and critical assumptions are discussed in this section.

Stages of Change

The stage construct is important in part because it represents a temporal dimension. Change implies phenomena occurring over time, but, surprisingly, none of the leading theories of therapy contained a core construct representing time. Behavior change was often construed as an event, such as quitting smoking, drinking, or overeating. The Transtheoretical Model construes change as a process that unfolds over time and involves progress through a series of six stages.

Precontemplation is the stage in which people are not intending to take action in the foreseeable future, a time frame usually measured as the next 6 months. People may be in this stage because they are uninformed or underinformed about the consequences of their behavior. Alternatively, they may have tried to change a number of times and become demoralized about their abilities to change. Both groups tend to avoid reading, talking, or thinking about their high-risk behaviors. They are often characterized in other theories as "noncompliant," "resistant" or "unmotivated," or "not ready" for therapy or health promotion programs. The fact is that traditional health promotion programs were not ready for such individuals and were not motivated to match their needs.

Contemplation is the stage in which people are intending to change in the next 6 months. They are more aware of the pros of changing but are also acutely aware of the cons. This balance between the costs and benefits of changing can produce profound ambivalence that can keep people stuck in this stage for long periods of time. We often characterize this phenomenon as chronic contemplation or behavioral procrastination. These folks are also not ready for traditional action-oriented programs.

Preparation is the stage in which people are intending to take action in the immediate future, usually measured as the next month. They have typically taken some significant action in the past year. These individuals have a plan of action, such as joining a health education class, consulting a counselor, talking to their physician, buying a self-help book, or relying on a self-change approach. These are the people we should recruit for action-oriented programs in smoking cessation, weight loss, or exercise.

Action is the stage in which people have made specific overt modifications in their lifestyles within the past 6 months. Since action is observable, behavior change often has been equated with action. In the Transtheoretical Model, however, action is only one of six stages. Not all modifications of behavior count as action in this model. People must attain a criterion that scientists and professionals agree is sufficient to reduce risks for disease. In smoking, for example, the field used to count reduction in the number of cigarettes or a switch to low-tar and -nicotine cigarettes as action. Now the consensus is clear: only total abstinence counts.

Maintenance is the stage in which people are working to prevent relapse but do not apply change processes as frequently as do people in the action stage. They are less tempted to relapse and increasingly are more confident that they can continue their changes. On the basis of temptation and self-efficacy data, we estimated that maintenance lasts from 6 months to about 5 years. While this estimate may seem somewhat pessimistic, longitudinal data in the 1990 Surgeon General's report gave some support to this temporal estimate (U.S. Department of Health and Human Services, 1990). After 12 months of continuous abstinence, the percentage of individuals who returned to regular smoking was 43%. It was not until 5 years of continuous abstinence that the risk for relapse dropped to 7%.

Termination is the stage in which individuals have zero temptation and 100% self-efficacy. No matter whether they are depressed, anxious, bored, lonely, angry, or stressed, they are sure they will not return to their old unhealthy habit as a way of coping. It is as if they had never acquired the habit in the first place. In a study of former smokers and alcoholics, we found that less than 20% of each group had reached the criteria of zero temptation and total self-efficacy (Snow, Prochaska, & Rossi, 1992). These criteria may be too strict, or it may be that this stage is an ideal goal for the majority of people. In other areas, like exercise and weight control, the realistic goal may be a lifetime of maintenance. Since termination may not be a practical reality for a majority of people, this stage has not been given as much emphasis in our research.

Processes of Change

These are the covert and overt activities that people use to progress through the stages. Processes of change provide important guides for intervention programs, since the processes are like the independent variables that people need to apply to move from stage to stage. Ten processes have received the most empirical support in our research to date.

Consciousness raising involves increased awareness about the causes, consequences, and cures for a particular problem behavior. Interventions that can increase awareness include feedback, education, confrontation, interpretation, bibliotherapy, and media campaigns.

Dramatic relief initially produces increased emotional experiences, followed by reduced affect if appropriate action can be taken. Psychodrama, role playing, grieving, personal testimonies, and media campaigns are examples of techniques that can move people emotionally.

Self-reevaluation combines both cognitive and affective assessments of one's self-image with and without a particular unhealthy habit, for example, as a couch potato and as an active person. Value clarification, healthy role models, and imagery are techniques that can move people evaluatively.

Environmental reevaluation combines both affective and cognitive assessments of how the presence or absence of a personal habit affects one's social environment, for example, the effect on others of smoking. It can also include the awareness that one can serve as a positive or negative role model for others. Empathy training, documentaries, and family interventions can lead to such reassessments.

As an example, here is a brief television spot from California's antitobacco campaign, designed to help smokers in precontemplation to progress. A middle-aged man clearly in grief says, "I always worried that my smoking would cause lung cancer. I was always afraid that my smoking would lead to an early death. But I never imagined that it would happen to my wife." Then on the screen is flashed the message, "50,000 deaths per year due to passive smoking—California Department of Health."

There are no action directives in this intervention, but there is (1) consciousness raising—"50,000 deaths per year"; (2) dramatic relief—around the grief, guilt, and fear that can be reduced if appropriate action is taken; (3) self-reevaluation—examination of how individuals think and feel about themselves as smokers; and (4) environmental reevaluation—how individuals feel and think about the effects of their smoking on their environment.

Self-liberation is both the belief that one can change and the commitment and recommitment to act on that belief. New Year's resolutions, public testimonies, and multiple, rather than single, choices can enhance what the public calls "willpower." Motivative research indicates that people with two choices have greater commitment than people with one choice; those with three choices have even greater commitment; but having four choices doesn't enhance willpower (Miller, 1985). So, for smokers, for example, three excellent action choices are quitting cold turkey, nicotine fading, and nicotine replacement.

Social liberation requires an increase in social opportunities or alternatives especially for people who are relatively deprived or oppressed. Advocacy, empowerment procedures, and appropriate policies can produce increased opportunities for minority health promotion, gay health promotion, and health promotion for impoverished people. These same procedures can also be used to help all people change, for example, by offering smoke-free zones or salad bars in school cafeterias and by providing provision of easy access to condoms and other contraceptives.

Counterconditioning requires the learning of healthier behaviors that can substitute for problem behaviors. Relaxation can counter stress; assertion can counter peer pressure; nicotine replacement can substitute for cigarettes, and fat-free foods can be safe substitutes for high-fat foods.

Stimulus control removes cues for unhealthy habits and adds prompts for healthier alternatives. Avoidance, environmental reengineering, and self-help groups can provide stimuli that support change and reduce risks for relapse. Planning parking lots that require a 2-minute walk to the office and putting art displays in stairwells are examples of reengineering that can encourage more exercise.

Contingency management provides consequences for taking steps in a particular direction. While contingency management can include the use of punishments, we found that self-changers rely on rewards much more than on punishments. Consequently, reinforcements are emphasized, since the philosophy of the stage model requires that it work in harmony with how people change naturally. Contingency contracts, overt and covert reinforcements, positive self-statements, and group recognition are procedures for increasing reinforcement and the probability that healthier responses will be repeated.

Helping relationships combine caring, trust, openness, and acceptance as well as support for the healthy behavior change. Rapport building, a therapeutic alliance, coaching calls, and buddy systems can be sources of social support.

Decisional Balance

This core construct reflects the individual's relative weighing of the pros and cons of changing. Originally, we relied on Janis and Mann's (1977) model of decision making that included four categories of pros (instrumental gains for self and others and approval for self and others). The four categories of cons were instrumental costs to self and others and disapproval from self and others. In a long series of studies attempting to produce this structure of eight factors, we always found a much simpler structure—just the pros and cons of changing.

Self-Efficacy

This is the situation-specific confidence that people have when they can cope with high-risk situations without relapsing to their unhealthy or high-risk habit. This construct was integrated from Bandura's (1982) self-efficacy theory.

Temptation

This core construct reflects the intensity of urges to engage in a specific habit when in the midst of difficult situations. In our research, we typically find that three factors account for the most common types of tempting situations: negative affect or emotional distress, positive social situations, and craving.

Critical Assumptions

The following are a set of assumptions that drive our theory, research, and practice:

1. No single theory can account for all of the complexities of behavior change. Therefore, a more comprehensive model will likely emerge from an integration across major theories.
2. Behavior change is a process that unfolds over time through a sequence of stages.
3. Stages are both stable and open to change, just as chronic behavioral risk factors are both stable and open to change.
4. Without planned interventions, most populations will remain stuck in the early stages. There is no inherent motivation to progress through the stages of intentional change as there seems to be in stages of physical and psychological development.
5. The majority of at-risk populations are not prepared for action and will not be served by traditional action-oriented prevention programs. Health promotion can have much greater impacts if it shifts from an action paradigm to a stage paradigm.
6. Specific processes and principles of change need to be applied at specific stages if progress through the stages is to occur. In the stages of change, paradigm intervention programs must be matched to each individual's stage of change.
7. Chronic behavior patterns are under usually some combination of biological, social, and self-control. Stage-matched interventions have been designed primarily to enhance self-controls.

Empirical Support: Basic Research

Stage Distribution

If we are to match the needs of entire populations, we need to know the stage distributions of specific high-risk behaviors. Results from a series of studies on smoking have clearly demonstrated that less than 20% of smokers in the United States are in the preparation stage in most populations (e.g., Velicer et al., 1995). Approximately 40% of smokers are in the contemplation stage, and another 40% are in precontemplation. The stage distribution in other countries are even more dramatic, with 70% of smokers in precontemplation in Germany, 70% in China, and 85% in Japan (Etter, Perneger, & Ronchi, 1997). These results show that action-oriented cessation programs will not match the needs of the vast majority of smokers.

Pros and Cons Structure Across 48 Behaviors

As indicated earlier, the pros and cons of decisional balance have a much simpler structure than Janis and Mann's (1977) theory suggests. Across 135 studies from 10 countries of 50 different behaviors (e.g., ceasing smoking, quitting cocaine, controlling weight, reducing dietary fat, managing stress, using condoms, acquiring exercise, using sunscreen, testing for radon, reducing delinquency, using mammography screening, and practicing preventive medicine), the two-factor structure was remarkably stable (Hall & Rossi, 2008).

Integration of Pros and Cons and Stages of Change Across 48 Health Behaviors

Stage is not a theory; it is a variable. A theory requires systematic relationships among a set of variables, ideally culminating in mathematical relationships. Figure 4.1 presents systematic relationships between stages and pros and cons of changing from the meta-analysis on 48 behaviors (Hall & Rossi, 2008). One might expect that, given the variability across so many problems and populations, there would be too much noise for a clear signal to emerge. Instead, very predictable and clear patterns were found.

As predicted from a previous study on 12 behaviors (Prochaska et al., 1994a), the meta-analysis of 48 behaviors found that the cons of changing are higher than the pros for people in precontemplation. The pros and cons are about equal

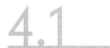

The pros and cons (in T scores) by stages of change for 48 problem behaviors.

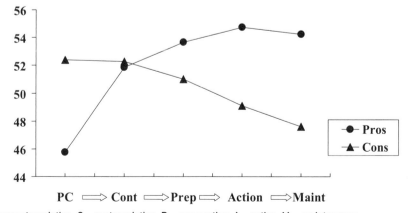

PC = precontemplation; C = contemplation; P = preparation; A = action; M = maintenance

for people in contemplation. The pros increase as people move from precontemplation to action. In contrast, as they go from contemplation to maintenance, the cons of changing are reduced. The pros of changing are higher than the cons for people in preparation through maintenance.

These basic findings suggest principles for progressing through the stages (Prochaska et al., 1994b). For people to progress from precontemplation to contemplation, the pros of changing must increase. To them to progress from contemplation to action, the cons of changing must decrease. So, for people in precontemplation, we would target the pros for intervention and save the cons until after they progress to contemplation. Before progressing to action, we would want to see the pros and cons crossing over, taking a pattern where the pros are higher than the cons as a sign that the person is well prepared for action. Having the pros high enough and the cons low enough is part of what it takes to be well prepared to progress to maintenance with a low chance of relapsing.

Strong and Weak Principles of Progress

Across the original behaviors, mathematical relationships were found between the pros and cons of changing and progress across the stages. The Strong Principle is:

$$PC \rightarrow A \cong 1 \text{ S.D. } \uparrow PROS$$

Progress from precontemplation to action involves approximately one standard deviation (S.D.) increase in the pros of changing. On intelligence tests, a one-S.D. increase would equal 15 points, which is a substantial increase. In the meta-analysis of 48 behaviors, the pros were found to increase exactly 1.00 S.D. (Hall & Rossi, 2008).

The Weak Principle is:

$$PC \rightarrow A \cong .5 \text{ S.D. } \downarrow CONS$$

Progress from precontemplation to action involves an approximately .5 S.D. decrease in the cons of changing. Across 48 behaviors, the cons decreased .53 S.D. In an analysis of two studies relating positive and negative expectancies from Social Cognitive Theory to the Stages of Change (Dijkstra et al., 1999, 2006), it was found that from precontemplation to action, positive expectancies increased 1.12 and 1.17 S.D. (Prochaska, 2006). From contemplation to action, the negative expectancies decreased .49 and .45 S.D. This is an example of how constructs from other theories can be integrated even mathematically by the stages of change (Prochaska, 2006).

One practical implication of these principles is that the pros of changing must increase twice as much as the cons must decrease. Perhaps twice as much emphasis should be placed on raising the benefits as on reducing the costs or barriers. For example, if couch potatoes in precontemplation can list only 5 pros of exercise, then being too busy will be a big barrier to change. But if program participants come to appreciate that there can be more than 50 benefits for 60 minutes a week, being too busy becomes a relatively smaller barrier.

Processes of Change Across Behaviors

One of the assumptions of the Transtheoretical Model is that there is a common set of change processes that people can apply across a broad range of behaviors. The higher-order structure of the processes (experiential and behavioral) has been replicated across problem behaviors better than specific processes have (Rossi, 1992a). Typically, we have found support for our standard set of 10 processes across such behaviors as smoking, diet, cocaine use, exercise, condom use, and sun exposure. But the structure of the processes across studies has not been as consistent as the structure of the stages and the pros and cons of changing. In some studies, we find fewer processes, and occasionally we find evidence for one or two more. It is also very possible that with some behaviors, fewer change processes may be used. With an infrequent behavior like a yearly mammogram, for example, fewer processes may be required to progress to long-term maintenance (Rakowski et al., 1998).

Relationship Between Stages and Processes of Change

One of our earliest empirical integrations was the discovery of systematic relationships between the stage people were in and the processes they were applying. This discovery allowed us to integrate processes from theories that were typically seen as incompatible and in conflict. For example, Freudian theory, which relied almost entirely on consciousness raising for producing change, was viewed as incompatible with Skinnerian theory, which relied entirely on contingency management for modifying behavior. But self-changers did not know that these processes were theoretically incompatible, and they taught us that processes from very different theories needed to be emphasized at different stages of change. Table 4.1 presents our current theoretical integration (Prochaska, DiClemente, & Norcross, 1992). This integration suggests that in the early stages of behavior change, people emphasis cognitive, affective, and evaluative processes to help them progress through the stages. In later stages, people rely more on commitments, conditioning, contingencies, environmental controls, and support to support their progress toward termination.

Table 4.1 has important practical implications. To help people progress from precontemplation to contemplation, we need to apply such processes as consciousness raising and dramatic relief. Applying processes like contingency management, counterconditioning, and stimulus control to people in precontemplation would represent a theoretical, empirical, and practical mistake. But for people in action, such strategies represent an optimal matching.

As with the structure of the processes, the integration of the processes and stages has not been as consistent as the integration of the stages and the pros and cons of changing. While part of the problem may be the greater complexity

4.1 Stages of Change in Which Change Processes Are Most Emphasized

	Stages of change				
	Precontemplation	Contemplation	Preparation	Action	Maintenance
Processes	Consciousness raising Dramatic relief Environmental reevaluation	Self-reevaluation	Self-liberation	Contingency management Helping relationship Counterconditioning Stimulus control	

of integrating 10 processes across five stages, the processes of change need more basic research.

Applied Studies

Within a large and diverse body of applied studies utilizing TTM, several trends can be identified. The most common application involves TTM-tailored expert system communications, which match intervention messages to an individual's particular needs (e.g., Kreuter, Strecher, & Glassman, 1999; Skinner, Campbell, Rimer, Curry, & Prochaska, 1999) across all TTM constructs. For example, individuals in precontemplation could receive feedback designed to increase their pros of changing to help them progress to contemplation. These interventions have most commonly been printed either on site or mailed to participants at home (Velicer et al., 1993); however, a growing range of applications is developing and evaluating more immediate multimedia expert system programs (Redding et al., 1999) that can be delivered onsite or online.

The largest number of TTM-related intervention studies have involved smoking (Aveyard et al., 1999; Curry et al., 1995; Dijsktra et al., 1999, 2006; O'Neill, Gillespie, & Slobin, 2000; Pallonen et al., 1998; Prochaska et al., 1993, 2001a; Strecher et al., 1994), diet (Beresford et al., 1997; Brug et al., 1998; Campbell et al., 1994; Glanz et al., 1998; Horwath, 1999), and exercise (Cardinal & Sachs, 1996; Marcus et al., 1998). Recent randomized clinical trials (RCT) outcome studies have looked at stress management (Evers, Prochaska, Mauriello,

Padula, & Prochaska, 2006), medication adherence (Johnson et al., 2006a, 2006b), and bullying prevention (Prochaska, Evers, Prochaska, Van Marter, & Johnson, 2007). There is a growing range of applications, from alcohol abuse (Carbonari & DiClemente, 2000), to condom use (Centers for Disease Control, 1999; Parsons, Huszti, Crudder, Rich, & Mendoza, 2000; Redding et al., 2007, Schneider, Wolitski, & Corby, 1997), to domestic violence offenders (Levesque et al., 2008), to organ donation (Robbins et al., 2001), to multiple behavior changes (Gold, Anderson, & Serxner, 2000; Kreuter & Strecher, 1996; Steptoe, Kerry, Rink, & Hilton, 2001).

A recent meta-analysis of tailored print communications found that TTM was the most commonly used theory across a broad range of behaviors (Noar et al., 2007). TTM or Stage of Change Models were used in 35 of the 53 studies. In terms of effectiveness, significantly greater effects were produced when tailored communications included each of the following TTM constructs: stages of change, pros and cons of changing, self-efficacy, and processes of change (Noar et al., 2007). In contrast, interventions that included the non-TTM construct of perceived susceptibility had significantly worse outcomes. Tailoring on non-TTM constructs like social norms and behavioral intentions produced no significant differences (Noar et al., 2007).

While each of the major TTM constructs (stage, pros and cons, self-efficacy, and processes) produces greater effects when each is included in tailored communications, what happens when only some of the constructs are used? Spencer, Pagell, Hallion, & Adams (2002) systematically reviewed 23 interventions that used one or more of the TTM variables for achieving smoking cessation. Most of the studies used just stage of change, and, of these, only about 40% produced significant effects. Five used stage plus pros and cons or self-efficacy, and, of these, 60% produced significant effects. Another five used all of the TTM variables, and 80% of these yielded significant results. This analysis raises the important dissemination question of what it means for practice and applied research to be theory-driven. Most of these studies were variable driven (e.g., they used the stage variable). Future research is needed to determine whether applied research is most effective when a full theory like TTM is applied or whether there is an optimal number of theoretical variables that can produce the same effect sizes, while placing fewer demands on participants and practitioners.

Challenging Studies

As with any model, not all of the research is supportive. Here are samples of some of the more challenging studies. Farkas et al. (1996) and then Abrams, Herzog, Emmons, & Linnan (2000) compared addiction variables to TTM variables as predictors of cessation over 12 to 24 months. Addiction variables, like number of cigarettes smoked and duration of prior quits (e.g., more than 100 days) outpredicted TTM variables, suggesting that addiction models were preferable to TTM. Responses to these comparative studies included concerns that Farkas et al. (1996) compared 14 addiction type variables to just the single-stage variable from TTM (Prochaska & Velicer, 1996; Prochaska, 2006). The Abrams et al.

(2000) study included self-efficacy and the contemplation ladder measure of stage as part of the addiction model, but these are part of TTM. Also, from an intervention perspective, the amount of variance accounted for by predictor variables is less important than the amount of variance that can be controlled or changed. Duration of previous quits (e.g., 100 days) may outpredict stage, but there is little that can be done to change this historical variable, while a dynamic variable like stage is open to interventions.

In the first of a series of studies, Herzog, Abrams, Emmons, Linnan, & Shadel (1999) found that six processes of change were not adequate predictors of stage progress over a 12-month period. In a second report, the processes did predict stage progress, but only when the contemplation ladder was used (Herzog, Abrams, Emmons, & Linnan, 2000). In the third report, TTM measures did predict 12-month outcomes, but, as indicated, earlier self-efficacy and the contemplation ladder were not counted as TTM variables (Abrams et al., 2000). Other research has found that change processes and other TTM variables do predict stage progress (e.g., Prochaska, DiClemente, Velicer, Ginpil, & Norcross, 1985; Prochaska, Velicer, Prochaska, & Johnson, 2004; DiClemente et al., 1991; Dijkstra et al., 2006; Johnson et al., 2000; Sun, Prochaska, Velicer, & Laforge, 2007; Velicer et al., 2007a). Johnson et al. (2000) in their study explained some of the inconsistencies in the previous research, such as predictions over 6 months and those over 12 months and use of all 10 processes of change instead of a subset.

One of the productive responses to critical studies is to do more research. In response to the criticism that addiction levels are better predictors of long-term outcomes than stage of change, a series of studies has been done to determine which types of effects predict long-term outcomes across multiple behaviors. To date, four such effects have been found (Prochaska et al., 2008). The first is severity effect in which individuals with less severe behavior risks at baseline are more likely to progress to action or maintenance and 24-month follow-up for smoking, diet, and sun exposure. This effect includes the level of addiction that Farkas et al. (1996) and Abrams et al. (2000) preferred.

The second is stage effect, in which participants in preparation at baseline have better 24-month outcomes for smoking, diet, and sun exposure than those in contemplation, who in turn do better than those in precontemplation. This effect is what Farkas et al. (1996) and Abrams et al. (2000) criticized.

The third is treatment effect, in which participants in treatment do better at 24 months than those randomly assigned to control groups for smoking, diet, and sun exposure. The fourth is effort effects, in which participants in both treatment and control groups who progressed to action and maintenance at 24 months were making better efforts with TTM variables like pros and cons, self-efficacy, and processes at baseline. There were no consistent demographic effects across the three behaviors indicating that no one demographic group did better across these multiple behaviors. What these results indicate is that either/or thinking, like relying on either severity or stage, is not as helpful as a more inclusive approach that seeks to identify the most important effects, whether they are based on TTM or on an addiction or severity model.

Applying innovative dynamic typologies, Sun et al. (2007) were able to analyze longitudinal relationships of all 14 of the TTM processes and principles of change to three dynatypes (maintenance, relapse, and no change) within a representative sample of 4,144 smokers in both TTM-tailored treatment and control groups. Assessments at every 6 months over 2 years demonstrated that the stable smokers who failed to progress to action at any assessment were applying the TTM variables least effectively at baseline and continued to apply the process variables similarly for the full 2 years. The maintainers, on the other hand, decreased their use of experiential processes like consciousness raising and self-reevaluation and decisional balance variables like the pros and cons of smoking. They increased their use of behavioral processes like counterconditioning and stimulus control and applied other processes like dramatic relief, environmental reevaluation, social liberation, and reinforcement management in a curvilinear pattern of increases followed by decreases. The relapsers paralleled the maintainers in their initial use of the TTM variables but over time ended up between the maintainers and stable smokers. What was particularly striking was that, even though the treatment group outperformed the control group in terms of the percentage who remained abstinent at 2-year follow-up, the successful quitters in both the intervention and the control groups applied the 14 TTM variables in the same manner and followed common pathways to change. This research may help answer the original question that generated TTM: how very different treatments like Cognitive Behavior Therapy, Motivational Interviewing, and 12-step treatments in Project MATCH (1997) can produce such similar outcomes. The answer might well be that successful changes in different treatments and in control groups apply processes and principles of change in very similar ways.

Applications of the Transtheoretical Model: Smoking Cessation Interventions as Protocol Examples

Smoking is costly to individual smokers and to society. In the United States, approximately 45,000,000 Americans continue to smoke. More than 400,000 preventable deaths per year are attributable to smoking (U.S. Department of Health and Human Services, 1990). Globally, the problem promises to be catastrophic. Of the people alive in the world today, 500,000,000 are expected to die from this single behavior, losing approximately 5,000,000,000 years of life to tobacco use (Peto & Lopez, 1990). If we can make even modest gains in our science and practice of smoking cessation, we can prevent millions of premature deaths and help preserve billions of years of life.

Currently, smoking cessation clinics have little impact. When offered for free by HMOs in the United States, such clinics recruit only about 1% of subscribers who smoke. When state health departments contract for free action-oriented quit lines, they typically budget for less than 1% of smokers to call each year. Such behavior health services simply cannot make much difference if they treat such a small percentage of the problem (Orleans et al., 1985).

Startled by such statistics, behavioral scientists took health promotion programs into communities and worksites. The results are now being reported, and, in the largest trials ever attempted, the outcomes are discouraging. In the Minnesota Heart Health project, for example, $40 million was spent with 5 years of intervention in four communities totaling 400,000 people. There were no significant differences between treatment and control communities on smoking, diet, cholesterol, weight, blood pressure, and overall risks for cardiovascular disease (Luepker et al., 1994).

What went wrong? The investigators speculate that maybe they diluted their programs by targeting multiple behaviors. But the COMMIT (COMMIT Research Group, 1995) trial had no effects with its primary target of heavy smokers and only a small effect with light smokers. Similarly, the largest work-site cessation program produced no significant differences between intervention and comparison sites (Glasgow, Terborg, Hollis, Severson, & Boles, 1995). Part of the problem is that the control populations were improving, making it more difficult for the intervention groups to outperform them.

A closer look at participation rates may explain some of the disappointing results. In the Minnesota study, nearly 90% of smokers in both the treatment and the control communities had processed media information about smoking in the past year. But only about 10% had been advised to quit by their physicians (Lando et al., 1995). And only about 3% had participated in the most powerful behavioral programs, such as individualized and interactive clinics, classes, and contests. In one of the Minnesota Heart Health studies, smokers were randomly assigned to one of three recruitment methods for home-based cessation programs (Schmidt, Jeffrey, & Hellerstedt, 1989). These announcements generated 1% to 5% participation rates, with a personalized letter generating the best results. We cannot have much impact on the health of our communities if we interact with only a small percentage of those populations that are at high risk for disease and early death.

Such disappointing impacts have led governments, health plans, and employers to rely on bans in public places, increased taxes on cigarettes and health insurance for smokers, and mass-media counteradvertising. These interventions are population-based, while cessation treatments were designed only for motivated smokers. The most recent U.S. Clinical Guidelines for the Treatment of Tobacco (Fiore et al., 2000) identified a broad range of evidence-based treatments for motivated smokers, defined as those in the preparation stage. There were no evidence-based treatments for the 80% or more of smokers who were not motivated or prepared to quit.

Our TTM alternative was to shift from an action paradigm to a stage paradigm in order to increase reach and interact with a much higher percentage of populations at risk. Let us examine how the stage paradigm has been applied to five of the most important phases of planned interventions.

Recruitment

Recall that cessation programs falter in this first phase of intervention and produce low participation rates. Stage distributions can help explain such low rates. Across four different samples, 20% or less of smokers were in the preparation stage (Velicer et al., 1995). When we advertised or announced programs, we were explicitly or implicitly targeting less than 20% of a population. The other 80% plus were left on their own.

In two home-based programs with approximately 5,000 smokers in each study, we reached out either by telephone alone or by personal letters followed by telephone calls if needed and recruited smokers to stage-matched interventions. For each of five stages, these interventions included self-help manuals, individualized computer feedback reports based on assessments of the pros and cons, processes, self-efficacy, and temptations and/or counselor protocols based on the computer reports. Using these proactive recruitment methods and stage-matched interventions, we were able to generate participation rates of 82% to 85%, respectively (Prochaska, Velicer, Fava, Rossi, & Tsoh, 2001a; Prochaska et al., 2001b). Such large increases in participation rates provide the potential to generate unprecedented impacts with entire populations of smokers.

Population impact equals participation rate times the rate of efficacy or action. If a program produced 30% efficacy (such as long-term abstinence), historically it was judged to be better than a program that produced 25% abstinence. But a program that generates 30% efficacy but only 5% participation has an impact of only 1.5% (30% × 5%). A program that produces only 25% efficacy but 60% participation has an impact of 15%. With health promotion programs, this would mean a 1000% greater impact on a high-risk population.

The stage paradigm would shift our outcomes from efficacy alone to impact. To achieve such high impact, we needed to shift from reactive recruitment, where we advertised or announced our programs and reacted when people reach us to proactive recruitments where we reached out to interact with all potential participants.

Proactive recruitment alone doesn't work. In the most intensive recruitment protocol to date, Lichtenstein and Hollis (1992) had physicians spend up to 5 minutes with each smoker just to get the person to sign up for an action-oriented cessation clinic. If that didn't work, a nurse spent 10 minutes to persuade each smoker to sign up, followed by 12 minutes with a videotape and health educator and even a proactive call from a counselor if necessary. The base rate was 1% participation. This proactive protocol led 35% of smokers in precontemplation to sign up. But only 3% showed up, and 2% finished the program. When smokers in contemplation and preparation are combined, 65% signed up, 15% showed up, and 11% finished the program.

To optimize our impacts, we need to use proactive protocols to recruit participants to programs that match the stage they are in. Once we generate high recruitment rates, we then have to be concerned about high retention rates, lest we lose many of the initial participants in our health promotion programs.

Retention

One of the skeletons in the closet of psychotherapy and behavior change interventions is their relatively poor retention rates. Across 125 studies, the average retention rate was only about 50% (Wierzbicki & Pekarik, 1993). Furthermore, this meta-analysis found few consistent predictors of which participants would drop out prematurely and which would continue in therapy. In studies on smoking, weight control, substance abuse, and a mixture of DSM-III disorders, stage-of-change measures proved to be the best predictors of premature termination. For example, when we look at stage profiles of groups of therapy participants, we find that the pretreatment stage profile of the entire 40% who dropped out prematurely as judged by their therapists was that of patients in precontemplation. The 20% who terminated quickly but appropriately had a profile of patients in action. Using pretreatment-stage-related measures, we were able to correctly classify 93% of the groups (Brogan, Prochaskam, & Prochaska, 1999).

We simply cannot treat people with a precontemplation profile as if they were ready for action interventions and expect them to stay in treatment. Relapse prevention strategies are indicated with smokers who are taking action. But those in precontemplation are more likely to need drop-out-prevention strategies.

The best strategy we have found to promote retention is to match our interventions to stage of change. In four smoking cessation studies using such matching strategies, we found that we were able to retain smokers in the precontemplation stage at the same high levels as those who started in the preparation stage (Prochaska et al., 2001a).

Progress

The amount of progress participants make following health promotion programs is directly related to the stage they were in at the start of the interventions. This *stage effect* is illustrated where smokers initially in precontemplation show the smallest amount of abstinence over 18 months and those in preparation progress the most. Across 66 different predictions of progress, we found that smokers starting in contemplation were about two-thirds more successful than those in precontemplation at 6-, 12-, and 18-month follow-ups. Similarly, those in preparation were about two-thirds more successful than those in contemplation at the same follow-ups (Prochaska, Velicer, Prochaska, & Johnson, 2004).

These results can be used clinically. A reasonable goal for each therapeutic intervention with smokers is to help them progress one stage. If over the course of brief therapy they progress two stages, they will be about 2.66 times more successful at longer-term follow-ups (Prochaska et al, 2004).

Process

To help populations progress through the stages, we need to understand the processes and principles of change. One of the fundamental principles for progress is that different processes of change need to be applied at different stages of change. Classic conditioning processes like counterconditioning, stimulus control, and contingency control can be highly successful for participants who are ready to take action but can produce resistance in individuals in precontemplation. More experiential processes, such as consciousness raising and dramatic relief, can move these people cognitively and affectively and help them shift to contemplation (Prochaska, Norcross, & DiClemente, 1994a).

After 15 years of research, we have identified 14 variables on which to intervene in order to accelerate progress across the first five stages of change (Prochaska et al., 1994b). At any particular stage, we need to intervene with a maximum of six variables. To help guide individuals at each stage of change, we have developed computer-based expert systems that can deliver individualized and interactive interventions to entire populations (Velicer et al.,

1993). These computer programs can be used alone or in conjunction with counseling.

Outcomes

In our first large-scale clinical trial, we compared four treatments: one of the best home-based action-oriented cessation programs (standardized); stage-matched manuals (individualized); expert system computer reports plus manuals (interactive); and counselors plus computers and manuals (personalized). We randomly assigned by stage 739 smokers to one of the four treatments (Prochaska, DiClemente, Velicer, & Rossi, 1993).

In the computer condition, participants answered by mail or telephone interview 40 questions, and their responses were entered in our central computers and generated feedback reports. These reports informed participants about their stage of change, their pros and cons of changing, and their use of change processes appropriate to their stages. At baseline, participants were given positive feedback on what they were doing correctly and guidance on which principles and processes they needed to apply more in order to progress. In two progress reports delivered over the next 6 months, participants also received positive feedback on any improvement they made on any of the variables relevant to progressing. This way, demoralized and defensive smokers could begin progressing without having to quit and without having to work too hard. Smokers in the contemplation stage could begin taking small steps, like delaying their first cigarette in the morning for an extra 30 minutes. They could choose small steps that would increase their self-efficacy and help them become better prepared for quitting.

In the personalized condition, smokers received four proactive counselor calls over the 6-month intervention period. Three of the calls were based on the computer reports. Counselors reported much more difficulty in interacting with participants without any progress data. Without scientific assessments, it was much harder for both clients and counselors to tell whether any significant progress had occurred since their last interaction.

Figure 4.2 presents point prevalence abstinence rates for each of the four treatment groups over 18 months with treatment ending at 6 months (Prochaska et al., 1993). Those in the two self-help-manual groups paralleled each other for 12 months. At 18 months, the group with the stage-matched manuals had moved ahead. This is an example of a *delayed action effect,* which we often observe with stage-matched programs specifically and which others have observed with self-help programs generally (Glynn, Anderson, & Schwarz, 1992). It takes time for participants in the early stages to progress all the way to action. Therefore, some treatment effects as measured by action will be observed only after considerable delay. But it is encouraging to find treatments producing therapeutic effects months and even years after treatment ended.

The computer-alone group and the computer-plus-counselor group paralleled each other for 12 months. Then, the effects of the counselor condition flattened out, while the computer-condition effects continued to increase. We can only speculate as to the delayed differences between these two conditions. Participants in the personalized-condition group may have become somewhat de-

4.2

Point prevalence abstinence (%) for four treatment groups at pretest and at 6, 12, and 18 months.

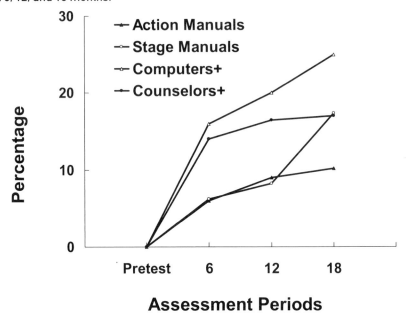

ALA + = standardized manuals; TTT = individualized stage-matched manuals; ITT = interactive computer reports; PITT = personalized counselor calls.

pendent on the social support and social control provided by the calls from the counselor. The last call came after the 6-months assessment and benefits were observed at 12 months. Termination of the contact with the counselors might have led to the cessation of progress because of the loss of social support and control. The classic pattern in smoking-cessation clinics is that rapid relapse begins as soon as the treatment is terminated. Some of this rapid relapse may well be the result of the sudden loss of social support or social control provided by the counselors and other participants in the clinic.

In this clinical trial, smokers were recruited reactively. They called us in response to advertisements, announcements, and articles. How did their results compare to those of smokers proactively recruited to our programs? Most people would predict that smokers who call us for help would be more successful than smokers whom we called to help.

In fact, the results of a comparison between smokers in a study who called (reactive) (Prochaska et al., 1993) and those in a study whom we called (proactive) (Prochaska, Velicer, Fava, Rossi, & Tsoh, 2001a) were remarkable. Both groups received the same home-based expert system computer reports delivered over a 6-month period. While the reactively recruited subjects were slightly more successful at each follow-up, what was striking was how similar were the abstinence curves over long-term follow-up.

Outcomes With Diverse Groups

In a small pilot study of a multimedia TTM-tailored smoking cessation expert system in urban primary-care medical clinics, good rates of participation and quitting among a group composed primarily of African American, older smokers were found (Hoffman et al., 2006). These promising data led us to offer a comparable interactive smoking-cessation system to women at risk for or infected with HIV. Although we cannot yet evaluate quit rates, early participation rates have been good in this sample with multiple comorbidities and health challenges (Goldberg, Weber, Redding, & Cohen, 2006).

Outcomes with diverse groups were part of an analysis that combined data from five effectiveness trials in which 2,622 smokers were proactively recruited and all received the same TTM-tailored intervention plus stage-matched manuals. The intervention produced a consistent 22%–26% long-term cessation rate across the five studies with a mean of about 24% (Velicer, Redding, Sun, & Prochaska, 2007b). There were no significant differences in abstinence rates between females (24.6%) and males (23.6%). There were no significant differences between African Americans (26.3%) and Whites (24.9%) or between Hispanics and non-Hispanics. The oldest smokers (65 and older) had abstinence rates (35.2%) that were 45% higher than the mean. College graduates had abstinence rates (30.1%) that were significantly higher than average.

The Surgeon General's Report (U.S. Department of Health and Human Services, 1994) on Adolescent Smoking basically concluded that teenage smokers would not participate in treatment, and if they did, they would not quit. Hollis et al. (2005) were able to proactively recruit 65% of teens in primary care to a smoking-cessation program based on our TTM tailored communications. At long-term follow-up, the regular smokers receiving treatment had significantly higher cessation rates (23.9%) than the randomized control group (11.4%). Furthermore, their quit rate of 23.9% was essentially the same as the average quit rate in our adult treatment groups (Hollis et al., 2005).

The Clinical Guidelines for the Treatment of Tobacco (Fiore et al., 2000) identified no evidence-based treatments for smokers with mental illness, even though such smokers consume nearly 50% of all cigarettes in the U.S. Hall and colleagues (2006) reached out to smokers who were being treated for depression in clinics at UC San Francisco. Those randomized to treatment received our TTM-tailored program plus counseling and nicotine replacement therapy. At 24-month follow-up, the treatment group had significantly higher abstinence rates (24.6%) than the controls (19.1%), and its quit rates were remarkably similar to those of our average treated adults (Hall et al., 2006).

These outcomes with diverse groups receiving similar TTM-tailored treatments challenge stereotypes that assume that some groups do not have the same ability to change. Minorities, the elderly, adolescents, and mentally ill groups are often assumed not to have the same ability to change as other populations. These results suggest that the issue may not be their ability to change. The issue may be their accessibility to quality change programs.

If these results continue to be replicated, health promotion programs will be able to produce unprecedented impacts on entire populations. We believe that such unprecedented impacts require scientific and professional shifts:

1. From an action paradigm to a stage paradigm;
2. From reactive to proactive recruitment;
3. From expecting participants to match the needs of our programs to having our programs match participants' needs;
4. From efficacy trials for select samples to more inclusive population trials;
5. From clinic-based to community-based behavioral health programs that apply the field's most powerful individualized and interactive intervention strategies.

With these types of shifts in health promotion, we may be better prepared to respond to the huge unmet needs and the great opportunities related to the prevention of chronic diseases and premature death (Prochaska, 2008).

Future Research

While we are encouraged by the research results to date, much still needs to be done to advance the Transtheoretical Model. Basic research needs to be done with other theoretical variables, such as perceived risk, subjective norms, and severity of the problem, to determine whether such variables relate systematically to the stages and whether they predict progress across particular stages. More research is needed on the structure of the processes and on the stages of change across a broad range of health behaviors. What modifications are most needed for specific types of behavior (e.g., having fewer processes for infrequent behaviors, such as annual mammograms)? What additional behaviors, beyond the 50 already studied, can be understood from a stage perspective?

Can the stage model be useful in describing, explaining, and predicting changes beyond the individual level, such as changes in couples, families, organizations, and communities? What happens when two or more people are trying to change together and they are in different stages? Can social policies be made more effective by matching policies to a community's stage of readiness to change? Are there particular types of public health campaigns, such as media campaigns, that can best produce progress in communities in the early stages of change?

At the individual level, much more research needs to be done on the most cost-effective interventions for producing progress through the stages across a variety of health behaviors. What are the minimum interventions needed to accelerate progress at each stage?

The Transtheoretical Model is a dynamic theory of change, and it must remain open to modification as more students, scientists, and practitioners apply the stage model to a growing number of theoretical and public health problems.

Summary

Research to date supports the Transtheoretical perspective that the adoption and maintenance of health behavior change involves progress through a series of stages. Such progress can be accelerated and facilitated by tailoring particular processes and principles of change to populations and individuals at each stage of change. Proactively applying TTM tailoring interventions for multiple behaviors can greatly increase participation, retention, progress, and impact rates in entire populations at risk for chronic disease and premature death.

References

Abrams, D. B., Herzog, T. A., Emmons, K. M., & Linnan, L. (2000). Stages of change versus addiction: A replication and extension. *Nicotine & Tobacco Research, 2,* 223–229.

Aveyard, P., Cheng, K. K., Almond, J., Sherratt, E., Lancashire, R., Lawrence, T., et al. (1999). Cluster randomised controlled trial of expert system based on the transtheoretical ("stages of change") model for smoking prevention and cessation in schools. *British Medical Journal, 319,* 948–953.

Bandura, A. (1982). Self-efficacy mechanism in human agency. *American Psychologist, 37,* 122-147.

Beresford, S. A. A., Curry, S. J., Kristal, A. R., Lazovich, D., Feng, Z., & Wagner, E. H. (1997). A dietary intervention in primary care practice: The eating patterns study. *American Journal of Public Health, 87,* 610–616.

Brogan, M. M., Prochaska, J. O., & Prochaska, J. M. (1999). Predicting termination and continuation status in psychotherapy using the transtheoretical model. *Psychotherapy, 36,* 105–113.

Brug, J., Glanz, K., Van Assema, P., Kok, G., & van Breukelen, G. J. P. (1998). The impact of computer-tailored feedback and iterative feedback on fat, fruit, and vegetable intake. *Health Education & Behavior, 25,* 517–531.

Campbell, M. K., DeVellis, B. M., Strecher, V. J., Ammerman, A. S., DeVellis, R. F., & Sandler, R. S. (1994). Improving dietary behavior: The effectiveness of tailored messages in primary care settings. *American Journal of Public Health, 84,* 783–787.

Carbonari, J. P., & DiClemente, C. C. (2000). Using Transtheoretical Model profiles to differentiate levels of alcohol abstinence success. *Journal of Consulting and Clinical Psychology, 68,* 810–817.

Cardinal, B. J., & Sachs, M. L. (1996). Effects of mail-mediated, stage-matched exercise behavior change strategies on female adults leisure-time exercise behavior. *Journal of Sports Medicine and Physical Fitness, 36,* 100–107.

Centers for Disease Control, AIDS Community Demonstration Projects Research Group. (1999). Community-Level HIV intervention in 5 cities: Final outcome data from the CDC AIDS Community Demonstration Projects. *American Journal of Public Health, 89*(3), 336–345.

The COMMIT Research Group. (1995). Community intervention trial for smoking cessation (COMMIT): I. Cohort results from a four-year community intervention. *American Journal of Public Health, 85*(2), 183–192.

Curry, S. J., McBride, C., Grothaus, L. C., Louie, D., & Wagner, E. H. (1995). A randomized trial of self-help materials, personalized feedback, and telephone counseling with nonvolunteer smokers. *Journal of Consulting and Clinical Psychology, 63,* 175–180.

DiClemente, C. C., Prochaska, J. O., Fairhurst, S. K., Velicer, W. F., Valesquez, M. M., Rossi, J. S., et al. (1991). The processes of smoking cessation: An analysis of precontemplation, contemplation, and preparation stages of change. *Journal of Consulting and Clinical Psychology, 59,* 295–304.

Dijkstra, A., Conijm B., & De Vries, H. (2006). A match-mismatch test of a stage model of behavior change in tobacco smoking. *Addiction, 101,* 1035–1043.

Dijkstra, A., DeVries, H., & Roijackers, J. (1999). Targeting smokers with low readiness to change with tailored and non-tailored self-help materials. *Preventive Medicine, 28,* 203–211.

Etter, J.-F., Perneger, T. V., & Ronchi, A. (1997). Distributions of smokers by stage: International comparison and association with smoking prevalence. *Preventive Medicine, 26,* 580–585.

Evers, K. E., Prochaska, J. O., Mauriello, L. M., Padula, J. A., & Prochaska, J. M. (2006). A randomized clinical trial of a population and transtheoretical-based stress management intervention. *Health Psychology, 25*(4), 521–529.

Farkas, A. J., Pierce, J. P., Zhu, S. H., Rosbrook, B., Gilpin, E. A., Berry, C., et al. (1996). Addiction versus stages of change models in predicting smoking cessation. *Addiction, 91,* 1271–1280.

Fiore, M. C., Bailey, W. C., Cohen, S. J., et al. (2000). *Treating tobacco use and dependence: Clinical practice guideline.* Rockville, MD: U.S. Department of Health and Human Services, Public Health Service.

Glanz, K., Patterson, R. E., Kristal, A. R., Feng, Z., Linnan, L., Heimendinger, J., et al. (1998). Impact of work site health promotion on stages of dietary change: The working well trial. *Health Education & Behavior, 25,* 448–463.

Glasgow, R. E., Terborg, J. R., Hollis, J. F., Severson, H. H., & Boles, M. (1995). Take heart: Results from the initial phase of a work-site wellness program. *American Journal of Public Health, 85*(2), 209–216.

Glynn, T. J., Anderson, D. M., & Schwarz, L. (1992). Tobacco use reduction among high risk youth: Recommendations of a National Cancer Institute Expert Advisory Panel. *Preventive Medicine, 24,* 354–362.

Gold, D. B., Anderson, D. R., & Serxner, S. A. (2000). Impact of telephone-based intervention on the reduction of health risks. *American Journal of Health Promotion, 15*(2), 97–106.

Goldberg, D., Weber, K., Redding, C., & Cohen, M. (2006, October). *Use of an interactive multimedia computer system to reduce smoking among HIV infected and at risk women: Preliminary data, the 10th International Conference on Malignancies in AIDS and Other Acquired Immunodeficiencies.* Washington, DC.

Hall, J. S., & Rossi, J. S. (2008). Meta-analytic examination of the strong and weak principles across 48 health behaviors. *Preventive Medicine, 46*(3), 266–274.

Hall, S. M., Tsoh, J., Prochaska, J., Eisendrath, S., Rossi, J. S., Redding, C. A., et al. (2006). Treatment of depressed mental health outpatients for cigarette smoking: A randomized clinical trial. *American Journal of Public Health, 96*(10), 1808–1814.

Herzog, T. A., Abrams, D. B., Emmons, K. A., & Linnan, L. (2000). Predicting increases in readiness to quit smoking: A prospective analysis using the contemplation ladder. *Psychology & Health, 15,* 369–381.

Herzog, T. A., Abrams, D. B., Emmons, K. A., Linnan, L., & Shadel, W. G. (1999). Do processes of change predict stage movements? A prospective analysis of the transtheoretical model. *Health Psychology, 18,* 369–375.

Hoffman, A., Redding, C. A., Goldberg, D. A., Añel, D., Prochaska, J. O., Meyer, P. M., et al. (2006). Computer expert systems for African American smokers in physicians' offices: A feasibility study. *Preventive Medicine, 43*(3), 204–211.

Hollis, J. F., Polen, M. R., Whitlock, E. P., Lichtenstein, E., Mullooly, J., Velicer, W. F., et al. (2005). Teen REACH: Outcomes from a randomized controlled trial of a tobacco reduction program for teens seen in primary medical care. *Pediatrics, 115*(4), 981–989.

Horwath, C. C. (1999). Applying the transtheoretical model to eating behaviour change: Challenges and opportunities. *Nutrition Research Review, 12,* 281–317.

Janis, I. L., & Mann, L. (1977). *Decision making: A psychological analysis of conflict, chance and commitment.* London: Cassil & Collier Macmillan.

Johnson, J. L., Regan, R., Maddock, J. E., Fava, J. L., Velicer, W. F., Rossi, J. S., et al. (2000). What predicts stage of change for smoking cessation? *Annals of Behavioral Medicine, 22,* S173. (Abstract).

Johnson, S. S., Driskell, M. M., Johnson, J. L., Dyment, S. J., Prochaska, J. O., Prochaska, J. M., et al. (2006a). Transtheoretical Model intervention for adherence to lipid-lowering drugs. *Disease Management, 9*(2), 102–114.

Johnson, S. S., Driskell, M., Johnson, J. L, Prochaska, J. M., Zwick, W., & Prochaska, J. O. (2006b). Efficacy of a Transtheoretical Model based expert system for antihypertensive adherence. *Disease Management, 9*(5), 291–301.

Kreuter, M., & Strecher, V. J. (1996). Do tailored behavior change messages enhance the effectiveness of health risk appraisal? Results from a randomized trial. *Health Education Research, 11,* 97–105.

Kreuter, M. W., Strecher, V. J., & Glassman, B. (1999). One size does not fit all: The case for tailoring print materials. *Annals of Behavioral Medicine, 21*(4), 276–283.

Lando, H. A., Pechacek, T. F., Pirie, P. L., Murray, D. M., Mittelmark, M. B., Lichtenstein, E., et al. (1995). Changes in adult cigarette smoking in the Minnesota Heart Health Program. *American Journal of Public Health, 85*(2), 201–208.

Levesque, D. A., Driskell, M., Prochaska, J. M., & Prochaska, J. O. (2008). Acceptability of a stage-matched expert system intervention for domestic violence offenders. *Violence and Victims, 23,* 433–446.

Lichtenstein, E., & Hollis, J. (1992). Patient referral to smoking cessation programs: Who follows through? *The Journal of Family Practice, 34,* 739–744.

Luepker, R. V., Murray, D. M., Jacobs, D. R., Mittelmark, M. B., Bracht, N., Carlaw, R., et al. (1994). Community education for cardiovascular disease prevention: Risk factor changes in the Minnesota Heart Health Program. *American Journal of Public Health, 84*(9), 1383–1393.

Marcus, B. H., Bock, B. C., Pinto, B. M., Forsyth, L. H., Roberts, M. B., & Traficante, R. M. (1998). Efficacy of an individualized, motivationally-tailored physical activity intervention. *Annals of Behavioral Medicine, 20,* 174–180.

Miller, W. R. (1985). Motivation for treatment: A review with special emphasis on alcoholism. *Psychological Bulletin, 98,* 84–107.

Noar, S. M., Benac, C., & Harris, M. (2007). Does tailoring matter? Meta-analytic review of tailored print health behavior change interventions. *Psychological Bulletin, 133*(4), 673–693.

O'Neill, H. K., Gillespie, M. A., & Slobin, K. (2000). Stages of change and smoking cessation: A computer administered intervention program for young adults. *American Journal of Health Promotion, 15*(2), 93–96.

Orleans, C. T., George, L. K., Houpt, J. L., & Brodie, H. K. H. (1985). Health promotion in primary care: A survey of U.S. family practitioners. *Preventive Medicine, 14,* 636–647.

Pallonen, U. E., Velicer, W. F., Prochaska, J. O., Rossi, J. S., Bellis, J. M., Tsoh, J. Y., et al. (1998). Computer-based smoking cessation interventions in adolescents: Description, feasibility, and six-month follow-up findings. *Substance Use & Misuse, 33,* 935–965.

Parsons, J. T., Huszti, H. C., Crudder, S. O., Rich, L., & Mendoza, J. (2000). Maintenance of safer sexual behaviours: Evaluation of a theory-based intervention for HIV seropositive men with haemophilia and their female partners. *Haemophilia, 6,* 181–190.

Peto, R., & Lopez, A. (1990). World-wide mortality from current smoking patterns. In B. Durstone & K. Jamrogik (Eds.), *The global war: Proceedings of the Seventh World Conference on Tobacco and Health* (pp. 62–68). East Perth, Western Australia: Organizing Committee of Seventh World Conference on Tobacco and Health.

Prochaska, J. O. (1979). *Systems of psychotherapy: A transtheoretical analysis* (2nd ed.). Pacific Grove, CA: Brooks-Cole, 1984.

Prochaska, J. O. (2006). Is Social Cognitive Theory becoming a Transtheoretical Model? *Addiction, 101*(7), 916–917.

Prochaska, J. O. (2008). Multiple Health Behavior Research represents the future of preventive medicine. *Preventive Medicine, 46,* 281–285.

Prochaska, J. O., & DiClemente, C. C. (1983). Stages and processes of self-change of smoking: Toward an integrative model of change. *Journal of Consulting and Clinical Psychology, 51,* 390-395.

Prochaska, J. O., DiClemente, C. C., & Norcross, J. C. (1992). In search of how people change: Applications to the addictive behaviors. *American Psychologist, 47,* 1102–1114.

Prochaska, J. O., DiClemente, C. C., Velicer, W. F., Ginpil, S., & Norcross, J. C. (1985). Predicting change in smoking status for self-changers. *Addictive Behaviors, 10,* 395–406.

Prochaska, J. O., DiClemente, C. C., Velicer, W. F., & Rossi, J. S. (1993). Standardized, individualized, interactive, and personalized self-help programs for smoking cessation. *Health Psychology, 12,* 399–405.

Prochaska, J. O., Evers, K. E., Prochaska, J. M., Van Marter, D., & Johnson J. L. (2007). Efficacy and effectiveness trials: Examples from smoking cessation and bullying prevention. *Journal of Health Psychology, 12*(1), 170–178.

Prochaska, J. O., Norcross, J. C., & DiClemente, C. C. (1994a). *Changing for good.* New York: William Morrow.

Prochaska, J. O., & Velicer, W. F. (1996). On models, methods and premature conclusions. *Addictions, 91,* 1281–1283.

Prochaska, J. O., Velicer, W. F., Fava, J. L., Rossi, J. S., & Tsoh, J. Y. (2001a). Evaluating a population-based recruitment approach and a stage-based expert system intervention for smoking. *Addictive Behaviors, 26,* 583–602.

Prochaska, J. O., Velicer, W. F., Fava, J., Ruggiero, L., Laforge, R., Rossi, J. S., et al. (2001b). Counselor and stimulus control enhancements of a stage matched expert system for smokers in a managed care setting. *Preventive Medicine, 32,* 23–32.

Prochaska, J. O., Velicer, W. F., Prochaska, J. M., & Johnson, J. L. (2004). Size, consistency and stability of stage effects for smoking cessation. *Addictive Behaviors, 29,* 207–213.

Prochaska, J. O., Velicer, W. F., Redding, C. A., et al. (2008). *Treatment, stage, severity and effort effects predict long-term changes in multiple behaviors.* Submitted for publication.

Prochaska, J. O., Velicer, W. F., Rossi, J. S., Goldstein, M. G., Marcus, B. H., Rakowski W., et al. (1994b). Stages of change and decisional balance for twelve problem behaviors. *Health Psychology, 13,* 39–46.

Rakowski, W. R., Ehrich, B., Goldstein, M. G., Rimer, B. K., Pearlman, D. N., Clark, M. A., et al. (1998). Increasing mammography among women aged 40–74 by use of a stage-matched, tailored intervention. *Preventive Medicine, 27,* 748–756.

Redding, C. A., Morokoff, P. J., Rossi, J. S., & Meier, K. S. (2007). A TTM-tailored condom use intervention for at-risk women and men. In T. Edgar, S. Noar, & V. Friemuth (Eds.), *Communication perspectives on HIV/AIDS for the 21st century* (pp. 423–428). Mahwah, NJ: Erlbaum.

Redding, C. A., Prochaska, J. O., Pallonen, U. E., Rossi, J. S., Velicer, W. F., Rossi, S. R., et al. (1999). Transtheoretical individualized multimedia expert systems targeting adolescents' health behaviors. *Cognitive & Behavioral Practice, 6*(2), 144–153.

Robbins, M. L., Levesque, D. A., Redding, C. A., Johnson, J. L., Prochaska, J. O., Rohr, M. S., et al. (2001). Assessing family members' motivational readiness and decision making for consenting to cadaveric organ donation. *Journal of Health Psychology, 6,* 523–536.

Rossi, J. S. (1992). *Stages of change for 15 health risk behaviors in an HMO population.* Paper presented at 13th meeting of the Society for Behavioral Medicine, New York, NY.

Schmidt, T. L., Jeffrey, R. W., & Hellerstedt, W. L. (1989). Direct mail recruitment to house-based smoking and weight control programs: A comparison of strengths. *Preventive Medicine, 18,* 503–551.

Schneider Jamner, M., Wolitski, R. J., & Corby, N. H. (1997). Impact of a longitudinal community HIV intervention targeting injecting drug users' stage of change for condom use and bleach use. *American Journal of Health Promotion, 12,* 15–24.

Skinner, C. S., Campbell, M. D., Rimer, B. K., Curry, S., & Prochaska, J. O. (1999). How effective is tailored print communication? *Annals of Behavioral Medicine, 21*(4), 290–298.

Snow, M. G., Prochaska, J. O., & Rossi, J. S. (1992). Stages of change for smoking cessation among former problem drinkers: A cross-sectional analysis. *Journal of Substance Abuse, 4,* 107–116.

Spencer, L., Pagell, F., Hallion, M. E., & Adams, T. B. (2002). Applying the Transtheoretical Model to tobacco cessation and prevention: A review of the literature. *American Journal of Health Promotion, 17*(1), 7–71.

Steptoe, A., Kerry, S., Rink, E., & Hilton, S. (2001). The impact of behavioral counseling on stages of change in fat intake, physical activity, and cigarette smoking in adults at increased risk of coronary heart disease. *American Journal of Public Health, 91*(2), 26.

Strecher, V. J., Kreuter, M., Boer, D. J., Kobrin, S., Hospers, H. J., & Skinner, C. S. (1994). The effects of computer tailored smoking cessation messages in family practice settings. *The Journal of Family Practice, 39,* 262–270.

Sun, X., Prochaska, J. O., Velicer, W. F., & Laforge, R. G. (2007). Transtheoretical principles and processes for quitting smoking: A 24-month comparison of a representative sample of quitters, relapsers and non-quitters. *Addictive Behaviors, 32*(12), 2707–2726.

U.S. Department of Health and Human Services. (1990). *The health benefits of smoking cessation: A report of the Surgeon General* (DHHS Publication No. CDC 90–8416). Washington, DC: U.S. Government Printing Office.

U.S. Department of Health and Human Services. (1994). *Preventing tobacco use among young people: A report of the Surgeon General.* Atlanta, GA. USDHHS, PHS, CDCP, NCCDPHP Office on Smoking and Health.

Velicer, W. F., & DiClemente, C. C. (1993). Understanding and intervening with the total population of smokers. *Tobacco Control, 2,* 95–96.

Velicer, W. F., Fava, J. L., Prochaska, J. O., Abrams, D. B., Emmons, K. M., & Pierce, J. (1995). Distribution of smokers by stage in three representative samples. *Preventive Medicine, 24,* 401–411.

Velicer, W. F., Prochaska, J. O., Bellis, J. M., DiClemente, C. C., Rossi, J. S., Fava, J. L., et al. (1993). An expert system intervention for smoking cessation. *Addictive Behaviors, 18,* 269–290.

Velicer, W. F., Redding, C. A., Anatchkova, M. D., Fava, J. L., & Prochaska, J. O. (2007a). Identifying cluster subtypes for the prevention of adolescent smoking acquisition. *Addictive Behaviors, 32,* 228–247.

Velicer, W. F., Redding, C. A., Sun, X., & Prochaska, J. O. (2007b). Demographic variables, Smoking variables, and outcome across five studies. *Health Psychology, 26*(3), 278–287.

Wierzbicki, M., & Pekarik, G. (1993). A meta-analysis of psychotherapy dropout. *Professional Psychology: Research and Practice, 29,* 190–195.

Multilevel Theories of Behavior Change: A Social Ecological Framework

5

Margaret Schneider
and Daniel Stokols

Social ecological analyses of health and health behavior have gained increasing prominence in the fields of health education, behavioral medicine, and public health from the 1990s onward (cf. Green, Richard, & Potvin, 1996; McLeroy, Bibeau, Steckler, & Glanz, 1988; Sallis & Owen, 1997; Smedley & Syme, 2001; Stokols, Allen, & Bellingham, 1996; Winnett, King, & Altman, 1989). The emergence of ecological models of health, behavior, and disease has been fueled by a growing recognition among scientists and practitioners that the etiology of contemporary public health problems is jointly influenced by diverse causative factors situated at multiple levels of analysis (e.g., ranging from molecular and genetic to behavioral, environmental, and societal levels). It is now widely acknowledged among health scholars and professionals that chronic diseases including diabetes, cardiovascular disease, cancer, and the threats to public health posed by community violence must be approached from a multilevel, ecological systems perspective to adequately understand their diverse etiologic underpinnings and to develop effective strategies for preventing or ameliorating them (Abrams, 2006; Best et al., 2003; Breslow, 1996; Glass & McAtee, 2006; Schneider & Stokols, 2000; Stokols, Grzywacz, McMahan, & Phillips, 2003).

The present chapter highlights the core assumptions and principles of multilevel ecological analyses of health and health-behavior change. Unlike earlier *biomedical* and *biopsychosocial* models that focus on the interplay among genetic, physiological, psychological, and social factors in health and illness, *social ecological* analyses place greater emphasis on the role of environmental conditions that influence an individual's or group's health status (Schwartz, 1982; Stokols, 2000). Environmental influences on health and health behavior are found both in the immediate, *micro-level settings* of everyday life (e.g., in one's home or workplace) and in the more distal, *macro-level conditions* that are pervasive in one's community (e.g., levels of unemployment, social capital, and income disparities existing within a particular society (cf. Kaplan, 1998; Kawachi & Berkman, 2003; Macintyre, 2003). Moreover, contextual influences on health behavior and illness symptoms include features of *built* as well as *natural* environments (e.g., exposure to urban traffic congestion vs. living in a rural wilderness area). *Objective* attributes of these environments (e.g., the spatial and social density of a dwelling measured in terms of its square footage and the number of residents living there), as well as individuals' *perceptions* of them (e.g., perceived crowding and related feelings of stress), must be considered in ecological analyses, since both have the capacity to influence health behaviors and outcomes (Lazarus, 1966; Lepore, Evans, & Palsane, 1991; Stokols, 1972). Thus, the environmental contexts of health are multifaceted, encompassing objective and subjective features of built and natural settings, and distributed across different levels of geographic scale; they influence well-being both directly and through their interaction with biogenetic and psychological factors.

Social ecological analyses also emphasize *systems processes* in health and illness, such as the ways in which chronic exposure to environmental stressors and coping challenges can undermine immunologic functioning and deplete the individual's capacity to resist or recover from a variety of health threats (McEwen, 2006; Miller, 1978; Seeman, McEwen, Rowe, & Singer, 2001). Systems processes of *adaptation, homeostasis,* and *coping behavior* regulate individuals' interactions with their everyday surroundings and are a major facet of ecological analyses of human resistance and vulnerability to disease (Antonovsky, 1987; Lazarus & Folkman, 1984; Selye, 1956).

The social ecological perspective on health behavior is also inherently *interdisciplinary* in its approach to scientific research and its translation into practice. Social Ecology spans several different fields, including neuroscience, medicine, epidemiology, health psychology, sociology, anthropology, health education, and community health promotion. Moreover, social ecological analyses emphasize not only *personal* health decisions and behavior but also *other-directed* behaviors enacted by physicians, case managers in health maintenance organizations, corporate managers, and elected officials that have a direct bearing on the well-being of hundreds and sometimes thousands of other people (Stokols, 1996).

In the following sections of the chapter, social ecological principles of health and behavior change are illustrated in relation to a variety of health risks, behaviors, and illnesses including obesity, smoking, diabetes, cardiovascular disease, cancer, and the common cold. Implications of social ecological analyses of these health problems for disease prevention, wellness promotion, and public policy are also discussed. Finally, we discuss unresolved conceptual and methodological issues and identify high-priority directions for future social ecological research on health behavior formation, maintenance, and change.

Foundations of the Social Ecological Framework

A 1993 report by McGinnis and Foege (1993), replicated and updated in 2004 by Mokdad and colleagues (2004), showed that the top causes of death in the United States are tobacco use, poor nutrition, physical inactivity, and alcohol consumption. This report represented a paradigm shift, in which causes of mortality were depicted not in terms of the diseases that lead to organ failure (i.e., cancer, heart disease, stroke) but in terms of the behaviors that contribute to the development of disease. Moreover, these behaviors were recognized as calling for comprehensive intervention strategies that integrate medical, psychological, organizational, cultural, and regulatory perspectives. The Social Ecological Framework (SEF) has emerged as an approach toward behavior change that encourages researchers to incorporate these disparate influencing factors into a causative web that spans multiple disciplines and extends across levels from the microscopic (i.e., cellular) to the global (i.e., economic and environmental). Research in the area of tobacco use, for example, has demonstrated that smoking behavior is influenced by genetic susceptibility to nicotine addiction (MacLeod & Chowdhury, 2006); stress, social influence, and depression (Schepis & Rao, 2005); and the consumer price of cigarettes (Ding, 2005; Siegel, 2002).

The danger inherent in this inclusive approach is that the causative web becomes so unwieldy that its very complexity reduces its utility. Thus, there is a tension between the practitioner's desire to identify an intervention target and the theorist's drive to delineate all possible avenues of influence. In recognition of this tension, the SEF has as its aim the goal of detecting "high-impact leverage points" (Stokols, 1992). These targets of intervention represent especially promising pathways for stimulating positive health behavior change. An assumption, then, of the SEF is that each element in a model should be examined with respect to its relative utility for affecting behavior change as compared to other elements in the model.

Bronfenbrenner's (1992) Bioecological Systems Theory of child development illustrates both the promise and the pitfalls of an expansive approach to model building. Bronfenbrenner's theory features multiple "layers" of environment, each of which influence child development (see Figure 5.1). In this model, the *microsystem* includes structures with which the child has direct contact, such as family, school, or neighborhood environments. These structures shape the child's behavior and, in turn, may be shaped by the child's behavior. There are also connections between the various structures within the child's microsystem, which Bronfenbrenner designates as the *mesosystem*. The *exosystem* is the larger social system with which the child does not interact directly but by which the microsystem may be influenced, such as parent worksite policies that

5.1

Depiction of Bronfenbrenner's Bioecological Systems Theory.

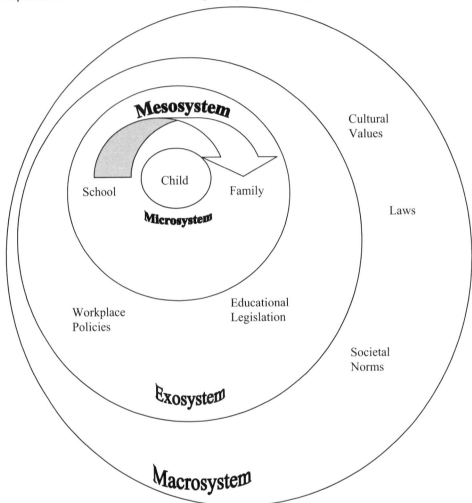

may limit a parent's availability to the child during work hours. The outermost layer of the child's environment is the *macrosystem,* composed of cultural values, customs, and laws. The effect of these distal influences on the child is mediated by the micro-, meso-, and exosystems. Overall, Bronfenbrenner's model is an elegant example of incorporating multiple levels, yet it also demonstrates the downside to complex model building: the potential for becoming overwhelmed by its very complexity, and the unanswered question as to which of the model's variables offer the greatest potential for improving health.

Recently, Glass and McAtee (2006) proposed an even more elaborate depiction of the "society-behavior-biology nexus" (p. 1653). Their representation of

the many influences on human behavior features several layers of factors residing within the individual (the genomic substrate, the subcellular/molecular
level, the cellular level, and the multi-organ system level), as well as a temporal
dimension from conception to old age. These additional dimensions of complexity serve simultaneously to expand the range of theoretically significant
pathways of influence and to emphasize the critical importance of seeking out
pathways of greater potential influence.

Both Bronfenbrenner's and Glass and McAtee's models embody the SEF
in that they include influences from the immediate to the more distal environment and emphasize the bidirectional nature of the relationships between the
individual and the environment. Both models also emphasize the role that the
social environment plays in influencing health behavior. The Glass and McA-
tee (2006) representation, however, goes further in terms of acknowledging
the physical environment as a contextual variable that should be considered.
They point out, for example, the contribution that both the built environment
and the local food environment make to the behaviors that lead to obesity. In
this recognition of the physical environment as an integral part of the forces
shaping health behavior, Glass and McAtee's model exemplifies the approach
of the SEF.

The Impact of Environmental Context on Health

The concept that individual susceptibility to disease is influenced by both the
social and the physical environment has long been recognized. Cassel (1976)
posited that the social context within which an individual resides has a nonspecific impact on health; that is, the social environment can increase or reduce
susceptibility to a wide array of chronic diseases (cf. Kawachi & Berkman, 2003;
Smedley & Syme, 2001). More recently, Cohen's research on the moderating effect of life stress on susceptibility to colds (Cohen et al., 1998; Cohen, Tyrrell,
& Smith, 1991) showed that, indeed, individuals exposed to a cold virus under
controlled conditions are more likely to develop viral infections and more severe cold symptoms if they have recently been experiencing great amounts of
psychological stress, thus demonstrating that viral susceptibility is contextually
moderated rather than absolute.

The Impact of Environmental Context
on Health Behavior

It has taken some time and accumulated experience, however, for behavior
change researchers to begin including contextual variables into their conceptual models and empirical studies. The accumulation of a number of failed
large-scale behavioral interventions (e.g., Multiple Risk Factor Intervention
Trial Research Group [MRFIT], 1982; The COMMIT Research Group, 1995)
has starkly illustrated how difficult it is to influence individual health behavior through interventions that ignore context. The MRFIT trial, for example,

delivered a resource-intensive lifestyle change program to high-risk men over 6 years. Despite the enormous effort put into helping the men change their behavior, little actual behavior change occurred, and at the end of the trial there was no statistical difference in heart disease rates between the intervention and the control groups.

The lessons learned from this and other disappointing efforts to target individual health behavior on a large scale have inspired a new wave of studies that highlight community and environmental influences on health and behavior (cf. Macintyre, 2003; Woods, Montgomery, Herring, Gardner, & Stokols, 2006; Yen & Syme, 1999). A recent study demonstrates the contextual approach and identifies neighborhood safety as a crucial intervention target for changing urban children's health behavior (Wilson, Syme, Boyce, Battistich, & Selvin, 2005). Moreover, efforts to understand and address the low levels of physical activity characteristic of the majority of Americans have turned toward the pervasive and influential role of the built environment (cf. Frank, Engelke, & Schmid, 2003; Frumkin, Frank, & Jackson, 2004; Jackson & Kochtitzky, 2002; Killingsworth, 2003). This emphasis on the physical and social context within which behavioral choices are made is characteristic of the SEF.

Overview of Social Ecological Theory

Definition of Social Ecology

Social ecology is a *meta-theoretical perspective* that encompasses several interrelated themes and research strategies for understanding illness etiology, health behavior, and well-being: namely *contextualist, systems-oriented, interdisciplinary, multilevel action research* analyses incorporating both qualitative and quantitative research methods and a variety of experimental and nonexperimental research designs. In lay terms, social ecology is based on the assumption that the answer to questions such as "how do we get people to wear sunscreen?" is, in essence, "it depends" (cf. English et al., 2005; Milne, Johnston, Cross, Giles-Corti, & English, 2002). The answers to such questions depend upon the physical and social environment within which the target population lives and works, upon the genetic and phenotypic predispositions that individuals bring to the situation, upon the institutional, legislative, and economic constraints that envelop the persons we are interested in influencing, and even upon the disciplinary perspective of those who are trying to answer these questions. Finally, and perhaps most essential to the SEF, the answers to these types of questions depend upon the ways in which all of these multiple factors interact with one another.

It is important to note that the SEF represents a heuristic device that is intended to stimulate the formation of specific models or theories of health behavior in which multiple levels of influence and interactions between theoretical components are considered. At each level, existing theories may be used or new theories posited to select salient variables. Many theories already exist to guide investigators in the identification of critical variables at the level of the individual. Far fewer models are available to inform variable selection at the environmental levels, and there is much work to be done in terms of coming up with conceptual and operational definitions of factors that operate at the meso and macro levels. Thus, one function of the SEF is to provide the impetus for researchers to measure, test, and compare alternative theories and influencing factors at the meso and macro levels.

Historical Context of Social Ecology

Baranowski and colleagues (2003) provide an overview of the evolution of behavior change models that places social ecology within an historical context. As depicted in this review, the SEF represents an attempt to respond to the inadequate explanatory power of primarily cognitive models of behavior change (e.g., the Knowledge-Attitude-Behavior model and the Health Belief Model) and social-cognitive models of behavior change (e.g., Social-Cognitive Theory, the Theory of Planned Behavior, and the Transtheoretical Model), all of which focus primarily on the individual as the unit of analysis and yield recommendations for intervention that are limited in scope and impact (Breslow, 1996; Glanz, Rimer, & Lewis, 2002; National Cancer Institute, 2005; Sallis & Owen, 1997). The innovation of the SEF lies in its attention to etiologic influences on health and behavior ranging from molecular and cellular to global levels, *and on the interactions among these factors.*

Core Assumptions of the SEF

Social ecological models of health and health behavior change are guided by a number of underlying assumptions (Stokols, 1992):

1. Social ecological models are multiplicative rather than simply additive. That is, they provide a conceptualization of *interactions* among variables situated at multiple analytic levels, from the micro to the macro. For instance, Rashad and Grossman's (2004) analysis of the obesity epidemic in the United States highlights the synergistic influence of multiple physical and social environmental factors on levels of obesity in the population, including economic determinants of food supply in the United States, the increasing participation of women in the U.S. labor force, technological changes such as the advent of microwave ovens, the presence of fast-food restaurants in a family's neighborhood, and the social characteristics of households, including the number of working adults residing at the same address.
2. The relative scale and complexity of environments that influence health behaviors and outcomes can be characterized in terms of their physical and social attributes, objective versus perceived qualities, and relative immediacy to individuals and groups (ranging from proximal to distal settings). Independent attributes of environments are relevant, such as lighting, temperature, noise, space arrangement, and group size. Furthermore, these independent attributes may combine to result in a characteristic behavior setting or social climate (cf. Barker, 1968; Moos, 1979). The impact of such a composite may go beyond a simple adding together of the independent effects of each attribute.
3. The SEF takes into account both the interdependencies that exist among immediate and more distant environments and the dynamic interrelations between people and their environments (Miller, 1978; Von Bertalanffy, 1950).

That is, people-environment transactions are characterized by cycles of mutual influence, whereby the physical and social features of settings directly influence their occupant's behavior, and concurrently the participants modify the healthfulness of their surroundings through their individual and collective actions (Lazarus & Folkman, 1984; Stokols & Shumaker, 1981).

4. Elements of the micro-, meso-, exo-, and macrosystems facilitate and/or impede individual behaviors and, therefore, individuals' ability to "choose" their behavior can be substantially determined by the social and environmental context. In the MRFIT trial (Multiple Risk Factor Intervention Trial Research Group, 1982), it was assumed that lifestyle behavior could be changed by providing individuals with skills training, such as instruction in how to prepare low-fat meals, combined with health education. This approach failed, perhaps because participants remained in the same environment that had shaped their original (unhealthy) behavior to begin with, and their ability to "choose" a healthier lifestyle was limited by this environment. Acknowledging the limited power of choice that individuals have over their own health behavior opens the door to interventions that are less focused on changing health behavior and more oriented toward facilitating healthful behavior. These interventions may include entirely passive approaches that require no decision making on the part of the individual, such as adding fluoride to the water supply (Williams, 1982). They may include regulatory approaches that make certain behavioral choices very costly, as when legislation is passed to increase the penalties for drunk driving or the cost of cigarettes (Breslow & Johnson, 1993; Siegel, 2002). There can also be a combination of behavioral restrictions plus opportunities for obtaining support in behavior change, as when companies establish worksite nonsmoking policies in conjunction with smoking cessation classes. All of these approaches have in common an acceptance of the premise that simply targeting the individual with persuasive communication is seldom an effective method for achieving health behavior change.

5. The wide range of individual behavioral responses that typically occur within a given physical and/or social environment are evidence for the importance of individual differences in physiology, personality, and cognitions as mediators of environmental influences on behavior. Taking these individual differences into account lays the foundation for more finely tuned designs of intervention programs or materials. In the area of tobacco use, social influences may play a significant role in determining the likelihood that an adolescent will experiment with smoking cigarettes (Bricker, Peterson, Sarason, Andersen, & Rajan, 2007), whereas individual genetic susceptibility to nicotine addiction may be instrumental in determining whether experimentation leads to regular smoking (Koopmans, Slutske, Heath, Neale, & Boomsma, 1999). Understanding individual differences can facilitate advances in creating tailored interventions that are targeted toward specific subgroups of a population (cf., Kreuter et al., 2006; Kreuter et al., 2005; Noar, Benac, & Harris, 2007; Strecher & McPheeters, 2006). The SEF incorporates individual level differences along with contextual factors in order to identify the most promising avenues of intervention for a given population.

6. The SEF acknowledges the multifaceted and dynamic nature of behavior itself. At times, behaviors may cluster, so a change in one behavior may

facilitate a change in a related behavior. This may be the case for the association between drinking coffee and smoking cigarettes (Fernandez et al., 1997). Moreover, behavioral choices are played out in continuous interaction with and adaptation to a changing environment. Therefore, efforts to influence behavioral choices cannot be static or "one size fits all" (Noar, Benac, & Harris, 2007). Behaviors also cannot be described as all-or-none phenomena; an individual may pass through a series of "stages" or behavioral approximations on the way to adopting a new behavior (Prochaska & Velicer, 1997). A useful model of behavior change, then, must be flexible enough to reflect that the behavioral target is likely to be neither fixed nor isolated.

These core assumptions of the SEF provide a conceptual basis for constructing models of health behavior that feature diverse influencing factors spanning multiple levels as well as reciprocal lines of causation connecting the model components. Key principles that guide the translation of social ecological theory into health-enhancing policies and programs are summarized in the next section.

Translating Social Ecological Theory Into Effective Strategies for Health Promotion

A distinguishing feature of the SEF is its emphasis on identifying "high-leverage" intervention targets that have the greatest potential for bringing about positive health behavior change (Stokols, 1996). Beyond simply highlighting the great variety of influencing factors that should be considered in determining how best to intervene to promote healthful behavior, the SEF encourages researchers to examine the relative utility of targeting each of the variables in the model. In this emphasis, the SEF is consistent with "solution-oriented research" (Robinson & Sirard, 2005). Solution-oriented research is characterized by studies that have clear implications for intervention and are likely to lead to changes in clinical practice or public health policy. In the imagery of Krieger (1994), rather than being content with simply identifying the causative web, researchers should strive to unmask the spider behind its pattern.

The SEF also stresses the implementation of health-promotive interventions that involve the coordination of individuals and groups acting at different levels. Thus, leverage points at different levels of analysis should be targeted simultaneously in order to achieve a synergistic effect. School-based interventions are a good illustration of this point. A classroom-based educational program that teaches students the benefit of eating well is likely to have a much greater impact if it is accompanied by changes in the school food service at the same time. That is, an educational intervention may be effective if delivered in the context of environmental change that facilitates the targeted behavior.

It should be noted that in order to effectively identify the most salient influencing factors, appropriate assessment tools and analytic methods must be developed that enable investigators to examine not only the relative impact of individual factors but also their joint and/or interactive effects (Glass & McAtee, 2006). Currently available assessment tools are inadequate to describe potentially relevant dimensions of the social and physical environment.

Similarly, traditional linear analytic models are insufficient for capturing the nested relationships and complex interactions that may typify a fully elaborated model of any health behavior (Ockene et al., 2007).

Applications of the SEF to Contemporary Health Problems

An illustrative and timely example of a behavior-based health problem that calls out for multilevel, cross-disciplinary, and interactive explanatory models is childhood obesity. Childhood obesity has traditionally been depicted as the result of an imbalance between energy in and energy out. That is, excessive body fat accumulates when the calories burned are outnumbered by the calories ingested. This reductionist perspective results in attempts to correct the imbalance by engaging in health education, specifically, "planned learning experiences that facilitate voluntary changes in behavior" (Green, 1999). These attempts may be made clinically, as in the case of physician-based counseling interventions (cf. Patrick et al., 2006) or on a public health scale, as in the case of mass-media communication campaigns (e.g., Huhman, Potter, & Wong, 2005). Whether applied on an individual or a group level, however, the health education approach fails to address the contextual factors that to a large degree shape the behaviors that directly influence childhood obesity, namely dietary intake and physical activity.

More recent analyses of the factors contributing to the contemporary unprecedented increase in childhood obesity have emphasized environmental influences and have focused attention on facets of the "obesogenic environment" (Rashad & Grossman, 2004; Swinburn, Caterson, Seidell, & James, 2004). This relatively new term refers to the elements in the environment that contribute to the development or maintenance of obesity. While still acknowledging that individual behavior is at the crux of the obesity problem and is therefore central to its solution, many researchers are pointing out and finding evidence for the contextual factors that curtail both the likelihood that individuals will engage in recommended dietary and activity practices and their ability to do so. More specifically, recent reviews have highlighted physical environmental factors that are more distal from the target behavior, such as urban design and transportation infrastructure (Brug, van Lenthe, & Kremers, 2006; Papas et al., 2007), as well as social environmental influences that are more proximal to the target behavior, such as supportive home and school environments (Swinburn et al., 2004). These multilevel models of obesity identify promising intervention leverage points both in the political arena (e.g., modifying children's food preferences by changing food marketing) and in the personal arena (e.g., reducing children's sedentary behavior by removing TVs from their bedrooms) (Anderson & Butcher, 2006).

Encouraged by several theoretical articles published in the 1990s (Breslow, 1996; O'Donnell, 1996; Sallis & Owen, 1997; Stokols, 1996), the field of obesity prevention has embraced the SEF. Initially, this perspective was reflected in a wave of correlational studies examining the multilevel environmental and psychosocial influences on obesity (Blanchard et al., 2005; Fleury & Lee, 2006). That is, researchers have conducted cross-sectional studies in which they have shown that obesity is related to a variety of influences, including urban design (Sallis, Kraft, & Linton, 2002), food marketing (Anderson & Butcher, 2006), and television watching (Marshall, Biddle, Gorely, Cameron, & Murdey, 2004). As the utility of the SEF for identifying relevant sources of influence on obesity has been confirmed, recommendations and models for adopting this approach to the development of health promotive interventions have emerged (Best et al., 2003; Nigg et al., 2005; Whittemore, Melkus, & Grey, 2004). As a result, recent interventions targeting childhood obesity are more likely to employ a "combination of educational and environmental supports for action and conditions of living conducive to health" (Green, 1999). For example, an NIH-funded trial intended to promote physical activity among adolescent females (Elder et al., 2007) was designed to "create environments at school and in the community that facilitate physical activity, enhance social support in those environments, and provide the girls with the motivation and skills to seek out activity in all settings" (p. 162).

A provocative article addressing the causes of childhood obesity (Lustig, 2006) provides a clear illustration of the explanatory value that can be added by combining a biomedical understanding of a disease process with an appreciation for the environmental context. Lustig discusses a biochemical theory of obesity in which an individual's hormonal signaling may be inappropriately triggering a starvation response (see Figure 5.2). This response causes the body to move energy into adipose tissue and reduce energy expenditure while simultaneously stimulating an appetitive drive. Thus, a child may be gaining weight because of a biochemical imbalance that is causing her to experience hunger and sluggishness even though she is ingesting more calories than should be required to meet her metabolic needs.

This biochemical explanation for childhood obesity takes on new resonance when described in the context of the environmental factors that may trigger this metabolic imbalance. Lustig theorizes that the dysfunctional biochemistry is related to chronic hyperinsulinemia brought about by a combination of: (1) stress; (2) low physical activity (associated with the sedentary lifestyle that has emerged within the context of car-centered urban design, individual reliance on the automobile, and the popularity of sedentary forms of entertainment); and (3) a food environment that is characterized by high-energy-density foods (i.e., foods that contain relatively few essential nutrients per calorie), foods with significant fat and fructose, and foods low in fiber. As a model, this multilevel, multidisciplinary, and interactive theory of childhood obesity illustrates the promise of expanding upon a biomedical model of a disease process by examining the context within which people reside and within which people make behavioral choices. In this way, Lustig offers a demonstration of how the SEF can be employed to yield a number of potential leverage points for intervention that can be explored in future research.

Physical activity is one of the behaviors that has been extensively studied in response to the rise in obesity. Many different models have been applied to gain insight into why some people are more active than others. Much of the past work in this area has focused on characteristics of the individual, such as Body Mass Index or perceived self-efficacy. These studies have resulted in the identification of a large number of behavioral mediators that have generally been found to explain a small percentage of the variance in physical activity

5.2

Postulated algorithm describing the vicious cycle wherein stress, poor diet, and low
physical activity all contribute to hyperinsulinemia and obesity, which then feeds back,
via impaired leptin sensitivity, to further exacerbate the cycle.

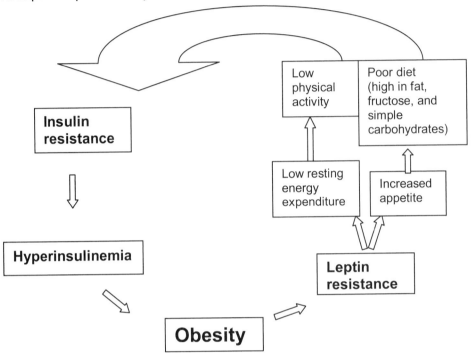

Note: Adapted with permission from image originally from American Heart Association.

levels (King, Stokols, Talen, Brassington, & Killingsworth, 2002). The past decade has seen an increasingly contextual paradigm being adopted in this area,
as researchers have looked to the environment to help explain physical activity
behavior (cf. Sallis & Owen, 1999). One discipline that has emerged as a fruit-
ful partner in this endeavor is that of urban planning (Dannenberg et al., 2003;
Frank et al., 2003; Hoehner, Brennan, Brownson, Handy, & Killingsworth, 2003).
Initial evidence supports an association between urban form (indexed in terms
of residential density, intersection density, land use mix, commercial and recreational space, and urban sprawl) and physical activity (Frank, Kerr, Chapman, &
Sallis, 2007; Frumkin et al., 2004; Saelens, Sallis, & Frank, 2003).

It is worth noting that an individual study may yet embody social ecological
principles, even in the absence of environmental variables. Individual studies
can contribute toward a social ecological analysis of behavior by examining a
particular slice of what, in its more elaborated form, would be a model that included environmental influence. For instance, a recent study on the factors that
influence voluntary exercise participation (Bryan, Hutchison, Seals, & Allen,
2007) exemplifies certain principles of social ecology even though it does not
include the social or physical environment as measured variables. This study

employs a multidisciplinary model that integrates genetic, physiological, and psychological correlates of voluntary exercise. The authors hypothesized that "the physiological effects (e.g., changes in body temperature, heart rate) of exercise influence the subjective experience of exercise (e.g., changes in mood, perceived exertion, perceived reward), which in turn are important determinants of motivation to exercise (e.g., higher self-efficacy for exercise behavior and higher intentions to exercise) and of future exercise behavior" (p. 30). The authors further explain that the model is "both circular and dynamic [and that] genetic factors are included in the model as potential mediators or determinants of the physiological effects of exercise as well as the subjective experience of exercise" (p. 30).

This multidisciplinary study, then, exemplifies several of the underlying principles of the social ecological approach. By incorporating a genetic component, the research speaks directly to the importance of understanding the etiology of a behavior and appreciating the importance of individual differences. If, in fact, there are certain genotypes that are associated with having a negative affective response to exercise, this dynamic could inform strategies designed to increase physical activity. Moreover, the investigators have incorporated concepts from systems theory in their depiction of the relationships between these different influencing factors as both iterative and interactive. The inclusion of factors derived from multiple levels (genetic, physiological, psychological) and the use of diverse methodologies (genetic analysis, experimental manipulation of mood and heart rate) further exemplifies some of the principles that are central to the SEF.

Although this study lacks the contextual component, it is important to recognize that pragmatic limits exist on the number and scope of variables that can be included in a single study and that the SEF can be applied to an entire field of study, such that the cumulative results of many studies will yield a more comprehensive model incorporating elements from the level of genetics to the level of global economic policy. Thus, the SEF can provide overarching guiding principles for a field of study which, if they are consistently applied, should reveal useful avenues for intervention in the quest to modify health behavior and promote well-being.

Future Directions of Social Ecological Research on Health Behavior Change

In ecological studies of health and health behavior change, a basic unit of analysis is the *environment(E)-behavior(B)-physiology(P)-health outcomes(H) pathway*.

Each category within the EBPH pathway can be further differentiated (e.g., in terms of objective vs. perceived, built vs. natural, micro vs. macro features of the environment; personal vs. other directed health behaviors). In some cases, the effects of environmental factors on health outcomes are direct (e.g., exposure to environmental asbestos induces pulmonary symptoms and increases one's susceptibility to lung cancer), whereas, in other instances, environmental influences on health status are mediated or moderated by behavioral factors (e.g., exposure to environmental asbestos combined with smoking cigarettes on a regular basis increases the individual's susceptibility to lung cancer in a multiplicative fashion [Grunberg, 1991]). Moreover, behavioral influences on health are sometimes direct, as in cases of lethal behavior directed toward one-self (suicide) or toward others (homicide); in other cases, behavioral impacts on health are mediated in a more gradual fashion through cumulative physi-ological processes (e.g., high cholesterol intake precipitating atheroslerotic pro-cesses that eventually lead to acute myocardial infarction).

Each individual's or group's ecology of health is uniquely made up of cer-tain highly influential EBPH pathways. For instance, one family may live close to exercise facilities and neighborhood parks, which enables them to engage in physical activity regularly, whereas another may reside far from such facili-ties or parks and, instead, live close to several fast-food restaurants, which may encourage frequent consumption of high-fat, low-fiber meals (Corti, Donovan, & Holman, 1997; Rashad & Grossman, 2004). A particular challenge in ecologi-cal analyses of health and health behavior is to identify the *effective context* of health, or those EBPH pathways that exert the greatest influence on an individ-ual's or group's health behaviors and outcomes (cf. Stokols, 1987). An important strength of the SEF is that it provides a broad conceptualization of environmen-tal and behavioral factors, physiological processes, and health outcomes within each segment of the EBPH pathway. At the same time, however, a major chal-lenge facing ecological analyses of health is to pare down potentially lengthy lists of etiologic factors within the E, B, P, and H categories and to develop more parsimonious and powerful conceptualizations of *high-leverage* variables in those categories (and situated at multiple levels of analysis) that have the great-est bearing on important health behaviors and outcomes.

The EBPH pathway is a useful analytic tool for examining both the prog-ress that has been made to date toward developing broad conceptualizations of ecological influences on health, as well as the conceptual, methodological, and translational challenges inherent in the SEF that remain to be addressed in future research. These issues are outlined in the next sections.

Development of the SEF: Progress to Date

Important strides have been made in identifying and measuring environmental influences on health behavior and outcomes at micro-, meso-, and macrosys-tem levels.

At the macrosystem level, for example, operational measures of urban sprawl have been developed and the impact of sprawl on levels of physical activity and body mass index (BMI) in the population have been demonstrated empirically (Frank, Kerr, Chapman, & Sallis, 2007; Frumkin, Frank, & Jackson, 2004). Similarly, a recent study by O'Neill and colleagues (2007) indicates that exposure to elevated levels of ambient air pollution exacerbates inflammatory processes among diabetic individuals, thereby heightening their susceptibility to cardiovascular events. Also, research by Jerrett and colleagues has linked air pollution exposure to higher rates of cancer and atherosclerosis (Jerrett & Burnett, 2007; Jerrett et al., 2005; Krewski et al., 2005; Künzli et al., 2005). At the micro- and mesosystem levels of analysis, as well, a wide range of environmen-tal stressors and their effects on individuals' health risk behaviors and physiol-ogy have been documented (Evans, 1999).

At the same time, pivotal health risk behaviors have been identified and shown to exert significant impacts on disease etiology, from Belloc & Breslow's (1972) early studies of healthy and unhealthy lifestyles to more recent reports identifying the major causes of chronic illness in developed countries (McGinnis & Foege, 1993; Mokdad et al., 2004). After several decades of research, poor nutrition, physical inactivity, consumption of alcohol and tobacco, and sleep disturbances have emerged as high-risk behaviors that exert a disproportionate impact on premature morbidity and mortality. What is distinctive about the more recent studies, however, is that we now know much more about the physiological processes that are triggered by these pivotal health risk behaviors. For instance, sleep deprivation in adolescents has been found to be associated with elevated levels of C-reactive protein and leptin, which are physiological precursors of inflammation and hyperinsulinemia (Larkin et al., 2005; Prinz, 2004). Moreover, it is becoming increasingly clear that chronic processes of inflammation, metabolic syndrome, and hyperinsulinemia are common precursors of multiple illnesses, including diabetes, heart disease, and cancer. Thus, in addition to classifying and measuring important environmental, behavioral, and physiological influences on health, ecologically oriented research is now beginning to document the empirical links between environmental and behavioral variables, on the one hand, and physiological processes and health outcomes, on the other.

Another indicator of progress in ecologically oriented research on health behavior and outcomes is the recent emphasis on identifying *synergistic processes* involving multiple environmental and behavioral factors that have a multiplicative or interactive impact on health outcomes. One example of this synergistic orientation is Evans's (2004) analysis of the "environment of childhood poverty," which emphasizes multiple and closely interrelated environmental factors (e.g., poor housing quality, substandard school environments, frequent exposures to toxins and environmental stressors, food insecurity) that jointly undermine the health outcomes of children and their parents. Chronic exposure to these multiple contextual dimensions of poverty result in elevated levels of allostatic load—that is, cumulative environmental demands that jeopardize health status when experienced over an extended period (McEwen, 2006; Seeman et al., 2001).

A synergistic orientation also is reflected in recent studies of the interactive health impacts of multiple risky behaviors. For instance, the combination of sleep deprivation and unhealthy diet increases adolescents' susceptibility to early-adult phase cardiovascular disease beyond the risks associated with poor nutrition and obesity alone (Larkin et al., 2005). Similarly, the synergistic influence of environmental and behavioral factors is reflected in a recent study of heath outcomes in mice and primate populations, which demonstrated that chronic exposure to environmental stressors amplifies the obesogenic influence of a high fat, high sugar diet (Kuo, Abe, & Zukowska, 2007; Kuo, Kitlinska, et al., 2007).

Refinement of the SEF: Priorities for Future Research

Clearly, substantial progress has been made in recent decades toward identifying and measuring multiple environmental, behavioral, and physiological determinants of health and the interrelationships among them. At the same time, ecological research on health behaviors and outcomes face at least three kinds of challenges in the coming years: *conceptual, methodological, and translational.* At a conceptual level, analyses that are broad-gauged (i.e., span macroenvironmental through microphysiological levels) as well as parsimonious and powerful (i.e., identify the highest-leverage influences on health situated at each analytic level) are needed. The tradeoffs between broad conceptual scope and theoretical parsimony remain to be better balanced or resolved in future research. As well, ecological analyses of health must continue to identify and document the most powerful synergies among multiple environmental, behavioral, and physiological factors that have the greatest cumulative influence on personal and aggregate indicators of well-being.

At a methodological level, broader-gauged research designs are needed to document the empirical links among all segments of the EBPH pathways for a particular individual or group. This is not to say that all ecological studies must encompass the full array of EBPH categories and their interrelations. As noted earlier, studies focusing on the links among more limited subsets of E, B, P, and H factors have been instrumental in advancing the SEF. Nonetheless, a larger number of broad-gauged studies encompassing the full range of hypothesized variables within a particular EBPH pathway should be designed and supported by health research funding agencies and foundations in the future. More expansive field-experimental studies that address all segments of the EBPH pathway are essential for documenting their empirical links and for moving the study of ecology and health forward in future years.

A major translational challenge facing ecological research on health is the design and evaluation of multilevel, multicomponent programs and policies that explicitly modify high-leverage environmental, behavioral, and physiological precursors of health status among individuals and groups. To date, broadly conceived disease prevention and health promotion programs that target facets of the macro-, meso-, and microenvironment and their effects on health behaviors, physiological processes, and well-being have been lacking, partly because these kinds of studies are notoriously labor- and time-intensive and financially costly to implement and sustain. Those constraints notwithstanding, the design, implementation, and evaluation of more comprehensive health improvement interventions that encompass the full range of factors within the EBPH pathway remain as important and valuable goals for future research.

Finally, broad-gauged studies of health enhancement and disease prevention programs will require close collaboration among cross-disciplinary teams of scientists, clinicians, and community decision-makers (Abrams, 2006; Stokols, 2006). Earlier studies of team science suggest that the effectiveness of cross-disciplinary collaboration in health research, training, and the translation of scientific knowledge into clinical practices and policies is highly variable and depends on several contextual factors that either facilitate or constrain teamwork (Kessel & Rosenfield, 2006; Stokols, Harvey, Gress, Fuqua, & Phillips, 2005) and influence the impact and sustainability of evidence-based community interventions (Altman, 1995; Kerner, Rimer, & Emmons, 2005). Strategies for sustaining effective collaboration extending across multiple academic and professional fields will need to be implemented and refined as a basis for advancing social ecological research on health out-comes and health behavior in future years.

References

Abrams, D. B. (2006). Applying transdisciplinary research strategies to understanding and eliminating health disparities. *Health Education & Behavior, 33*(4), 515–531.

Altman, D. (1995). Sustaining interventions in community systems: On the relationship be-tween researchers and communities. *Health Psychology, 14,* 526–536.

Anderson, P., & Butcher, K. (2006). Childhood obesity: Trends and potential causes. *The Future of Children, 16*(1), 19–45.

Antonovsky, A. (1987). *Unraveling the mystery of health: How people manage stress and stay well.* San Francisco: Jossey-Bass.

Baranowski, T., Cullen, K. W., Nicklas, T., Thompson, D., & Baranowski, J. (2003). Are current health behavioral change models helpful in guiding prevention of weight gain efforts? *Obesity Research, 11 Suppl.,* 23S–43S.

Barker, R. G. (1968). *Ecological psychology: Concepts and methods for studying the environment of human behavior.* Stanford: Stanford University Press.

Belloc, N. B., & Breslow, L. (1972). Relationship of physical health status and health practices. *Preventive Medicine, 1*(3), 409–421.

Best, A., Stokols, D., Green, L. W., Leischow, S., Holmes, B., & Buchholz, K. (2003). An integrative framework for community partnering to translate theory into effective health promotion strategy. *American Journal of Health Promotion, 18*(2), 168–176.

Blanchard, C. M., McGannon, K. R., Spence, J. C., Rhodes, E., Nehl, E., Baker, F., et al., (2005). Social ecological correlates of physical activity in normal weight, overweight, and obese individuals. *International Journal of Obesity, 29*(6), 720–726.

Breslow, L. (1996). Social ecological strategies for promoting healthy lifestyles. *American Journal of Health Promotion, 10*(4), 253–257.

Breslow, L., & Johnson, M. (1993). California's proposition 99 on tobacco, and its impact. *Annual Review of Public Health, 14,* 585–604.

Bricker, J. B., Peterson, A. V., Jr., Sarason, I. G., Andersen, M. R., & Rajan, K. B. (2007). Changes in the influence of parents' and close friends' smoking on adolescent smoking transitions. *Addictive Behaviors, 32*(4), 740–757.

Bronfenbrenner, U. (1992). Ecological systems theory. In R. Vasta (Ed.), *Six theories of child de-velopment: Revised formulations and current issues* (pp. 187–249). London: Jessica Kingsley.

Brug, J., van Lenthe, F. J., & Kremers, S. P. (2006). Revisiting Kurt Lewin: How to gain insight into environmental correlates. *American Journal of Preventive Medicine, 31*(6), 525–529.

Bryan, A., Hutchison, K. E., Seals, D. R., & Allen, D. L. (2007). A transdisciplinary model inte-grating genetic, physiological, and psychological correlates of voluntary exercise. *Health Psychology, 26*(1), 30–39.

Cassel, J. (1976). The contribution of the social environment to host resistance: The fourth Wade Hampton Frost Lecture. *American Journal of Epidemiology, 104*(2), 107–123.

Cohen, S., Frank, E., Doyle, W. J., Skoner, D. P., Rabin, B. S., & Gwaltney, J. M. (1998). Types of stressors that increase susceptibility to the common cold in healthy adults. *Health Psy-chology, 17,* 214–223.

Cohen, S., Tyrrell, D. A., & Smith, A. P. (1991). Psychological stress and susceptibility to the com-mon cold. *New England Journal of Medicine, 325*(9), 606–612.

COMMIT Research Group. (1995). Community Intervention Trial for Smoking Cessation (COMMIT): I. Cohort results from a four-year community intervention. *American Journal of Public Health, 85,* 183–192.

Corti, B., Donovan, R., & Holman, D. (1997). Factors influencing the use of physical activity fa-cilities: Results from qualitative research. *Health Promotion Journal of Australia, 7,* 16–21.

Dannenberg, A. L., Jackson, R. J., Frumkin, H., Schieber, R. A., Pratt, M., Kochtitzky, C., et al., (2003). The impact of community design and land-use choices on public health: A scien-tific research agenda. *American Journal of Public Health, 93*(9), 1500–1508.

Ding, A. (2005). Curbing adolescent smoking: A review of the effectiveness of various policies. *Yale Journal of Biological Medicine, 78*(1), 37–44.

Elder, J., Lytle, L., Sallis, J., Young, D., Steckler, A., Simons-Morton, D., et al. (2007). A description of the social-ecological framework used in the trial of activity for adolescent girls (TAAG). *Health Education Research, 22*(2), 155–165.

English, D. R., Milne, E., Jacoby, P. Giles-Corti, B., Cross, D., & Johnston, R. (2005). The effect of a school-based sun protection intervention on the development of melanocytic nevi in children: 6-year follow-up. *Cancer Epidemiology Biomarkers & Prevention, 14*(4), 977–980.

Evans, G. W. (1999). Measurement of the physical environment as a stressor. In S. L. Friedman & T. D. Wachs (Eds.), *Measuring environment across the lifespan: Emerging methods and concepts* (pp. 249–277). Washington, DC: American Psychological Association.

Evans, G. W. (2004). The environment of childhood poverty. *American Psychologist, 59*(2), 77–92.

Fernandez, E., La Vecchia, C., D'Avanzo, B., Braga, C., Negri, E., & Franceschi, S. (1997). Quitting smoking in northern Italy: A cross-sectional analysis of 2,621 subjects. *European Journal of Epidemiology, 13*(3), 267–273.

Fleury, J., & Lee, S. M. (2006). The social ecological model and physical activity in African American women. *American Journal of Community Psychology, 37*(1–2), 129–140.

Frank, L., Kerr, J., Chapman, J., & Sallis, J. F. (2007). Urban form relationships with walk trip frequency and distance among youth. *American Journal of Health Promotion, 21*(4), 305–311.

Frank, L. D., Engelke, P. O., & Schmid, T. L. (2003). *Health and community design: The impact of the built environment on physical activity.* Washington, DC: Island Press.

Frumkin, H., Frank, L., & Jackson, R. (2004). *Urban sprawl and public health: Designing, planning, and building for health communities.* Washington, DC: Island Press.

Glanz, K., Rimer, B. K., & Lewis, F. M. (2002). *Health behavior and health education: Theory, research, and practice* (3rd ed.). San Francisco, CA: Jossey-Bass.

Glass, T. A., & McAtee, M. J. (2006). Behavioral science at the crossroads in public health: Extending horizons, envisioning the future. *Social Science & Medicine, 62*(7), 1650–1671.

Green, L. (1999). *Health promotion planning: An educational and ecological approach* (3rd ed.). Mountain View, CA: Mayfield.

Green, L. W., Richard, L., & Potvin, L. (1996). Ecological foundations of health promotion. *American Journal of Health Promotion, 10*(4), 270–281.

Grunberg, N. E. (1991). Cigarette smoking at work: Data, issues, and models. In S. M. Weiss, J. E. Fielding, & A. Baum (Eds.), *Perspectives in behavioral medicine: Health at work* (pp. 75–98). Hillsdale, NJ: Erlbaum.

Hoehner, C. M., Brennan, L. K., Brownson, R. C., Handy, S. L., & Killingsworth, R. (2003). Opportunities for integrating public health and urban planning approaches to promote active community environments. *American Journal of Health Promotion, 18*(1), 14–20.

Huhman, M., Potter, L., & Wong, F. (2005). Effects of a mass media campaign to increase physical activity among children: Year-1 results of the verb campaign. *Pediatrics, 116,* 277–284.

Jackson, R. J., & Kochtitzky, C. (2002). *Creating a healthy environment: The impact of the built environment on public health* (Sprawl Watch Clearinghouse Monograph Series). Washington, DC: Sprawl Watch Clearinghouse.

Jerrett, M., & Burnett, R. T. (2007). Air pollution and cardiovascular events. *New England Journal of Medicine, 356*(20), 2104–2105.

Jerrett, M., Burnett, R. T., Ma, R., Pope III, C. A., Krewski, D., Newbold, K. B., et al., (2005). Spatial analysis of air pollution and mortality in Los Angeles. *Epidemiology, 16*(6), 727–736.

Kaplan, G. A. (1998). Socioeconomic considerations in the health of urban areas. *Journal of Urban Health, 75*(2), 228–235.

Kawachi, I., & Berkman, L. F. (2003). *Neighborhoods and health.* New York: Oxford University Press.

Kerner, J., Rimer, B., & Emmons, K. (2005). Introduction to the special section on dissemination: Dissemination research and research dissemination: How can we close the gap? *Health Psychology, 24*(5), 443–446.

Kessel, F., & Rosenfield, P. (2006, October 30–31). *Lessons learned from earlier case studies of transdisciplinary scientific collaboration.* Paper presented at the NCI/NIH Conference on the Science of Team Science: Assessing the Value of Transdisciplinary Research, Bethesda, MD.

Killingsworth, R. E. (2003). Health promoting community design: A new paradigm to promote healthy and active communities. *American Journal of Health Promotion, 17*(3), 169–170.

King, A. C., Stokols, D., Talen, E., Brassington, G. S., & Killingsworth, R. (2002). Theoretical approaches to the promotion of physical activity: Forging a transdisciplinary paradigm. *American Journal of Preventive Medicine, 23*(2 Suppl.), 15–25.

Koopmans, J. R., Slutske, W. S., Heath, A. C., Neale, M. C., & Boomsma, D. I. (1999). The genetics of smoking initiation and quantity smoked in Dutch adolescent and young adult twins. *Behavioral Genetics, 29*(6), 383–393.

Kreuter, M. W., Black, W. J., Friend, L., Booker, A. C., Klump, P., Bobra, S., et al. (2006). Use of computer kiosks for breast cancer education in five community settings. *Health Education and Behavior, 33*(5), 625–642.

Kreuter, M. W., Sugg-Skinner, C., Holt, C. L., Clark, E. M., Haire-Joshu, D., Fu, Q., et al. (2005). Cultural tailoring for mammography and fruit and vegetable intake among low-income African-American women in urban public health centers. *Preventive Medicine, 41*(1), 53–62.

Krewski, D., Burnett, R., Jerrett, M., Pope, C. A., Rainham, D. G., Calle, E. E., et al. (2005). Mortality and long-term exposure to ambient air pollution: Ongoing analyses based on the American Cancer Society cohort. *Journal of Toxicology and Environmental Health A, 68,* 1093–1109.

Krieger, N. (1994). Epidemiology and the web of causation: Has anyone seen the spider? *Social Science & Medicine, 39*(7), 887–903.

Künzli, N., Jerrett, M., Mack, W. J., Beckerman, B., LaBree, L., Gilliland, F., et al. (2005). Ambient air pollution and atherosclerosis in Los Angeles. *Environmental Health Perspectives, 113*(2), 201–206.

Kuo, L. E., Abe, K., & Zukowska, Z. (2007). Stress, NPY and vascular remodeling: Implications for stress-related diseases. *Peptides, 28*(2), 435–440.

Kuo, L. E., Kitlinska, J. B., Tilan, J. U., Li, L., Baker, S. B., Johnson, M. D., et al. (2007). Neuropeptide Y acts directly in the periphery on fat tissue and mediates stress-induced obesity and metabolic syndrome. *Nature Medicine, 13,* 803–811.

Larkin, E. K., Rosen, C. L., Kirchner, H. L., Storfer-Isser, A., Emanxipator, J. L., Johnson, N. L., et al. (2005). Variation of C-reactive protein levels in adolescents associated with sleep-disordered breathing and sleep duration. *Circulation, 111*(15), 1978–1984.

Lazarus, R. S. (1966). *Psychological stress and the coping process.* New York: McGraw Hill.

Lazarus, R. S., & Folkman, S. (1984). *Stress, appraisal, and coping.* New York: Springer Publishing Company.

Lepore, S. J., Evans, G. W., & Palsane, M. N. (1991). Social hassles and psychological health in the context of chronic crowding. *Journal of Health and Social Behavior, 32*(4), 357–367.

Lustig, R. H. (2006). The "skinny" on childhood obesity: How our western environment starves kids' brains. *Pediatric Annals, 35*(12), 898–902, 905–897.

Macintyre, S. & Ellaway, A. (2003). Neighborhoods and health: Overview. In I. Kawachi & L. Berkman (Eds.), *Neighborhoods and health* (pp. 20–42). Oxford: Oxford University Press.

MacLeod, S. L., & Chowdhury, P. (2006). The genetics of nicotine dependence: Relationship to pancreatic cancer. *World Journal of Gastroenterology, 12*(46), 7433–7439.

Marshall, S., Biddle, S., Gorely, T., Cameron, N., & Murdey, I. (2004). Relationships between media use, body fatness and physical activity in children and youth: A meta-analysis. *International Journal of Obesity, 28,* 1238–1246.

McEwen, B. S. (2006). Protective and damaging effects of stress mediators: Central role in the brain. *Dialogues In Clinical Neuroscience, 8*(4), 283–297.

McGinnis, J. M., & Foege, W. H. (1993). Actual causes of death in the United States. *Journal of the American Medical Association, 270*(18), 2207–2212.

McLeroy, K. R., Bibeau, D., Steckler, A., & Glanz, K. (1988). An ecological perspective on health promotion programs. *Health Educator Quarterly, 15*(4), 351–377.

Miller, J. G. (1978). *Living systems.* New York: McGraw-Hill.

Milne, J. G., Johnston, R., Cross, D., Giles-Corti, B., & English, D. R. (2002). Effect of a school-based sun-protection intervention on the development of melanocytic nevi in children. *American Journal of Epidemiology, 155*(8), 739–745.

Mokdad, A. H., Marks, J. S., Stroup, D. F., & Gerberding, J. L. (2004). Actual causes of death in the United States, 2000. *Journal of the American Medical Association, 291*(10), 1238–1245.

Moos, R. H. (1979). Social ecological perspectives on health. In G. C. Stone, F. Cohen, & N. E. Adler (Eds.), *Health psychology: A handbook* (pp. 523–547). San Francisco, CA: Jossey-Bass.

Multiple Risk Factor Intervention Trial Research Group. (1982). Multiple risk factor intervention trial. Risk factor changes and mortality results. *Journal of the American Medical Association, 248*(12), 1465–1477.

National Cancer Institute. (2005). *Theory at a glance: A guide for health promotion practice* (2nd ed.). Retrieved July 1, 2007, from http://www.cancer.gov/PDF/481f5d53-63df-41bc-bfaf-5aa48ee1da4d/TAAG3.pdf

Nigg, C., Maddock, J., Yamauchi, J., Pressler, V., Wood, B., & Jackson, S. (2005). The healthy Hawaii initiative: A social ecological approach to promoting healthy communities. *American Journal of Health Promotion, 19*(4), 310–313.

Noar, S. M., Benac, C. N., & Harris, M. S. (2007). Does tailoring matter? Meta-analytic review of tailored print health behavior change interventions. *Psychological Bulletin, 133*(4), 673–693.

Ockene, J. K., Edgerton, E. A., Teutsch, S. M., Marion, L. N., Miller, T., Genevro, J. L., et al. (2007). Integrating evidence-based clinical and community strategies to improve health. *American Journal of Preventive Medicine, 32*(3), 244–252.

O'Donnell, M. P. (1996). Social ecological approach to health promotion. *American Journal of Health Promotion, 10*(4), 244.

O'Neill, M. S., Veves, A., Sarnat, J. A., Zanobetti, A., Gold, D. R., Economides, P. A., et al. (2007). Air pollution and inflammation in type 2 diabetes: A mechanism for susceptibility. *Occupational and Environmental Medicine, 64,* 373–379.

Papas, M. A., Alberg, A. J., Ewing, R., Helzlsouer, K. J., Gary, T. L., & Klassen, A. C. (2007). The built environment and obesity. *Epidemiology Review, 29,* 129–143.

Patrick, K., C. K., Norman, G. J., Zabinski, M. F., Sallis, J. F., Rupp, J., Covin, J., et al. (2006). Randomized controlled trial of a primary care and home-based intervention for physical activity and nutrition behaviors: Pace+ for adolescents. *Archives of Pediatric Adolescent Medicine, 160*(2), 128–136.

Prinz, P. (2004). Sleep, appetite, and obesity: What is the link? *Public Library of Science Medicine, 1*(3), 186–187.

Prochaska, J. O., & Velicer, W. F. (1997). The transtheoretical model of health behavior change. *American Journal of Health Promotion, 12*(1), 38–48.

Rashad, I., & Grossman, M. (2004). The economics of obesity. Retrieved July 2, 2007, from https://wfs.gc.cuny.edu/PAnderson1/www/Papers/public interest published version 6–04.pdf?uniq=vxuadc

Robinson, T. N., & Sirard, J. R. (2005). Preventing childhood obesity: A solution-oriented research paradigm. *American Journal of Preventive Medicine, 28*(2 Suppl. 2), 194–201.

Saelens, B. E., Sallis, J. F., & Frank, L. D. (2003). Environmental correlates of walking and cycling: Findings from the transportation, urban design, and planning literatures. *Annals of Behavioral Medicine, 25*(2), 80–91.

Sallis, J. F., Kraft, K., & Linton, L. S. (2002). How the environment shapes physical activity: A transdisciplinary research agenda. *American Journal of Preventive Medicine, 22*(3), 208.

Sallis, J. F., & Owen, N. (1997). Ecological models. In K. Glanz, F. M. Lewis, & B. K. Rimer (Eds.), *Health behavior and health education: Theory, research and practice* (2nd ed., pp. 403–424). San Francisco, CA: Jossey-Bass.

Sallis, J. F., & Owen, N. (1999). *Physical activity & behavioral medicine.* Thousand Oaks, CA: Sage.

Schepis, T. S., & Rao, U. (2005). Epidemiology and etiology of adolescent smoking. *Current Opinion in Pediatrics, 17*(5), 607–612.

Schneider, M., & Stokols, D. (Eds.). (2000). *Promoting human wellness: New frontiers for research, practice, and policy.* Berkeley: University of California Press.

Schwartz, G. E. (1982). Testing the biopsychosocial model: The ultimate challenge facing behavioral medicine? *Journal of Consulting and Clinical Psychology, 50*(6), 1040–1053.

Seeman, T. E., McEwen, B. S., Rowe, J. W., & Singer, B. H. (2001). Allostatic load as a marker of cumulative biological risk: MacArthur studies of successful aging. *Proceedings of the National Academy of Sciences, 98*(8), 4770–4775.

Selye, H. (1956). *The stress of life.* New York: McGraw-Hill.

Siegel, M. (2002). The effectiveness of state-level tobacco control interventions: A review of program implementation and behavioral outcomes. *Annual Review of Public Health, 23*, 45–71.

Smedley, B. D., & Syme, S. L. (2001). Promoting health: Intervention strategies from social and behavioral research. *American Journal of Health Promotion, 15*(3), 149–166.

Stokols, D. (1972). On the distinction between density and crowding: Some implications for future research. *Psychological Review, 79*(3), 275–277.

Stokols, D. (1987). Conceptual strategies of environmental psychology. In D. Stokols & I. Altman (Eds.), *Handbook of environmental psychology* (pp. 41–70). New York: Wiley.

Stokols, D. (1992). Establishing and maintaining healthy environments. Toward a social ecology of health promotion. *American Psychologist, 47*(1), 6–22.

Stokols, D. (1996). Translating social ecological theory into guidelines for community health promotion. *American Journal of Health Promotion, 10,* 282–298.

Stokols, D. (2000). The social ecological paradigm of wellness promotion. In M. Schneider Jamner & D. Stokols (Eds.), *Promoting human wellness: New frontiers for research, practice, and policy* (pp. 21–37). Berkeley: University of California Press.

Stokols, D. (2006). Toward a science of transdisciplinary action research. *American Journal of Community Psychology, 38*(1), 63–77.

Stokols, D., Allen, J., & Bellingham, R. L. (1996). The social ecology of health promotion: Implications for research and practice. *American Journal of Health Promotion, 10*(4), 247–251.

Stokols, D., Grzywacz, J. G., McMahan, S., & Phillips, K. (2003). Increasing the health promotive capacity of human environments. *American Journal of Health Promotion, 18*(1), 4–13.

Stokols, D., Harvey, R., Gress, J., Fuqua, J., & Phillips, K. (2005). In vivo studies of transdisciplinary scientific collaboration: Lessons learned and implications for active living research. *American Journal of Preventive Medicine, 28*(2S2), 202–213.

Stokols, D., & Shumaker, S. (1981). People in places: A transactional view of settings. In J. Harvey (Ed.), *Cognition, social behavior, and the environment* (pp. 441–488). Hillsdale, NJ: Erlbaum.

Strecher, V., & McPheeters, M. (2006). The potential role of tailored messaging. *Behavioral Healthcare, 26*(10), 24–26.

Swinburn, B., Caterson, I., Seidell, J., & James, W. (2004). Diet, nutrition and the prevention of excess weight gain and obesity. *Public Health Nutrition, 7*(1A), 123–146.

Von Bertalanffy, L. (1950). The theory of open systems in physics and biology. *Science, 3,* 23–29.

Whittemore, R., Melkus, G. D. E., & Grey, M. (2004). Applying the social ecological theory to type 2 diabetes prevention and management. *Journal of Community Health Nursing, 21*(2), 87–99.

Williams, A. F. (1982). Passive and active measures for controlling disease and injury: The role of health psychologists. *Health Psychology, 1,* 399–409.

Wilson, N., Syme, S. L., Boyce, W. T., Battistich, V. A., & Selvin, S. (2005). Adolescent alcohol, tobacco, and marijuana use: The influence of neighborhood disorder and hope. *American Journal of Health Promotion, 20*(1), 11–19.

Winnett, R. A., King, A. C., & Altman, D. G. (1989). *Health psychology and public health: An integrative approach.* New York: Pergamon Press.

Woods, V. D., Montgomery, S. B., Herring, R. P., Gardner, R. W., & Stokols, D. (2006). Social ecological predictors of prostate-specific antigen blood test and digital rectal examinations in black American men. *Journal of the National Medical Association, 98*(4), 492–504.

Yen, I. H., & Syme, S. L. (1999). The social environment and health: A discussion of the epidemiologic literature. *Annual Review of Public Health, 20,* 287–308.

Models of Provider-Patient Interaction and Shared Decision Making

6

Michael G. Goldstein,
Judith DePue, and
Alessandra N. Kazura

Health care providers have the potential to play a central role in influencing and supporting their patients' efforts to adopt, change, or maintain health behaviors. Data from the 2000–2001 U.S. National Health Interview Survey indicate that 83% of adults 18–64 years of age report that they have a usual source of care, a place where they usually go when they are "sick or . . . need advice about health"(National Center for Health Statistics, 2003). Moreover, there is increasing evidence that clinical interventions to address health risk behaviors and support patient self-management of chronic illnesses are efficacious (Bodenheimer, Lorig, Holman, & Grumbach, 2002; M. G. Goldstein, Whitlock, & DePue, 2004; Whitlock, Orleans, Pender, & Allan, 2002). In addition, patients report that their physicians have considerable influence regarding their health behaviors (Davis et al., 2002). The behaviors that may be influenced by providers fall along a very broad spectrum and include health risk behaviors (e.g., risky drinking, cigarette smoking, sedentary behavior); chronic illness self-management behaviors (e.g., monitoring symptoms and test results and adjusting regimens appropriately, medication taking, pacing, coping with emotional changes); preventive behaviors (e.g., participating in screening tests, wearing seat belts, practicing safer sex); and health-promoting behaviors (e.g., healthy diet, stress management).

Despite the evidence for effectiveness of health behavior counseling interventions in primary care, several population-based surveys have reported relatively low rates of provider intervention to address health risk behaviors. For example, results from the 2001–2003 National Ambulatory Medical Care Surveys (NAMCS) indicate that smoking cessation counseling was received by only 20% of patients who smoke (Thorndike, Regan, & Rigotti, 2007). Surveys of patients with chronic conditions suggest that providers are regularly missing opportunities to offer and provide tests and referrals recommended by practice guidelines (Committee on Quality of Health Care in America, 2001; Davis et al., 2002).

In this chapter, we first briefly describe barriers to delivery of health behavior change interventions in health care settings. Then, we describe several conceptual models of provider-patient interactions that have generated effective or promising provider-delivered health behavior change interventions. These include patient-centered models, approaches that focus on supporting self-management, models of shared decision making, and the 5 As approach to health behavior counseling. The provider-patient interaction models discussed here have been derived and informed by a variety of health behavior change theories and models that are comprehensively addressed in other chapters of this volume and are only touched upon here. Though we refer to Motivational Interviewing (MI) (Miller & Rollnick, 2002) and brief motivational strategies based on MI (Rollnick, Miller, & Butler, 2008), the reader is referred to chapter 8, on MI, for a more complete discussion of these approaches.

After reviewing these conceptual models of provider-patient interactions, we broaden our focus and briefly describe a conceptual model, the Chronic Care Model, that focuses on the organizational level of health care delivery. This system-level model integrates patient and provider factors with health care delivery system and organizational factors that influence the delivery of care and patient outcomes.

Barriers to Provider Delivery of Effective Health Behavior Change Interventions

Barriers to provider involvement in health behavior change interventions can be categorized as deficits in knowledge, deficits in skill, attitudinal barriers, and organizational barriers. These are listed in Table 6.1.

While many clinicians recognize the importance of health risk behavior change, they often have limited knowledge of effective communication, behavior change counseling, and self-management support skills and strategies (Bodenheimer, Lorig, et al., 2002). Until recently, physicians also had little exposure to organizational models and strategies for improving the effectiveness

6.1 Barriers to Provider Involvement in Behavior Change Interventions

Physician barriers

Knowledge deficit

    Behavior change principles

    Effectiveness of physician intervention

    Intervention methods

    Resources for patients—materials and referrals

    Organizational and system models for supporting behavior change and self-management

Skill deficit

    Interviewing/assessment/diagnostic skills

    Patient education skills

    Behavioral counseling skills

    Maintenance/relapse prevention skills

Beliefs and attitudes

    Belief that patients don't want to change or can't change

    Perceived ineffectiveness in helping patients follow through with treatment or change

    Lack of confidence in helping patents adhere or change

    Emphasis on final outcomes

    Disease-oriented biomedical approach

    Provider-centered, directive style

    Moralistic view of behavior problems

Poor personal health habits

Dearth of role models practicing preventive care

Organizational barriers

Limited use of reminder systems, tracking logs

Little or no reimbursement for patient education, counseling, or preventive services

Poor coordination with self-help and behavioral treatment programs

Limited involvement of office staff in patient education and health promotion activities

Note. From "Behavioral Medicine Strategies for Medical Patients" by M. G. Goldstein, L. Ruggiero, B. J. Guise, & D. B. Abrams, in *Clinical Psychiatry for Medical Students* (2nd ed., pp. 671–693), A. Stoudemire (Ed.), 1994, Philadelphia: J. B. Lippincott.

and quality of care (Wagner, Glasgow, et al., 2001). Knowledge is a prerequisite to learning these skills and organizing care to provide effective and efficient health behavior change interventions. Lack of specific skills in health behavior counseling and self-management support is a second important barrier to provider effectiveness. Training in these skills during professional training has been neglected, particularly in medical schools (Waldstein, Neumann, Drossman, & Novack, 2001). Many providers manifest attitudinal barriers, such as low confidence or self-efficacy to engage in health behavior counseling (Orleans, George, Houpt, & Brodie, 1985). Lack of confidence is related to lack of knowledge and the presence of other attitudes, such as perceived lack of effectiveness and a tendency to measure their success by final outcomes, such as abstinence from smoking, rather than recognizing that lasting behavior change occurs only after multiple trials and through intermediate steps (Bandura, 2004). Perceived lack of effectiveness fuels the attitude that patients don't want to change or can't change. Provider attitudes are also shaped by the prevailing model in medicine, the biomedical model, which emphasizes a focus on diagnosis and treatment of disease and undervalues the role of psychological, behavioral, and social factors in health and disease (Waldstein et al., 2001). Despite an increased emphasis in recent years on the teaching of prevention, there are very few role models who emphasize patient education and counseling, contributing to the belief that health promotion activities are outside providers' role. Providers may also harbor negative or moralistic attitudes toward patients who exhibit problematic behaviors or who don't follow their recommendations. These attitudes may interfere with their willingness or capacity to assist these patients to change. Finally, providers with negative personal health practices are less likely to counsel patients regarding prevention (Frank, Rothenberg, Lewis, & Belodoff, 2000).

Organizational barriers to provider involvement in behavior change counseling and self-management are also listed in Table 6.1. Organizational factors are key factors in determining the success of interventions to address health risk behaviors and self-management and can undermine or enhance the efforts of individual providers. The effectiveness of reminders on the delivery of preventive services by physicians and other health care providers has been conclusively demonstrated in multiple studies (Grimshaw et al., 2001). Despite the promise of information technology for enhancing the delivery of high-quality medical care, most medical care settings have not yet adopted integrated platforms that support the delivery of educational and health behavior change interventions across multiple health behaviors and conditions (Pronk, Peek, & Goldstein, 2004). In the following sections, we review models for provider-patient interaction that may be employed to develop and test interventions to address and overcome these barriers to delivering effective health behavior change interventions in health care settings.

Models of Provider-Patient Interaction

The Patient-Centered Model

The landmark 2000 Institute of Medicine (IOM) report, "Crossing the Quality Chasm: A New Health System for the 21st Century," suggested that a redesigned quality health care system must be patient centered as well as safe, effective, timely, efficient, and equitable (Committee on Quality of Health Care in America, 2000). The IOM defined patient-centered care as care that is respectful of and responsive to individual patient preferences, needs, and values; care that ensures that patient values guides all clinical decisions (Committee on Quality of Health Care in America, 2001). Thus, the delivery of patient-centered care is considered to be a core value or principle of high-quality care.

Stewart and colleagues at the University of Western Ontario, Canada, have described a Patient-Centered Model that embodies the principles of patient-centered care as defined in the IOM report (Stewart et al., 1995). This patient-centered approach has origins in the work of Carl Rogers (1951). A number of other educators and researchers have described models of clinician-patient communication (Makoul, 2001), patient education and counseling (Grueninger, Duffy, & Goldstein, 1995; Ockene & Zapka, 2000), and self-management support (Roter & Kinmonth, 2002) that are closely aligned with the Patient-Centered Model.

The Patient-Centered Model emphasizes a collaborative process of provider-patient interaction: developing a common, shared understanding of the problem or illness; addressing the patient's feelings, beliefs, expectations, and concerns; knowing the "whole person" and his family and social context; and collaboratively choosing among options for treatment, behavior change, and follow-up (Stewart et al., 1995). These elements reflect a process characterized by partnership, collaboration, and respect; a process that seeks to understand the meaning of the patient's experiences, needs, values, and preferences; and a process that shares control and responsibility for decision making.

Substantial research supports the relationships between these patient-centered provider-patient communication principles and a wide range of outcomes, including diagnostic accuracy, symptom control, patient satisfaction, patient follow-through with treatment recommendations, and health behavior change (DiMatteo, 1994; Ockene & Zapka, 2000; Roter & Kinmonth, 2002; Safran, Taira, Rogers, Kosinski, & Tarlov, 1998; Stewart et al., 2000; Whitlock et al., 2002).

Self-Management Support: A Patient-Centered Approach for Enhancing Chronic Illness Care

Self-management has emerged as a central concept in chronic illness care and has become a core component of interventions to improve the outcomes for patients with chronic conditions (Bodenheimer, Lorig et al., 2002; Lorig & Holman, 2003). Self-management is broadly defined as *all* that a patient does to manage her chronic condition and to live her life as fully and as productively as possible (Bodenheimer, Lorig et al., 2002; Lorig & Holman, 2003). Lorig and Holman have described three general domains of self-management: (1) managing symptoms and disease activity (medical management); (2) carrying out normal activities as a parent, worker, student, and so on (role management); and (3) coping with emotions (emotional management) (Lorig & Holman, 2003). To address these general domains, patients must engage in a wide variety of self-management behaviors and activities. The American Association of Diabetes Educators (AADE) has specified seven sets of self-management behaviors, the "AADE 7 Self-Care Behaviors™": Healthy Eating, Being Active, Monitoring, Taking Medication, Problem Solving, Healthy Coping, and Reducing Risks. It has also proposed standards and outcome measures for each (American Association of Diabetes Educators, 2003).

Note that the term "adherence" is not listed among the tasks of self-management, while medication taking is included. Many educators, clinicians, and researchers in chronic illness care have moved away from describing patient behavior as adherent or nonadherent (Anderson & Funnell, 2000; Glasgow

& Anderson, 1999), terms that appraise patient behavior from the provider point of view. "Nonadherence" to provider prescriptions and recommendations is a rather judgmental or pejorative way to describe patient behavior, especially in light of evidence that providers frequently fail to adequately educate patients and enlist them in a process of informed decision making (Braddock, Edwards, Hasenberg, Laidley, & Levinson, 1999; Street, Gordon, Ward, Krupat, & Kravitz, 2005). Though the term "adherence" is less objectionable than "compliance," we prefer to use terms that simply describe patient behavior (e.g., medication taking).

As proponents of the self-management concept point out, all patients self-manage, though some manage more effectively than others (Bodenheimer, Lorig et al., 2002; Lorig & Holman, 2003). Competence in self-management does not happen overnight; developing competence is a developmental process that evolves over the course of a patient's illness (Hibbard, Mahoney, Stockard, & Tusler, 2005; Hibbard & Tusler, 2007; Lorig & Holman, 2003). Hibbard has described four developmental levels or stages of "patient activation" that reflects a patient's capacity to self-manage: (1) unaware of the value or importance of taking an active role in self-management; (2) aware, but with limited knowledge, skills, and confidence to self-manage; (3) has knowledge and is beginning to take action, but has limited confidence; (4) has adopted new behaviors and is gaining confidence in sustaining behavior change (Hibbard et al., 2005; Hibbard & Tusler, 2007). As many as 40% of patients with a chronic illness are in the first two stages of patient activation; these patients are less likely to engage in a wide variety of self-management behaviors (Hibbard et al., 2005; Hibbard & Tusler, 2007) and have poorer health (Mosen et al., 2007). On the other hand, longitudinal studies have found that patients who progress to a higher stage of patient activation are more likely to adopt self-management behaviors (Hibbard, Mahoney, Stock, & Tusler, 2007). Strategies that are tailored to a patient's stage of activation have the potential to accelerate movement to the next stage and increase effective self-management behaviors, though this has yet to be demonstrated in controlled trials (Hibbard et al., 2007; Hibbard & Tusler, 2007). Research by other investigators has demonstrated links between chronic illness outcomes and concepts related to patient activation, including patient autonomy (Williams, McGregor, Zeldman, Freedman, & Deci, 2004), empowerment (Anderson et al., 1995) and more active participation in a medical visit (Greenfield, Kaplan, Ware, Yano, & Frank, 1988). In the next section, we discuss approaches that providers may employ to support and enhance patient self-management and movement through the stages of patient activation.

Self-management support is the term used to delineate efforts to assist patients to become more effective self-managers (Bodenheimer, Lorig, et al., 2002; Lorig & Holman, 2003). According to the Institute of Medicine, self-management support is the systematic provision of education and supportive interventions to increase patients' skills and confidence in managing their health problems, including regular assessment of progress and problems, goal setting, and problem-solving support (Adams, Corrigan, & Committee on Identifying Priority Areas for Quality Improvement, 2003). Self-management support is best characterized as a *process* for educating and empowering patients that is quite different from more traditional information-focused educational strategies. Though self-management support interventions are often delivered by clinicians or other health care staff within clinical settings, elements of self-management support may also be delivered in community settings by lay educators, peer counselors, or other community-based workers (Fisher et al., 2005; Glasgow, Strycker, Toobert, & Eakin, 2000; Lorig & Holman, 2003). Controlled trials of self-management support interventions have produced improvements in clinical outcomes across a number of other chronic conditions (Bodenheimer, Lorig, et al., 2002; Lorig & Holman, 2003; Warsi, Wang, LaValley, Avorn, & Solomon, 2004). Systematic reviews of educational interventions in diabetes care have documented the clear superiority of self-management-based approaches to diabetes education over more traditional didactic-information-only educational interventions (Norris, Engelgau, & Narayan, 2001; Renders et al., 2001).

What are the elements of health behavior counseling and self-management support that are necessary to produce improved patient health outcomes? Recent efforts to integrate self-management support into general health care settings suggest that the following elements are critical to individual patient and program success: (1) assessment of patient beliefs, behavior, and knowledge; (2) collaborative goal setting; (3) identification of personal barriers and supports; (4) skills teaching, including problem-solving to address barriers; (5) increasing access to resources and supports; and (6) developing a personal action plan that is based on the previous steps (Fisher et al., 2005; Glasgow et al., 2002).

Provider Communication Behaviors That Are Associated With Effective Self-Management Support

One may also look more granularly and consider the specific provider communication behaviors that are associated with effective self-management support. In a review of evidence-based self-management support interventions in diabetes care, Roter and Kinmonth identified several specific communication and counseling elements that were linked to successful outcomes: (1) hear the patients perspective; (2) provide information that is useful and relevant and check for accuracy; (3) negotiate a plan and anticipate problems; (4) offer ongoing monitoring and follow-up; (5) find problems and renegotiate solutions; and (6) offer emotional support (Roter & Kinmonth, 2002). A remarkably similar constellation of clinician-patient communication variables has been associated with increased patient follow-through with clinician recommendations (DiMatteo et al., 1993; Safran et al., 1998; Squier, 1990). Of particular note is the strong association between clinician empathy (defined behaviorally as responding to, supporting, and respecting patients' feelings and concerns) and patient follow-through (Squier, 1990). Supporting patient autonomy, for example, by offering treatment options in a patient-centered and noncontrolling way, also appears to promote follow-through and successful behavior change (Williams, McGregor, King, Nelson, & Glasgow, 2005). Note the alignment between these communication elements, the elements of the Patient-Centered Model and the elements of successful self-management support interventions described earlier. A distillation of the effective components of self-management support may be found in the list of "Core Competencies for Self-Management Support" that

6.2 Core Competencies for Self-Management Support

- Relationship building
- Exploring patients' needs, expectations, and values
- Information sharing
- Collaborative goal setting
- Action planning
- Skills building and problem solving
- Following up on progress

Note. From New Health Partnerships: Improving Care by Engaging Patients, a quality improvement project funded by the Robert Wood Johnson Foundation. Retrieved January 6, 2008, from www.newhealth partnerships.org.

were developed by New Health Partnerships, a quality improvement project funded by the Robert Wood Johnson Foundation. (See Table 6.2 and www.ne whealthpartnerships.org.)

Motivational Interviewing and Brief Motivational Approaches

Motivational Interviewing (MI) (Miller & Rollnick, 2002) is covered in depth in chapter 8. MI is compatible with the patient-centered models and self-management support principles described earlier and is particularly useful for the large percentage of individuals who are in the early "stages" of motivational readiness (Prochaska & DiClemente, 1986). Initially developed as an intervention for alcohol and substance use problems, the efficacy of MI has been demonstrated across multiple behavioral targets (Britt, Hudson, & Blampied, 2004; Rubak, Sandbaek, Lauritzen, & Christensen, 2005).

Brief versions of MI have been developed for use by clinicians in primary care and other health care settings (Keller & White, 1997; Rollnick et al., 2008). These versions emphasize patient-centered strategies including eliciting patient priorities, needs, and values; building rapport (i.e., reflective listening and empathy); supporting autonomy and resisting the temptation to recommend or prescribe prematurely; and tailoring counseling to address two dimensions of motivation: (1) the patient's *conviction* (or level of importance) regarding the need for change; and (2) the patient's *confidence (or self-efficacy)* about successfully changing. Assessment remains the key step of brief versions of MI, permitting clinicians to provide more efficient, tailored interventions that are matched to patients' levels of readiness and commitment to change. When both conviction and confidence are low, the primary focus of brief MI is to build conviction. To enhance conviction, clinicians may offer a menu of options (including simply thinking about change); support patient choice among options; explore ambivalence; and provide information and feedback to enhance knowledge and awareness about the value of change and the risk of not changing (Keller & White, 1997; Rollnick et al., 2008). When a patient's confidence is low, brief MI includes reviewing past experience, especially successes; encouraging small steps that are likely to lead to initial success; and teaching problem-solving and coping skills. For all patients, a follow-up plan is essential.

Shared Decision Making

According to Frosch and Kaplan (1999), shared medical decision making is a process by which patients and providers consider outcome probabilities and patient preferences and reach a health care decision based on mutual agreement. Though definitions of shared decision making (SDM) vary, virtually all emphasize a collaborative process that actively engages patients in decisions about prevention, treatment, and self-management (Makoul & Clayman, 2006). Most descriptions and definitions of SDM also incorporate the broader principles of patient-centered communication described earlier. On the basis of an extensive review of the literature, Makoul and Clayman (2006) identified several "essential elements" of SDM in behavioral terms: define/explain the problem; present options; discuss pros/cons (benefits/risks/costs); elicit patients' values/preferences; discuss patient ability/self-efficacy; offer knowledge/recommendations; check/clarify patient understanding; make or explicitly defer a decision; and arrange follow-up.

As Makoul and Clayman note, patients and providers must come to a shared understanding of the problem, disease, and condition or preventive activity (e.g., immunization, screening test, regular physical activity) as a prerequisite to making an informed decision. Patients, and providers for that matter, also require access to evidence-informed knowledge about the risks and benefits of interventions, as well as the risks and consequences of not taking action (Epstein, Alper, & Quill, 2004; O'Connor et al., 2007). Clarifying patients' values and preferences regarding outcomes, symptoms, side effects, and so on is another key aspect of the SDM process, as values and preferences vary considerably between patients as well as within patients over the course of a condition (Levinson, Kao, Kuby, & Thisted, 2005). As Entwhistle and Watt have argued, clinicians need to explore not only what patients know but also how they feel about their role in the decision-making process (Entwistle & Watt, 2006). In a large population-based sample of patients, 96% preferred to be offered choices and to be asked about their opinions. However, 44% preferred to rely on physicians for medical knowledge rather than seeking out information themselves, and about half (52%) preferred to leave final decisions to their physicians (Levinson et al., 2005). Results of this survey also found that preferences for an active role in decision making increased with age up to 45 years and then declined, while women, more educated, and healthier people were more likely to prefer an active role in decision making. Preferences for participation in decision making also varies across cultural and ethnic subgroups (Charles, Gafni, & Whelan, 1999; Levinson et al., 2005). The wide variability in preferences for participation in decision making that has been documented in these studies supports the view that providers must assess individual patient preferences and tailor their approach to decision making accordingly (Charles et al., 1999; Levinson et al., 2005).

Decision-making aids can assist providers to meet the requirements of fully informed SDM (O'Connor et al., 2007), but aids alone are insufficient to ensure that patients have an opportunity to participate in the process of decision making at the level of involvement they need or desire (Epstein et al., 2004). Patients' age, cognitive capacity, educational level, and literacy also impact their capacity to fully participate in SDM (Bastiaens, Van Royen, Pavlic, Raposo, & Baker, 2007; Epstein et al., 2004).

The 5 As of Health Behavior Counseling: A Unifying Framework

The U.S. Preventive Services Task Force Counseling and Behavioral Interventions Work Group has recommended the 5 As framework (i.e., Assess, Advise, Agree, Assist, Arrange follow-up) as a unifying conceptual framework for evaluating and describing health behavior counseling interventions in primary and general health care settings (Whitlock et al., 2002). The 5 As have been applied to a wide variety of individual health behavioral counseling targets (Goldstein et al., 2004) as well as the self-management component of chronic illness care (Glasgow, Davis, Funnell, & Beck, 2003; Glasgow et al., 2002). See Table 6.3 for a summary of the 5 As construct, adapted from the

6.3 The 5 As for Behavioral Counseling and Health Behavior Change

Assess
- Assess behavioral risk factors to identify patients in need of intervention
- Assess beliefs, behaviors, knowledge, motivation, and past experience

Advise
- Offer clear, specific, personalized behavior change advice
- Link to patient's expressed concerns, values, beliefs, experiences
- Adapt to level of health literacy

Agree
- Offer options for behavior change goals and methods to achieve goals
- Collaboratively choose specific behavior change goals and methods

Assist
- Provide motivational interventions when needed
- Offer self-help resources and materials and links to community resources
- Review options for formal treatment programs
- Develop a specific action plan to accomplish goals
- Identify and address barriers using problem-solving strategies
- Teach skills for achieving behavior change (including problem-solving skills)

Arrange follow-up
- Specify a follow-up plan including when, how, and with whom

Note. From "Assessing Delivery of the Five 'As' for Patient-Centered Counseling," by R. E. Glasgow, S. Emont, & D. C. Miller et al., 2006, *Health Promotion International, 21*(3), pp. 245–255; "Multiple Behavioral Risk Factor Interventions in Primary Care; Summary of Research Evidence," by M. G. Goldstein, E. P. Whitlock, & J. DePue, 2004, *American Journal of Preventive Medicine, 27*(2 Suppl), 61–79; "Evaluating Primary Care Behavioral Counseling Interventions: An Evidence-Based Approach," by E. P. Whitlock, C. T. Orleans, N. Pender, & J. Allan, 2002, *American Journal of Preventive Medicine, 22*(4), 267–284.

USPSTF Counseling and Behavioral Interventions Work Group report and other publications (Glasgow, Emont, & Miller, 2006; Goldstein et al., 2004; Whitlock et al., 2002).

A notable and important difference between the Patient-Centered Model and the 5 As is the absence of a specific relationship building component among the 5 As. As previously discussed, provider use of empathy is strongly linked to positive outcomes of communication and counseling interventions (Roter & Kinmonth, 2002; Squier, 1990). However, the easily remembered and concise 5 As framework has advantages as a tool for learning and dissemination.

Interventions that have included training providers in the 5 As counseling approach have been shown to be effective across multiple health behavior targets (Ockene et al., 1999; Whitlock et al., 2002). However, provider training alone is not sufficient to produce significant changes in patients' health behaviors; system-based strategies to prompt, document, and support provider interventions are required to produce benefits at the patient and population levels (Glasgow, Goldstein, Ockene, & Pronk, 2004; Ockene & Zapka, 2000; Pronk et al., 2004).

In the next section, we briefly discuss the Chronic Care Model (CCM), a model that addresses the organizational or system-level elements and factors that influence and support provider-patient interactions.

An Organizational Model of Provider-Patient Interaction

The Chronic Care/Planned Care Model

The Chronic Care Model (CCM), also known as the Planned Care Model, was developed by Edward Wagner and colleagues at the MacColl Institute for the Robert Wood Johnson Foundation-funded Improving Chronic Illness Care (ICIC) program (Wagner, 1998). (See Figure 6.1 and the ICIC website:http://www.improvingchroniccare.org.)

Since its introduction, in the mid-1990s, the CCM has emerged as a key evidence-based conceptual model for understanding how forces at the community, organizational, provider, and patient levels interact to influence health care quality (Wagner, 1998; Wagner, Glasgow, et al., 2001). More recently, the CCM model has also been applied to preventive care (Glasgow, Orleans, & Wagner, 2001). The CCM, depicted graphically in Figure 6.1, posits that "productive interactions" between "informed activated patients" and a "prepared, proactive practice team" are the basis for generating positive health outcomes (Bodenheimer, Wagner, & Grumbach, 2002; Wagner, 1998; Wagner, Glasgow, et al., 2001). Productive interactions, in turn, are supported by several essential elements at the health care organizational level: (1) self-management support (see section of this chapter on self-management support for a definition and description); (2) delivery system design (e.g., planned regularly scheduled visits for patients with chronic illnesses, follow-up telephone contact for patients making a behavioral change); (3) decision support (e.g., care guidelines available at the point of care, provider training); (4) clinical information systems (e.g., patient registries, computerized reminder systems for patients and clinicians); (5) the overall organization of health care (e.g., leadership, support for quality improvement at all levels); and (6) community linkages and resources (Bodenheimer, Wagner, et al., 2002;

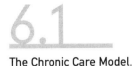

The Chronic Care Model.

The Chronic Care Model

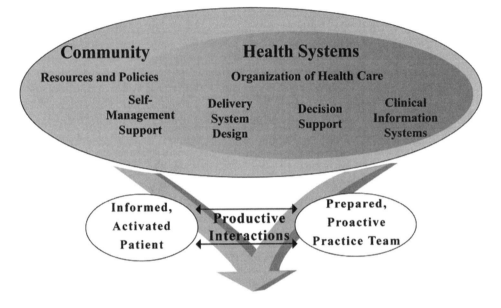

Improved Outcomes

Note. From "Chronic Disease Management: What Will it Take to Improve Care for Chronic Illness?" by E. H. Wagner. 1998. *Effective Clinical Practice, 1,* pp. 2–4. Copyright 1998 by ACP-ASIM Journals and Books. Reprinted with permission.

Wagner, 1998; Wagner, Glasgow, et al., 2001). The overarching principles that cut across all six CCM elements include planned care, rather than responding only to issues that are raised; proactive care (e.g., outreach to identifying needs and encourage regular contact); population-based care (i.e., focused on an entire panel of patients rather than only those who appear in the exam room); and patient-centered care (informed by patient needs and priorities and individually relevant assessment data) (Wagner, 1998; Glasgow, Goldstein, et al., 2004).

The elements of the CCM interact in a complex and synergistic manner to produce positive health outcomes (Bodenheimer, Wagner, et al., 2002; Wagner, 1998; Wagner, Glasgow, et al., 2001). For example, to consistently provide high-quality self-management support, providers need training in self-management support core competencies (decision support); information systems that identify and track patients with chronic conditions through registries and provide a means for clinicians to document outcomes and self-management goals in the health record (information systems); provider teams that determine which team member will provide patients with follow-up to determine progress toward goals (delivery system design); organizational leaders who provide incentives and rewards for provider delivery of self-management support interventions (organizational support); and a way to help patients identify community resources that will support and enable achievement of self-management goals (community linkages).

Through a variety of quality improvement projects, ICIC has developed, tested, and refined a package of *change strategies* that link to each of the key elements of the CCM. System and organizational strategies derived from the CCM that link most directly to supporting patient self-management and health behavior change have been documented in a number of publications (Bodenheimer, 2005; Fisher et al., 2007; Fisher et al., 2005; Glasgow & Toobert, 2000) and can also be found at the RWJF-funded New Health Partnerships Web site, http://www.newhealthpartnerships.org.

When considering the *delivery system design* element of the CCM, it is important to specify the role that each member of the clinical team will have in delivering elements of self-management support, both within specific types of visits (e.g., routine planned care visits) and over the course of a patient's illness over time (Bodenheimer, 2005; Bodenheimer, Wagner, et al., 2002; Glasgow et al., 2003). To efficiently utilize office staff and resources to meet patient needs and deliver comprehensive care, some have advocated adopting a "microsystem" approach that focuses on organizing and redesigning care within small units of providers, office staff, and patients (Wasson, Godfrey, Nelson, Mohr, & Batalden, 2003). For example, medical assistants might take on the Assess element of the 5A, the primary-care clinician might accomplish the Advise and Agree steps, and a medical assistant, nurse, or health educator (if available) might complete the Assist and Arrange steps of the 5 As, which might include referral to outside resources if intensive support is needed and desired by the patient (Goldstein et al., 2004; Wasson et al., 2003; Whitlock et al., 2002). Specifying and systematizing a follow-up plan, including identifying the member of the team who provides follow-up, by what method and when, is crucial to achieving positive outcomes of health behavior change and self-management support interventions (Bodenheimer, 2005; Bodenheimer, Wagner, et al., 2002; R. E. Glasgow et al., 2003).

Innovations in delivery system design also include group medical visits for patients with a specific chronic condition that allow various members of the heath care team (e.g., medical assistant, physician, nurse, nutritionist, peer educator) to efficiently provide education and self-management support while also providing patients with an opportunity to support and learn from one another (Clancy, Huang, Okonofua, Yeager, & Magruder, 2007; Wagner, Grothaus, et al., 2001). Another promising delivery system design innovation is a "previsit" conducted by a medical assistant (MA) following standard orders signed by a practice physician (Langford, Sawyer, Gioimo, Brownson, & O'Toole, 2007).

Clinical information systems, another key element of the CCM, can also be employed to enhance the system's capacity to address patient needs. The use of previsit health risk appraisal instruments, questionnaires, or interactive computer-based systems may be employed to reduce burden on the primary-care clinician (Glasgow, Bull, Piette, & Steiner, 2004; Pronk et al., 2004). Computer-based information systems and some electronic health records permit questionnaire data that are collected in the office to be rapidly analyzed and fed back to the provider and patient to aid tailoring of patient education and counseling interventions (Glasgow, Bull, et al., 2004). The integrated use of patient assessments also provides a useful way of prompting both the patient and the provider to address health behaviors and self-management during the subsequent clinical interaction (Bodenheimer, 2003; Grimshaw et al., 2001; Ockene & Zapka, 2000; Walsh & McPhee, 1992).

Tools (e.g., assessments, action plans), training, technology, and delivery system design strategies derived from the CCM (e.g., group visits, educational programs) can support a clinical team to promote self-management and health behavior change. For example, a completed action plan not only prompts, reminds, and supports patients to work on progress toward goals; it also serves as a useful format for sharing information among providers across multiple visits over time (Bodenheimer, MacGregor, & Sharifi, 2005; Glasgow et al., 2002; Glasgow, Goldstein, et al., 2004). See Figure 6.2 for a graphic depiction of how the core competencies of self-management support can be translated into a cyclical process that centers around the creation of a living, evolving action plan that is shared with both patients and providers over multiple encounters over time (Bodenheimer et al., 2005; Glasgow et al., 2002; Glasgow, Goldstein, et al., 2004).

Recent adaptations of the CCM have emphasized the importance of expanding, strengthening, and deepening linkages between the health care systems and these other potential sources of support (i.e., family, social networks, community, and the local environment) (Fisher et al., 2007; Fisher et al., 2005). (See chapter 37 for further discussion of the effect of the environment on behavior.)

The CCM and a specific strategy for driving quality improvement through rapid-cycle testing and collaborative learning networks, developed in collaboration with the Institute for Healthcare Improvement (Glasgow et al., 2002; Wagner,

6.2

Self-management support: An ongoing process.

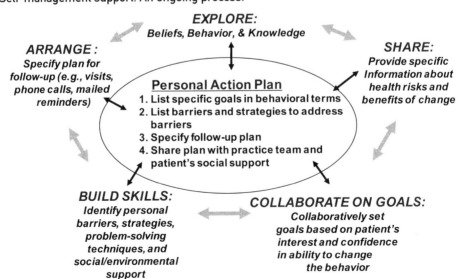

EXPLORE:
Beliefs, Behavior, & Knowledge

ARRANGE :
Specify plan for follow-up (e.g., visits, phone calls, mailed reminders)

SHARE:
Provide specific Information about health risks and benefits of change

Personal Action Plan
1. List specific goals in behavioral terms
2. List barriers and strategies to address barriers
3. Specify follow-up plan
4. Share plan with practice team and patient's social support

BUILD SKILLS:
Identify personal barriers, strategies, problem-solving techniques, and social/environmental support

COLLABORATE ON GOALS:
Collaboratively set goals based on patient's interest and confidence in ability to change the behavior

Note. From "Self-Management Aspects of the Improving Chronic Illness Care Breakthrough Series: Implementation With Diabetes and Heart Failure Teams," by R. E. Glasgow, M. M. Funnell, A. E. Bonomi, C. Davis, V. Beckham, & E. H. Wagner, 2002, *Annals of Behavioral Medicine, 24*(2), 80–87.

Glasgow, et al., 2001), have produced positive effects on process measures (e.g., performing recommended blood tests, documenting self-management goals), though there is less evidence for an effect on disease outcomes (Landon et al., 2007). Emerging results of an ongoing comprehensive evaluation of ICIC collaboratives can be found at http://www.rand.org/health/projects/icice/. The reader is referred to the ICIC Web site, http://www.improvingchronic care.org, for links to the CCM "Change Package" and other resources that health care organizations may utilize to implement the CCM.

In summary, the Chronic Care Model offers useful ways to consider how to integrate and organize care to support productive, patient-centered interactions between clinical teams and patients and families. The CCM emphasizes teamwork, organizational systems, and tools to support counseling and the important roles multiple members of the office staff team can play in the delivery of health behavior counseling and self-management support. Moreover, the CCM features elements that extend the influence of the provider-patient interaction beyond the exam or consultation room, both within and between visits. The CCM includes links between the health care system and myriad potential sources of care and support within spheres of influence that exist outside the health care system within the community (Fisher et al., 2007; Fisher et al., 2005).

As depicted in the Chronic Care Model, the final pathway to effective clinical and functional outcomes rests on effective and productive interactions between prepared proactive provider teams and activated informed patients and families (Wagner, 1998). As noted in the sections of this chapter on the Patient Centered Model, Brief Motivational Interviewing, Self-Management Support, the 5 As, and Shared Decision Making, each of these provider-patient interaction models offer principles and strategies that providers may employ to maximize the impact of their interactions with patients and families. The integration of these patient-provider interaction models and strategies with systems, tools, and strategies at the organizational level shows the greatest promise for achieving desirable changes in health behavior outcomes.

References

Adams, K., Corrigan, J., & Committee on Identifying Priority Areas for Quality Improvement, Institute of Medicine. (2003). *Priority areas for national action: Transforming health care quality.* Washington, DC: National Academies Press.

American Association of Diabetes Educators. (2003). Standards for outcomes measurement of diabetes self-management education. *The Diabetes Educator, 29*(5), 804, 808–810, 813–816.

Anderson, R., Funnell, M., Butler, P., Arnold, M., Fitzgerald, J., & Feste, C. (1995). Patient empowerment: Results of a randomized controlled trial. *Diabetes Care, 18*(7), 943–949.

Anderson, R. M., & Funnell, M. M. (2000). Compliance and adherence are dysfunctional concepts in diabetes care. *The Diabetes Educator, 26*(4), 597–604.

Bandura, A. (2004). Health promotion by social cognitive means. *Health Education & Behavior, 31*(2), 143–164.

Bastiaens, H., Van Royen, P., Pavlic, D. R., Raposo, V., & Baker, R. (2007). Older people's preferences for involvement in their own care: A qualitative study in primary health care in 11 European countries. *Patient Education and Counseling, 68*(1), 33–42.

Bodenheimer, T. (2003). Interventions to improve chronic illness care: Evaluating their effectiveness. *Disease Management, 6*(2), 63–71.

Bodenheimer, T. (2005). Helping patients improve their health-related behaviors: What system changes do we need? *Disease Management, 8*(5), 319–330.

Bodenheimer, T., Lorig, K., Holman, H., & Grumbach, K. (2002). Patient self-management of chronic disease in primary care. *Journal of the American Medical Association, 288*(19), 2469–2475.

Bodenheimer, T., MacGregor, K., & Sharifi, C. (2005). *Helping patients manage their chronic conditions.* Oakland, CA: California Health Care Foundation.

Bodenheimer, T., Wagner, E. H., & Grumbach, K. (2002). Improving primary care for patients with chronic illness: The chronic care model, Part 2. *Journal of the American Medical Association, 288*(15), 1909–1914.

Braddock, C. H., III, Edwards, K. A., Hasenberg, N. M., Laidley, T. L., & Levinson, W. (1999). Informed decision making in outpatient practice: time to get back to basics. *Journal of the American Medical Association, 282*(24), 2313–2320.

Britt, E., Hudson, S. M., & Blampied, N. M. (2004). Motivational interviewing in health settings: a review. *Patient Education and Counseling, 53*(2), 147–155.

Charles, C., Gafni, A., & Whelan, T. (1999). Decision-making in the physician-patient encounter: Revisiting the shared treatment decision-making model. *Social Science Medicine, 49*(5), 651–661.

Clancy, D. E., Huang, P., Okonofua, E., Yeager, D., & Magruder, K. M. (2007). Group visits: Promoting adherence to diabetes guidelines. *Journal of General Internal Medicines, 22*(5), 620–624.

Committee on Quality of Health Care in America. (2001). *Crossing the quality chasm: A new health system for the 21st century.* Washington, DC: National Academy Press.

Davis, D., Schoenbaum, S. C., Collins, K. S., Teeney, K., Hughes, D. L., & Audet, A.-M. J. (2002). *Room for improvement: Patients report on the quality of their health care* (Publication no. 534). New York: The Commonwealth Fund.

DiMatteo, M. R. (1994). Enhancing patient adherence to medical recommendations. *Journal of the American Medical Association, 271*(1), 79, 83.

DiMatteo, M. R., Hays, R. D., Gritz, E. R., Bastani, R., Crane, L., Elashoff, R., et al. (1993). Patient adherence to cancer control regimens: Scale development and initial validation. *Psychological Assessment, 5,* 102–112.

Entwistle, V. A., & Watt, I. S. (2006). Patient involvement in treatment decision-making: The case for a broader conceptual framework. *Patient Education and Counseling, 63*(3), 268–278.

Epstein, R. M., Alper, B. S., & Quill, T. E. (2004). Communicating evidence for participatory decision making. *Journal of the American Medical Association, 291*(19), 2359–2366.

Fisher, E. B., Brownson, C. A., O'Toole, M. L., Shetty, G., Anwuri, V. V., Fazzone, P., et al. (2007). The Robert Wood Johnson Foundation Diabetes Initiative: Demonstration projects emphasizing self-management. *The Diabetes Educator, 33*(1), 83–84, 86–88, 91–82, passim.

Fisher, E. B., Brownson, C. A., O'Toole, M. L., Shetty, G., Anwuri, V. V., & Glasgow, R. E. (2005). Ecological approaches to self-management: The case of diabetes. *American Journal of Public Health, 95,* 1523–1535.

Frank, E., Rothenberg, R., Lewis, C., & Belodoff, B. F. (2000). Correlates of physicians' prevention-related practices. Findings from the Women Physicians' Health Study. *Archives of Family Medicine, 9*(4), 359–367.

Frosch, D. L., & Kaplan, R. M. (1999). Shared decision making in clinical medicine: Past research and future directions. *American Journal of Preventive Medicine, 17*(4), 285–294.

Glasgow, R., & Toobert, D. (2000). Brief, computer-assisted diabetes dietary self-management counseling: Effects on behavior, physiologic outcomes, and quality of life. *Medical Care, 38*(11), 1062–1073.

Glasgow, R. E., & Anderson, R. M. (1999). In diabetes care, moving from compliance to adherence is not enough. Something entirely different is needed. *Diabetes Care, 22*(12), 2090–2092.

Glasgow, R. E., Bull, S. S., Piette, J. D., & Steiner, J. F. (2004). Interactive behavior change technology. A partial solution to the competing demands of primary care. *American Journal of Preventive Medicine, 27*(2 Suppl.), 80–87.

Glasgow, R. E., Davis, C. L., Funnell, M. M., & Beck, A. (2003). Implementing practical interventions to support chronic illness self-management. *Joint Commission Journal on Quality and Safety, 29*(11), 563–574.

Glasgow, R. E., Emont, S., & Miller, D. C. (2006). Assessing delivery of the five 'As' for patient-centered counseling. *Health Promotion International, 21*(3), 245–255.

Glasgow, R. E., Funnell, M. M., Bonomi, A. E., Davis, C., Beckham, V., & Wagner, E. H. (2002). Self-management aspects of the improving chronic illness care breakthrough series: Implementation with diabetes and heart failure teams. *Annals of Behavioral Medicine, 24*(2), 80–87.

Glasgow, R. E., Goldstein, M. G., Ockene, J. K., & Pronk, N. P. (2004). Translating what we have learned into practice. Principles and hypotheses for interventions addressing multiple behaviors in primary care. *American Journal of Preventive Medicine, 27*(2 Suppl), 88–101.

Glasgow, R. E., Orleans, C. T., & Wagner, E. H. (2001). Does the chronic care model serve also as a template for improving prevention? *Milbank Q, 79*(4), 579–612, iv–v.

Glasgow, R. E., Strycker, L. A., Toobert, D. J., & Eakin, E. (2000). A social-ecologic approach to assessing support for disease self-management: The Chronic Illness Resources Survey. *Journal of Behavioral Medicine, 23*(6), 559–583.

Goldstein, M. G., Ruggiero, L., Guise, B. J., & Abrams, D. B. (1994). Behavioral medicine strategies for medical patients. In A. Stoudemire (Ed.), *Clinical Psychiatry for Medical Students* (2nd ed., pp. 671–693). Philadelphia: Lippincott.

Goldstein, M. G., Whitlock, E. P., & DePue, J. (2004). Multiple behavioral risk factor interventions in primary care; Summary of research evidence. *American Journal of Preventive Medicine, 27*(2 Suppl), 61–79.

Greenfield, S., Kaplan, S. H., Ware, J. E., Jr., Yano, E. M., & Frank, H. J. (1988). Patients' participation in medical care: Effects on blood sugar control and quality of life in diabetes. *Journal of General Internal Medicine, 3*(5), 448–457.

Grimshaw, J. M., Shirran, L., Thomas, R., Mowatt, G., Fraser, C., Bero, L., et al. (2001). Changing provider behavior: An overview of systematic reviews of interventions. *Medical Care, 39*(8 Suppl 2), II2–45.

Grueninger, U., Duffy, F., & Goldstein, M. (1995). Patient education in the medical encounter: How to facilitate learning, behavior change and coping. In M. J. Lipkin, S. Putnam, & A. Lazare (Eds.), *The medical interview: Clinical care, education, research* (pp. 122–133). New York: Springer-Verlag.

Hibbard, J. H., Mahoney, E. R., Stock, R., & Tusler, M. (2007). Do increases in patient activation result in improved self-management behaviors? *Health Services Research, 42*(4), 1443–1463.

Hibbard, J. H., Mahoney, E. R., Stockard, J., & Tusler, M. (2005). Development and testing of a short form of the patient activation measure. *Health Services Research, 40*(6 Pt 1), 1918–1930.

Hibbard, J. H., & Tusler, M. (2007). Assessing activation stage and employing a "next steps" approach to supporting patient self-management. *The Journal of Ambulatory Care Management, 30*(1), 2–8.

Keller, V., & White, M. (1997). Choices and changes: A new model for influencing patient health behavior. *Journal of Clinical Outcomes Management, 4*(6), 33–36.

Landon, B. E., Hicks, L. S., O'Malley, A. J., Lieu, T. A., Keegan, T., McNeil, B. J., et al. (2007). Improving the management of chronic disease at community health centers. *New England Journal of Medicine, 356*(9), 921–934.

Langford, A. T., Sawyer, D. R., Gioimo, S., Brownson, C. A., & O'Toole, M. L. (2007). Patient-centered goal setting as a tool to improve diabetes self-management. *The Diabetes Educator, 33*(Suppl. 6), 139S–144.

Levinson, W., Kao, A., Kuby, A., & Thisted, R. A. (2005). Not all patients want to participate in decision making. A national study of public preferences. *Journal of General Internal Medicine, 20*(6), 531–535.

Lorig, K. R., & Holman, H. R. (2003). Self-management education: History, definition, outcomes, and mechanisms. *Annals of Behavioral Medicine, 26*(1), 1–7.

Makoul, G. (2001). Essential elements of communication in medical encounters: The Kalamazoo consensus statement. *Academic Medicine, 76*(4), 390–393.

Makoul, G., & Clayman, M. L. (2006). An integrative model of shared decision making in medical encounters. *Patient Education Counseling, 60*(3), 301–312.

Miller, W. R., & Rollnick, S. (2002). *Motivational interviewing: Preparing people for change* (2nd ed.). New York: Guilford Press.

Mosen, D. M., Schmittdiel, J., Hibbard, J., Sobel, D., Remmers, C., & Bellows, J. (2007). Is patient activation associated with outcomes of care for adults with chronic conditions? *The Journal of Ambulatory Care Management, 30*(1), 21–29.

National Center for Health Statistics. (2003). *Health, United States, 2003* (DHHS Publication No. 2003-1232). Hyattsville, MD: National Center for Health Statistics.

Norris, S. L., Engelgau, M. M., & Narayan, K. M. V. (2001). Effectiveness of self-management training in type 2 diabetes: A systematic review of randomized controlled trials. *Diabetes Care, 24*(3), 561–587.

Ockene, I. S., Hebert, J. R., Ockene, J. K., Saperia, G. M., Stanek, E., Nicolosi, R., et al. (1999). Effect of physician-delivered nutrition counseling training and an office-support program on saturated fat intake, weight, and serum lipid measurements in a hyperlipidemic population: Worcester Area Trial for Counseling in Hyperlipidemia (WATCH). *Archives of Internal Medicine, 159*(7), 725–731.

Ockene, J. K., & Zapka, J. G. (2000). Provider education to promote implementation of clinical practice guidelines. *Chest, 118*(2 Suppl), 33S–39S.

O'Connor, A. M., Wennberg, J. E., Legare, F., Llewellyn-Thomas, H. A., Moulton, B. W., Sepucha, K. R., et al. (2007). Toward the "tipping point": Decision aids and informed patient choice. *Health Affairs (Millwood), 26*(3), 716–725.

Orleans, C. T., George, L. K., Houpt, J. L., & Brodie, K. H. (1985). Health promotion in primary care. A survey of U.S. family practitioners. *Preventive Medicine, 14,* 636–647.

Prochaska, J. O., & DiClemente, C. C. (1986). Towards a comprehensive model of change. In W. R. Miller & N. Heather (Eds.), *Treating addictive disorders: Processes of change* (pp. 3–27). New York: Plenum Press.

Pronk, N. P., Peek, C. J., & Goldstein, M. G. (2004). Addressing multiple behavioral risk factors in primary care: A synthesis of current knowledge and stakeholder dialogue sessions. *American Journal of Preventive Medicine, 27*(2 Suppl), 4–17.

Renders, C. M., Valk, G. D., Griffin, S. J., Wagner, E. H., Eijk Van, J. T., & Assendelft, W. J. (2001). Interventions to improve the management of diabetes in primary care, outpatient, and community settings: A systematic review. *Diabetes Care, 24*(10), 1821–1833.

Rogers, C. (1951). *Client-centered therapy: Its current practice, implications, and theory.* Cambridge, MA: Riverside.

Rollnick, S., Miller, W. R., & Butler, C. C. (2008). *Motivational interviewing in health care: Helping patients change behavior.* New York: Guilford Press.

Roter, D., & Kinmonth, A.-L. (2002). What is the evidence that increasing participation of individuals in self-management improves the processes and outcomes of care? In R. Williams, A. Kinmonth, N. Wareham, & W. Herman (Eds.), *The evidence base for diabetes care* (pp. 679–700). New York: Wiley.

Rubak, S., Sandbaek, A., Lauritzen, T., & Christensen, B. (2005). Motivational interviewing: A systematic review and meta-analysis. *The British Journal of General Practice, 55*(513), 305–312.

Safran, D., Taira, D., Rogers, W., Kosinski, M., & Tarlov, A. (1998). Linking primary care performance to outcomes of care. *The Journal of Family Practice, 47,* 213–220.

Squier, R. W. (1990). A model of empathic understanding and adherence to treatment regimens in practitioner-patient relationships. *Social Science & Medicine, 30*(3), 325–339.

Stewart, M., Brown, J., Donner, A., McWhinney, I., Oates, J., Weston, W., et al. (2000). The impact of patient-centered care on outcomes. *The Journal of Family Practice, 49*(9), 805–807.

Stewart, M., Brown, J., Weston, W., McWhinney, I., McWilliam, C., & Freeman, T. (1995). *Patient-centered medicine: Transforming the clinical method.* Thousand Oaks, CA: Sage.

Street, R. L., Jr., Gordon, H. S., Ward, M. M., Krupat, E., & Kravitz, R. L. (2005). Patient participation in medical consultations: Why some patients are more involved than others. *Medical Care, 43*(10), 960–969.

Thorndike, A. N., Regan, S., & Rigotti, N. A. (2007). The treatment of smoking by U.S. physicians during ambulatory visits: 1994–2003. *American Journal of Public Health, 97*(10), 1878–1883.

Wagner, E. H. (1998). Chronic disease management: What will it take to improve care for chronic illness? *Effective Clinical Practice, 1*(1), 2–4.

Wagner, E. H., Glasgow, R. E., Davis, C., Bonomi, A. E., Provost, L., McCulloch, D., et al. (2001). Quality improvement in chronic illness care: A collaborative approach. *The Joint Commission Journal on Quality Improvement, 27*(2), 63–80.

Wagner, E. H., Grothaus, L. C., Sandhu, N., Galvin, M. S., McGregor, M., Artz, K., et al. (2001). Chronic care clinics for diabetes in primary care: A system-wide randomized trial. *Diabetes Care, 24*(4), 695–700.

Waldstein, S. R., Neumann, S. A., Drossman, D. A., & Novack, D. H. (2001). Teaching psychosomatic (biopsychosocial) medicine in United States medical schools: Survey findings. *Psychosomatic Medicine, 63*(3), 335–343.

Walsh, J. M., & McPhee, S. J. (1992). A systems model of clinical preventive care: An analysis of factors influencing patient and physician. *Health Education Quarterly, 19*(2), 157–175.

Warsi, A., Wang, P. S., LaValley, M. P., Avorn, J., & Solomon, D. H. (2004). Self-management education programs in chronic disease: A systematic review and methodological critique of the literature. *Archives of Internal Medicine, 164*(15), 1641–1649.

Wasson, J. H., Godfrey, M. M., Nelson, E. C., Mohr, J. J., & Batalden, P. B. (2003). Microsystems in health care: Part 4. Planning patient-centered care. *Joint Commission Journal on Quality and Safety, 29*(5), 227–237.

Whitlock, E. P., Orleans, C. T., Pender, N., & Allan, J. (2002). Evaluating primary care behavioral counseling interventions: An evidence-based approach. *American Journal of Preventive Medicine, 22*(4), 267–284.

Williams, G. C., McGregor, H. A., King, D., Nelson, C. C., & Glasgow, R. E. (2005). Variation in perceived competence, glycemic control, and patient satisfaction: Relationship to autonomy support from physicians. *Patient Education and Counseling, 57*(1), 39–45.

Williams, G. C., McGregor, H. A., Zeldman, A., Freedman, Z. R., & Deci, E. L. (2004). Testing a self-determination theory process model for promoting glycemic control through diabetes self-management. *Health Psychology, 23*(1), 58–66.

Relapse Prevention and the Maintenance of Optimal Health

7

Christian S.
Hendershot,
G. Alan Marlatt, and
William H. George

Relapse prevention (RP) is a tertiary intervention strategy for reducing the likelihood and severity of relapse following the cessation or reduction of problematic behavior. This chapter reviews RP as a method for facilitating health behavior change. We begin with a concise overview of the historical and theoretical foundations of the RP model and a brief summary of intervention strategies. Next, we review the major theoretical, methodological, and applied developments related to RP that have transpired since the last iteration of this chapter (Marlatt & George, 1998). A large portion of the current chapter is devoted to describing recent empirical findings that coincide with key tenets of

Acknowledgment: The authors thank Katie Witkiewitz for her helpful
feedback on earlier drafts of this chapter.

the RP model. We conclude by summarizing current and future directions in the study and prevention of relapse.

Overlaying these topics are two themes unique to the present version of this chapter. First, emphasis is placed on the reformulated cognitive-behavioral model of relapse (Witkiewitz & Marlatt, 2004) as a framework for conceptualizing relapse as a dynamic process. Second, consistent with the theme of this book, we focus our empirical review on studies investigating health behavior or its antecedents. Predictably, the prime focus is on addictive behaviors, for which RP was initially conceived. However, findings from health domains such as diet, exercise, and HIV are also incorporated. In emphasizing health behavior, we forgo a detailed discussion of other behaviors and disorders to which RP approaches have been extended (e.g., sexual offending, depression, gambling) and refer readers to other sources (Marlatt & Donovan, 2005; Witkiewitz & Marlatt, 2007a) for further detail on the growing range of RP applications.

Relapse as a Barrier to Health Behavior Change

Definitions of relapse are varied, ranging from a dichotomous treatment outcome to an ongoing, transitional process (Brownell, Marlatt, Lichtenstein, & Wilson, 1986; Witkiewitz & Marlatt, 2004). As a testament to the complexity of relapse, a sizable volume of research has yielded no consensus operational definition of the term (Maisto & Connors, 2006; Piasecki, 2006). For present purposes we define *relapse* as a setback that occurs during the behavior change process, such that progress toward the initiation or maintenance of a behavior change goal (for instance, abstinence from drug use) is interrupted by a reversion to the target behavior. However defined, relapse poses a fundamental barrier to health maintenance by constituting the modal outcome of behavior change efforts (Orleans, 2000; Polivy & Herman, 2002).

Originating from early research with alcohol-dependent individuals (Marlatt, 1978), RP has been studied and applied largely in the context of addictive behaviors. However, the implications of RP for health maintenance extend well beyond this domain. Initial formulations of RP stressed its relevance to the emergent field of health psychology (Marlatt, 1982), and the seminal overview of the model appeared in a behavioral medicine text (Marlatt & Gordon, 1980). Subsequently, RP principles have been extended to a widening range of health domains, including diet, exercise, diabetes, and sexual risk taking. Clinical applications will inevitably vary across health behaviors owing to differences in the definition, rates, correlates, and implications of relapse. Nonetheless, the universal difficulty of sustaining modifications to long-standing behaviors (Polivy & Herman, 2002) renders RP a fundamental and broadly applicable approach for most researchers and clinicians with interests in health behavior change.

Relapse Prevention: Overview of the Model

The RP model developed by Marlatt and Gordon (1980, 1985) provides both a conceptual framework for understanding relapse and a set of treatment strategies designed to limit relapse likelihood and severity. Detailed accounts of the model's historical background and theoretical underpinnings have been published elsewhere (e.g., Cummings, Gordon, & Marlatt; 1980; Dimeff & Marlatt, 1998; Marlatt, 1996; Marlatt & Gordon, 1985). The following section offers a concise review of the model's history, core concepts, and clinical applications. For simplicity, RP theory and approaches are discussed specifically in relation to substance use behavior.

Historical Foundations

RP was initially conceived as an outgrowth and augmentation of traditional behavioral approaches to studying and treating addictions. Based on the cognitive-behavioral model of relapse, the RP model was distinctive in its blending of basic learning principles with emerging theory from social psychology, cognitive psychology, and stress-and-coping perspectives. The evolution of cognitive-behavioral theories of substance use witnessed notable changes in the conceptualization of relapse, many of which departed from traditional (i.e., disease-based) models of addiction. For instance, whereas traditional models often attribute relapse to endogenous factors like cravings or withdrawal (construed as symptoms of an underlying disease state), cognitive-behavioral theories emphasize contextual factors (e.g., environmental stimuli, cognitive processes) as proximal relapse antecedents.

Cognitive-behavioral theories also diverged from disease models in rejecting the notion of relapse as a dichotomous outcome. Whereas disease models tend to view relapse as a state or endpoint signaling treatment failure, cognitive-behavioral theories consider relapse as a fluctuating process that begins prior to and extends beyond the return to the target behavior (Larimer, Palmer, & Marlatt, 1999). From this stance, the initial return to a problematic behavior after a period of volitional abstinence (a *lapse*) is seen not as a dead end but as a fork in the road. Though an initial lapse can prompt a full-blown relapse, another possible outcome is that the problem behavior is corrected and the desired behavior re-instantiated—an event referred to as *prolapse*. A key implication is that lapses, rather than signaling a breakdown or failure in the behavior change process, can be considered temporary setbacks that present opportunities for new learning. In viewing relapse as a common (albeit undesirable) event, emphasizing contextual antecedents over internal causes, and asserting that relapse does not amount to treatment failure, RP introduced a comprehensive, flexible, and optimistic alternative to traditional models.

Theoretical Basis

Marlatt and Gordon (1985) proposed that relapse is influenced both by *immediate precipitants* and *covert antecedents*. In terms of immediate precipitants, the RP model assumes that lapses typically occur during *high-risk situations*, broadly defined as any context that confers increased vulnerability for engaging in the target behavior. High-risk contexts can include emotional or cognitive states (e.g., negative affect, diminished self-efficacy), environmental contingencies (e.g., interpersonal events, exposure to conditioned drug cues), or physiological states (e.g., acute withdrawal). Although some high-risk situations appear nearly universal across addictive behaviors (e.g., negative affect; Marlatt, 1978;

Baker, Piper, McCarthy, Majeskie, & Fiore, 2004), high-risk situations are likely to vary across behaviors, across individuals, and within the same individual over time (Witkiewitz & Marlatt, 2007a). Whether a high-risk situation culminates in a lapse depends largely on another situational factor: the individual's capacity to enact an effective *coping response,* globally defined as any compensatory strategy (cognitive or behavioral) that reduces the likelihood of lapsing.

While emphasizing situational antecedents, the RP model also posits that the relapse process begins prior to the onset of a high-risk situation. *Covert antecedents* refer to ongoing factors that influence one's overall risk for relapse. A significant distal influence is one's overall level of lifestyle balance, defined as the equilibrium between day-to-day activities perceived as external demands ("shoulds") and those activities perceived as voluntary or pleasurable ("wants") (Marlatt and Gordon, 1985). For instance, a lifestyle encumbered with perceived "shoulds" may foster a sense of self-deprivation and a corresponding desire for gratification, which can manifest as urges or cravings. Covert antecedents can also take the form of subtle decision-making tendencies. Apparently Irrelevant Decisions (AIDs) refer to seemingly innocuous choices that serve to set up a relapse (e.g., purchasing alcohol "just in case guests drop by"). Overall, covert antecedents can contribute to relapse by facilitating exposure to high-risk situations and/or undermining one's motivation to cope with them (Larimer, Palmer, & Marlatt, 1999).

The RP model further stresses the role of cognitive factors as proximal and/or distal influences. For example, successful navigation of high-risk situations may increase *self-efficacy* (one's perceived capacity to cope with an impending situation or task; Bandura, 1997), in turn decreasing relapse probability. Conversely, a return to the prohibited behavior can undermine self-efficacy, increasing the risk of future lapses. *Outcome expectancies* (e.g., anticipated effects of substance use; Goldman, Darkes, & Del Boca, 1999) also figure prominently in the RP model. Finally, attitudes or beliefs about the causes and meaning of a lapse may influence whether a full relapse ensues. Viewing a lapse as a personal failure may lead to feelings of guilt, perceived helplessness, and abandonment of the behavior change goal (Larimer, Palmer, & Marlatt, 1999). This reaction, termed the Abstinence Violation Effect (AVE) (Marlatt and Gordon, 1980, 1985), may be more likely when one holds a dichotomous view of relapse and/or neglects to consider situational explanations for lapsing. In sum, the RP framework emphasizes high-risk contexts, coping responses, self-efficacy, affect, expectancies, and the AVE as primary relapse influences.

Intervention Strategies

The RP approach assumes that the initiation and maintenance of behavior change represent separate processes governed by unique contingencies (e.g., Brownell et al., 1986; Rothman, 2000). Thus, specific cognitive and behavioral strategies are often necessary to maintain initial treatment gains and minimize relapse likelihood. RP strategies fall into two broad categories: specific intervention techniques, often designed to help the patient anticipate and cope with high-risk situations, and global self-control approaches, intended to reduce relapse risk by promoting positive lifestyle change. It should be noted that this emphasis on posttreatment maintenance and overall lifestyle balance renders

RP a potentially useful adjunct to various treatment modalities (e.g., cognitive-behavioral therapy, 12-step programs, pharmacotherapy), irrespective of the strategies used to enact initial behavior change.

An essential starting point to treatment is a thorough assessment of the client's substance use patterns, high-risk situations, and coping skills. Other important targets of assessment include the client's self-efficacy, outcome expectancies, and readiness to change, along with concomitant factors that may complicate treatment (e.g., comorbid disorders, neuropsychological deficits). Using high-risk situations as a starting point, the therapist works backward to identify immediate precipitants and distal lifestyle factors related to relapse and forward to evaluate coping responses (Larimer, Palmer, & Marlatt, 1999; Marlatt & Gordon, 1985). Ideally, this approach helps clients to (a) recognize high-risk situations as discriminative stimuli signaling relapse risk, and (b) identify possible cognitive and behavioral strategies to obviate these situations or minimize their impact. Examples of specific intervention strategies include enhancing self-efficacy (e.g., by setting achievable goals) and eliminating myths and placebo effects (e.g., challenging misperceptions about the effects of substance use). The client's postlapse reaction also serves as a pivotal intervention point, since it can determine whether a lapse escalates or desists. Establishing lapse management plans can aid the client in self-correcting soon after a slip, and cognitive restructuring can help clients to reframe the meaning of the event and minimize the AVE (Larimer, Palmer, & Marlatt, 1999).

The final thrust in the RP program is the global intervention of lifestyle balancing, designed to target more pervasive factors that can function as relapse antecedents. To reiterate, relapse risk is often heightened when individuals perceive their lifestyle as predominated by obligations and lacking in commensurate pleasurable activities. A useful way to assess lifestyle imbalance is for clients to monitor their behavior, keeping a daily log of both obligations and indulgences, to highlight disequilibrium between "shoulds" and "wants." Clients are encouraged to integrate pleasurable activities and "positive addictions," like exercise or meditation, into their daily routine. The psychological and health benefits derived from positive addictions may enhance self-efficacy, in turn reducing relapse risk. As implied by the strategies discussed, RP is characterized by a highly ideographic treatment approach, a contrast to the "one size fits all" perspective typical of other treatments (e.g., 12-step programs).

Recent Developments in Relapse Prevention

The decade since the last edition of this volume (Shumaker, Schron, Ockene, & McBee, 1998) has seen several noteworthy developments related to RP. A significant milestone was the publication of *Relapse Prevention,* 2nd ed. (Marlatt & Donovan, 2005). This updated volume reflects the expanding range of RP applications, with new chapters devoted to specific drugs (stimulants, opioids, cannabis, and "club" drugs) and nonsubstance-use behaviors (gambling, eating disorders/obesity, sexual offending, and sexual risk behavior). The volume was developed in tandem with *Assessment of Addictive Behaviors,* 2nd ed. (Donovan & Marlatt, 2005), which serves as its companion text.

The continual influence of RP is evident in its broad dissemination and increasing accessibility. RP modules are standard to virtually all psychosocial interventions for substance use (McGovern, Wrisley, & Drake, 2005) and an increasing number of self-help manuals are available to assist both therapists and clients. A new text designed for practicing clinicians discusses RP techniques across a range of behavior domains (Witkiewitz & Marlatt, 2007a). RP strategies have been disseminated using simple but effective methods; for instance, mail-delivered RP booklets are shown to reduce smoking relapse (Brandon, Collins, Juliano, & Lazev, 2000). Researchers and clinicians continue to extend RP applications by tailoring treatment approaches to specific populations (Witkiewitz & Marlatt, 2007a). Finally, the broad influence of RP is evident in the clinical vernacular, as "relapse prevention" has evolved into an umbrella term synonymous with most skills-based interventions addressing high-risk situations and coping responses.

Conceptualizing Relapse as a Dynamic Process

Greater efforts to develop, test, and refine theoretical models are critical to enhancing the understanding and treatment of relapse (Maisto & Connors, 2006; Orleans, 2000). A noteworthy development in this respect was the reformulation of Marlatt's cognitive-behavioral relapse model to emphasize dynamic processes (Witkiewitz & Marlatt, 2004).

Whereas most theories presume linear relationships among constructs, the dynamic model views relapse as a complex, nonlinear process in which various factors act jointly and interactively to affect relapse timing and severity. Similar to the original RP model, the dynamic model centers on the high-risk situation. Against this backdrop, both tonic (stable) and phasic (fluctuating) influences can act to determine relapse likelihood. Tonic processes include *distal risks,* or stable background factors that determine an individual's "set point" or initial threshold for relapse (Hufford, Witkiewitz, Shields, Kodya, & Caruso 2003; Witkiewitz & Marlatt, 2004). Personality, genetic or familial risk factors, drug sensitivity and metabolism, and physical withdrawal profiles are examples of distal variables that may influence one's a priori relapse liability. Tonic processes also include cognitive factors showing stability over time, such as outcome expectancies, global self-efficacy, and personal beliefs about abstinence or relapse. Whereas tonic processes may dictate relapse susceptibility, its occurrence is determined largely by *phasic responses*—proximal or transient factors that serve to actuate (or prevent) a lapse. Phasic responses include cognitive and affective processes that can fluctuate across time and contexts—such as urges and cravings, mood, situational self-efficacy, and motivation—as well as momentary coping responses. Substance use and its immediate consequences (e.g., impaired decision making, the AVE) are additional phasic processes that are set into motion once a lapse occurs. To summarize, tonic processes usually determine *who* is vulnerable for relapse, whereas phasic processes determine *when* relapse occurs (Hufford et al., 2003; Witkiewitz & Marlatt, 2004).

A key feature of the dynamic model is its emphasis on the complex interplay between tonic and phasic processes. As indicated in Figure 7.1, distal risks may influence relapse either directly or indirectly (via phasic processes). The model also predicts feedback loops among hypothesized constructs. For instance, the return to substance use can have reciprocal effects on the same

7.1

Dynamic model of relapse.

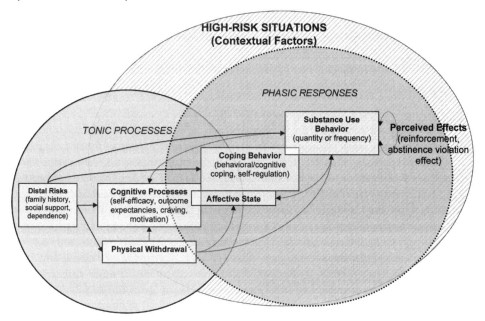

Note. From "Relapse Prevention for Alcohol and Drug Problems: That was Zen, This is Tao," by K. Witkiewitz & G. A. Marlatt, 2004, *American Psychologist, 59,* pp. 224–235. Copyright 2004 by American Psychological Association. Reprinted with permission.

cognitive or affective factors (motivation, mood, self-efficacy) that contributed to the lapse. Lapses may also evoke physiological (e.g., alleviation of withdrawal) and/or cognitive (e.g., the AVE) responses that in turn determine whether use escalates or desists. The dynamic model further emphasizes the importance of nonlinear relationships and timing/sequencing of events. For instance, in a high-risk context, a slight and momentary drop in self-efficacy can have a disproportionate impact on other relapse antecedents (negative affect, expectancies) (Witkiewitz & Marlatt, 2004, 2007a). Furthermore, the strength of proximal influences on relapse may vary based on distal risk factors, with these relationships becoming increasingly nonlinear as distal risk increases (Hufford et al., 2003). This notion assumes that relapse can take the form of sudden and unexpected returns to the target behavior, a prediction that concurs both with clinical observations and with contemporary learning models stipulating that recently modified behavior is inherently unstable and easily swayed by context (Bouton, 2000). While maintaining its footing in cognitive-behavioral theory, the dynamic model also draws from nonlinear dynamical systems theory (NDST) and catastrophe theory, both approaches for understanding the operation of complex systems (Witkiewitz & Marlatt, 2007a, b). Detailed discussions of relapse in relation to NDST and catastrophe theory are available elsewhere (Hufford et al., 2003; Witkiewitz, van der Maas, Hufford, & Marlatt, 2007; Witkiewitz & Marlatt, 2007a, b).

Empirical Support for the RP Model

Driven by methodological and theoretical advances, the literature on relapse has grown substantially over the past decade. Since the volume and scope of this work preclude an exhaustive review, the following section summarizes a select body of findings reflective of the overall literature. First, major review studies and large-scale clinical outcome trials are summarized. Next, findings from smaller studies are presented, with an emphasis on recent findings pertinent to the dynamic model's predictions and theoretical assumptions.

Systematic Reviews and Large-Scale Treatment Outcome Studies

As of the preceding edition of this volume (Shumaker et al., 1998), the most comprehensive review of RP studies was Carroll's (1996) descriptive account of 24 treatment outcome studies focusing on substance use. This review found consistent support for the superiority of RP over no treatment, inconsistent support for its superiority over discussion control conditions, and consistent evidence that RP was as efficacious as other active treatments. Carroll concluded that RP, though not consistently superior to other active treatments, showed particular promise in three areas: reducing relapse severity, enhancing durability of treatment gains, and matching treatment strategies to client characteristics. RP also showed delayed emergence effects in some studies, suggesting that it may outperform other treatments during the maintenance stage of behavior change (Carroll, 1996).

Appearing shortly after Carroll's review was a meta-analysis of 26 RP treatment outcome studies totaling 9,504 participants (Irvin, Bowers, Dunn, & Wang, 1999). The authors examined two primary outcomes, substance use and psychosocial functioning, and evaluated several treatment moderators. Effect sizes indicated that RP was generally successful in reducing substance use ($r = .14$) and improving psychosocial functioning ($r = .48$), consistent with its purpose as both a specific and global intervention approach. Moderation analyses suggested that RP was consistently efficacious across treatment modalities (individual vs. group) and settings (inpatient vs. outpatient). RP was most effective for reducing alcohol and polysubstance use and less effective for tobacco and cocaine use—a contrast to Carroll's (1996) finding of comparable efficacy across drug classes. In addition, RP was more effective when delivered in conjunction with pharmacotherapy, when compared to wait-list (vs. active) comparison conditions, and when outcomes were assessed soon after treatment. Though some findings were considered tentative due to sample sizes, the authors concluded that RP was broadly efficacious (Irvin et al., 1999).

An increasing number of large-scale trials have allowed for statistically powerful evaluations of psychosocial interventions for alcohol use. Project MATCH (Project MATCH Research Group, 1997) evaluated the efficacy of three interventions—Motivational Enhancement Therapy (MET), 12-Step Facilitation (TSF), and Cognitive Behavioral Therapy (CBT)—for treating alcohol dependence. The CBT intervention was a skills-based treatment containing elements of RP. Spanning nine data collection sites and following more than

1,700 participants for up to 3 years, Project MATCH was the largest psycho-therapy trial ever conducted. Multiple "matching hypotheses" were tested to see whether treatments showed differential efficacy as a function of theoretically relevant client attributes. Only 1 of 16 primary matching hypotheses was supported: outpatients with less severe psychiatric diagnoses fared better in TSF than in CBT during the year following treatment (Project MATCH Research Group, 1997). Though impressive in its design and implementation, the study provided relatively little justification for tailoring alcohol treatments on the basis of the client attributes examined.

More recently, the COMBINE Study (Anton et al., 2006) tested the individual and joint efficacy of two pharmacological treatments (naltrexone and acamprosate) and a combined behavioral intervention (CBI) for alcohol dependence. CBI represented a blending of established behavioral approaches including RP. A total of 1,383 individuals with alcohol dependence were randomly assigned to conditions crossing medication (naltrexone, acamprosate, naltrexone plus acamprosate, placebo) and behavioral (CBI vs. none) interventions. Participants in these eight groups also received medication management in a primary-care format. A ninth group received CBI without medication management. Interventions were delivered in a 16-week outpatient program, and drinking was assessed for 1 year posttreatment. Both CBI and naltrexone reduced drinking, but results showed no incremental efficacy of combined treatments, and those receiving CBI alone actually fared worse than those in the placebo condition. Although overall treatment effects diminished over time, some trends emerged in the 1 year follow-up period: those receiving naltrexone were less likely to return to heavy drinking, and the CBI groups showed marginally greater abstinence than the medical management groups, suggesting that both naltrexone and CBI may reduce relapse occurrence prospectively (Anton et al., 2006).

Recent Findings in Support of RP Model Components

The following section reviews selected empirical findings that support or co-incide with tenets of the RP model. We emphasize findings relevant to the dynamic model of relapse, building upon other such reviews (Witkiewitz & Marlatt, 2004, 2007a) by including studies from several health behavior domains and by providing an expanded discussion of neurocognitive and genetic factors as components of distal relapse risk. Sections are organized in accordance with major model constructs. It should be noted that, although dynamic processes likely play a role in relapse for most or all health behavior domains, the specific constructs and findings discussed here may vary in relevance across behaviors. Researchers and clinicians should consult current theory and research to determine the constructs and processes that are likely to be most relevant for any given health behavior.

Psychiatric Comorbidity

A well-established risk factor for relapse is the presence of a psychiatric disorder (Drake, 2005). Comorbid disorders are exceedingly common (McGovern et al., 2005) and can be conceptualized from various etiological perspectives (Mueser, Drake, & Wallach 1998). For instance, co-occurring disorders may reflect common genetic, personality, and/or neurobiological risk factors. Comorbidity may also influence relapse indirectly by introducing other biopsychosocial risk factors (e.g., cognitive deficits, lack of housing, low social support) (Drake, Wallach, & McGovern, 2005). Some research suggests that relapse antecedents (i.e., high-risk situations) differ for those with dual diagnoses compared to those without such diagnoses (Tate, Brown, Unrod, & Ramo, 2004). Additionally, substance use and other behavior disorders can be reciprocally maintained over time. For example, indicators of conduct disorder in adolescence predict later substance use (Myers, Brown, & Mott, 1995), which in turn can serve to maintain antisocial behavior in adulthood (Hussong, Curran, Moffitt, Caspi, & Carrig, 2004).

Both static and dynamic processes may contribute to relapse among individuals with comorbid disorders. One study of adolescents examined baseline psychiatric diagnoses as well as symptom changes preceding relapses (McCarthy, Tomlinson, Anderson, Marlatt, & Brown, 2005). Proximal symptom severity predicted relapse to certain drugs, and relapse in some cases predicted subsequent psychiatric symptoms, suggesting reciprocal relationships. A similar study with adults also found that relapse tended to exacerbate psychiatric symptoms (Tomlinson, Tate, Anderson, McCarthy, & Brown, 2006). Effects of psychiatric disorders on substance use may also be mediated by cognitive-behavioral constructs. For example, the influence of preadolescent indicators of conduct disorder on substance use may be explained by coping skills and lifestyle factors (Myers et al., 1995). Detailed reviews of theory and interventions for co-occurring disorders are available (Drake, 2005; Mueser et al., 1998).

Neurocognitive and Genetic Factors

Predominating models of health behavior derive largely from social-cognitive perspectives; therefore, an important goal is to augment existing theoretical models by including relevant biological variables (Bryan, Hutchison, Seals, & Allen 2007). Although neurocognitive and genetic factors are historically acknowledged by the RP model, only recently have such variables been studied in relation to relapse and its antecedents. Neurocognitive functioning is relevant to relapse insofar as it can affect one's ability to appraise high-risk situations and enact effective coping responses (Tapert, Brown, Myers, & Granholm, 1999). Prospective research suggests that neurocognitive performance can interact with coping skills to predict relapse (Tapert et al., 1999). Also, recent theory and research suggest that *cognitive control* processes are critical for the ability to resist well-rehearsed, appetitive responses in favor of novel and adaptive behaviors, a concept with clear implications for relapse (Curtin, McCarthy, Piper, & Baker, 2006).

Functional magnetic resonance imaging (fMRI) techniques have been instrumental in identifying neural correlates of substance use. Several studies indicate differential patterns of cue-elicited neural activation among individuals with and without substance use disorders (e.g., Tapert, Brown, Baratta, & Brown, 2004; Tapert et al., 2003). Patterns of neural responding have also been linked to phenomena implicated in drinking behavior, including alcohol expectancies (Anderson, Schweinsburg, Paulus, Brown, & Tapert, 2005), level of response to alcohol (Tapert, Pulido, Paulus, Schuckit, & Burke, 2004), and craving (Hommer, 1999). A recent study of treatment-seeking methamphetamine users provided initial evidence that fMRI can be used to predict relapse (Paulus, Tapert, and Schuckit, 2004). In this study, researchers examined fMRI activation during a decision-making task and obtained information on relapse more than 1 year later. On the basis of activation patterns in several cortical regions, they were able to correctly identify 17 of 18 participants who relapsed and 20 of 22 who did not.

It is likely that distal relapse risk is influenced largely by genetic factors. Accumulating evidence suggests that genetic polymorphisms (variations at a given allele) can influence relapse-related phenomena. Among the genes receiving the most attention to date are the dopamine regulatory genes *DRD4* and *DRD2* and the μ-opioid receptor gene (*OPRM1*). One study found that after exposure to smoking cues, individuals with the long-repeat version of the *DRD4* VNTR polymorphism (*DRD4* L) reported elevated craving and arousal, greater attention to smoking cues, and lower positive affect than those homozygous for the short-repeat version (*DRD4* S) (Hutchison, LaChance, Niaura, Bryan, & Smolen, 2002). Another study linked *DRD4* L to cue-induced craving for food (Sobik, Hutchison, & Craighead, 2005). The *OPRM1* Asp40 allele has been linked to increased alcohol-related craving (van den Wildenberg et al., 2007). Notably, this study found that the Asp40 allele predicted cue-elicited craving among individuals low in baseline craving but not in those high in initial craving, suggesting that tonic craving could interact with genotype to predict phasic responses to drug cues. Collectively, these studies provide a basis for inferring genetic influences on craving in natural contexts.

Genetic variations may also influence relapse by moderating the effects of pharmacotherapy. Olanzapine (a dopamine antagonist) has been found to reduce alcohol-related craving in *DRD4* L individuals but not in *DRD4* S individuals (Hutchison et al., 2003, 2006), and in a randomized trial olanzapine led to significantly improved drinking outcomes in the former but not in the latter group (Hutchison et al., 2006). Studies of pharmacotherapy for smoking have found that *DRD2* variations predict withdrawal symptoms, medication response, and time to relapse (e.g., Lerman et al., 2003). A placebo-controlled trial of naltrexone for alcohol use found that *OPRM1* gene status moderated pharmacotherapeutic response such that individuals with the Asp40 allele had a longer time until the first heavy drinking day and were half as likely to relapse as those homozygous for the Asn40 variant (Oslin et al., 2003). In a study of smoking cessation, those with the Asp40 variant had higher rates of abstinence, less weight gain, and reduced negative affect compared to Asn40 individuals (Lerman et al., 2004). In this study, post hoc analyses indicated that Asp40 carriers were more likely to regain abstinence following a lapse than those without the variant, suggesting a possible role of genotype in predicting prolapse.

In addition to modulating craving and pharmacotherapy response, genetic factors could influence relapse in part via cognitive-affective processes. For instance, variants of the *DRD2* and *GABRB3* genes have been associated with alcohol expectancies and drinking-related self-efficacy (Young, Lawford, Feeney, Ritchie, & Noble, 2004). A study of physical exercise showed that *BDNF* gene variation moderated cognitive and physiological responses during physical exertion and that these responses in turn predicted motivation for future exercise (Bryan et al., 2007). Overall, these findings provide initial evidence that genetic variations can influence health behavior and relapse-related outcomes. Notably, human laboratory studies offer early indication that these variations can influence phasic relapse processes, supporting examination of genetic factors in the context of the dynamic model. Further characterizing the role of neuro-cognitive and genetic factors in relapse stands as an intriguing and important research direction (McKay et al., 2006; Piasecki, 2006), and integration of these factors within existing psychosocial theories will aid in bridging biological and behavioral perspectives on relapse.

Withdrawal

Withdrawal typically develops early in the course of addiction (Baker et al., 2004) and symptom profiles can vary based on stable intra-individual factors (Piasecki, Jorenby, Smith, Fiore, & Baker, 2003), suggesting the involvement of tonic processes. Despite serving as a chief diagnostic criterion, withdrawal often does not predict relapse, perhaps partly explaining its de-emphasis in contem-porary motivational models of addiction (Piasecki et al., 2000). However, recent studies show that withdrawal profiles are complex, multifaceted, and idiosyn-cratic and that, in the context of fine-grained analyses, withdrawal indeed can predict relapse (Piasecki, Fiore, & Baker, 1998; Piasecki et al., 2000). Such find-ings have contributed to renewed interest in negative reinforcement models of drug use (Piasecki et al., 2003).

Although withdrawal is usually viewed as a physiological process, recent theory emphasizes the importance of behavioral withdrawal processes (Baker, Japuntich, Hogle, McCarthy, & Curtin, 2006). Whereas physiological withdrawal symptoms tend to abate in the days or weeks following drug cessation, the un-availability of a conditioned *behavioral* coping response (e.g., the ritual of drug administration) may leave the former user ill equipped to cope with ongoing stressors, thus exacerbating and/or prolonging symptoms (Baker et al., 2006). Current theory and research indicate that physiological components of drug withdrawal may be motivationally inert, with the core motivational constituent of withdrawal being negative affect (Baker et al., 2004, 2006). Thus, examining withdrawal in relation to relapse may only prove useful to the extent that nega-tive affect is assessed adequately (Piasecki et al., 2000).

Outcome Expectancies

Expectancies (anticipated outcomes of a given behavior or experience) are cen-tral to the RP model and have been studied extensively in the domain of alcohol use (Goldman et al., 1999). Alcohol expectancies are shown to anticipate drink-ing initiation (Christiansen, Smith, Roehling, & Goldman, 1989) and to predict drinking prospectively (Sher, Wood, Wood, & Raskin, 1996). Further supporting a causal process, expectancy manipulations can produce changes in drinking behavior (Darkes & Goldman, 1993). In theory, expectancies are shaped by vari-ous distal factors (e.g., environment, culture, personality, genetics) and mediate these antecedent influences on drinking (Goldman et al., 1999). Research sup-ports that expectancies partially mediate influences of personality factors (Katz, Fromme, & D'Amico, 2000), familial risk for alcohol dependence (Sher, Walitzer, Wood, & Brent, 1991), genetic variations (McCarthy et al., 2000), and negative affect (Cohen, McCarthy, Brown, & Myers, 2002) on drinking. Expectancies have been linked to a range of health behaviors and outcomes outside the domain of addictions, including exercise, diet, and HIV symptom progression.

Studies have historically shown that expectancies can undergo changes over long periods (e.g., Sher et al., 1996). However, there is increasing interest in studying dynamic expectancy processes over shorter intervals. One study found that participants engaged in a behavioral intervention for obesity lost more weight during weeks in which outcome expectancies for weight loss were more positive (Carels et al., 2005). In the first study to examine how daily fluctuations in expectancies predict relapse, Gwaltney, Shiffman, Balabanis, & Paty (2005) assessed positive outcome expectancies for smoking (POEs) among participants during a tobacco cessation attempt. Lower POEs on the quit day were associated with greater abstinence likelihood, and POEs decreased in the days following the quit day. Lapses were associated with higher POEs on the preceding day, and, in the days following a lapse, those who avoided a full relapse showed decreases in POEs, whereas those who relapsed did not (Gwaltney, Shiffman, Balabanis, & Paty 2005).

Expectancy research is increasingly focusing on implicit cognitive processes (i.e., those that can operate outside conscious awareness) (Wiers & Stacy, 2006). Implicit measures of alcohol-related cognitions can discriminate among light and heavy drinkers (Kramer & Goldman, 2003) and predict drinking above and beyond explicit measures (McCarthy & Thompsen, 2006). One study found that smokers' attention to tobacco cues predicted early lapses during a quit attempt, but this relationship was not evident among people receiving nicotine replacement therapy, who showed reduced attention to cues (Waters et al., 2003). Research on implicit cognitions stands to enhance understanding of dynamic relapse processes (Curtin et al., 2006) and could ultimately aid in predicting lapses during high-risk situations.

Self-Efficacy

Self-efficacy (SE), the perceived ability to execute a given behavior in a specified context (Bandura, 1997), is a principal determinant of health behavior according to social-cognitive theories. In theory, SE is a fluctuating and dynamic construct (Bandura, 1997). However, most studies rely on static measures of SE, preventing evaluation of within-person changes over time or contexts (Shiffman et al., 2000). Shiffman, Gwaltney, and colleagues have used ecological momentary assessment (EMA; Stone & Shiffman, 1994) to examine temporal variations in SE in relation to smoking relapse. Findings from these studies suggested that participants' SE was lower on the day before a lapse and that lower SE in the days following a lapse in turn predicted progression to relapse (Gwaltney et al., 2005a; Shiffman et al., 2000). One study reported increases in daily SE during abstinent intervals, perhaps indicating mounting confidence as treatment goals were maintained (Gwaltney, Shiffman, Balabanis, & Paty 2005).

The first study to examine relapse in relation to phasic changes in SE (Gwaltney, Shiffman, & Sayette, 2005) found results that appear consistent with the dynamic model of relapse. During a smoking cessation attempt, participants reported on SE, negative affect, and urges at random intervals. Findings indicated nonlinear relationships between SE and urges, such that momentary SE decreased linearly as urges increased but dropped abruptly as urges peaked. Moreover, this finding appeared attributable to individual differences in baseline (tonic) levels of SE. When urge and negative affect were low, individuals with low, intermediate, or high baseline SE were similar in their momentary

SE ratings. However, these groups' momentary ratings diverged significantly at high levels of urges and negative affect, such that those with low baseline SE had large drops in momentary SE in the face of increasingly challenging situations. These findings support that higher distal risk can result in bifurcations (divergent patterns) of behavior as the level of proximal risk factors increase, consistent with predictions from nonlinear dynamic systems theory (e.g., Hufford et al., 2003; Witkiewitz & Marlatt, 2007b).

Negative Affect

A large literature attests to the role of negative affect (NA) in the etiology and maintenance of addictive behaviors. NA is consistently cited as a relapse trigger in retrospective reports (e.g., Marlatt, 1978; Shiffman, Paty, Gnys, Kassel, & Hickcox, 1996a), although participants may sometimes misattribute lapses to negative mood states (Piasecki, 2006; Shiffman et al., 1997). In one study, individuals who were unable to sustain a smoking cessation attempt for more than 24 hours reported greater depressive symptoms and NA in response to stress and displayed less perseverance during experimental stress inductions than did those with a sustained quit attempt (Brown, Lejuez, Kahler, & Strong 2002). Supporting the dynamic influence of NA on relapse, Shiffman and Waters (2004) found that smoking lapses were not associated with NA in the preceding days but were associated with rising NA in the hours leading up to a lapse. Evidence further suggests that negative affect can promote positive outcome expectancies (Cohen et al., 2002) or undermine situational self-efficacy (Gwaltney et al., 2001), outcomes which could in turn promote a lapse. Moreover, Baker and colleagues propose that high levels of negative affect can interfere with controlled cognitive processes, such that adaptive coping and decision making may be undermined as negative affect peaks (Baker et al., 2004; Curtin et al., 2006).

Knowledge about the role of NA in drinking behavior has benefited greatly from daily process studies in which participants provide regular reports of mood and drinking. Such studies have shown that both positive and negative moods show close temporal links to alcohol use (Armeli, Tennen, Affleck, & Kranzler, 2000). Hussong, Hicks, Levy, and Curran (2001) found evidence suggesting a feedback cycle of mood and drinking whereby elevated daily levels of NA predicted alcohol use, which in turn predicted spikes in NA. These findings were moderated by gender, social context, and time of week. Other studies have similarly found that relationships between daily events and/or mood and drinking can vary based on intra-individual or situational factors (Armeli et al., 2000), suggesting dynamic interplay between these influences. Research also indicates that relationships among daily events, mood and drinking are moderated by naltrexone (Armeli, Feinn, Tennen, & Kranzler, 2006). The sophisticated methods evidenced in these studies could serve as a model for researchers investigating the effects of NA on other health behaviors.

Coping Responses and Abstinence Violation Effects

Strengthening coping skills is a goal of virtually all cognitive-behavioral interventions for substance use (Morgenstern & Longabaugh, 2000). Several studies have used ecological momentary assessment (EMA) to examine coping responses in real time. O'Connell, Hosein, Schwartz, and Leibowitz (2007) found that momentary coping differentiated smoking lapses from temptations, such that coping responses were reported in 91% of successful resists but only 24% of lapses. Similarly, a study of dieters found that momentary coping responses distinguished temptations from lapses (Carels, Douglass, Cacciapaglia, & O'Brien, 2004). Shiffman and colleagues (1996b) found that restorative coping following a smoking lapse decreased the likelihood of a second lapse the same day. Exactly how coping responses reduce the likelihood of lapsing remains unclear. One study found that momentary coping reduced urges among smokers, suggesting a possible mechanism (O'Connell et al., 2007). Some studies find that the number of coping responses is more predictive of lapses than the specific type of coping used (Litt, Kadden, & Stephens, 2005; O'Connell et al., 2007). However, despite findings that coping can prevent lapses, there is scant evidence to show that skills-based interventions in fact lead to improved coping (Morgenstern & Longabaugh, 2000).

Several studies have examined abstinence violation effects (AVEs) following lapses. Shiffman and colleagues (1996a) found no evidence for AVEs after smoking lapses, though a subsequent study reported decreased self-efficacy after lapses (Shiffman et al., 2000). A study of binge eating found clear evidence for AVEs, with prospective analyses suggesting that attributing lapses to internal, global causes predicted subsequent binges (Grilo & Shiffman, 1994). Similarly, Carels and colleagues (2004) found evidence for AVEs among women engaged in a weight-loss intervention.

Some researchers propose that the self-control required to maintain behavior change strains motivational resources and that this "fatigue" can undermine subsequent self-control efforts (Muraven & Baumeister, 2000). Consistent with this idea, EMA studies have shown that social drinkers report greater alcohol consumption and violations of self-imposed drinking limits on days when self-control demands are high (Muraven, Collins, Shiffman, & Paty, 2005). Limit violations were predictive of AVE responses the following day, and greater distress about violations in turn predicted greater drinking (Muraven et al., 2005). Findings also suggested that these relationships varied based on individual differences, suggesting the interplay of static and dynamic factors in AVE responses.

Using Nonlinear Methods to Model Relapse

Most studies of relapse rely on statistical methods that assume continuous linear relationships, but these methods may be inadequate for studying a behavior characterized by discontinuity and abrupt changes (Witkiewitz et al., 2007). Several studies suggest advantages of nonlinear statistical approaches for studying relapse. In one, researchers used catastrophe models to examine proximal and distal predictors of posttreatment drinking among individuals with alcohol use disorders (Hufford et al., 2003). Catastrophe models accounted for more than double the amount of variance in drinking than that predicted by linear models. Similar results have been found using the much larger Project MATCH dataset (Witkiewitz & Marlatt, 2007b).

Another recent analysis of the MATCH dataset showed that nonlinear approaches can detect processes that may go unobserved in the context of linear models. Witktiewitz and colleagues (2007) used catastrophe modeling and latent growth mixture modeling to reassess one of the matching hypotheses that was not supported in the original study—that individuals low in baseline self-efficacy would respond more favorably to cognitive-behavioral therapy (CBT) than to motivational enhancement therapy (MET) (Project MATCH Research Group, 1997). Catastrophe models provided the best fit to the data, and latent growth analyses confirmed the predicted interaction: frequent drinkers with low initial self-efficacy had better outcomes in CBT than in MET, while those high in self-efficacy fared better in MET (Witkiewitz et al., 2007).

Critiques of the RP Model

The widespread application of RP in the 1980s and 1990s largely outpaced efforts to systematically validate the model and test its underlying assumptions. Recognizing this limitation, NIAAA sponsored the Relapse Replication and Extension Project (RREP), a multisite study aiming to test the reliability and validity of Marlatt's original relapse taxonomy. Efforts to evaluate the construct validity (Maisto, Connors, & Zywiak, 1996) and predictive validity (Stout, Longabaugh, & Rubin 1996) of the taxonomy failed to generate supportive data. However, these findings were qualified by methodological and conceptual limitations of the RREP. In focusing on the relapse taxonomy, the RREP failed to provide a comprehensive evaluation of the full RP model (Donovan, 1996). Furthermore, the study defined relapse in a way that violates a crucial assumption of the RP model. Whereas RP is designed for individuals making a volitional attempt at behavior change, the RREP made no effort to verify whether periods of abstinence represented voluntary quit attempts. Nevertheless, these studies were useful in identifying limitations and qualifications of the RP taxonomy and generated valuable suggestions for improving the model (Donovan, 1996).

The recently introduced dynamic model of relapse (Witkiewitz & Marlatt, 2004) takes many of the RREP criticisms into account. Still, some have suggested limitations to the revised model. Stanton (2005) criticized the model for not emphasizing interpersonal factors as proximal or phasic influences. Other critiques include that nonlinear dynamic systems approaches are not refined enough to be of clinical utility (McKay et al., 2006) and that the theory and statistical methods characterizing these approaches are too esoteric to be of use for most researchers (Maisto & Connors, 2006). Rather than signaling weaknesses of the model, these issues likely reflect methodological challenges that researchers must overcome in order to better understand dynamic aspects of behavior (e.g., Gwaltney, Shiffman, Balabanis, & Paty 2005).

Future Directions

Characterizing Dynamic Relapse Processes

As the foregoing discussion suggests, researchers are only beginning to evaluate dynamic relapse processes. Currently, the dynamic model can be viewed as a hypothetical, theory-driven framework that awaits empirical evaluation. Testing the model's components will require that researchers avail themselves of innovative assessment techniques (such as EMA) and pursue cross-disciplinary collaboration in order to integrate appropriate statistical methods. It should also be noted that experimental paradigms (e.g., Hutchison et al., 2002, 2003) have shown considerable early promise in identifying dynamic processes relevant for relapse but have likely been underutilized overall. Even sophisticated approaches like EMA cannot effectively address causal relationships in the absence of random assignment. Experiments are therefore necessary to complement correlational studies, which presently dominate the health behavior literature (Weinstein, 2007). Irrespective of study design, greater integration of distal and proximal variables will aid in modeling the interplay of tonic and phasic influences on relapse outcomes.

Mechanisms of Treatment Effects

Elucidating the "active ingredients" of CBT treatments remains an important and challenging goal. Changes in coping skills, self-efficacy, and/or outcome expectancies are the primary putative mechanisms by which CBT-based interventions work (Longabaugh et al., 2005). However, few studies support these presumptions. One study, in which substance-abusing individuals were randomly assigned to RP or 12-step (TS) treatments, found that RP participants showed increased self-efficacy, which accounted for unique variance in outcomes (Brown, Seraganian, Tremblay, and Annis, 2002). Despite isolated findings like this, most studies fail to show that theoretical mediators account for salutary effects of CBT on health behavior, indicating that researchers should strive to consider alternative mechanisms, improve assessment methods, and/or revise theories about how CBT-based interventions work (Litt et al., 2005; Morgenstern & Longabaugh, 2000).

Mindfulness-Based Relapse Prevention

Mindfulness-based intervention approaches are receiving increasing popular and empirical attention (Lau & Segal, 2007). The merging of mindfulness and cognitive-behavioral approaches holds both theoretical and practical appeal; many Buddhist principles are highly compatible with cognitive-behavioral perspectives (Marlatt, 2002), and mindfulness-based interventions can be simple and cost-effective. Mindfulness interventions have been examined in various patient populations, including individuals coping with eating disorders, heart disease, multiple sclerosis, cancer, and HIV. Data supporting the efficacy of mindfulness interventions is growing, particularly in the areas of chronic pain and relapse of depression (Lau & Segal, 2007). Encouraged by these findings, research on mindfulness-based relapse prevention (MBRP) for substance use is gaining momentum. In contrast to cognitive restructuring, MBRP stresses nonjudgmental attention to thoughts or feelings, such that urges and cravings are labeled as transient events that need not be acted upon reflexively. This stance is exemplified by the "urge surfing" technique (Marlatt, 2002), whereby clients are taught to view urges as analogous to an ocean wave that rises, crests, and diminishes. Rather than being overwhelmed by the wave, the goal is to "ride" its crest as if on a surfboard, attending to thoughts and sensations as the urge peaks and invariably subsides. Results from a preliminary, nonrandomized trial at the University of Washington support the potential utility of MBRP for reducing substance use. In this study, incarcerated individuals were offered the chance to participate in an intensive 10-day course in Vipassana meditation (VM); those participating in VM were compared to a treatment-as-usual (TAU) group on measures of postincarceration substance use and psychosocial functioning. At follow-up, the VM group reported significantly lower levels of substance use and alcohol-related consequences, as well as improved psychosocial functioning compared to the TAU group. (Bowen et al., 2006). A larger, randomized trial is currently under way at the University of Washington to evaluate the efficacy of MBRP for substance use.

Conclusion

Relapse prevention is a cognitive-behavioral approach designed to help individuals anticipate and cope with setbacks during the behavior change process. The broad aim of RP, to reduce the incidence and the severity of relapse, subsumes two basic goals: to minimize the impact of high-risk situations through increasing awareness and building coping skills and to limit relapse proneness by promoting a healthy and balanced lifestyle. Given its ideographic approach and emphasis on maintaining treatment gains, RP is applicable to most health behaviors for which there is a need to establish and sustain long-term change. Over the past decade, RP principles have been incorporated across an increasing array of health domains. Many of the model's basic tenets have received support, and findings regarding its clinical effectiveness have generally been supportive. While these developments encourage confidence in the RP model, additional research is needed to test its predictions and limitations and to evaluate its applicability across health behaviors. Continued refinement of the model's theoretical assumptions and clinical applications will further enhance its utility for understanding and facilitating the maintenance of optimal health.

References

Anderson, K. G., Schweinsburg, A., Paulus, M. P., Brown, S. A., & Tapert, S. (2005). Examining personality and alcohol expectancies using functional magnetic resonance imaging (fMRI) with adolescents. *Journal of Studies on Alcohol, 66,* 323–331.

Anton, R. F., O'Malley, S. S., Ciraulo, D. A., Cisler, R. A., Couper, D., Donovan, D. M., et al. (2006). Combined pharmacotherapies and behavioral interventions for alcohol dependence: The combined study: A randomized controlled trial. *Journal of the American Medical Association, 295,* 2003–2017.

Armeli, S., Feinn, R., Tennen, H., & Kranzler, H. R. (2006). The effects of naltrexone on alcohol consumption and affect reactivity to daily interpersonal events among heavy drinkers. *Experimental and Clinical Psychopharmacology, 14,* 199–208.

Armeli, S., Tennen, H., Affleck, G., & Kranzler, H. R. (2000). Does affect mediate the association between daily events and alcohol use? *Journal of Studies on Alcohol, 61,* 862–871.

Baker, T. B., Japuntich, S. J., Hogle, J. M., McCarthy, D. E., & Curtin, J. J. (2006). Pharmacologic and behavioral withdrawal from addictive drugs. *Current Directions in Psychological Science, 15,* 232–236.

Baker, T. B., Piper, M. E., McCarthy, D. E., Majeskie, M. R., & Fiore, M. C. (2004). Addiction motivation reformulated: An affective processing model of negative reinforcement. *Psychological Review, 111,* 33–51.

Bandura, A. (1997). *Self-efficacy: The exercise of control.* New York: Freeman.

Bouton, M. E. (2000). A learning theory perspective on lapse, relapse, and the maintenance of behavior change. *Health Psychology, 19*(Suppl 1), 57–63.

Bowen, S., Witkiewitz, K., Dillworth, T. M., Chawla, N., Simpson, T. L., Ostafin, B. D., et al. (2006). Mindfulness meditation and substance use in an incarcerated population. *Psychology of Addictive Behaviors, 20,* 343–347.

Brandon, T. H., Collins, B. N., Juliano, L. M., & Lazev, A. B. (2000). Preventing relapse among former smokers: A comparison of minimal interventions through telephone and mail. *Journal of Consulting and Clinical Psychology, 68,* 103–113.

Brown, R. A., Lejuez, C. W., Kahler, C. W., & Strong, D. R. (2002). Distress tolerance and duration of past smoking cessation attempts. *Journal of Abnormal Psychology, 111,* 180–185.

Brown, T. G., Seraganian, P., Tremblay, J., & Annis, H. (2002). Process and outcome changes with relapse prevention versus 12-step aftercare programs for substance abusers. *Addiction, 97,* 677–689.

Brownell, K. D., Marlatt, G. A., Lichtenstein, E., & Wilson, G. T. (1986). Understanding and preventing relapse. *American Psychologist, 41,* 765–782.

Bryan, A., Hutchison, K. E., Seals, D. R., & Allen, D. L. (2007). A transdisciplinary model integrating genetic, physiological, and psychological correlates of voluntary exercise. *Health Psychology, 26,* 30–39.

Carels, R. A., Darby, L. A., Rydin, S., Douglass, O. M., Cacciapaglia, H. M., & O'Brien, W. H. (2005). The relationship between self-monitoring, outcome expectancies, difficulties with eating and exercise, and physical activity and weight loss treatment outcomes. *Annals of Behavioral Medicine, 30,* 182–190.

Carels, R. A., Douglass, O. M., Cacciapaglia, H. M., & O'Brien, W. H. (2004). An ecological momentary assessment of relapse crises in dieting. *Journal of Consulting and Clinical Psychology, 72,* 341–348.

Carroll, K. M. (1996). Relapse prevention as a psychosocial treatment: A review of controlled clinical trials. *Experimental and Clinical Psychopharmacology, 4,* 46–54.

Christiansen, B. A., Smith, G. T., Roehling, P. V., & Goldman, M. S. (1989). Using alcohol expectancies to predict adolescent drinking behavior after one year. *Journal of Consulting and Clinical Psychology, 57,* 93–99.

Cohen, L. M., McCarthy, D. M., Brown, S. A., & Myers, M. G. (2002). Negative affect combines with smoking outcome expectancies to predict smoking behavior over time. *Psychology of Addictive Behaviors, 16,* 91–97.

Cummings, C., Gordon, J. R., & Marlatt, G. A. (1980). Relapse: Strategies of prevention and prediction. In W. R. Miller (Ed.), *The addictive behaviors: Treatment of alcoholism, drug abuse, smoking, and obesity* (pp. 291–321). Oxford: Pergamon.

Curtin, J. J., McCarthy, D. E., Piper, M. E., & Baker, T. B. (2006). Implicit and explicit drug motivational processes: A model of boundary conditions. In R. W. Wiers & A. W. Stacy (Eds.), *Handbook of implicit cognition and addiction* (pp. 233–250). Thousand Oaks, CA: Sage.

Darkes, J., & Goldman, M. S. (1993). Expectancy challenge and drinking reduction: Experimental evidence for a mediational process. *Journal of Consulting and Clinical Psychology, 61,* 344–353.

Dimeff, L. A., & Marlatt, G. A. (1998). Preventing relapse and maintaining change in addictive behaviors. *Clinical Psychology: Science and Practice, 5,* 513–525.

Donovan, D. M. (1996). Marlatt's classification of relapse precipitants: Is the emperor still wearing clothes? *Addiction, 91,* S131–S137.

Donovan, D. M., & Marlatt, G. A. (Eds.) (2005). *Assessment of addictive behaviors* (2nd ed.). New York: Guilford Press.

Drake, R. E. (2005). Section special section on relapse prevention: Introduction to the special section. *Psychiatric Services, 56,* 1269.

Drake, R. E., Wallach, M. A., & McGovern, M. P. (2005). Future directions in preventing relapse to substance abuse among clients with severe mental illnesses. *Psychiatric Services, 56,* 1297–1302.

Goldman, M. S., Darkes, J., & Del Boca, F. K. (1999). Expectancy mediation of biopsychosocial risk for alcohol use and alcoholism. In I. Kirsch (Ed.), *How expectancies shape experience* (pp. 233–262). Washington, DC: American Psychological Association.

Grilo, C. M., & Shiffman, S. (1994). Longitudinal investigation of the abstinence violation effect in binge eaters. *Journal of Consulting and Clinical Psychology, 62,* 611–619.

Gwaltney, C. J., Shiffman, S., Normal, G. J., Paty, J. A., Kassel, J. D., Gnys, M., et al. (2001). Does smoking abstinence self-efficacy vary across situations? Identifying context-specificity within the relapse situation efficacy questionnaire. *Journal of Consulting and Clinical Psychology, 69,* 516–527.

Gwaltney, C. J., Shiffman, S., Balabanis, M. H., & Paty, J. A. (2005). Dynamic self-efficacy and outcome expectancies: Prediction of smoking lapse and relapse. *Journal of Abnormal Psychology, 114,* 661–675.

Gwaltney, C. J., Shiffman, S., & Sayette, M. A. (2005). Situational correlates of abstinence self-efficacy. *Journal of Abnormal Psychology, 114,* 649–660.

Hommer, D. W. (1999). Functional imaging of craving. *Alcohol Research & Health, 23,* 187–196.

Hufford, M. R., Witkiewitz, K., Shields, A. L., Kodya, S., & Caruso, J. C. (2003). Relapse as a nonlinear dynamic system: Application to patients with alcohol use disorders. *Journal of Abnormal Psychology, 112,* 219–227.

Hussong, A. M., Curran, P. J., Moffitt, T. E., Caspi, A., & Carrig, M. M. (2004). Substance abuse hinders desistance in young adults' antisocial behavior. *Development and Psychopathology, 16,* 1029–1046.

Hussong, A. M., Hicks, R. E., Levy, S. A., & Curran, P. J. (2001). Specifying the relations between affect and heavy alcohol use among young adults. *Journal of Abnormal Psychology, 110,* 449–461.

Hutchison, K. E., LaChance, H., Niaura, R., Bryan, A., & Smolen, A. (2002). The DRD4 VNTR polymorphism influences reactivity to smoking cues. *Journal of Abnormal Psychology, 111,* 134–143.

Hutchison, K. E., Ray, L., Sandman, E., Rutter, M.-C., Peters, A., Davidson, D., et al. (2006). The effect of olanzapine on craving and alcohol consumption. *Neuropsychopharmacology, 31,* 1310–1317.

Hutchison, K. E., Wooden, A., Swift, R. M., Smolen, A., McGeary, J., Adler, L., et al. (2003). Olanzapine reduces craving for alcohol: A DRD4 VNTR polymorphism by pharmacotherapy interaction. *Neuropsychopharmacology, 28,* 1882–1888.

Irvin, J. E., Bowers, C. A., Dunn, M. E., & Wang, M. C. (1999). Efficacy of relapse prevention: A meta-analytic review. *Journal of Consulting and Clinical Psychology, 67,* 563–570.

Katz, E. C., Fromme, K., & D'Amico, E. J. (2000). Effects of outcome expectancies and personality on young adults' illicit drug use, heavy drinking, and risky sexual behavior. *Cognitive Therapy and Research, 24,* 1–22.

Kramer, D. A., & Goldman, M. S. (2003). Using a modified Stroop task to implicitly discern the cognitive organization of alcohol expectancies. *Journal of Abnormal Psychology, 112,* 171–175.

Larimer, M. E., Palmer, R. S., & Marlatt, G. A. (1999). Relapse prevention: An overview of Marlatt's cognitive-behavioral model. *Alcohol Research & Health, 23,* 151–160.

Lau, M.A., & Segal, Z.V. (2007). Mindfulness-based cognitive therapy as a relapse prevention approach to depression. In K. Witkiewitz & G. A. Marlatt (Eds.), *Therapist's guide to evidence-based relapse prevention.* London: Academic Press.

Lerman, C., Shields, P. G., Wileyto, E. P., Audrain, J., Hawk, L. H., Jr., Pinto, A., et al. (2003). Effects of dopamine transporter and receptor polymorphisms on smoking cessation in a bupropion clinical trial. *Health Psychology, 22,* 541–548.

Lerman, C., Wileyto, E. P., Patterson, F., Rukstalis, M., Audrain-McGovern, J., et al. (2004). The functional mu opioid receptor (OPRM1) Asn40Asp variant predicts short-term response to nicotine replacement therapy in a clinical trial. *Pharmacogenetics Journal, 4,* 184–192.

Litt, M. D., Kadden, R. M., & Stephens, R. S. (2005). Coping and self-efficacy in marijuana treatment: Results from the Marijuana Treatment Project. *Journal of Consulting and Clinical Psychology, 73,* 1015–1025.

Longabaugh, R., Donovan, D. M., Karno, M. P., McCrady, B. S., Morgenstern, J., & Tonigan, J. S. (2005). Active ingredients: How and why evidence-based alcohol behavioral treatment interventions work. *Alcoholism: Clinical and Experimental Research, 29,* 235–247.

Maisto, S. A., & Connors, G. J. (2006). Relapse in the addictive behaviors: Integration and future directions. *Clinical Psychology Review, 26,* 229–231.

Maisto, S. A., Connors, G. J., & Zywiak, W. H. (1996). Construct validation analyses on the Marlatt typology of relapse precipitants. *Addiction, 91,* S89-S97.

Marlatt, G. A. (1978) Craving for alcohol, loss of control, and relapse: A cognitive-behavioral analysis. In P. E. Nathan, G. A. Marlatt, & T. Loberg (Eds.), *Alcoholism: New directions in behavioral research and treatment* (pp. 271–314). New York: Plenum.

Marlatt, G. A. (1982). Relapse prevention: A self-control program for the treatment of addictive behaviors. In R. B. Stuart (Ed.), *Adherence, compliance, and generalization in behavioral medicine* (pp. 329–378). New York: Brunner/Mazel.

Marlatt, G. A. (1996). Taxonomy of high-risk situations for alcohol relapse: Evolution and development of a cognitive-behavioral model. *Addiction, 91,* S37–S49.

Marlatt, G. A. (2002). Buddhist philosophy and the treatment of addictive behavior. *Cognitive and Behavioral Practice, 9,* 44–49.

Marlatt, G. A., & Donovan, D. M. (Eds.) (2005). *Relapse prevention: Maintenance strategies in the treatment of addictive behaviors* (2nd ed.). New York: Guilford.

Marlatt, G. A., & George, W. H. (1984). Relapse prevention: Introduction and overview of the model. *British Journal of Addiction, 79,* 261–273.

Marlatt, G. A., & George, W. H. (1998). Relapse prevention and the maintenance of optimal Health. In S. A. Shumaker, E. B. Schron, J. K. Ockene, & W. L. McBee (Eds.), *The handbook of health behavior change* (2nd ed.). New York: Springer Publishing Company.

Marlatt, G. A., & Gordon, J. R. (1980). Determinants of relapse: Implications for the maintenance of behavior change. In P. O. Davidson & S. M. Davidson (Eds.), *Behavioral medicine: Changing health lifestyles* (pp. 410–452). New York: Brunner/Mazel.

Marlatt, G. A., & Gordon, J. R. (Eds.). (1985*). Relapse prevention: Maintenance strategies in the treatment of addictive behaviors.* New York: Guilford Press.

McCarthy, D. M., & Thompsen, D. M. (2006). Implicit and explicit measures of alcohol and smoking cognitions. *Psychology of Addictive Behaviors, 20,* 436–444.

McCarthy, D. M., Tomlinson, K. L., Anderson, K. G., Marlatt, G. A., & Brown, S. A. (2005). Relapse in alcohol- and drug-disordered adolescents with comorbid psychopathology: Changes in psychiatric symptoms. *Psychology of Addictive Behaviors, 19,* 28–34.

McCarthy, D. M., Wall, T. L., Brown, S. A., & Carr, L. G. (2000). Integrating biological and behavioral factors in alcohol use risk: The role of ALDH2 status and alcohol expectancies in a sample of Asian Americans. *Experimental and Clinical Psychopharmacology, 8,* 168–175.

McGovern, M. P., Wrisley, B. R., & Drake, R. E. (2005). Relapse of substance use disorder and its prevention among persons with co-occurring disorders. *Psychiatric Services, 56,* 1270–1273.

McKay, J. R., Franklin, T. R., Patapis, N., & Lynch, K. G. (2006). Conceptual, methodological, and analytical issues in the study of relapse. *Clinical Psychology Review, 26,* 109–127.

Morgenstern, J., & Longabaugh, R. (2000). Cognitive-behavioral treatment for alcohol dependence: A review of evidence for its hypothesized mechanisms of action. *Addiction, 95,* 1475–1490.

Mueser, K. T., Drake, R. E., & Wallach, M. A. (1998). Dual diagnosis: A review of etiological theories. *Addictive Behaviors, 23,* 717–734.

Muraven, M., & Baumeister, R. F. (2000). Self-regulation and depletion of limited resources: Does self-control resemble a muscle? *Psychological Bulletin, 126,* 247–259.

Muraven, M., Collins, R. L., Morsheimer, E. T., Shiffman, S., & Paty, J. A. (2005). The morning after: Limit violations and the self-regulation of alcohol consumption. *Psychology of Addictive Behaviors, 19,* 253–262.

Muraven, M., Collins, R. L., Shiffman, S., & Paty, J. A. (2005). Daily fluctuations in self-control demands and alcohol intake. *Psychology of Addictive Behaviors, 19,* 140–147.

Myers, M. G., Brown, S. A., & Mott, M. A. (1995). Preadolescent conduct disorder behaviors predict relapse and progression of addiction for adolescent alcohol and drug abusers. *Alcoholism: Clinical and Experimental Research, 19,* 1528–1536.

O'Connell, K. A., Hosein, V. L., Schwartz, J. E., & Leibowitz, R. Q. (2007). How does coping help people resist lapses during smoking cessation? *Health Psychology, 26,* 77–84.

Orleans, C. T. (2000). Promoting the maintenance of health behavior change: Recommendations for the next generation of research and practice. *Health Psychology, 19,* 76–83.

Oslin, D. W., Berrettini, W., Kranzler, H. R., Pettinati, H., Gelernter, J., Volpicelli, J. R., et al. (2003). A functional polymorphism of the μ-opioid receptor gene is associated with naltrexone response in alcohol-dependent patients. *Neuropsychopharmacology, 28,* 1546–1552.

Paulus, M. P., Tapert, S. F., & Schuckit, M. A. (2004). Neural activation patterns of methamphetamine-dependent subjects during decision making predict relapse. *Archives of General Psychiatry, 62,* 761–768.

Piasecki, T. M. (2006). Relapse to smoking. *Clinical Psychology Review, 26,* 196–215.

Piasecki, T. M., Fiore, M. C., & Baker, T. B. (1998). Profiles in discouragement: Two studies of variability in the time course of smoking withdrawal symptoms. *Journal of Abnormal Psychology, 107,* 238–251.

Piasecki, T. M., Jorenby, D. E., Smith, S. S., Fiore, M. C., & Baker, T. B. (2003). Smoking withdrawal dynamics: III. Correlates of withdrawal heterogeneity. *Experimental and Clinical Psychopharmacology, 11,* 276–285.

Piasecki, T. M., Niaura, R., Shadel, W. G., Abrams, D., Goldstein, M., Fiore, M. C., et al. (2000). Smoking withdrawal dynamics in unaided quitters. *Journal of Abnormal Psychology, 109,* 74–86.

Polivy, J., & Herman, C. P. (2002). If at first you don't succeed: False hopes of self-change. *American Psychologist, 57,* 677–689.

Project MATCH Research Group. (1997). Matching alcoholism treatments to client heterogeneity: Project MATCH posttreatment drinking outcomes. *Journal of Studies on Alcohol, 58,* 7–29.

Rothman, A. J. (2000). Toward a theory-based analysis of behavioral maintenance. *Health Psychology, 19,* 64–69.

Sher, K. J., Walitzer, K. S., Wood, P. K., & Brent, E. E. (1991). Characteristics of children of Alcoholics: Putative risk-factors, substance use and abuse, and psychopathology. *Journal of Abnormal Psychology, 100,* 427–448.

Sher, K. J., Wood, M. D., Wood, P. K., & Raskin, G. (1996). Alcohol outcome expectancies and alcohol use: A latent variable cross-lagged panel study. *Journal of Abnormal Psychology, 105,* 561–574.

Shiffman, S., Balabanis, M. H., Paty, J. A., Engberg, J., Gwaltney, C. J., Liu, K. S., et al. (2000). Dynamic effects of self-efficacy on smoking lapse and relapse. *Health Psychology, 19,* 315–323.

Shiffman, S., Hickcox, M., Paty, J. A., Gnys, M., Kassel, J. D., & Richards, T. J. (1996b). Progression from a smoking lapse to relapse: Prediction from abstinence violation effects, nicotine dependence, and lapse characteristics. *Journal of Consulting and Clinical Psychology, 64,* 993–1002.

Shiffman, S., Hufford, M., Hickcox, M., Paty, J. A., Gnys, M., & Kassel, J. D. (1997). Remember that? A comparison of real-time versus retrospective recall of smoking lapses. *Journal of Consulting and Clinical Psychology, 65,* 292–300.

Shiffman, S., Paty, J. A., Gnys, M., Kassel, J. A., & Hickcox, M. (1996a). First lapses to smoking: Within-subjects analysis of real-time reports. *Journal of Consulting and Clinical Psychology, 64,* 366–379.

Shiffman, S., & Waters, A. J. (2004). Negative affect and smoking lapses: A prospective analysis. *Journal of Consulting and Clinical Psychology, 72,* 192–201.

Shumaker, S. A., Schron, E. B., Ockene, J. K., & McBee, W. L. (Eds.) (1998). *The handbook of health behavior change* (2nd ed.). New York: Springer Publishing Company.

Sobik, L., Hutchison, K., & Craighead, L. (2005). Cue-elicited craving for food: A fresh approach to the study of binge eating. *Appetite, 44,* 253–261.

Stanton, M. (2005). Relapse prevention needs more emphasis on interpersonal factors. *American Psychologist, 60,* 340–341.

Stone, A. A., & Shiffman, S. (1994). Ecological momentary assessment (EMA) in behavorial medicine. *Annals of Behavioral Medicine, 16,* 199–202.

Stout, R. L., Longabaugh, R., & Rubin, A. (1996). Predictive validity of Marlatt's relapse taxonomy versus a more general relapse code. *Addiction, 91,* S99-S110.

Tapert, S. F., Brown, G. G., Baratta, M. V., & Brown, S. A. (2004). FMRI bold response to alcohol stimuli in alcohol dependent young women. *Addictive Behaviors, 29,* 33–50.

Tapert, S. F., Brown, S. A., Myers, M. G., & Granholm, E. (1999). The role of neurocognitive abilities in coping with adolescent relapse to alcohol and drug use. *Journal of Studies on Alcohol, 60,* 500–508.

Tapert, S. F., Pulido, C., Paulus, M. P., Schuckit, M. A., & Burke, C. (2004). Level of response to alcohol and brain response during visual working memory. *Journal of Studies on Alcohol, 65,* 692–700.

Tapert, S. F., Schweinsburg, A.D., Barlett, V. C., Brown, S. A., Frank, L. R., Brown, G. G., et al. (2004). Blood oxygen level dependent response and spatial working memory in adolescents with alcohol use disorders. *Alcoholism: Clinical and Experimental Research, 28,* 1577–1586.

Tate, S. R., Brown, S. A., Unrod, M., & Ramo, D. E. (2004). Context of relapse for substance-dependent adults with and without comorbid psychiatric disorders. *Addictive Behaviors, 29,* 1707–1724.

Tomlinson, K. L., Tate, S. R., Anderson, K. G., McCarthy, D. M., & Brown, S. A. (2006). An examination of self-medication and rebound effects: Psychiatric symptomatology before and after alcohol or drug relapse. *Addictive Behaviors, 31,* 461–474.

van den Wildenberg, E., Wiers, R. W., Dessers, J., Janssen, R. G. J. H., Lambrichs, E. H., Smeets, H. J. M., et al. (2007). A functional polymorphism of the μ-opioid receptor gene (OPRM1) influences cue-induced craving for alcohol in male heavy drinkers. *Alcoholism: Clinical and Experimental Research, 31,* 1–10.

Waters, A. J., Shiffman, S., Sayette, M. A., Paty, J. A., Gwaltney, C. J., & Balabanis, M. H. (2003). Attentional bias predicts outcome in smoking cessation. *Health Psychology, 22,* 378–387.

Weinstein, N. D. (2007). Misleading tests of health behavior theories. *Annals of Behavioral Medicine, 33,* 1–10.

Wiers, R. W., & Stacy, A. W. (Eds.) (2006). *Handbook of implicit cognition and addiction.* Thousand Oaks, CA: Sage.

Witkiewitz, K., & Marlatt, G. A. (2004). Relapse prevention for alcohol and drug problems: That was Zen, this is Tao. *American Psychologist, 59,* 224–235.

Witkiewitz, K., & Marlatt, G. A. (Eds.) (2007a). *Therapist's guide to evidence-based relapse prevention.* London: Academic Press.

Witkiewitz, K., & Marlatt, G. A. (2007b). Modeling the complexity of post-treatment drinking: It's a rocky road to relapse. *Clinical Psychology Review, 27,* 724–738.

Witkiewitz, K., van der Maas, H. L. J., Hufford, M. R., & Marlatt, G. A. (2007). Nonnormality and divergence in posttreatment alcohol use: Reexamining the project MATCH data "another way." *Journal of Abnormal Psychology, 116,* 378–394.

Young, R. M., Lawford, B. R., Feeney, G. F. X., Ritchie, T., & Noble, E. P. (2004). Alcohol-related expectancies are associated with the D₂ dopamine receptor and GABAA receptor ß3 subunit genes. *Psychiatry Research, 127,* 171–183.

Motivational Interviewing

8

Claire A. Lane and
Stephen Rollnick

Patients usually understand that they need to make changes to improve their health, yet time and again they return to see their clinicians having not implemented any of the changes discussed in the consultation. Others may choose not to return, feeling that they have failed and thinking that they "cannot face another lecture" about what they should be doing. For these reasons, talking with patients about making changes to the unhealthier aspects of their lifestyles can often be a difficult, sometimes frustrating experience.

This chapter provides an overview of Motivational Interviewing (MI) (Miller and Rollnick, 2002). Following some background information about the situations in which MI might be useful, the rationale behind the method is described, and examples of how MI can be incorporated into clinical practice are provided. The evidence that MI can facilitate behavior change also is discussed.

Ambivalence in Health Behavior Change

Before addressing MI, it is important to consider one reason why behavior change may be challenging (for practitioners and patients alike) within health care settings. In many cases, patients may be ambivalent about making changes to their lifestyles.

What Is Ambivalence?

In relation to behavior change, the term "ambivalence" refers to the notion of having mixed feelings and therefore feeling unsure or indecisive. Many people can think of a time in their lives when they have had to make a decision and have felt torn between taking one course of action or another. This may have led to feelings of inner conflict about which course of action is the best or a sense of hopelessness when neither path seems to lead to a satisfactory outcome—"I'm damned if I do, and I'm damned if I don't."

Discussions About Behavior Change
With Ambivalent Patients

Many clinicians consult with ambivalent patients on a daily basis. Most can see the damage patients are doing to themselves through behaviors such as smoking, drinking too much alcohol, eating unhealthy foods, and not getting enough exercise. It is natural to want to stop patients from taking part in these harmful activities—after all, it is often the desire to help and to improve the health of others that draws people into careers in health care in the first place. The practitioner may try to persuade patients to live a healthier life by telling them about the damage a particular behavior is doing to their body and in turn prescribing a course of action to "rescue" them from such harm.

If the patient does not implement the advice that has been given to them, it is understandable that the clinician may feel a number of different emotions—ranging from worry and concern, through to frustration and helplessness. Many may feel that the patient is apathetic about his health or is unmotivated.

In reality, however, the patient may feel several different ways about making those changes. They can see how changing will be beneficial to their health and will improve their overall quality of life. Conversely, however, they may also see that it will be hard to change. Such changes may affect other family members and have a perceived negative impact on their social life. They may not enjoy some of the things they have been told they should do or feel unhappy about giving up a behavior that until now has been pleasurable or enjoyable. This is the essence of ambivalence about making changes to health behaviors, which often makes the decision to change a difficult one.

Readiness, Importance, and Confidence

For change to occur, patients need to be ready, willing, and able to make the change (Miller & Rollnick, 2002).

The first question to ask is how ready the patient is to make changes to her lifestyle. Is changing her behavior her number one priority, or are there more pressing issues in her life at the moment? (For further discussion on readiness, please see the chapter "The Transtheoretical Model of Behavior Change.") The next question that needs to be asked is how willing the patient is to make changes to her lifestyle? Does she want to make changes, or is she happy to remain as she is (importance)? One final question concerns how able the patient feels to succeed with these changes (confidence)? Does she truly believe she can make the changes she needs to make? The importance of these two questions has been illustrated by one study that involved interviews with smokers in a primary-care setting (Rollnick, Butler, & Stott, 1997). The researchers asked smokers how ready they were to make changes to their smoking and asked them if they could describe what factors influenced their readiness. *Importance* (or "willingness") and *confidence* (or "ability") were two major themes that emerged in this data in regard to readiness. This supports other research in the field (Keller & White, 1997), showing that, in general, if importance and confidence are both high, the patient will feel more ready to make changes. If importance and confidence are both low, the patient will not feel at all ready to make changes. If importance and confidence are somewhere in between high and low, or if one factor is high but the other is low, the patient is likely to be *ambivalent* about making changes. Having the confidence to achieve change is recognized as a major factor in making lifestyle changes. If an individual believes she cannot change, she may not even try (Bandura, 1995).

Motivation

In the guidelines developed within Motivational Interviewing, the degree of importance and confidence individuals attribute to making changes can influence how motivated they are to change (Rollnick et al., 1997). Most practitioners recognize that some patients are more motivated than others and that this apparent motivation is related to whether they succeed in changing their lifestyle. The more patients increases the weight they allocate to the importance of changing, and the greater their confidence about making changes, the more motivated they will be (Rollnick, Mason, & Butler, 1999). Motivational Interviewing incorporates a number of skills that a practitioner can utilize in helping patients explore their own reasons for why they might make changes. These are described later in the chapter.

Resistance

Resistance to change is often seen by health care providers as the patient being difficult. It is often associated with concrete behaviors that the patient may exhibit in the consulting room, such as denial, arguing, objecting, disengagement, defensiveness, and reluctance. Most clinicians can recall a patient who claims that his great uncle smoked until he was 107 years old and was never ill, presenting this as a rationale for refusing to give up smoking.

Why does this resistance occur? Both the patient and the practitioner can contribute to the degree of resistance encountered. Patients may feel under pressure to change their behavior before they even enter the consulting room and may perceive talking about such issues to be a threat. Equally, other patients may not object to talking about these matters in the clinical environment but may become resistant if the topic is dealt with insensitively. Perhaps the practitioner has wrongly assumed that the patient is more ready to make changes than he actually is.

In either case, resistance should be a signal to practitioners that the rapport they have with the patient has broken down. Confrontational behavior is likely to worsen this relationship and in turn lead to an increase in resistance. A skillful practitioner can take measures to reduce resistance in the consultation, should it occur, by avoiding confrontation or by "rolling with the resistance." This is discussed in more detail later.

Communication Styles and the Role of Guiding

How does a method like Motivational Interviewing fit into the everyday practice of a psychologist, counselor, nurse, or other health care practitioner? One answer to this question lies in the recent construction of a simple three-styles model for understanding how practitioners approach problem-solving in everyday practice (Rollnick et al., 2007):

- Directing
- Guiding
- Following

Practitioners, it seems, shift quite naturally between the three styles according to need. A *directing* style is widely used in health and social work to solve problems. It involves the delivery of expert advice and help and, done skillfully, is well timed, personally relevant, and based on good rapport with the patient or client. A *following* style is also used naturally in many situations, for example, when responding to someone who is upset. Listening is a core skill here, where the agenda of the practitioner is not to solve a problem immediately but to follow the other as a means of providing support and encouragement. Breaking bad news is probably the most common scenario in health care which this style is used. A third, perhaps less well-used style is *guiding*, where the two parties work collaboratively to help the patient identify solutions to a problem. It's this style that is particularly well suited to addressing problems like skill acquisition or difficult health behavior change challenges, and this is where Motivational Interviewing fits in; it has been defined as a refined form of guiding, enabling practitioners to understand how it might fit into their everyday practice. Shifting between styles according to need is a marker of skillfulness, and a focus on guiding when it comes to health behavior change is likely to be most effective.

Motivational Interviewing

Motivational Interviewing is "a client-centered, directive style for enhancing intrinsic motivation to change by exploring and resolving ambivalence" (Miller and Rollnick, 2002). It evolved from the work of the psychologist Carl Rogers (Rogers, 1959) on the client-centered counseling framework. In delivering psychotherapy to his patients, Rogers found that his clients often had improved results if he listened more and allowed them to determine the rate of treatment.

In turn, he believed that a flexible attitude to treatment was important. By encouraging clients to be self-aware and to make independent choices, he enabled them to gain a better understanding of the problem at hand.

MI is similar to the client-centered counseling framework in that it "does not focus on teaching new coping skills, reshaping cognitions or excavating the past. It is quite focused on the person's present interests and concerns. Whatever discrepancies are explored and developed have to do with incongruities among aspects of the person's own experiences and values" (Miller & Rollnick, 2002, p. 25). Motivation for change is drawn from the client, rather than imposed. However, MI differs from the client-centered counseling framework in that it is purposely directive in nature: "Motivational interviewing involves selective responding to speech in a way that resolves ambivalence and moves the person toward change" (Miller & Rollnick, 2002, p. 25). It has thus been described as a refined form of the naturally used guiding style (Rollnick et al., 2007).

Why Might MI Help With Ambivalent Patients?

Miller and Rollnick (2002) argue that as ambivalence can be a barrier to making changes, resolving ambivalence can in turn be a key to change. Instead of approaching patients as individuals who do not want to change, MI focuses on trying to elicit what patients do want and how they think they might be able to achieve it.

Background

MI has traditionally been conducted within specialist, help-seeking clinical settings, with consultation times ranging from approximately 30 minutes to an hour in length. In recent times, however, MI has been adapted for use in briefer consultations in a range of other environments, including general health care.

When patients are talking about their ambivalence, they are likely to produce two main kinds of talk regarding changing their behavior. If patients talk about the costs of changing their behavior or the benefits of not changing, this is referred to as *sustain talk*. On the other hand, they may produce *change talk*, which is talk about the benefits of changing their behavior or the costs of not changing. In using MI, the practitioner uses a number of skills to encourage the production of patient change talk, which in turn helps patients increase their motivation to change their behavior. This is accomplished through a variety of means, such as asking open-ended questions, making summaries, and skillfully using reflective listening to both express empathy and to direct the patient in producing change talk. This does not mean however, that sustain talk is avoided in MI. Patient autonomy is respected throughout, and sustain talk is accepted as part of the process of exploring ambivalence to change. However, unlike change talk, sustain talk is not purposely elicited by the practitioner.

One common misconception about MI is that it is a set of techniques that can be inflicted on a patient without genuine empathy and understanding. MI is a clinical skill, rather than a tool. To further define the nature of MI, Miller and Rollnick (2002) describe the *spirit* of MI (or a "way of being" with a patient), and present four *principles* (or "conventions guiding practice") behind the method.

Spirit

MI spirit is divided into three components. These are:

- Collaboration
- Evocation
- Autonomy

Collaboration refers to the patient and practitioner working together in partnership, not against each other (for example, with the practitioner advocating for change and the patient arguing why change is not a good idea). *Evocation* describes the process whereby the practitioner elicits the patient's goals, thoughts, and feelings about behavior change, rather than providing information as to how and what the patient should feel about change. *Autonomy* signifies the practitioner's respect for the patient's rights as an individual. Patients know their own mind and should be allowed to choose what to do about their behavior—there is recognition that any changes that patients do decide to make are entirely their choice and that the practitioner is not there to force them to do anything. Should the patient decide that he does not want to make any changes to his behavior, the practitioner in turn has to respect this decision.

Principles

The four principles to be followed while conducting MI are as follows:

1. Express empathy
2. Roll with resistance
3. Support self-efficacy
4. Develop discrepancy

Expressing empathy describes how the practitioner should demonstrate her understanding of the patient's perspective. This is mainly achieved through the use of active, reflective listening techniques, which demonstrate that the practitioner understands what the patient has told her (for example, "It sounds like you have had enough of people telling you what you should do"). *Rolling with resistance* is the approach taken to avoid confrontation with a patient. It could be described as "going along with what the patient says for a bit" while demonstrating understanding of the resistance as a means of reducing it (for example, "You think I'm going to try to force you to do things you're not happy with"). As well as eliciting the patient's motivation to change, the practitioner should *support* the patient's *self-efficacy* (a person's belief that he has the ability to do something) and build on the patient's confidence in achieving change without telling him what to do (for example, "So, despite finding it really tough this week, you've still managed to lose a few pounds. That must feel pretty good"). *Developing discrepancy* is the most complex of the principles underlying Motivational Interviewing. It requires the practitioner to listen carefully to what patients say about their personal values and to illustrate how this is at odds with their current behavior. This is often achieved by highlighting how the behavior in question does not fit in with patients' perception of how they would like to be (for example "So, on the one hand, smoking is a big thing in your life, and you can't imagine not doing it. Yet you love your family, and you hate feeling that you are letting them down by smoking").

Using an MI Approach to Health Behavior Change

As mentioned earlier, MI is a clinical skill, rather than a set of magic-bullet techniques for making people change. When using an MI approach to discuss health behavior change with a patient, it is important to remember the following.

You Cannot *Make* Somebody Change

The decision to change lies ultimately with the individual. A practitioner cannot force a patient to change. That decision is, and always will be, the patient's to make. As Pascal noted, "People are generally better persuaded by the reasons which they themselves discovered, than by those which have come into the mind of others" (Pascal, 1623–1662). Theories such as "reactance theory" suggest that trying to take away another person's personal choice may have a counteractive effect and may indeed motivate patients to choose to perform the behavior they are being told not to do (Brehm, 1966). This can also increase the degree of resistance encountered in the consultation. Reasons for change should be elicited from, rather than imposed on, the patient.

The Patient Is the Expert

Closely related to the preceding point is the idea that patients are the ones who are considering making changes. They know best about what changes they feel they are able to make, what changes will fit in with their life, and how to cope in difficult situations. This therefore puts them in the role of the expert in changing their own behavior. If patients can find ways in which they can make small changes and can imagine doing this in their daily lives, this may in turn help them to succeed (Bem, 1972).

Establish a Good Rapport

If the practitioner builds a good rapport with patients, helping them to feel at ease to talk about their behavior, free of coercion and judgment, patients will find it easier to explore and resolve their ambivalence about change.

Dance, Don't Wrestle!

MI should be a collaborative partnership between the patient and the clinician working together, rather than a fight with one side advocating for change and the other for staying the same. MI trainers often explain to trainees that the consultation should feel like a dance between the practitioner and the patient, rather than a wrestling match. The second a practitioner feels like he is wrestling, he should take it as a signal that the rapport with the patient is taking a turn for the worse, and steps should be taken to remedy this (see the discussion of "rolling with resistance").

MI Inside the Consultation

To explore ambivalence about behavior change with patients, the practitioner needs to take on a curious mind-set. To be able to demonstrate that she understands how patients feel about change, the clinician needs to listen effectively to them, to encourage them to describe their feelings, and to avoid the urge to prescribe a course of action without their permission.

Building on the spirit and principles of MI, the practitioner can make use of a number of skills in the consultation to help patients explore and resolve their ambivalence about behavior change. These are outlined in this following sections. For more detailed descriptions of these skills, the reader should consult Miller and Rollnick (2002) and/or Rollnick et al. (1999).

Open vs. Closed Questioning

Closed questions are those that encourage brief answers, whereas open questions encourage longer answers. For example, a closed question might be "Do you enjoy exercising?" whereas an open question would be "How do you feel about exercising?" Throughout the consultation, the practitioner should use mainly open, rather than closed, questions, because they encourage patients to explore how they feel about a particular behavior and help the practitioner to gain a deeper understanding of how patients feel about making changes.

This is not to say that closed questions should not be used ever, under any circumstances! In the real world, there may be occasions where closed questions are necessary and can be asked skillfully. However, given that the aim of MI is to help patients explore and resolve ambivalence, closed questions should be kept to a minimum to encourage this exploration.

The Importance of Listening

Asking open questions is an excellent way of gathering information from the patient. However, asking too many questions could lead patients to feel a little interrogated and thus increase resistance in the consultation. Another way of demonstrating understanding and encouraging patients to elaborate without asking questions is through the use of *reflective listening,* one of the most important skills used in MI. Miller and Rollnick (2002) recommend that a ratio of one question to two or three reflective listening statements should be used, as this may help to prevent resistance or confrontational behavior within the consultation.

Listening is generally a passive process—the listener remains quiet and hears what the other person has said. By contrast, reflective listening is an active process and involves making a statement in reply to what the patient has just said. Figure 8.1, adapted from the work of Gordon (1970), shows how the process of reflective listening works. It involves making a statement that bridges the gap between the practitioner's understanding and what the patient is saying or meaning.

Reflective listening is done through a series of statements, not questions (i.e., the practitioner's intonation must go *down* at the end of a statement, not up as at the end of a question). It takes practice to get used to making these

8.1

Reflective listening.

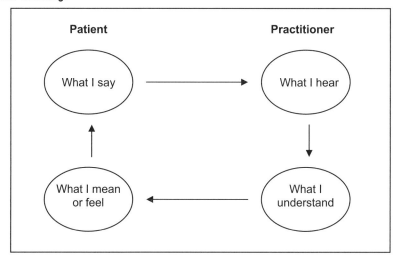

Patient	Practitioner
What I say	What I hear
What I mean or feel	What I understand

statements, but statements have the advantage of being less interrogative and in turn reduce the risk of confrontation.

Miller and Rollnick (2002) describe a number of different forms of reflective listening statements that could be used. For the purposes of this chapter, two broad kinds of reflection are described (Dr. Gary Rose, personal communication, 2004):

- *Content reflections*—short summaries of what the patient has said
- *Meaning reflections*—reflections of what the patient has meant

For example, if a patient said something like "I want to give up smoking because I don't want another heart attack; I want to see my kids grow up," a *content reflection* of this statement would be something like "You see a connection between your smoking and the possibility of having another heart attack." A possible *meaning reflection* could be "Your children are important to you, and you'll go to great lengths to be there for them." Both statements encourage the patient to elaborate further about her reasoning and in turn to explore her ambivalence about change.

In addition to reflections, another way to demonstrate understanding and encourage exploration of ambivalence is through the use of *summaries*. These are lengthier than reflections and are conducted periodically through the consultation. They can be used to bring together all the things the patient has said regarding a particular issue, to link some things a patient has said with other things he has said at another point in the session, or to bring a discussion to a close.

Reflections and summaries are useful tools in the elicitation of change talk, as they can be used to highlight what patients perceive to be the benefits of changing and the costs of staying the same are and then encouraging them to elaborate on these further. They can also be used to affirm patients by demonstrating appreciation and supporting their achievements.

Rolling With Resistance

When talking about behavior change, from time to time a patient may disagree with the practitioner or become defensive about their behavior. One of the principles of MI is to "roll with resistance," or rather to respond to resistance without confrontation.

Rolling with resistance can be done in several ways. The use of reflective listening statements usually helps, as they encourage patients to tell the practitioner how they are feeling and why, which in itself can lower resistance.

Resistance often occurs when patients feel that their freedom is being taken away (Brehm, 1966). Therefore, reassuring patients that they are free to make their own choices and that they are under no obligation to make changes to their behavior can also be helpful (for example, "I'm not here to force you to change. The decision to change is and always will be entirely yours"). It can also help to shift focus by acknowledging that patients are obviously not happy to talk about the particular issue in hand at the moment and asking them if there is anything else they would prefer talk about, instead, again emphasizing personal freedom and choice (for example, "It sounds like you aren't really very happy to talk about your smoking at the moment. What would you prefer to talk about instead?").

Another factor that may evoke resistance from patients is a sense that the practitioner has misunderstood how ready they are to change. Should this be the case, it can be useful to go back and reassess the patient's readiness.

If a patient is becoming resistant, this may reflect that the practitioner and the patient have different views on the subject at hand, and a different approach may be needed to resume the "dance."

Setting the Agenda, and Asking Permission to Talk About Behavior Change

Choosing to talk about behavior change should ultimately be the patient's choice. Given the importance of patient choice in lowering resistance, the practitioner should always ask permission to talk about the behavior with patients, rather than just telling them that today there will be a discussion about their health behavior.

In Motivational Interviewing, patients are encouraged to set the agenda for talking about behavior change. This is particularly important if there are a number of different lifestyle issues to be addressed. For example, a cardiac rehabilitation patient may have been identified as having a number of risk factors that may have contributed to a myocardial infarction. He may need to make dietary changes, do more exercise, and cut down on the amount of alcohol consumed to try to reduce his risk of having another heart attack. It is often easier to make changes gradually, rather than trying to make a number of substantial changes all at one time.

Individuals may even be at different stages of readiness to change different aspects of one health behavior (Rollnick et al., 1999), or they may have other issues that are more important for them to talk about and that are affecting their readiness to change, such as worries in other aspects of their life.

Achieving small changes can increase self-efficacy (Bandura, 1995) and make patients feel more able to make other small changes. It is therefore important to start where patients feel most comfortable and encourage them to suggest what area they would like to talk about, rather than selecting what the health care practitioner feels is the most important issue to talk about first.

Encouraging patients to set the agenda can be initiated through the use of open questions, such as "There are a number of different things we can talk about today. I'm just wondering what aspect of your lifestyle you would like to talk about?" One clinical tool that can help with this task is an agenda setting chart (Rollnick et al., 1999), which contains a number of circles containing picture representations of various different lifestyle factors and some blank circles for other factors to be inserted by the patient. Practitioners should be prepared for the patient to raise issues that they may not have anticipated—for example, a newly diagnosed type-2 diabetic patient may be most worried about what the diagnosis might mean for her family, rather than for her personal health, at that moment.

Exploring How the Patient Feels About Change

Given the role that readiness plays in motivation to change behavior, it can be useful to gain an understanding of this. One way this can be achieved within clinical practice is by exploring how important patients feel it is to change their behavior and how confident they feel about achieving such change.

In exploring importance and confidence, many practitioners find it useful to use scaling questions. This involves asking patients, on a scale of 0–10, how important is it for them to change a particular behavior and then asking, on the same scale, how confident they feel of success in changing that behavior. Following on from this, the practitioner can ask patients why they have given themselves this score and not a higher or lower number and what they think would help them to move up the scale in terms of importance and/or confidence.

Of course, the use of scaling questions like this is not compulsory. This technique has only been described, as many practitioners find it a useful way of understanding where patients are at a particular point in time. Importance and confidence could equally be assessed by the use of skillful open-ended questions, such as "How important would you say it is for you to make changes?" and "If you made the decision that you were going to change, how confident are you that you would succeed?"

Closely related to the importance/confidence strategy is exploration of what patients like and dislike like about their current behavior, including what they feel they would gain or lose from making changes. This can also help the practitioner to understand patients' barriers to change and also offers a valuable opportunity to elicit change talk from patients.

Exchanging Information

Within health care consultations, there often comes a point where patients need information. Perhaps patients need to know something for their safety or well-being, perhaps they have asked you for information on what they should do, or perhaps they have misunderstood something with regard to their care or recovery.

Information giving within health care is usually a process in which the patient is a passive recipient. A typical example might be "You are eating too much of x. This means that you are at a much higher risk of developing x. What I suggest you do is x." This has the advantage of being direct and to the point. However, it has the disadvantage of possibly telling the patient something she knows already or that may be misunderstood in terms of its personal relevance. It also makes the assumption that the patient will just take the advice and do as she is told, which is unlikely in the case of the ambivalent patient.

Within Motivational Interviewing, information is exchanged with patients, rather than simply provided to them. This involves the use of the "elicit-provide-elicit" method: first finding out what the patient knows already, providing information (after asking if the patient is happy for you to do this), and then finding out what the patient has made of that information. An example of this might be:

- *Elicit:* "What do you know about the complications of diabetes?"
- *Provide:* "Would it be OK if I told you a little bit more about that?"
- *Elicit:* "So, what do you think that might mean for you?"

This means that information is given in a neutral manner, building on what the patient already knows, and the interpretation of the facts is left to the patient.

Exchanging information in this way can encourage patients to actively think of how the information given applies to themselves as individuals and can even save the practitioner time, as it prevents the provision of redundant information, or "telling the patient what he knows already."

Talking About Making Changes

If patients indicate that they are ready to make changes, the most useful course of action is to elicit from them what changes they feel they would like to make. The practitioner no doubt has years of experience in clinical practice and knows exactly what the patient needs to do to achieve better health. However, as the patient is the individual who has to make these changes, it is argued that the patient is the expert in knowing what will work best for her. This process can be initiated through the use of open-ended questions such as "What sorts of things do you think you might be able to do?"

This does not mean that the practitioner cannot offer possible courses of action to the patient—the patient may indeed ask for advice about what to do. However, the practitioner should ask permission before making a suggestion, and it should be made clear to the patient that he is not obliged to follow this suggestion if he does not feel it will suit him. The patient should be an active decision maker, rather than a passive recipient of information and instruction.

It can be helpful to encourage patients to think about previous attempts to change their behavior. For example, what has worked well before, what kinds of things did not work, and why? How has the patient dealt with other life challenges before?

The focus should be on small changes that feel achievable for the patient. If patients succeed with one change, they may feel more able to face others (Bandura, 1995). If a major changes need to be made, it may be easier for patients to break these changes down into smaller tasks. This may make change feel more achievable than if they try to do everything at once.

Adaptations of MI

MI has been used in several different contexts, including (but not limited to) addictions, primary and secondary health care, and criminal justice settings. There are a number of systemic differences among these settings, which have resulted in adaptations of the method described by Miller and Rollnick (2002). To try to protect against confusion as to what is and what is not MI (Miller 2000), researchers have developed a number of different adaptations of MI (AMIs) (Rollnick & Miller, 1995; Rollnick et al., 2002).

Examples of Adaptations of MI

Examples of AMIs described in the literature include the "Drinker's Check-up" (Miller & Sovereign, 1989), and Motivational Enhancement Therapy (MET) (Miller, Zweben, DiClemente, & Rychtarik, 1992). The Drinker's Checkup is a two-session assessment and feedback of a client's drinking, delivered in an MI style. MET is also delivered as an intervention of assessment and feedback on drinking in an MI style, but it was implemented across four sessions as part of Project MATCH (Project MATCH Research Group, 1993).

In health settings, Rollnick and colleagues developed a "menu of strategies" approach based on MI for use with non-help-seeking heavy drinkers in primary care, which they termed "brief motivational interviewing," with an emphasis on utilizing MI skills in practice (Rollnick et al., 1992). Building on this, Rollnick et al. (1999) adapted MI for use with general health behaviors in health care settings, termed "behavior change counseling" (Rollnick et al., 2002), which differs slightly from traditional MI, although the skills and spirit between behavior change counseling and MI are very similar. There is less emphasis on the strategic elicitation of change talk and less elicitation of deeply held patient values but generally more elicitation of patient information needs and exchanging of information than would typically be found in an MI session.

What's in a Label?

Several AMIs have taken on different names, to try to explicitly illustrate that they contain qualitative differences from the original parent method. This has both advantages and disadvantages. It makes it clear that the intervention delivered differs from Miller and Rollnick (2002) in some way, but at the same time it can be confusing when one is trying to establish whether the study in question has drawn on the skills and spirit of MI in any way, and to what extent.

Using a different label to describe an AMI is less important than actually describing how it was designed, how it differs from MI, and which of its characteristics are consistent with MI. The importance of defining the components of behavioral interventions has been highlighted by research guidance documents, such as the Medical Research Council's guidelines on the study of complex interventions (Medical Research Council, 2002). Failure to do so can make it difficult to interpret the implications about the efficacy and effectiveness of MI as an intervention.

Evidence for MI in Health Care Settings

Systematic Reviews and Meta-Analyses

A number of recent systematic reviews have presented growing evidence for the effectiveness of MI as an intervention. The strongest evidence is in the treatment of drug and alcohol misuse (Burke, Arkowitz, & Dunn, 2002; Burke, Arkowitz, & Menchola, 2003; Dunn, Deroo, & Rivara, 2001; Hettema, Steele, & Miller, 2005). As MI is still a relatively new method, and as it entered the general health care arena much later than the addictions field, the evidence for MI within health care settings is still somewhat limited, although the technique has shown much promise.

Rubak and colleagues conducted a systematic review of 72 randomized controlled trials in health care settings (Rubak, Sandboek, Lauritzen, & Christensen, 2005) and found that MI interventions had a significant effect on reducing BMI, cholesterol, systolic BP, blood alcohol content, and standard ethanol content, although not on the number of cigarettes smoked per day in smokers or on HbA1c in people with diabetes. Vasilaki and colleagues systematically reviewed studies that used brief alcohol interventions based on MI and concluded that MI was effective in reducing alcohol consumption in the short term with mainly risky (rather than alcohol-dependent) drinkers (Vasilaki, Hosier, & Cox, 2006). Another more recent systematic review (Knight, McGowan, Dickens, & Bundy, 2006) into the effects of MI interventions on physical activity concluded that these interventions do appear to increase exercise uptake among patients, although the poor quality of trials made this hard to determine, with just eight studies being included in the review as a result—mirroring the findings of previous reviews that have attempted to look at MI in relation to specific health behaviors (Dunn et al., 2001; Burke et al., 2002; Burke et al., 2003; Hettema et al., 2005). To date, there are more than 150 published trials of motivational interviewing (see Rollnick et al., 2007).

One salient aspect of patient behavior during an MI session that has been shown to correlate with outcomes is the amount of *commitment language* patients produce in a consultation (Amrhein, Miller, Yahne, Palmer, & Fulcher, 2003). Commitment language is a kind of change talk in which the patient indicates that he is committed to taking particular courses of action (for example, "I'm definitely going to give that a try"). It should be emphasized that commitment language is elicited from, rather than imposed upon, the patient.

Issues in the Reporting of Trials of MI

Although most studies of MI exhibit high levels of external validity, reviews of research papers have indicated that the internal validity of these trials is often poor. Dunn and colleagues found that the evaluation of the efficacy of AMIs was difficult because of the lack of information regarding the training and skill level of practitioners who delivered the intervention (Dunn et al., 2001). Of 29 studies, only 10 reported the number of hours training given, 11 reported that training was provided but gave no indication of how much training was given, and 8 did not mention training at all. No studies mentioned practitioner skill level in delivering AMIs and how much training produced how much skill in using AMIs. Each AMI was different from the next, making it difficult to compare like with like. Burke and colleagues also highlight a lack of adequate specification of the intervention used; there is often no detail regarding the amount or nature of the training delivered, the background and credentials of the intervention providers, and the nature of the intervention delivered (Burke et al., 2002). They also state that there has been no indication of how the intervention was delivered to patients. Indeed, one earlier review of 11 clinical trials of MI questioned whether it was fair to describe the intervention delivered in some trials as an AMI (Noonan & Moyers, 1997).

To enhance the quality of such trials, more attention is being focused on the quality of the intervention actually delivered by practitioners in a number of different contexts, resulting in the development of instruments to measure practitioner skill in delivering MI (Barsky & Coleman, 2001; Lane et al., 2005; Madson, Campbell, Barrett, Brondino, & Melchert, 2005; Moyers, Martin, Manuel, Hendrickson, & Miller, 2005). Several trials of MI interventions are now using instruments and qualitative analyses to assess practitioner skill level posttraining and the fidelity of AMI delivery in practice. It is anticipated that this will contribute greatly to the interpretation of results of trials of MI and its adaptations and increase the understanding of how different features of MI might work best with individual patients.

Summary

MI is a clinical skill that has been used in a range of different contexts involving behavior change. It aims to help patients explore and resolve ambivalence to change. There are a number of microskills that can be used in consultations with patients, but it is important to adhere to the spirit of MI when employing these techniques. Evidence shows that MI is effective in the drug and alcohol field, and it has shown potential in encouraging patient behavior change in health care settings. Studies that define the intervention delivered and attempt to assess the fidelity of the intervention delivered will provide more information about what aspects of MI seem to work best in helping patients to achieve changes in their behavior.

References

Amrhein, P. C., Miller, W. R., Yahne, C. E., Palmer, M., & Fulcher, L. (2003). Client commitment language during motivational interviewing predicts drug use outcomes. *Journal of Consulting and Clinical Psychology, 71,* 862–878.
Bandura, A. E. (1995). *Self-efficacy in changing societies.* New York: Cambridge University Press.

Barsky, A., & Coleman, H. (2001). Evaluating skill acquisition in motivational interviewing: The development of an instrument to measure practice skills. *Journal of Drug Education 31*, 69–82.

Bem, D. J. (1972). Self-perception theory. In L. Berkowitz (Ed.), *Advances in experimental social psychology*. New York: Academic Press.

Brehm, J. W. (1966). *A theory of psychological reactance*. New York: Academic Press.

Burke, B., Arkowitz, H., & Dunn, C. (2002). The efficacy of motivational interviewing and its adaptations: What we know so far. In W. Miller & S. Rollnick (Eds.), *Motivational interviewing: Preparing people for change* (pp. 217–250). New York: Guilford Press.

Burke, B., Arkowitz, H., & Menchola, M. (2003). The efficacy of motivational interviewing: A meta-analysis of controlled clinical trials. *Journal of Consulting and Clinical Psychology, 71*, 843–861.

Dunn, C., Deroo, L., & Rivara, F. (2001). The use of brief interventions adapted from motivational interviewing across behavioral domains: A systematic review. *Addiction, 96*, 1725–1742.

Gordon, T. (1970). *PET: Parent Effectiveness Training*. New York: Wyden.

Hettema, J., Steele, J., & Miller, W. R. (2005). Motivational interviewing. *Annual Review of Clinical Psychology, 1*, 91–111.

Keller, V., & White, M. (1997). Choices and changes: A new model for influencing patient health behavior. *Journal of Clinical Outcomes Management, 4*, 33–36.

Knight, K., McGowan, L., Dickens, C., & Bundy, C. (2006). A systematic review of motivational interviewing in physical health care settings. *British Journal of Health Psychology, 11*, 319–332.

Lane, C., Huws-Thomas, M., Hood, K., Rollnick, S., Edwards, K., & Robling, M. (2005). Measuring adaptations of motivational interviewing: The development and validation of the Behavior Change Counseling Index. *Patient Education and Counseling, 56*, 166–173.

Madson, M. B., Campbell, T. C., Barrett, D. E., Brondino, M. J., & Melchert, T. P. (2005). Development of the Motivational Interviewing Supervision and Training Scale. *Psychology of Addictive Behaviors, 19*, 303–310.

Medical Research Council. (2002). *A framework for the development of complex interventions to improve health*. Retrieved August 1, 2005, from www.mrc.ac.uk/pdf-mrc_cpr.pdf

Miller, W., & Rollnick, S. (2002). *Motivational interviewing: Preparing people for change*. New York: Guilford Press.

Miller, W. R., & Sovereign, R. G. (1989). The check-up: A model for early intervention in addictive behaviors. In T. Løberg, W. R. Miller, P. E. Nathan, & G. A. Marlatt (Eds.), *Addictive behaviors: Prevention and early intervention*. Amsterdam: Swets & Zeitlinger.

Miller, W. R., Zweben, A., DiClemente, C. C., & Rychtarik, R. G. (1992). *Motivational Enhancement Therapy manual: A clinical research guide for therapists treating individuals with alcohol abuse and dependence,* Rockville, MD: National Institute on Alcohol Abuse and Alcoholism.

Moyers, T., Martin, T., Manuel, J., Hendrickson, S., & Miller, W. (2005). Assessing competence in the use of motivational interviewing. *Journal of Substance Abuse Treatment, 28*, 19–26.

Noonan, W., & Moyers, T. (1997). Motivational Interviewing: A review. *Journal of Substance Misuse, 2*, 8–16.

Pascal, B. (1623–1662). *Pensées*. Retrieved August 20, 2008, from http://books.google.co.uk/books?id=hUvBsaMWOU8C

Project Match Research Group. (1993). Project MATCH: Rationale and methods for a multisite clinical trial matching patients to alcoholism treatment. *Alcoholism: Clinical and Experimental Research, 17*, 1130–1145.

Rogers, C. (1959). A theory of therapy, personality and interpersonal relationships as developed in the client-centered framework. In S. Koch (Ed.), *Psychology: The study of a science*. New York: McGraw-Hill.

Rollnick, S., Allison, J., Ballasiotes, S., Barth, T., Butler, C., Rose, G., et al. (2002). Variations on a theme: Motivational Interviewing and its adaptations. In W. Miller & S. Rollnick (Eds.), *Motivational Interviewing: Preparing people for change*. New York: Guilford Press.

Rollnick, S., Butler, C. C., & Stott, N. (1997). Helping smokers make decisions: The enhancement of brief intervention for general medical practice. *Patient Education and Counseling, 31*, 191–203.

Rollnick, S., Heather, N., & Bell, A. (1992). Negotiating behavior change in medical settings: The development of brief motivational interviewing. *Journal of Mental Health 1,* 25–39.

Rollnick, S., Mason, P., & Butler, C. (1999). *Health behaviour change: A guide for practitioner.* Edinburgh: Harcourt Brace.

Rollnick, S., Miller, W., & Butler, C. (2007). *Motivational interviewing in healthcare.* New York: Guilford Press.

Rollnick, S., & Miller, W. R. (1995). What is motivational interviewing? *Behavioural and Cognitive Psychotherapy, 23,* 325–334.

Rubak, S., Sandboek, A., Lauritzen, T., & Christensen, B. (2005). Motivational Interviewing: A systematic review and meta-analysis. *British Journal of General Practice, 55,* 305–312.

Vasilaki, E., Hosier, S., & Cox, W. (2006). The efficacy of Motivational Interviewing as brief intervention for excessive drinking: A meta-analytic review. *Alcohol and Alcoholism, 41,* 328–335.

E-Health Strategies to Support Adherence

9

Patricia D. Franklin,
Ramesh Farzanfar, and
Deborah D. Thompson

Defining E-Health and Its Proposed Contribution to Health Care

A commonly cited definition of e-health describes the emerging field as "the intersection of medical informatics, public health and business, referring to health services and information delivered or enhanced through the Internet and related technologies" (Eysenbach, 2001). For clinicians, the benefits of e-health applications include improved patient information management, co-ordination of longitudinal care, and symptom monitoring. For patients, e-health tools have the potential to improve communication with clinicians, access to personal health information, and health education with the goal of preparing patients to take a more active role in their care. E-health developers and be-havioral researchers and clinicians are challenged to develop easy-to-use, ac-cessible, and engaging technology that employs interactive strategies to attract and retain diverse patient users. If these goals are attained, it is plausible that e-health technologies will assume a significant future role in supporting pa-tient adherence.

Why Incorporate E-Health Strategies in Health Care?

Developing and deploying effective e-health strategies to promote adherence to healthy behaviors are priorities now because these technologies are able to reach broad numbers of people simultaneously, Web access is growing, and the demand for additional health promotion interventions persists.

E-Health Tools Have Broad Reach

Strategies are needed to increase the *reach* and *impact* of effective health pro-motion programs. Traditional prevention and chronic disease management pro-grams are labor intensive and time consuming and reach only the minority of individuals who attend in-person sessions. Thus, despite the efficacy, the cost to reach the at-risk population is often disproportionate to the small numbers of people who benefit. In contrast, the Internet, cell phones, and other e-health tools span geographic and time differences, sustain relationships, and build links between people and information (Wellman, 2001). E-mail and Internet access is available 24 hours a day, seven days a week, and information can be customized to serve the individual characteristics of the user. These technology attributes may serve the goals of both broad reach and effective impact.

Users Have Growing Access to the Internet

During the past decade, both health care providers and payers have increas-ingly incorporated information technology into their practices to serve pa-tients directly, through information and education, and indirectly through clinical data management. In addition, patients and consumers have rapidly adopted electronic technologies to obtain information, education, and disease management tools. Between 2000 and 2005, it is estimated that the number of U.S. Internet users seeking health information more than doubled, reaching 88.5 million people (Ahern, Phalen, & Mockenhaupt, 2003). Sixty-eight percent of U.S. adults, including seniors, now have access to the Internet. The Pew Study on "Older Americans and the Internet" reports that the percentage of seniors online increased by 27% between 2000 and 2004, as 8 million adults over 65 years of age (22% of those in this age group) reported Web access (Rainie & Horrigan, 2005). Furthermore, the Pew Study reports, "As Internet users in their 50's get older and retire, they are unlikely to give up their wired [Web use] ways and therefore will transform the wired senior stereotype." A recent study of health e-mails delivered to working adults with uniform computer access offers further evidence that adults readily accept Internet-delivered health information. More than 80% of 345 employee participants opened more than half of the daily health e-mails they received during a 6 month period. Importantly, e-mail open rates did not vary by employee gender, age, income, education, ethnicity, or baseline health behavior (Franklin, Rosenbaum, Carey, & Roizen, 2006). Recent data report that Hispanic consumers report spending more time online at home than other U.S. online consumers (9.5 vs. 8.4 hours), and 43% of online Hispanics are interested in or already use the Internet for health care reasons ("Hispanics Going Online in Record Numbers," 2003). Finally, *Healthy People 2010* includes a goal of facilitating Internet access in 80% of U.S. homes by the year 2010 to support its health promotion goals (U.S. Department of Health & Human Services, 2000). Thus, as computer and Internet access spreads, widespread use of electronic technology offers an opportunity to integrate e-health technology in support of medical and self-care.

Demand for Alternative Health Promotion and Self-Care Strategies

In parallel to the emergence of electronic communication tools, the demand for health promotion and chronic disease management among an aging U.S. population is growing. It is estimated that chronic disease costs account for more than 70% of all health care expenditures and the majority of disability (Bodenheimer, 2005). Furthermore, health promotion behaviors lag behind *Healthy People 2010* goals despite targeted efforts. For example, 77% of adults report diets that include less than the recommended daily intake of fruits, vegetables, and vitamins, and more than 80% of adults are overweight or obese (National Center for Chronic Disease Prevention and Health Promotion, 2005). E-health tools offer a relatively untested mechanism to deliver patient-centered health promotion and self-management strategies widely among the U.S. population. While improving health is the primary goal of technology, significant cost savings may be possible if effective adherence strategies improve behavioral choices. In this context, it is critical to define and evaluate the appropriate roles for e-health interventions to improve adherence to health-promoting behaviors.

User-Centered Design of E-Health Interventions

E-health interventions vary in design, technology application, delivery, and content. A sample of the wide variety of e-health applications developed and in evaluation are summarized here to illustrate design, delivery, and content considerations in e-health adherence interventions. Definitive research to define the most effective formats and delivery strategies is limited at this time. Thus, each section identifies some of the relevant unanswered questions.

The nature of health promotion, disease prevention, and chronic disease management involves ongoing, consistent patient participation. Thus, it follows that e-health programs targeting health behaviors depend on repeat patient use over extended periods of time. As a result, user adherence to the e-health intervention schedule is central to effective results. Identification of the factors that contribute to regular or appropriate use of e-health programs is critical to achieve desired health outcomes. Research is needed to both measure adherence to e-health programs and to clearly understand the essential attributes of e-health programs associated with patient and consumer use and acceptance.

User-Defined Specifications

The most important factor in the success of an e-health system is design informed by user's needs and perceptions of what works best for them, that is, a system's usability and helpfulness. In fact, an effective user evaluation of an e-health program may provide an early indication of a technology's worth and ultimate viability. Varied research methods may be used to obtain user input during the development of e-health applications. The specific method may vary depending on the nature of the application and availability of resources. Evaluation objectives may be achieved through controlled and structured methodologies (e.g., formalized and structured instruments), heuristic analyses, or cognitive walkthroughs (Nielsen, 1992; Vitalari, 1985). The most useful methods tend to be those through which users communicate their likes and dislikes directly to the designers and developers, including qualitative studies and ethnography (Beyer & Holtzblatt, 1999; Forsythe, 1995; Prasad, 1997). Focus groups, workshops, in-depth face-to-face interviews, and short- and long-duration participant observations are commonly employed. Evaluations should solicit a rich description of the users' opinions, as well as the context of use to ensure user-centered systems (Geertz, 1973). For example, clinicians and teens were asked to pretest a phone text messaging system to deliver reminders to diabetic teens to enhance self-management (Waller, Franklin, Pagliari, & Greene, 2006). Early feedback resulted in a reliable system that effectively fit into the daily life of a teen.

Should E-Health Systems Be Designed to Be Humanlike?

A common evaluation standard for e-health systems asks whether the intervention emulates an interaction with a human health professional. Anthropomorphism is enhanced in systems that are voice-based, using either a human voice or a synthesized, computerized voice. Users' tendency to anthropomorphize is higher in voice-based systems than in those that are only text based (e.g., Internet applications that use only written words). In addition, many e-health systems replicate users' typical interactions with health care professionals, including specific wording, tone, and style. Similarly, humor, concern, and expressions of support and encouragement intensify users' tendency to anthropomorphize the e-health system. Anthropomorphism is a deliberate design strategy to enhance the system's impact, as users who anthropomorphize a system tend to feel more positively toward it (Farzanfar, Finkelstein, & Friedman, 2004). Anthropomorphic attributions offer patients a useful reference to describe their experience and facilitate comparison of the system to a human health care professional.

Conversely, some evaluations of an automated telephone linked call system (TLC) have demonstrated that enhancing human-like characteristics of a system may have unintended negative consequences. Users who are not comfortable with a human health care professional will extrapolate these feelings to the system. For example, when the health topic is one that addresses sensitive topics such as diet or mental health disorders, humanlike systems may not be an advantage (Farzanfar et al., 2004; Farzanfar, 2006). In fact, some users prefer interacting with computers rather than with health care professionals when sensitive or personal issues are involved and report that automated systems are less judgmental. Whether anxiety is caused by personal or societal factors, nonjudgmental technology is less threatening to some users. For example, some sexual behaviors were more accurately reported on private questionnaires, on computer or paper, than in face-to-face interviews (Durant & Carey, 2000). Importantly, when users are not anxious, they are more receptive to the educational health messages communicated by the system.

Alleviating User Anxiety With E-Health Systems

E-health system components, including word selection, must be cautiously designed to ensure that systems do not unintentionally promote feelings of inadequacy or anxiety. For example, an automated telephone messaging system that is based on goal setting might be threatening among users who fail to achieve a goal (Farzanfar, Frishkopf, Migneault, & Friedman, 2005). We have noted that fear of criticism adversely impacts the utilization regimen specific to a system. This indicates that e-health systems that target modification of an unhealthy behavior must take into consideration users' sensitivities to words and surveillance. These findings might be extrapolated to Web-based programs using relational agents. Relational agents are animated software that imitate human-to-human communication style and interact with users in intelligent and sometimes affective ways (Bickmore, 2003). Depending on their sophistication, these intelligent software agents can function as both advisers and support systems.

In summary, to reach the design objectives, e-health programs need to be well designed and to meet users' needs and sensitivities. This can be achieved only by exploring potential users' perceptions and their understanding of an e-health program through formal evaluations.

Targeting and Tailoring Health Strategies

The power of e-health applications arises from the computer's ability to target user groups with similar needs or tailor strategies to individual attributes and context. Targeted communication is designed to reach a *group* of individuals who share a similar attribute. E-health targeting is based on stored information that the user provides. For example, in contrast to televised advertisements for antihypertensive medications that reach all viewers, with and without high blood pressure, computer-based targeting can direct messages to reach those with known prescriptions for high blood pressure treatment. Users of one popular health promotion Web site complete a health risk assessment and identify priority behaviors they would like to improve. This Web site then delivers regular health messages to all Web site users who have identified certain suboptimal health behaviors. Targeting the e-health program to those who are most likely to benefit from the message enhances the efficiency of the message delivery.

Tailoring refers to feedback or guidance designed to address an *individual's* personal characteristics, thereby increasing the personal relevance and enhancing the potential effectiveness. Well-designed tailored programs have the potential to simulate an individualized counseling session (DeVries & Brug, 1999). Message tailoring adds greatest value when significant variability exists among the users on key attributes that will influence the intervention outcome (Kreuter, Strecher, & Glassman, 1999). Tailoring also assumes the ability to collect information about the key user attributes to be considered in refining the tailored message. Researchers have reported effective use of computer-tailored, individual feedback message programs for behaviors ranging from asthma management to alcohol use in emergency room patients to physical activity and diet (Blow et al., 2006; Kroeze, Werkman, & Brug, 2006).

Alternate Delivery Technologies for Health Interventions

Effective methods for reaching large populations of people with health-promoting messages are needed. Computers, the Internet, personal communication devices, and electronic games are being tested to meet these needs, and all offer promising results. This section briefly reviews promising e-health delivery technologies and their early evidence of success and identifies further research needs.

Studies of telephone counseling have used structured clinician phone calls to successfully modify behavior (Eakin, Lawler, Vanderlanotte, & Owen, 2007). Computer-Assisted Telephone Interviewing (CATI) technologies, in conjunction with telephone counseling, display consistent interviewer questions on a computer screen and allow the interviewer to enter the patient's responses into a database. Experience with scripted, nonlocal telephone counseling supported by computer data collection has informed the design of e-health interventions where computer protocols deliver tailored or targeted health information to patients through electronic devices, replacing one-to-one patient-provider interactions.

Internet

In the span of a few short years, the Internet has become an essential part of life for many Americans, reshaping the ways in which we communicate, locate information, and entertain ourselves (Rainie & Horrigan, 2005). Because of its familiarity, broad availability, and accessibility, the Internet is being investigated as a channel for delivering e-health programs. A review of the e-health literature reveals a wide variety of Internet-based health behavior programs have been developed and tested. Examples include programs based on a one-time Internet session (Shegog et al., 2005), structured programs with multiple contacts over time (Baranowski et al., 2003; Block, Block, Wakimoto, & Block, 2004; Jago et al., 2006; Napolitano et al., 2003; Plotnikoff, McCargar, Wilson, & Loucaides, 2005; Tate, Wing, & Winett, 2001; Tate, Jackvony, & Wing, 2003; Winett, Tate, Anderson, Wojcik, & Winett, 2005); self-paced programs offering access to tailored Web sites (Woolf et al., 2006); programs combining in-person and Internet sessions (Baranowski et al., 2003; Jago et al. , 2006; Tate et al., 2001, 2003); virtual coaches (Tate et al., 2001, 2003; Winett et al., 2005); and e-mail messages or prompts alone plus Internet resources (Block et al., 2004; Franklin et al., 2006; Plotnikoff et al., 2005) or in combination with other electronic programs (Napolitano et al., 2003; Tate et al., 2001, 2003; Winett et al., 2005). Emerging evidence indicates that Internet-based e-health programs show promising results. These programs are able to reach broad audiences, both adults and youth, sustain participation, and address a variety of health behaviors, ranging from changing diet and physical activity to smoking cessation and asthma management.

Personal Communication Devices

Personal digital assistants (PDAs) have been investigated both as educational aids and as a method for collecting self-report data (Trapl et al., 2005; Wang, Kogashiwa, Ohta, & Kira, 2002; Wang, Kogashiwa, & Kira, 2006; Yon, Johnson, Harvey-Berino, & Gold, 2006; Yon, Johnson, Harvey-Berino, Gold, & Howard, 2007). Advantages to collecting data through PDA include simplicity of use, transportability (Jaspan et al., 2007), and immediate transferability of responses to a central database (Dale & Hagen, 2007). When compared to pen-and-paper measures, data collected via PDA appear to be more complete and to have fewer errors (Dale & Hagen, 2007). A systematic review comparing PDAs to pen-and-paper measures concluded that PDAs outperformed pen-and-paper measures in most areas and that participants generally preferred PDAs over pen and paper. The primary disadvantage was technical malfunction resulting in loss of data (Dale & Hagen, 2007). PDAs, enhanced with digital video, have successfully delivered patient education (Brock & Smith, 2006). Patients taking HIV/AIDS medication watched a 25-minute digital video on a PDA to review information about the disease, medications, and adherence. Patients liked the PDA video, suggesting that PDAs may be an effective educational method in a clinical setting. Audio-enhanced PDA data collection has also been tested; although the results were promising, more work is needed to overcome deficits in data quality across different groups (Trapl et al., 2005). PDAs containing a camera and phone cards have been investigated as a novel method for recording dietary intake (Wang et al., 2002, 2006). In one study, participants took digital photographs of foods entered in a daily diary. The data were then transmitted digitally to registered dietitians for review. Results indicate that digital photos taken on a PDA may be an effective method for recording dietary intake.

Cellular phones and "smart phones" (a handheld device that combines the features of a cellular phone, PDA, and personal computer) have also been investigated for their ability to influence health outcomes. Diabetes management appears to be an area of particular interest for this methodology. In children with type 1 diabetes, mobile phones were tested as a way to promote self-care and parental monitoring (Gammon et al., 2005). Text messages, sent via a cellular phone, have also been tested as a component of diabetes management, with promising results (Ferrer-Roca, Cardenas, Diaz-Cardama, & Pulido, 2004; Wangberg, Arsand, & Andersson, 2006).

Finally, extensive application of interactive voice response (IVR) systems that use telephones to communicate computer-generated health messages to patients have been found to be well accepted and effective. The Telephone-Linked Communication (TLC) system has been used to educate and advise patients and to reinforce or change varied health-related behaviors, including medication management (Friedman, 1996, 1998), diet (Delichatsios et al., 2001), exercise (Jarvis, Friedman, Heeren, & Cullinane, 1997), and smoking cessation (Ramelson, Friedman, & Ockene, 1999).

Electronic Health Records and Web Portals

In the future, electronic health records (EHR) with patient portals may offer enhanced patient involvement, quality of care, and efficiency of service (Ford, Menachemi, & Phillips, 2006). Web portals allow patients to obtain access to their electronic health records and to communicate electronically with their providers (Hassol et al., 2004). A recent survey found that patients generally have positive attitudes toward use of portals and electronic communication with their provider. However, some patients expressed concerns about confidentiality and privacy. Interestingly, while patients preferred e-mail or in-person communication, physicians preferred telephone communication over e-mail (Hassol et al., 2004). A randomized controlled trial comparing a Web portal with usual care found that portal patients reported greater overall satisfaction than the usual-care patients (Lin, Wittevrongel, Moore, Beaty, & Ross, 2005). Additionally, patients indicate a willingness to pay for e-mail correspondence with their provider (Adler, 2006; Lin et al., 2005) and online access to their electronic health records, suggesting that patient portals may become important to future health care delivery.

Electronic Games

Youth enjoy electronic games (computer and video) and play them often. In a recent survey of media use among 8–18-year-olds, 59% of youth reported playing electronic games for an average of 1 hour 8 minutes each day (Roberts, Foehr, & Rideout, 2005). A 2006 report on gaming found that adults spend more time each week playing games than youth. Among 25–34-year-olds, more females than males played video games, dispelling the myth that gamers are mostly young males. For the health field, this suggests that electronic games may be a method for reaching a large proportion of the population by using a familiar, enjoyable method.

Emerging evidence suggests that electronic games can be effective at achieving desirable health outcomes. An evaluation of Squire's Quest!, a 10-session computer game to increase fruit-vegetable consumption among elementary school youth, found that children who played the game achieved a one-serving-a-day increase in intake over those who did not play the game (Baranowski et al., 2003). Elementary school youth who played nutrition knowledge games had improvements in knowledge, practices, and consumption (Turnin et al., 2001). Paradoxically, games promoting active game play have also been effective at enhancing energy expenditure (Lanningham-Foster et al., 2006; Tan, Aziz, Chua, & Teh, 2002) although declining interest and use over time remains a concern (Madsen, Yen, Wlasiuk, Newman, & Lustig, 2007). Interim results of an action-adventure game where children were required to wear pedometers as part of game play revealed a general increase in activity after 1 week of game play (Southard & Southard, 2006). Electronic games have also shown positive effects in treatment and self-management of chronic diseases such as asthma and diabetes (Lieberman, 2001). Preliminary evidence also suggests that games can be used to decrease anxiety prior to surgery (Patel et al., 2006) and to assist in lung function measurement among young children (Vilozni et al., 2005). Not all game effects have produced the expected outcomes (Homer et al., 2000; Huss et al., 2003; McPherson, Glazebrook, Forster, James, & Smyth, 2006), suggesting that more research is needed to determine features of effective games. The ideal design of games to achieve optimal health effects is not known. It is likely that increased realism will enhance generalization of behaviors taught in a game environment to the external world (Funk, 2005). Creating game environments, story lines, characters, situations, and barriers that players are likely to encounter in real life may provide them with a protected environment within which to practice self-management skills.

Future Technologies

The sciences of artificial intelligence, robotics, and natural language processing will converge to create smart, automated entities that interact with users in various capacities. Intelligent agents have been created to help consumers with their health-related lifestyle choices, such as enhanced physical activity (Bickmore 2003), or to help clinicians with their monitoring and diagnostic tasks (Mabry, Schneringer, Etters, & Edwards, 2003). The future holds great promise for these smart entities as multiagent systems to enhance patient health, including provision of remote care for the elderly, dissemination of health information, and monitoring of diagnostic tests.

Finally, there is a great deal of enthusiasm for the deployment of personal health records (PHR) that can incorporate many of the technologies discussed. A PHR integrates and organizes a broad array of health information and is managed by the patient. Using e-health devices ensures broad access to the information (i.e., data stored on the Web or easily transferred to phone for transmission and review by multiple parties without geographic limitations). Table 9.1 summarizes the current user and design attributes of the e-health strategies discussed in this chapter. As users become more familiar with these strategies and the developers enhance the functions, all of these technologies have the potential to broadly deliver tailored, interactive health messages to support patient behaviors.

9.1 Comparison of Attributes of E-Health Strategies

	Interactive voice telephony	Web	E-mail	Smart phone/PDA	Games
User					
Acceptance					
Familiar technology	✓✓✓	✓✓	✓✓	✓	✓
Anonymity	✓	✓✓✓	✓	✓	✓
Humanlike	✓✓✓	✓✓	✓	✓✓✓	✓✓✓
Access	✓✓✓	✓✓	✓✓	✓	✓
Interactive	✓✓	✓✓	✓	✓✓	✓✓
Cost	✓	✓✓	✓✓	✓✓✓	✓✓✓
Designer					
Reach	✓✓✓	✓✓	✓✓	✓	✓
Tailored	✓✓	✓	✓✓	✓✓	✓✓
Cost	✓✓✓	✓✓	✓✓	✓✓✓	✓✓✓

Key: ✓ = Low   ✓✓ = Moderate   ✓✓✓ = High

Theory to Guide Content

Behavioral science theory can guide e-health intervention efforts to target key forces that govern behavior patterns, increasing the probability of behavior change. For example, Fishbein et al. (2001) reviewed five leading theories of health behavior change and identified eight overlapping variables that explain most of the variance in health behavior change: intention, environmental constraints, skills, anticipated outcomes (or attitude), norms, self-standards, emotion, and self-efficacy. The first three variables are viewed as necessary and sufficient for behavior change, whereas the remaining five influence the strength and direction of the change. Thus, a theory-based e-health Internet program may include a structured self-assessment of skills and intention, motivational information to emphasize anticipated outcomes, self-monitoring tools to gauge environmental constraints and self-efficacy, and individualized feedback in response to progress. An e-health Behavior Management Model has been proposed and applied to Internet applications addressing varied chronic conditions (Bensley et al., 2004). The model combines the Transtheoretical Model, aspects of the Theory of Planned Behavior, and persuasive communication and advocates matching user stage of readiness to change with existing Internet information. Although technology constraints may modify some aspects of the theoretical model, behavior change programs based on theory appear to have a greater likelihood of success (Baranowski et al., 2003). Further research is needed to clarify how current behavior change theories explain and support individual e-health interventions. Finally, at a health care system level, the application of e-health tools in chronic disease care is supported by the Chronic Care Model (CCM) that includes both self-management support and clinical information systems as two of its key elements. The CCM hypothesizes that informed, activated patients, together with proactive health care providers, will lead to improved health outcomes (Bodenheimer, Wagner, & Grumbach, 2002; Wagner, Austin, Davis, Hindmarsh, Schaefer, & Bonomi, 2001).

Health Applications for Specific Populations

E-health applications have been tested to support self-care and adherence among patients with varied chronic diseases and health behavior challenges. A general trend toward patient acceptance, sustained use, and positive behavioral effects has been documented. The following illustrate the variation in content and delivery technology.

Diabetes Care

A wide variety of e-health applications have been successfully tested among diabetic patients. A 2005 review of diabetes self-management Web sites found 87 publicly available Internet sites hosted by a variety of institutions (Bull, Gaglio, McKay, & Glasgow, 2005). While the majority of Web sites disseminated information, few sites offered interactive assessments, social supports, or problem-solving assistance. Although the diabetes Web sites reach a broad audience, Web site designs mimic paper education and do not fully employ the power of electronic technology to individualize the material (Blonde & Parkin, 2006; Glasgow, Boles, McKay, Feil, & Barrera, 2003). In contrast, one Internet diabetes comanagement program offered patient access to its EHR, tools to upload glucose readings, an online diary for entry and tracking of medications, nutrition, and physical activity, communication with its clinicians, and educational information (Goldberg, Raston, Hirsch, Hoath, & Ahmed, 2003). This model illustrates the creative

9.1

User interaction intensity.

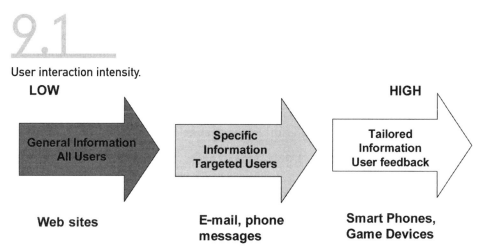

Continuum of interaction intensity between the e-health device and the user. At the low-intensity end, all users have open access to Web sites providing general health information. At the high end, select users receive tailored messages and provide individual feedback to the system. Depending upon the design, devices can function at different points along the continuum.

integration of multiple e-health technologies (i.e., EHR, e-mail, and Internet), behavioral strategies (i.e., self-monitoring, skills development), and self-care targets (i.e., medication, diet, and nutrition) to support diabetic patients over time (see Figure 9.1).

Asthma Care

Tailored self-monitoring and educational asthma Web sites have been evaluated in teen patients and their parents with relative success. A randomized trial of a school-based, tailored, 6 month Web program for African American teens with asthma found that participants had significantly fewer symptom days, school absences, and hospitalizations for asthma at 12 months after intervention. The authors estimated that the cost to deliver the Web program was $6.66 per participant. If these results are generalizable, e-health may play an important role in achieving significant health benefits for asthmatic teens. School and workplace delivery of health interventions also can support uniform Web access. Another team directed a tailored asthma education and self-monitoring Web site to parents of children with asthma. The Internet site was paired with monthly nurse case manager education phone calls to improve adherence to daily medication management, asthma control, and parent quality of life (Krishna et al., 2003; Wise et al., 2007; Yawn et al., 2000).

Arthritis Care

Home-based Internet interventions are well suited for persons with limited mobility due to advanced arthritis. Thus, successful face-to-face arthritis programs have been translated to Internet delivery. One-year outcome data for *both* face-to-face groups and Internet programs showed significantly lower disability, health distress, and limitations in daily activities among the intervention groups (Lorig, 2001; Lorig, Ritter, Laurent, & Plant, 2006).

Depression and Psychological Health

The high prevalence of untreated depression is a public health concern in the United States. E-health strategies may contribute to depression screening, support treatment adherence, and broaden the delivery of therapeutic interventions. Early trials of Internet interventions for depression (without therapist contact) did not successfully improve depressed mood in those studied. Thus, Clark and colleagues added periodic telephone or postcard reminders to study participants to prompt use of the "Overcoming Depression on the Internet" (ODIN) program at Kaiser Permanente. The addition of the prompts resulted in significantly improved mood among ODIN users when compared to controls. Of importance, participants with severely depressed affect at baseline reported the greatest improvement (Clark et al., 2005). Because of the relatively small number of participants from among a large pool of eligible adults, the generalizability of these findings must be tested. Others found the integration of telephone cognitive-behavioral psychotherapy with computer-based care management and medications improved treatment outcomes (Tutty, Ludman,

& Simon, 2005). Finally, an Australian Internet-based depression care program offered e-consultations, surveys to assess treatment progress, and psychoeducation. Both e-mail and telephone reminders were used to support ongoing participation. Participants reported medication adherence of more than 90% and clinical improvement from severe to mild depression following eight sessions (Robertson, Smith, Castle, & Tannenbaum, 2006). These encouraging results suggest that further evaluation of innovative e-health tools is warranted in this patient population.

Generic Chronic Disease Conditions

After an in-person chronic disease self-management program demonstrated sustained improvement in exercise, self-reported health, health distress, fatigue, disability, and role limitations, the program was adapted for Internet delivery. At 1 year, intervention participant health status was significantly improved over that of controls; results were similar to those for face-to-face group programs (Lorig et al., 2006). Of note, all participants were computer and Internet literate, and both intervention and control patients accessed health-related Web sites at a similar rate.

Dietary Modifications

Campbell (1994) found that subjects who received individually tailored computer messages had decreases in total fat and saturated fat intake greater than those of subjects in two comparison conditions. Glanz and colleagues (1998) also found that providing subjects with individualized computer-generated nutrition information and personally tailored feedback led to reduced fat intake and increased fruit and vegetable intake. A third study reported that a multimedia computer game for elementary school students was associated with those students' eating an average of 1.0 more serving per day of fruit, juice, and vegetables (Baranowski et al., 2003). These studies suggest a future role for e-health systems in efforts to facilitate improved dietary choices.

Weight Management

Wing randomly assigned patients to receive a face-to-face or an Internet-delivered weight loss maintenance program of daily weighing and self-regulation or to a control group. After 18 months, those in the face-to-face program had the smallest weight gain. However, when compared to those in the control group, fewer people in the groups that received either intervention, face-to-face or Internet, regained more than 2.3 kg (Wing et al., 2006). Importantly, this research evaluated the relative effectiveness of clinician-delivered and electronic-delivered behavioral support. Other research tested PDAs as tools for self-monitoring of diet and exercise (Yon et al., 2006, 2007) and Internet programs (Williamson et al., 2006) and obesity prevention games as tools for promoting diet and physical activity (Goran & Reynolds, 2005). The latter study found gender differences in game effect, suggesting the need to evaluate e-health intervention acceptance in demographic subgroups.

Substance Abuse

Both nicotine and alcohol abuse have been addressed with e-health programs. For example, Pallonen et al. (1998) found that use of interactive expert-system computerized reports along with a traditional intervention was more effective in promoting smoking cessation than noncomputer based interventions. In addition, a randomized trial using a computer-based survey to screen for at-risk drinkers seen in an emergency department found that tailored information plus brief direct advice was associated with a 48% reduction in average weekly alcohol consumption during the 12-month study (Blow et al., 2006). The latter study illustrates the model of computer-based screening and messaging to augment brief clinical intervention in a busy, acute environment. Additional research on mechanisms to integrate e-health supports into acute medical settings is needed.

Pharmaceutical Adherence and Biological Self-Monitoring

Medication adherence and associated errors are key quality issues for the U.S. health system. Correct dosing and timing are significant challenges for aging adults taking multiple medications. To serve aging veterans, the Veterans Affairs health system integrated its computerized pharmacy and patient records systems to create a visual medication profile to facilitate efficient and effective management of patient medications (Hornick et al., 2006). Digital photographs are used to identify individual pills for patients. Early pilots suggest that clinician-patient communication about medication changes will be improved using this system. Technology to assess and transfer a series of digital blood pressure measurements to clinicians via the Internet have been developed and shown to improve management of hypertension between physician office visits (Gardiner, 2006; Nakajima, 2006).

Issues of Participation and Delivery of E-Health Programs

A limitation of traditional health behavior programs is that the participant must make the initial contact, thus skewing participation to those already motivated to consider health behavior change. Similarly, Web-based health information requires a motivated and technically literate user to seek, find, and use Internet health tools. However, "electronic outreach" and e-mail reminders have been successfully integrated into e-health programs to reach broader populations and to sustain active participation. For example, a worksite health promotion program translated existing Web-based information to brief daily emails that were delivered to employee computers. This "push" method of delivering Web information eliminated the need for the user to initiate the search for information or to contact a health professional. Employee participants reported varied health behaviors, stages of change, and intentions to adopt health behaviors at the beginning of the program. Importantly, no variation in email opening was observed across stages of change or self-reported intention to change during the 6 month program (Franklin et al., 2006). These findings indicate the potential for e-health promotion programs to reach less motivated adults with suboptimal behaviors. In addition, Web and email-delivery allow low-cost, yet ongoing regular delivery of health messages for sustained periods of time. The optimal length of behavioral support programs delivered through e-technology is not known. Finally, some initial attempts to integrate e-health systems into medical practice have failed, suggesting that the current organization of medical offices is not prepared to incorporate computer based behavioral systems (Sciamanna et al., 2004). However, acute care hospitals and ambulatory care offices are not designed to support self-care in chronic disease or health promotion. It is unclear whether future e-health systems will reach patients within the health care system or directly, in their homes, workplaces, and schools.

Future Research Needed to Clarify the Roles of E-Health in Adherence

Carefully designed research to identify the ideal design, content, and delivery of effective e-health adherence interventions is beginning to emerge. Ahern and colleagues (2006) report a notable lack of consensus among e-health developers regarding intervention designs, user evaluations, and health outcome measures. Under the auspices of the Health-e-Technology Initiative funded by the Robert Wood Johnson Foundation (hetinitiative.org), research studies are systematically addressing tools, delivery mechanisms, user acceptance, and health benefits of a variety of electronic technologies designed to support behavior change and adherence. Despite the early state of research in the field, clinicians and technology experts are optimistic about the potential value and efficiency of e-health interventions serving both current and traditionally underserved patient populations. Future research should include multiple perspectives of patients, clinicians, and technology experts.

Evaluation of e-health systems typically revolves around the system's acceptability to users, its impact (helpfulness and effectiveness), and whether it fulfills the vision of the designers. Depending on the evaluation question(s), however, quantitative or qualitative methods of investigation may provide different types of information about a system. Quantitative structured instruments provide useful insight into users' overall perceptions but may not adequately address the complex dimensions of system utilization (Farzanfar et al., 2004). Qualitative methods, on the other hand, explore users' perceptions in depth and detail and enable designers to uncover the meaning users make of their experience with a system, that is, information from their point of view (Guba & Lincoln, 1981; Weiss, 1994). Qualitative methods, including one-on-one in-depth interviews, periodic focus groups, and, at times, ethnography, can also address system enhancements and redesign. An alternative method is "contextual inquiry," which is commonly used for evaluating information systems (Beyer & Holtzblatt, 1997). In "contextual inquiry," the emphasis is on the researcher's presence in the user's environment while exploring and understanding the context in which a system is used through in-depth interviews and participant observation. This method can be easily employed in evaluating e-health systems to more comprehensively identify user needs and acceptance of e-health systems.

Unanswered Questions About E-Health Design, Delivery, and Content

Several areas of research are needed to elucidate the potential effectiveness of e-health programs. First, research is needed to determine appropriate behavioral theories to guide design and delivery of e-health behavior change programs to achieve optimal results.

- Do the same theories and mediating constructs guide behavior change in e-health programs as in face-to-face programs?
- Does the delivery technology alter effectiveness? Evaluations of the relative benefits of varying delivery modes (PC, video game, video phone, or MP3 player), including comparisons to traditional clinician delivery, are needed.
- What are the optimal uses of tailored information? Are targeted and generic information adequate to foster certain behavior changes or in particular populations?

Second, methods for enhancing and quantifying e-health program dose (i.e., log-on rate and time on tasks) need to be identified. Methods are needed to define and achieve log-on rates at desirable intervals to ensure that participants receive an intervention dose needed to facilitate and sustain behavior change (Danaher, Boles, Akers, Gordon, & Severson, 2006; Thompson et al., 2007). In addition, more sophisticated use measures are needed to ascertain the depth and user benefits at each log-on session. Unanswered questions include these:

- What is the optimal interval between log-ons? Optimal length of engagement at each log-on? Optimal total number of log-ons?
- What is the role for reminders and strategies to enhance active participation?
- What measures capture understanding, depth, and benefits at each session?

Third, methods for providing equal access to e-health programs and services must be identified. Even with increasing connectivity, there is evidence of a digital divide (Fox, 2005). Only 26% of those 65 years and older use the Internet, and slightly more than half (57%) of African Americans are online, as opposed to nearly three-fourths of Whites (70%). Internet use among Hispanics varies, depending on how the data are collected. Disparities also exist by educational level. Because it is possible that populations without traditional access to medical care may benefit significantly from Internet-based applications, uniform Web connectivity is an important goal. Research may address these questions:

- Will uneven access to and comfort with e-health tools contribute to health disparities?
- Are users of e-health interventions representative of the general patient population? If not, how are nonusers engaged in e-health programs?

Finally, future evaluations should incorporate the evaluation of e-health program costs, including both the development and delivery costs, direct costs to health care systems and indirect costs to users, such as effects on their social networks (Griffiths, Lindenmeyer, Powell, Lowe, & Thorogood, 2006). E-health programs will not realize their full potential for delivering cost-effective, convenient health programs until issues such as these are resolved. However, experiences with a variety of e-health interventions to date suggest a future role for technology to support self-care behaviors and adherence to health promotion and chronic disease management.

References

Adler, K. G. (2006, October). Web portals in primary care: An evaluation of patient readiness and willingness to pay for online services. *Journal of Medical and Internet Research, 8*(4), e26. Retrieved October 18, 2007, from http://www.jmir.org/2006/4/e26/

Ahern, D. K., Kreslake, J. M., & Phalen, J. (2006, March). What is e-health? (6): Perspectives on the evolution of e-health research. *Journal of Medical and Internet Research, 8*(1): e4. Retrieved October 18, 2007, from http://www.jmir.org/2006/1/e4

Ahern, D. K, Phalen, J. M., & Mockenhaupt, R. E. (2003, January). Science and the advancement of e-health: A call to action. *American Journal of Preventive Medicine, 24,* 108–109.

Baranowski, T., Baranowski, J., Cullen, K.W., Marsh, T., Islam, N., Zakeri, I., Honess-Morreale, L., et al. (2003). Squire's Quest! Dietary outcome evaluation of a multimedia game. *American Journal of Preventive Medicine, 24*(1), 52–61.

Baranowski, T., Baranowski, J., Cullen, K. W., Thompson, D. I., Nicklas, T., Zakeri, I. E., et al. (2003, Winter). The Fun, Food, and Fitness Project (FFFP): The Baylor GEMS pilot study. *Ethnicity & Disease, 13*(Suppl. 1), S30–S39.

Baranowski, T., Cullen, K. W., Nicklas, T., Thompson, D., & Baranowski, J. (2003, October 11). Are current health behavioral change models helpful in guiding prevention of weight gain efforts? *Obesity Research* (Suppl.) 23S–43S.

Bensley, R. J., Mercer, N., Brusk, J. J., Underhile, R., Rivas, J., Anderson, J., et al. (2004, October). The e-health Behavior Management Model: A stage based approach to behavior change and management. *Preventing Chronic Disease, 1*(4), A14. Retrieved October 19, 2007, from http://www.pubmedcentral.nih.gov/articlerender.fcgi?tool=pubmed&pubmedid=15670446

Beyer, H., & Holtzblatt, K. (1997). *Contextual design: A customer-centered approach to systems design (Interactive Technologies).* San Francisco: Morgan Kaufmann Publishers.

Beyer, H., & Holtzblatt, K. (1999). Contextual design. *Interactions, 6*(1), 32–42.

Bickmore, T. (2003). *Relational agents: Effecting change through human-computer relationships.* Ph.D. Thesis, MIT Media Arts and Sciences.

Block, G., Block, T., Wakimoto, P., & Block, C. H. (2004, October). Demonstration of an e-mailed worksite nutrition intervention program. *Preventing Chronic Disease, 1*(4), A06. Retrieved October 19, 2007, from PubMed Central.

Blonde, L., & Parkin, C. G. (2006, January-February). Internet resources to improve health care for patients with diabetes. *Endocrine Practice, 12* (Suppl. 1), 131–137.

Blow, F. C., Barry, K. L., Walton, M. A., Maio, R. F., Chermack, S. T., Bingham, C. R., et al. (2006, July). The efficacy of two brief intervention strategies among injured, at risk drinkers in the emergency department: Impact of tailored messaging and brief advice. *Journal of Studies on Alcohol, 67,* 568–578.

Bodenheimer, T. (2005, November). High and rising health care costs. Part 1: Seeking an explanation. *Annals of Internal Medicine, 143* (10), 759.

Bodenheimer, T., Wagner, E. H., & Grumbach, K. (2002, October 16). Improving primary care for patients with chronic illness. The chronic care model, part 2. *Journal of the American Medical Association, 288,* 1909–1914.

Brock, T. P., & Smith, S. R. (2006, November 16). Using digital videos displayed on personal digital assistants (PDAs) to enhance patient education in clinical settings. *International Journal of Medical Informatics.* Retrieved October 19, 2007, from http://www.sciencedirect.com/science?_ob=ArticleURL&_udi=B6T7S-4MC71XJ-1&_user=115184&_coverDate=12%2F31%2F2007&_rdoc=1&_fmt=&_orig=search&_sort=d&view=c&_acct=C000009258&_version=1&_urlVersion=0&_userid=115184&md5=37e500022807d92fede243e7a08e6817

Bull, S. S., Gaglio, B., McKay, H. G., & Glasgow, R. E. (2005, June). Harnessing the potential of the internet to promote chronic illness self-management: Diabetes as an example of how well we are doing. *Chronic Illness, 1,* 143–155.

Campbell, M. K., DeVellis, B. M., Strecher, V. J., Ammerman, A. S., DeVellis, R. F., & Sandler, R. S. (1994). Improving dietary behavior: The effectiveness of tailored messages in primary care settings. *American Journal of Public Health, 84*(5), 783–787.

Clarke, G., Eubanks, D., Reid, E., Kelleher C., O'Connor, E., DeBar, L.L., et al. (2005, June). Overcoming depression on the Internet (ODIN) (2): A randomized trial of a self-help depression skills program with reminders. *Journal of Medical and Internet Research, 7(2),* e16. Retrieved October 22, 2007, from http://www.jmir.org/2005/2/e16/

Dale, O., & Hagen, K. B. (2007, January). Despite technical problems personal digital assistants outperform pen and paper when collecting patient diary data. *Journal of Clinical Epidemiology, 60*(1), 8–17.

Danaher, B. G., Boles, S. M., Akers, L., Gordon, J. S., & Severson, H. H. (2006, August 30). Defining participant exposure measures in Web-based health behavior change programs. *Journal of Medical and Internet Research 8*(3), e15. Retrieved October 22, 2007, from http://www.pubmedcentral.nih.gov/articlerender.fcgi?tool=pubmed&pubmedid=16954125

Delichatsios, H., Glanz, K., Tennstedt, S., Smigelski, S., Pinto, B. M., Kelley, H., et al. (2001). Randomized trial of a "talking computer" to improve adults' eating habits. *American Journal of Health Promotion, 15,* 215–224.

DeVries, H., & Brug, J. (1999, February). Computer-tailored interventions motivating people to adopt health promoting behaviors: Introduction to a new approach. *Patient Education and Counseling, 36*(2), 99–105.

Durant, L. E., & Carey, M. P. (2000, August). Self-administered questionnaires versus face-to-face interviews in assessing sexual behavior in young women. *Archives of Sexual Behavior, 29,* 309–322.

Eakin, E., Lawler, S., Vanderlanotte, C., & Owen, N. (2007, May). Telephone interventions for physical activity and dietary behavior change: A systematic review. *American Journal of Preventive Medicine, 32*(5), 419–434.

Eysenbach, G. (2001, April-June). What is e-health? *Journal of Medical and Internet Research. 3*(2), e20. Retrieved October 22, 2007, from http://www.jmir.org/2001/2/e20

Farzanfar, R. (2006, September). When computers should remain computers: A qualitative look at the humanization of health care technology. *Health Informatics, 12,* 239–254.

Farzanfar, R., Finkelstein, J., & Friedman, R. (2004, April 28). Testing the usability of two automated home-based patient-management systems. *Journal of Medical Systems, 28*(2), 143–153.

Farzanfar, R., Frishkopf, S., Migneault, J., & Friedman, R. (2005, June). Telephone linked care for physical activity: A qualitative evaluation of the use patterns of an information technology program for patients. *Journal of Biomedical Informatics, 38,* 220–228.

Ferrer-Roca, O., Cardenas, A., Diaz-Cardama, A., & Pulido, P. (2004). Mobile phone text messaging in the management of diabetes. *Journal of Telemedicine and Telecare, 10*(5), 282–285.

Fishbein, M., Hennessy, M., Kamb, M., Bolan, G. A., Hoxworth, T., Iatesta, M., et al. (2001). Using intervention theory to model factors influencing behavior change Project RESPECT. *Evaluation and the Health Professions, 24*(4), 363–384.

Ford, E. W., Menachemi, N., & Phillips, M. T. (2006, January-February). Predicting the adoption of electronic health records by physicians: When will health care be paperless? *Journal of the American Medical Informatics Association, 13*(1), 106–112.

Forsythe, D. (1995). Using ethnography in the design of an explanation system. Expert systems with applications. *Bulletin of the American Library Association, 8,* 403–417.

Fox, S. (2005, October 5). Digital divisions. Pew Internet and American Life Project: Washington, DC. Retrieved October 22, 2007, from http://www.pewinternet.org/pdfs/PIP_Digital_Divisions_Oct_5_2005.pdf

Franklin, P. D., Rosenbaum, P. F., Carey, M. P., & Roizen, M. F. (2006, March). Using sequential e-mail messages to promote health behaviors: Evidence of feasibility and reach in a worksite sample. *Journal of Medical and Internet Research, 8*(1), e3. Retrieved October 22, 2007, from http://www.jmir.org/2006/1/e3/

Friedman, R. H. (1998). Automated telephone conversations to assess health behavior and deliver behavioral interventions. *Journal of Medical Systems, 22,* 95–102.

Friedman R., Kazis, L. E., Jette, A., Smith, M. B., Stollerman, J., Torgerson, J., et al. (1996). A tele-communication system for monitoring and counseling patients with hypertension: Impact on medication adherence and blood pressure control. *American Journal of Hypertension, 9,* 285–292.

Funk, J. B. (2005). Video games. *Adolescent Medicine Clinics, 16*(2), 395–411, ix.

Gammon, D., Arsand, E., Walseth, O. A., Andersson, N., Jenssen, M., & Taylor, T. (2005). Parent-child interaction using a mobile and wireless system for blood glucose monitoring. *Journal of Internet Research, 7*(5), e57.

Gardiner, C., Williams, K., Mackie, I. J., Machin, S. J., & Cohen, H. (2006, April). Can oral antico-agulation be managed using telemedicine and patient self-testing? A pilot study. *Clinical and Laboratory Haematology, 28*(2), 122–125.

Geertz, C. (1973). *The interpretation of cultures: Selected essays by Clifford Geertz.* New York: Basic Books.

Glanz, K., Basil, M., Maibach, E., Goldberg, J., & Snyder, D. (1998). Why Americans eat what they do: Taste, nutrition, cost, convenience, and weight control concerns as influences on food consumption. *Journal of the American Dietetic Association, 98*(10), 1118–1126.

Glasgow, R. E., Boles, S. M., McKay, H. G., Feil, E. G., & Barrera, M., Jr. (2003, April). The D-Net diabetes self-management program: Long-term implementation, outcomes, and generalization results. *Preventive Medicine, 36*(4), 410–419.

Goldberg, H. I., Raston, J. D., Hirsch, I. B., Hoath, J. I., & Ahmed, K. I. (2003, September). Using an Internet comanagement module to improve the quality of chronic disease care. *Joint Commission Journal on Quality and Safety, 29,* 443–451.

Goran, M. I., & Reynolds, K. (2005 April). Interactive multimedia for promoting physical activity (IMPACT) in children. *Obesity Research, 13*(4), 762–771.

Griffiths, F., Lindenmeyer, A., Powell, J., Lowe, P., & Thorogood, M. (2006, June 3). Why are health care interventions delivered over the internet? A systematic review of the published literature. *Journal of Medical and Internet Research, 8*(2), e10. Retrieved October 22, 2007, from http://www.jmir.org/2006/2/e10/

Guba, E. G., & Lincoln Y. S. (1981). *Effective evaluation: Improving the usefulness of evaluation results through responsive and naturalistic approaches.* San Francisco: Jossey-Bass.

Hassol, A., Walker, J. M., Kidder, D., Rokita, K., Young, D., Pierdon, S., et al. (2004, November–December). Patient experiences and attitudes about access to a patient electronic health care record and linked web messaging. *Journal of the American Medical Informatics Association, 11*(6), 505–513.

Hispanics going online in record numbers, according to America Online/RoperASW's First Annual U.S. Hispanic Cyberstudy. (2003, January 27). Retrieved June 16, 2008, from http://www.timewarner.com/corp/newsroom/pr/0,20812,669698,00.html

Homer, C., Susskind, O., Alpert, H. R., Owusu, M., Schneider, L., Rappaport, L. A., et al. (2000, July). An evaluation of an innovative multimedia educational software program for asthma management: Report of a randomized, controlled trial. *Pediatrics, 106*(1 Pt. 2), 210–215.

Hornick, T. R., Higgins, P. A., Stollings, C., Wetzel, L., Barzilai, K., & Wolpaw, D. (2006, March). Initial evaluation of a computer-based medication management tool in a geriatric clinic. *American Journal of Geriatrics and Pharmacotherapy, 4,* 62–69.

Huss, K., Winkelstein, M., Nanda, J., Naumann, P. L., Sloand, E. D., & Huss, R. W. (2003, March-April). Computer game for inner-city children does not improve asthma outcomes. *Journal of Pediatric Health Care, 17*(2), 72–78.

Jago, R., Baranowski, T., Baranowski, J. C., Thompson, D., Cullen, K. W., Watson, K., et al. (2006, March). Fit for Life Boy Scout badge: Outcome evaluation of a troop and Internet intervention. *Preventive Medicine, 42,* 181–187.

Jarvis, K., Friedman, R. H., Heeren, T., & Cullinane, P. M. (1997). Older women and physical activity: Using the telephone to walk. *Women's Health Issues, 4,* 413–425.

Jaspan, H. B., Flisher, A. J, Myer, L., Mathews C., Seebreqts, C., Berwick, J. R., et al. (2007, April). Methods for collecting sexual behavior information from South African adolescents—a comparison of paper versus personal digital assistant questionnaires. *Journal of Adolescence, 30*(2), 353–359.

Kreuter, M. W., Strecher, V. J., & Glassman, B. (1999, Fall). One size does not fit all: The case for tailoring print materials. *Annals of Behavioral Medicine, 21*(4), 276–283.

Krishna, S., Francisco, B. D., Balas, E. A., Konig, P., Graff, G. R., & Madsen, R. W. (2003). Internet-enabled interactive multimedia asthma education program: A randomized trial. *Pediatrics, 111*(3), 503–510.

Kroeze, W., Werkman, A., & Brug, J. (2006, June). A systematic review of randomized trials on the effectiveness of computer-tailored education on physical activity and dietary behaviors. *Annals of Behavioral Medicine, 31,* 205–223.

Lanningham-Foster, L., Jensen, T. B., Foster, R. C., Redmond, A. B., Walker, B. A., Heinz, D., et al. (2006, December). Energy expenditure of sedentary screen time compared with active screen time for children. *Pediatrics, 118*(6), e1831–1835.

Lieberman, D. A. (2001, January). Management of chronic pediatric diseases with interactive health games: Theory and research findings. *Journal of Ambulatory Care Management, 24*(1), 26–38.

Lin, C. T., Wittevrongel, L., Moore, L., Beaty, B. L., & Ross, S. E. (2005, August). An Internet-based patient-provider communication system: Randomized controlled trial. *Journal of Medical and Internet Research, 7*(4), e47.

Lorig, K. R., Ritter, P. L., Laurent, D. D., & Plant, K. (2006, November). Internet-based chronic disease self-management: A randomized trial. *Medical Care, 44,* 964–971.

Lorig, K. R., Sobel, D. S., Ritter, P. L., Laurent, D., & Hobbs, M. (2001). Effect of self-management program on patients with chronic disease. *Effective Clinical Practice, 4*(6), 256–262.

Mabry, S. L., Schneringer, T., Etters, T., & Edwards, N. (2003). *Intelligent agents for patient monitoring and diagnostics. Proceedings of the 2003 ACM symposium on applied computing.* Retrieved October 22, 2007, http://portal.acm.org/citation.cfm?id=952532.952585

Madsen, K. A., Yen, S., Wlasiuk, L., Newman, T. B., & Lustig, R. (2007, January). Feasibility of a dance videogame to promote weight loss among overweight children and adolescents. *Archives of Pediatrics & Adolescent Medicine, 161*(1), 105–107.

McPherson, A. C., Glazebrook, C., Forster, D., James, C., & Smyth, A. (2006, April). A randomized, controlled trial of an interactive educational computer package for children with asthma. *Pediatrics, 117*(4), 1046–1054.

Nakajima, K., Nambu, M., Kiryu, T., Tamura, T., & Sasaki, K. (2006). Low-cost e-mail-based system for self blood pressure monitoring at home. *Journal of Telemedicine and Telecare, 12,* 203–207.

Napolitano, M. A., Fotheringham, M., Tate, D., Sciamanna, C., Leslie E., Owen N., et al. (2003, Spring). Evaluation of an internet-based physical activity intervention: A preliminary investigation. *Annals of Behavioral Medicine, 25*(2), 92–99.

National Center for Chronic Disease Prevention and Health Promotion. (2005, November 17). *Preventing chronic diseases: Investing wisely in health preventing obesity and chronic diseases through good nutrition and physical activity.* Retrieved June 16, 2008, from http://www.webcitation.org/query?snapshotid=3023

Nielsen, J. (1992). *Usability engineering.* San Diego: Academic Press.

Pallonen, U. E., Velicer, W. F., Prochaska, J. O., Rossi, J. S., Bellis, J. M., Tsoh, J. Y., et al. (1998). Computer-based smoking cessation interventions in adolescents: Description, feasibility, and six-month follow-up findings. *Substance Use and Misuse, 33*(4), 935–965.

Patel, A., Schieble, T., Davidson, M., Tran, M. C., Schoenberg, C., Delphin, E., et al. (2006, October). Distraction with a hand-held video game reduces pediatric preoperative anxiety. *Pediatric Anesthesia, 16*(10), 1019–1027.

Plotnikoff, R. C., McCargar, L. J., Wilson, P. M., & Loucaides, C. A. (2005, July-August). Efficacy of an e-mail intervention for the promotion of physical activity and nutrition behavior in the workplace context. *American Journal of Health Promotion, 19*(6), 422–429.

Prasad, P. (1997). Systems of meaning: Ethnography as a methodology for the study of information technologies. In A. S. Lee, J. Leibenau, & J. I. DeGross, *Information systems and qualitative research* (pp. 101–118). London: Chapman & Hall.

Rainie, L., & Horrigan, J. (2005). *The mainstreaming of online life. Pew Internet and American Life Project.* Retrieved February 27, 2007, from http://www.pewinternet.org/pdfs/Internet_Status_2005.pdf

Ramelson, H. Z., Friedman, R. H., & Ockene, J. K. (1999). An automated telephone-based smoking cessation education and counseling system. *Patient Education and Counseling, 36*(2), 131–144.

Roberts, D., Foehr, U., & Rideout, V. (2005, March 9). Generation M: Media in the lives of 8–18 year-olds. Publication no. 7251, The Henry Kaiser Family Foundation, Washington, DC. Retrieved October 22, 2007, from http://www.kff.org/entmedia/upload/Generation-M-Media-in-the-Lives-of-8-18-Year-olds-Report.pdf

Robertson, L., Smith, M., Castle, D., & Tannenbaum, D. (2006, December). Using the Internet to enhance the treatment of depression. *Australas Psychiatry, 14,* 413–417.

Sciamanna, C. N., Marcus, B. H., Goldstein, M. G., Lawrence, K., Swartz, S., Bock, B., et al. (2004). Feasibility of incorporating computer-tailored health behavior communications in primary care settings. *Informatics in Primary Care, 12,* 40–48.

Shegog, R., McAlister, A. L., Hu, S., Ford, K. C., Meshack, A. F., & Peters, R. J. (2005, May–June). Use of interactive health communication to affect smoking intentions in middle school students: A pilot test of the "Headbutt" risk assessment program. *American Journal of Health Promotion, 19*(5), 334–338.

Southard, D. R., & Southard, B. H. (2006, October). Promoting physical activity in children with MetaKenkoh. *Clinical and Investigative Medicine, 29*(5), 293–297.

Tan, B., Aziz, A. R., Chua, K., & Teh, K. C. (2002, February). Aerobic demands of the dance simulation game. *International Journal of Sports Medicine, 23*(2), 125–129.

Tate, D. F., Jackvony, E. H., & Wing, R. R. (2003, April). Effects of Internet behavioral counseling on weight loss in adults at risk for type 2 diabetes. *Journal of the American Medical Association, 289,* 1833–1836.

Tate, D. F., Wing, R. R., & Winett, R. A. (2001). Using Internet technology to deliver a behavioral weight loss program. *Journal of the American Medical Association, 285*(9), 1172–1177.

Thompson, D., Baranowski, T., Cullen, K., Watson, K., Canada, A., Bhatt, R., et al. (2007, June 25). Food, Fun, and Fitness Internet Program for Girls: Influencing log-on rate. *Health Education Research.* Retrieved October 22, 2007, from http://her.oxfordjournals.org/cgi/content/full/cym020v1

Trapl, E. S., Borawski, E. A., Stork, P. P., Lovegreen, L. D., Colabianchi, N., Cole, M. L., et al. (2005, October). Use of audio-enhanced personal digital assistants for school-based data collection. *Journal of Adolescent Health, 37*(4), 296–305.

Turnin, M. C., Tauber, M. T., Couvaras, O., Jouret, B., Bolzonella, C., Bourgeois, O., et al. (2001, September). Evaluation of microcomputer nutritional teaching games in 1,876 children at school. *Diabetes and Metabolism, 27*(4 Pt. 1), 459–464.

Tutty, S., Ludman, E. J., & Simon, G. (2005). Feasibility and acceptability of a telephone psychotherapy program for depressed adults treated in primary care. *General Hospital Psychiatry, 27*(6), 400–410.

U.S. Department of Health and Human Services. (2000). *Healthy People 2010: Understanding and improving health.* Washington, DC: U.S. Government Printing Office. Retrieved October 22, 2007, from http://www.healthypeople.gov/Document/

Vilozni, D., Barak, A., Efrati, O., Springer, C., Yahav, Y., & Bentur, L. (2005, September). The role of computer games in measuring spirometry in healthy and "asthmatic" preschool children. *Chest, 128*(3), 1146–1155.

Vitalari, N. (1985). The need for longitudinal designs in the study of computing environment. In E. Mumford et al. (Eds.), *Research methods in information systems* (pp. 243–265). North-Holland, Amsterdam: Elsevier.

Wagner, E. H., Austin, B. T., Davis, C., Hindmarsh, M., Schaefer, J., & Bonomi, A. (2001, November-December). Improving chronic illness care: Translating evidence into action. *Health Affairs (Millwood), 20,* 64–78.

Waller, A., Franklin, V., Pagliari, C., & Greene, S. (2006, December). Participatory design of a text message scheduling system to support young people with diabetes. *Health Informatics Journal, 12,* 304–318.

Wang, D. H., Kogashiwa, M., & Kira, S. (2006, October). Development of a new instrument for evaluating individuals' dietary intakes. *Journal of the American Dietetic Association, 106*(10), 1588–1593.

Wang, D. H., Kogashiwa, M., Ohta, S., & Kira S. (2002, December). Validity and reliability of a dietary assessment method: The application of a digital camera with a mobile phone card attachment. *Journal of Nutritional Science and Vitaminology (Tokyo), 48*(6), 498–504.

Wangberg, S. C., Arsand, E., & Andersson, N. (2006). Diabetes education via mobile text messaging. *Journal of Telemedicine and Telecare, 12*(Suppl. 1), 55–56.

Weiss, R. (1994). *Learning from strangers: The art and method of qualitative interview studies.* New York, The Free Press.

Wellman, B. (2001, September). Computer networks as social networks. *Science, 293*(5537), 2031–2034.

Williamson, D. A., Walden, H. M., White, M. A., York-Crowe, E., Newton, R. L., Jr., Alfonso, A., et al. (2006 July). Two-year Internet-based randomized controlled trial for weight loss in African-American girls. *Obesity (Silver Spring), 14*(7), 1231–1243.

Winett, R. A., Tate, D. F., Anderson, E. S., Wojcik, J. R., & Winett, S. G. (2005, August). Long-term weight gain prevention: A theoretically based Internet approach. *Preventive Medicine, 41*(2), 629–641.

Wing, R. R., Tate, D. F., Gorin, A. A., Raynor, H. A., & Fava, J. L. (2006 October). A self-regulation program for the maintenance of weight loss. *New England Journal of Medicine, 355*(15), 1563–1571.

Wise, M., Gustafson, D. H., Sorkness, C. A., Molfenter, T., Staresinic, A., Meis, T., et al. (2007, July). Internet tele-health for pediatric asthma case management: Integrating computerized and case manager features for tailoring a Web-based asthma education program. *Health Promotion Practice, 8*(3), 282–291.

Woolf, S. H., Krist, A. H., Johnson, R. E., Wilson, D. B., Rothemich, S. F., Norman, G. J., et al. (2006 March-April). A practice-sponsored Web site to help patients pursue healthy behaviors: An ACORN study. *Annals of Family Medicine, 4*(2), 148–152.

Yawn, B. P., Algatt-Bergstrom, P. J., Yawn, R. A., Wollan, P., Greco, M., Gleason, M., et al. (2000, April). An in-school CD-ROM asthma education program. *The Journal of School Health, 70*(4), 153–159.

Yon, B. A., Johnson, R. K., Harvey-Berino, J., & Gold, B. C. (2006, August). The use of a personal digital assistant for dietary self-monitoring does not improve the validity of self-reports of energy intake. *Journal of the American Dietetic Association, 106,* 1256–1259.

Yon, B. A., Johnson, R. K, Harvey-Berino, J., Gold, B. C., & Howard, A. B. (2007, April). Personal Digital Assistants are comparable to traditional diaries for dietary self-monitoring during a weight loss program. *Journal of Behavioral Medicine, 30*(2), 165–175.

Section 2

Interventions for Lifestyle Change

Judith K. Ockene
Editor

As was emphasized in chapter 1, "Theories of Prevention," the message in medicine and public health is strong: many acute and chronic diseases can be prevented, or at least have their impact lessened, by increased attention to the adoption and maintenance of health-promoting behaviors. This recognition grows out of the many epidemiologic investigations that demonstrate the existence of a strong relationship between the onset, progression, and exacerbation of disease and subsequent quality of life and alterable health-related behaviors such as smoking, diet, physical activity, sexual practices, and stress management. Using the theories and models presented in Section I, as well as theories addressing factors at the organizational and community levels that we'll read about in Section VII, chapters in this section focus on intervention strategies designed to facilitate change in health-promoting and disease-preventing behaviors and the maintenance of these behaviors. The strategies provided demonstrate the important translation from theory and research to application in practice.

A chapter now included in Section II and not included in previous editions of this book, "Multiple Risk Behavior Change: What Most Individuals Need," is an important addition. It addresses the integration of interventions for working with individuals who have multiple risk behaviors or comorbidities. Providers in all disciplines are faced each day with patients who have a clustering of disease-promoting or comorbid behaviors. Health practitioners need integrated approaches that can be applied to patients, rather than a collection of disparate single-behavior interventions. The chapters in Section II demonstrate that, while we have learned much in the last several decades about facilitating the maintenance of healthy behaviors, such endeavors are still a challenge to health practitioners and researchers.

Researchers Jolicoeur and colleagues, in "Addressing Tobacco Use and Dependence," stress the importance of a multifaceted approach to tobacco. McCann and Bovbjerg, in "Promoting Dietary Change," stress the importance of community and organizational change for facilitating nutritional and other health-related interventions and the complementarity of individual and organizational change. Marcus and colleagues, in discussing "Adherence to Physical Activity Recommendations and Interventions," ask us to give strong consideration to patient-treatment matching models as a way of responding to the differences patients bring with them. Naughton and Rhodes, in "Adoption and Maintenance of Safer Sexual Practices," emphasize that the diversity of the population groups affected by unsafe sexual practices makes developing effective strategies for this population challenging and that societal norms and interpersonal relationships play a strong role in this behavior. The state of the science in this area is younger than for the other behaviors that are addressed in this section, and the authors suggest directions for future research. Salmon and colleagues remind us in "Intervention Elements Promoting Adherence to Mindfulness-Based Stress Reduction (MBSR) Programs in a Clinical Behavioral Medicine Setting," that we must be ever mindful of the point of view of patients when caring for them. Judith Prochaska and Janice Prochaska, in their chapter on multiple risk behavior change (MRBC), note that MRBC research is "at an early stage, with its boundaries still being defined" and with much research still to be implemented.

The authors of each of the chapters agree that long-term change is yet another challenge, one that often feels elusive.

Addressing Tobacco Use and Dependence

10

Denise G. Jolicoeur,
Beth M. Ewy,
Judith K. Ockene,
Lori Pbert, and
David B. Abrams

At the national level, over the past several decades, a wide variety of tobacco control efforts have been implemented in the United States in a relatively unsystematic manner. Nevertheless, the net impact of all strategies resulted in a 50% decrease in the prevalence of smoking, from 42.4% in 1965 to 20.8% in 2006 (Centers for Disease Control and Prevention, 2006c). A population level drop in prevalence of tobacco use behavior of this magnitude within the short time span of 40 years (less than one to two generations) is an astounding public health success. Thun and Jamal (2006) estimate that the decline in tobacco-related cancers is so large as to contribute more than 40% of the variance attributable to the much-publicized reversal in the overall cancer mortality rate in the United States that has occurred for the first time since the war on cancer was declared in 1971 (Thun & Jemal, 2006). While the mortality rate attributable to smoking has declined as a result of the reduction in smoking prevalence (Rodu & Cole, 2007), tobacco use still accounted for more than 435,000 deaths in 2000 (Mokdad, Marks, Stroup, & Gerberding, 2004, 2005).

Much urgent work remains to be completed because there were still more than 40 million current smokers in the United States in 2006 and more than a billion worldwide. Tobacco use behavior remains the leading preventable cause of premature death, disability, and unnecessary expense, despite the rise of other pressing public health challenges such as the obesity, type 2 diabetes, and HIV-AIDS epidemics. It is estimated that as many as half the current smokers, more than 20 million human beings, will die prematurely of a smoking-related disease (Camenga & Klein, 2004) unless more effective, efficient, and compre-hensive tobacco use prevention, treatment, and policy initiatives are developed and aggressively deployed.

Treatment services for nicotine dependence are recommended as an in-tegral component of the multipronged approach that has contributed to the decline in smoking (Centers for Disease Control and Prevention, 1999; U.S. Pre-ventive Services Task Force, 2006). The Clinical Practice Guideline for Treat-ing Tobacco Use and Dependence, published by the Public Health Service, has compiled the available research demonstrating that effective smoking cessation interventions exist, including behavioral and pharmacological treatment (Fiore et al., 2008). Using evidence-based treatment significantly increases success, from almost double to as much as fourfold the cessation rate among those who quit on their own. Despite the social climate that is making it more difficult to smoke (e.g., bans in worksites, higher taxes on cigarettes), effective cessation programs are greatly underutilized. We are at a critical junction in the journey to further reduce smoking rates. The Institute of Medicine has recommended a "comprehensive, coordinated system of care management for cessation treat-ment" that includes five key elements: (1) motivating tobacco users to make more frequent quit attempts, (2) educating tobacco users to use evidence-based treatments when they try to quit, (3) reducing the very high rates of relapse to tobacco use after successful quitting, (4) ensuring that all tobacco users have access to the best care available and full insurance coverage for treatment ser-vices, and (5) structuring the system of care to provide additional levels of more intensive/specialized treatment (i.e., stepped care) for tobacco users who need them (Institute of Medicine, 2007).

This chapter provides an overview of the multifaceted nature of tobacco use behavior and cessation, including biological, psychological, and social factors. We review the major components of effective individual-level interventions, including behavioral and pharmacological options ranging from minimal (e.g., self-help) to maximal (e.g., inpatient treatment) in intensity and cost. Finally, system-level interventions are addressed.

The Nature of Nicotine Dependence

Defining Dependence

Dependence as defined by the American Psychiatric Association's Diagnostic and Statistical Manual (American Psychiatric Association, 2000) (DSM-IV-R) involves key signs and symptoms, including an inability to discontinue use despite the presence of harm, tolerance to nicotine, and withdrawal symptoms. Withdrawal symptoms are often a primary factor in the inability to quit and relapse; they include (1) dysphoric or depressed mood; (2) insomnia; (3) irritability, frustration, or anger; (4) anxiety; (5) difficulty concentrating; (6) restlessness; (7) decreased heart rate; and (8) increased appetite or weight gain (American Psychiatric Association, 2000). The appearance of withdrawal symptoms may occur very early in the life of some smokers and in the presence of intermittent smoking (DiFranza et al., 2007). Estimates of the percentage of dependent smokers can be as high as 87% (Hale et al., 1993). Greater tobacco dependence and the ability to quit are influenced by the interaction of genetic, neurobiological, psychological, social, and cultural factors.

Neurobiology of Nicotine Dependence

Nicotine produces subtle, short-term, pleasurable effects, and cigarettes in particular are a highly efficient nicotine delivery system. Carried on the tar droplets produced by cigarette smoke, nicotine is passed from lungs to heart to brain in 7–10 seconds. The physiologic effects of nicotine play a major role in the establishment and maintenance of tobacco use. The short half-life of nicotine (2 hours) drives the frequent dosing of a regular smoker in order to achieve the desired positive effects and to stave off withdrawal symptoms.

As with many other drugs of abuse, the role of the mesolimbic system of the brain appears to be the most significant and so far the best understood in nicotine dependence. Nicotine's stimulation of this system hijacks the reward pathway whose primary purpose is to ensure survival by associating pleasure with natural stimulants such as food, water, sex, and nurturing. Nicotine binds to nicotinic acetylcholine receptors (nAChRs), stimulating the release of dopamine and the sensation of pleasure (Balfour, 2004; Dani, 2001). The noradrenergic system, including the locus ceruleus, is thought to play a major role in the mediation of withdrawal symptoms.

Stimulation of nAChRs by nicotine also results in an increase in glutamate (Lambe, Picciotto, & Aghajanian, 2003), which contributes to reinforcement of the pleasurable memory. By contrast, the inhibitory effect of GABA, whose function is to regulate the amount of available dopamine, is reduced. Thus these complementary functions serve to increase and reinforce the pleasurable effects of nicotine (Kalivas & Volkow, 2005).

The role of these neurobiological processes is significant in understanding the underpinning of dependence and has led to the development of pharmacologic treatments that are beneficial in assisting with cessation (Harris & Anthenelli, 2005). Recent research is also revealing more specific genetic or cellular mechanisms involved in dependence and in individual differences in patterns of use, such as the role of $\alpha_4\beta_2$ nicotinic receptors and allelic variation in the CYP2D6 gene related to differential rates of nicotine to cotinine metabolism. Thus, new discoveries in basic science may lead to better understanding of differential use and effectiveness of cessation aids and possible gender or racial differences in addiction susceptibility, and this in turn may lead to even more effective and efficient use of genetically tailored pharmacotherapies (Lerman & Niaura, 2002).

Psychological Aspects of Dependence

Tobacco users report myriad benefits from its use. Paradoxical effects such as stress reduction and relaxation and stimulation and arousal point to the ability of the tobacco user to control its effects. It is not entirely clear if improved cognitive functioning (e.g., memory and concentration) are direct effects of tobacco use or the result of relief of withdrawal (Heishman, 2000). It is, however, very clear that the pleasurable effects of nicotine become intricately linked to daily activities, emotions, and situations (e.g., talking on the phone, driving, coping with anger). These links become "triggers" for the urge to use tobacco and strongly reinforce its habitual use. Tobacco use becomes essential to daily functioning even in the absence of conscious forethought. Identification of the triggers and the perceived benefits of tobacco use are essential during the cessation process.

For those with psychiatric and substance use comorbidities, the psychological benefits appear to be more pronounced and even more intricately linked with daily functioning. Depression, alcohol, and other substance use disorders, adult attention deficit/hyperactivity problems, psychotic disorders, and anxiety disorders are associated with increased prevalence of smoking and lower rates of cessation (J. Hughes, 1995; J. Hughes et al., 1996; J. R. Hughes, 1993). One recent population-based study estimated that 44% of cigarettes sold are consumed by persons suffering from current mental illness (Lasser et al., 2000). Smoking rates of more than 85% are observed in alcoholics, opiate addicts, and poly-drug users (Fertig & Allen, 1995) and, because of this, smoking can be considered a marker of other substance use. It is encouraging to note, however, that abstinence from tobacco appears to enhance recovery and reduce relapse to other substance use (Prochaska, Delucchi, & Hall, 2004). Although use of evidence-based interventions improves cessation outcomes for all tobacco users across the board, those who do have comorbidity and smoke more heavily are likely to require more intensive interventions in order achieve a tobacco-free status.

Social and Cultural Factors Associated With Dependence

There are a number of important individual and population-level smoker characteristics associated with differences in smoking prevalence, motivation to quit, and some cessation outcomes. Some of these factors are important in considering how best to reach more smokers, motivate them to try to stop smoking, and encourage them to use the best interventions available to increase the likelihood of success and to reduce the high rates of relapse after quit attempts. Factors include gender, education, income, age, and racial and ethnic background.

Women differ from men in their biological responses to nicotine (Perkins, Donny, & Caggiula, 1999); however, there are mixed data regarding whether women have more difficulty quitting than men (Killen, Fortmann, Varady, & Kraemer, 2002; Wetter et al., 1999). Concerns about weight gain, stress reduction, and the need for social support may contribute to differences between men and women smokers.

Educational attainment, income level, and age are among the strongest predictors of smoking, 43.2% of those with a GED, 29.9% of those living below the poverty level (Centers for Disease Control and Prevention, 2004), and 29.0% of those 44 years of age or younger (but only 12.0% of those older than 65) are identified as smokers (Centers for Disease Control and Prevention, 1998).

There is also wide variation among cultural and ethnic groups. For example, the aggregate smoking rate for Asians/Pacific Islanders is reported as 13.3%, while community-level surveys report that 36%–56% of Vietnamese men smoke (Centers for Disease Control and Prevention, 2004; U.S. Department of Health and Human Services, 1998). The smoking rate for American Indians and Alaska Natives is 40.8% but only 16.7% for Hispanics (Centers for Disease Control and Prevention, 2004). In addition, there appear to be some biological differences between African Americans and Chinese on one hand and Whites on the other; the former metabolize nicotine at a slower rate than Whites (Benowitz, Perez-Stable, Herrera, & Jacob, 2002; Centers for Disease Control and Prevention, 1998; Perez-Stable, Herrera, Jacob, & Benowitz, 1998).

Smoking patterns among adolescents are more variable than those among adults, with many adolescents smoking intermittently rather than daily. Factors such as parental smoking and socioeconomic stress affect smoking rates among adolescents, and the most significant predictor is peer smoking (Milton et al., 2004). Ethnic and cultural differences can be seen here, as well, with the highest rates of smoking among American Indian and Alaska Native teens, followed by White teens (Centers for Disease Control and Prevention, 2006b) (see Section IV, chapter 22, for additional information about tobacco use among adolescents).

While few generalizations can be made regarding effective treatment strategies for subgroups, whenever possible both behavioral and pharmacologic treatment should be tailored and monitored in order to best meet the needs of the individual. Smokers who are at higher risk due to certain biobehavioral or socioeconomic vulnerabilities may indeed benefit from more intensive, longer, or specialized clinical interventions. The following section provides the foundation upon which effective treatment strategies at the individual and systems level are based.

Individual-Level Interventions

The vast majority of smokers who make quit attempts do so without any form of assistance, and more than 95% relapse (National Institutes of Health, State-of-the-Science Panel, 2006). Few smokers know about treatment efficacy, few use any treatments at all, and those who do use an evidence-based program may not use or have access to the best programs to address their individual requirements. Consequently, there is a need to increase the interest and motivation of smokers to make more quit attempts and to use evidence-based interventions when quitting to improve the likelihood of cessation and to reduce the likelihood of relapse (Orleans & Slade, 1993; Orleans & Alper, 2003).

Implementation of comprehensive-care management systems can ensure that each smoker receives continuity and the appropriate level of care based on screening and triage into a level and type of treatment that meets his needs (e.g., a stepped-care approach) (Abrams et al., 2003). Treatments can range from minimal/brief intensity (e.g., over-the-counter nicotine replacement,

Internet-based interventions, and brief primary care) to moderate intensity (e.g., proactive telephone) to maximum intensity (e.g., outpatient and inpatient multisession clinical care delivered by specialists trained to treat severe tobacco addiction). This should not be interpreted as an indication that a novice quitter should have access only to minimal treatment, rather that this range of treatment should be available to best meet the needs and interest of the tobacco user at the time of her quit attempt. Even a first-time quitter should have access to intensive treatment if interested in order to reduce the recycling so common among tobacco users.

Generally, there is broad consensus that smokers who use proven tobacco dependence interventions (either behavioral or pharmacologic) have roughly double the quit rate of users who do not. Combined behavioral and pharmacologic treatments can result in as much as a three- to fourfold increase in cessation outcomes. In addition to the PHS guideline (Fiore et al., 2008) that details best-practice recommendations, there are resources available to assist practitioners in developing evidence-based treatment protocols, including a comprehensive handbook for the assessment and treatment of smokers that covers program planning, assessment, and a range of treatment options, from brief motivational intervention to intensive treatment for smokers with co-morbid psychiatric conditions (Abrams et al., 2003), as well as several other manuals (McEwen, Hajek, McRobbie, & West, 2006; Perkins, Conklin, & Levine, 2007).

Recommendations for treating special populations such as adolescents (Sussman, Sun, & Dent, 2006), pregnant smokers (Lumley, Oliver, Chamberlain, & Oakley, 2004), and those with mental health disorders (Williams & Ziedonis, 2004) also have been published. In addition, a number of tobacco treatment specialist training programs now exist (see www.attud.org). All evidence-based treatment protocols address both pharmacologic treatment (except where contraindicated) and psychosocial components that are based upon many of the behavior change theories described elsewhere in this book (see Section I). A brief summary of the application of psychosocial and pharmacologic strategies for tobacco treatment is presented here.

Psychosocial Treatment Theories and Models

Cognitive Social Learning Theory (CSLT) (Bandura, 1986) describes many of the elements of behavior change that serve as the foundation of skills training considered to be key components of tobacco treatment (Vidrine, Cofta-Woerpel, Daza, Wright, & Wetter, 2006). Together with the principle of reciprocal determinism (what we think influences what we do and vice versa), self-efficacy and outcome expectancies are common pathways leading to the initiation of behavior change (Bandura, 1986, 1995). The relationship between self-efficacy and outcome expectancies may play a critical role in the response to urges and craving related to tobacco addiction (Niaura, 2000). Other self-regulatory mechanisms, such as goal setting and corrective feedback, provide intermediary steps that can serve to facilitate the process of change (Abrams, Elder, Carleton, Lasater, & Artz, 1986; Abrams, Emmons, Niaura, Goldstein, & Sherman, 1991). Integration of skills training also includes a strong focus on relapse prevention, based on the work of Marlatt and Gordon (1985).

Motivation is important for making the initial decision to change behavior, as well as for carrying out the tasks (i.e., meeting the goals) required to complete the behavior change. For example, a smoker not only needs to make the decision about whether he is ready to quit but also needs to set goals consistent with this objective, such as increasing knowledge, changing attitudes, or setting a quit day. Motivation for smoking cessation refers to both smokers' reasons for quitting and to the strength of their desire to quit (Curry, Wagner, & Grothaus, 1990). Miller and Rollnick (Rollnick, Miller, & Butler, 2007) have developed Motivational Interviewing (MI), a method that uses client-centered techniques designed to increase motivation, primarily among substance abuse patients, who are often ambivalent about stopping or decreasing their addictive behavior(s) (see Section I, chapter 8, for additional details). While the body of evidence regarding the effectiveness of MI for tobacco treatment is limited (Burke, Arkowitz, & Menchola, 2003), a combination of MI techniques and skills training is common practice. Patient-centered counseling is a similar intervention style that has demonstrated significant results when implemented by physicians as part of programs to combat smoking, poor nutrition, and alcohol use (I. S. Ockene et al., 1999; J. Ockene et al., 1994; J. Ockene et al., 1988; J. Ockene, Wheeler, Adams, Hurley, & Hebert, 1997).

Prochaska and colleagues, using a stage of change model (Prochaska, DiClemente, Velicer, & Rossi, 1993), have suggested that tailoring interventions to motivational level may increase smoking cessation among less motivated smokers. The stages-of-change model (Prochaska & Velicer, 2004) lends itself to the development of interventions tailored to the smoker's motivational readiness to change (see Section I, Chapter 4 for additional details). It also provides a useful roadmap for smokers in that it provides milestones (precontemplation, contemplation, preparation, action, maintenance) and guidelines for processes used at every phase of the journey, from smoking initiation to various patterns of use to efforts at cessation, relapse, and recycling to the ultimate success of permanent maintenance of cessation. There is some debate over the ultimate utility of a stage model of change, especially regarding its ability to accurately assess readiness to change and its prospective predictive value (e.g., Herzog & Blagg, 2007; Sutton, 2001; West, 2005). Continuous measures to assess motivation, such as the Contemplation Ladder, have also been used as an alternative to a categorical staging algorithm (Herzog & Blagg, 2007). Despite the potential limitations, outcomes research has supported some components of this model when applied to written and electronic materials for smoking cessation (Becona & Vazquez, 2001; Etter & Perneger, 2001; Prochaska, Velicer, Fava, Rossi, & Tsoh, 2001).

Behavioral Treatment Strategies

In general, greater intensity of treatment (duration and number of contacts, more modalities of intervention) improves cessation outcomes, and delivery of treatment via in-person (1:1 or group) and proactive telephone counseling are all equally effective (Fiore et al., 2008). Although the following classification is an oversimplification, for many purposes intervention intensity can be classified into three categories: (1) minimal or brief; (2) moderate; and (3) maximal. For the clinical setting, these levels can be described in relation to the Public

Health Service–recommended 5A model: *Ask* about tobacco use, *Advise* tobacco users about the risks of smoking and benefits of quitting, *Assess* readiness to change, *Assist* with cessation, *Arrange* follow-up.

Ask and *Advise,* combined with *Referral* to more intensive treatment, are the components of a brief intervention (level 1) and should be the minimum provided to all tobacco users seen in a clinical setting (see http://smokingcessation leadership.ucsf.edu). The addition of *Assess, Assist,* and *Arrange* components is consistent with moderate (level 2) and maximal service (level 3). Strategies for addressing these components are reviewed briefly in the following sections.

Assessing Motivation to Quit

Patient-Centered Counseling (PCC) using techniques such as Motivational Interviewing (MI) techniques and an understanding of stages of change help the clinician assess the tobacco user's willingness and confidence in quitting. However, despite the appeal of the stages-of-change model, it should also be noted that some smokers suddenly decide to quit smoking in an unpredictable fashion that does not follow the rational and sequential flow of a stages of change theory (West, 2006). As many as 49% of smokers may quit without any advance planning.

Tobacco users vary widely in their motivation to quit and initial interventions are most effective when clinicians take the time to actively listen to their clients and encourage them to articulate the pros and cons of tobacco use and quitting. For the tobacco user who is not ready to quit (precontemplation), this exploration may begin to open the door for future consideration of a cessation attempt. For those considering or preparing to quit (contemplation and preparation), this discussion will begin to uncover the facilitators and barriers to change that will be faced by the client. As mentioned earlier, the level of self-efficacy or confidence expressed by the client may strongly influence readiness to change. Low confidence is often a barrier, and increasing confidence will be a proximal goal. The basic PCC skills of using open-ended questions and asking the smoker to identify his own strengths, challenges, and resources are essential at this stage of the process. For a more detailed discussion of the tools available to address motivation to quit, see Emmons et al. in Abrams et al. (2003).

Assisting With Cessation

As the tobacco user moves into preparation and action, a more thorough assessment of current and past use patterns is relevant. This assessment includes reviewing the motivation and strategies related to past quit attempts and factors that contributed to relapse. Exploration of current use patterns reveals what situations, moods, and routines trigger smoking. These triggers are often identified during a period of behavioral self-monitoring, which involves recording time, place, situation, mood, thoughts, and need level associated with each instance of tobacco use.

Skill training in specific cognitive-behavioral techniques assists the tobacco user to develop strategies to address identified triggers and anticipated problems. Practical counseling focuses on developing coping strategies such as identifying and avoiding or removing oneself from high-risk situations; replacing tobacco use with other, incompatible behaviors; using cognitive strategies and restructuring to reshape positive beliefs about smoking, counteract irrational thinking, and reduce negative moods; and developing refusal skills and other skills necessary to effectively manage triggers. For an evidence-based guide to the behavioral tools for intensive treatment and for treating smokers with co-morbid psychiatric conditions, see Brown in Abrams et al. (2003).

Pharmacotherapy

The Public Health Service Guideline recommends that all patients who are try-ing to quit be offered pharmacotherapy, unless medically contraindicated or in the presence of other special situations such as pregnancy, lactation, adoles-cence, or smoking fewer than 10 cigarettes per day. As of this writing, there are seven first-line medications approved by the FDA for use in smoking cessation: five nicotine replacement therapy (NRT) products (transdermal patch, gum, lozenge, inhaler, and nasal spray) and two non-nicotine medications (bupro-pion SR and varenicline). In this section, we discuss the role of NRT, bupropion SR, and varenicline in promoting smoking cessation and also look at the factors that facilitate or impede adherence to each form of therapy. See Table 10.1 for specific precautions, dosing instructions, and adverse effects of each product.

Determining Appropriate Medications

When recommending medication, one must assess the level of dependence, especially in relation to the use of NRT products or combination therapy. A simple assessment can include time to first cigarette (<30 minutes indicates high dependence), which has been found to be an accurate predictor of level of nicotine dependence (Heatherton, Kozlowski, Frecker, & Fagerstrom, 1991) and number of cigarettes per day. The final determination of which type of medi-cation a particular patient should use depends upon such factors as patient preference, prior experience, cost and/or insurance coverage, patient ability to comply with usage and dosing instructions, side effects, availability, and access. For additional details on the management of pharmacotherapies for smoking cessation, see Goldstein in Abrams et al. (2003).

Nicotine Replacement Therapy (NRT)

The goal of using nicotine replacement therapy (NRT) is to gradually wean the tobacco user by replacing the nicotine from tobacco products and blunting nic-otine withdrawal symptoms. There are several barriers to more widespread use of NRT products. Many smokers are not aware of the effectiveness of NRT or believe that these products are harmful. Less than 22% of smokers trying to quit used any pharmacologic aide in 2000 (Cokkinides, Ward, Jemal, & Thun, 2005). The products are relatively expensive and are not available in small quanti-ties, resulting in a high out-of-pocket expense that is particularly burdensome for low- and middle-income smokers. Many smokers do not know that NRT is available in less expensive generic forms and is legally available at lower cost online. Some health plans do not cover the cost of NRT, although in recent years coverage has been improving.

Pharmacologic Product Guide: FDA-Approved Medications

Nicotine replacement therapy (NRT) formulations

	Gum	Lozenge	Transdermal Preparations[a]		Nasal Spray	Oral Inhaler	Bupropion SR	Varenicline
Product	Nicorette[b], Generic OTC 2 mg, 4 mg: original, mint, fruit, orange, cinnamon	Commit[b], Generic OTC 2 mg, 4 mg mint, cherry	Nicoderm CQ[b] OTC 24-hour release 7 mg, 14 mg, 21 mg	Generic Patch OTC/ Rx (formerly Habitrol) 24-hour release 7 mg, 14 mg, 21 mg	Nicotrol NS[c] Rx Metered spray 0.5 mg nicotine in 50 μL aqueous nicotine solution	Nicotrol Inhaler[c] Rx 10 mg cartridge delivers 4 mg inhaled nicotine vapor	Zyban[b], Generic Rx 150 mg sustained-release tablet	Chantix[c] Rx 0.5 mg, 1 mg tablet
Precautions	▪ Pregnancy category: Not applicable for OTC formulations ▪ Recent (≤2 weeks) myocardial infarction ▪ Serious underlying arrhythmias ▪ Serious or worsening angina pectoris ▪ Temporomandibular joint disease	▪ Pregnancy category: Not applicable for OTC formulations ▪ Recent (≤2 weeks) myocardial infarction ▪ Serious underlying arrhythmias ▪ Serious or worsening angina pectoris	▪ Pregnancy category: D for prescription patch, not applicable for OTC formulations ▪ Recent (≤2 weeks) myocardial infarction ▪ Serious underlying arrhythmias ▪ Serious or worsening angina pectoris		▪ Pregnancy category: D ▪ Recent (≤2 weeks) myocardial infarction ▪ Serious underlying arrhythmias ▪ Serious or worsening angina pectoris ▪ Underlying chronic nasal disorders (rhinitis, nasal polyps, sinusitis)	▪ Pregnancy category: D ▪ Recent (≤2 weeks) myocardial infarction ▪ Serious underlying arrhythmias ▪ Serious or worsening angina pectoris ▪ Bronchospastic disease	▪ Pregnancy category: C ▪ Concomitant therapy with medications or medical conditions known to lower the seizure threshold ▪ Severe hepatic cirrhosis Contraindications: ▪ Seizure disorder ▪ Concomitant bupropion (e.g., Wellbutrin) therapy ▪ Current or prior diagnosis of bulimia or anorexia nervosa	▪ Pregnancy category: C ▪ Severe renal impairment (dosage adjustment is necessary)

	Nicotine Gum	Nicotine Lozenge	Nicotine Patch	Nicotine Patch	Nicotine Nasal Spray	Nicotine Inhaler	Bupropion SR	Varenicline
					■ Simultaneous abrupt discontinuation of alcohol or sedatives (including benzodiazepines) ■ MAO inhibitor therapy in previous 14 days	■ Severe reactive airway disease		
Dosing	≥25 cigarettes/day: 4 mg <25 cigarettes/day: 2 mg Week 1–6: 1 piece q 1–2 hours Week 7–9: 1 piece q 2–4 hours Week 10–12: 1 piece q 4–8 hours ■ Maximum, 24 pieces/day ■ Chew each piece slowly ■ Park between cheek and gum when peppery or tingling sensation appears (~15–30 chews) ■ Resume chewing when taste or tingle fades ■ Repeat chew/park steps until most of the nicotine is gone (taste or tingle does not return: generally 30 min)	1st cigarette ≤30 minutes after waking: 4 mg 1st cigarette >30 minutes after waking: 2 mg Week 1–6: 1 lozenge q 1–2 hours Week 7–9: 1 lozenge q 2–4 hours Week 10–12: 1 lozenge q 4–8 hours ■ Maximum, 20 lozenges/day ■ Allow to dissolve slowly (20–30 minutes) ■ Nicotine release may cause a warm, tingling sensation ■ Do not chew or swallow	>10 cigarettes/day: 21 mg/day x 6 weeks 14 mg/day x 2 weeks 7 mg/day x 2 weeks ≤10 cigarettes/day: 14 mg/day x 6 weeks 7 mg/day x 2 weeks ■ May wear patch for 16 hours if patient experiences sleep disturbances (remove at bedtime)	>10 cigarettes/day: 21 mg/day x 4 weeks 14 mg/day x 2 weeks 7 mg/day x 2 weeks ≤10 cigarettes/day: 14 mg/day x 6 weeks 7 mg/day x 2 weeks ■ May wear patch for 16 hours if patient experiences sleep disturbances (remove at bedtime)	1–2 doses/hour (8–40 doses/day) One dose = 2 sprays (one in each nostril): each spray delivers 0.5 mg of nicotine to the nasal mucosa ■ Maximum 5 doses/hour 40 doses/day ■ For best results, initially use at least 8 doses/day ■ Patients should not sniff, swallow, or inhale through the nose as the spray is being administered ■ Duration: 3–6 months	6–16 cartridges/day Individualize dosing: initially use 1 cartridge q 1–2 hours ■ Best effects with continuous puffing for 20 minutes ■ Nicotine in cartridge is depleted after 20 minutes of active puffing ■ Patient should inhale into back of throat or puff in short breaths ■ Do NOT inhale into the lungs (like a cigarette) but "puff" as if lighting a pipe	150 mg po q AM x 3 days, then increase to 150 mg po bid ■ Do not exceed 300 mg/day ■ Treatment should be initiated while patient is still smoking ■ Set quit date 1–2 weeks after initiation of therapy ■ Allow at least 8 hours between doses ■ Avoid bedtime dosing to minimize insomnia ■ Dose tapering is not necessary ■ Can be used safely with NRT ■ Duration: 7–12 weeks, with maintenance up to 6 months in selected patients	Days 1–3: 0.5 mg po q AM Days 4–7: 0.5 mg po bid Weeks 2–12: 1 mg po bid ■ Patients should begin therapy 1 week prior to quit date ■ Take dose after eating with a full glass of water ■ Dose tapering is not necessary ■ Nausea and insomnia are side effects that are usually temporary ■ Duration: 12 weeks; an additional 12 week course may be used in selected patients

(continued)

Nicotine replacement therapy (NRT) formulations

	Gum	Lozenge	Transdermal Preparations[a]		Nasal Spray	Oral Inhaler	Bupropion SR	Varenicline
Product	Nicorette[b]. Generic OTC 2 mg. 4 mg: original. mint. fruit. orange. cinnamon	Commit[b]. Generic OTC 2 mg. 4 mg. mint. cherry	Nicoderm CQ[b] OTC 24-hour release 7 mg. 14 mg. 21 mg	Generic Patch OTC/Rx (formerly Habitrol) 24-hour release 7 mg. 14 mg. 21 mg	Nicotrol NS[c] Rx Metered spray 0.5 mg nicotine in 50 μL aqueous nicotine solution	Nicotrol Inhaler[c] Rx 10 mg cartridge delivers 4 mg inhaled nicotine vapor	Zyban[b]. Generic Rx 150 mg sustained-release tablet	Chantix[c] Rx 0.5 mg. 1 mg tablet
Dosing	▪ Park in different areas of mouth ▪ No food or beverages 15 min before or during use ▪ Duration: up to 12 weeks	▪ Occasionally rotate to different areas of the mouth ▪ No food or beverages 15 minutes before or during use ▪ Duration: up to 12 weeks	▪ Duration: 8–10 weeks	▪ Duration: 8 weeks		▪ Open cartridge retains potency for 24 hours ▪ Duration: up to 6 months		
Adverse Effects	▪ Mouth/jaw soreness ▪ Hiccups ▪ Dyspepsia ▪ Hypersalivation ▪ Effects associated with incorrect chewing technique: ▪ Lightheadedness ▪ Nausea/vomiting ▪ Throat and mouth irritation	▪ Nausea ▪ Hiccups ▪ Cough ▪ Heartburn ▪ Headache ▪ Flatulence ▪ Insomnia	▪ Local skin reactions (erythema. pruritus. burning) ▪ Headache ▪ Sleep disturbances (insomnia) or abnormal/vivid dreams (associated with nocturnal nicotine absorption)		▪ Nasal and/or throat irritation (hot. peppery. or burning sensation) ▪ Rhinitis ▪ Tearing ▪ Sneezing ▪ Cough ▪ Headache	▪ Mouth and/or throat irritation ▪ Unpleasant taste ▪ Cough ▪ Rhinitis ▪ Dyspepsia ▪ Hiccups ▪ Headache	▪ Insomnia ▪ Dry mouth ▪ Nervousness/difficulty concentrating ▪ Rash ▪ Constipation ▪ Seizures (risk is 1/1.000 [0.1%])	▪ Nausea ▪ Sleep disturbances (insomnia. abnormal dreams) ▪ Constipation ▪ Flatulence ▪ Vomiting

Advantages	■ Gum use might satisfy oral cravings ■ Gum use might delay weight gain ■ Patients can titrate therapy to manage withdrawal symptoms	■ Lozenge use might satisfy oral cravings ■ Lozenge use might delay weight gain ■ Patients can titrate therapy to manage withdrawal symptoms	■ Provides consistent nicotine levels over 24 hours ■ Easy to use and conceal ■ Once-a-day dosing associated with fewer compliance problems	■ Patients can titrate therapy to more rapidly manage withdrawal symptoms	■ Patients can titrate therapy to manage withdrawal symptoms ■ Mimics hand-to-mouth ritual of smoking	■ Easy to use: oral formulation might be associated with fewer compliance problems ■ Can be used with NRT ■ Might be beneficial in patients with depression	■ Easy to use: oral formulation might be associated with fewer compliance problems ■ Offers a new mechanism of action for patients who have failed other agents
Disadvantages	■ Gum chewing may not be socially acceptable ■ Gum is difficult to use with dentures ■ Patients must use proper chewing technique to minimize adverse effects	■ Gastrointestinal side effects (nausea, hiccups, heartburn) might be bothersome	■ Patients cannot titrate the dose ■ Allergic reactions to adhesive might occur ■ Patients with dermatologic conditions should not use the patch	■ Nasal/throat irritation may be bothersome ■ Dependence can result ■ Patients must wait 5 minutes before driving or operating heavy machinery ■ Patients with chronic nasal disorders or severe reactive airway disease should not use the spray	■ Initial throat or mouth irritation can be bothersome ■ Cartridges should not be stored in very warm conditions or used in very cold conditions ■ Patients with underlying bronchospastic disease must use the inhaler with caution	■ Seizure risk is increased ■ Several contraindications and precautions preclude use (see PRECAUTIONS, above)	■ May induce nausea in up to one third of patients ■ Post-marketing surveillance data not yet available

(continued)

10.1 Pharmacologic Product Guide: FDA-Approved Medications (Continued)

Nicotine replacement therapy (NRT) formulations

	Gum	Lozenge	Transdermal Preparations[a]		Nasal Spray	Oral Inhaler	Bupropion SR	Varenicline
			Nicoderm CQ[b]	Generic Patch OTC/Rx				
Product	Nicorette[b]. Generic OTC 2 mg. 4 mg: original. mint. fruit. orange. cinnamon	Commit[b]. Generic OTC 2 mg. 4 mg mint. cherry	OTC 24-hour release 7 mg. 14 mg. 21 mg	Generic Patch OTC/Rx (formerly Habitrol) 24-hour release 7 mg. 14 mg. 21 mg	Nicotrol NS[c] Rx Metered spray 0.5 mg nicotine in 50 μL aqueous nicotine solution	Nicotrol Inhaler[c] Rx 10 mg cartridge delivers 4 mg inhaled nicotine vapor	Zyban[b]. Generic Rx 150 mg sustained-release tablet	Chantix[c] Rx 0.5 mg. 1 mg tablet
Web site	www.nicorette.com	www.commitlozenge.com	www.nicodermcq.com	www.habitrol.com	www.nicotrol.com	www.nicotrol.com	- - - -	www.chantix.com
Cost/day[d]	2 mg: $3.28–$6.57 (9 pieces) 4 mg: $4.31–$6.57 (9 pieces)	2 mg: $3.66–$5.26 (9 pieces) 4 mg: $3.66–$5.26 (9 pieces)	$2.24–$3.89 (1 patch)	$1.90–$2.94 (1 patch)	$3.67 (8 doses)	$5.29 (6 cartridges)	$3.62–$6.04 (2 tablets)	$4.00–$4.22 (2 tablets)

Note. From Rx for Change: Clinician-Assisted Tobacco Cessation program. The Regents of the University of California. University of Southern California. and Western University of Health Sciences. Copyright © 1999–2008 by Rx for Change. Reprinted with permission.

[a]Transdermal patch formulations previously marketed. but no longer available: Nicotrol 5 mg. 10 mg. 15 mg delivered over 16 hours (Pfizer) and generic patch (formerly Prostep) 11 mg and 22 mg delivered over 24 hours.
[b]Marketed by GlaxoSmithKline.
[c]Marketed by Pfizer.
[d]Average wholesale price from 2007 Drug Topics Redbook. Montvale. NJ: Medical Economics Company. Inc.. June 2007.

A factor that may reduce the effectiveness of NRT is the fact that the rec-ommended dosages of NRT deliver only about half the amount of nicotine a smoker would typically receive by smoking a pack of cigarettes under typical conditions. The rate at which nicotine is delivered also varies by NRT product. For instance, the patch delivers nicotine continuously over 24 hours, whereas the nicotine nasal spray raises nicotine levels the most rapidly of all products and may be more effective in reducing acute cravings in highly dependent smokers (Pbert, Luckmann, & Ockene, 2004). Another factor affecting the effectiveness of NRT is compliance. The patch has been found to have the highest compli-ance rates (Henningfield, Fant, Buchhalter, & Stitzer, 2005) and can be combined with acute therapies (gum, lozenge, inhaler, spray) on an ad lib basis to manage breakthrough cravings in heavy smokers. The gum, lozenge, inhaler, and spray require multiple dosing regimens and may cause irritating side effects that may lessen compliance and require careful explanation about proper usage.

While the evidence for using NRT products in combination is mixed, the use of gum and patch together seems to do a better job of alleviating withdrawal symptoms than use of either one alone (Institute of Medicine, 2007). In practice, NRT products are frequently used in combination with no evidence of nicotine toxicity or other adverse events. In addition, NRT (all forms) and bupropion can be used together, and this combination has been found to be effective, at least in the short term (Jorenby et al., 1999).

There are few contraindications to the use of NRT (see Table 10.1). Smok-ing while on NRT is discouraged, but there is no evidence that persons who smoke while on the patch are at greater risk of any serious adverse event than those who do not. In fact, the Cut Down then Stop protocol approved by the British National Health Service in 2005 recommends that smokers initiate nico-tine gum or inhaler use while still smoking, then gradually reduce intake to 50% of baseline at 6 weeks, aiming for cessation by 6 months and discontinuation of NRT within 12 months. Other studies (Schuurmans, Diacon, van Biljon, & Bol-liger, 2004) report that smokers who used the nicotine patch for 2 weeks before quitting had higher sustained quit rates at 6 months than smokers who were not pretreated with NRT.

The *transdermal nicotine patch (TNP)* delivers nicotine at a relatively steady rate and has few barriers to adherence. A tobacco user simply puts a new patch on a different nonhairy part of the upper body every day. Generic brands are less expensive and generally work as well as name brands. The TNP does not appear to prevent postcessation weight gain, which may be of concern to many smokers. Combination therapy (patch plus gum) may be indicated in this case, as use of nicotine gum has been found to delay postcessation weight gain (Allen, Hatsukami, Brintnell, & Bade, 2005).

Nicotine gum (NG) has been shown to be effective in helping smokers quit, but there are several barriers in adhering to nicotine gum use. First, smokers may not chew enough gum for it to be effective in countering cravings. Chew-ing 12–15 pieces per day on a fixed schedule is recommended by the manufac-turer. Second, smokers may experience uncomfortable side effects, which may cause noncompliance, although some side effects may be alleviated by using the proper "chew and park" technique. The *nicotine lozenge* is easier to use than the gum. Beginning dose is determined by time to first cigarette. Using this index, most smokers in the United States require the 4 mg lozenge (Henningfield et al., 2005). The lozenge should not be chewed but allowed to dissolve slowly in the mouth.

The *nicotine inhaler* consists of a mouthpiece and a cartridge that contains 10 ml of nicotine. The name may be misleading since it is "puffed," not inhaled, in order to draw nicotine into the mouth through the mouthpiece. The nicotine is then absorbed through the oral mucosa, much like the nicotine gum. The *nicotine nasal spray* delivers nicotine the most rapidly of all NRTs and therefore has a greater potential for abuse and dependence. The multiple side effects, including nasal and/or throat irritation, are extremely unpleasant and may serve as a disincentive to use.

Non-Nicotine Medications

Sustained-release bupropion (Trade names Zyban, Wellbutrin, Buproban, and Budeprion) is an antidepressant demonstrated to be effective in helping smokers manage withdrawal and cravings when quitting smoking. The major contraindication for bupropion is a history of seizures or being at risk for seizures. Bupropion SR potentially postpones weight gain and reduces relapse rates, making it a good alternative for smokers with multiple failed quit attempts or those who fear weight gain (Hays et al., 2001). It has been approved for use up to 12 months following smoking cessation. Bupropion is begun 7–10 days before quit date, which appeals to many smokers.

Varenicline (Chantix), the most recently approved FDA medication, addresses nicotine dependence by stimulating dopamine release while simultaneously blocking nicotine receptors. This serves to blunt withdrawal, reduce cravings, and reduce the rewarding effects of nicotine (Foulds, Steinberg, Williams, & Ziedonis, 2006). Varenicline is an $\alpha4\beta2$ nicotinic receptor partial agonist that is believed to aid smoking cessation by moderately increasing the release of dopamine. Varenicline has been found to be safe, effective, and well tolerated in most people (Niaura, Jones, & Kirkpatrick, 2006). However, the FDA issued a Public Health Advisory in February 2008 urging careful monitoring for possible adverse psychiatric effects (i.e. agitation, depression, suicidal thoughts and attempted/completed suicide). As with bupropion, use is started approximately 1 week before quit date to achieve steady-state blood levels. If a person has successfully quit smoking after 12 weeks, long-term abstinence can be improved by continuing varenicline for an additional 12 weeks. Because varenicline works at the nicotinic receptor sites, adjuvant use of NRT is not recommended. Varenicline has not yet been studied in populations with medical or psychiatric comorbidities, so recommendations cannot be made at this time regarding its use in higher-risk populations.

Summary

In general, all seven first-line FDA-approved smoking cessation medications produce similar efficacy rates. The one exception to this may be varenicline, which has been found to have higher quit rates in three randomized control trials (Keating & Siddiqui, 2006). The effectiveness of NRT has been demonstrated even when it is used in the absence of counseling (West & Zhou, 2007), and it is likely that bupropion and varenicline have similar effects. However, the combination of counseling plus pharmacotherapy has been found to be superior in helping tobacco users quit and should be utilized if available.

Assisting Special Populations

Some evidence supports the concept that tailoring of interventions to individual smoker characteristics or targeting of intervention to group characteristics (e.g., race or ethnic background, gender, age) improves outcomes. Using proven behavioral and pharmacologic methods may be especially important for tobacco users with comorbidity (e.g., psychiatric problems, alcohol, substance abuse). Persons with a history of mental health or substance use disorders may need higher levels of medications for longer periods of time and require more monitoring (Hughes, 2008). Persons suffering from depression or a history of depression may do well with bupropion because of its antidepressant qualities.

Behavioral strategies should be considered the preferred treatment approach for pregnant women. Use of pharmacotherapy in pregnant women is usually not recommended unless the woman and her physician agree that the risks of continuing to smoke outweigh the possible risks of using pharmacotherapy (Fiore et al., 2008). Note that all the first-line prescription medications are FDA-rated C or D, so caution is warranted.

Additionally, while pharmacotherapy has been found to be safe in adolescents, studies to date have not found it to be particularly effective (Grimshaw & Stanton, 2006).

Relapse Prevention

Interventions for smoking typically consist of discreet periods of treatment leading to abstinence or relapse. Relapse is all too common: between 65% and 95% of quit attempts end in relapse (Pierce & Gilpin, 2003), with the greatest proportion of relapse (44%) occurring within 14 days (Garvey, Bliss, Hitchcock, Heinold, & Rosner, 1992) of a serious quit attempt.

Although repeated quit attempts are common, overall results of studies encouraging repeat quit attempts (recycling) have been discouraging. Lando and colleagues (1996) reported that a telephone support intervention significantly increased recycling but not long-term abstinence. Tonneson and colleagues (1996) found that introducing nicotine replacement after 1 year did not appreciably increase abstinence (6% for nasal spray and 0% for patch). Relapse prevention and recycling represent a huge public health opportunity, but the research base to inform effective and efficient recycling/relapse prevention intervention is sparse (Brandon, Herzog, & Webb, 2003).

Relapse should be regarded as part of the learning experience along the pathway to cessation. Just as with learning to ride a bicycle for the first time, persistent effort, practice, and openness to the correction of past mistakes will lead to eventual mastery and success (Bandura, 1997). If one falls off the bicycle, one has to get back on and try again to become proficient at negotiating the curves and the bumps in the road. Thus, the idea of recycling smokers who have slipped back into smoking should be included in the treatment planning process. The Internet may be an especially useful new modality of intervention to reduce relapse and improve recycling because those who are engaged in the quitting process or have recently quit can have 24/7/365-day-a-year access to online resources. Such resources include social support and self-help coping-skills programs available through interactive computer expert systems. In one preliminary study, a very strong correlation was reported between use of chat rooms for support and successful maintenance of cessation at 3-month follow-up (Cobb, Graham, Bock, Papandonatos, & Abrams, 2005).

Systems-Level Interventions

Smoking prevalence is lower than the national average (20.8%) in those states with strong, visible, comprehensive, and sustained antismoking programs (e.g., 14.9% in California and 17.8% in Massachusetts) (Institute of Medicine, 2007). Access to effective tobacco treatment resources is a key component of such comprehensive programs. The full impact of cessation interventions on the intended target population is a product of the proportion of the population reached and the efficacy and fidelity of implementation of the intervention delivered (Impact = Reach x Efficacy) (see Abrams et al., 2003; Abrams et al., 1993, for details). Thus, in addition to trying to motivate more smokers to make quit attempts, there is an enormous opportunity to further increase cessation outcomes by implementing systems-level interventions that reach more smokers and increase access to treatment. Diverse strategies that include clinical, medical, and community interventions can contribute significantly to improving the health of the public (Ockene et al., 2007).

Interventions by health care providers are among the factors related to smokers' interest in receiving counseling to help with a quit attempt (Weber et al., 2007). Despite this, the national rate at which physicians provide advice and assistance to their patients who smoke has remained low (Thorndike, Regan, & Rigotti, 2007). A common rationale for this includes physicians' lack of time and resources. However, studies have demonstrated the feasibility of developing linkages between clinical settings and community-level services (Bentz et al., 2006; Perry, Keller, Fraser, & Fiore, 2005). An example of such a program is QuitWorks, currently operating in Massachusetts through collaboration between the Massachusetts Tobacco Control Program and major health plans in the commonwealth. QuitWorks coordinates clinical and community-based efforts by linking patients, clinicians, and a proactive telephone counseling quitline through the use of faxed referrals forms (Centers for Disease Control and Prevention, 2006a). Linking quitline services with free NRT also has proved to be an effective method of reaching large numbers of smokers. Frieden and colleagues (2005) reported on the effectiveness of a large-scale distribution of free NRT patches in New York City. Using a conservative intent-to-treat (ITT) analysis (all nonrespondents were considered to be smoking at 6-month follow-up), the cessation rate was 20%. Those who received counseling were also more likely to quit than those who did not (38% vs. 27%). A study of the Minnesota QUITPLAN Helpline before and after the availability of free NRT found that participation in counseling, use of medications, and abstinence rates all increased (An et al., 2006). Easy access to free NRT cessation medication in diverse populations can help large numbers of smokers to quit.

The Internet can reach millions of smokers cost-effectively. Many cessation Web sites exist, but few have been evaluated, and of more than 300 Web sites, fewer than 10 met criteria for having content outlined as effective in the PHS guideline (Bock et al., 2004). In a European study, 3,501 purchasers of a nicotine patch who proactively logged on to use a free Internet program and then consented to participate in a research study (76%) were randomly assigned to a tailored or an untailored program (Strecher, Shiffman, & West, 2005). At 3-month follow-up, using ITT analysis of continuous abstinence for 10 weeks, the tailored condition (22.8%) outperformed the untailored condition (18.1%). A preliminary large-scale evaluation of a broadly disseminated smoking cessation Web site reported cessation at 3 months in the range of 7% (ITT) to 30% (responders only) (Cobb et al., 2005). It is noteworthy from a comprehensive systems perspective that approximately 30% of those surveyed indicated they had already quit smoking at registration and were using the Web site for relapse prevention. Collectively, these studies are a promising start in evaluating Internet-based smoking cessation programs.

Interventions that are translated from clinical to community settings to proactively reach more smokers in a cost-effective manner vary widely in outcome effectiveness. This is because of variability in the factors that are present in real-world settings; for example, target groups have more heterogeneous characteristics, and there are differences among programs, providers, delivery systems, and other contextual or setting factors. Channels of intervention delivery must also be factored in, such as whether the setting is a health care organization or a medical setting, from hospitals to private offices, a worksite, a school, a telephone quit lines, the Internet, or other print and electronic media.

Systems-level models are needed to address the diversity of channels and of populations of users. Models such as stepped care, the tailoring of interventions to motivational readiness to quit (e.g., stages-of-change model, Motivational Interviewing), and the targeting of interventions to channels of delivery (e.g., primary-care offices, managed-care organizations, worksites, schools, the Internet, telephone quit lines) or to population groups (e.g., younger or older smokers, underserved or uninsured groups, women and minorities) will need to be evaluated empirically to demonstrate their utility and cost-effectiveness.

The role of private payers (i.e., health plans, employers) must be considered in this discussion as well. State and local departments of health cannot be expected to bear the burden of providing accessible treatment services to all comers. Medicare and, in some states, Medicaid programs are setting the example in covering pharmacologic and counseling services for its beneficiaries, and private insurers are slowly increasing their coverage, as well (Centers for Disease Control and Prevention: Morbidity and Mortality Weekly Report, 2006; Curry & Orleans, 2005; Curry, Orleans, Keller, & Fiore, 2006).

Conclusion

The fact that there are still more than 40 million smokers in the United States alone in the early part of the 21st century points to the urgent need for a redoubling of efforts to adopt a nationwide comprehensive approach to addressing tobacco use. The most effective and efficient evidence-based interventions and policies must be adopted and incorporated into a comprehensive plan of policy and practice. The political will is needed to adopt this comprehensive approach, as recommended by the prestigious National Academy of Sciences, because such a policy ought to be a part of the very fabric of quality public health and health care delivery systems in the United States (Institute of Medicine, 2007). While smoke-free laws and ordinances are increasing, media campaigns have decreased. The most dramatic recent declines in smoking rates have occurred in states where residents have easy access to medications and counseling (Centers for Disease Control and Prevention, 2007). Institutionalizing tobacco treatment within the health care system is one way to ensure that all smokers are aware of and have the ability make use of treatment services available. Programs such as QuitWorks offer a step in the right direction by providing treatment resources to the health care system and their patients.

The Institute of Medicine includes this compelling summary in the appendix entitled *Comprehensive Smoking Cessation Policy* (see D. Abrams in Institute of Medicine [2007]):

> *For a smoker it is a long and arduous journey from starting to smoke to enjoying smoking in one's carefree youth to wanting to stop to actually stopping for good. For much of that journey the smoker is not motivated to quit and does not make any quit attempts at all. Somewhere along the way the smoker may change, either suddenly or gradually over time. Smokers can move from being unmotivated and not making any quit attempts to wanting to quit (over 70% say they want to quit) and then to making serious quit attempts (about 45% try seriously to quit each year). If at first a smoker is not successful at quitting (over 90% are not), the arduous journey continues from cycles of trying to quit but relapsing to trying again. Some smokers may give up trying to quit and withdraw out of fear of failure, shame or embarrassment. Sometimes the smoker may use unproven treatments or will power to quit (over 75% do that) and perhaps the smoker may use an effective product or service. Finally the journey ends when the smoker either quits for good or suffers and dies from a smoking related cause (about a third to a half of lifetime smokers will die of a smoking related disease). A comprehensive approach must also provide aggressive, direct to consumer marketing and education campaigns to improve their health literacy about the dangers of smoking and the best tools for quitting (Cokkinides et al., 2005). An approach that covers the entire smoker's journey and provides interventions tailored to the smoker's needs. This can be achieved through cessation policies that support a comprehensive care management network with aligned financial incentives at federal state and local levels across both the health care industry and the public health system. (p. 373)*

References

Abrams, D., Elder, J., Carleton, R., Lasater, T., & Artz, L. (1986). Social learning principles for organizational health promotion: An integrated approach. In M. Cataldo & T. Coates (Eds.), *Health & industry: A behavioral medicine perspective.* New York: Wiley.

Abrams, D., Emmons, K., Niaura, R., Goldstein, M., & Sherman, C. (1991). Tobacco dependence: An integration of individual and public health perspectives. In P. Nathan, J. Langenbucher,

B. McCrady, & W. Frankenstein (Eds.), *Annual review of addictions treatment and research* (Vol. 1, pp. 391–436). New York: Pergamon Press.

Abrams, D., Niaura, R., Brown, R., Emmons, K. A., Goldstein, M., & Monti, P. (2003). *The tobacco dependence treatment handbook: A guide to best practices.* New York: Guilford Press.

Abrams, D., Orleans, C. T., Niaura, R., Goldstein, M., Velicer, W., & Prochaska, J. O. (1993). Treatment issues: Towards a stepped care model. *Tobacco Control, 2*(Suppl.), S17–S37.

Allen, S. S., Hatsukami, D., Brintnell, D. M., & Bade, T. (2005). Effect of nicotine replacement therapy on post-cessation weight gain and nutrient intake: A randomized controlled trial of postmenopausal female smokers. *Addictive Behaviors, 30*(7), 1273–1280.

American Psychiatric Association. (2000). *Diagnostic and statistical manual of mental disorders: DSM-IV-TR* (4th ed.). Washington, DC: American Psychiatric Association.

An, L. C., Schillo, B. A., Kavanaugh, A. M., Lachter, R. B., Luxenberg, M. G., Wendling, A. H., et al. (2006). Increased reach and effectiveness of a statewide tobacco quitline after the addition of access to free nicotine replacement therapy. *Tobacco Control, 15*(4), 286–293.

Balfour, D. J. (2004). The neurobiology of tobacco dependence: A preclinical perspective on the role of the dopamine projections to the nucleus accumbens [corrected]. *Nicotine & Tobacco Research, 6*(6), 899–912.

Bandura, A. (1986). *Social foundation of thought and action: A social cognitive theory.* Englewood Cliffs, NJ: Prentice-Hall.

Bandura, A. (1995). *Moving in forward gear in health promotion and disease prevention.* Paper presented at the Society of Behavioral Medicine, 16th Annual Scientific Sessions, March 15–19, San Diego, CA.

Bandura, A. (1997). *Self-efficacy: The exercise of control.* New York: W. H. Freeman.

Becona, E., & Vazquez, F. L. (2001). Effectiveness of personalized written feedback through a mail intervention for smoking cessation: A randomized-controlled trial in Spanish smokers. *Journal of Consulting and Clinical Psychology, 69*(1), 33–40.

Benowitz, N. L., Perez-Stable, E. J., Herrera, B., & Jacob, P., III. (2002). Slower metabolism and reduced intake of nicotine from cigarette smoking in Chinese-Americans. *Journal of the National Cancer Institute, 94*(2), 108–115.

Bentz, C., Bayley, K., Bonin, K., Fleming, L., Hollis, J., & McAfee, T. (2006). The feasibility of connecting physician offices to a state-level tobacco quit line. *American Journal of Preventive Medicine, 30*(1), 31–37.

Bock, B., Graham, A., Sciamanna, C., Krishnamoorthy, J., Whiteley, J., Carmona-Barros, R., et al. (2004). Smoking cessation treatment on the Internet: Content, quality, and usability. *Nicotine & Tobacco Research, 6*(2), 207–219.

Brandon, T. H., Herzog, T. A., & Webb, M. S. (2003). It ain't over till it's over: The case for offering relapse-prevention interventions to former smokers. *American Journal of the Medical Sciences, 326*(4), 197–200.

Burke, B. L., Arkowitz, H., & Menchola, M. (2003). The efficacy of motivational interviewing: A meta-analysis of controlled clinical trials. *Journal of Consulting and Clinical Psychology, 71*(5), 843–861.

Camenga, D. R., & Klein, J. D. (2004). Adolescent smoking cessation. *Current Opinion in Pediatrics, 16*(4), 368–372.

Centers for Disease Control and Prevention. (1998). Tobacco use among high school students—United States, 1997. *Morbidity and Mortality Weekly Report, 47*(12), 229–233.

Centers for Disease Control and Prevention. (1999). *Best practices for comprehensive tobacco control programs.* Atlanta: U.S. Department of Health and Human Services, Centers for Disease Control and Prevention, National Center for Chronic Disease Prevention and Health Promotion, Office on Smoking and Health.

Centers for Disease Control and Prevention. (2004). Cigarette smoking among adults—United States, 2002. *Morbidity and Mortality Weekly Report, 53,* 427–431.

Centers for Disease Control and Prevention. (2006a). *A practical guide to working with health-care systems on tobacco-use treatment.* Atlanta: U.S. Department of Health and Human Services.

Centers for Disease Control and Prevention. (2006b). Racial/ethnic differences among youths in cigarette smoking and susceptibility to start smoking—United States, 2002–2004. *Morbidity and Mortality Weekly Report, 55*(47), 1275–1277.

Centers for Disease Control and Prevention. (2006c). Smoking prevalence among U.S. adults, 2006. *Morbidity and Mortality Weekly Report, 56*(44), 1157–1161.

Centers for Disease Control and Prevention. (2007). Decline in smoking prevalence—New York City, 2002–2006. *Morbidity and Mortality Weekly Report, 56*(24), 604–608.

Centers for Disease Control and Prevention: Morbidity and Mortality Weekly Report. (2006). State Medicaid coverage for tobacco-dependence treatments—United States, 2005. *Journal of the American Medical Association, 296*(24), 2917–2919.

Cobb, N. K., Graham, A. L., Bock, B.C., Papandonatos, G., & Abrams, D. B. (2005). Initial evaluation of a real-world Internet smoking cessation system. *Nicotine & Tobacco Research, 7*(2), 207–216.

Cokkinides, V. E., Ward, E., Jemal, A., & Thun, M. J. (2005). Under-use of smoking-cessation treatments: Results from the National Health Interview Survey, 2000. *American Journal of Preventive Medicine, 28*(1), 119–122.

Curry, S., & Orleans, C. T. (2005). Addressing tobacco treatment in managed care. *Nicotine & Tobacco Research, 7 (Suppl. 1),* s5–s8.

Curry, S., Wagner, E. H., & Grothaus, L. C. (1990). Intrinsic and extrinsic motivation for smoking cessation. *Journal of Consulting and Clinical Psychology, 58*(3), 310–316.

Curry, S. J., Orleans, C. T., Keller, P., & Fiore, M. (2006). Promoting smoking cessation in the healthcare environment: 10 years later. *American Journal of Preventive Medicine, 31*(3), 269–272.

Dani, J. A. (2001). Overview of nicotinic receptors and their roles in the central nervous system. *Biological Psychiatry, 49*(3), 166–174.

DiFranza, J. R., Savageau, J. A., Fletcher, K., O'Loughlin, J., Pbert, L., Ockene, J. K., et al. (2007). Symptoms of tobacco dependence after brief intermittent use: The Development and Assessment of Nicotine Dependence in Youth-2 study. *Archives of Pediatric and Adolescent Medicine, 161*(7), 704–710.

Etter, J. F., & Perneger, T. V. (2001). Effectiveness of a computer-tailored smoking cessation program: A randomized trial. *Archives of Internal Medicine, 161*(21), 2596–2601.

Fertig, J., & Allen, J. (1995). *Alcohol and tobacco: From basic science to policy:* National Institute on Alcohol Abuse and Alcoholism Monograph.

Fiore, M. C., Jaen, C. R., Baker, T. B., et al. (2008). *Treating tobacco use and dependence: 2008 update.* Clinical practice guideline. Rockville, MD: US Department of Health and Human Services, Public Health Services.

Foulds, J., Steinberg, M. B., Williams, J. M., & Ziedonis, D. M. (2006). Developments in pharmacotherapy for tobacco dependence: Past, present and future. *Drug and Alcohol Review, 25*(1), 59–71.

Frieden, T. R., Mostashari, F., Kerker, B. D., Miller, N., Hajat, A., & Frankel, M. (2005). Adult tobacco use levels after intensive tobacco control measures: New York City, 2002–2003. *American Journal of Public Health, 95*(6), 1016–1023.

Garvey, A., Bliss, R., Hitchcock, J., Heinold, J., & Rosner, B. (1992). Predictors of smoking relapse among self-quitters: A report from the normative aging study. *Addictive Behaviors, 17*(4), 367–377.

Grimshaw, G. M., & Stanton, A. (2006). Tobacco cessation interventions for young people. *Cochrane Database of Systematic Reviews, 4,* CD003289.

Hale, K., Hughes, J., Oliveto, A., Helzer, J., Higgins, S., Bickel, W., et al. (1993). Nicotine dependence in a population-based sample: Problems of drug dependence. In L. Harris (Ed.), *NIDA Research Monograph Series.* Washington: U.S. Government Printing Office.

Harris, D. S., & Anthenelli, R. M. (2005). Expanding treatment of tobacco dependence. *Current Psychiatry Reports, 7*(5), 344–351.

Hays, J. T., Hurt, R. D., Rigotti, N. A., Niaura, R., Gonzales, D., Durcan, M. J., et al. (2001). Sustained-release bupropion for pharmacologic relapse prevention after smoking cessation. A randomized, controlled trial. *Annals of Internal Medicine, 135*(6), 423–433.

Heatherton, T., Kozlowski, L., Frecker, R., & Fagerstrom, K. (1991). The Fagerstrom Test for Nicotine Dependence: A revision of the Fagerstrom Tolerance Questionnaire. *British Journal of Addiction, 86*(9), 1119–1127.

Heishman, S. (2000). Cognitive and behavioral effects of nicotine. In R. Ferrence, J. Slade, R. Room & M. Pope (Eds.), *Nicotine and public health* (pp. 93–113). Washington, DC: American Public Health Association.

Henningfield, J. E., Fant, R. V., Buchhalter, A. R., & Stitzer, M. L. (2005). Pharmacotherapy for nicotine dependence. *CA: A Cancer Journal for Clincians, 55*(5), 281–299; quiz 322–283, 325.

Herzog, T. A., & Blagg, C. O. (2007). Are most precontemplators contemplating smoking cessation? Assessing the validity of the stages of change. *Health Psychology, 26*(2), 222–231.

Hughes, J. (1995). Clinical implications of the association between smoking and alcoholism. In J. Fertig & R. Fuller (Eds.), *Alcohol and tobacco: From basic science to policy. NIAAA Research Monograph 30* (pp. 171–181). Washington, DC: U.S. Government Printing Office.

Hughes, J., Fiester, S., Goldstein, M., Resnick, M., Rock, N., & Ziedonis, D. (1996). American Psychiatric Association Practice Guideline for the treatment of patients with nicotine dependence. *American Journal of Psychiatry, 153*(10 Suppl), S1–S31.

Hughes, J. N. (2008). An algorithm for choosing among smoking cessation treatments. *Journal of Substance Abuse Treatment, 34*(4), 426–432.

Hughes, J. R. (1993). Pharmacotherapy for smoking cessation: Unvalidated assumptions, anomalies, and suggestions for future research. *Journal of Consulting and Clinical Psychology, 61*(5), 751–760.

Institute of Medicine. (2007). *Ending the tobacco problem: A blueprint for the nation.* Washington, DC: National Academies Press.

Jorenby, D., Leischow, S., Nides, M., Rennard, S., Johnston, J., Hughes, A., et al. (1999). A controlled trial of sustained-release bupropion, a nicotine patch, or both for smoking cessation. *New England Journal of Medicine, 340*(9), 685–691.

Kalivas, P. W., & Volkow, N. D. (2005). The neural basis of addiction: A pathology of motivation and choice. *American Journal of Psychiatry, 162*(8), 1403–1413.

Keating, G. M., & Siddiqui, M. A. (2006). Varenicline: A review of its use as an aid to smoking cessation therapy. *CNS Drugs, 20*(11), 945–960.

Killen, J. D., Fortmann, S. P., Varady, A., & Kraemer, H. C. (2002). Do men outperform women in smoking cessation trials? Maybe, but not by much. *Experimental and Clinical Psychopharmacology, 10*(3), 295–301.

Lambe, E. K., Picciotto, M. R., & Aghajanian, G. K. (2003). Nicotine induces glutamate release from thalamocortical terminals in prefrontal cortex. *Neuropsychopharmacology, 28*(2), 216–225.

Lando, H. A., Pirie, P. L., Roski, J., McGovern, P. G., & Schmid, L. A. (1996). Promoting abstinence among relapsed chronic smokers: The effect of telephone support. *American Journal of Public Health, 86*(12), 1786–1790.

Lasser, K., Boyd, J. W., Woolhandler, S., Himmelstein, D. U., McCormick, D., & Bor, D. H. (2000). Smoking and mental illness: A population-based prevalence study. *Journal of the American Medical Association, 284*(20), 2606–2610.

Lerman, C., & Niaura, R. (2002). Applying genetic approaches to the treatment of nicotine dependence. *Oncogene, 21*(48), 7412–7420.

Lumley, J., Oliver, S. S., Chamberlain, C., & Oakley, L. (2004). Interventions for promoting smoking cessation during pregnancy. *Cochrane Database of Systematic Review, 4,* CD001055.

Marlatt, G., & Gordon, J. (Eds.). (1985). *Relapse prevention.* New York: Guilford Press.

McEwen, A., Hajek, P., McRobbie, H., & West, R. (2006). *Manual of smoking cessation: A guide for counsellors and practitioners.* Oxford: Blackwell.

Milton, B., Cook, P. A., Dugdill, L., Porcellato, L., Springett, J., & Woods, S. E. (2004). Why do primary school children smoke? A longitudinal analysis of predictors of smoking uptake during pre-adolescence. *Public Health, 118*(4), 247–255.

Mokdad, A. H., Marks, J. S., Stroup, D. F., & Gerberding, J. L. (2004). Actual causes of death in the United States, 2000. *Journal of the American Medical Association, 291*(10), 1238–1245.

Mokdad, A. H., Marks, J. S., Stroup, D. F., & Gerberding, J. L. (2005). Correction: Actual causes of death in the United States, 2000. *Journal of the American Medical Association, 293*(3), 293–294.

Niaura, R. (2000). Cognitive social learning and related perspectives on drug craving. *Addiction, 95 Suppl 2,* S155–S163.

Niaura, R., Jones, C., & Kirkpatrick, P. (2006). Varenicline. *Nature Reviews Drug Discovery, 5*(7), 537–538.

NIH State-of-the-Science Panel. (2006). National Institutes of Health State-of-the-Science conference Statement: Tobacco use: Prevention, cessation, and control. *Annals of Internal Medicine, 145,* 839–844.

Ockene, I. S., Hebert, J. R., Ockene, J. K., Saperia, G. M., Stanek, E., Nicolosi, R., et al. (1999). Effect of physician-delivered nutrition counseling training and an office-support program on saturated fat intake, weight, and serum lipid measurements in a hyperlipidemic population: Worcester Area Trial for Counseling in Hyperlipidemia (WATCH). *Archives of Internal Medicine, 159*(7), 725–731.

Ockene, J., Kristeller, J., Pbert, L., Hebert, J., Luippold, R., Goldberg, R., et al. (1994). The PDSIP: Can short-term interventions produce long-term effects for a general outpatient population. *Health Psychology, 13*(3), 278–281.

Ockene, J., Quirk, M., Goldberg, R., Kristeller, J., Donnelly, G., Kalan, K., et al. (1988). A residents' training program for the development of smoking intervention skills. *Archives of Internal Medicine, 148,* 1039–1045.

Ockene, J., Wheeler, E., Adams, A., Hurley, T., & Hebert, J. (1997). Provider training for patient-centered alcohol counseling in a primary care setting. *Archives of Internal Medicine, 157,* 2334–2341.

Ockene, J. K., Edgerton, E. A., Teutsch, S. M., Marion, L. N., Miller, T., Genevro, J. L., et al. (2007). Integrating evidence-based clinical and community strategies to improve health. *American Journal of Preventive Medicine, 32*(3), 244–252.

Orleans, C., & Slade, J. (1993). *Nicotine addiction: Principles and management.* New York: Oxford University Press.

Orleans, C. T., & Alper, J. (2003). Helping addicted smokers quit. In S. Issacs & J. Knickman (Eds.), *To improve health and health care* (Vol. 6, pp. 125–148). San Francisco: Jossey Bass.

Pbert, L., Luckmann, R., & Ockene, J. K. (2004). Smoking cessation treatment. In L. J. Haas (Ed.), *Handbook of primary care psychology* (pp. 527–549). New York: Oxford University Press.

Perez-Stable, E. J., Herrera, B., Jacob III, P., & Benowitz, N. L. (1998). Nicotine metabolism and intake in black and white smokers. *Journal of the American Medical Association, 280*(2), 152–156.

Perkins, K., Conklin, C., & Levine, M. (2007). *Cognitive-behavioral therapy for smoking cessation: A practical guidebook to the most effective treatments.* New York & London: Routledge.

Perkins, K. A., Donny, E., & Caggiula, A. R. (1999). Sex differences in nicotine effects and self-administration: Review of human and animal evidence. *Nicotine & Tobacco Research, 1*(4), 301–315.

Perry, R., Keller, P., Fraser, D., & Fiore, M. (2005). Fax to quit: A model for delivery of tobacco cessation services to Wisconsin residents. *Wisconsin Medical Journal, 104*(4), 37–44.

Pierce, J. P., & Gilpin, E. A. (2003). A minimum 6-month prolonged abstinence should be required for evaluating smoking cessation trials. *Nicotine & Tobacco Research, 5*(2), 151–153.

Prochaska, J., DiClemente, C., Velicer, W., & Rossi, J. (1993). Standardized, individualized, interactive and personalized self-help programs for smoking cessation. *Health Psychology, 12,* 399–405.

Prochaska, J. J., Delucchi, K., & Hall, S. M. (2004). A meta-analysis of smoking cessation interventions with individuals in substance abuse treatment or recovery. *Journal of Consulting and Clinical Psychology, 72*(6), 1144–1156.

Prochaska, J. O., & Velicer, W. F. (2004). Integrating population smoking cessation policies and programs. *Public Health Reports, 119*(3), 244–252.

Prochaska, J. O., Velicer, W. F., Fava, J. L., Rossi, J. S., & Tsoh, J. Y. (2001). Evaluating a population-based recruitment approach and a stage-based expert system intervention for smoking cessation. *Addictive Behaviors, 26*(4), 583–602.

Rodu, B., & Cole, P. (2007). Declining mortality from smoking in the United States. *Nicotine & Tobacco Research, 9*(7), 781–784.

Rollnick, S., Miller, W., & Butler, C. (2007). *Motivational Interviewing in health care: Helping patients change behavior.* New York: Guilford Press.

Schuurmans, M. M., Diacon, A. H., van Biljon, X., & Bolliger, C. T. (2004). Effect of pre-treatment with nicotine patch on withdrawal symptoms and abstinence rates in smokers subsequently quitting with the nicotine patch: A randomized controlled trial. *Addiction, 99*(5), 634–640.

Strecher, V. J., Shiffman, S., & West, R. (2005). Randomized controlled trial of a Web-based computer-tailored smoking cessation program as a supplement to nicotine patch therapy. *Addiction, 100*(5), 682–688.

Sussman, S., Sun, P., & Dent, C. W. (2006). A meta-analysis of teen cigarette smoking cessation. *Health Psychology, 25*(5), 549–557.

Sutton, S. (2001). Back to the drawing board? A review of applications of the transtheoretical model to substance use. *Addiction, 96*(1), 175–186.

Thorndike, A. N., Regan, S., & Rigotti, N. A. (2007). The treatment of smoking by U.S. physicians during ambulatory visits: 1994–2003. *American Journal of Public Health, 97*(10), 1878–1883.

Thun, M. J., & Jemal, A. (2006). How much of the decrease in cancer death rates in the United States is attributable to reductions in tobacco smoking? *Tobacco Control, 15*(5), 345–347.

Tonneson, P., Mikkelson, K., Norregaard, J., & Jorgenson, S. (1996). Recycling hard core smokers with nicotine nasal spray. *European Respiratory Journal, 9,* 1619–1623.

U.S. Department of Health and Human Services. (1998). *Tobacco use among U.S. racial/ethnic minority groups—African Americans, American Indians, and Alaska Natives, Asian Americans and Pacific Islanders, and Hispanics: A report of the Surgeon General.* Atlanta, GA: U.S. Department of Health and Human Services, Centers for Disease Control and Prevention, National Center for Chronic Disease Prevention and Health Promotion, Office on Smoking and Health.

U.S. Preventive Services Task Force. (2006). *Guide to community preventive services: Tobacco.* Atlanta: Centers for Disease Control.

Vidrine, J. I., Cofta-Woerpel, L., Daza, P., Wright, K. L., & Wetter, D. W. (2006). Smoking cessation 2: Behavioral treatments. *Behavioral Medicine, 32*(3), 99–109.

Weber, D., Wolff, L. S., Orleans, T., Mockenhaupt, R. E., Massett, H. A., & Vose, K. K. (2007). Smokers' attitudes and behaviors related to consumer demand for cessation counseling in the medical care setting. *Nicotine & Tobacco Research, 9*(5), 571–580.

West, R. (2005). Time for a change: Putting the Transtheoretical (Stages of Change) Model to rest. *Addiction, 100*(8), 1036–1039.

West, R. (2006). "Catastrophic" pathways to smoking cessation: Findings from national survey. *British Medical Journal, 332*(7539), 458–460.

West, R., & Zhou, X. (2007). Is nicotine replacement therapy for smoking cessation effective in the "real world"? Findings from a prospective multinational cohort study. *Thorax, 62*(11), 998–1002.

Wetter, D. W., Kenford, S. L., Smith, S. S., Fiore, M. C., Jorenby, D. E., & Baker, T. B. (1999). Gender differences in smoking cessation. *Journal of Consulting and Clinical Psychology, 67*(4), 555–562.

Williams, J. M., & Ziedonis, D. (2004). Addressing tobacco among individuals with a mental illness or an addiction. *Addictive Behaviors, 29*(6), 1067–1083.

Promoting Dietary Change

11

Barbara S. McCann
and Viktor E.
Bovbjerg

In the decade since the publication of the second edition of the *Handbook of Health Behavior Change*, it has become increasingly apparent that obesity is the single most important diet-related condition affecting the health of individuals in first world or industrialized countries. In the United States in 2003–2004, 17% of children and adolescents were overweight, and an astonishing 32% of adults were obese (Ogden et al., 2006). Obesity is a risk factor for many serious medical conditions, including cardiovascular disease, diabetes, certain types of cancer, gallbladder disease, and osteoarthritis (Field et al., 2002). Long-term studies of dietary interventions for weight loss show that modest weight loss can be achieved and is associated with reduced risk of diabetes and cardiovascular disease in at-risk individuals (Diabetes Prevention Program Research Group,

2002; Douketis, Macie, Thabane, & Williamson, 2005). For this reason, much of the following discussion of strategies for dietary change draws examples from the literature on weight loss.

Dietary interventions generally target the individual, with the intervention delivered in a variety of formats, including one-on-one, face-to-face delivery, delivery in groups or classes, and delivery through other formats, such as the Internet. Herein we refer to all such interventions as individual-level approaches to dietary change. Interventions may also target change at the level of the community, in which community may mean entire towns, schools, churches, or worksites. In this chapter, these interventions and perspectives are referred to as public health approaches to dietary change. While a review of all individual and public health intervention targets is beyond the scope of this chapter, we will attempt to highlight some of the more promising approaches to promoting dietary change in individuals and communities.

Individual-Level Approaches to Dietary Change

Clinical lore and research experience have repeatedly demonstrated that it is difficult for people to follow dietary recommendations. The problem of dietary adherence grows out of a wide range of biopsychosocial issues, including intra- and interpersonal factors, economic constraints (food insecurity), cultural preference, social influences, environmental conditions, and myriad psychological factors. Health delivery systems also impact patients' ability to follow health providers' dietary recommendations.

Barriers to Making Dietary Changes

All modifications in eating patterns for the purpose of losing weight require one or both of the following: decreasing the quantity of food consumed (e.g., smaller portions, fewer servings) and making less-preferred food choices on the basis of caloric density (e.g., choosing vegetables instead of cookies). A combination of these approaches reduces total daily caloric intake. Increased energy expenditure, often in the form of planned physical activity, is also helpful in facilitating weight loss. The problems associated with exercise adherence are addressed in chapter 12.

Barriers to dietary adherence may be a result of environmental factors, internal states, or social factors. A common environmental barrier is limited food selection. For example, grocery stores in low-income areas often have a more restricted range of products from which to choose than stores in more affluent areas, and this is reflected in poorer-quality diets among shoppers in those areas (Laraia, Siega-Riz, Kaufman, & Jones, 2004; Rose & Richards, 2004). The most common internal barrier to good dietary adherence is hunger, and the interplay between diet composition and satiety is complex (Hill, 2007). Emotional factors often contribute to poor adherence, with patients reporting that they ignore dietary guidelines in the face of emotional extremes. Social factors, such as holidays or other cultural influences, also pose barriers to people attempting to exert control over their intake (McCann, 2006).

Enhancing Dietary Adherence

Most approaches to individual-level dietary change incorporate several key components to achieve initial dietary change and long-term maintenance. We previously identified several common components used in dietary intervention programs to promote dietary change and maximize long-term maintenance (Mc-Cann & Bovbjerg, 1998). These include nutrition education, use of Motivational Interviewing and readiness to change, careful assessment of "baseline" diet practices, goal setting, self-monitoring, training in stimulus control, problem-solving training, enhancing social support for changes, enhancing self-efficacy through cognitive control strategies, relapse prevention training, and ongoing program contact to facilitate maintenance of changes. These treatment elements are grounded in principles of behavioral self-management (Kanfer, 1977; McFall, 1977; Watson & Tharp, 1997), social cognitive theory (Bandura, 1977), motivational interviewing (Miller & Rollnick, 2002), and the Transtheoretical Model of Change (Prochaska & Velicer, 1997). Several clinical trials of diet or lifestyle (diet plus exercise) interventions have used these treatment components to maximize weight loss (Diabetes Prevention Program Research Group, 2002; Funk et al., 2006; Lin et al., 2007; Pi-Sunyer et al., 2007) and to achieve reductions in sodium and alcohol intake (Funk et al., 2006; Lin et al., 2007). Specific examples of these components and their practical application have been described elsewhere (McCann, 2006). However, we will provide a brief update on the use of these components over the past decade.

Nutrition Education

Adequate nutrition information is an important ingredient for success in dietary interventions. Greater nutrition knowledge is associated with healthier diets (Wardle, Parmenter, & Waller, 2000). In a study of low-income mothers of young children, women in a weight-loss program who lost at least 2.27 kg over the course of 8 weeks had higher scores on a 25-item nutrition knowledge test than those who did not lose as much weight (Klohe-Lehman et al., 2006).

Motivational Interviewing and Readiness to Change

Motivational Interviewing (Miller & Rollnick, 2002) has emerged as an important component in both initiating and maintaining individuals' involvement in dietary interventions. Individuals vary in their willingness to accept recommendations to make dietary changes (McCann et al., 1996). Several studies have used Motivational Interviewing both at the initiation stage of dietary changes and at various points during treatment in order to enhance participants' involvement in lifestyle interventions (Carels et al., 2007; Diabetes Prevention Program Research Group, 2002; Funk et al., 2006).

Problem-Solving Training

Another important treatment component for improving the efficacy of individual-level interventions is training in problem solving. Problem-solving therapy addresses patients' approaches to dealing with obstacles through the use of cognitive and behavioral techniques (D'Zurilla, 1999). Patients are trained to identify problems, generate alterative solutions to solving them, decide which solution to try, make plans for implementing the solution, and evaluate the outcome (Nezu, Nezu, & Perri, 2006). Problem-solving therapy has been shown to facilitate greater weight loss as a component of a stepped-care approach to treatment (Carels et al., 2005) and to be more effective than relapse prevention training during the maintenance phase of weight-loss treatment (Perri et al., 2001).

Goal Setting

Goal setting remains an important component of interventions designed to promote dietary adherence. Goal setting can refer to the setting of specific weight-loss goals. In the Diabetes Prevention Program and the Look AHEAD trial, the weight-loss goal was expressed in terms of a percentage of weight loss (7%) from each participant's starting weight (Diabetes Prevention Program Research Group, 2002; Pi-Sunyer et al., 2007). In the PREMIER study of blood pressure control, the weight-loss goal was expressed in terms of absolute pounds (15) for participants who entered the study with a body mass index of 25 kg/m² or greater (Lin et al., 2007).

Importantly, goal setting is not limited to establishing clear expectations for outcome goals. Participants in the Diabetes Prevention Program and the Look AHEAD trial were also provided with specific goals for daily intake of grams of fat or total calories, as well as goals for weekly amounts of exercise expressed in minutes per week (Diabetes Prevention Program Research Group, 2002; Pi-Sunyer et al., 2007). Likewise, participants in PREMIER were given specific goals regarding exercise minutes per week, daily sodium intake, and daily alcohol intake (Funk et al., 2006).

Self-Monitoring

Frequent self-monitoring of dietary intake has emerged as perhaps the single most important ingredient to successful dietary change efforts. Survey studies of people who have successfully lost weight find that regular self-monitoring of weight and food intake are common and appear to be critical to successful weight loss (Kruger et al., 2006; Wing & Phelan, 2005). Several studies have shown that weight gains typically associated with significant holidays can be avoided through careful self-monitoring during these periods (Baker & Kirschenbaum, 1998; Boutelle, Kirschenbaum, Baker, & Mitchell, 1999).

Ongoing Program Contact

Ongoing program contact is now recognized as a key component of maintenance of initial dietary changes—sometimes referred to as the continuing care model (Latner et al., 2000). Long-term maintenance of changes in obesity treatment appears to be best met by continued program contact (Perri & Corsica, 2002).

Social Support

Just as inadequate social support can be seen as a barrier to making and maintaining dietary changes, interventions that enhance social support among program participants or otherwise promote social support may have an advantage over those that do not (Latner et al., 2006). For example, participants encouraged to bring weight-loss partners with them to programs may have an overall advantage (Wing & Jeffery, 1999).

Stepped-Care Approaches to Dietary Change

Stepped-care approaches to the delivery of these interventions have become increasingly common (Carels et al., 2005; Carels et al., 2007). In the traditional stepped-care approach, all individuals receive a basic intervention considered to be of sufficient intensity to achieve reasonable gains in the majority of its recipients. Efforts are intensified for individuals who have difficulty making reasonable progress. These approaches are generally more successful than "one size fits all" programs where all participants receive the same treatment "package." The "toolbox" approaches employed in the Diabetes Prevention Program and the Look AHEAD study are stepped-care approaches in that participants who were not achieving weight-loss goals were offered additional tools, resources, and contacts with program staff in order to optimize their chances for success (Diabetes Prevention Program Research Group, 2002; Pi-Sunyer et al., 2007).

In summary, virtually all programs designed to produce dietary changes in individuals include nutrition education. The use of various self-monitoring and goal-setting tools is generally introduced early on. This is often sufficient for a significant number of individuals to make changes in their diet that produce sufficient significant improvements in health.

Additional assessment is often introduced if individuals are struggling to make significant changes in diet without success. This may include evaluation by a dietitian or by someone trained in more advanced behavioral issues, such as a psychologist. Intensification of efforts may include more frequent meetings between the patient and the health care provider, meetings with another specialist, use of new self-monitoring tools, or use of motivational enhancement strategies. Techniques and topics including stimulus control strategies, problem-solving training, cognitive strategies, and relapse prevention may be introduced.

Maintenance of initial dietary changes generally requires ongoing program contact. Longer treatment programs are associated with better maintenance of new dietary behaviors. Extended contact can be achieved via telephone contact, mail, or e-mail. In-person contact may be face-to-face or in groups, even in some instances having patients form their own support networks for ongoing monitoring of dietary changes.

Public Health Approaches to Dietary Change

The late psychologist George W. Albee often noted, "No mass disorder afflicting humankind is ever brought under control or eliminated by attempts at treating the individual." While the "mass disorder" Albee was referring to is mental illness, his comment is relevant to the worldwide epidemic of diet- and activity-related disorders. Individual-level approaches to diet change will not by themselves stem the tide of overweight and obesity (Mann et al., 2007) and face an uphill struggle when attempted in "obesogenic" environments and societies (Caballero, 2007). Individual-level approaches to dietary change—very useful in clinical settings—have not focused on environmental factors promoting dietary choices, except to promote changes in the immediate environment of individuals (e.g., limiting household food options, promoting social support). Increasingly, there is recognition that a wide range of genetic, personal, interpersonal, and environmental factors influence dietary intake and that interventions at all levels may be needed to effectively change population-level health outcomes (Sallis & Owen, 2002). Clearly, approaches that take into account the traditional triad of person, behavior, and environment provide the greatest promise of success (Caballero, 2007; Glanz, 2002).

Community-Level Dietary Change

Community-level approaches to dietary change have incorporated elements of mass marketing and mass communication to spread the intended health-promoting messages. Some critical elements of mass-marketing approaches to health promotion have been enumerated. It is essential to obtain the means to disseminate the message—characterized as "pay for exposure" (buy airtime and print space), "beg for exposure" (ask for donations), and "earn exposure" (make the cause newsworthy in its own right) (Hornik & Kelly, 2007). Community members or target populations must be exposed to the relevant messages. In several well-known community-level health-promotion efforts, exposure to study-specific health-promotion measures was nearly as great in control as in intervention communities (Hornik & Kelly, 2007). Diet interventions also face a challenge unlike other health-promotion campaigns (e.g. tobacco use), in that there is no simple, single message that can be communicated that implies an obvious course of action (e.g., don't smoke). Furthermore, it is not always clear through which pathway(s) mass-communication approaches may work to effect dietary behavior change: direct persuasion, changing social and community norms, or modifying institutional or policymaker behavior. No matter how well funded, mass-communication campaigns to promote dietary change also have the potential to be drowned out in an advertising and media environment that promotes behavior opposite to that encouraged by the campaign. Finally, like any other intervention, the message must be tailored to the target audience. Dietary-change messages may differ depending on whether the need is for information or motivation and on whether the message is simple or complex; decisions regarding whether to use a celebrity spokesperson or dietitian, whether to present information undermining competing messages, and whether to use fear of disease as a motivator can be important in presenting appealing and effective messages (Wilson, 2007). In tailoring strong behavior-change messages to target audiences, however, it is crucial that such messages not overstate their case and inadvertently reinforce the already strong stereotype that disease prevention is largely the result of individual behavior (Sankofa & Johnson-Taylor, 2007).

In addition to the large-scale community and mass-communication projects—which are difficult to mount, methodologically challenging, and open to substantial influences of secular trends external to the study—many smaller community interventions have been carried out in grocery stores, restaurants, schools, and worksites. Though many effective interventions combine population and individual approaches, the discussion that follows focuses on community-*level* interventions, in which a primary focus of the intervention is at the population level, separate from the conceptually distinct community-*based* but primarily individual-level interventions.

Community-Level Dietary Change in Organizations

Schools

Schools are natural venues for promoting healthful eating, but school interventions face several challenges. First, institutional resources may be constrained, making it difficult to institute school- or system-level changes in food purchases or vending-machine policy. Second, outcomes of school-based interventions may include changes in attitude, individual behavior, institutional behavior, the physical and social environment, and markers of excess weight and it may be difficult to demonstrate effects on BMI or disease risk (French, 2005). Third, many school-based studies use multicomponent approaches—a combination of individual, institutional, and sometimes family-level interventions, often incorporating additional interventions to increase physical activity. Such approaches gain synergy, but may not be of sufficient scope to disentangle the effects of the individual components (French, 2005). Fourth, school-based initiatives may not carry over outside school, where children get the majority of their food energy. Finally, if substantial external (e.g., school district or statewide) efforts are made to modify pupils' dietary behavior, the ability to detect treatment effects may be compromised by larger secular trends. Nonetheless, studies to date suggest that interventions at the school level can influence dietary intake, at least while children are at school.

Multicomponent approaches, combining individual-level behavioral interventions, family involvement, and changes in school environment or policy, are most likely to observe changes in both behavior and the environment (French, 2005; French & Wechsler, 2004). Such interventions are popular and have been successfully implemented and evaluated outside more controlled academic research activities (Stables et al., 2005).

Food availability has been examined in a number of settings. Making healthful choices available, through school meal programs or vending machines, may influence some students to select those options more frequently (French, 2005). For example, increasing low-fat and decreasing high-fat options in one school led purchasers to make low-fat selections 32% of the time, whereas low-fat options were picked only 14% of the time in a comparison school (Bartholomew & Jowers, 2006).

One attractive intervention may be to simply provide healthful food to children, rather than merely encourage their purchase or consumption. Providing a salad bar has been shown to increase consumption of fruits and vegetables among low-income children eligible for free or subsidized meals (Slusser,

Cumberland, Browdy, Lange, & Neumann, 2007). Recently, a school-level randomized trial in 98 schools demonstrated that offering a daily fruit or vegetable to young students increased intake during the program period and that the effect waned after program cessation (Ransley et al., 2007). Such interventions are likely to be modest, and ongoing support is needed to maintain changes long enough to develop lasting health benefits or substantial changes in school or community norms.

The influence of food pricing in schools has been relatively well documented. Adding low-fat snack items to school vending machines and pairing that with varying levels of discount for purchasing low-fat options can lead to large proportional (but small absolute) increases in low-fat snack purchases (French et al., 2001). Similar significant but small effects have been observed by subsidizing low-fat options and "taxing" high-fat options in school cafeterias (Hannan, French, Story, & Fulkerson, 2002). Even substantial discounts have modest effects on choice—adolescents cite price as important in food choices but cite taste substantially more often (Shannon, Story, Fulkerson, & French, 2002), so effective interventions must address acceptability and taste, in addition to cost.

Promoting healthful eating, either through broad or individually targeted methods, is effective in increasing consumption of health-promoting foods. General promotion activities, either school-wide or at the point of purchase (i.e., school cafeteria, vending machines), such as informational or motivational signs and posters, seem to have small but independent effects on food choices by students (French, 2005).

Worksites

Like schools, worksites offer a tempting venue for dietary change efforts but there are important differences between the two. Worksite interventions, though not reaching the entire population, have the potential to change not only individual behavior but social norms both in surrounding communities and other businesses. The physical and social variation in worksites that makes it difficult to say "what works" is compounded by the heterogeneity of interventions and outcomes in worksite research (Katz et al., 2005). Unlike school pupils, employees often have a say in working conditions. Like schools, worksites may be loath to introduce changes that divert time from business activities or decrease profits or wages. If there is substantial dropout or workforce turnover, as was common in many early worksite studies (French, 2005), generalizability and validity can suffer. Nonetheless, changes in dietary behavior can be promoted at worksites, using many of the same techniques that have been effective in school settings.

Many of the more successful efforts have employed multicomponent interventions (French, 2005), typically pairing individual educational efforts with some combination of mass media, labeling and other point-of-purchase information, product promotion, and, often, an employee advisory board. Worksite-level trials have generally shown modest but significant improvements in target behaviors, according to measures ranging from fruit and vegetable intake to intake of calories and fat calories. The Working Healthy Project (WHP), for example, combined individual-level dietary change education, changes to vending-machine signage, modifications to catering policies, general promotional materials, incentives for participation, and the formation of an employee advisory board, and found small but significant increases in fruit and vegetable and fiber intake (Emmons, Linnan, Shadel, Marcus, & Abrams, 1999). It is difficult, however, to disentangle the effects of individual-level interventions from the collective and environmental interventions unless that is an explicit part of the study design. Multicomponent approaches will continue to be popular, in the hope that the synergy between individual and environmental approaches will result in greater, more robust effects.

Pricing influences purchases in worksites, as well. Discounts appear to promote selection of targeted items at worksites (Seymour, Yaroch, Serdula, Blanck, & Khan, 2004), hardly surprising given that cost is second only to taste in determining food purchases (Popkin, Duffey, & Gordon-Larsen, 2005). Pricing approaches, while promoting healthful food choices, must be implemented carefully to avoid unintended consequences. In the CHIPS project (French et al., 2001), 10% price reductions on low-fat vending snacks had little influence on purchases, but discounts of 25% and 50% showed not only strong associations with increased selection of low-fat snacks but increased purchases, suggesting that employees may have been using the discounts to buy extra snacks. Future investigations should determine whether eating habits modified by price changes generalize to other settings and whether sustained change requires sustained discounts.

Promotional approaches have had mixed success in apparently similar settings, with the pairing of promotional items and nutritional information reducing selection of higher-fat options and promoting lower-fat choices in some settings (Zifferblatt, Wilbur, & Pinsky, 1980) but not others (Mayer, Brown, Heins, & Bishop, 1987). Multiple promotional and informational approaches— for instance, posters, brochures, table-top information, inserts in paychecks, flyers, newsletters, tip sheets, and message cards—can be combined to reinforce a central interventional theme or message (Beresford et al., 2001).

The work climate is important in fostering success. Company leadership is important in carrying out and supporting interventions (Sorensen, Linnan, & Hunt, 2004). Advisory boards are a common way of involving both management and employees in worksite nutrition interventions. Such boards take responsibility for tailoring interventions to their specific worksites, for implementing intervention activities, and for involving other employees in intervention activities (Beresford et al., 2001) and are crucial to success and sustainability.

The Built Environment

Built environments are associated with overweight and obesity. There is evidence that body mass index may be associated with the density of fast-food outlets, the presence of convenience stores, a relative lack of supermarkets, and higher costs for fruits and vegetables (Papas et al., 2007), but the field is only now emerging, and both methods and results have been mixed. The growth of investigations on diet and environment, along with improving research methods, suggests that the field will contribute substantially to community-level dietary change efforts.

While neighborhood characteristics may be used to assess associations with eating patterns, they can also be used to identify barriers to healthful eating and to promote dietary change. For instance, community members have combined physical neighborhood surveys with previously published work to successfully identify barriers to healthful eating, such as relative lack of supermarkets in some areas, high fast-food outlet density, and relative paucity of produce markets (Jilcott, Laraia, Evenson, Lowenstein, & Ammerman, 2007). Using neighborhood assessments allows interventions to be tailored to specific settings and is compatible with both individual and community-level approaches. Two important sources of food and therefore potential venues for promoting community-level dietary change in every community are grocery stores and restaurants. Because grocery stores and restaurants are ubiquitous and similar, interventions developed locally have the potential to be relatively easily translatable across settings and populations.

Grocery Stores

The availability of healthful food items at grocery stores, and their placement within stores, may influence shopping and, in turn, eating habits and therefore affect our ability to prevent or control disease. If healthful items are not available, they cannot be purchased and consumed, and stores located in low SES settings have been shown to be less likely to stock healthful items (Horowitz, Colson, Hebert, & Lancaster, 2004). Grocery stores, while an attractive venue for interventions to promote more healthful eating, must balance commercial and marketing considerations against the desire to promote healthful items and provide nutrition education (Winett et al., 1992), and it will be difficult to mount successful efforts to promote health eating in commercial stores if they require staff or management time, interfere with the volume or variety of products on display, or discourage purchase of entire types of foods.

In general, diet change interventions in grocery stores employ point-of-purchase information; coupons or price reductions, increased access or availability, or promotions (Glanz & Yaroch, 2004). All grocery stores use information, advertisements, and product placement to promote items—the placement of energy dense confections near checkout stands to encourage impulse purchases is well documented (Dixon, Scully, & Parkinson, 2006). Despite this, there have been relatively few published results of such interventions specifically to promote healthful food choices. A recent review (Seymour et al., 2004) suggested that information strategies were the most common approach to promoting healthful items, while multiple avenues of information, incentives, and improved access and availability were used less frequently. Outcomes of grocery store interventions were mixed, however, with 5 of 10 studies showing no effect and the others showing modest effects on targeted foods. Price may be one of the most powerful incentives for modifying behavior but is based on the cost of production, storage, and transportation rather than on the healthfulness of the product. In many settings, this means that health-promoting foods are more expensive than less-healthful choices, and price has been shown to be second only to taste in the consideration of food purchases (Popkin et al., 2005). Providing free access to reduced-calorie foods has proven effective in experimental settings (Weststrate et al., 1998), but it is not clear how such findings translate into environments with inexpensive high-calorie foods.

Overcoming some methodological challenges may also promote evaluation of grocery store interventions. For instance, the advent of extensive and identifiable purchase information makes it possible—with appropriate privacy safeguards—to examine individual-level purchasing over time (Ni Mhurchu et al., 2007), as a complement to established environmental methods of characterizing community shopping habits (Cheadle et al., 1993).

Restaurants

With approximately one-third of U.S. calories consumed in or prepared by restaurants, the potential for public health impact through changes in restaurant eating practices is great. However, like grocery stores, commercial restaurants may be reluctant to allow dietary change efforts that result in substantial management or employee effort, disruption to efficient operations or increased costs, and potential for diminished sales or dissatisfied customers. Diners are confronted with the fact that the same amount of money used to purchase a several-hundred-calorie salad at an upscale restaurant can buy a several-thousand-calorie meal at a fast-food outlet.

Restaurant interventions often use some combination of information, availability or access, pricing, and advertising and promotion (Glanz & Hoelscher, 2004). Restaurants often respond to perceived consumer demand by identifying health-promoting menu items. Unless these items are appealing and competitively priced, there will be little reason to eliminate the pricing incentives for larger portions of energy-dense foods (French, 2005). Health-promoting interventions to date in restaurant settings suggest that informational strategies—labeling certain menu items to suggest healthfulness within a general promotional campaign—are the most common approach (Seymour et al., 2004), though there is concern that labeling healthful foods connotes poorer taste quality (Seymour et al., 2004) or invokes unfavorable stereotypes of healthful eating (Fries & Croyle, 1993). Nevertheless, these informational approaches have proven generally successful in the short term, though their long-term influences have not been documented. Increasing availability or access to health-promoting items in restaurants—for instance, by offering side dishes that feature fruits and vegetables—is an understudied approach (Glanz & Hoelscher, 2004), and efforts to modify availability of healthful foods and to reduce portion sizes may have to overcome norms and standards in both the food service industry and among food service workers (Condrasky, Ledikwe, Flood, & Rolls, 2007).

Looking to the Future

It is clear at this point that the epidemic of diseases related to diet and energy imbalance will be solved only through concerted efforts at both the individual and the collective level. However, there have been relatively few demonstrated community-level and environmental interventions to modify dietary intake, in contrast to the wealth of documentation of individual-level interventions. Diet change at the community, environmental, and organizational levels is likely to remain focused on multimodal approaches combining individual interventions with multiple environmental or organizational interventions. Researchers must focus on identifying those combinations of interventions that are most effective—and cost-effective—while at the same time identifying the individual contribution of each intervention component. Research to date suggests that point-of-purchase interventions hold a great deal of promise in communities, worksites, and schools, though the long-term effectiveness of such interventions has not been demonstrated (Matson-Koffman, Brownstein, Neiner, & Greaney, 2005). Translational research is needed to determine the settings in which economic incentives, information, and promotions not only have an impact on behavior but can do so in ways that are acceptable to consumers and businesses. Similarly, the role of the environment—whether community, worksite, or school—in shaping food choices is only now being fully explored, and this is reflected in the sometimes mixed results of studies to date. Research in the area is already moving away from merely associating physical aspects of the environment to characteristics of people in those environments and is exploring the dynamic person-environment interaction (Sallis & Owen, 2002). Both research and practice will continue to be improved by the involvement of interdisciplinary teams of researchers, clinicians, policymakers, business leaders, and citizens. Only such a widespread, concerted effort will be able to overcome the huge global challenge we face in combating diseases related to one of the most fundamental of all human behaviors—eating.

References

Baker, R. C., & Kirschenbaum, D. S. (1998). Weight control during the holidays: Highly consistent self-monitoring as a potentially useful coping mechanism. *Health Psychology, 17,* 367–370.

Bandura, A. (1977). *Social learning theory.* Englewood Cliffs, NJ: Prentice-Hall.

Bartholomew, J. B., & Jowers, E. M. (2006). Increasing frequency of lower-fat entrees offered at school lunch: An environmental change strategy to increase healthful selections. *Journal of the American Dietetic Association, 106,* 248–252.

Beresford, S. A., Thompson, B., Feng, Z., Christianson, A., McLerran, D., & Patrick, D. L. (2001). Seattle 5-a-Day worksite program to increase fruit and vegetable consumption. *Preventive Medicine, 32,* 230–238.

Boutelle, K. N., Kirschenbaum, D. S., Baker, R. C., & Mitchell, M. E. (1999). How can obese weight controllers minimize weight gain during the high risk holiday season? By self-monitoring very consistently. *Health Psychology, 18,* 364–368.

Caballero, B. (2007). The global epidemic of obesity: An overview. *Epidemiology Review, 29,* 1–5.

Carels, R. A., Darby, L., Cacciapaglia, H. M., Douglass, O. M., Harper, J., Kaplar, M. E., et al. (2005). Applying a stepped-care approach to the treatment of obesity. *Journal Psychosomatic Research, 59,* 375–383.

Carels, R. A., Darby, L., Cacciapaglia, H. M., Konrad, K., Coit, C., Harper, J., et al. (2007). Using motivational interviewing as a supplement to obesity treatment: A stepped-care approach. *Health Psychology, 26,* 369–374.

Cheadle, A., Psaty, B. M., Curry, S., Wagner, E., Diehr, P., Koepsell, T., et al. (1993). Can measures of the grocery store environment be used to track community-level dietary changes? *Preventive Medicine, 22,* 361–372.

Condrasky, M., Ledikwe, J. H., Flood, J. E., & Rolls, B. J. (2007). Chefs' opinions of restaurant portion sizes. *Obesity, 15,* 2086–2094.

Diabetes Prevention Program Research Group. (2002). The Diabetes Prevention Program (DPP): Description of lifestyle intervention. *Diabetes Care, 25,* 2165–2171.

Dixon, H., Scully, M., & Parkinson, K. (2006). Pester power: Snackfoods displayed at supermarket checkouts in Melbourne, Australia. *Health Promotion Journal of Australia, 17,* 124–127.

Douketis, J. D., Macie, C., Thabane, L., & Williamson, D. F. (2005). Systematic review of long-term weight loss studies in obese adults: Clinical significance and applicability to clinical practice. *International Journal of Obesity (Lond), 29,* 1153–1167.

D'Zurilla, T. J. (1999). *Problem-solving therapy: A social competence approach to clinical intervention.* New York: Springer Publishing Company.

Emmons, K. M., Linnan, L. A., Shadel, W. G., Marcus, B., & Abrams, D. B. (1999). The Working Healthy Project: A worksite health-promotion trial targeting physical activity, diet, and smoking. *Journal of Occupational and Environmental Medicine, 41,* 545–555.

Field, A. E., Barnoya, J., & Colditz, G. A. (2002). Epidemiology and health consequences of obesity. In T. A. Wadden & A. J. Stunkard (Eds.), *Handbook of obesity treatment* (pp. 3–18). New York: Guilford Press.

French, S. A. (2005). Population approaches to promote healthful eating behaviors. In D. Crawford & R. W. Jeffery (Eds.), *Obesity prevention and public health* (pp. 101–127). Oxford: Oxford University Press.

French, S. A., Jeffery, R. W., Story, M., Breitlow, K. K., Baxter, J. S., Hannan, P., et al. (2001). Pricing and promotion effects on low-fat vending snack purchases: The CHIPS Study. *American Journal of Public Health, 91,* 112–117.

French, S. A., & Wechsler, H. (2004). School-based research and initiatives: Fruit and vegetable environment, policy, and pricing workshop. *Preventive Medicine, 39*(Suppl. 2), S101–S107.

Fries, E., & Croyle, R. T. (1993). Stereotypes associated with a low-fat diet and their relevance to nutrition education. *Journal of the American Dietetic Association, 93,* 551–555.

Funk, K. L., Elmer, P. J., Stevens, V. J., Harsha, D. W., Craddick, S. R., Lin, P. H., et al. (2006). PREMIER—A trial of lifestyle interventions for blood pressure control: Intervention design and rationale. *Health Promotion Practice, 9,* 271–280.

Glanz, K. (2002). Perspectives on group, organization, and community interventions. In K. Glanz, B. K. Rimer, & F. M. Lewis (Eds.), *Health behavior and health education* (3rd ed., pp. 389–403). San Francisco: Wiley.

Glanz, K., & Hoelscher, D. (2004). Increasing fruit and vegetable intake by changing environments, policy and pricing: Restaurant-based research, strategies, and recommendations. *Preventive Medicine, 39*(Suppl. 2), S88–S93.

Glanz, K., & Yaroch, A. L. (2004). Strategies for increasing fruit and vegetable intake in grocery stores and communities: Policy, pricing, and environmental change. *Preventive Medicine, 39* (Suppl. 2), S75–S80.

Hannan, P., French, S. A., Story, M., & Fulkerson, J. A. (2002). A pricing strategy to promote sales of lower fat foods in high school cafeterias: Acceptability and sensitivity analysis. *American Journal of Health Promotion, 17,* 1–6, ii.

Hill, A. J. (2007). The psychology of food craving. *The Proceedings of the Nutrition Society, 66,* 277–285.

Hornik, R., & Kelly, B. (2007). Communication and diet: An overview of experience and principles. *Journal of Nutrition Education and Behavior, 39,* S5–S12.

Horowitz, C. R., Colson, K. A., Hebert, P. L., & Lancaster, K. (2004). Barriers to buying healthy foods for people with diabetes: Evidence of environmental disparities. *American Journal of Public Health, 94,* 1549–1554.

Jilcott, S. B., Laraia, B. A., Evenson, K. R., Lowenstein, L. M., & Ammerman, A. S. (2007). A guide for developing intervention tools addressing environmental factors to improve diet and physical activity. *Health Promotion Practice, 8,* 192–204.

Kanfer, F. H. (1977). The many faces of self-control, or behavior modification changes its focus. In R. B. Stuart (Ed.), *Behavioral self-management: Strategies, techniques and outcome* (pp. 1–48). New York: Brunner/Mazel.

Katz, D. L., O'Connell, M., Yeh, M. C., Nawaz, H., Njike, V., Anderson, L. M., et al. (2005). Public health strategies for preventing and controlling overweight and obesity in school and worksite settings: A report on recommendations of the Task Force on Community Preventive Services. *Morbidity and Mortality Weekly Reports. Recommendations and Reports, 54,* 1–12.

Klohe-Lehman, D. M., Freeland-Graves, J., Anderson, E. R., McDowell, T., Clarke, K. K., Hanss-Nuss, H., et al. (2006). Nutrition knowledge is associated with greater weight loss in obese and overweight low-income mothers. *Journal of the American Dietetic Association, 106,* 65–75.

Kruger, J., Blanck, H. M., & Gillespie, C. (2006). Dietary and physical activity behaviors among adults successful at weight loss maintenance. *The International Journal of Behavioral Nutrition and Physical Activity, 3,* 17.

Laraia, B. A., Siega-Riz, A. M., Kaufman, J. S., & Jones, S. J. (2004). Proximity of supermarkets is positively associated with diet quality index for pregnancy. *Preventive Medicine, 39,* 869–875.

Latner, J. D., Stunkard, A. J., Wilson, G. T., & Jackson, M. L. (2006). The perceived effectiveness of continuing care and group support in the long-term self-help treatment of obesity. *Obesity, 14,* 464–471.

Latner, J. D., Stunkard, A. J., Wilson, G. T., Jackson, M. L., Zelitch, D. S., & Labouvie, E. (2000). Effective long-term treatment of obesity: A continuing care model. *International Journal of Obesity and Related Metabolic Disorders, 24,* 893–898.

Lin, P. H., Appel, L. J., Funk, K., Craddick, S., Chen, C., Elmer, P., et al. (2007). The PREMIER intervention helps participants follow the dietary approaches to stop hypertension dietary pattern and the current dietary reference intakes recommendations. *Journal of American Dietetic Association, 107,* 1541–1551.

Mann, T., Tomiyama, A. J., Westling, E., Lew, A.M., Samuels, B., & Chatman, J. (2007). Medicare's search for effective obesity treatments: Diets are not the answer. *American Psychologist, 62,* 220–233.

Matson-Koffman, D. M., Brownstein, J. N., Neiner, J. A., & Greaney, M. L. (2005). A site-specific literature review of policy and environmental interventions that promote physical activity and nutrition for cardiovascular health: What works? *American Journal of Health Promotion, 19,* 167–193.

Mayer, J. A., Brown, T. P., Heins, J. M., & Bishop, D. B. (1987). A multi-component intervention for modifying food selections in a worksite cafeteria. *Journal of Nutrition Education, 19,* 277–280.

McCann, B. S. (2006). Adherence to dietary recommendations. In W. T. O'Donohue & E. R. Levensky (Eds.), *Promoting treatment adherence: A practical handbook for health care providers* (pp. 321–330). Thousand Oaks, CA: Sage.

McCann, B. S., & Bovbjerg, V. E. (1998). Promoting dietary change. In S. A. Shumaker, E. B. Schron, J. K. Ockene, & W. L. McBee (Eds.), *The handbook of health behavior change* (2nd ed., pp. 166–188). New York: Springer Publishing Company.

McCann, B. S., Bovbjerg, V. E., Curry, S. J., Retzlaff, B. M., Walden, C. E., & Knopp, R. H. (1996). Predicting participation in a dietary intervention to lower cholesterol among individuals with hyperlipidemia. *Health Psychology, 15,* 61–64.

McFall, R. M. (1977). Parameters of self-monitoring. In R. B. Stuart (Ed.), *Behavioral self-management: Strategies, techniques and outcome* (pp. 196–214). New York: Brunner/Mazel.

Miller, W. R., & Rollnick, S. (2002). *Motivational Interviewing: Preparing people for change* (2nd ed.). New York: Guilford Press.

Nezu, A.M., Nezu, C. M., & Perri, M. G. (2006). Problem solving to promote treatment adherence. In W. T. O'Donohue & E. R. Levensky (Eds.), *Promoting treatment adherence: A practical handbook for health care providers* (pp. 135–148). Thousand Oaks, CA: Sage.

Ni Mhurchu, C., Blakely, T., Wall, J., Rodgers, A., Jiang, Y., & Wilton, J. (2007). Strategies to promote healthier food purchases: A pilot supermarket intervention study. *Public Health Nutrition, 10,* 608–615.

Ogden, C. L., Carroll, M. D., Curtin, L. R., McDowell, M. A., Tabak, C. J., & Flegal, K. M. (2006). Prevalence of overweight and obesity in the United States, 1999–2004. *Journal of the American Medical Association, 295,* 1549–1555.

Papas, M. A., Alberg, A. J., Ewing, R., Helzlsouer, K. J., Gary, T. L., & Klassen, A. C. (2007). The built environment and obesity. *Epidemiology Review, 29,* 129–143.

Perri, M. G., & Corsica, J. A. (2002). Improving the maintenance of weight lost in behavioral treatment of obesity. In T. A. Wadden & A. J. Stunkard (Eds.), *Handbook of obesity treatment* (pp. 357–379). New York: Guilford Press.

Perri, M. G., Nezu, A.M., McKelvey, W. F., Shermer, R. L., Renjilian, D. A., & Viegener, B. J. (2001). Relapse prevention training and problem-solving therapy in the long-term management of obesity. *Journal of Consulting and Clinical Psychology, 69,* 722–726.

Pi-Sunyer, X., Blackburn, G., Brancati, F. L., Bray, G. A., Bright, R., Clark, J. M., et al. (2007). Reduction in weight and cardiovascular disease risk factors in individuals with type 2 diabetes: One-year results of the Look AHEAD trial. *Diabetes Care, 30,* 1374–1383.

Popkin, B. M., Duffey, K., & Gordon-Larsen, P. (2005). Environmental influences on food choice, physical activity and energy balance. *Physiology Behavior, 86,* 603–613.

Prochaska, J. O., & Velicer, W. F. (1997). The transtheoretical model of health behavior change. *American Journal of Health Promotion, 12,* 38–48.

Ransley, J. K., Greenwood, D. C., Cade, J. E., Blenkinsop, S., Schagen, I., Teeman, D., et al. (2007). Does the school fruit and vegetable scheme improve children's diet? A non-randomised controlled trial. *Journal of Epidemiology and Community Health, 61,* 699–703.

Rose, D., & Richards, R. (2004). Food store access and household fruit and vegetable use among participants in the U.S. Food Stamp Program. *Public Health Nutrition, 7,* 1081–1088.

Sallis, J. F., & Owen, N. (2002). Ecological models of health behavior. In K. Glanz, B. K. Rimer, & F. M. Lewis (Eds.), *Health behavior and health education* (3rd ed., pp. 462–484). San Francisco: Wiley.

Sankofa, J., & Johnson-Taylor, W. L. (2007). News coverage of diet-related health disparities experienced by black Americans: A steady diet of misinformation. *Journal of Nutrition Education and Behavior, 39,* S41–S44.

Seymour, J. D., Yaroch, A. L., Serdula, M., Blanck, H. M., & Khan, L. K. (2004). Impact of nutrition environmental interventions on point-of-purchase behavior in adults: A review. *Preventive Medicine, 39* (Suppl. 2), S108–S136.

Shannon, C., Story, M., Fulkerson, J. A., & French, S. A. (2002). Factors in the school cafeteria influencing food choices by high school students. *Journal of School Health, 72,* 229–234.

Slusser, W. M., Cumberland, W. G., Browdy, B. L., Lange, L., & Neumann, C. (2007). A school salad bar increases frequency of fruit and vegetable consumption among children living in low-income households. *Public Health Nutrition,* 1–7.

Sorensen, G., Linnan, L., & Hunt, M. K. (2004). Worksite-based research and initiatives to increase fruit and vegetable consumption. *Preventive Medicine, 39* (Suppl. 2), S94–S100.

Stables, G. J., Young, E. M., Howerton, M. W., Yaroch, A. L., Kuester, S., Solera, M. K., et al. (2005). Small school-based effectiveness trials increase vegetable and fruit consumption among youth. *Journal of the American Dietetic Association, 105,* 252–256.

Wardle, J., Parmenter, K., & Waller, J. (2000). Nutrition knowledge and food intake. *Appetite, 34,* 269–275.

Watson, D. L., & Tharp, R. G. (1997). *Self-directed behavior: Self-modification for personal adjustment* (7th ed.). Pacific Grove, CA: Brooks/Cole.

Weststrate, J. A., van het Hof, K. H., van den Berg, H., Velthuis-te-Wierik, E. J., de Graaf, C., Zimmermanns, N. J., Westerterp, K. R., Westerterp-Plantenga, M. S., Verboeket-van de Vente, W. P. (1998). A comparison of the effect of free access to reduced fat products or their full fat equivalents on food intake, body weight, blood lipids and fat-soluble antioxidants levels and haemostasis variables. *European Journal of Clinical Nutrition, 52,* 389–395.

Wilson, B. J. (2007). Designing media messages about health and nutrition: What strategies are most effective? *Journal of Nutrition Education and Behavior, 39,* S13–S19.

Winett, R. A., Moore, J. F., Wargerg-Rankin, J., Hite, L. A., Neubauer, T. E., & Lombard, D. (1992). Conceptual and strategic considerations effective supermarket interventions. In M. M. Henderson, D. J. Bowen, & K. K. DeRoos (Eds.), *Promoting dietary change in communities: Applying existing models of dietary change to population-based interventions* (p. 172). Seattle: Fred Hutchinson Cancer Research Center.

Wing, R. R., & Jeffery, R. W. (1999). Benefits of recruiting participants with friends and increasing social support for weight loss and maintenance. *Journal of Consulting and Clinical Psychology, 67,* 132–138.

Wing, R. R., & Phelan, S. (2005). Long-term weight loss maintenance. *American Journal of Clinical Nutrition, 82,* 222S–225S.

Zifferblatt, S. M., Wilbur, C. S., & Pinsky, J. L. (1980). A new direction for public health care: Changing cafeteria eating habits. *Journal of the American Dietetic Association., 76,* 15–20.

Adherence to Physical Activity Recommendations and Interventions

12

Bess H. Marcus,
Joseph T. Ciccolo,
Dori Whitehead,
Teresa K. King, and
Beth C. Bock

Understanding how to facilitate the maintenance of health-promoting behaviors represents a major challenge for health practitioners and researchers. Physical activity is particularly challenging to support as it takes more time and effort than most other preventive health behaviors. The difficulty of adhering to regular physical activity is reflected in the high proportion of individuals who are sedentary or irregularly active and thus not physically active at the level needed to achieve health benefits (Haskell et al., 2007). Difficulty adhering to a physical activity regimen also is reflected by the high relapse rates from physical activity programs, which have been estimated at approximately 50% (Castro & King, 2002). However, regular participation in physical activity yields tremendous benefits, and additional benefits continue to be discovered. Therefore, adherence to physical activity is a critical issue.

Adherence is difficult to define, as it can be discussed in very specific or very general terms and can apply to all phases of the physical activity continuum from the initiation of physical activity behavior to the early adoption of the physical activity habit to the maintenance phase and then periodically to the relapse phase and, one hopes, to recovery and the resumption of the physical activity habit. Thus, there is much inconsistency in the literature as to how physical activity adherence is defined. One definition of adherence that is often used is the fulfillment of predetermined goals (Dubbert, Rappaport, & Martin, 1987). This definition is a useful one, as it can be adapted to include goals set by public health initiatives such as *Healthy People 2010* (U.S. Department of Health and Human Services [USDHHS], 2000). In this chapter, adherence is considered more broadly to include the amount of physical activity one participates in relative to the amount that the participant was asked to perform. In this chapter we will typically use the phrase *physical activity,* rather than *exercise.* The American College of Sports Medicine (ACSM, 2000) defines exercise as "planned, structured and repetitive bodily movement done to improve or maintain one or more components of physical fitness" (p. 4), whereas physical activity is defined as "bodily movement that is produced by the contraction of skeletal muscle and that substantially increases energy expenditure" (ACSM, 2000, p. 4).

This chapter focuses on recent studies that examine the impact of various interventions on the physical activity patterns of healthy adults. Many of these studies utilize psychological theories as an organizing framework, and therefore, several of these theories are presented. Next, specific intervention studies organized by the channel utilized (i.e., provider, home-based, worksite, community) are discussed. It should be noted that the discussion of interventions is not an exhaustive review, which would go beyond the scope of this chapter (see Hillsdon, Foster, & Thorogood, 2005).

Physical Activity Recommendations

Despite the fact that it is now well known that regular participation in physical activity helps to reduce mortality rates (Schnohr, Lange, Scharling, & Jensen, 2006), approximately 70% of the U.S. population remain sedentary (USDHHS, 2006). Sedentary individuals are classified as those who do not consistently meet the minimum public health physical activity recommendations set forth by a joint recommendation from the American College of Sports Medicine and the American Heart Association (ACSM, 2000; Haskell et al., 2007). To maintain health, individuals should accumulate 30 minutes or more of at least moderate-intensity aerobic physical activity five or more days per week, or they should accumulate 20 minutes or more of vigorous-intensity aerobic physical activity, on three or more days per week. In addition, individuals should perform activities that maintain or increase muscular strength and endurance at least two days per week. Combinations of moderate and vigorous intensity physical activity can also be done to meet the recommendations (for more specific examples, see Haskell et al., 2007). These guidelines have important implications for adherence, as research has demonstrated that individuals are more likely to adopt and maintain moderate intensity physical activity than more vigorous activity (Perri et al., 2002).

Useful Psychological Frameworks

Understanding complex behavior, such as physical activity behavior, is facilitated through theories and models identifying important constructs. Theories such as learning theory (Skinner, 1953), social-cognitive theory (Bandura, 1977, 1986), the Transtheoretical Model (Prochaska & DiClemente, 1983) and the relapse prevention model (Marlatt & Gordon, 1980) are especially useful because of their inclusion of both personal and environmental factors and their explicit implications for interventions (Marcus & Sallis, 1997; USDHHS, 1996). Two additional frameworks that have become more popular recently include Motivational Interviewing (Miller & Rollnick, 2002) and ecological approaches (e.g., Spence & Lee, 2003) that explicitly change the environmental factors to increase physical activity.

Learning Theory

Applications of operant learning have been widely used in physical activity interventions. Physical activity is conceived as a response that can be acquired and maintained by controlling or modifying the antecedents and consequences associated with exercise participation. "Behavior modification" is a term used to denote strategies derived from learning theory, such as stimulus control and contingency management. Stimulus control involves increasing the cues for physical activity and/or decreasing the cues that prompt sedentary behavior. Contingency management utilizes reinforcements to increase physical activity adherence and may include strategies such as contracts, incentives, lotteries, and competitions. Behavior modification strategies have been found to increase physical activity adherence 10%–75% above that found in control groups that receive no treatment (e.g., Marcus et al., 2006). Overall, reviews of behavior modification strategies support their effectiveness in improving adherence; however, the particular strategy utilized does not appear important (e.g., Marcus et al., 2000).

Social-Cognitive Theory

Social-Cognitive Theory (SCT) (Bandura, 1977, 1986) focuses on the importance of the interaction between the person and her environment and stresses an individual's ability to control her behavior. Self-efficacy is a central concept within social-cognitive theory (Bandura, 1977, 1986) and involves individuals' degree of confidence that they can perform a particular behavior. Self-efficacy is one of the most frequently identified psychosocial determinants of adherence to physical activity among adults, and numerous studies demonstrate that high levels of self-efficacy prospectively predict physical activity behavior (e.g., Petosa, Suminski, & Hortz, 2003). In addition, recent exercise intervention studies have shown that increases in exercise self-efficacy mediate not only exercise behavior (Lubans & Sylva, 2006) but also health-related quality-of-life benefits (Anderson, King, Stewart, Camacho, & Rejeski, 2005). Another major component of SCT, self-regulation, includes many behavior modification strategies such as goal setting, planning, and self-monitoring and is frequently applied in exercise interventions (e.g., Hortz & Petosa, 2006).

Transtheoretical Model

The Transtheoretical or stage-of-change model integrates a person's current behavior with his intention to maintain or change this pattern of behavior (Prochaska & DiClemente, 1983). According to the model, individuals progress through a series of stages of readiness for change. As applied to physical activity, precontemplation includes individuals who do not participate in physical activity and do not intend to start. People in the contemplation stage do not participate in physical activity but intend to start. Those in preparation participate in some physical activity, but not regularly. The action stage includes individuals who currently participate in regular activity but have done so for less than six months, and the maintenance stage includes those who have been regularly active for 6 or more months (Marcus & Forsyth, 2003). Interventions based on the Transtheoretical Model utilize the concept of tailoring treatment to the individual's stage of readiness for change (e.g., Marcus et al., 2007b). A recent review concluded that stage-matched physical activity interventions appear effective at improving short- but not long-term physical activity adherence (Adams & White, 2003). However, more recently published studies show efficacy through 1 year (Marcus et al., 2007a; Marcus et al., 2007b). Additional research is needed, however, to determine how best to maintain physical activity among different populations.

Relapse Prevention

The relapse-prevention model (RPM) posits that maintenance of a new behavior is influenced by an individual's ability to cognitively and behaviorally cope with relapses to the undesirable behavior (Marlatt & Gordon, 1980). One concept from the RPM, the abstinence violation effect (AVE), applies to a broad range of behaviors and is a maladaptive belief that, once the abstinence rule has been broken, total relapse is inevitable. One goal of the model is to teach individuals to distinguish a lapse from a relapse in order to prevent a lapse from physical activity (e.g., missing a physical activity session) from escalating into a complete relapse (e.g., return to a sedentary lifestyle). The individual is encouraged to identify situations that are likely to lead to a lapse and then receives training in appropriate cognitive and behavioral skills to cope with the lapse. Data suggest that physical activity relapsers have fewer strategies for coping with high-risk situations than do physical activity maintainers (Simkin & Gross, 1994) and that relapse-prevention strategies are effective for increasing adherence to a physical activity program (Belisle, Roskies, & Levesque, 1987).

Motivational Interviewing

Motivational Interviewing (MI) is a client-centered approach to bringing about behavior change. According to Miller and Rollnick (2002), four general principles underlie this approach: expressing empathy, developing discrepancy, rolling with resistance, and supporting self-efficacy (for more information on this theory see chapter 8 of this book). A recent meta-analysis of MI-controlled clinical trials found that MI approaches were equivalent to other active treatments and superior to placebo or no-treatment controls in bringing about behavior change with regard to substance use and improvements in diet and exercise

(Burke, Arkowitz, & Menchola, 2003). More recently, Resnicow and colleagues found that MI did not add to the effectiveness of culturally tailored self-help materials designed to increase physical activity (Resnicow et al., 2005). Given the demonstrated effectiveness of MI for other behaviors and its initial promise with physical activity, more research is needed to determine the true value of MI for increasing physical activity.

Ecological Models

Ecological or social-ecological models add to social cognitive theory by recognizing that environments directly influence physical activity by promoting certain behaviors (e.g., commuting to work on bike paths) and restricting other behaviors (e.g., a lack of sidewalks discourages walking). Sallis and Owen (1996) define "ecological" activities as transactions between people and their physical and sociocultural environments. Ecological models take account of intra-individual factors such as physiology, self-efficacy, and attitudes, as well as extra-individual influences such as community, policy, and culture (McLeroy, Bibeau, Steckler, & Glanz, 1988). Ecological models conceive of these influences as interdependent and as exerting direct effects on each other (Kelly, 1990). A key feature of the ecological models is the belief that multiple levels of influence determine individual behavior. Thus, the most effective means of increasing physical activity would be to intervene on both the intra-individual and the extra-individual levels. Sallis and colleagues (2006) propose that the most powerful ecological interventions would include the provision of safe and attractive places to exercise, the introduction of strategies to increase motivation and self-efficacy, and the use of the mass media to bring about change in social norms for exercising. Because of its specification of numerous determinants of behavior, the ecological model provides a useful framework for understanding barriers to physical activity (e.g., Fleury & Lee, 2006).

Group-Based Interventions

Historically, physical activity adherence research focused on the identification of individual factors that were predictive of activity level (King, 1994). However, in light of the prevalence of a sedentary lifestyle and the time and effort required to deliver individualized treatments, more effective strategies need to be identified that can be applied at a group level. Some group interventions have merely tried to apply techniques obtained from research on individual behavior to a group setting. However, group interventions can differ from individual treatment on a number of dimensions. Group interventions can focus on social support, peer groups, or observational learning.

For example, Project Active was a randomized clinical trial comparing the efficacy of lifestyle and traditional structured group programs among 235 healthy, sedentary adults (Dunn et al., 1999). Participants received 6 months of intensive intervention based on Social-Cognitive Theory and the Transtheoretical Model. The structured group received an exercise prescription (50%–85% of maximal aerobic power for 20–60 minutes) and attended three exercise sessions per week with the goal of gradually increasing to five sessions. The lifestyle group received exercise prescriptions emphasizing 30 minutes of moderate lifestyle activity on most (preferably all) days of the week, along with monthly stage-matched manuals and weekly homework assignments for behavioral skill building and problem solving. In addition, small groups on cognitive and behavioral strategies were held weekly for 16 weeks and then biweekly through month 6. After 6 months, an 18-month maintenance intervention began, which involved regular meetings, monthly activities calendars, and quarterly newsletters. Results show that both the lifestyle and the structured exercise group programs produced significant (and equivalent) increases in physical activity and cardiorespiratory fitness from baseline to 24 months, along with reductions in blood pressure and individuals' percentage of body fat. Thus, the results from Project Active support the efficacy of structured group-based interventions for increasing physical activity.

However, group-based programs can be costly, and researchers have now begun to reexamine lower-cost strategies to enhance the adoption and maintenance of physical activity. As such, the future of studies utilizing a group-based design for physical activity adherence research will require researchers to weigh the costs and benefits of using this particular strategy in comparison to other designs. It may be that healthy individuals can be appropriately treated with lower-cost interventions, such as printed materials, phone calls, and computerized prompts. Newer studies will ultimately determine how the results from group-based interventions can most effectively be applied or generalized to a larger audience.

Public Health Approaches to Physical Activity Promotion

Individual and small-group approaches to enhancing adherence to physical activity have met with some success. However, these approaches, while important, are unlikely to make a significant impact on the achievement of the national physical activity goals outlined in *Healthy People 2010* (USDHHS, 2000). A primary goal of these objectives is to increase the proportion of adults who engage in regular moderate or vigorous intensity physical activity. Individual and small-group approaches reach only a small segment of the population, particularly those who may be self-selected and somewhat motivated to change their behavior. Therefore, higher-level and more macro-level approaches may be needed to achieve these goals. Public health interventions extend their reach to the 20%–30% of the population who are most sedentary and are at greatest risk for diseases preventable by increases in physical activity. These more macro approaches utilize worksites, primary care settings, and communities as both the target of intervention and the unit of analysis and aim for environmental, organizational, and policy changes. Thus, public health approaches widen the scope of intervention delivery by proactively targeting at-risk groups, often through preexisting channels. In the following section, we discuss the role of public health interventions in enhancing adherence to physical activity in whole communities and in special subgroups within communities, such as in the home, at worksites, and in physician's offices. We also discuss the policy and environmental changes that can facilitate the adoption and maintenance of the behavior change.

Provider-Delivered Interventions

Physicians play an important role in the promotion of healthy lifestyle behaviors such as physical activity. The U.S. Preventive Services Task Force has recommended that physicians counsel all patients to engage in a program of regular physical activity (Task Force on Community Prevention Services, 2002). The Task Force noted that there remains uncertainty about the effectiveness of provider-delivered physical activity counseling since most studies have tested brief, minimal, and low-intensity interventions, such as three- to five-minute counseling sessions in the context of a routine clinical visit. However, multicomponent interventions that combine provider advice with behavioral interventions appear promising. Such interventions often include patient goal setting, written exercise prescriptions, individually tailored physical activity regimens, and mailed or telephone follow-up assistance. Linking primary care patients with community-based fitness programs may enhance the effectiveness of primary care clinician counseling.

Although physicians are likely to have a positive effect on patients' level of activity, the rate of physical activity counseling by physicians is generally low (Rogers et al., 2006). For example, in one study, only 34% of physicians surveyed reported that they usually counsel on physical activity during a preventive checkup (Wee, McCarthy, Davis, & Phillips, 1999.) However, there is growing evidence suggesting that physician-delivered counseling can change patients' activity levels. A review of studies in which physical activity counseling in family practice was evaluated among adults (Petrella & Lattanzio, 2002) concluded that exercise prescriptions in family practice can help patients initiate physical activity. Positive results also have been obtained in other studies.

For example, a recent 5-year, multicenter trial, the Activity Counseling Trial (ACT), showed that the addition of a 30-minute counseling session ("Assistance") and counseling plus telephone follow-up ("Counseling") did better than physician advice alone (Anderson et al., 2005). At the 24-month follow-up, fitness test results were significantly higher in the Assistance and Counseling groups than in the Advice group. Overall, both the Assistance and Counseling treatment approaches were equally effective, although the Assistance approach appeared more effective for men and the Counseling approach seemed more effective for women.

In summary, the efficacy of brief physician-delivered counseling interventions enhanced by interventions delivered by nonphysician interventionists in physical activity hold great promise from a public health perspective. Trials examining the minimal and optimal doses of physician and other allied health professionals' time that produce the desired behavior change in patients are extremely important at this time.

Home-Based Interventions

A large number of home-based physical activity interventions have been conducted, and many have been done with specialized populations, such as older adults or those with known disease. Describing the various types of interventions utilized and the populations targeted is beyond the scope of this chapter, however. We therefore focus on two very recent home-based interventions that were done with a broad reach, utilizing mail and Internet-based interventions, and an apparently healthy population.

Recently, investigators tested the efficacy of a 1-year home-based individually tailored intervention using print and phone delivery channels and compared these to a contact control condition. At 6 months, results showed that the groups that received the print and the phone interventions showed significantly greater increases in number of weekly minutes of at least moderate intensity exercise than did the controls (Marcus et al., 2007a, 2007b). However, at 12 months, participants in the print condition continued to increase their exercise relative to those in the control group, while participants in the phone condition decreased to a level of exercise that was not significantly different from that of the control group. The print intervention was also shown to be more cost-effective than the phone intervention (Sevick et al., 2007).

The study just cited is an example of the recent advances in computer technology that have enabled health care delivery services to provide low-cost, yet highly individualized interventions. Computer "expert systems" have been developed to deliver professional-level counseling and interventions for the adoption of physical activity (e.g., Marcus et al., 2007a). An expert system is a computer program that mimics the reasoning or advice-giving capabilities of a human expert (Negotia, 1985). These systems can be used to supplement behavioral treatments and can enhance interventions delivered to the home. Expert systems can provide inexpensive, tailored interventions and are capable of modifying their intervention to match the needs and interests of the user (Slack, Safran, Kowaloff, Pearce, & Delbanco, 1995).

For example, a recent study randomized 249 sedentary adults to one of three physical activity interventions: (1) Internet intervention motivationally tailored to the individual (Tailored Internet); (2) print intervention motivationally tailored to the individual (Tailored Print; shown to be effective previously); and (3) six researcher-selected Web sites currently available to the public (Standard Internet). Results indicated that there were no significant differences among the three arms; however, all three arms significantly increased from baseline to 6 months and from baseline to 12 months (Marcus et al., 2007). Since the result for the group reached via the Internet was not different from that for the group reached via the print-based intervention, it appears that Internet-delivered physical activity interventions may provide a way to reach a larger proportion of sedentary adults in a more cost-effective way.

In sum, the utilization of computerized tailored reports that can be delivered to the home via the mail or the Internet has become an exciting new and important area for physical activity promotion and adoption (e.g., Marcus et al., 2007). With the increased number of home computers and the spread of Internet use in this country, home-based designs will likely continue to provide researchers with multiple opportunities to deliver effective physical activity interventions in the future.

Worksite-Based Interventions

One approach to increasing participation in physical activity has been to provide programs at the worksite. Worksites offer an accessible and often diverse population base, convenience, potential avenues for group support, and existing communication and health care delivery channels (Bull, Gillette, & Glasgow, 2003). Companies that sponsor these programs often hope to reduce costs to their business, such as those associated with absenteeism, sick leave, and low productivity levels (Marshall, 2004).

Although some worksite-based physical activity programs have been successful in increasing rates of physical-activity participation among employees (Proper, Hildebrandt, Van der Beek, Twisk, & Van Mechelen, 2003), many programs offering onsite fitness facilities or referrals to worksite fitness programs have showed little efficacy and were attended mostly by those who were either already exercising or highly motivated to do so (Marshall, 2004). Across a number of studies, higher socioeconomic status, based on level of education and income level and type of job (white-collar), is positively associated with participation in leisure-time physical activity (Seefeldt, Malina, & Clark, 2002). For instance, a recent review described the imbalances that exist among worksite wellness programs, with white-collar employees tending to utilize these programs more frequently than blue-collar employees (Thompson, Smith, & Bybee, 2005) and men tending to utilize worksite programs more frequently than women (Dishman, Oldenburg, O'Neal, & Shephard, 1998). However, worksite physical activity programs that have specifically targeted traditionally hard-to-reach blue-collar workers have shown improvements in the targeted group's participation in physical activity (Campbell et al., 2002). For example, a New Zealand study of low-income, blue-collar men found that after, attending a 30-minute worksite workshop once a month for 6 months, the men showed a significant increase in physical activity behavior at 12 months and when compared to a control group (Cook, Simmons, Swinburn, & Stewart, 2001). Thus, future worksite physical activity interventions may be more successful if they are tailored to meet the specific needs of the employees (e.g., Griffin-Blake & DeJoy, 2006).

In conclusion, worksite health promotion and physical activity campaigns have been somewhat successful in promoting physical activity adoption among employees. However, additional work is needed to determine the most effective methods for increasing physical activity among employees. The future of effective worksite interventions will require innovative programs that can reach the largest number of employees. Thus far, the majority of studies in these settings have enrolled self-selected samples of people who volunteer to participate in a physical activity program. This does not reach the majority of individuals who are sedentary, and would stand to benefit most from these interventions. Finally, there is currently a lack of evidence regarding the impact of increased physical activity on absenteeism, job stress, turnover rates, productivity levels, and job satisfaction (Marshall, 2004), and future research is needed to assess these and other outcomes that are hypothesized to occur with physical activity worksite interventions.

Randomized Community Trials

Few large-scale national trials have focused exclusively on the promotion of physical activity. Rather, physical activity promotion has often been embedded within larger multiple risk-factor interventions. For example, previous community-based research such as the Stanford Five-City Multiple

Risk Reduction Project sought to reduce cardiovascular disease risk factors through community organizations. Residents in the treatment cities were encouraged to build physical activity into their daily routines (e.g., walk to the store, take stairs), to increase participation in recreational activities, and to enroll in exercise classes. Overall mortality and cardiovascular disease risk were significantly reduced in intervention communities (Farquhar et al., 1990); however, changes in knowledge, attitudes, and behavior regarding physical activity were only modest. While these results were encouraging at the time, research like this ultimately fell short of achieving national goals for levels of physical activity. One possible explanation may be that previous community-based studies utilized broad approaches and took little account of differences among individual segments of the population. For instance, it may be necessary to penetrate the population at a variety of different levels vertically (from micro-level face-to-face interventions to the macro level of mass-media interventions), as well as horizontally (using sociodemographic, psychosocial, and biobehavioral parameters).

More recent research addresses some of these issues. For example, Active for Life (Wilcox et al., 2006), an ongoing physical activity intervention, has been developed in order to determine whether previously established evidence-based physical activity programs can be successfully and effectively translated into a community setting. One of the primary goals of the program is to determine the impact these interventions have on specific quality-of-life outcomes related to physical activity. Currently, the first-year results are promising, with statistically significant increases in moderate-to-vigorous physical activity and total physical activity, decreases in depressive symptoms and stress, increases in satisfaction with body appearance and function, and decreases in body mass index (Wilcox et al., 2006).

As such, it appears that effective community-level physical activity campaigns may need to first utilize evidenced-based, theoretically grounded programs previously established as efficacious. Second, they may need to account for individual differences in sociodemographic and psychosocial variables. Third, they may need to segment populations according to these differences, and, fourth and finally, develop interventions that target these specific subgroups and accelerate the acceptance of behavior change.

Ecological Interventions

Recent reviews of ecological interventions (e.g., Badland & Schofield, 2005; Foster & Hillsdon, 2004) have found evidence to support a relationship between the physical environment and physical activity. For example, researchers have consistently found neighborhood design and recreational environment (i.e., quality of sidewalks, walking/cycling facilities) to be significantly associated with participation in moderate and vigorous physical activity (De Bourdeadhuij, Sallis, & Saelens, 2003). Other studies have focused on changing the environment in order to bring about a change in physical activity behavior. For instance, Peel and Booth (2001) assessed physical changes to the work environment (e.g., the installation of weight training equipment and treadmills) in the Royal Australian Air Force (RAAF). The authors found that the proportion of RAAF participants reporting regular vigorous physical activity increased from 46% to 55% over a 6-year period, which was significantly greater than increases found in the control sample, whose activity increased from 44% to 48%.

Numerous other studies have examined the use of health education posters to increase physical activity (i.e., to prompt stair use; Boutelle, Jeffery, Murray, & Schmitz, 2001; Titze, Martin, Seiler, & Marti, 2001). While the settings (e.g., public transportation, commercial, worksite, and university) of these studies and the messages included on the posters varied widely, most of these interventions produced a short-term improvement in stair use that was maintained for up to 3 months, with one study demonstrating an effect lasting up to 6 months. Visible and cheerful reminder signs have also been used to promote the use of sidewalks and walking paths. For instance, Rhode Island is the first state in the United States to introduce the Paths to Health program. Paths to Health have already been established in 11 Rhode Island communities. The paths are generally in downtown areas near attractive historic sites, parks, or schools. A recent study (Napolitano, Lerch, Papandonatos, & Marcus, 2006) examined the impact of a 1-month promotional campaign on the use of paths in Providence, Rhode Island. The promotional materials included flyers, e-mail, Web site postings, and informational booths. Observations of path use revealed that the number of walkers tripled from baseline to postcampaign.

In a general review of the effectiveness of physical activity interventions, Kahn and colleagues (2002) located 10 studies involving ecological approaches to promoting physical activity, such as creating walking trails, building exercise facilities, or providing access to existing nearby facilities. These studies also typically offered training on how to use equipment, health behavior education, risk-factor screening, and referrals to physicians, fitness programs, and support systems. These studies suggest that ecological interventions produce a median 25% increase in the proportion of people who exercise at least three times per week. Thus, the Task Force on Community Prevention Services (2002) described the evidence in support of their effectiveness in increasing activity levels as "strong."

In sum, ecological interventions show promise as a public health intervention for promoting physical activity, but there have been few published studies in this area. Most of the research currently available is cross-sectional in design. Future researchers should consider prospective studies in settings other than the military and address methodological flaws (i.e., quasi-experimental design) common to this literature.

Targeting Underserved Populations

The term "underserved populations" typically refers to individuals with low incomes and/or minority racial or ethnic status. Despite their increased risk for sedentary behavior, there has been little physical activity research conducted among such groups. Early intervention studies in this area often lacked a theoretical background and were plagued with methodological flaws. However, recent studies with more rigorous designs have shown promising results among underserved populations.

For example, the Increasing Motivation for Physical ACTivity (IMPACT) Project (Albright et al., 2005) was designed to promote physical activity among low-income (73% had yearly incomes <$20,000) healthy Latinas in vocational training programs. The study began with eight weekly behavioral skills classes, which were run by Latina health educators and focused on local parks and community events and discussed barriers common to Latinas, such as family responsibilities. Participants were randomly assigned to receive stage-matched phone and mail counseling or standardized mail support materials. The phone and mail counseling group reported significantly greater increases in estimated total energy expenditure than did the mail support group at 10 months.

Another study, "Moms on the Move," also utilized a combination of provider and home-based approaches among low-income mothers enrolled in the Women, Infants, and Children (WIC) program. The intervention group received Transtheoretical Model (TTM)–based provider counseling supplemented by an interactive brochure and four telephone follow-ups over 8 weeks (Fahrenwald, Atwood, Walker, Johnson, & Berg, 2004). Two weeks after completing the program, the intervention group reported significantly greater increases in physical activity than the attention control group.

While results from these two studies support the use of combined (home and provider based) approaches among underserved populations, interventions have also been delivered entirely through mediated approaches (i.e., mail, telephone, Internet). Results from two studies suggest that theory-based (TTM) print materials produced short-term increases in physical activity among a sample of predominantly African American healthy female clerical staff (Cardinal & Sachs, 1996) and low-income primary care patients with high rates of chronic illnesses (Whitehead, Bodenlos, Cowles, Jones, & Brantley, 2007). However, rates of attrition were high and gains had attenuated by 6 months in one study (Whitehead et al., 2007).

Most efforts to promote physical activity among underserved populations have been combined with nutritional interventions. For example, the WISE-WOMAN projects funded by the Centers for Disease Control provide culturally and regionally appropriate cardiovascular disease prevention services based upon social cognitive and socioecological theories to low-income, multiethnic, middle-aged women with no insurance. A total of 12 state and tribal health agencies currently operate WISEWOMAN projects, and approximately 8,164 participants were screened by 2002. Available results from three studies suggest that WISEWOMAN interventions produced significant increases in activity levels (Staten et al., 2004; Stoddard, Palombo, Troped, Sorensen, & Will, 2004).

Similar multicomponent interventions have also been delivered through churches. For example, the Healthy Body Healthy Spirit Trial was delivered through African American churches in an attempt to promote physical activity, along with the consumption of fruits and vegetables (Resnicow et al., 2005). A total of 16 churches (1,056 participants) were randomly assigned to three conditions: standard education materials (exercise videos, cookbooks, pamphlets), culturally targeted self-help materials, or culturally targeted self-help materials plus four telephone calls using Motivational Interviewing techniques. At the end of 1 year, participants who received the culturally targeted self-help materials reported significantly greater increases in physical activity than the control group, but the additional telephone contacts did not enhance the impact of the intervention.

In sum, few studies have targeted or even included substantial numbers of those in underserved populations; however, the research available suggests that members of racial or ethnic minorities and low-income individuals do increase their physical activity levels in response to intervention. These groups can be hard to reach and often report more barriers to being active, such as child care problems and monetary costs. Future studies may wish to consider interventions delivered via mediated approaches, as they can be mass distributed and do not require clinic visits.

Discussion

While physical activity is positively associated with numerous physiological and psychological benefits, a large part of the population continues to be sedentary or irregularly active and therefore is at increased risk for morbidity and mortality. While research on the health benefits of physical activity was once concerned with vigorous exercise, current evidence shows that moderate intensity physical activity is also positively associated with improvements in health. The ACSM/AHA physical activity guidelines recommending moderate and/or vigorous activity are flexible, and, given that research suggests improved adherence to moderate activity, these guidelines may help to eventually increase the proportion of individuals who are regularly active.

Sedentary behavior is more characteristic of minorities, the elderly, and individuals with low levels of education and low income levels (USDHHS, 2006). Therefore, physical activity interventions need to accommodate the current needs of these individuals and address potential barriers to their participation in physical activity, recognizing that different individuals may have different needs and face different barriers to becoming physically active. For example, while certain barriers, such as time, money, and access to child care, are frequently cited by both genders (Seefeldt, Malina, & Clark, 2002), these barriers tend to have a greater impact among women and low-income individuals (Bennett, Wolin, Puleo, & Emmons, 2006; Weiss, O'Loughlin, Platt, & Paradis, 2007). Programs should be designed with these potential barriers in mind.

Worksite-based physical activity programs have the potential to reduce several common barriers to physical activity participation, such as inconvenience of facilities, financial costs, and both work and child care schedules. In addition, the most frequently cited barriers to participation, time and accessibility (Seefeldt, Malina, & Clark, 2002), may be most readily addressed by providing interventions in the workplace.

The issue of physical activity adherence, independent of initiation, has gained attention in large-scale community and public health studies. However, public health interventions need to deliver interventions at all levels of analysis (from micro individual to macro policy changes), while accounting for psychosocial and demographic factors within each level of analysis. In this way, matching treatments to specific patients does not have to lie exclusively within the realm of clinic-based programs.

In conclusion, research on physical activity interventions highlights the importance of increasing our understanding of the factors related to physical activity adherence so that more effective interventions can be developed. Research on behavior change has identified the importance of individual factors, and there is an increased interest in the environmental and policy factors. The Transtheoretical Model and Social-Cognitive Theory are particularly useful in matching treatments to individuals, as they provide a framework for tailoring interventions to the motivation level of the individual, as well as addressing the environmental and policy factors that may contribute to physical activity adherence.

References

Adams, J., & White, M. (2003). Are activity promotion interventions based on the transtheoretical model effective? A critical review. *British Journal of Sports Medicine, 37,* 106–114.

Albright, C. L., Pruitt, L., Castro, C., Gonzalez, A., Woo, S., & King, A. C. (2005). Modifying physical activity in a multiethnic sample of low-income women: One-year results from the IMPACT (Increasing Motivation for Physical ACTivity) Project. *Annals of Behavioral Medicine, 30*(3), 191–200.

American College of Sports Medicine. (2000). *ACSM's guidelines for exercise testing and prescription* (6th ed.). Philadelphia: Lippincott Williams & Wilkins.

Anderson, R. T., King, A., Stewart, A. L., Camacho, F., & Rejeski W. J. (2005). Physical activity counseling in primary care and patient well-being: Do patients benefit? *Annals of Behavioral Medicine, 30*(2), 146–154.

Badland, H. M., & Schofield, G. M. (2005). Posters in a sample of professional worksites have no effect on objectively measured physical activity. *Health Promotion Journal of Australia, 16*(1), 78–81.

Bandura, A. (1977). Self-efficacy: Toward a unifying theory of behavioral change. *Psychological Review, 84*(2), 191–215.

Bandura, A. (1986). *Social foundations of thought and action: A social cognitive theory.* Englewood Cliffs, NJ: Prentice-Hall.

Belisle, M., Roskies, E., & Levesque, J. M. (1987). Improving adherence to physical activity. *Health Psychology, 6*(2), 159–172.

Bennett, G. G., Wolin, K. Y., Puleo, E., & Emmons, K. M. (2006). Pedometer-determined physical activity among multiethnic low-income housing residents. *Medicine Science in Sports and Exercise, 38*(4), 768–773.

Boutelle, K. N., Jeffery, R. W., Murray, D. M., & Schmitz, K. H. (2001). Using signs, artwork and music to promote stair use in a public building. *American Journal of Public Health, 91,* 2004–2006.

Bull, S. S, Gillette, C., & Glasgow, R. E. (2003). Work site health promotion research: To what extent can we generalize the results and what is needed to translate research to practice? *Health Education & Behavior, 30*(5), 537–549.

Burke, B. L., Arkowitz, H., & Menchola, M. (2003). The efficacy of motivational interviewing: A meta-analysis of controlled clinical trials. *Journal of Consulting and Clinical Psychology, 71*(5), 843–861.

Campbell, M. K., Tessaro, I., DeVellis, B., Benedict, S., Kelsey, K., Belton, L., & Sanhueza, A. (2002). Effects of a tailored health promotion program for female blue-collar workers: Health works for women. *Preventive Medicine, 34,* 313–323.

Cardinal, B. J., & Sachs, M. (1996). Effects of mail-mediated, stage-matched exercise behavior change strategies on female adults' leisure-time exercise behavior. *Journal of Sports Medicine and Physical Fitness, 36*(2), 100–107.

Castro, C. M., & King, A. C. (2002). Telephone-assisted counseling for physical activity. *Exercise and Sport Science Reviews, 30*(2), 64–68.

Cook, C., Simmons, G., Swinburn, B., & Stewart, J. (2001). Changing risk behaviours for noncommunicable disease in New Zealand working men—is workplace intervention effective? *New Zealand Medical Journal, 114,* 175–178.

De Bourdeaudhuij, I., Sallis, J. F., & Saelens, B. E. (2003). Environmental correlates of physical activity in a sample of Belgian adults. *American Journal of Health Promotion, 18*(1), 83–92.

Dishman, R. K, Oldenburg, B., O'Neal, H., & Shephard, R. J. (1998). Worksite physical activity interventions. *American Journal of Preventive Medicine, 15,* 344–361.

Dubbert, P. M., Rappaport, N. B., & Martin, J. E. (1987). Exercise in cardiovascular disease. *Behavior Modification, 11*(3), 329–347.

Dunn, A. L., Marcus, B. H., Kampert, J. B., Garcia, M. E., Kohl, H. W., III, & Blair, S. N. (1999). Comparison of lifestyle and structured interventions to increase physical activity and cardiorespiratory fitness: A randomized trial. *Journal of the American Medical Association, 281,* 327–334.

Fahrenwald, N. L., Atwood, J. R., Walker, S. N., Johnson, D. R., & Berg, K. (2004). A randomized pilot test of "Moms on the Move": A physical activity intervention for WIC mothers. *Annals of Behavioral Medicine, 27,* 82–90.

Farquhar, J. W., Fortmann, S. P., Flora, J. A., Taylor, C. B., Haskell, W. L., Williams, P. T., et al. (1990). Effects of communitywide education on cardiovascular disease risk factors. The Stanford Five-City Project. *Journal of the American Medical Association, 264*(3), 359–365.

Fleury, J., & Lee, S. M. (2006). The social ecological model and physical activity in African American women. *American Journal of Community Psychology, 37,* 129–140.

Foster, C., & Hillsdon, M. (2004). Changing the environment to promote health enhancing physical activity. *Journal of Sports Sciences, 22,* 755–769.

Griffin-Blake, C. S., & DeJoy, D. M. (2006). Evaluation of social-cognitive versus stage-matched, self-help physical activity interventions at the workplace. *American Journal of Health Promotion, 20,* 200–209.

Haskell, W. L., Lee, I. M., Pate, R. R., Powell, K. E., Blair, S. N., Franklin, B. A., et al. (2007). Physical activity and public health: Updated recommendation for adults from the American College of Sports Medicine and the American Heart Association. *Medicine and Science in Sports and Exercise, 39*(8), 1423–1434.

Hillsdon, M., Foster, C., & Thorogood, M. (2005). Interventions for promoting physical activity. *Cochrane Database of Systematic Reviews, 25*(1), CD003180. Review.

Hortz, B., & Petosa, R. (2006). Impact of the "Planning to be Active" leisure time physical exercise program on rural high school students. *Journal of Adolescent Health, 39,* 530–535.

Kahn, E. B., Ramsey, L. T., Brownson, R. C., Heath, G. W., Howze, E. H., Powell, K. E., et al. (2002). The effectiveness of interventions to increase physical activity: A systematic review. *American Journal of Preventive Medicine, 22*(4S), 73–107.

Kelly, J. G. (1990). Changing contexts and the field of community psychology. *American Journal of Community Psychology, 18,* 769–792.

King, A. C. (1994). Clinical and community interventions to promote and support physical activity participation. In R. Dishman (Ed.), *Advances in exercise adherence* (pp. 183–212). Champaign, IL: Human Kinetics.

Lubans, D., & Sylva, K. (2006). Controlled evaluation of a physical activity intervention for senior school students: Effects of the Lifetime Activity Program. *Journal of Sport & Exercise Psychology, 28*(3), 252–268.

Marcus, B. H., Dubbert, P. M., Forsyth, L. H., McKenzie, T. L., Stone, E. J., Dunn, A. L., et al. (2000). Physical activity behavior change: Issues in adoption and maintenance. *Health Psychology, 19,* 32–41.

Marcus, B. H., & Forsyth, L. A. (2003). *Motivating people to be physically active.* Champaign, IL: Human Kinetics.

Marcus, B. H., Lewis, B. A., Williams, D. M., Dunsiger, S., Jakicic, J. M., Whiteley, J. A., et al. (2007). A comparison of Internet and print-based physical activity interventions. *Archives of Internal Medicine, 167*(9), 944–949.

Marcus, B. H., Napolitano, M. A., King, A. C., Lewis, B. A., Whiteley, J. A., Albrecht, A., et al. (2007a). Examination of print and telephone channels for physical activity promotion: Rationale, design, and baseline data from Project STRIDE. *Contemporary Clinical Trials, 28,* 90–104.

Marcus, B. H., Lewis B. A., Williams, D. M., Whiteley, J. A., Albrecht, A. E., Jakicic, J. M., et al. (2007b). Telephone versus print delivery of an individualized motivationally tailored physical activity intervention: Project STRIDE. *Health Psychology, 26*(4), 401–409.

Marcus, B. H., & Sallis, J. F. (1997). Determinants of physical activity behavior and implication for intervention. In A. S. Lean (Ed.), *Physical activity and cardiovascular health* (pp. 192–201). Champaign, IL: Human Kinetics.

Marcus, B. H., Williams, D. M., Dubbert, P. M., Sallis, J. F., King, A. C., Yancey, A. K., et al. (2006). Physical activity intervention studies: What we know and what we need to know: A scientific statement from the American Heart Association Council on Nutrition, Physical Activity, and Metabolism (Subcommittee on Physical Activity); Council on Cardiovascular Disease in the Young; and the Interdisciplinary Working Group on Quality of Care and Outcomes Research. *Circulation, 114* (24), 2739–2752.

Marlatt, G. A., & Gordon, J. R. (1980). Determinants of relapse: Implications for the maintenance of behavior change. In P. O. Davidson (Ed.), *Behavioral medicine: Changing health lifestyles* (pp. 410–452). Elmsford, NY: Pergamon.

Marshall, A. L. (2004). Challenges and opportunities for promoting physical activity in the workplace. *Journal of Science and Medicine in Sport, 7*(1 Suppl.), 60–66.

McLeroy, K. R., Bibeau, D., Steckler, A., & Glanz, K. (1988). An ecological perspective on health promotion programs. *Health Education Quarterly, 15,* 351–377.

Miller, W. R., & Rollnick, S. (2002). *Motivational interviewing: Preparing people for change* (2nd ed.). New York: Guilford Press.

Napolitano, M. A., Lerch, H. L., Papandonatos, G., & Marcus, B. H. (2006). Worksite and communications-based promotion of a local walking path. *Journal of Community Health, 31*(4), 326–342.

Negotia, U. N. (1985). *Expert systems and fuzzy systems.* Menlo Park, CA: Benjamin/Cummings.

Peel, G. R., & Booth, M. L. (2001). Impact evaluation of the Royal Australian Air Force health promotion program. *Aviation, Space and Environmental Medicine, 72,* 44–51.

Perri, M. G., Anton, S. D., Durning, P. E., Ketterson, T. U., Sydeman, S. J., Berlant, N. E., et al. (2002). Adherence to exercise prescriptions: Effects of prescribing moderate versus higher levels of intensity and frequency. *Health Psychology, 21*(5), 452–458.

Petosa, R. L., Suminski, R., & Hortz, B. (2003). Predicting vigorous physical activity using social cognitive theory. *American Journal of Health Behavior, 27,* 301–310.

Petrella, R. J, & Lattanzio, C. N. (2002). Does counseling help patients get active? Systematic review of the literature. *Canadian Family Physician, 48,* 72–80.

Prochaska, J. O., & DiClemente, C. C. (1983). Stages and processes of self-change of smoking: Toward an integrative model of change. *Journal of Consulting and Clinical Psychology, 51*(3), 390–395.

Proper, K. I., Hildebrandt, V. H., Van der Beek, A., Twisk, J. W., & Van Mechelen, W. (2003). Effect of individual counseling on physical activity fitness and health: A randomized controlled trial in a workplace setting. *American Journal of Preventive Medicine, 24*(3), 218–226.

Resnicow, K., Jackson, A., Blissett, D., Wang, T., McCarty, F., Rahotep, S., et al. (2005). Results of the Healthy Body Healthy Spirit trial. *Health Psychology, 24*(4), 339–348.

Rodgers, W. M., & Brawley, L. R. (1993). Using both self-efficacy theory and the theory of planned behavior to discriminate adherers and dropouts from structured programs. *Journal of Applied Social Psychology, 5,* 195–206.

Rogers, L. Q., Gutin, B., Humphries, M. C., Lemmon, C. R., Waller, J. L., Baranowski, T., et al. (2006). Evaluation of internal medicine residents as exercise role models and associations with self-reported counseling behavior, confidence, and perceived success. *Teaching and Learning in Medicine, 18*(3), 215–221.

Sallis, J. F., Cervero, R. B., Ascher, W., Henderson, K. A., Kraft, M. K., & Kerr, J. (2006). An ecological approach to creating active living communities. *Annual Reviews of Public Health, 27,* 297–322. Review.

Sallis, J. F., & Owen, N. (1996). Ecological models. In K. Glanz, F. M. Lewis, & B. K. Rimer (Eds.), *Health behavior and health education: Theory, research, and practice* (2nd ed.). San Francisco: Jossey-Bass.

Schnohr, P., Lange, P., Scharling, H., & Jensen, J. S. (2006). Long-term physical activity in leisure time and mortality from coronary heart disease, stroke, respiratory diseases, and cancer. The Copenhagen City Heart Study. *European Journal of Cardiovascular Preventive Rehabilitation, 13*(2), 173–179.

Seefeldt, V., Malina, R. M., & Clark, M. A. (2002). Factors affecting levels of physical activity in adults. *Sports Medicine, 32*(3), 143–168. Review.

Sevick, M. A., Napolitano, M. A., Papandonatos, G. D., Gordon, A. J., Reiser, L. M., & Marcus, B. H. (2007). Cost-effectiveness of alternative approaches for motivating activity in sedentary adults: Results of Project STRIDE. *Preventive Medicine, 45*(1), 54–61.

Simkin, L. R., & Gross, A. M. (1994). Assessment of coping with high-risk situations for exercise relapse among healthy women. *Health Psychology, 13*(3), 274–277.

Skinner, B. F. (1953). *Science and human behavior.* New York: Macmillan.

Slack, W. V., Safran, C., Kowaloff, H. B., Pearce, J., & Delbanco, T. L. (1995). A computer-administered health screening interview for hospital personnel. *MD Computing, 12*(1), 25–30.

Spence, J. C., & Lee, R. E. (2003). Toward a comprehensive model of physical activity. *Psychology of Sport & Exercise, 4,* 7–24.

Staten, L. K., Gregory-Mercado, K.Y., Ranger-Moore, J., Will, J.C., Giuliano, A.R., & Ford, E.S. (2004). Provider counseling, health education, and community healthworkers: The Arizona WISEWOMAN project. *Journal of Women's Health, 13,* 547–556.

Stoddard, A. M., Palombo, R., Troped, P. J., Sorensen, G., & Will, J. C. (2004). Cardiovascular disease risk reduction: The Massachusetts WISEWOMAN project. *Journal of Women's Health, 13,* 539–546.

Task Force on Community Prevention Services. (2002). Recommendations to increase physical activity in communities. *American Journal of Preventive Medicine, 22,* 67–72.

Thompson, S. E., Smith, B. A., & Bybee, R. F. (2005). Factors influencing participation in worksite wellness programs among minority and underserved populations. *Family and Community Health, 28,* 267–273.

Titze, S., Martin, B. M., Seiler, R., & Marti, B. (2001). A worksite intervention module encouraging the use of stairs: Results and evaluation issues. *Social and Preventive Medicine, 46,* 13–19.

U.S. Department of Health and Human Services. (2006). *Health behaviors of adults: United States, 2002–04.* Hyattsville, MD: Centers for Disease Control and Prevention, National Center for Health Statistics. Vital Health Stat 10(230). DHHS Publication No. (PHS) 2006–1558.

U.S. Department of Health and Human Services. (2000). *Healthy People 2010: Understanding and improving health and objectives for improving health* (2nd ed., 2 *vols.*). Washington, DC: U.S. Government Printing Office.

U.S. Department of Health and Human Services. (1996). *Physical activity and health: A report of the Surgeon General.* Atlanta: Centers for Disease Control and Prevention, National Center for Chronic Disease Prevention and Health Promotion.

Wee, C. C., McCarthy, E. P., Davis, R. B., & Phillips, R. S. (1999). Physician counseling about exercise. *Journal of the American Medical Association, 282,* 1583–1588.

Weiss, D. R., O'Loughlin, J. L., Platt, R. W., & Paradis, G. (2007). Five-year predictors of physical activity decline among adults in low-income communities: A prospective study. *International Journal of Behavioral Nutrition and Physical Activity, 18*(4), 2.

Whitehead, D., Bodenlos, J. S., Cowles, M. L., Jones, G. N., & Brantley, P. J. (2007). A stage-targeted physical activity intervention among a predominantly African-American low-income primary care population. *American Journal of Health Promotion, 21*(3), 160–163.

Wilcox, S., Dowda, M., Griffin, S. F., Rheaume, C., Ory, M. G., Leviton, L., et al. (2006). Results of the first year of active for life: translation of 2 evidence-based physical activity programs for older adults into community settings. *American Journal of Public Health, 96*(7), 1201–1209.

Adoption and Maintenance of Safer Sexual Practices

13

Michelle J. Naughton
and Scott D. Rhodes

Sexual risk behavior is a leading cause of morbidity in the United States and the world. Consequences of sexual risk behavior include exposure to and transmission of sexually transmitted infections (STIs), including HIV infection. Worldwide, more than 1 million people become infected with an STI each day. In the United States, 19 million new STIs occur each year, and about half of these infections occur in people ages 15–24 years.

HIV, which has multiple modes of transmission but most often is sexually transmitted (Heymann, 2005), continues its impact, with an estimated 40 million people living with HIV/AIDS worldwide, and 4.3 million people are newly infected each year. In the United States, an estimated 1 million people are living with HIV/AIDS currently, and 40,000 new infections occur each year (Centers for Disease Control and Prevention [CDC], 2006a). Rates of HIV infection in the United States have been decreasing over the past decade, although the rate of HIV diagnosis among African Americans and Hispanics/Latinos remains disproportionately high compared to that for non-Hispanic/non-Latino Whites (CDC, 2005a). Approximately 50% of new HIV infections occur among 13–24-year-olds, usually through sexual behavior. Approximately 60% of new cases in youth occur in females, and 75% are in racial or ethnic minorities (CDC, 2003; Futterman, 2005).

Unintended pregnancy is another outcome of unsafe sexual behaviors. More than one-third of all pregnancies worldwide, 80 million each year, are unintended. In the United States, approximately 95% of the 1 million pregnancies each year among U.S. teenagers are unplanned (Finer, 2007; Klima, 1998). Recent changes in contraceptive and sexual behaviors have resulted in significant declines in adolescent pregnancy rates (Ventura, Abma, Mosher, & Henshaw, 2004), although it is estimated that up to one-third of teenagers experience a pregnancy by age 20 (Hillard, 2005).

Because of the profound impact of STIs, there is a need for further implementation of existing interventions to reduce sexual risk behaviors that lead to negative sexual health consequences. In addition, the further development and evaluation of innovative strategies to prevent STIs and HIV infection and re-infection among multiple populations and subgroups are needed. Barrier methods of contraception, particularly latex male condoms and polyurethane female condoms, have been shown to be effective in reducing the spread of STIs and in preventing unintended pregnancies (Anonymous, 2005; CDC, 2005b; Sheroff & Darney, 2005; Winer et al., 2006). Therefore, the majority of safer sex programs have been designed to increase condom use and to decrease high-risk sexual behaviors among persons who are sexually active. Among teenagers not yet sexually active, efforts have focused on delaying the initiation of sexual behaviors.

In this chapter, we present an overview of the epidemiology of sexual risk, its predictors, and safer sexual intervention strategies that have been used with men who have sex with men (MSM), adolescents and young adults, and women who have sex with women (WSW). We also recommend directions for future research that may be necessary to reduce the morbidity and mortality associated with STIs and HIV.

Men Who Have Sex With Men

Risk Among MSM

National and international studies have found rates of same-sex sexual behavior among men ranging from 2.7% to 9.8% (Analyse des Comportements Sexuels en France ACSF Investigators, 1992; Laumann, Gagnon, Michael, & Michaels, 1994; Rhodes, McCoy, Hergenrather, Omli, & DuRant, 2007). HIV continues to disproportionately affect gay men, with an estimated 365,000–535,000 men currently infected with HIV in the United States (Blair, Fleming, & Karon, 2002; Wolitski, Valdiserri, Denning, & Levine, 2001). A 1997 study of urban MSM found HIV prevalence of 17% overall, with the prevalence ranging from 29% among African American MSM to 40% among MSM who reported injecting drugs (Catania et al.,

2001). Although there has been a decline in the prevalence and incidence of HIV infection among MSM in the United States during the past 10–15 years, MSM still account for a significant proportion of new infections (Karon, Fleming, Steketee, & De Cock, 2001), and recent reports suggest that the rates of new HIV infections among MSM may be on the rise (CDC, 2001; Rhodes & Yee, 2006). Moreover, African American and Hispanic/Latino MSM made up 53% of all MSM diagnosed with AIDS in 1999 (CDC, 2001; Malebranche, 2003; Rhodes, Yee, & Hergenrather, 2006; Wolitski et al., 2001). HIV is important in the MSM community not only among young men but across many age groups of MSM. In a probability sample of 2,881 MSM over the age of 50 years from several urban centers in the United States (New York, Los Angeles, Chicago, and San Francisco), the prevalence of HIV observed was 19% for men in their 50s and 3% for men in their 60s (Dolcini, Catania, Stall, & Pollack, 2003).

In addition to HIV, recent trends suggest an increased incidence of gonorrhea and syphilis among MSM (CDC, 2002a; Fox et al., 2001), indicating that increased risk is eclipsing the safer sex practices promoted in the 1980s and early 1990s. Consistent condom use remains low among MSM. Studies have found use rates during anal intercourse to range from about 30% among MSM in U.S. urban centers (Koblin et al., 2006) up to 60% among a multiethnic sample of young self-identifying gay men in the rural southern United States (Rhodes et al., 2006). Condom use varies by sexual activity, too; it is much higher for anal sex than for oral sex (Hunt et al., 1993; Rhodes et al., 2006). Studies of condom use among international populations of MSM suggest even lower rates of condom use in less well-resourced communities and higher condom use in more well-resourced communities (Herbst et al., 2005).

Predictors of Risk and Condom Use

A lack of consensus about the predictors of condom use among MSM exists because of often contradictory results from various studies and the complexity of condom use behavior. Among the many variables that have been identified as predictive, consistent condom use has been found to be associated with higher levels of social support from informal sources of help, the perception that condom use is the community norm, expectations that condoms will have positive interpersonal and personal consequences, increased condom-use self-efficacy, and HIV-positive serostatus. Inconsistent condom use has been found to be associated with substance use, including use of alcohol, methamphetamines, and medications designed to treat sexual dysfunction (i.e., Viagra, Levitra, and Cialis) used recreationally to enhance sexual satisfaction; injecting-drug use; negative attitudes and expectations about condoms; sex in public venues; perceiving oneself or one's partner as "low risk," condoms as decreasing sensation, and condom use as an inconvenience and interruption of intimacy; indifference about condom use; lack of control over initiating or negotiating safer sex; commercial sex work; and meeting partners on vacation and online through the Internet (Bull, Piper, & Rietmeijer, 2002; Carballo-Dieguez & Dolezal, 1996; Koblin et al., 2006; Rhodes, 2004; Rhodes, DiClemente, Cecil, Hergenrather, & Yee, 2002; Rhodes et al., 2006; Whittier, Lawrence, & Seeley, 2005).

Although some studies indicate that alcohol use is associated with unsafe sexual behaviors (Semple, Patterson, & Grant, 2003; Stone et al., 1999;

Tawk, Simpson, & Mindel, 2004), other research has not found this association (Clutterbuck, Gorman, McMillan, Lewis, & Macintyre, 2001; Seage et al., 1998; Smith, Grierson, Pitts, & Pattison, 2006). Alcohol use may be associated with indiscriminate forms of sexual behavior or risk taking (e.g., having multiple partners or engaging in "casual" sexual intercourse) but is not negatively associated with protective behaviors such as condom use (Cooper, 2002; Rhodes et al., 2006; Vanable et al., 2004). This hypothesis, which requires further theoretical exploration and testing, suggests that the decision to engage in sexual intercourse is affected by alcohol use, but protective behaviors during sexual intercourse are not (Rhodes et al., 2006b). More research is needed to untangle the associations between substance use and risk behavior (e.g., having multiple partners) and prevention behaviors (e.g., condom use). These associations also may differ by population subgroup.

Cultural and social factors also affect condom use (Bajos, 1997; Bakeman & Peterson, 2007; Diaz, 1998; Rhodes & Yee, 2006). For example, Hispanic/Latino and African American MSM may have less social support, and therefore lower condom use, because of the stigma associated with same-sex behavior within some communities. Furthermore, sex holds different meanings. MSM who consistently have unprotected anal intercourse have been found to be less likely to approve of sex without love (Crosby, Stall, Paul, Barrett, & Midanik, 1996). Thus, for these men, sex may hold meanings associated with intimacy, trust, and commitment. Condom promotion contradicts these meanings.

Intervention Research

Because publicly funded risk reduction interventions were slow to address prevention among MSM (Miller, 1995), significant resources within the gay community enabled gay community-initiated and community-based interventions early on during the epidemic. These interventions concentrated on risk counseling with HIV testing, eroticizing safer sex among men, modeling social and behavior change through community organizing and peer leadership, and training in condom skills (Miller, 1995; Rhodes & Yee, 2006). Because of the urgency of the epidemic, little time was available for determining efficacy prior to the implementation of interventions (Valdiserri, Lyter, Leviton, Stoner, & Silvestre, 1987), and thorough evaluation of many interventions remains rare (Chesney et al., 2003; Gay and Lesbian Medical Association, 2001; Herbst et al., 2005; Rhodes, 2004; Rhodes, Hergenrather, Duncan, Ramsey, Yee, & Wilkin, 2007; Rhodes & Yee, 2006; Wolitski et al., 2001).

However, since the 1980s, much has been tried and learned about preventing HIV and STIs among MSM. Characteristics of effective interventions include the provision of facts and information to increase HIV and/or STI knowledge, as well as to change cognitive factors such as attitudes, perceptions, or beliefs of MSM about HIV, STDs, and protection (e.g., condoms). Effective interventions develop technical skills, including the correct use of condoms; personal skills, including safer sex eroticization; and interpersonal skills, including negotiating safer sex and assertiveness. Most effective interventions are delivered in small groups by trained peers or counselors during multiple sessions (Herbst et al., 2005).

Effective interventions for MSM also are based on scientifically derived theoretical models. For example, the Popular Opinion Leader (POL) intervention

(Kelly et al., 1992) is based on theories of peer influence (Hallinan, 1982), social support (House, 1981), and diffusion of innovations (Rogers, 1983). A bar-based, HIV-prevention intervention using natural helpers, POL intervention has been found to be effective in HIV risk behavior reduction, including decreasing unprotected anal intercourse among gay bar patrons (Kelly et al., 1992). As it was originally tested using the naturally occurring social network of the bar, natural helpers known as "popular opinion leaders" were selected on the basis of their popularity. They attended four weekly 90-minute sessions that led them through a process of exploring and thoroughly understanding HIV prevention, both facts and skills, and practicing effective communication and leadership strategies. The training of these popular opinion leaders covered basic epidemiology and transmission of HIV/AIDS, behavioral strategies for risk reduction, misconceptions about HIV/AIDS, characteristics of effective health promotion messages, and role plays of conversations endorsing safer sex. Community-level triggers such as posters within the bar and buttons worn by popular opinion leaders promoted the intervention and encouraged dialogue between bar patrons and opinion leaders; often, these popular opinion leaders were bartenders. Bartenders have been found to be successful as opinion leaders because they have more and less busy moments, are often casual yet well-trusted confidantes, and are "on-site" regularly.

The use of this type of a natural helper approach is especially appropriate for STI and HIV prevention because opinion leaders can reach populations not easily accessed by health professionals. For example, harnessing the Internet, Chat Room-Based Education and Referral/Men for Men (CyBER/M4M) is an ongoing intervention to increase STI and HIV knowledge and testing within local existing chat rooms designed to facilitate social and sexual networking among MSM (Rhodes et al., 2007). CyBER/M4M educators, who are trained individuals from the MSM community and are familiar with the chat room culture, participate in the development and distribution of culturally relevant chat room dialogue triggers and educational materials that use culturally relevant channels (i.e., chat rooms). They provide information and skills building around safer sex and risk reduction and affect the norms regarding sexual risk within online social networks. Implicit in this approach is the exchange of social support (Eng & Parker, 2002). From a public health perspective, the empirical associations found between social support and health (Berkman, Glass, Brissette, & Seeman, 2000; Broadhead et al., 1983; Cassel, 1976; Kaplan, Cassel, & Gore, 1977) hold substantial potential for translating the health-enhancing effects of social support into interventions (Heaney & Israel, 2002).

Adoption and adherence to safer sex behaviors among MSM, as among all populations, is complex. The diversity among MSM mirrors the expansive diversity of society as a whole. Whether exploring needs through basic behavioral and epidemiologic research or planning, offering, providing, or evaluating one-on-one counseling or support services, referrals, clinical services, or group- or community-level interventions designed to affect sexual risk behavior, it is key to move beyond assumptions about MSM men. As with any population or subgroup, a comprehensive understanding of the individual as he exists within a variety of influencing contexts is key to successful intervention. These contexts include a variety of partnerships and family systems, spatial neighborhoods and social networks, institutions (schools, workplaces, and religious organizations), racial and ethnic communities, and other influencing contexts from the larger society. These contexts have unique norms and cultures and impose expectations that create and interact with the individual's sense of self and identity. These influencing contexts vary in the messages, overtly and covertly, relayed about being MSM. These messages are internalized and affect each individual differently.

Adolescents and Young Adults

Risk Among Adolescents and Young Adults

In general, participation in sexual activity increases with age during adolescence and young adulthood. Adolescent males are likely to initiate sexual behaviors at younger ages than adolescent females, as African American males and females are more likely than Hispanic/Latino or non-Hispanic/Latino White males and females to do so (CDC, 2002b). From the 1970s until the mid-1990s, the initiation of sexual behaviors among teenagers occurred at increasingly younger ages (Forrest & Singh, 1990; Zelnick & Kantner, 1980). Between 1991 and 2003, however, the percentages of 9th-grade through 12th-grade students who had had sexual intercourse decreased from 54% to 47%, and there were corresponding decreases among African American, Hispanic/Latino, and non-Hispanic/Latino White adolescents (CDC, 2002b; Grunbaum et al., 2004). A 2003 study found that by 12th grade, 61.6% of males and females had had vaginal intercourse (Grunbaum et al., 2004). Between 1991 and 2003, the number of adolescents having had four or more sex partners in their lifetime decreased, and the number who had made use of a condom at last sexual intercourse increased (Biddlecom, 2004; CDC, 2002b; Grunbaum et al., 2004). These improvements in health outcomes are attributed to multiple efforts by parents, schools, community organizations, health care providers, religious organizations, the media, and governments agencies to reduce sexual risk among adolescents and young adults (CDC, 2005b).

Rates of participation in oral sexual activities were not assessed in adolescents and young adults until recently (Mosher, Chandra, & Jones, 2005). In 2002, cross-sectional data of males ages 15–24 years indicated that rates of participating in any oral sexual contact with a member of the opposite sex were approximately 25% at age 15, 63.5% at age 17, 74% at age 19, and 82% ages 22–24. Rates for females were comparable at 26% at age 15, 55.5% at age 17, 74% at age 19, and 85% at ages 22–24. STI prevention efforts have not always focused on safer sexual practices for those participating in oral sexual activities, either alone or in combination with other sexual behaviors, suggesting a need to enhance intervention strategies to include oral sexual acts among adolescents and young adults.

In general, those who initiate sexual intercourse at younger ages report a higher number of sexual partners in their lifetime and are at greater risk for an unintended pregnancy and/or sexually transmitted infection, largely due to higher rates of unprotected sexual encounters. Thus, safer sex interventions in adolescents and young adults are aimed primarily at delaying the initiation of sexual activity for those not yet sexually active and, among those already sexually active, reducing the incidence of STIs and unplanned pregnancies. Although the behaviors to be initiated or sustained are somewhat similar for either the prevention of STIs or pregnancy (e.g., condom use, reduction in the number of sexual partners), the focus of the interventions and the information provided vary.

Barriers to Safer Sexual Practices

Many studies have investigated barriers to condom use among adolescents and young adults. Some of the most frequently mentioned barriers are the cost of condoms; their interference with pleasure and spontaneity; embarrassment about purchasing condoms; difficulty negotiating condom use with partners; and/or lack of partner support (Crosby et al, 2004; Kline & Van Landingham, 1994; Pulerwitz, Amaro, DeJong, Gortmaker, & Rudd, 2002; Smith, 2003); alcohol and other substance use (Chesson, Harrison, & Stall, 2003; Fortenberry, 1995; Kline & Van Landingham, 1994; Santelli et al., 2004); younger age (DiClemente et al., 2003; Santelli et al., 1999); greater number of sexual partners (DiClemente et al., 2003); and low perceived need (DiClemente, Wingood, & Crosby, 2003; Wendt & Solomon, 1995). Factors not predictive of condom use consistently are fears of contracting HIV, knowledge about STIs, and a prior history of STIs (Crosby et al., 2004; Diamond & Buskin, 2000; Fortenberry, Brizendine, Katz, & Orr, 2002). Sexual coercion may also play a more significant role in younger women's sexual behavior than has been thought previously (Shrier, Pierce, Emans, & DuRant, 1998). Incidents of rape, sexual assault, and emotional coercion place women at increased risk for negative health outcomes.

Among adolescents and college students, the consistent use of condoms, although increasing, is lower than desired. Condom use also appears to be higher in casual relationships or those of shorter duration than in long-term and/or exclusive sexual relationships (Doval, Duran, O'Donnell, & O'Donnell, 1995). The movement away from consistent use of condoms in long-term relationships may reflect the progression to a more stable, exclusive status, where there is perceived trust in the partner, as well as a decision to use an unobtrusive or more effective method of contraception, such as oral contraceptives. The higher use of nonbarrier methods of contraception, particularly oral or other hormonally based contraceptives, has increased the risk of acquiring a STI among young adults who are not in exclusive sexual relationships and do not also use condoms for the prevention of disease (Wendt & Solomon, 1995). These data suggest that condoms are viewed primarily as a means of contraception, not as protection against STIs.

Despite increasing knowledge of the transmission of STIs and HIV, many individuals underestimate their vulnerability to contracting a STI. Adolescents and young adults who are just becoming sexually active are particularly likely to believe they are invincible to these risks (DiClemente et al., 2003). The need for education and intervention with adolescents and young adults is particularly crucial during this period of life as patterns of sexual behavior are tried and adopted and may frame subsequent behavior and practices during adulthood.

Intervention Research

A variety of different interventions have been used with adolescents and young adults to encourage condom use, safer sex, and effective methods of contraception for those persons who are sexually active. Strategies that have been developed include peer education programs, didactic lectures, patient education in student health or community health centers, school-based clinics, school-based classroom educational programs, brochures, increasing condom availability, skills training, and presentations by print and broadcast media.

Informational programs have been the most widely used interventions in this population, with some varying degree of success. Education alone has not always been related to behavior change without also teaching skills training and modifications in attitudes or beliefs about sexual activity and STI contractions. Skills training aimed at addressing social interactions provides young adults with methods to increase interpersonal competencies to resist coercion and peer pressure and increase skills to manage and negotiate their preferences successfully (St. Lawrence et al., 1995).

In general, providing safer sex interventions to adolescents is a socially sensitive issue. Concerns have been expressed that providing explicit information or skills training may serve to condone or promote sexual activity. Others, however, have advocated a more explicit and interactive approach because of the high rates of sexual activity among adolescents and the fact that sexual activity is rarely followed by a return to abstinence once it has been initiated (DiClemente, 1993; DiClemente et al., 2003). In addition, federal funding for educational programs has largely been restricted to abstinence-only programs in the past decade, which has limited the range of acceptable prevention strategies in school-based interventions (Landry, Darroch, Singh, & Higgins, 2003). Such programs often focus on abstinence as the best or only option for pregnancy prevention, rather than presenting abstinence as the best among multiple contraceptive choices. Focusing on the ineffectiveness of contraceptive methods, except for abstinence, and not providing students with information on how to use methods effectively may contribute to sexually active adolescents' and young adults' poor use of contraceptive methods or failure to use any at all (Bearman & Bruckner, 2001; Jemmott et al., 1998). Abstinence-focused programs are also not as effective or practical among those youth who are already sexually active, so it is necessary that a range of information be included in effective prevention materials and programs (Aten, Siegel, Enaharo, & Auinger, 2002).

Although there has been some progress in recent years in delaying the onset of sexual activity in adolescents and in increasing condom use, the prevalence of STIs and unplanned pregnancy still necessitates the development and long-term evaluation of effective prevention strategies for adolescents and young adults. These programs should be tailored to address specific needs for information about pregnancy and STI prevention, as well as to take into account the specific needs of the subgroups to be addressed (e.g., minority populations, women, poor individuals, well-educated persons). Tailoring the information to the developmental stages and transitions that occur during adolescence and young adulthood has also been identified as an important component (Pedlow & Carey, 2004). In addition, sexual behavior is a social activity, and, thus, the social context in which sexual behavior occurs and is negotiated and managed needs to be considered in effective prevention efforts.

Women Who Have Sex With Women (WSW)

Risk Among WSW

Research on STI rates and prevention strategies for women who have sex with women (WSW) and bisexual women is lacking. It is often assumed that WSW are at low risk for the contraction of STIs, which may lead to unsafe sexual practices. However, the actual lifetime rates of STIs between WSW have been found to be roughly equivalent to those of heterosexual women (10%–20%; Diamant, Lever, & Schuster, 2000; Skinner, Stokes, Kirlew, Kavanagh, & Forster, 1996).

Part of the difficulty in examining safer sexual practices among women who are not exclusively heterosexual is in how terms such as "lesbian" or "bisexual" are defined in research investigations or survey tools (McNair, 2005). In fact, in most behavioral and epidemiologic studies, including those studies that are population based, measures of sexual orientation are not included routinely (Gay and Lesbian Medical Association, 2001; Greenwood et al., 2005; Marrazzo, 2004; Rhodes & Yee, 2006; Sell & Becker, 2001). Research in this area is often based on very small sample sizes, such as convenience samples of clinic attendees or volunteers, and there is a lack of uniformity and clarity regarding women's sexual history and practices (Marrazzo, 2004).

Predictors of Risk

It has been reported that approximately 80% of women who may now engage in sexual activities exclusively with women have had sex with a man at some point in their lifetime (Diamant, Schuster, McGuigan, & Level, 1999). Thus, a women's sexual history regarding the sex of her partners can be an important determinant in establishing her lifetime STI and HIV risk.

In general, STI risk has been found to increase among WSW who have a higher number of female partners and independently among those with a higher number of male sexual partners (Diamant et al., 2000). Sexual practices involving digital-vaginal or digital-anal contact and the use of penetrative sex toys have been reported as a means for STI contraction (Bailey, Farquhar, Owen, & Whittaker, 2003; Fethers, Marks, Mindel, & Estcourt, 2000). Sexual practices that involve the transmission of cervicovaginal secretions may also be related to higher rates of bacterial vaginosis, which can be related to problems in the upper genital tract, such as pelvic inflammatory disease, as well as greater risks of acquiring other STIs, such as gonorrhea and HIV (Marrazzo, 2004; Marrazzo, Coffey, & Bingham, 2005; McNair, 2005). WSW and bisexual women have also been found to have higher rates of behavioral risk factors, such as alcohol and illicit drug use (Friedman et al., 2003; Hillier, De Visser, Kavanagh, & McNair, 2003), sexual risk tasking, sexual abuse (McNair, 2005), and lower levels of social support and self-esteem (Jordan and Deluty, 1998), all of which have been found to be negatively related to safer sexual practices. One of the more problematic factors, however, is the perception that WSW have lower rates of STIs.

This leads to an inaccurate perception that they have a low STI risk and that they therefore do not need knowledge about how to protect themselves in sexual activity with other women (Diamant et al., 2000; Morrow et al., 2000).

Intervention Research

Although it is clear that many WSW do not know how to engage in safer sex behaviors (Fishman & Anderson, 2003), at present, there is a lack of tested interventions that have been used with WSW populations to increase their knowledge of their STI risk and to teach them how to prevent risky sexual behaviors. Part of the difficulty has been the lack of knowledge about rates of STIs among exclusively female partners and how specific STIs are transmitted between women. Clinical screening guidelines for annual cervical cancer screening are meant to apply to all women, regardless of their sexual orientation, and can serve as a mechanism to detect and treat STIs among WSW (Marrazzo, 2004). The CDC has also provided brief STI/HIV prevention guidelines for WSW (CDC, 2006b). In addition, the CDC Web site regarding gay, lesbian, bisexual, and transsexual health issues is also updated on a periodic basis to provide information regarding preventive health behaviors (http://www.cdc.gov/lgbthealth). Other types of written materials are increasingly being developed for WSW (Booth, 2002), which can also serve as a guide for practicing preventive behaviors among WSW.

Information regarding effective interventions for the prevention of STIs among WSW has not been reported in the published literature to date. The development, implementation, and evaluation of interventions targeting WSW should be a priority in the coming years in order to reduce the incidence of STIs among these individuals.

Conceptual Considerations

The adoption and maintenance of safer sexual behaviors and STI prevention strategies is of critical importance. Intervention strategies must largely focus on the modification of very intimate behaviors between individuals, which in themselves are shaped by the larger interpersonal and social environment. Personal meanings attached to sex, societal norms and expectations for behavior, and attitudes strongly influence sexual behaviors and the adoption and maintenance of preventive strategies. In addition, the diverse population groups affected by unsafe sexual practices make devising effective strategies extremely challenging.

The majority of research regarding safer sex has been completed in the past several decades. Research across many subgroups is still focused on delineating predictors of safer sexual practices and developing and testing effective strategies to modify behavior. The state-of-the science has not progressed to where there are multiple, effective interventions that are being widely disseminated and used in the population.

Several cross-cutting themes exist that deserve consideration:

■ Sexual activities are often viewed as individual acts, rather than as social acts engaged in by two or more individuals. Interventions that have focused on changing the behavior of individuals without regard to the social relationship inherent in sexual behavior have been relatively ineffective. Condom use should be viewed as an attribute of a relationship, rather than as an individual attribute.

■ Sexual behavior is often viewed as monosemic. However, sexual behavior has different meanings in different contexts, and, consequently, different codes of behavior apply in different situations. Attention should be focused on the type of relationship in which sex is shared (e.g., casual or primary partner; the exchange of sex for money, shelter, food, or drugs) and the factors that promote or reduce safer sexual practices in each of these contexts.

■ Power imbalances in relationships are often ignored. Across all categories, the less powerful, whether they be uneducated, young, women, or economically or psychologically dependent on their partners, seem to be the least successful in changing their behavior. These individuals are often at a disadvantage in negotiating safer sexual practices, because they have less power and control than their partners in their sexual relationships. These observations suggest the need for intervention efforts that target the empowered partner separately from, and in equal proportion to, the disempowered partner in the relationship.

■ Social norms and gender roles strongly influence the ability to implement and maintain safer sexual practices. Beliefs about appropriate behavior for males and females are strongly ingrained across subgroups of the population and need to be considered in intervention efforts. Gender-specific interventions may be required.

■ Ethnic and cultural differences influence the adoption of safer sexual practices. Ethnicity is a category that glosses a complex set of political, economic, and social interactions. Poverty is highly correlated with ethnicity and the increased risk of disease, but cultural or ethnic differences should not be confused with differences engendered by political and economic forces. For interventions to be effective, they must incorporate ethnic values and priorities, as well as specific attitudes and behaviors toward the adoption and maintenance of safer sexual practices.

■ Results from many of the studies suggest that greater success in adopting and maintaining safer sexual behaviors is obtained when action is taken early. It may be easier and more efficient to prevent unsafe sex than it is to attempt to modify existing patterns of unsafe behavior. For instance, middle-aged women who initiated sexual activity when the primary focus was on pregnancy prevention may have used oral contraceptives primarily. These women who are now in new sexual relationships at midlife have to reorient their view of "protected" intercourse to include not only contraception but also the prevention of STIs.

Research Needs

Future research needs and priorities include the following:

■ Because researchers have relied on cross-sectional data to infer trends in sexual behaviors and success in modifying and maintaining safer sexual behaviors, more research is needed to follow cohorts of individuals in order to understand trends and evaluate the effectiveness of intervention programs over time.

- More research regarding how the dynamic environment through changing social norms, medical advances, and technology, affect risk is needed. For instance, AIDS fatigue, methamphetamine use, medications used for sexual dysfunction and sexual satisfaction enhancement (i.e., Viagra, Levitra, and Cialis), barebacking, migration and immigration trends, and the Internet contribute to risk among various populations and subgroups in profound ways. Furthermore, emerging technologies such as microbicides hold promise and further challenges for pregnancy and disease prevention.
- A thorough understanding and a comprehensive operationalization of masculinity are absent from much of the sexual health literature. Research utilizing constructs and measures that assess endorsement of beliefs and values about manhood are needed to test and build models that embed masculinity within a risk-reduction framework.
- With the increase in oral sexual behaviors among adolescents and young adults, intervention strategies may need to be broadened and re-evaluated among heterosexual populations to include more specific information about sexual risks associated with these types of sexual activities.
- Research that is authentic and explores the health and sexual well-being of women who have sex with women (WSW) is needed. WSW may in fact be one of the most understudied groups in the STI and HIV literature.
- Studies of the sexual practices and intervention needs for middle-aged and older adults are necessary in order to reduce the sexual risk of these persons, who are often neglected in STI prevention efforts.
- Studies focused on identifying effective strategies to change the negative attitudes toward condoms, particularly among males, may prove to increase condom use across people in all age and ethnic groups.

Conclusion

Research designed to increase and promote the maintenance of safer sexual behaviors is of paramount importance but is extremely challenging to complete. Research efforts in recent decades have provided needed information that can be used to guide the development, implementation, evaluation, and refinement of intervention efforts. Targeted future research that builds on what is currently known and understood will serve to enhance public health efforts to reduce the spread of undesirable health consequences associated with unsafe sexual practices.

References

Analyse des Comportements Sexuels en France ACSF Investigators. (1992). AIDS and sexual behaviour in France. *Nature, 360*(6403), 407–409.

Anonymous. (2005). More use of female condom recommended. *AIDS Patient Care and STDS,* *19*(2), 132.

Aten, M. J., Siegel, D. M., Enaharo, M., & Auinger, P. (2002). Keeping middle school students abstinence: Outcomes of a primary prevention intervention. *Journal of Adolescent Health,* *31,* 70–78.

Bailey, J. V., Farquhar, C., Owen, C., & Whittaker, D. (2003). Sexual behaviour of lesbians and bisexual women. *Sexually Transmitted Infections, 79*(2), 147–150.

Bajos, N. (1997). Social factors and the process of risk construction in HIV sexual transmission. *AIDS Care, 9*(2), 227–237.

Bakeman, R., & Peterson, J. L. (2007). Do beliefs about HIV treatments affect peer norms and risky sexual behaviour among African-American men who have sex with men? *International Journal of STD and AIDS, 18*(2), 105–108.

Bearman, P. S., & Bruckner, H. (2001). Promising the future: Virginity pledges and first intercourse. *American Journal of Sociology, 106*(4), 859–912.

Berkman, L. F., Glass, T., Brissette, I., & Seeman, T. E. (2000). From social integration to health: Durkheim in the new millennium. *Social Science and Medicine, 51*(6), 843–857.

Biddlecom, A. E. (2004). Trends in sexual behaviors and infections among young people in the United States. *Sexually Transmitted Infections, 80*(Suppl. 2), ii71–ii79.

Blair, J. M., Fleming, P. L., & Karon, J. M. (2002). Trends in AIDS incidence and survival among racial/ethnic minority men who have sex with men, United States, 1990–1999. *Journal of Acquired Immune Deficiency Syndrome, 31*(3), 339–347.

Booth, C. (2002). *Woman to woman: A guide to lesbian sexuality.* Sydney: Simon & Schuster.

Broadhead, W. E., Kaplan, B. H., James, S. A., Wagner, E. H., Schoenbach, V. J., Grimson, R., et al. (1983). The epidemiologic evidence for a relationship between social support and health. *American Journal of Epidemiology, 117*(5), 521–537.

Bull, S. S., Piper, P., & Rietmeijer, C. (2002). Men who have sex with men and also inject drugs-profiles of risk related to the synergy of sex and drug injection behaviors. *Journal of Homosexuality, 42*(3), 31–51.

Carballo-Dieguez, A., & Dolezal, C. (1996). HIV risk behaviors and obstacles to condom use among Puerto Rican men in New York city who have sex with men. *American Journal of Public Health, 86*(11), 1619–1622.

Cassel, J. C. (1976). The contribution of the social environment to host resistance: The fourth Wade Hampton Frost lecture. *American Journal of Epidemiology, 104,* 107–123.

Catania, J. A., Osmond, D., Stall, R. D., Pollack, L., Paul, J. P., Blower, S., et al. (2001). The continuing HIV epidemic among men who have sex with men. *American Journal of Public Health, 91*(6), 907–914.

Centers for Disease Control and Prevention. (2001). HIV incidence among young men who have sex with men—seven U.S. cities, 1994–2000. *Morbidity and Mortality Weekly Report, 50*(21), 440–444.

Centers for Disease Control and Prevention. (2002a). Primary and secondary syphilis among men who have sex with men—New York City, 2001. *Morbidity and Mortality Weekly Report, 51,* 853–856.

Centers for Disease Control and Prevention. (2002b). Trends in sexual risk behaviors among high school students—United States, 1991–2001. *Morbidity and Mortality Weekly Report, 51*(38), 856–859.

Centers for Disease Control and Prevention. (2003). HIV/AIDS surveillance report, 2003, vol. 15. Retrieved February 28, 2008, from http://www.cdc.gov/hiv/stats/hasrlink.htm

Centers for Disease Control and Prevention. (2005a). Trends in HIV/AIDS Diagnosis—33 States, 2001–2004. *Morbidity and Mortality Weekly Report, 54*(45), 1149–1153.

Centers for Disease Control and Prevention. (2005b). *Trends in reportable sexually transmitted diseases in the United States, 2004. National surveillance data for chlamydia, gonorrhea, and syphilis.* Retrieved February 28, 2008, from http://www.cdc.gov/std/stats

Centers for Disease Control and Prevention. (2006a). Twenty-five years of HIV/AIDS—United States, 1981–2006. *Morbidity and Mortality Weekly Report, 55*(21), 585–589.

Centers for Disease Control and Prevention. (2006b). *HIV and AIDS: Are you at risk?* Retrieved September 17, 2007, from http://www.cdc.gov/hiv/pubs/brochure/atrisk.htm

Chesney, M. A., Koblin, B. A., Barresi, P. J., Husnik, M. J., Celum, C. L., Colfax, G., et al. (2003). An individually tailored intervention for HIV prevention: Baseline data from the explore study. *American Journal of Public Health, 93*(6), 933–938.

Chesson, H. W., Harrison, P., & Stall, R. (2003). Changes in alcohol consumption and in sexually transmitted disease incidence rates in the United States: 1983–1998. *Journal of Studies on Alcohol, 64*(5), 623–630.

Clutterbuck, D. J., Gorman, D., McMillan, A., Lewis, R., & Macintyre, C. C. (2001). Substance use and unsafe sex amongst homosexual men in Edinburgh. *AIDS Care, 13*(4), 527–535.

Cooper, M. L. (2002). Alcohol use and risky sexual behavior among college students and youth: Evaluating the evidence. *Journal of Studies on Alcohol,* (14)(Suppl.), 101–117.

Crosby, G. M., Stall, R. D., Paul, J. P., Barrett, D. C., & Midanik, L. T. (1996). Condom use among gay/bisexual male substance abusers using the timeline follow-back method. *Addictive Behavior, 21*(2), 249–257.

Crosby, R. A., DiClemente, R. J., Wingood, G. M., Salazar, L. F., Rose, E., Levine, D., et al. (2004). Associated between sexually transmitted disease diagnosis and subsequent sexual risk and sexually transmitted disease incidence among adolescents. *Sexually Transmitted Diseases, 31*(4), 205–208.

Diamond, C., & Buskin, S. (2000). Continued risky behavior in HIV-infected youth. *American Journal of Public Health, 90,* 115–118.

Diamont, A. L., Schuster, M. A., McGuigan, K., & Level, J. (1999). Lesbians' sexual history with men: Implications for taking a sexual history. *Archives of Internal Medicine, 159,* 2730–2736.

Diamont, A. L., Lever, J., & Schuster, M. A. (2000). Lesbians' sexual activities and efforts to reduce risks for sexually transmitted diseases. *Journal of the Gay and Lesbian Medical Association, 4*(2), 41–48.

Diaz, R. M. (1998). *Latino gay men and HIV: Culture, sexuality and risk behavior.* New York: Routledge.

DiClemente, R. J. (1993). Preventing HIV/AIDS among adolescents: Schools as agents of behavior change. *Journal of the American Medical Association, 270,* 760–762.

DiClemente, R. J., Wingood, G. M., & Crosby, R. A. (2003). A contextual perspective for understanding and preventing STD/HIV among adolescents. In D. Romer (Ed.), *Reducing adolescent risk: Toward an integrated approach* (pp. 366–373). Thousand Oaks, CA: Sage.

Dolcini, M. M., Catania, J. A., Stall, R. D., & Pollack, L. (2003). The HIV epidemic among older men who have sex with men. *Journal of Acquired Immune Deficiency Syndromes, 33*(2 Suppl.), S115–S121.

Doval, A. S., Duran, R., O'Donnell, L., & O'Donnell, C. R. (1995). Barriers to condom use in primary and nonprimary relationships among Hispanic STD clinic patients. *Hispanic Journal of Behavioral Sciences, 17,* 385–397.

Eng, E., & Parker, E. A. (2002). Natural helper models to enhance a community's health and competence. In R. J. DiClemente, R. A. Crosby, & M. C. Kegler (Eds.), *Emerging theories in health promotion practice and research: Strategies for improving public health* (pp. 126–156). San Francisco: Jossey-Bass.

Fethers K., Marks C., Mindel, A., & Estcourt, C. S. (2000). Sexually transmitted infections and risk behaviours in women who have sex with women. *Sexually Transmitted Infections, 76*(5), 345–349.

Finer, L. B. (2007). Trends in premarital sex in the United States, 1954–2003. *Public Health Reports, 122*(1), 73–78.

Fishman, S. J., & Anderson, E. H. (2003). Perception of HIV and safer sexual behaviors among lesbians. *Journal of the Association of Nurses in AIDS Care, 14*(6), 48–55.

Forest, J. D., & Singh, S. (1990). The sexual and reproductive behavior of American women, 1982–1988. *Family Planning Perspectives, 22,* 206–214.

Fortenberry, J. D. (1995). Adolescent substance use and sexually transmitted diseases risk: A review. *Journal of Adolescent Health, 16,* 304–308.

Fortenberry, J. D., Brizendine, E. J., Katz, B. P., & Orr, D. P. (2002). Post-treatment sexual and prevention behaviours of adolescents with sexually transmitted infections. *Sexually Transmitted Infections, 78,* 365–368.

Fox, K. K., del Rio, C., Holmes, K. K., Hook, E. W., III, Judson, F. N., Knapp, J. S., et al. (2001). Gonorrhea in the HIV era: A reversal in trends among men who have sex with men. *American Journal of Public Health, 91*(6), 959–964.

Friedman, S. R., Ompad, D. C., Maslow, C., Young, R., Case, P., Hudson, S. M., et al. (2003). HIV prevalence, risk behaviors, and high-risk sexual and injection networks among young women injectors who have sex with women. *American Journal of Public Health, 92*(6), 902–906.

Futterman, D. (2005). HIV in adolescents and young adults: Half of all new infections in the United States. *Topics in HIV Medicine, 13*(3), 101–105.

Gay and Lesbian Medical Association. (2001). *Healthy People 2010: Companion document for lesbian, gay, bisexual, and transgender (LGBT) health.* San Francisco: Gay and Lesbian Medical Association.

Greenwood, G. L., Paul, J. P., Pollack, L. M., Binson, D., Catania, J. A., Chang, J., et al. (2005). Tobacco use and cessation among a household-based sample of us urban men who have sex with men. *American Journal of Public Health, 95*(1), 145–151.

Grunbaum, J., Kann, L., Kinchen, S., Ross, J., Hawkins, J., Lowry, R., et al. (2004). Youth Risk Behavior Surveillance—United States, 2003 (Abridged). *Journal of School Health, 74*(8), 307–324.

Hallinan, M. T. (1982). The peer influence process. *Studies in Educational Evaluation, 7*(3), 285–306.

Heaney, C. A., & Israel, B. A. (2002). Social networks and social support. In K. Glanz, B. K. Rimer, & F. M. Lewis (Eds.), *Health behavior and health education: Theory, research and practice* (pp. 185–209). San Francisco: Jossey-Bass.

Herbst, J. H., Sherba, R. T., Crepaz, N., Deluca, J. B., Zohrabyan, L., Stall, R. D., et al. (2005). A meta-analytic review of HIV behavioral interventions for reducing sexual risk behavior of men who have sex with men. *Journal of Acquired Immune Deficiency Syndrome, 39*(2), 228–241.

Heymann, D. L. (2005). *Control of communicable diseases manual* (18th ed.). Washington, DC: American Public Health Association.

Hillard, P. J. A. (2005). U.S. adolescent pregnancy rates: Declining, but more progress is needed. *Current Opinion in Obstetrics and Gynecology, 17,* 453–455.

Hillier, L., De Visser, R., Kavanagh, A., & McNair, R. (2003). The association between licit and illicit drug use and sexuality in young Australian women. *Medical Journal of Australia, 179*(6), 326–327.

House, J. S. (1981). *Work stress and social support.* Reading, MA: Addison-Wesley.

Hunt, A. J., Weatherburn, P., Hickson, F. C., Davies, P. M., McManus, T. J., & Coxon, A. P. (1993). Changes in condom use by gay men. *AIDS Care, 5*(4), 439–448.

Jemmott, J. B., Jemmott, L. S., & Fong, G. T. (1998). Abstinence and safer sex HIV risk-reduction interventions for African American adolescents: A randomized controlled trial. *Journal of the American Medical Association, 279*(19), 1529–1536.

Jordan, K. M., & Deluty, R. H. (1998). Coming out for lesbian women: Its relation to anxiety, positive affectivity, self-esteem, and social support. *Journal of Homosexuality, 35*(2), 41–63.

Kaplan, B. H., Cassel, J. C., & Gore, S. (1977). Social support and health. *Medical Care, 15*(5 Suppl.), 47–58.

Karon, J. M., Fleming, P. L., Steketee, R. W., & De Cock, K. M. (2001). HIV in the United States at the turn of the century: An epidemic in transition. *American Journal of Public Health, 91*(7), 1060–1068.

Kelly, J. A., St. Lawrence, J. S., Stevenson, L. Y., Hauth, A. C., Kalichman, S. C., Diaz, Y. E., et al. (1992). Community AIDS/HIV risk reduction: The effects of endorsements by popular people in three cities. *American Journal of Public Health, 82*(11), 1483–1489.

Klima, C. S. (1998). Unintended pregnancy. Consequences and solutions for a worldwide problem. *Journal of Nurse Midwifery, 43*(6), 483–491.

Kline, A., & Van Landingham, M. (1994). HIV-infected women and sexual risk reduction: The relevance of existing models of behavior change. *AIDS Education and Prevention, 6,* 390–402.

Koblin, B. A., Husnik, M. J., Colfax, G., Huang, Y., Madison, M., Mayer, K., et al. (2006). Risk factors for HIV infection among men who have sex with men. *AIDS, 20*(5), 731–739.

Landry, D. J., Darroch, J. E., Singh, S., & Higgins, J. (2003). Factors associated with the content of sex education in U.S. public secondary schools. *Perspectives on Sexual Reproductive Health, 35*(6), 261–269.

Laumann, E. O., Gagnon, J. H., Michael, R. T., & Michaels, S. (1994). *The social organization of sexuality: Sexual practices in the United States.* Chicago: University of Chicago Press.

Malebranche, D. J. (2003). Black men who have sex with men and the HIV epidemic: Next steps for public health. *American Journal of Public Health, 93*(6), 862–865.

Marrazzo, J. M. (2004). Barriers to infectious disease care among lesbians. *Emerging Infectious Diseases, 10*(11), 1974–1978.

Marrazzo, J. M., Coffey, P., & Bingham, A. (2005). Sexual practices, risk perception and knowledge of sexually transmitted disease risk among lesbian and bisexual women. *Perspectives on Sexual and Reproductive Health, 37*(1), 6–12.

McNair, R. (2005). Risks and prevention of sexually transmissible infections among women
who have sex with women. *Sexual Health, 2,* 209–217.

Miller, R. L. (1995). Assisting gay men to maintain safer sex: An evaluation of an AIDS service
organization's safer sex maintenance program. *AIDS Education and Prevention, 7*(5 Suppl.),
48–63.

Morrow, K. M., & Allsworth, J. E. (2000). Sexual risk in lesbians and bisexual women. *Journal of
the Gay and Lesbian Medical Association, 4*(4), 159–165.

Mosher, W. D., Chandra, J., & Jones, J. (2005). *Sexual behavior and selected health measures: Men
and women 15–44 years of age, United States, 2002.* U.S. Department of Health and Human
Services, Centers for Disease Control and Prevention, National Center for Health Statistics, No. 362 (September 15).

Pedlow, C. T., & Carey, M. P. (2004). Developmentally appropriate sexual risk reduction interventions for adolescents: Rationale, review of interventions, and recommendations for
research and practice. *Annals of Behavioral Medicine, 27*(3), 172–184.

Pulerwitz, J., Amaro, H., DeJong, W., Gortmaker, S. L., & Rudd, R. (2002). Relationship power,
condom use and HIV risk among women in the USA. *AIDS Care, 14*(6), 789–800.

Rhodes, S. D. (2004). Hookups or health promotion? An exploratory study of a chat room-based
HIV prevention intervention for men who have sex with men. *AIDS Education and Prevention, 16*(4), 315–327.

Rhodes, S. D., DiClemente, R. J., Cecil, H., Hergenrather, K. C., & Yee, L. J. (2002). Risk among
men who have sex with men in the United States: A comparison of an internet sample and
a conventional outreach sample. *AIDS Education and Prevention, 14*(1), 41–50.

Rhodes, S. D., Hergenrather, K. C., Duncan, J., Ramsey, B., Yee, L. J., & Wilkin, A. M. (2007). Using
community-based participatory research to develop a chat room-based HIV prevention
intervention for gay men. *Progress in Community Health Partnerships; Research, Education, and Action, 1*(2), 175–184.

Rhodes, S. D., Hergenrather, K. C., Yee, L. J., Knipper, E., Wilkin, A. M., & Omli, M. R. (2007).
Characteristics of a sample of men who have sex with men, recruited from gay bars and
internet chat rooms, who report methamphetamine use. *AIDS Patient Care and STDs,
21*(8), 575–583.

Rhodes, S. D., McCoy, T., Hergenrather, K. C., Omli, M. R., & DuRant, R. H. (2007). Exploring the
health behavior disparities of gay men in the United States: Comparing gay male university students to their heterosexual peers. *Journal of LGBT Health Research, 3*(1), 15–23.

Rhodes, S. D., McCoy, T., Omli, M. R., Cohen, G., Champion, H., & DuRant, R. H. (2006). Who really uses condoms? Findings from a large internet-recruited random sample of unmarried
heterosexual college students in the southeastern U.S. *Journal of HIV/AIDS Prevention in
Children and Youth, 7*(2), 9–27.

Rhodes, S. D., & Yee, L. J. (2006). Public health and gay and bisexual men: A primer for practitioners, clinicians, and researchers. In M. Shankle (Ed.), *The handbook of lesbian, gay,
bisexual, and transgender public health: A practitioner's guide to service* (pp. 119–143).
Binghamton, NY: Haworth.

Rhodes, S. D., Yee, L. J., & Hergenrather, K. C. (2006). A community-based rapid assessment of
HIV behavioural risk disparities within a large sample of gay men in southeastern USA: A
comparison of African American, Latino and white men. *AIDS Care, 18*(8), 1018–1024.

Rogers, E. M. (1983). *Diffusion of innovations.* New York: Free Press.

Santelli, J. S., DiClemente, R., Mikker, K., & Kirby, D. (1999). Sexually transmitted diseases, unintended pregnancy, and adolescent health promotion. *Adolescent Medicine, 10,* 87–108.

Santelli, J. S., Kaiser, J., Hirsch, L., Radosh, A., Simkin, L., & Middlestadt, S. (2004). Initiation of
sexual intercourse among middle school adolescents: The influence of psychosocial factors. *Journal of Adolescent Health, 34,* 200–208.

Seage, G. R., Mayer, K. H., Wold, C., Lenderking, W. R., Goldstein, R., Cai, B., et al. (1998). The social context of drinking, drug use, and unsafe sex in the Boston young men study. *Journal
of Acquired Immune Deficiency Syndrome and Human Retrovirology, 17*(4), 368–375.

Sell, R. L., & Becker, J. B. (2001). Sexual orientation data collection and progress toward *Healthy
People 2010. American Journal of Public Health, 91*(6), 876–882.

Semple, S. J., Patterson, T. L., & Grant, I. (2003). HIV-positive gay and bisexual men: Predictors of unsafe sex. *AIDS Care, 15*(1), 3–15.

Sheroff, L., & Darney, P. D. (2005). *A clinical guide for contraception* (4th ed.). Philadelphia: Lippincott, Williams, & Wilkin.

Shrier, L. A., Pierce, J. D., Emans, S. J., & DuRant, R. H. (1998). Gender differences in risk behaviors associated with forced or pressured sex. *Archives of Pediatric and Adolescent Medicine, 152,* 57–63.

Skinner, C. J., Stokes, J., Kirlew, Y., Kavanagh, J., & Forster, G. E. (1996). A case-controlled study of the sexual health needs of lesbians. *Genitourinary Medicine, 72,* 277–280.

Smith, A. M., Grierson, J., Pitts, M., & Pattison, P. (2006). Individual characteristics are less important than event characteristics in predicting protected and unprotected anal intercourse among homosexual and bisexual men in Melbourne, Australia. *Sexually Transmitted Infections, 82*(6), 474–477.

Smith, L. A. (2003). Partner influence on noncondom use: Gender and ethnic differences. *Journal of Sex Research, 40*(4), 346–350.

St. Lawrence, J. S., Brasfield, T. L., Jefferson, K. W., Alleyne, E., O'Bannon, R. E., & Shirley, A. (1995). Cognitive-behavioral intervention to reduce African-American adolescents' risk for HIV infection. *Journal of Consulting and Clinical Psychology, 62,* 221–237.

Stone, E., Heagerty, P., Vittinghoff, E., Douglas, J. M., Jr., Koblin, B. A., Mayer, K. H., et al. (1999). Correlates of condom failure in a sexually active cohort of men who have sex with men. *Journal of Acquired Immune Deficiency Syndrome and Human Retrovirology, 20*(5), 495–501.

Tawk, H. M., Simpson, J. M., & Mindel, A. (2004). Condom use in multi-partnered males: Importance of HIV and hepatitis B status. *AIDS Care, 16*(7), 890–900.

Valdiserri, R. O., Lyter, D. W., Leviton, L. C., Stoner, K., & Silvestre, A. (1987). Applying criteria for the development of health promotion and education programs to AIDS risk reduction programs for gay men. *Journal of Community Health, 12,* 199–212.

Vanable, P. A., McKirnan, D. J., Buchbinder, S. P., Bartholow, B. N., Douglas, J. M., Jr., Judson, F. N., et al. (2004). Alcohol use and high-risk sexual behavior among men who have sex with men: The effects of consumption level and partner type. *Health Psychology, 23*(5), 525–532.

Ventura, S. J., Abma, J. C., Mosher, W. D., & Henshaw, S. (2004). Estimated pregnancy rates for the United States, 1990–2000: An update. *National Vital Statistics Reports, 52*(23), 1–9.

Wendt, S. J., & Solomon, L. J. (1995). Barriers to condom use among heterosexual male and female college students. *Journal of American College Health, 44*(3), 105–110.

Whittier, D. K., Lawrence, J. S., & Seeley, S. (2005). Sexual risk behavior of men who have sex with men: Comparison of behavior at home and at a gay resort. *Archives of Sexual Behavior, 34*(1), 95–102.

Winer, R. L., Hughes, J. P., Feng, Q., O'Reilly, S., Kiviat, N. B., Holmes, K. K., et al. (2006). Condom use and the risk of genital human papillomavirus infection in young women. *New England Journal of Medicine, 354*(25), 2645–2654.

Wolitski, R. J., Valdiserri, R. O., Denning, P. H., & Levine, W. C. (2001). Are we headed for a resurgence of the HIV epidemic among men who have sex with men? *American Journal of Public Health, 91*(6), 883–888.

Zelnik, M., & Kantner, J. F. (1980). Sexual activity, contraceptive use and pregnancy among metropolitan-area teenagers: 1971–1979. *Family Planning Perspectives, 12,* 230–237.

Intervention Elements Promoting Adherence to Mindfulness-Based Stress Reduction (MBSR) Programs in a Clinical Behavioral Medicine Setting

14

Paul G. Salmon,
Saki F. Santorelli,
Sandra E. Sephton,
and Jon Kabat-Zinn

This chapter describes recent applications of *mindfulness meditation* in clinical health care settings centered on the Mindfulness-Based Stress Reduction (MBSR) program established at the Stress Reduction Clinic and its umbrella institute, the Center for Mindfulness in Medicine, Health Care, and Society (CFM) at the University of Massachusetts Medical School (UMMS). Since the previous edition of this chapter, there has been an explosion of interest in mindfulness, evident in the proliferation of programs in mindfulness-based stress reduction (MBSR) and close derivatives involving cognitive and other forms of psychotherapy (Germer, Siegel, & Fulton, 2005; Teasdale et al., 2000), eating awareness training, art therapy for cancer patients, and childbirth and parenting education. It is also evident in the range of conceptual and construct analyses (Bishop, 2002; Brown & Ryan, 2003), operational definitions (Kabat-Zinn, 2003; Bishop et al., 2004), and empirical investigations of mindfulness-based interventions reviewed by Baer (2003) and Salmon et al. (2004). This literature underscores not only the increasing number and sophistication of clinical outcome studies but also the increasing breadth of applications in medicine, health care, and psychology (Walsh and Shapiro, 2006). Mindfulness- and acceptance-based therapy models are referred to as the "third wave" of Cognitive-Behavior Therapy (Hayes, Follette, & Linehan, 2004). Moreover, mindfulness-based approaches are now cited in medical journals as empirically validated health care interventions in their own right (Astin, Shapiro, Eisenberg, & Forys, 2003).

The growing interest in mindfulness in clinical medicine itself, the context in which MBSR developed, is related to the fact that medical practice is by necessity rapidly becoming far more participatory than its 20th-century counterpart (Epstein, Alper, & Quill, 2004; Kabat-Zinn, 2000). While medical care has always been participatory to some degree because of the primacy of the doctor-patient relationship within the Hippocratic calling, it is also true that in large measure, most 20th-century medicine has been characterized by authoritarian, paternalistic physician-patient relationships. In this context, the patient's point of view has historically been less relevant to treatment than that of the physician or even unacknowledged (Toombs, 1993) because of the tacit habits and dictates of medicine itself (Epstein, 1999).

While the biopsychosocial perspective (Engel, 1977) and increased understanding of suffering and illness (Cassell, 1999) in patients seeking medical treatment have improved patient-practitioner relationships, mindfulness-based approaches offer an even broader entrée and perspective into these relational dynamics. When patients *and* practitioners practice mindfulness, *both* may begin to experience more directly their own suffering *from the inside out.* Often overlooked or undervalued, the process of learning to "own" these inborn, archetypal dimensions of humanness can alter the physician-patient relationship and the entire healing enterprise. Adherence may be affected by the mutually shared honoring of these interpenetrating realities and set the stage for a more authentic patient-practitioner relationship (Santorelli, 1999).

The process of caring for people in times of both health and illness increasingly involves active listening to the patient's experience, collaborative problem solving, and negotiated decision making. This entails recognizing and respecting the patient as a person, rather than just an interesting problem or case. In turn, this necessitates sensitivity to the actual *lived experience* (Toombs, 1993) of the patient and an appreciation for its first-person manifestations, embodiment, and meaning. Connecting with people in this way is a powerful stimulus for mobilizing inner resources to promote healing and coping with chronic medical conditions and other life-altering stressors. Making this connection is fundamental to the MBSR program, a factor we believe is directly relevant to high-level adherence (Santorelli, 1999; Kabat-Zinn, 2005).

One early manifestation of the trend toward greater participatory health and medical care was the rapid proliferation of hospital- and clinic-based MBSR programs. Currently, more than 240 hospitals and clinics nationwide and abroad offer MBSR programs, in which compliance rates are typically high (Kabat-Zinn and Chapman-Waldrop 1988). The program originated with the founding of the Stress Reduction Clinic at the University of Massachusetts Medical Center in 1979. Since 1995, it has been embedded within the larger

Center for Mindfulness (CFM) in Medicine, Health Care, and Society, within the Department of Medicine, Division of Preventive and Behavioral Medicine. As originally conceived, MBSR was an outpatient service, based on a patient education model emphasizing self-care as a complement to traditional medical treatment (Kabat-Zinn, 1990; Kabat-Zinn, 1993). Since its inception, more than 17,000 medical patients and other participants have completed the program, consisting of weekly sessions based on intensive training in mindfulness meditation. Between 1979 and 2000, more than 90% of all referrals to the program were from physicians, with the remainder coming from other health professionals. However, in recent years, there has been a steady increase in self-referrals to the Stress Reduction Program, to the point that over the 4-year period 2002–2006, the majority of enrollments (51%) were self-referrals, with only 49% from within the medical system (S. Santorelli, 2007, personal communication).

Despite changes in referral sources at UMMS and modification of the pre- and post-program assessment procedures described in this chapter, program completion rates remained unchanged (S. Santorelli, 2007, personal communication). Overall completion rates for a one-year period in 2002, based on 1,254 program participants, remains high (median completion rate > 80%). Data for enrolled participants for the period 2002–2006 (N = 1,520) revealed a comparable 85% completion rate. This pattern of high adherence is consistent with results of early outcome studies (Kabat-Zinn, 1982; Kabat-Zinn, Lipworth, & Burney 1985; Kabat-Zinn, Lipworth, Burney, & Sellers, 1987; Kabat-Zinn & Chapman-Waldrop, 1988; Kabat-Zinn et al., 1992; Miller, Fletcher, & Kabat-Zinn, 1995). The UMMS-based MBSR program is the prototype for clinically oriented mindfulness-based group interventions that have been widely adapted for use in other clinical settings. In this chapter, we focus on elements of the UMMS program that, on the basis of 29 years of clinical experience, we believe are particularly potent in both engaging and sustaining active participant involvement.

Mindfulness-Based Stress Reduction (MBSR)

MBSR is based on intensive training in mindfulness meditation, the systematic cultivation of nonjudgmental, moment-to-moment attention (Kabat-Zinn, 2003).

The following description and discussion are based on the MBSR Program at UMMS. Following orientation and enrollment in the program, participants are immersed in eight weekly 2.5–3.5 hour-long, instructor-taught classes for approximately 30 individuals with a wide range of medical and psychological conditions. This heterogeneity is deliberate, for several reasons. First, it is a practical acknowledgment that stress and suffering accompany all forms of medical and psychiatric maladies. Second, it bypasses the inherent tendency of groups sharing a particular diagnosis to focus primarily on specifics of the disease burden itself. Third, being surrounded by fellow participants with a wide range of diagnoses encourages perspective taking and an immediate shift of focus onto what is "right" with them, rather than what is "wrong." Finally, the program encourages an investigation and sharing of basic life experiences that individually and collectively contribute to a sense of integrity and wholeness, akin to the salutatory perspective on health (Antonovsky, 1987). This sense of shared humanity is underscored by a day-long retreat held on the weekend following the sixth session and attended by all participants in the current program cycle (four per year), and prior program graduates, as well. As many as 150 participants attend these day-long retreats, which reinforce and deepen mindfulness through extended practice. They also serve as "booster sessions" for graduates to help sustain, deepen, and further integrate mindfulness into their everyday lives. Current participants benefit from seeing program graduates return to engage in a day of "non-doing" that may at first seem daunting and from hearing others speak and share their experiences toward the end of the day (Kabat-Zinn, 1990; Santorelli, 1999).

Prior to 2001, extended individual interviews were conducted with virtually all potential participants referred to the Stress Reduction Clinic to evaluate their suitability and to provide an overview of the program (Kabat-Zinn and Chapman-Waldrop, 1988; Santorelli & Kabat-Zinn, 2002). Since then, group-based orientation sessions have replaced the original individual interview model. During these sessions, baseline assessment questionnaires are administered, and essential information about the 8-week program and an introduction to mindfulness are presented to groups of 15–40 individuals. An additional brief screening interview is also conducted to further ensure the appropriateness of each candidate, augmented by further assessment if warranted. This format is highly cost-effective, resulting in a 30% saving in operating expenses (S. Santorelli, 2007, personal communication) while ensuring that participants are appropriately screened and well informed about the program. These orientation sessions were phased in over time, making it possible to compare the impact of both pre-admission formats on program outcome. Between 2001 and 2006, symptoms and global measures of distress using the Medical Symptom Checklist (MSCL) and SCL-90-R inventories showed comparable and significant reductions in these outcome measures for both models (S. Santorelli, 2007, personal communication).

During the program itself, participants are exposed to four primary mindfulness practices: (1) the Body Scan Meditation; (2) Sitting Meditation; (3) Mindful Hatha Yoga; and (4) Mindful Walking. These formal mindfulness practices and the rationale for their use are described in detail elsewhere (Kabat-Zinn, 1990, 1994b, 2005; Santorelli, 1999). Other structural elements of the program include (a) home practice (45–60 minutes per day, 6 days per week) using CDs; (b) a workbook with daily awareness exercises; (c) the all-day retreat; and (d) a post-program assessment.

Home practice, an integral element of the program (Kabat-Zinn, 1990; Santorelli, 1999) is structured using CDs to guide participants through the Body Scan, Sitting Meditation, and two Mindful Hatha Yoga sequences, each approximately 45 minutes in duration. These sessions emphasize noticing (without becoming preoccupied with) sensations associated with the body in stillness and in movement, as well as transient thoughts and emotions that inevitably come and go. In addition, "informal" mindfulness practices are also assigned each week involving aspects of daily living, such as breathing, walking, driving, cooking, eating, cleaning, showering, talking, listening, working, parenting, and playing. This aspect of the practice emphasizes and builds on (1) awareness of body sensations and carriage of the body cultivated in formal practice; (2) awareness of emotional states, thoughts, and perceptions that arise during daily activities; and (3) awareness of stressful situations, the events that trigger them, and possible responses that might serve as alternatives to habitual, automated reactions. Because informal practice is woven into the fabric of daily life, it requires little extra time and is viewed as highly useful by a majority of responders in follow-up studies (Miller, Fletcher, & Kabat-Zinn, 1995).

In addition to practicing formal meditation during class sessions, participants spend considerable time in dialogue with course instructors and with each other about their personal experiences with meditation practice. These interactions constitute another means of integrating mindfulness into common aspects of everyday life (e.g., mindfulness of speech). The dialogue can be extremely animated, cogent, sensitive, and emotionally moving, while reinforcing the sense that participants and instructors alike share in common expertise and creativity in facing life's challenges.

MBSR and Adherence: Descriptive Factors

Outcome studies noted earlier assessing the impact of the MBSR program tend to report high rates of program completion and substantial participant engagement in the formal and informal class- and home-based mediation practices. We believe the following characteristics of MBSR contribute to this pattern of strong commitment:

1. A time-limited, group format of sufficient duration to foster lifestyle changes
2. An educational orientation to elicit active participation and self-inquiry
3. A range of mindfulness practices to accommodate individual temperaments
4. Highly developed instructor competencies, including a personal meditation practice
5. Recognition of how suffering and wholeness unite participants and instructors
6. Meditation practices that foster sensitivity to mind-body interactions
7. Heterogeneous group composition
8. An all-day silent retreat
9. Emphasis on growth and learning via coping, sharing with others, and even unwanted distress.

We now consider adherence in relation to (1) entry into the MBSR program; (2) initial, intermediate, and end-stage sessions; and (3) post-program assessment and relapse.

Referral Procedures and Pre-Program Orientation

The intention of the original MBSR individualized screening interview was to provide outpatient clinical services with minimal exclusionary criteria—primarily active suicidality, severe psychopathology, or both (Santorelli & Kabat-Zinn, 2002). It also introduced participants to mindfulness, as taught in the program. The current procedure streamlines this procedure, via group orientations and briefer personal interviews.

Historically, a network of referral sources was developed throughout the medical center and surrounding community. Various referring physicians even participated in the MBSR program themselves, attended in-service programs, or developed a feeling for referrals based on patients they had referred in the past and from periodic updates sent by the clinic. Since the original focus of the program was on medical patients, the incidence of severe psychiatric symptomatology was relatively low and remains so, although symptomatic anxiety and depression were (and continue to be) common.

Referral procedures always exert some degree of influence on program adherence by selecting potential candidates likely to do well in the program. However, since 2001, entry has shifted from being primarily physician-based to self-referrals (S. Santorelli, 2007, personal communication). Although this eliminates one screening level, it capitalizes on the heightened motivation of those who actively seek out the program. This shift appears to reflect several factors, including the momentum that has developed over years of operation, with thousands of participants from the immediate geographic region who serve as a potent word-of-mouth referral source. Second, the program increasingly appeals to clients facing a broader range of challenging life circumstances, not just those of a medical nature. Third, this trend reflects a broader social movement toward a participatory model of health care, health maintenance, and disease prevention to which MBSR has contributed. Fourth, meditation has become a more common and accepted aspect of experience in contemporary society. Finally, and perhaps most important, the philosophical basis of this intervention model extends beyond medicine to other facets and strata of society.

Orientation sessions address this increasing diversity by providing a broad overview of factors that create stress and emphasize the importance of taking personal responsibility for one's behavior. This helps distinguish the program from traditional medicine, which emphasizes predictable diagnostic and treatment procedures.

The fact that prospective participants are provided with a detailed explanation of the program may have at least two potential effects on adherence. First, it discourages enrollment by individuals who are not up to the challenges posed by the program. Second, some may decline to participate at a particular point in time because they are not able or willing to make the necessary commitment of time and energy.

Participants are exposed from the very start to an orientation that explicitly and somewhat paradoxically emphasizes nondoing and nonstriving, consistent with the nondualistic meditative approach underlying mindfulness (Kabat-Zinn, 1994b, 2003, 2005). Participants are cautioned from the start against becoming overly invested in setting goals or obtaining "results," such as an end to pain or relief from anxiety. Instead, emphasis is placed on simply doing what is required from day to day in keeping with the present moment orientation of mindfulness. It is further recommended that one suspend judgment about the program until the very end.

In keeping with this orientation, the various aspects of mindfulness are practiced in a manner that slows things down, minimizes extraneous stimulation, and encourages an increasingly intimate relationship with whatever is

encountered internally or externally. The purpose of this is to enhance perceptual clarity ("bare attention"), regardless of what one may experience in a given
moment: relaxation, tension, or any other state.

The typical emphasis on behavior change characteristic of most cognitive-
behavioral interventions is absent. Rather, careful self-observation and appreciation for the experience of one's life from moment to moment is encouraged.
Somewhat paradoxically, such acceptance constitutes a positive attitudinal shift
for those who struggle constantly with the desire for things to be somehow
different than they are (Hayes, Follette, & Linehan, 2004; Hayes, Strosahl, &
Wilson, 1999; Williams, Teasdale, Segal, & Kabat-Zinn, 2007).

Initial Program Stage and Adherence

During the first 20 years of the MBSR program, the use of preliminary individual interviews resulted in an enrollment rate of approximately 90% and a
subsequent 85% program completion rate among those who attended the first
class (Kabat-Zinn & Chapman-Waldrop, 1988). Nine percent of those who enrolled did not attend any classes (no shows), and 15% dropped out before the
program was over. "Completers" were those who attended at least five classes
and were present for the final class, the post-program interview, or both. As
already noted, switching to group-based orientations and brief screening interviews has not significantly affected completion rates.

During the program, participants are expected to notify their course instructor or administrative support personnel if they miss a class and to make it
up if possible in a concurrent group. Participants who do not call are contacted
within a day by the instructor as an immediate expression of concern. Moreover,
since 2001, group members have had the option of communicating with instructors via e-mail.

The first class frequently progresses spontaneously to a substantial and
striking level of self-disclosure, as participants are invited to share their reasons for entering the program. Importantly, this is not intentionally elicited by
the instructor but appears to emerge out of the collective sense of affirming
one's commitment to doing something for oneself in a supportive therapeutic and social context. The willingness of most participants to openly express
grief, fear, and pain has several effects. First, it highlights the broad range of
human suffering represented within the room, counterbalanced by the courage
embodied by participants in the face of such suffering. At the very least, this is
inspiring to other class members; at best, it illuminates the possibility inherent
within each individual to bring full-hearted attention to stress, pain, and illness. In turn, this places any one person's story or problems in a broader context. Some people, no matter how severe their own problems, feel they do not
belong because others' problems seem more serious, a reaction addressed by
emphasizing the unique qualities of each individual's situation. Second, powerful emotional forces are often generated as people begin to share with each
other—many for the first time ever—burdens that may have accumulated for
years, along with more recent stressors that may have catalyzed referral to the
program. One participant, who could speak in class and feel accepted and supported subsequently remarked that, while riding the subway, he came to see the
entire world was "a community of the afflicted" (Kabat-Zinn, 1994a).

In the first class, participants are provided with a more detailed context and framework for the program, based on the preliminary orientation session. The cultivation of a nongoal orientation and nonjudgmental, moment-to-moment attention to experience is emphasized. Common misconceptions about meditation as an esoteric or mysterious practice are addressed early on. To help counter such views, the first meditation typically involves eating one or two raisins mindfully over a period of several minutes. The sheer novelty and intensity of the experience, coupled with highly focused attention directed at so seemingly mundane a task, typically evokes a range of responses from astonishment to insightful laughter. This simple exercise helps illustrate the nature of mindfulness meditation as a systematic form of attention training, a way of learning to consciously attend to even the most mundane aspects of everyday life. It helps emphasize the pervasive range of opportunities to practice mindfulness. Instructors describe their role as guides or coaches and do not assume an authoritarian stance or tone.

Ongoing Participation and Adherence

As suggested in a qualitative study of participants in an MBSR class (Santorelli, 1992), as well as in our clinical experience with MBSR over almost 30 years, one of the most powerful elements promoting strong engagement in home practice is the deep sense of well-being that can arise from regular exposure to the various "formal" mindfulness practices. This is related to an intentional willingness to reside in stillness and silence, observing the unfolding of one's experience from moment to moment, while assuming a nonreactive, nonjudgmental stance through even difficult and troubling experiences. Sitting meditation in particular emphasizes nonjudgmental, open awareness of whatever arises in body or mind as a natural part of the landscape of consciousness. Such unrestricted awareness is related to feelings of ease, calmness, and perhaps self-efficacy that can develop within the observational process.

It should be noted that meditation and its effects are neither romanticized nor idealized in MBSR. Rather, the emphasis is simply on nondoing and being and *resting in awareness* of whatever arises in the present moment, rather than trying to achieve any particular mind state that might seem desirable. This novel feature of mindfulness training may contribute to long-term engagement, since the core message is that one is already *whole* in the most fundamental way and possessed of inner resources to draw upon even when facing aversive experiences, thoughts, and feelings.

As the program continues, new factors potentially related to adherence come into play as well. The required daily home practice becomes embedded in daily life, drawing on the body scan, sitting meditation, and mindful yoga (using guided-practice CDs), and teaching members to treat life circumstances as opportunities to cultivate focused attention and skillful response patterns. The constant repetition of these elements all emphasizes the same thing: cultivating and sustaining focused attention and familiarity with awareness *itself*. Elements of Western cognitive psychotherapy, including "self-monitoring" and "nonreinforced exposure" (Linehan, 1994), are clearly evident within this orientation, both of which involve selectively directed attention: "self-monitoring" helps clients track thoughts, emotions, and behaviors associated with negative emotions, whereas "'nonreinforced exposure" encourages confronting anxiety-provoking circumstances as a means of reducing their impact. However, both forms of awareness are intended to enact change in emotions or behavior. "Being mindful" offers an alternative: rather than attempting to fix or alter, deny or subdue unwanted mental or behavioral events, it advocates cultivating *hospitality*—sometimes referred to as generosity or basic warmth—toward whatever arises in the field of awareness. Paradoxically, this more acceptance-oriented stance experience seems to slowly and radically dismantle strong, conditioned behaviors associated with fight, flight, or denial. Simply acknowledging, rather than attempting to change, unwanted thoughts or feelings appears to have positive implications for living one's life more fully (Santorelli, 1999).

Nonjudgmental attention is key to this process, the foundation of an attitudinal framework that makes it less likely that doubts or feelings of inadequacy about how one is doing in the program will adversely impact adherence. "Being mindful" not only makes it more likely that thoughts and feelings that could adversely affect practice motivation will be detected but also provides a conceptual framework and practical strategy for limiting the impact of such thoughts and feelings on adherence when they occur.

This capacity to dispassionately notice and track potentially stressful, anxiety-provoking, or depressive thoughts has been fruitfully incorporated in other recent clinical applications. For example, Teasdale and colleagues (Teasdale, Segal, & Williams, 1995) proposed employing attention regulation (mindfulness) as a method for preventing relapse from clinical depression by teaching participants to detect and respond nonjudgmentally to recurring depressive thoughts or emotions that, if left unacknowledged, might result in full-blown relapse. The positive impact of this theorizing was documented in a large-scale study (Teasdale et al., 2002) in which patients with three or more lifetime episodes of major depression showed a significantly reduced rate of relapse. These results were replicated in a second trial (Ma and Teasdale, 2004), providing further empirical validation of what is now termed mindfulness-based cognitive therapy (MBCT) (Segal, Williams, & Teasdale, 2002; Williams, Teasdale, Segal, & Kabat-Zinn, 2007).

In addition to formal mindfulness practice, participants are encouraged to take advantage of episodic practice opportunities in the context of daily life that provide a means of generalizing treatment effects in a manner consistent with psychotherapeutic "exposure" or "inoculation" (Santorelli, 1992). Both formal and informal mindfulness practices are intended to foster nonattachment, self-acceptance, compassion for others and for oneself, and deepening insight into the nature of "self" and self-in-relationship (Gunaratana, 1991; Kabat-Zinn, 1990; Santorelli 1999; Thera, 1962). Informal practice is especially noteworthy, because it encompasses experiences that may be more challenging than those encountered in the classroom or during quiet practice at home. Teaching basic skills in the context of formal meditation and encouraging their development through daily practice helps bridge the gap between in-class and real-life experiences (Kabat-Zinn and Chapman-Waldrop, 1988; Santorelli, 1992). The time between classes serves as an *in-vivo* laboratory for practicing *a way of being,* not just reducing stress.

Yet another factor potentially related to high program completion rates is a progressive shift from prescriptive adherence to the program to gradually "making the practice your own." Self-exploration and self-responsibility are increasingly encouraged to help translate program requirements into personal terms concerning both formal and informal practice. For example, participants are encouraged to "mix and match" home practice elements (body scan, sitting meditation, yoga) in personally meaningful ways as the program progresses, within a 45-minute daily practice framework.

Overall, this process-oriented approach to education, growth, and change contrasts markedly with more goal or "end-oriented" models, with important implications for adherence. In essence, participants learn to cultivate an awareness of what they are already doing, thinking, or experiencing in any particular moment, whatever it may be, rather than focusing on trying to change things. Given a willingness to cultivate nonjudgmental awareness in the present moment, there is really little else that one might do or say or think that would somehow *not* reflect inherent adherence. The invitation to simply "pay attention" creates a relatively permissive context within which change can occur, a characteristic now embodied in emerging acceptance-based psychotherapy (Germer, Siegel, & Fulton, 2005; Hayes, Strosahl, & Wilson, 1999; Linehan, 1994). Mindfulness reduces potential resistance because it can be directed toward resistance itself, thereby narrowing the range of what would otherwise be considered nonadherent behaviors.

Finally, the all-day meditation retreat certainly stands out as a key element affecting adherence. The challenge of an entire day (approximately 8 hours) of predominantly silent practice guided by teachers in the presence of other current and past participants provides a rich experiential laboratory for sustained practice of the principal components of MBSR training. It might be described as "quasi *in vivo*," because it entails the shared experience of an environment that is less intimate than the regular classes because of the size (up to 150 people) but is at the same time very different from one's day-to-day living environment. There is a strong sense of a shared community ("*sangha*") common to both the classes themselves and the larger all-day meditation session (Santorelli, 1999).

Prior participants in the MBSR program also benefit from the all-day sessions, which serve as booster sessions to deepen mindfulness practice. They also offer an opportunity to reconnect with teachers and other participants in a setting that may evoke recollections of their reasons for taking the program and of the internal resources they developed at that time. As best we can determine, combining current and former participants in a large practice setting is unique to mindfulness-based interventions. Current participants benefit in part simply from seeing people come back to practice intensively after finishing the program, as well as from reflections that graduates often share during a group dialogue near the day's end (Kabat-Zinn, 1990; Santorelli, 1999).

Adherence and Concluding Weeks of the MBSR Program

As noted, participants are encouraged to devise their own home meditation practice as the program progresses. This feature of MBSR may positively affect end-stage adherence in several ways. First, the element of choice reinforces the importance of personal responsibility emphasized throughout the course.

Second, many participants develop strong preferences for specific techniques by this time (Kabat-Zinn, Chapman, & Salmon, 1997) and are motivated to continue practicing. Finally, this phase serves a preparatory function with respect to closure at a time when participants still have the benefit of contact with each other and their instructors. The last 2 weeks provide opportunities for participants to explore and reinforce individual inclinations and initiatives, and to tailor the program to their own present and anticipated needs. The eighth week (following the eighth and final class) is characteristically termed "the rest of your life," implying that as people prepare to leave the security and structure of the program, the momentum they have developed can continue indefinitely if they make a commitment to maintain the practice.

Post-Program Assessment and Advanced Training

The original MBSR program concluded with participants completing assessment measures and a personal interview with the course instructor at post-program interviews following the last class. Since initiation of the Group Orientation Model, the post-program assessment is now conducted during the final (8th class) session itself. In both models, the purpose of the assessment serves two functions: First, it provides participants with an opportunity to reflect on their experience in the program in terms of meeting their needs and intentions. Second, repeating the assessment measures administered prior to the program provides data for program outcome studies.

Currently, all participants continue to be assessed pre- and post-intervention using the Medical Symptom Checklist (MSCL) and the General Severity Index (GSI) of the SCL-90-R. In the first teaching cycle using the group assessment model, the mean reduction on the MSCL was 30.2% (N = 134), and the mean reduction in the GSI was 51.6% (N = 118) (S. Santorelli, 2007, personal communication). These findings are comparable to those obtained using the individual interview model. Similar reductions were also found for a larger sample of consecutive program participants enrolled in the period 2002–2006; the mean MSCL reduction was 28.7% (N = 724) and the mean GSI reduction, 42.3% (N = 674). Thus, symptom reductions have been sustained despite changes in the intake and post-program assessment procedures, while completion rates across the two models have remained virtually identical (Individual Interview Model = 86%; Group Orientation Model = 85%), using data collected between 2002–2006. Significantly, in the period 1979–2001, virtually all program referrals came from the medical system. Since initiation of the group orientation and assessment model, medical referrals now constitute 49% of the program participants, and self-referrals make up the other 51%. Of those who actually enroll, 38% are medically referred, while the majority (62%) are self-referred. Thus, while referral patterns and assessment procedures have changed, adherence and outcome figures have remained consistently high over 28 years of continuous operation of the MBSR program.

In addition to ongoing all-day retreats, participants may attend "graduate programs" offered periodically to further deepen their meditation practice by applying skills learned during the initial MBSR experience. Focusing on various program themes such as interpersonal mindfulness, coping with holiday stress, mindfulness and cinema themes, or mindful aging, these sessions meet weekly, biweekly, or bimonthly for several months and incorporate extended periods of meditation practice using methods taught in the basic course, with an overarching focus on application of mindfulness not only to stress and illness but also to health and well-being. Home practice is augmented with additional materials and assignments mailed to participants midway between sessions to encourage ongoing engagement and to help keep the focus on continuously bringing mindfulness to the unfolding of daily life experience. Also, these programs offer those whose practice has relapsed an opportunity to recommit to it, and encourages those who have maintained the practice to explore deeper implications of mindfulness.

Relapse

Relapse to pretreatment mind-states or behavior constitutes a significant impediment to long-term adherence, even following "successful" behavior change interventions. The MBSR program addresses relapse (faltering engagement in and implementation of what one has learned in the program) in several ways. First, the nonjudgmental, nonstriving orientation tends to reframe ideas of "relapse" (and other comparably judgmental terms) in a more benign way that emphasizes acceptance. This idea is increasingly prominent in contemporary cognitive therapies that view acceptance as a fundamental starting point for meaningful change (Germer, Siegel, & Fulton, 2005; Hayes, Follette, & Linehan, 2004). Periodic relapses—ceasing to sustain the meditation practices in one form or another—are treated as a natural part of learning, worthy of attention and curiosity. It is also remediable in any moment simply by re-establishing mindfulness. Thus, one is always only one breath, one moment, one thought away from being fully in the practice, especially if this shift in attention is sustained over time.

Second, meditation practice emphasizes that the present moment is continuously unfolding, presenting itself in new and unique configurations. One comes to appreciate that no two moments are identical, and that there is always the potential to see a new opening, a new choice, and to allow change to occur out of one's deliberately cultivated awareness. A common self-statement describing relapse, such as "I've fallen back into my old patterns again," implies that one is at the mercy of old behaviors, simply repeated without variation. However, this is not only improbable but virtually impossible, owing to the dynamic and fluid nature of experience itself. The words "I" "have fallen back" "into my old patterns" "again" are linguistic labels describing a unique experience that cannot duplicate the past. Attending systematically to present-moment experience, rather than merely thinking about an experience or a moment, loosens "the dominance of evaluative languaging" (Hayes, 1994; Hayes, Barnes-Holmes, & Roche, 2001).

Third, within this framework, a relapse incident can be viewed with generosity and compassion, rather than as a setback. Missing daily practice sessions or feelings of panic, anxiety, or depression can all be seen as simply new opportunities for practice. By framing events in this manner, mindfulness, along with contemporary contextualist thought (Hayes, 1994; Hayes, Strosahl, & Wilson,

1999), cognitive and constructivist psychotherapies (Meichenbaum, 1993), and relapse prevention models (Marlatt, 1985) emphasizes taking a "fresh look" at linguistically driven interpretive biases. In a general sense, this encourages getting beyond linguistic terms like "relapse" used to describe experience (Hayes, 1994; Hayes, Strosahl, & Wilson, 1999; Hayes, Barnes-Holmes, & Roche, 2001) because they embody unconscious, habitual, reflexive, and often idiosyncratic associations that tend to inhibit seeing new possibilities for adaptation, growth, and change. By inviting participants to become more observant of the ebb and flow of beliefs and experiences and less attached to thoughts and self-statements, both voiced and silent, the program encourages moving beyond emotional-laden concepts capable of triggering distressful reactions commonly associated with the "slippery slope" of relapse.

Finally, of crucial importance with respect to relapse is the "phasic," nonlinear nature of human development and learning. Whereas relapse is commonly viewed as a discontinuity in a linear process of change, growth and change are dynamic, nonlinear processes that involve cycles of regression, restructuring, and reintegration. This cyclic progression, documented in a studies of meditation practitioners (Kornfield, 1979) and MBSR participants (Santorelli, 1992), suggests that what might be termed "relapse" or "regression" actually represents an inevitable aspect of learning and personal growth.

Summary and Conclusions

The MBSR program has stimulated considerable research in clinical, health, and experimental psychology. It has paved the way for the development of acceptance-based forms of psychotherapy that have been characterized as the "third wave" of cognitive behavior therapy (Hayes, Follette, & Linehan, 2004)—a clear testament to its impact. Mindfulness-based treatment protocols for depression (Segal, Williams, & Teasdale, 2002), anxiety (Orsillo & Roemer, 2005), and other conditions are becoming more prominent in clinical practice. Many, if not most, of these interventions show the influence of mindfulness meditation as initially conceptualized and developed at the University of Massachusetts Medical Center (Kabat-Zinn, 1990, 2005; Santorelli, 1999).

MBSR teaches participants to pay attention and be present with whatever arises in the field of experience, a message that is easily remembered and applicable in a variety of contexts, through both formal and informal mindfulness practices. The behavioral changes associated with MBSR are equally simple and direct, emphasizing being reflective and responsive rather than reactive, and focusing more on "being" and less on "doing." The orientation is attractive in its simplicity. Although maintaining the practice is both challenging and arduous, MBSR skills can be practiced with many degrees of persistence and awareness. Sitting quietly for a time or lying down and resting in awareness moment by moment with whatever arises in the domain of inner and outer experience is a capability native to all human beings and virtually universally accessible, even though internal associative mind and body states vary widely from person to person. Such mind-body patterns are observable by and profoundly amenable to nonreactive mindful attending (Goldstein & Kornfield, 1987; Gunaratana, 1991; Siegel, 2007; Thera, 1962; Wallace, 2006). MBSR may help provide access to a new dimension of one's own experience associated with nourishment and growth and stemming from the commitment to bring intentional awareness to the unfolding of one's life. It has been described as an "orthogonal rotation of consciousness" (Kabat-Zinn, 2005). In essence, mindfulness fosters both familiarity and intimacy with body and mind, with self and other, and with the world itself. As this intimacy becomes more fully integrated and embodied, the willingness to inhabit—to live fully inside—one's life becomes increasingly possible and palpably real. If what we are most drawn to as human beings is a direct, fully embodied experience of being alive, regardless of our circumstances, it may be that the connection with such aliveness is the most compelling motive for cultivating a mindful way of being.

References

Antonovsky, A. (1987). The salutogenic perspective: Toward a new view of health and illness. *Advances, 4*(1), 47–55.

Astin, J. A., Shapiro, S. L., Eisenberg, D. M., & Forys, K. L. (2003). Mind-body medicine: State of the science, implications for practice. *Journal of the American Board of Family Practice, 16*(2), 131–147.

Baer, R. (2003). Mindfulness training as a clinical intervention: A conceptual and empirical review. *Clinical Psychology: Science and Practice 10*, 125–143.

Bishop, S. (2002). What do we really know about mindfulness-based stress reduction? *Psychosomatic Medicine 64*(1), 71–83.

Bishop, S., Lau, M., Shapiro, S., Carlson, L., Anderson, N. D., Carmody, J., et al. (2004). Mindfulness: A proposed operational definition. *Clinical Psychology: Science and Practice, 11*, 230–241.

Brown, K., & Ryan, R. (2003). The benefits of being present: Mindfulness and its role in psychological well-being. *Journal of Personality and Social Psychology 84*, 822–848.

Cassell, E. J. (1999). Diagnosing suffering: A perspective. *Annals of Internal Medicine 131*, 531–539.

Engel, G. (1977). The need for a new medical model: a challenge for biomedicine. *Science, 196*(4286), 833–839.

Epstein, R. (1999). Mindful practice. *Journal of the American Medical Association, 282*(9), 833–839.

Epstein, R. M., Alper, B. S., & Quill, T. E. (2004). Communicating evidence for participatory decision making. *Journal of the American Medical Association 291*(19), 2359–2366.

Germer, C., Siegel, R., & Fulton, P. R. (2005). *Mindfulness and psychotherapy.* New York: Guilford Press.

Goldstein, J., & Kornfield, J. (1987). *Seeking the heart of wisdom: The path of insight meditation.* Boston: Shambhala.

Gunaratana, H. (1991). *Mindfulness in plain English.* Boston: Wisdom.

Hayes, S. (1994). Content, context, and the types of psychological acceptance. In S. Hayes, N. Jacobson, V. Follette, & M. Dougher (Eds.), *Acceptance and change: Content and context in psychotherapy* (pp. 13–32). Reno, NV: Context Press.

Hayes, S., Barnes-Holmes, D., & Roche, B. (Eds.). (2001). *Relational frame theory: A post-Skinnerian account of human language and cognition.* New York: Kluwer Academic/Plenum.

Hayes, S., Follette, V., & Linehan, M. (2004). *Mindfulness and acceptance: Expanding the cognitive-behavioral tradition.* New York: Guilford Press.

Hayes, S., Strosahl, K., & Wilson, K. G. (1999). *Acceptance and commitment therapy: An experiential approach to behavior change.* New York: Guilford Press.

Kabat-Zinn, J. (1982). An outpatient program in behavioral medicine for chronic pain patients based on the practice of mindfulness meditation: Theoretical considerations and preliminary results. *General Hospital Psychiatry 4*, 33–47.

Kabat-Zinn, J. (1990). *Full catastrophe living: Using the wisdom of your body and mind to face stress, pain, and illness.* New York: Delta.

Kabat-Zinn, J. (1993). Mindfulness meditation: Health benefits of an ancient Buddhist practice. In D. Goleman & J. Gurin (Eds.), *Mind/body medicine* (pp. 259–275). New York: Consumer Reports Books.

Kabat-Zinn, J. (1994a). *Wherever you go, there you are: Mindfulness meditation in everyday life.* New York: Hyperion.

Kabat-Zinn, J. (1994b). Foreword. In M. Lerner, *Choices in healing.* Cambridge, MA: MIT Press.

Kabat-Zinn, J. (2000). Participatory medicine. *Journal of the European Academy of Dermatology and Venereology 14*(4), 239–240.

Kabat-Zinn, J. (2003). Mindfulness-based interventions in context: Past, present, and future. *Clinical Psychology: Science and Practice, 10,* 144–156.

Kabat-Zinn, J. (2005). *Coming to our senses: Healing ourselves and the world through mindfulness.* New York: Hyperion.

Kabat-Zinn, J., & Chapman-Waldrop, A. (1988). Compliance with an outpatient stress reduction program: Rates and predictors of program completion. *Journal of Behavioral Medicine 11*(4), 333–352.

Kabat-Zinn, J., Chapman-Waldrop, A., & Salmon, P. (1997). The relationship of cognitive and somatic components of anxiety to patient preference for different relaxation techniques. *Mind-Body Medicine 2*(3), 101–109.

Kabat-Zinn, J., Lipworth, L., & Burney, R. (1985). The clinical use of mindfulness meditation for the self-regulation of chronic pain. *Journal of Behavioral Medicine 8*(2), 163–190.

Kabat-Zinn, J., Lipworth, L., Burney, R., & Sellers, W. (1987) Four-year follow-up of a meditation-based program for the self-regulation of chronic pain. *Clinical Journal of Pain 2,* 159–173.

Kabat-Zinn, J., Massion, A. O., Kristeller, J., Peterson, L. G., Fletcher, K. E., Pbert, L., et al. (1992). Effectiveness of a meditation-based stress reduction program in the treatment of anxiety disorders. *American Journal of Psychiatry 149*(7), 936–943.

Kornfield, J. (1979). Intensive insight meditation: A phenomenological study. *Journal of Transpersonal Psychology 11,* 41–58.

Linehan, M. (1994). Acceptance and change: The central dialectic in psychotherapy. In S. Hayes, N. Jacobson, V. Follette, & M. Dougher (Eds.), *Acceptance and change: Content and context in psychotherapy.* Reno, NV: Context Press.

Ma, S. H., & Teasdale, J. D. (2004). Mindfulness-based cognitive therapy for depression: Replication and exploration of differential relapse prevention effects. *Journal of Consulting And Clinical Psychology 72*(1), 31–40.

Marlatt, A. (1985). Cognitive assessment and intervention procedures for relapse prevention. In A. Marlatt & J. R. Gordon (Eds.), *Relapse prevention: Maintenance strategies in the treatment of addictive behaviors* (pp. 201–279). New York: Guilford Press.

Meichenbaum, D. (1993). Changing conceptions of cognitive behavior modification: Retrospect and prospect. *Journal of Consulting and Clinical Psychology 61,* 202–204.

Miller, J. J., Fletcher, K., & Kabat-Zinn, J. (1995). Three-year follow-up and clinical implications of a mindfulness meditation-based stress reduction intervention in the treatment of anxiety disorders. *General Hospital Psychiatry 17*(3), 192–200.

Orsillo, S., & Roemer, L. (2005). *Acceptance and mindfulness-based approaches to anxiety: Conceptualization and treatment.* New York: Springer Publishing Company.

Salmon, P. G., Sephton, S. E., Weissbecker, I., Hoover, K., Ulmer, C., & Studts, J. L. (2004). Mindfulness meditation in clinical practice. *Cognitive and Behavioral Practice 11,* 434–446.

Santorelli, S. F. (1992). *A qualitative case analysis of mindfulness meditation training in an outpatient stress reduction clinic and its implications for self-knowledge.* Kalamazoo, MI: University Microfilms International.

Santorelli, S., & Kabat-Zinn, J. (2002). *Heal thy self: Lessons on mindfulness in medicine.* New York: Random House/Crown.

Santorelli, S. F. (1999). *Mindfulness-based stress reduction. Qualifications and recommended guidelines for providers.* Worcester, MA: Center for Mindfulness in Medicine, Healthcare, and Society.

Segal, Z., Williams, M., & Teasdale, J. D. (2002). *Mindfulness-based cognitive therapy for depression: A new approach to preventing relapse.* New York: Guilford Press.

Siegel, D. (2007). *The mindful brain.* New York: Norton.

Teasdale, J., Segal, Z. V., & Williams, J. M. (1995). How does cognitive therapy prevent depressive relapse and how should attentional control (mindfulness) training help? *Behavior Research and Therapy 1,* 25–39.

Teasdale, J. D., Moore, R. G., Hayhurst, H., Pope, M., Williams, J., & Segal, Z. V. (2002). Meta-cognitive awareness and prevention of relapse in depression: Empirical evidence. *Journal of Consulting & Clinical Psychology 70*(2), 275–287.

Teasdale, J. D., Segal, Z. V., Williams, J., Ridgeway, V., Soulsby, J., & Lau, M. A. (2000). Prevention of relapse/reoccurrence in major depression by mindfulness-based cognitive therapy. *Journal of Consulting and Clinical Psychology 68*(4), 615–623.

Thera, N. (1962). *The heart of Buddhist meditation.* New York: Weiser.

Toombs, S. (1993). *The meaning of illness: A phenomenological account of the different perspectives of physician and patient.* Dordrecht (Netherlands): Kluwer.

Wallace, B. (2006). *The attention revolution: Unlocking the power of the focused mind.* Boston: Wisdom.

Walsh, R., & Shapiro, S. L. (2006). The meeting of meditative disciplines and Western psychology: A mutually enriching dialogue. *American Psychologist, 61*(3), 227–239.

Williams, J., Teasdale, J., Segal, Z., & Kabat-Zinn, J. (2007). *The mindful way through depression: Freeing yourself from chronic unhappiness.* New York: Guilford Press.

Multiple Risk Behavior Change: What Most Individuals Need

15

Judith J. Prochaska and
Janice M. Prochaska

The co-occurrence of risk behaviors—such as tobacco and other substance use, poor quality diet, physical inactivity, stress, and distress—predicts a heightened risk of morbidity and mortality, as well as increased health care costs (Edington, Yen, & Witting, 1997). The majority of U.S. adults meets criteria for two or more behavioral risk factors (Fine, Philogene, Gramling, Coups, & Sinha, 2004; Pronk et al., 2004); yet, to date, most health promotion research has addressed risk factors as categorically separate entities.

Given a window of intervention opportunity, a higher impact paradigm is to target multiple behaviors. Growing evidence suggests the potential for multiple risk behavior change (MRBC) interventions to have much greater impact on public health than single-behavior interventions. In this chapter, we discuss the need for and evidence base of interventions that target multiple risk behaviors. Recent innovative studies are presented, and methodological, analytic, and theoretical issues unique to MRBC interventions are discussed. We close with consideration of dissemination issues and our vision for this growing area of research.

Background and Rationale for Multiple Risk Behavior Change

Background and Rationale

The major causes of morbidity and premature mortality in the United States—heart disease, cancer, and stroke—are influenced by multiple health behaviors, including smoking, alcohol abuse, physical inactivity, and poor diet. The 52-nation INTERHEART study identified tobacco use, obesity, high lipids, and psychosocial factors as accounting for about 90% of the population-attributable risks for myocardial infarction; fruit and vegetable consumption and exercise were identified as protective (Lanas et al., 2007; Yusuf et al., 2004). Mental illness, or stress and distress more broadly, also place a significant burden on health and productivity in the United States and globally (U.S. Department of Health & Human Services, 1999).

Individuals often struggle with multiple unhealthful behaviors, and there is evidence of co-occurrence among the risk factors. Analysis of data from the 2001 National Health Interview Study indicated that the majority of adults in the United States met criteria for two or more risk behaviors (Fine et al., 2004; Pronk et al., 2004). Tobacco users, in particular, tended to have poor behavioral profiles, with about 92% of smokers having at least one additional risk behavior (Fine et al., 2004; Klesges, Eck, Isbell, Fulliton, & Hanson, 1990; Pronk et al., 2004). In the United States, only 3% of adults met all four health behavior goals of being a nonsmoker, having a healthy weight, being physically active, and eating five or more fruits and vegetables a day (Reeves & Rafferty, 2005).

Among youth, there is evidence of a clustering of dietary patterns and physical activity (Sallis, Prochaska, & Taylor, 2000); tobacco use increases the likelihood of experimentation with illicit drug use (Lai, Lai, Page, & McCoy, 2000), and tobacco and other substance use is highly predictive markers for youth engagement in multiple risk behaviors, including bicycling without a helmet, perpetrating violence and carrying a weapon, not using a seat belt, and having suicidal ideation (DuRant, Smith, Kreiter, & Krowchuk, 1999).

The health care burden is believed to multiply with an increasing number of risk factors in terms of both medical consequences and costs (Edington et al., 1997). Put simply, excess risks lead to excess costs. Figures 15.1 and 15.2 at the end of this chapter show the incremental gain in pharmaceutical and disability costs due to excess risks. Longitudinal data indicate that effectively treating two behaviors reduces medical costs by about $2,000 per year (Edington, 2001). Targeting multiple risk behaviors for change offers the potential of greater health benefits, maximized health promotion opportunities, and reduced health care costs.

Lifestyle behaviors also may serve as a gateway to intervention on behaviors for which individuals have low motivation to change. Confidence or self-efficacy gained from making changes in one behavior may serve to support changes in additional risks. In a 3-year prospective study, individuals who quit smoking significantly increased their physical activity, whereas continued smokers did not (Perkins et al., 1993). Similar changes were not observed for diet or alcohol use. The change process appears to be similar for different health behaviors, and it may be efficient to work on multiple behaviors at the same time in a single intervention.

Given limited opportunity for health promotion contacts, interventions would ideally address all behaviors relevant to an individual's health profile. Researchers have emphasized that opportunities for intervening on multiple behaviors abound in the applied setting and have reasoned that specifically targeted interventions, even if effective, will be limited in their impact (Hayes, Barlow, & Nelson-Gray, 1999). A science of multibehavioral change is needed.

Definitions

MRBC interventions can be defined as efforts to treat two or more risk behaviors effectively within a limited time period simultaneously or sequentially. By risk behaviors, we mean actions in which individuals engage that impact health. The impact can be negative, as with tobacco and other drug use and risky sexual behaviors, or positive, as with physical activity, fruit and vegetable consumption, and the wearing of helmets or seatbelts. Medical screening behaviors, such as mammography, colonoscopy, cholesterol testing, blood pressure screening, HIV tests, and glucose screening, also are clearly relevant to health and disease prevention and may be included as behavioral targets in MRBC interventions.

The field of MRBC research is at an early stage, with its boundaries still being defined. Historically, much of the research has focused on changing multiple risk behaviors within populations; fewer studies have targeted multiple risks within individuals; and the distinction is meaningful. When MRBC interventions are focused on populations, a program of interventions is offered to a community and community members receive intervention only on the behaviors for which they are identified as at risk. For example, only smokers in a community would receive the quit-smoking program, while individuals with high-fat diets would receive the nutrition intervention and individuals at risk for both smoking and high fat-diet would receive both intervention components. Changes are reported at the population level as a change in means or prevalence rates (e.g., smoking rates). With greater behavioral targets, the relevance of the intervention to the community and systems being served is increased as all members are likely to be at risk for at least one of the targeted behaviors.

When MRBC interventions target multiple risks in individuals, all individuals receive intervention on all targeted behaviors. The potential impact on an individual's health is increased, as are the behavior change demands. MRBC interventions within individuals may be relevant to only a select high-risk group, since participants need to be at risk for all targeted behaviors, though this may be less of an issue with behaviors that co-occur at high rates, such as alcohol and tobacco use or physical inactivity and poor diet. If the intervention promotes concurrent immediate action in multiple behaviors, it may be overwhelming and result in poor adherence. Sequencing change goals or matching intervention strategies to individuals' readiness to change may facilitate greater adherence and overall change.

To summarize, the main difference between MRBC interventions at the population level and similar interventions at the individual level is that the former matches the intervention strategies to the risk needs of the participants within the community, whereas the latter delivers all interventions to all participants. The former provides interventions more broadly to everyone in the community, while the latter focuses on a more select high-risk group.

Reviews of Multiple Risk Behavior Change Intervention Studies

Studies of MRBC Interventions in Populations

The concept of intervening on multiple risk behaviors concurrently became a focus of attention in the early 1970s and was targeted at preventing cardiovascular disease (CVD) (Labarthe, 1998). One early proposal was a factorial design to evaluate the independent contributions and the joint effects of targeting diet, physical activity, and smoking habits in a single trial, named "Jumbo." The proposal was deemed too costly, however, and the trial was never conducted. Large-scale multifactorial CVD risk factor interventions that were conducted include the Multiple Risk Factor Intervention Trial (MRFIT), the North Karelia Project, the Stanford Three-City and Five-City Projects, and the Pawtucket and Minnesota Heart Health Programs. Youth multifactor interventions also were developed, with a movement toward comprehensive school health programs.

The multibehavioral studies conducted over the past 30 years have had a range of outcomes, from favorable to unfavorable. The interventions have focused almost entirely on practitioner-based modalities such as health advice and counseling from a physician, dietician, or nurse; home visits; and group health education. Community-level promotional materials also have been incorporated. Significant changes were often seen in some but not all targeted behaviors (Emmons, Marcus, Linnan, Rossi, & Abrams, 1994; Sorensen et al., 1996). A Cochrane review of these large multifactor interventions estimated the net reduction in smoking prevalence at 20% (Ebrahim, Beswick, Burke, & Davey Smith, 2006). Changes in dietary and physical activity behaviors, unfortunately, were not reported in the review. The pooled effects suggested that the MRBC interventions had no effect on mortality.

Findings from 14 youth obesity prevention studies that targeted physical activity and dietary change were summarized in another Cochrane review (Summerbell et al., 2005). The studies were conducted in schools and communities, with children and adolescents, in the United States and Europe, representing a diversity of ethnic groups and socioeconomic levels. Most of the studies followed a social learning or environmental theoretical framework. Only 1 of the 14 studies achieved significant changes in both dietary and physical activity behaviors, with the finding significant only for girls and not for boys (Gortmaker et al., 1999). This same study was the only one to report significant reductions in youth body mass index; again, however, the finding was specific to girls.

A recent Dutch, school-based, obesity prevention intervention used individual and environmental components (Singh, Paw, Brug, & van Mechelen, 2007). The intervention yielded significant reductions in waist-to-hip ratio for girls and boys and in the sum of skin fold measurements for girls. Changes in body mass index and fitness, however, were not statistically significant, and changes in physical activity and dietary behaviors were not reported.

Recent Successes in Population-Based MRBC Interventions

While many of the attempts at achieving change in multiple risk behaviors within populations have met with limited success, the story does not end there. Here we describe several recent examples of innovative interventions that have succeeded in stimulating change in multiple risk behaviors and discuss some of the potential reasons for their successes.

Historically, researchers and practitioners have used an action paradigm, prescribing immediate action in a risk behavior. Pushing individuals to make behavioral changes in more than one area, however, can have negative effects. For example, less than 10% of smokers are prepared to take action on more than one risk behavior (Prochaska, Velicer, Prochaska, Delucchi, & Hall, 2006). When instructed to change multiple behavioral risks, individuals can become overwhelmed, disillusioned, and ineffective at making any behavior changes.

In contrast to action-oriented paradigms, which promote immediate action among all participants, the Transtheoretical Model (TTM) recommends tailoring of strategies to an individual's intention and readiness to change (Prochaska, DiClemente, & Norcross, 1992). Briefly, the TTM has identified five stages of change defined as *precontemplation,* not intending to change; *contemplation,* intending to change within the next 6 months; *preparation,* actively planning change within the next 30 days; *action,* overtly making changes; and *maintenance,* taking steps to sustain change and resist temptation to relapse. To be in action, individuals are required to meet some behavioral criterion for some minimal amount of time (e.g., quit smoking for 24 hours). With most behaviors, the action stage has been defined as lasting up to 6 months, at which time the individual enters maintenance. Other key TTM constructs are decisional balance, or the pros and cons of change, and self-efficacy, operationalized as situational confidence in changing a behavior and situational temptations to engage in a problem behavior. Using the TTM or stage-of-change paradigm, there is consistent evidence supporting multiple risk behavior change (e.g., Johnson et al., 2006; Jones et al., 2003; Prochaska et al., 2004; Prochaska et al., 2005).

Three parallel TTM population-based MRBC studies targeted smoking, high-fat diet, and high-risk sun exposure (Prochaska et al., 2005; Prochaska et al., 2004; Velicer et al., 2004). The studies were conducted with employees in worksites, parents of high school students, and patients in primary care. The interventions used computerized expert system interventions delivering tailored individualized feedback based on participants' responses to measures of the key TTM constructs. The expert system was repeated at three time points over a 6-month period, and feedback was provided on the basis of both normative data and participants' earlier responses. Combined, the studies included nearly 10,000 participants. Participants assigned to the TTM intervention group received treatment for the behavior(s) for which they were identified as being at risk on the basis of their baseline stage of change. In all three studies, across all three behaviors, treatment effects were significant at 12- and 24-month follow-up, with the exception of smoking in the worksite study, which had a relatively small number of smokers. Importantly, the smoking cessation effects obtained in these TTM-based MRBC studies were comparable to previously reported intervention effects for TTM studies focused on smoking alone (Prochaska et al., 2006). Further, among smokers in the three trials, treatment of one or two coexisting risk factors (diet and/or sun exposure) did not decrease the effectiveness of smoking cessation treatment, and treatment for the coexisting factors was effective, as well.

Targeting individuals with high cholesterol, another population-based TTM intervention reported significant effects on lipid medication adherence, physical activity, and dietary fat reduction. The treatment group was 50% more likely than the control group to make changes to reach the criterion for action on all three behaviors (Johnson et al., 2006).

The unique advantage of TTM interventions for multiple risk behavior change is that the likelihood of overwhelming participants is greatly reduced and the proportion of the at-risk population participating is likely to be greatly increased, since immediate action is not demanded. With proactive recruitment strategies such as random digit dialing, TTM studies have consistently reported participation rates of 80% or greater (Prochaska et al., 2004; Velicer et al., 2004). Importantly, strategies are matched to participants' readiness to change, and all participants at risk are supported through the change process.

Social cognitive theory, which focuses on the interaction of personal factors, behavior, and the environment, also has been applied to multiple risk behaviors with some success (Bandura, 1986). PREVENT, a telephone-delivered intervention plus tailored materials, based on motivation to change and social-cognitive theory, targeted six behavioral factors in determining colon cancer risk: red meat consumption, fruit and vegetable intake, multivitamin intake, alcohol, smoking, and physical inactivity (Emmons et al., 2005). Participants were 1,247 adults with recent diagnoses of adenomatous colorectal polyps. Intervention participants were more likely to change two or more risk behaviors than were those in the standard care condition. For the individual behaviors, intervention effects were significant for improved multivitamin intake and reduced red meat consumption, and there was less regression in physical activity levels among those receiving intervention over the course of the study. There were no between-condition differences in smoking, alcohol, or fruit and vegetable consumption.

The Mediterranean Lifestyle Program is another successful example of a population-level MRBC intervention (Toobert et al., 2007). This randomized clinical trial for postmenopausal women with type 2 diabetes employed social learning theory to guide intervention strategies to address healthful eating, physical activity, stress management, smoking cessation, and social support. At 12 and 24 months, intervention participants demonstrated improvements in all targeted lifestyle behaviors except smoking (there were too few smokers to analyze effects of the intervention on tobacco use). Additionally, significant treatment effects were seen in psychosocial measures of use of supportive resources, problem solving, self-efficacy, and quality of life.

Studies of MRBC Interventions in Individuals

Few studies have directly compared the effectiveness of multifactor interventions within individuals to that of single-factor interventions, and findings have been inconsistent. A recent review of MRBC interventions in primary care identified large gaps in the field's knowledge base (Goldstein, Whitlock, & DePue, 2004). The review emphasized the successes of interventions targeted on single risks, such as tobacco use, alcohol use, poor diet, and, to a lesser extent, physical inactivity, but acknowledged the dearth of studies in primary care aimed at treating multiple risks.

The strongest evidence for MRBC interventions in individuals has aimed at secondary rather than primary prevention, specifically interventions focused on individuals at high risk for or already diagnosed with CVD (Ketola, Sipila, & Makela, 2002) or diabetes (Norris, Engelgau, & Narayan, 2001). These interventions have targeted tobacco use, physical inactivity, and poor diet, as well as more specific disease management care, for example, adherence to lipid-lowering drugs and hypertensives for those with CVD and blood glucose monitoring and foot exams for those with diabetes. Even in these studies, while the evidence generally has been strong for short-term effects, sustained effects have been difficult to achieve.

A notable exception is the Lifestyle Heart Trial for patients with moderate to severe CVD. The intensive intervention promotes a 10% fat whole foods vegetarian diet, aerobic exercise, stress management, and smoking cessation and provides group psychosocial support. In a small efficacy trial (N = 48), program adherence was reported as excellent and significant intervention effects were seen at 1 and 5 years for reductions in weight and LDL cholesterol, as well as reduction in arterial diameter stenosis and cardiac events (Ornish et al., 1998).

Individuals with drug and alcohol problems are another high-risk patient group of interest for multibehavioral change. In particular, rates of tobacco use are high, and tobacco is a primary cause of death among individuals treated for substance abuse (Hser, McCarthy, & Anglin, 1994; Hurt et al., 1996). The health effects of tobacco and other substance use appear synergistic, 50% greater than the sum of each individually (Bien & Burge, 1990). Historically, clinical lore has discouraged smoking cessation efforts during addictions treatment out of concern that sobriety would be compromised. Tobacco has been viewed as the last remaining vice among those in recovery and a necessary behavioral crutch. A recent meta-analysis examined this issue in 12 randomized controlled smoking cessation interventions delivered to individuals in substance abuse treatment (Prochaska, Delucchi, & Hall, 2004). The interventions were built on a variety of theoretical frameworks, including stage-based or motivational enhancement, cognitive-behavioral therapy, relapse prevention, and pharmacological treatments. Smoking cessation effects were significant at post-treatment but were not sustained at long-term follow-up. Importantly, exposure to the smoking cessation interventions was associated with a 25% increased likelihood of long-term abstinence from alcohol and illicit drugs. The study concluded that, contrary to previous concerns, smoking cessation interventions delivered during addictions treatment appeared to enhance rather than compromise long-term sobriety.

Tobacco treatment studies also have examined the impact of incorporating strategies to prevent weight gain, a common side effect and a potential deterrent to quitting smoking. Efforts to integrate dietary restraint components within tobacco treatment interventions, however, have raised concerns about their potential deleterious effects on motivation to quit smoking (Hall, Tunstall, Vila, & Duffy, 1992). Clinical tobacco treatment guidelines even discourage weight control efforts through dieting so as not to detract from motivations to quit smoking (Fiore et al., 2000). As with tobacco cessation among substance users, the concern is with multiple intervention interference—that change in one behavior may negatively impact change in another.

When there is concern about multiple intervention interference, a sequential treatment approach may be undertaken. A recent study compared the effect of a dietary intervention implemented early in the quit attempt to those of an after-cessation effort and a no-diet control program (Spring et al., 2004). The study reported no difference in smoking cessation rates among the three groups, with some advantage in weight gain prevention among participants in the delayed diet group. Similarly, a recent study evaluating immediate and delayed smoking cessation among veterans in substance abuse treatment reported comparable quit smoking rates, with some apparent benefit to sobriety among participants treated for tobacco use in the delayed-treatment group (Joseph, Willenbring, Nugent, & Nelson, 2004).

Another study examining the impact of simultaneous and sequential targeting of multiple risks concluded that sequential targeting was not superior to, and may be inferior to, a simultaneous approach (Hyman, Pavlik, Taylor, Goodrick, & Moye, 2007). The intervention used stage-based counseling and promoted changes in physical activity, dietary sodium intake, and tobacco use. The theoretical model employed and the types of behaviors targeted certainly may influence the efficacy of a simultaneous and a sequential approach. More research is needed to address this key intervention design issue.

Health behaviors also may be used as a treatment strategy. For example, the effect of exercise for supporting smoking cessation has been tested. A Cochrane review concluded that while exercise promotion did not appear to harm smoking cessation efforts, there was limited evidence that it helped (Ussher, 2005). Only 1 of the 11 identified trials found evidence for exercise aiding smoking cessation at long-term follow-up (Marcus et al., 1999). Unfortunately, only two of the studies reported changes in physical activity, limiting our understanding of the feasibility of efforts to help smokers make changes in their tobacco use and exercise patterns concurrently. Of note, the one study that had significant effects for both quitting smoking and increasing fitness was based on the TTM and matched exercise and smoking cessation strategies to participants' readiness to quit, rather than prescribing immediate action (Marcus et al., 1999).

Co-occurring mental illness often is an exclusionary criterion for clinical trials, and, as a result, the field knows very little about intervening on multiple risks with those with mental problems. Two recent innovative studies, by separate research teams, evaluated tobacco treatments among smokers with current mental illness—one focused on clinically depressed outpatients (Hall et al., 2006) and the other on veterans with posttraumatic stress disorder (McFall et al., 2006). Both reported significant intervention effects for long-term smoking cessation with no adverse effects on mental health functioning (Prochaska, Hall, et al., 2008). The study with veterans demonstrated the value of integrating tobacco treatment into mental health services, rather than referring out to a separate system of care.

Two other trials examined exercise as a treatment for clinical depression and reported significant changes in physical activity with significant reductions in depressive symptoms (Blumenthal et al., 1999; Dunn, Trivedi, Kampert, Clark, & Chambliss, 2005). The immediate effects of exercise in treating depression were comparable to those of antidepressant medication, with a significantly lower likelihood of depression relapse over time (Babyak et al., 2000). Further, individuals with clinical depression rank exercise among the most commonly tried and effective self-help strategy for managing depression (Parker & Crawford, 2007).

Methodological Issues

Methodological challenges with multibehavioral interventions include the increased time and participant demands for intervention and evaluation components and the lack of direction in the field on how best to conceptualize and analyze multiple risk behavior change.

Measuring Changes in Multiple Risk Behaviors

Approaches taken to minimize assessment and participant burden include efforts to simplify assessment tools, while maintaining rigorous psychometrics, and movement toward more technologically sophisticated and, one hopes, more objective, assessment tools that ideally reduce the burden on participants for data collection. Health risk appraisals are one option for quickly assessing engagement in a wide range of risk behaviors (Smith, McKinlay, & McKinlay, 1989).

More objective behavioral measures include biochemical measures of dietary changes (e.g., plasma carotenoid concentrations), tobacco (e.g., cotinine, anabasine), and other drug use; biometric measures of physical activity (pedometers, accelerometers) and fitness (VO2max); and computerized innovations to assess medication adherence (e.g., MEMScaps). All measures, of course, have their limitations. With biometrics, a metabolite's half-life may be too short to detect sustained behavioral changes, research costs can be high, and participants may not adhere to assessment protocols. In the tobacco arena, consensus guidelines have been developed recommending when bio-information is and is not necessary (Society for Research on Nicotine and Tobacco, 2002).

Alternatively, rather than measuring changes separately for each targeted behavior, measures may be incorporated to conceptualize and assess overall health outcomes due to changes in multiple risks. Examples include changes in weight, blood pressure, cholesterol, or blood glucose due to changes in diet, exercise, and/or tobacco use. Self-report measures of overarching change may include health-related quality of life (Rasanen et al., 2006). The Mediterranean Life Program, for example, reported changes in behavioral, psychological, and quality of life measures (Toobert et al., 2007). Economic measures may include medical, pharmaceutical, and disability costs (see Figures 15.1 and 15.2). If MRBC interventions ultimately aim to maximize health outcomes, then measures should assess these gains. Longer follow-up periods, however, will likely be necessary to detect changes in these more distal outcomes.

15.1

Excess pharmaceutical costs due to excess risks, age and gender adjusted.

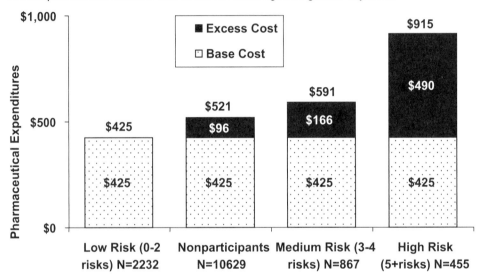

15.2

Excess disability costs due to excess risks.

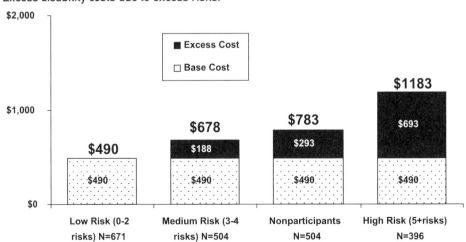

Analyzing Changes in Multiple Risk Behaviors

Use of overarching, integrative measures also would serve to simplify analysis of outcomes in MRBC interventions. Historically, MRBC interventions have included separate measures for each risk behavior targeted, sometimes incorporating multiple measures for each behavior. The consequence is multiple significance testing with the potential for inflating the type I error rate, as well as creating confusion by describing inconsistent findings across the different outcomes.

Indices of MRBC have been proposed as a way of combining changes in separate risk behaviors, although no standard exists and questions remain about whether behaviors should be weighted with respect to mortality risk. Examples include the Framingham Heart Study risk score; the Cooper Clinic mortality risk index; cancer risk indices; dietary quality indices; and an index of early problem behaviors (Janssen, Katzmarzyk, Church, & Blair, 2005; McGue, Iacono, & Krueger, 2006; Patterson, Haines, & Popkin, 1994; Wilson et al., 1998).

Another alternative is creating an index of behavior change scores. If the behavioral measures to be combined are on different scales—for example, minutes of physical activity and servings of fruits and vegetables—a statistical transformation will be necessary. Standardized change scores can be created by subtracting baseline scores from the follow-up scores and then dividing by the standard deviation of the difference (i.e., z-score). The scores can then be summed into a combined behavioral index, which indicates the amount of increase or decrease in the combined behaviors from baseline to follow-up. Alternatively, standardized residuals from linear regressions of follow-up scores on baseline measures provide a simple change score adjusted for baseline variance. Residualized change scores are referred to as "base-free" measures of change (Tucker, Damarin, & Messick, 1966) and are viewed as superior to simple pretest-posttest differences in scores (Veldman & Brophy, 1974).

Impact Factor

The significance of intervention effects is moderated by the generalizability of the individuals willing to participate. An important outcome measure that incorporates intervention efficacy and participation rates is impact. Impact is increased by greater intervention efficacy and greater participation among individuals in the target population. For interventions targeting single-risk behaviors, impact has been measured as intervention efficacy (E) times participation (P) or $I = E \times P$. In MRBC interventions, measures for assessing impact need to account for the number of behaviors treated effectively. In MRBC interventions, impact may be considered as intervention efficacy times participation summed over the multiple behavioral targets, $I = \Sigma_{\text{# of behaviors(n)}} (E_n \times P_n)$. Here, P is the proportion of at-risk individuals participating in the intervention for each behavior. E is the estimate of efficacy for each behavior. Use of a common metric, such as the percentage no longer at risk (i.e., the percent reaching Action or Maintenance), allows for summation across behaviors. This revised-impact equation provides a measure for assessing the impact of interventions for treating individuals and populations with multiple behavior risks.

Theory Testing Across Behaviors

Theories of behavior and behavior change have been applied across a wide variety of risk factors, demonstrating that the same skills can be applied to multiple behaviors. A model of lifestyle behavior change has suggested that with behaviors that co-occur (e.g., alcohol abuse and smoking), change in one may support change in the other (Wankel & Sefton, 1994). At this time, however, no theory of behavior change directly addresses the issue of how to intervene on more than one behavior simultaneously.

The Transtheoretical Model (TTM) of behavior change, discussed earlier, was developed in the area of smoking cessation and has demonstrated relevance to over 20 problem or target behaviors (Hall & Rossi, 2005; Prochaska et al., 1994). Across multiple health behaviors, significant cross-sectional associations have been found with the TTM mediators of change. Among adults, the pros and cons for smoking were inversely associated with the pros and cons of exercising (King, Marcus, Pinto, Emmons, & Abrams, 1996). That is, individuals rating the benefits of smoking highly were less likely to endorse the benefits of physical activity as self-important. Self-efficacy for smoking cessation also was significantly related to self-efficacy for exercise. While the data were cross-sectional in nature, the authors concluded that the associations provide preliminary evidence for how change in one behavior may be related to change in another. Individuals working on increasing their physical activity seem motivated and confident about decreasing their smoking and vice versa. Similarly, Unger (1996) observed that adults in the later stages of change for smoking cessation had more healthful levels of alcohol use and exercised more than subjects in the earlier stages of change, suggesting people changing on their own may make improvements in several health behaviors concurrently.

The PREVENT trial, which utilized social cognitive theory, broadened intervention goals to include raising participants' self-efficacy for changing multiple risks by helping them recognize the natural intersections among their risky health habits. General cognitive and behavioral skills also were taught for application in changing any of their risk behaviors (Emmons et al., 2005).

The National Institutes of Health, the American Heart Association, and the Robert Wood Johnson Foundation jointly funded a Behavior Change Consortium (BCC) focused on multiple risk behavior change. The BCC studies include assessment of the utility of different theoretical models for changing two or more health risk behaviors (Nigg, Allegrante, & Ory, 2002). The field looks forward to the findings from these theory-comparison and MRBC research studies.

Considerations for Dissemination

Most of the early successes in MRBC interventions were achieved in research clinics or specialty settings, and serious considerations need to be taken into account when planning for dissemination. From the practitioner's perspective, there are legitimate concerns about addressing more than one behavioral risk at a time. It can be very challenging for health care professionals to try to impact behavioral changes through counseling or other forms of intervention within short medical appointments. One recent clever health message for promoting changes in multiple risk behaviors is 0–5–10–25, indicating 0 cigarettes, 5 servings of fruits and vegetables, 10,000 steps, and a body mass index of less than 25 (Reeves & Rafferty, 2005).

In designing programs for dissemination, key considerations include: (1) involving the target population and organizations in intervention design and development; (2) reducing individual and organizational barriers to participation; and (3) being mindful of feasibility issues and the breadth of appeal of the intervention to the target system (Nigg et al., 2002).

Experts in the field have concluded that using interactive behavior change technologies and tailored feedback are the current best practices for addressing multiple risks in primary care (Glasgow, Bull, Piette, & Steiner, 2004; Goldstein et al., 2004). Interactive behavior change technologies have been praised for offering a viable solution to the otherwise overwhelming problem of addressing prevention effectively in primary care. Computer-delivered expert system interventions are self-directed, generate tailored feedback to participants, maintain treatment fidelity, and are an important dissemination option.

Moving beyond the clinic, schools and worksites are becoming important channels for distribution of multiple risk behavior changes. Expert systems can reside on a school's Web server with multimedia components provided on a CD-ROM to minimize download time. Teachers do not require additional training, as their main responsibility is to assist students in starting and completing the program. The programs provide a private interaction for youth to address sensitive issues such as experiences with bullying and experimentation with substance use. Because the programs are tailored to individuals' readiness to adopt or cease a risk behavior, they are broadly relevant to the populations served. Within a worksite, employees can take a comprehensive health risk appraisal online and then be guided to work on their identified risk behaviors. In addition to computer-tailored feedback, participants can be referred to a self-help interactive workbook with activities to increase engagement in effective change processes.

As one example of success with disseminating MRBC interventions to clinics, schools, and worksites, Pro-Change Behavior Systems, with funding from the National Institutes of Health, has focused on developing and disseminating evidence-based behavior change programs. The programs utilize stage-based expert system interventions to target multiple risk behaviors, including weight gain (physical inactivity and poor diet), substance use, tobacco use, bullying, interpersonal violence, and high cholesterol. The programs have been disseminated nationally to more than 500 schools, 100 worksites, and 200,000 adults and youths. The programs have been well received and well used and have delivered significant impacts on multiple behavioral risks (Evers, Prochaska, Van Marter, Johnson, & Prochaska, 2007; Mauriello et al., 2006; Mauriello, Sherman, Driskell, & Prochaska, 2007).

The Internet provides a convenient option for dissemination, but it still can be difficult to engage individuals. In the research literature, Internet-delivered intervention trials have reported participation rates as low as 2% to 10% and retention rates as low as 20% (Glasgow et al., 2007; Rothert et al., 2006). Through our research and dissemination practices, we have found that participation rates range greatly based on the types of incentives employed (see Table 15.1).

15.1 Recruitment Incentives and Participation Rates		
Recruitment incentives	Mechanism	Participation rate
Persuasive messages in letter or e-mails with or without a token incentive (e.g., T-shirt or $15 coupon)	social influence	20%–30%
Positive reinforcement in the form of $150 to $300	social influence	40%–50%
Personal outreach through face-to-face or phone call contact	social influence	60%–70%
Negative reinforcement by requiring all nonparticipants to face some increase in financial payment for their health care plan for not participating	social control	80%–90% (but do get negative reactions)

Vision for the Future

The need for multiple risk, transbehavioral research models and paradigms has been identified (Orleans, 2004). Specific research questions include "whether, or in which situations, multiple risk factor interventions are *more* effective or efficient at reducing risk than targeted single interventions" (Atkins & Clancy, 2004). For example, some attribute the success of tobacco-cessation initiatives to a narrowly focused research and policy agenda. Research is needed to determine under what conditions multiple risks can be targeted without diminishing the effectiveness on any single behavior (Atkins & Clancy, 2004). Other areas in need of greater research are interventions that integrate efforts to change multiple risk behaviors, as well as interventions that teach change strategies that can be generalized to multiple behavior change goals. With increased interest in MRBC interventions, the field will need ways to conceptualize and analyze the issue of overall behavior change (Prochaska, Velicer, et al., 2008).

    If the challenge of MRBC intervention is met, health promotion and disease management programs will significantly effect entire populations. Such impacts require scientific and professional shifts from:

1. An action paradigm to a stage paradigm;
2. Reactive recruitment to a public health approach of proactive recruitment (that is, reaching out proactively to individuals and populations to engage them in MRBC interventions, rather than waiting passively in the clinic to react to the small proportion of patients who will seek services);
3. The expectation that participants must match the needs of programs to the understanding that programs must match their needs;

4. Clinic-based to population-based programs that are able to apply the field's most powerful individualized and interactive intervention strategies;
5. Single-behavior-change programs to MRBC programs for entire populations.

If the health behavior change field makes these paradigm shifts, a behavior health delivery system could be developed to reach many more people with behaviors that are the major killers and cost drivers in the United States.

How can population approaches to health promotion be funded? Longitudinal data indicate that effectively treating two behaviors reduces health care costs by about $2,000 per year (Edington, 2001). For worksites, the return on investment (ROI) for employee participation in MRBC programs is estimated at 1.98 over 3 years' time, on the basis of reductions in absenteeism and workers compensation hours, nearly a two-fold return on investment (Schultz et al., 2002). Population-based behavioral medicine is one of the few opportunities for health care systems to increase services that improve health and reduce health care costs. Over time, population-based prevention programs could pay for themselves.

We can envision a health care system in the near future where interactive MRBC interventions will be to behavioral medicine what pharmaceuticals are to biological medicine: one of the most cost-effective methods to bring optimal amounts of science to bear on multiple behavior problems, in entire populations, in a relatively user-friendly manner, without many of the side effects seen with pharmaceuticals.

References

Atkins, D., & Clancy, C. (2004). Multiple risk factors interventions. Are we up to the challenge? *American Journal of Preventive Medicine, 27*(2 Suppl.), 102–103.

Babyak, M., Blumenthal, J. A., Herman, S., Khatri, P., Doraiswamy, M., Moore, K., et al. (2000). Exercise treatment for major depression: Maintenance of therapeutic benefit at 10 months. *Psychosomatic Medicine, 62*(5), 633–638.

Bandura, A. (1986). *Social foundations of thought and action: A social cognitive theory.* Englewood Cliffs, NJ: Prentice-Hall.

Bien, T. H., & Burge, R. (1990). Smoking and drinking: A review of the literature. *International Journal of Mental Health & Addiction, 25*(12), 1429–1454.

Blumenthal, J. A., Babyak, M. A., Moore, K. A., Craighead, W. E., Herman, S., Khatri, P., et al. (1999). Effects of exercise training on older patients with major depression. *Archives of Internal Medicine, 159*(19), 2349–2356.

Burton, W. N., Chen, C. Y., Conti, D. J., Schultz, A. B., & Edington, D. W. (2003). Measuring the relationship between employees' health risk factors and corporate pharmaceutical expenditures. *Journal of Occupational and Environmental Medicine, 45*(8), 793–802.

Burton, W. N., Chen, C. Y., Conti, D. J., Schultz, A. B., Pransky, G., & Edington, D. W. (2005). The association of health risks with on-the-job productivity. *Journal of Occupational and Environmental Medicine, 47*(8), 769–777.

Dunn, A. L., Trivedi, M. H., Kampert, J. B., Clark, C. G., & Chambliss, H. O. (2005). Exercise treatment for depression: Efficacy and dose response. *American Journal of Preventive Medicine, 28*(1), 1–8.

DuRant, R. H., Smith, J. A., Kreiter, S. R., & Krowchuk, D. P. (1999). The relationship between early age of onset of initial substance use and engaging in multiple health risk behaviors among young adolescents. *Archives of Pediatric & Adolescent Medicine, 153*(3), 286–291.

Ebrahim, S., Beswick, A., Burke, M., & Davey Smith, G. (2006). Multiple risk factor interventions for primary prevention of coronary heart disease. *Cochrane Database of Systematic Reviews* (4), CD001561.

Edington, D. W. (2001). Emerging research: A view from one research center. *American Journal of Health Promotion, 15*(5), 341–349.

Edington, D. W., Yen, L. T., & Witting, P. (1997). The financial impact of changes in personal health practices. *Journal of Occupational & Environmental Medicine, 39*(11), 1037–1046.

Emmons, K. M., Marcus, B. H., Linnan, L., Rossi, J. S., & Abrams, D. B. (1994). Mechanisms in multiple risk factor interventions: Smoking, physical activity, and dietary fat intake among manufacturing workers. Working Well Research Group. *Preventive Medicine, 23*(4), 481–489.

Emmons, K. M., McBride, C. M., Puleo, E., Pollak, K. I., Clipp, E., Kuntz, K., et al. (2005). Project PREVENT: A randomized trial to reduce multiple behavioral risk factors for colon cancer. *Cancer Epidemiology Biomarkers & Prevention, 14*(6), 1453–1459.

Evers, K. E., Prochaska, J. O., Van Marter, D., Johnson, J. L., & Prochaska, J. M. (2007). Transtheoretical-based bullying prevention effectiveness trial in middle schools and high schools. *Educational Research, 49,* 397–414.

Fine, L. J., Philogene, G. S., Gramling, R., Coups, E. J., & Sinha, S. (2004). Prevalence of multiple chronic disease risk factors. 2001 National Health Interview Survey. *American Journal of Preventive Medicine, 27*(2 Suppl.), 18–24.

Fiore, M. C., & the Tobacco Use and Dependence Clinical Practice Guideline Panel, Staff, and Consortium Representatives. (2000). A clinical practice guideline for treating tobacco use and dependence: A U.S. public health service report. *Journal of the American Medical Association, 283*(24), 3244–3254.

Glasgow, R. E., Bull, S. S., Piette, J. D., & Steiner, J. F. (2004). Interactive behavior change technology. A partial solution to the competing demands of primary care. *American Journal of Preventive Medicine, 27*(2 Suppl.), 80–87.

Glasgow, R. E., Nelson, C. C., Kearney, K. A., Reid, R., Ritzwoller, D. P., Strecher, V. J., et al. (2007). Reach, engagement, and retention in an Internet-based weight loss program in a multi-site randomized controlled trial. *Journal of Medical Internet Research, 9*(2), e11.

Goldstein, M. G., Whitlock, E. P., & DePue, J. (2004). Multiple behavioral risk factor interventions in primary care. Summary of research evidence. *American Journal of Preventive Medicine, 27*(2 Suppl.), 61–79.

Gortmaker, S. L., Peterson, K., Wiecha, J., Sobol, A. M., Dixit, S., Fox, M. K., et al. (1999). Reducing obesity via a school-based interdisciplinary intervention among youth: Planet Health. *Archives of Pediatric & Adolescent Medicine, 153*(4), 409–418.

Hall, K. L., & Rossi, J. S. (2005). A meta-analysis of the processes of change across 20 behaviors: Testing theory and informing interventions. *Annals of Behavioral Medicine, 29,* S162.

Hall, S. M., Tsoh, J. Y., Prochaska, J. J., Eisendrath, S., Rossi, J. S., Redding, C. A., et al. (2006). Treatment for cigarette smoking among depressed mental health outpatients: A randomized clinical trial. *American Journal of Public Health, 96*(10), 1808–1814.

Hall, S. M., Tunstall, C. D., Vila, K. L., & Duffy, J. (1992). Weight gain prevention and smoking cessation: Cautionary findings. *American Journal of Public Health, 82*(6), 799–803.

Hayes, S. C., Barlow, D. H., & Nelson-Gray, R. O. (1999). *The scientist practitioner: Research and accountability in the age of managed care* (2nd ed.). Boston: Allyn & Bacon.

Hser, Y. I., McCarthy, W. J., & Anglin, M. D. (1994). Tobacco use as a distal predictor of mortality among long-term narcotics addicts. *Preventive Medicine, 23*(1), 61–69.

Hurt, R. D., Offord, K. P., Croghan, I. T., Gomez-Dahl, L., Kottke, T. E., Morse, R. M., et al. (1996). Mortality following inpatient addictions treatment. Role of tobacco use in a community-based cohort. *Journal of the American Medical Association, 275*(14), 1097–1103.

Hyman, D. J., Pavlik, V. N., Taylor, W. C., Goodrick, G. K., & Moye, L. (2007). Simultaneous vs sequential counseling for multiple behavior change. *Archives of Internal Medicine, 167*(11), 1152–1158.

Janssen, I., Katzmarzyk, P. T., Church, T. S., & Blair, S. N. (2005). The Cooper Clinic Mortality Risk Index: Clinical score sheet for men. *American Journal of Preventive Medicine, 29*(3), 194–203.

Johnson, S. S., Driskell, M. M., Johnson, J. L., Dyment, S. J., Prochaska, J. O., Prochaska, J. M., et al. (2006). Transtheoretical model intervention for adherence to lipid-lowering drugs. *Disease Management, 9*(2), 102–114.

Jones, H., Edwards, L., Vallis, T. M., Ruggiero, L., Rossi, S. R., Rossi, J. S., et al. (2003). Changes in diabetes self-care behaviors make a difference in glycemic control: The Diabetes Stages of Change (DiSC) study. *Diabetes Care, 26*(3), 732–737.

Joseph, A.M., Willenbring, M. L., Nugent, S. M., & Nelson, D. B. (2004). A randomized trial of concurrent versus delayed smoking intervention for patients in alcohol dependence treatment. *Journal of Studies on Alcohol, 65*(6), 681–691.

Ketola, E., Sipila, R., & Makela, M. (2002). Effectiveness of individual lifestyle interventions in reducing cardiovascular disease and risk factors. *Annals of Medicine, 32*(4), 239–251.

King, T. K., Marcus, B. H., Pinto, B. M., Emmons, K. M., & Abrams, D. B. (1996). Cognitive-behavioral mediators of changing multiple behaviors: Smoking and a sedentary lifestyle. *Preventive Medicine, 25*(6), 684–691.

Klesges, R. C., Eck, L. H., Isbell, T. R., Fulliton, W., & Hanson, C. L. (1990). Smoking status: Effects on the dietary intake, physical activity, and body fat of adult men. *American Journal of Clinical Nutrition, 51*(5), 784–789.

Labarthe, D. R. (1998). *Epidemiology and prevention of cardiovascular disease: A global challenge.* Gaithersburg, MD: Aspen.

Lai, S., Lai, H., Page, J. B., & McCoy, C. B. (2000). The association between cigarette smoking and drug abuse in the United States. *Journal of Addictive Diseases, 19*(4), 11–24.

Lanas, F., Avezum, A., Bautista, L. E., Diaz, R., Luna, M., Islam, S., et al. (2007). Risk factors for acute myocardial infarction in Latin America: The INTERHEART Latin American study. *Circulation, 115*(9), 1067–1074.

Marcus, B. H., Albrecht, A. E., King, T. K., Parisi, A. F., Pinto, B. M., Roberts, M., et al. (1999). The efficacy of exercise as an aid for smoking cessation in women: A randomized controlled trial. *Archives of Internal Medicine, 159*(11), 1229–1234.

Mauriello, L. M., Driskell, M. M., Sherman, K. J., Johnson, S. S., Prochaska, J. M., & Prochaska, J. O. (2006). Acceptability of a school-based intervention for the prevention of adolescent obesity. *Journal of School Nursing, 22*(5), 269–277.

Mauriello, L. M., Sherman, K. J., Driskell, M. M., & Prochaska, J. M. (2007). Using interactive behavior change technology to intervene on physical activity and nutrition with adolescents. *Adolescent Medicine: State of the Art Reviews, 18,* 383–399.

McFall, M., Atkins, D. C., Yoshimoto, D., Thompson, C. E., Kanter, E., Malte, C. A., et al. (2006). Integrating tobacco cessation treatment into mental health care for patients with post-traumatic stress disorder. *American Journal of Addiction, 15*(5), 336–344.

McGue, M., Iacono, W. G., & Krueger, R. (2006). The association of early adolescent problem behavior and adult psychopathology: A multivariate behavioral genetic perspective. *Behavioral Genetics, 36*(4), 591–602.

Nigg, C. R., Allegrante, J. P., & Ory, M. (2002). Theory-comparison and multiple-behavior research: Common themes advancing health behavior research. *Health Education Research, 17*(5), 670–679.

Norris, S. L., Engelgau, M. M., & Narayan, K. M. (2001). Effectiveness of self-management training in type 2 diabetes: A systematic review of randomized controlled trials. *Diabetes Care, 24*(3), 561–587.

Orleans, C. T. (2004). Addressing multiple behavioral health risks in primary care. Broadening the focus of health behavior change research and practice. *American Journal of Preventive Medicine, 27*(2 Suppl.), 1–3.

Ornish, D., Scherwitz, L. W., Billings, J. H., Brown, S. E., Gould, K. L., Merritt, T. A., et al. (1998). Intensive lifestyle changes for reversal of coronary heart disease. *Journal of the American Medical Association, 280*(23), 2001–2007.

Parker, G., & Crawford, J. (2007). Judged effectiveness of differing antidepressant strategies by those with clinical depression. *Australian & New Zealand Journal of Psychiatry, 41*(1), 32–37.

Patterson, R. E., Haines, P. S., & Popkin, B. M. (1994). Diet quality index: Capturing a multidimensional behavior. *Journal of the American Dietetic Association, 94*(1), 57–64.

Perkins, K. A., Rohay, J., Meilahn, E. N., Wing, R. R., Matthews, K. A., & Kuller, L. H. (1993). Diet, alcohol, and physical activity as a function of smoking status in middle-aged women. *Health Psychology, 12*(5), 410–415.

Prochaska, J. J., Delucchi, K., & Hall, S. M. (2004). A meta-analysis of smoking cessation interventions with individuals in substance abuse treatment or recovery. *Journal of Consulting & Clinical Psychology 72*(6), 1144–1156.

Prochaska, J. J., Hall, S. M., Tsoh, J., Eisendrath, S., Rossi, J. S., Redding, C. A., et al. (2008). Treating tobacco dependence in clinically depressed smokers: Effect of smoking cessation on mental health functioning. *American Journal of Public Health, 98,* 446–448.

Prochaska, J. J., Velicer, W. F., Nigg, C. R., & Prochaska, J. O. (2008). Methods of quantifying change in multiple risk factor interventions. *Preventive Medicine, 46,* 260–265.

Prochaska, J. J., Velicer, W. F., Prochaska, J. O., Delucchi, K., & Hall, S. M. (2006). Comparing intervention outcomes in smokers treated for single versus multiple behavioral risks. *Health Psychology, 25*(3), 380–388.

Prochaska, J. O., DiClemente, C. C., & Norcross, J. C. (1992). In search of how people change. Applications to addictive behaviors. *American Psychologist, 47*(9), 1102–1114.

Prochaska, J. O., Velicer, W. F., Redding, C., Rossi, J. S., Goldstein, M., DePue, J., et al. (2005). Stage-based expert systems to guide a population of primary care patients to quit smoking, eat healthier, prevent skin cancer, and receive regular mammograms. *Preventive Medicine, 41*(2), 406–416.

Prochaska, J. O., Velicer, W. F., Rossi, J. S., Goldstein, M. G., Marcus, B. H., Rakowski, W., et al. (1994). Stages of change and decisional balance for 12 problem behaviors. *Health Psychology, 13*(1), 39–46.

Prochaska, J. O., Velicer, W. F., Rossi, J. S., Redding, C. A., Greene, G. W., Rossi, S. R., et al. (2004). Multiple risk expert systems interventions: Impact of simultaneous stage-matched expert system interventions for smoking, high-fat diet, and sun exposure in a population of parents. *Health Psychology, 23*(5), 503–516.

Pronk, N. P., Anderson, L. H., Crain, A. L., Martinson, B. C., O'Connor, P. J., Sherwood, N. E., et al. (2004). Meeting recommendations for multiple healthy lifestyle factors. Prevalence, clustering, and predictors among adolescent, adult, and senior health plan members. *American Journal of Preventive Medicine, 27*(2 Suppl.), 25–33.

Rasanen, P., Roine, E., Sintonen, H., Semberg-Konttinen, V., Ryynanen, O. P., & Roine, R. (2006). Use of quality-adjusted life years for the estimation of effectiveness of health care: A systematic literature review. *International Journal of Technology Assessment in Health Care, 22*(2), 235–241.

Reeves, M. J., & Rafferty, A. P. (2005). Healthy lifestyle characteristics among adults in the United States, 2000. *Archives of Internal Medicine, 165*(8), 854–857.

Rothert, K., Strecher, V. J., Doyle, L. A., Caplan, W. M., Joyce, J. S., Jimison, H. B., et al. (2006). Web-based weight management programs in an integrated health care setting: A randomized, controlled trial. *Obesity, 14*(2), 266–272.

Sallis, J. F., Prochaska, J. J., & Taylor, W. C. (2000). A review of correlates of physical activity of children and adolescents. *Medicine & Science in Sports & Exercise, 32*(5), 963–975.

Schultz, A. B., Lu, C., Barnett, T. E., Yen, L. T., McDonald, T., Hirschland, D., et al. (2002). Influence of participation in a worksite health-promotion program on disability days. *Journal of Occupational & Environmental Medicine, 44*(8), 776–780.

Singh, A. S., Paw, M. J., Brug, J., & van Mechelen, W. (2007). Short-term effects of school-based weight gain prevention among adolescents. *Archives of Pediatric & Adolescent Medicine, 161*(6), 565–571.

Smith, K. W., McKinlay, S. M., & McKinlay, J. B. (1989). The reliability of health risk appraisals: a field trial of four instruments. *American Journal of Public Health, 79*(12), 1603–1607.

Society for Research on Nicotine and Tobacco. (2002). Biochemical verification of tobacco use and cessation. *Nicotine & Tobacco Research, 4*(2), 149–159.

Sorensen, G., Thompson, B., Glanz, K., Feng, Z., Kinne, S., DiClemente, C., et al. (1996). Work site-based cancer prevention: Primary results from the Working Well Trial. *American Journal of Public Health, 86*(7), 939–947.

Spring, B., Pagoto, S., Pingitore, R., Doran, N., Schneider, K., & Hedeker, D. (2004). Randomized controlled trial for behavioral smoking and weight control treatment: Effect of concurrent versus sequential intervention. *Journal of Consulting & Clinical Psychology, 72*(5), 785–796.

Summerbell, C. D., Waters, E., Edmunds, L. D., Kelly, S., Brown, T., & Campbell, K. J. (2005). Interventions for preventing obesity in children. *Cochrane Database of Systematic Reviews* (3), CD001871.

Toobert, D. J., Glasgow, R. E., Strycker, L. A., Barrera, M., Jr., Ritzwoller, D. P., & Weidner, G. (2007). Long-term effects of the Mediterranean lifestyle program: A randomized clinical trial for postmenopausal women with type 2 diabetes. *International Journal of Behavioral Nutrition & Physical Activity, 4,* 1.

Tucker, L. R., Damarin, F., & Messick, S. (1966). A base-free measure of change. *Psychometrika, 31*(4), 457–473.

Unger, J. B. (1996). Stages of change of smoking cessation: Relationships with other health behaviors. *American Journal of Preventive Medicine, 12*(2), 134–138.

U.S. Department of Health & Human Services. (1999). *Mental health: A report of the Surgeon General.* Washington, DC: Department of Health and Human Services.

Ussher, M. (2005). Exercise interventions for smoking cessation. *Cochrane Database of Systematic Reviews* (1), CD002295.

Veldman, D. J., & Brophy, J. (1974). Measuring teacher effects on pupil achievement. *Journal of Educational Psychology, 66*(3), 319–324.

Velicer, W. F., Prochaska, J. O., Redding, C. A., Rossi, J. S., Sun, X., & Greene, G. W. (2004). Efficacy of expert system interventions for employees to decrease smoking, dietary fat, and sun exposure (Abstract). *International Journal of Behavioral Medicine, 11*(Suppl.), 277.

Wankel, L. M., & Sefton, J. M. (Eds.). (1994). *Physical activity, fitness, and health: International proceedings and consensus statement.* Champaign, IL: Human Kinetics.

Wilson, P. W., D'Agostino, R. B., Levy, D., Belanger, A. M., Silbershatz, H., & Kannel, W. B. (1998). Prediction of coronary heart disease using risk factor categories. *Circulation, 97*(18), 1837–1847.

Wright, D. W., Beard, M. J., & Edington, D. W. (2002). Association of health risks with the cost of time away from work. *Journal of Occupational and Environmental Medicine, 44*(12), 1126–1134.

Yusuf, S., Hawken, S., Ounpuu, S., Dans, T., Avezum, A., Lanas, F., et al. (2004). Effect of potentially modifiable risk factors associated with myocardial infarction in 52 countries (the INTERHEART study): Case-control study. *Lancet, 364*(9438), 937–952.

Section 3

Measurement

Kristin A. Riekert
Editor

Section III is new to this edition of the handbook and represents the growing attention given to the importance of reliable and valid measures of health behavior as well as appropriate analysis of behavioral data within clinical trials. If a clinician feels it is important to recommend a regimen, be it diet, exercise, or medication, it should be just as important to the clinician to know the extent to which the patient followed that recommendation. Unfortunately, few clinicians routinely incorporate valid protocols for assessing regimen adherence into their practice. Similarly, the measurement of participants' adherence to study protocols is a critical component of clinical trials research. If a trial is focused on drug development, then it is important to know if and how participants are using the drug to assess its efficacy and to understand the occurrence of adverse events. If the focus of the study is lifestyle change, then to appropriately evaluate the efficacy of the intervention, accurate and valid measures are needed that not only assess what behavior was performed and how often but one that is also sensitive to change over time. Unfortunately, the measurement of health behaviors is challenging.

Otsuki and colleagues (chapter 16, Medication Regimens), Wilcox and Ainsworth (chapter 17, Physical Activity) and Dougherty, Dawes, and Nouvion (chapter 18, Substance Use) discuss the various types of assessment methodologies for their respective behaviors and compare and contrast content of measures and their psychometric properties, as well as costs and benefits of each approach. The similarities of the measurement issues and limitations are quite notable considering the very different behaviors the chapters address. A take-home message is that no one measure is ideal for every purpose, so it is essential to carefully consider the trade-off between accuracy and comprehensiveness, as well as the ease and cost of administration. Often the optimal solution is to use multiple measures.

Finally, chapter 19 focuses on missing data and statistical methods. Even the best-designed and -managed studies will encounter missing data and, as Conway and colleagues discuss, if missing data are ignored, this can lead to biased estimates. The authors offer recommendations for selecting the optimal statistical approach for handling different types of missing data and incorporating strategies to minimize the occurrence of missing data.

Measuring Adherence to Medication Regimens in Clinical Care and Research

16

Michiko Otsuki,
Emmanuelle
Clerisme-Beaty,
Cynthia S. Rand, and
Kristin A. Riekert

When patients' therapies do not work, clinicians often adjust dosages, order more diagnostic tests, or switch to different, sometimes riskier treatments. When a clinical trial does not find a significant treatment effect for a promising investigative drug, that therapy may be judged inefficacious and abandoned as a possible treatment option. All too often, however, the cause of the ineffective therapy lies not with the drug or treatment but rather with patient or provider behavior. Clinicians and researchers who do not measure patient adherence appropriately are at risk of misjudging the causes of treatment ineffectiveness.

Patient adherence is the necessary intermediary between efficacious therapies and treatment effectiveness. Studies that have measured patient adherence to medication regimens have repeatedly documented the magnitude of medication nonadherence across all diseases and therapies. Estimates are that

50%–65% of all outpatients do not adhere appropriately to their medication regimens (DiMatteo, 2004b; Melnikow & Kiefe, 1994; Schaub, Steiner, & Vetter, 1993).

Nonadherence to prescribed treatment has implications for clinicians in several critical areas. Most obviously, a patient who does not adhere to a short- or long-term medical regimen may not get the complete therapeutic benefits (DiMatteo, Giordani, Lepper, & Croghan, 2002). A physician can often be misled by patient nonadherence to conclude that the prescribed treatment is inadequate or inappropriate. This, in turn, can lead to costly diagnostic procedures or even dangerous intensification of therapy, when the patient would have been served best by accurately following the originally prescribed regimen.

Another serious consequence of patient nonadherence is the compromise of clinical drug trials. A new treatment can easily be judged ineffective if participants do not adhere adequately to the treatment protocol. So critical is the issue of adherence to the evaluation of drug efficacy that some researchers have suggested that clinical studies are of only limited value without the inclusion of valid measures of adherence (Besch, 1995; Granger et al., 2005; Melnikow & Kiefe, 1994).

Defining and Classifying Adherence

"Adherence" or "compliance" may be broadly defined as the degree to which patient behaviors coincide with the clinical recommendations of health care providers. Despite the fact that clinicians and researchers alike categorize patients as being either complaint or noncompliant, such adherence is not inherently a dichotomous variable. There is no gold standard for what defines "satisfactory" or "poor" adherence across all health behaviors. Factors such as the dosage necessary for therapeutic effectiveness, the risks of nonadherence, and the clinical or research goals will all influence the criteria for good adherence. Appropriate adherence must be situationally defined, with parameters of good adherence explicitly delineated and appropriate to the medication regimen or health behavior under study. How one chooses to define good adherence is integrally related to the way in which adherence will best be measured. A broadly defined, flexible criterion of acceptable adherence may not need precise measurement methodology. In contrast, when detailed and exact adherence data are necessary, the measurement instruments should be comparably precise. Assessment of adherence in a clinical trial, for example, must be as rigorous as possible in order to ensure the fundamental integrity of the study's conclusions.

In both clinical care and research settings, measuring and classifying patients' patterns of medication uses is as necessary as assessing overall adherence level. Understanding patterns of medication use is important in the evaluation of treatment response and efficacy and in developing strategies to enhance adherence. The expected patient behavior is "appropriate adherence"—that is, using medications exactly as prescribed and consistently over time. The most obvious form of noncompliance is chronic "underuse," where a patient regularly uses less medication than is prescribed. Although underuse is most often considered a risk for poor disease control, for some patients, underuse may be an effective self-management or self-titration strategy when treatment has been overprescribed (Diette et al., 1999; Sale, Gignac, & Hawker, 2006). Patients also may have "erratic adherence," in which medication use alternates between adherent use (usually when symptomatic) and underuse or total nonuse (when asymptomatic). Patients with erratic adherence may present for treatment during symptom exacerbations with apparent complete adherence to their prescribed regimen. Erratic adherence may also reflect forgetfulness, stress, changed schedules, running out of medication, or other barriers to full adherence. The term "drug holiday" is sometimes used to describe multiday lapses in medication use. Finally, some patients using pain or symptom-relieving drugs on an as-needed basis (i.e., PRN), may be prone to "overuse" during exacerbations. This may cause a patient to delay seeking care or lead to complications associated with excessive medication use (Diette et al., 1999; Rand, Nides, Cowles, Wise, & Connett, 1995; Spitzer et al., 1992).

Methods for Measuring Medication Adherence

Several investigators have published excellent reviews of medication adherence measurement research, and the reader is referred to them for greater detail (Berg, Dischler, Wagner, Raia, & Palmer-Shevlin, 1993; Melnikow & Kiefe, 1994; Rand, 2002). As these reviewers have noted, various methods for assessing adherence have both strengths and weaknesses that must be considered in their use. Adherence measures can be divided into "indirect methods" (presumed used) and "direct methods" (confirmed use).

Indirect Measures

Clinician Judgment

In everyday clinical care, health care providers form thumbnail impressions of how well each of their patients is following their prescribed regimens. These judgments necessarily shape the patient-provider interaction, the selected therapy, and the follow-up plan. Results from the majority of published studies show that physicians generally greatly overestimate the degree to which their patients comply with their recommendations (Davis, 1966; Kasl, 1975; Paulson, Krause, & Iber, 1977; Sherman, Hutson, Baumstein, & Hendeles, 2000). Sherman et al. (2000) showed that, measured against a pharmacy database, physicians were able to accurately identify only 49% of subjects who obtained less than 50% of the refills of the medication prescribed for children with asthma. Another study by Miller et al. (2002) looking at the accuracy of clinicians' judgment regarding patients adherence to antiretroviral therapy, found that clinicians overestimated measured adherence using electronic monitors by 8.9% (86.2% vs. 77.3%).

Hamilton (2003) showed that although physician judgment and electronic monitoring had comparable rates of adherence, they were not correlated. Physicians not only overestimate patient adherence but are also poor predictors of which specific patients will be good or poor adherers. Steele, Jackson, and Gutmann (1990) found that physicians identified only 53% of the adherence problems in 38 critical-case encounters. Physicians who used indirect approaches to assessment (e.g., "have you noticed any changes since you started taking your medicine?") were the least successful in identifying adherence problems (0/9 correct); simple, direct questioning (e.g., "You've been taking your medications?") was moderately successful (8/13 correct); and information-intensive strategies (open-ended queries about patterns of medication use) was the most successful approach (8/10 correct). The investigators conclude that a "nonaccusatory, open-ended, information-intensive approach can be a sensitive and productive tool for the diagnosis of patient's adherence status" (Steele et al., 1990, p. 299). The lack of physician skill in identifying patients with adherence difficulties has been attributed to a medical education focus that neglects communication skills and attention to psychosocial issues. A study by Steiner and colleagues (1991), however, found that even nurse-practitioners (members of a profession that emphasizes patient education and communication) were poor judges of patient adherence, identifying only 23.1% of the poorly adherent patients and misclassifying 22.5% of the more adherent patients as partial compliers. Clinical judgments based on preconceived beliefs about the attributes of the "typical" compliant patient are destined to fail. Patient characteristics such as race, education, gender, socioeconomic status, and personality have not been found to be reliable predictors of adherence (see chapter 20). Physician interviewing skills and the qualities of the patient-provider interaction are more important in both measuring and facilitating adherence than stereotypical beliefs about adherence (DiMatteo et al., 1993; Dunbar-Jacob, 1993; Heszen-Klemens & Lapinska, 1984; Sackett & Haynes, 1976).

Self-Report

Self-report of medication use is a common measure of adherence in both clinical trials and behavioral intervention studies. Patient self-reports may be collected by interview, diaries, and questionnaires. No cross-disease, validated adherence-specific questionnaire is currently in common use, in part because most self-report questionnaires of adherence have been designed for specific diseases and studies or because they are often embedded in more general disease self-management measures (Dolce et al., 1991; Rand & Wise, 1994). Self-report is an inexpensive, simple measurement strategy that is applicable to different regimens, is generally brief, and has face validity (see Rand, 2000, for a review). In addition, self-report (particularly in the clinical setting) is the best measure for collecting information about patient beliefs, attitudes, and experiences with medication regimens. For example, the patient who misunderstands a dosing regimen or who has altered her regimen because of fear of side effects will not be identified by objective adherence assessments (Britten, 1994; Donovan & Blake, 1992).

Self-report is the most appropriate means for evaluating reasons for nonadherence, including health and attitudes as well as cultural variations that affect adherence to prescribed therapy (Rand, 2000). Several studies have shown that patients' dissatisfaction with therapy, their perceptions of treatment efficacy, inconvenience, fear of side effects, and self-efficacy are associated with nonadherence (Apter et al., 2003; Bosworth et al., 2006; Brown, Rehmus, & Kimball, 2006). As a quantitative measure of medication use, self-report has been found to have a highly variable degree of accuracy (Coutts, Gibson, & Paton, 1992;

Mason, Matsuyama, & Jue, 1995; Waterhouse, Calzone, Mele, & Brenner, 1993). Specifically, self-report has been shown to consistently overestimate medication adherence relative to objective measures in hypertension (Wang et al., 2004), HIV (Liu et al., 2001), asthma (Krishnan et al., 2004), cancer (Waterhouse et al., 1993), epilepsy (Cramer, Mattson, Prevey, Scheyer, & Oullette, 1989), and arthritis medications (Kraag, Gordon, Menard, Russell, & Kalish, 1994).

Self-reports of adherence are influenced by the demand characteristics on the setting in which the information is collected. The desire to please the physician or investigator can lead patients to exaggerate reports of medication use. Patients with memory impairment (related to illness, age, concurrent medications, or stress) may not be able to accurately self-report their usage pattern of any one medication (Levine et al., 2006). Patients' report regarding long-term medication use may be less reliable the longer the recall period becomes. Physicians' and investigators' sensitivity and skill in eliciting patients' self-reports will certainly influence the reliability and usefulness of the information they receive.

While self-report may not be a sufficient measure of adherence in many settings (particularly in research), it is probably a necessary measure in all settings. For, when carefully collected, this information can provide invaluable insight into the nature of patients' problems with adherence. Additionally, because there is no evidence to suggest that adhering patients will misrepresent themselves as nonadherers, when the patients report that they are non-adherent to the prescribed therapy, the information can be considered to be reliable and valid (Rand et al., 1995).

Medication Measurement

Medication measurement has frequently been used as a relatively simple, yet objective measure of adherence. Counting pills and weighing inhaler canisters or liquid mediation are examples of measures that allow researchers to infer the degree of medication adherence. This method requires that the clinician or investigator know exactly how much medication the patient began the measurement period with and how much medication should have been used during this period.

Medication measurement has been used to provide objective data on the relationship between adherence with therapy and disease exacerbations. Hilbrands and colleagues (1995) used pill counts to evaluate adherence with immunosuppressive and antihypertensive drugs among adult patients who had received a renal transplant in the previous year. They found that overall adherence was generally good (87% to 64% of patients were fully adherent); however, there was considerable variability, both within patients for different drugs, and among patients. Patients who experienced a subsequent rejection episode had lower adherence with immunosuppressive drugs than did patients without a rejection episode, and adherence appeared to improve in these patients after the rejection month.

In some settings, medication measurement can serve as both an adherence intervention tool and an outcome measure. Koch and colleagues (1993) contracted with 23 pediatric patients with thalassemia to improve adherence to desferrioxamine iron chelation therapy. Patients were asked to increase the number of days they used the subcutaneous pump delivery system, and the number of empty desferrioxamine vials served as a basis for reinforcement and adherence documentation. By the end of the 6-month program, patients' use of the pump had climbed from 4.5 to approximately 5.5 days per week. Koch and colleagues note that because of the need for parental supervision during therapy and the high cost of desferrioxamine, it was unlikely that patients would deceptively empty vials.

Medication measurement need not be confined to clinic visits. Cromer and colleagues (1989) studied adherence with therapy for iron deficiency among 71 adolescents using a home pill count (conducted by research staff), serum ferritin levels, and urinary assays for tracer riboflavin. Pill counts in this setting were found to be highly correlated with biochemical indices of compliance, suggesting that this measurement strategy is an accurate method for measuring adherence. Moss and colleagues (2004) examined adherence to highly active antiretroviral therapy (HAART) in the homeless population, a high-risk population for poor adherence to therapy and for developing drug-resistant HIV strains. In this special population, pill count was found to be a more feasible method of adherence monitoring than electronic measures.

While these adherence data are both objective and reasonably simple to collect, they are limited by several factors. Medication measures can easily be influenced by a patient's efforts to deceive the investigator. As discussed, some patients may discard medication to appear adherent. Participants' knowledge that medication will be measured may negatively affect its accuracy. For example, DuBard and colleagues (1993) evaluated adherence with low-dose aspirin therapy for the prevention of pre-eclampsia. They compared pill-count estimations of adherence with biochemical measure (serum thromboxane 2) and found that women with a pill count greater than 100% had lower biochemical levels of drug than did women with pill counts <95%, suggesting that pills may have been discarded. This phenomenon of medication "dumping" has been described by a number of investigators (Mawhinney et al., 1991; Rand et al., 1992; Urquhart, 1991) and appears to be a common occurrence when medication measurement is used in a clinical trial setting to confirm compliance. Medications are often shared within households, particularly when family members are on the same medication (i.e., tranquilizers, antibiotics, sleeping pills). Additionally, medication measures give no indication of the accuracy of dosages or the timing of medication. However, in situations where patients are unthreatened by the consequences of reporting nonadherence, the pattern of medication use is not critical, and where the likelihood of medication-sharing is low, medication measurement is a useful, objective, and valid means of assessing adherence.

Automated Pharmacy Database Review

As managed care has expanded and the technology for health care utilization data tracking and management has become more sophisticated, it has become increasingly feasible to monitor patients' medication adherence by examining insurance pharmacy databases. Pharmacy databases can provide information regarding prescription practices, the amount of medication dispensed, and the timing of refills. This data can be used to calculate roughly the average dose per day. In some health care data management systems, prescriptions written but never filled can also be monitored. Dispensing data also can be matched with medical record and health care utilization databases to provide integrated analyses of the antecedents and consequences of patient adherence behaviors.

Studies using this methodology have examined patient adherence across a wide range of regimens and diseases, including depression (Stein, Cantrell, Sokol, Eaddy, & Shah, 2006), glaucoma (Gurwitz et al., 1993), hypertension (Grant, Singer, & Meigs, 2005) hyperlipidemia (Parris, Lawrence, Mohn, & Long, 2005; Schectman, Hiatt, & Hartz, 1994), HIV (Laine et al., 2000), and asthma (Bender, Pedan, & Varasteh, 2006; Stempel et al., 2005). Review of automated pharmacy records also can allow large-scale population studies of patient adherence with medications. Nachega and colleagues (2006) used pharmacy claims to evaluate the association between HAART adherence and HIV-1 survival in South Africa and showed a relationship between medication adherence and survival. Another study by Spitzer and colleagues (1992) examined the relationship between beta-agonist use in pulmonary patients and the risk of death and near-death from asthma by examining computerized prescription-refill records. Their study, based on refill patterns, suggested that regular use or overuse of beta-agonist medications was associated with an increased risk of death or near-death. Although this provocative study could not determine if this increased risk results directly from toxic properties of the pharmacological agent itself or indirectly from the patient's delayed treatment, its publication sparked intense debate on the relationship between patient adherence patterns and asthma mortality.

Pharmacy data review can reveal refill-based adherence patterns for different classes of medication or dosing regimens (Dolder, Lacro, & Jeste, 2003). Using data from a pharmacy database, Marceau, Lemiere, Berbiche, Perreault, and Blais (2006) found that, although treatment adherence to inhaled corticosteroids (ICS) and long-acting beta-agonist (LABA) medication was overall poor, patients on a combination therapy were more persistent and adherent than those treated with ICSs and LABAs taken in two different inhalers. Review of pharmacy and medical records can also determine the risks associated with nonadherence. Maronde and colleagues (1989) reviewed records of patients being treated for hypertension after having been admitted to an acute-care hospital with a diagnosis of hypertension in the previous 6 months and found that poor compliance was associated with a higher risk of rehospitalization within a year. In contrast, Steiner and colleagues (1991) reviewed the automated pharmacy records of hypertensive patients enrolled in a medication step-down program in a VA hospital and found that patients with histories of partial compliance were more likely to be successful in reducing their antihypertensive medication regimens, suggesting that some patients may have been successfully self-regulating their medication doses. They note that the review of centralized pharmacy records to identify partial compliers with normal blood pressure would allow reductions in unnecessarily high doses of medication.

Pharmacy database review to identify nonadherence has several limitations. First, adherence estimates can be calculated only for patients who exclusively rely on the target pharmacy system for all prescriptions and refills. Patients who use "out-of-network" pharmacies will have incomplete refill data. Second, pharmacy data can determine when a prescription was filled; however, it provides no confirmation of consumption or appropriate consumption patterns. Pharmacy database review cannot determine if medications sit unused, are hoarded for future use, are shared or given to family and friends, or are taken inappropriately. However, Tamblyn and colleagues (1995), in a study of the accuracy and comprehensiveness of the prescription claims database in Quebec, found pharmacy databases to be an accurate measure of medication dispenses. As more pharmacy data go online, this adherence-measuring strategy has great potential to "be applied comprehensively, inexpensively and unobtrusively to a large number of individuals" (Steiner, Fihn, Blair, & Inui, 1991).

Electronic Medication Monitors

In the past 15 years, the increased availability of computer-based technology has introduced a new strategy for adherence monitoring. Electronic monitoring devices record and store the date (and, in the case of some devices, the time) of each medication use. Devices have been developed to monitor medication adherence behaviors including, but not restricted to, opening a pill bottle, releasing a blister-pak pill, discharging inhaled medications, and releasing eyedrops. Behaviors important to medical outcomes, such as home apnea monitoring for premature infants (Cordero, Morehead, & Miller, 1993), self-monitoring of blood glucose for patients with diabetes (Wysocki, Green, & Huxtable, 1989), and the use of removable appliance wear in orthodontic patients (Bartsch, Witt, Sahm, & Schneider, 1993), also have been targeted for electronic monitoring.

Three electronic devices that have been widely investigated are the Medication Event Monitoring System (MEMS-AARDEX, LTD, Switzerland), the Doser (Meditrack Products, Hudson, MA) and the MDILog (Westmed Technologies, Englewood, CO). The MEMS can be used in conjunction with any regimen that includes the use of pills or tablets. A microprocessor in the MEMS cap electronically records each time the bottle is opened and stores the date, time, and duration of opening for subsequent downloading and retrieval via computer. The Doser is made of a pressure-activated cap that is attached to the most commercially available Metered Dose Inhalers (MDIs). The Doser has a pre-programmable liquid crystal display that shows the number of remaining doses in the canister and the number of actuations for each day. The MDILog is a more recent model of Nebulizer Chronolog (NC-Medtrac Technologies, Lakewood, CO) that is attached to MDIs. The MDILog has an embedded computer chip that records the date and time of each actuation. Additionally, the MDILog evaluates whether the canister was shaken before use and an inhalation actually took place (see Riekert & Rand, 2002, for a detailed description of each medication monitor). Last, there is emerging technology concerning remote download of adherence data. This will enable clinicians to assess patients' adherence between clinic visits, as well as allow researchers the opportunity to minimize missing data in clinical studies.

These devices provide a unique opportunity to investigate long-term patterns of presumptive adherence that were heretofore unavailable in such detail. For example, using electronic monitors, Rand et al. (2007) were able to examine the effect of dosing frequency and mode of therapy delivery on both adherence and clinical outcome. The study consisted of 389 patients with mild intermittent asthma randomized to either a once-a-day oral medication (montelukast) or a twice-a-day inhaler (fluticasone). The authors found that although subjects were more likely to use their inhalers at least once a day, they were more likely to take the once-daily medication as prescribed. However, they failed to demonstrate any benefits of increased adherence on the clinical outcomes measured in the study.

Mason and colleagues (1995) used several measures of adherence in addition to the MEMS to determine which most closely assessed metabolic control in patients with noninsulin-dependent diabetes mellitus. Assessment of medication adherence by provider, patient, and pill count did not explain metabolic control as closely or as accurately as assessment by the MEMS. Adherence studies conducted as a part of the Lung Health Study (Rand et al., 1992) using the Nebulizer Chronolog also have demonstrated the limitations of self-report and medication measurement seen with many of the studies using the MEMS. However, the NC was better able to capture a phenomenon called "dumping." In the Lung Health Study, participant self-report and canister weighing overestimated participant adherence by more than 30%. In addition, this study indicated that there was a subset of participants who appeared to discard medication deliberately before follow-up visits. Dumping is nearly impossible to detect by traditional methods of adherence assessment, and inclusion of dumping data in a dose-response analysis can yield counterintuitive results; highly adherent subjects show poorer response than moderately adherent subjects.

In recent years, the number of published studies using electronic adherence-monitoring devices has increased dramatically. The primary benefit of this type of monitoring is clear: electronic monitoring methods can provide a continuous record of timing of presumptive doses over periods of months. Assessments of adherence made by provider, self-report, pill counts, or canister weights can be inaccurate because of recall, demand characteristics, deception, and provider biases. These methods, usually the "gold standards" of adherence, reveal medication ingestion but do not reveal the timing of doses.

While this trend toward high-tech computer-based monitoring devices continues, these systems are not without their limitations. The cost for wide-scale use can be prohibitive for a small practice and may be feasible only in a clinical trial setting. The up-front cost can be thousands of dollars. Additionally, there is a failure rate associated with the use of any type of electronic device. The failure rate in electronic devices can be caused by patient misuse, device failure, or computer hardware or software problems. In a study by Cramer and colleagues (1995), participants at 8 out of 10 sites did not use MEMS properly, thereby voiding their data for analyses. It also may be argued that the monitoring devices themselves, or the awareness that one is being monitored electronically, may alter adherence behavior. A detailed discussion of the benefits, issues, and precautions for using electronic medication monitors is found in Riekert and Rand (2002).

Direct Measures

Biochemical Analysis

Clinical analysis of blood, urine, or other bodily excretions has frequently been used to objectively measure medication or byproduct levels (Berg et al.,

1993; Gordis, 1976; Schaub et al., 1993). This is the only method of adherence measurement that confirms that medications have actually been taken by a patient, and for this reason biochemical analysis is one of the most valuable techniques available for assessing adherence. Unfortunately, this strategy is available for only a few drugs, and individual variations in absorption patterns may limit interpretation. Investigators can sometimes measure adherence with drugs that are not directly evaluable by biochemical assays by adding tracer substances that can be monitored. Riboflavin (Dubbert et al., 1985), digoxin (Maenpaa, Manninen, & Heinonen, 1992), phenobarbitone (Hatton, Allen, Vathenen, Feely, & Cooke, 1996), and deuterium oxide (Rodewald & Pichichero, 1993) have all been used as added biochemical adherence markers.

While biochemical analysis allows a very direct assessment of drug use, it also has some limitations. In order for the excretion pattern of the drug, tracer, or byproduct to be clearly understood, drug adherence is best assessed by repeated measures and analyses. This type of repeated assessment is probably clinically practical only when the monitoring is also necessary for determining appropriate therapeutic levels of medication (i.e., dilantin levels). Repeated measures solely for confirming adherence are usually impractical, particularly when biochemical analysis requires the use of an invasive procedure to collect a sample. Even when biochemical monitoring is feasible, not all medications can be easily detected or tagged with tracer substances. Biochemical analysis can provide a measure of adherence for a single test or for multiple tests, but it cannot realistically be used to measure day-to-day adherence with long-term medication. And, finally, even this technique can be compromised if a patient deliberately or inadvertently begins taking his or her medication just prior to the clinical analysis.

Directly Observed Therapy (DOT)

Other than biochemical analysis, observing therapy is the only direct measure of patient adherence to therapy. Directly observed therapy (DOT) requires that patients be monitored for each dose or treatment to confirm adherence. DOT was pioneered in the treatment of tuberculosis because (1) poor patient adherence had been identified as the major barrier to effective treatment; (2) as a highly infectious disease, TB posed a major public health threat, and (3) those populations with the highest incidence of TB (I.V. drug abusers, recent immigrants, homeless people) were historically the most transient and difficult to retain in conventional therapy (Volmink & Garner, 2000).

In addition to tuberculosis, recent data have shown DOT to be feasible and sustainable intervention to significantly improve patient adherence with treatment for active diseases like HIV (Jayaweera et al, 2004; Lucas, Weidle, Hader, & Moore, 2004), as well as prophylactic therapy for communicable diseases like pertussis (Purcell, Dooley, Gray, Hill, & Oliverson, 2004). Results of a clinical trial by Lucas et al. (2006) showed that directly administered antiretroviral therapy (DAART) was more effective at achieving viral suppression (74%) than medication self-administration (33%) in 82 subjects with HIV on methadone therapy. However, DOT is a potentially coercive strategy, particularly when used for society's most indigent, disenfranchised members, and, as such, it raises important issues of public health policy, medical ethics, and civil liberties (Bayer & Dupuis, 1995).

Issues in Adherence Measurement

No one measure of adherence is appropriate for all settings. When considering the most appropriate strategy to apply, the following issues should be considered.

Reactivity

When adherence behavior is monitored by methods that are known by both the clinician and the patient to be both accurate and revealing, there is a strong possibility that the patient's adherence behavior will meet the demand characteristics of the monitoring situation. Few existing studies have evaluated this concern, and the findings in this area have been mixed. In the aforementioned Lung Health Study, Rand et al. (1992) found no difference in adherence rates (as measured with canister weights) between those using a Nebulizer Chronolog and those without it. Similarly, Matsui et al. (1994) found no significant changes in adherence before and after the explanation of the purpose of MEMS. In contrast, other studies have shown that there can be a direct relationship between the detail and precision of any measurement strategy and its impact on adherence (Nides, Tashkin, Simmons, Wise, Li, & Rand, 1993). How troublesome reactivity is depends upon the goals of the study or clinical interaction. When the focus of a study is on the ability to generalize the study's conclusions (i.e., will most patients use enough bronchodilator to achieve therapeutic goals?) or clinical purposes, then the use of reactive measurement techniques may be desirable. It is therefore important to clarify the goals of adherence assessment in each research or clinical application and then to select the most appropriate measurement strategies.

Measuring Children's Adherence

Assessing medication adherence in children presents unique challenges that require evaluating and considering both the family context in which medication use occurs and the level of communication between the health care provider and the family (see DiMatteo, 2004b, for a review).

This communication starts with identifying the family member responsible for delivering medications to the child and who is the most reliable source of adherence information. Responsibility for medication administration generally shifts as a child grows, from total parent management for a young child, to shared medication management for the school-age child, to complete self-management for the adolescent. Caregivers' reports of medication adherence on behalf of their children are often discrepant from objective measures of adherence as obtained by pill counts and electronic medication monitor (e.g., Steele et al., 2001). As parents transfer responsibility for medication management, they generally become less accurate reporters of the child's medication adherence.

There can be great diversity among families in how medication management is implemented. Day care providers, grandparents, and siblings may assume responsibility for regular medication delivery in some households. Because of the highly variable and often shifting family responsibility for a child's medication use, it is necessary for the health care provider to review medication-use habits with both the caregiver and the child in order to develop an adherence profile.

Multiple Measures of Adherence

Because of the relative strengths and weaknesses of each of the adherence measures discussed, the optimal strategy for assessing adherence usually involves the use of multiple measures (DiMatteo, 2004b; Liu, Kaplan, & Wenger, 2002). In a longitudinal study of medication adherence to HAART using MEMS, pill count, and self-report, Golin and colleagues (2002) found that although all three measures tracked over time, they each had shortcomings that could be minimized by combining the different methods of assessment. Llabre et al. (2006) found that using at least two different methods of adherence measurement assessed at multiple times enhances reliability and validity of adherence measures.

Nevertheless, patient contacts in both clinical and research settings should almost certainly include eliciting self-report information. Skillfully collected, these data not only identify adherence difficulties and barriers but also provide the investigator with information about the circumstances of nonadherence. The correction of adherence difficulties may well depend upon the investigator understanding the "whys of nonadherence" and working with the patient toward a solution. The inclusion of one or more objective measures when assessing adherence will confirm patients' self-reports, but the potential reactive effect of the measures should be weighed. Self-report and an unannounced biochemical analysis of a urine sample are unlikely to have any impact on patients' adherence behavior, while self-report and electronic medication monitoring and repeated drug-screening urinalysis probably will alter the patient's adherence behavior, the self-report, or both.

The Use of Adherence Data

Clinicians interested in assessing patient adherence should clarify to themselves and then, in turn, to their patients why this information is being collected and how the information will be used. In a research context, where the value of a drug or therapeutic regimen is being evaluated, the purpose of adherence assessment may be well defined for the investigator but unclear to the participant. In clinical care, adherence assessment can easily be interpreted by patients as paternalistic intrusion, the doctor checking for who's been "naughty" or "nice." Unfortunately, for some clinicians, that is exactly the intent and tone of their adherence assessment, with patients categorized as "good" adherers or "bad" adherers. Such classifications fail to consider the barriers to patient adherence (Dunbar-Jacob, 1993; Ross, 1991; Waitzkin, 1984). If the goal of adherence determination is to evaluate a treatment's efficacy, rather than to judge the patient's reliability or trustworthiness, then this goal should be both explicit and implicit in the patient-physician interaction.

Future Directions for Adherence Research

The better a behavior can be observed, the more complete will be our understanding of that behavior. The recent explosion in microcomputer technology has opened up remarkable new opportunities to incorporate adherence-monitoring technology into everyday patient care. Similar opportunities are possible with the increased access to sophisticated, integrated pharmacy and health care databases. The possibility now exists for both the clinicians and the investigator to examine real-life adherence behavior and to directly correlate this behavior with patient response to therapy. While automated health care databases and specialized electronic adherence monitors are hardly a panacea for patient adherence difficulties, incorporating their use in both clinical and research settings would not only improve measurement precision but also offer increased opportunities for adherence-promoting interventions.

Whether sophisticated new technology or a simple clinical interview is used to measure and promote adherence, the patient or subject should be recognized as an active partner in the patient-provider exchange. No technology, now or in the future, will replace the good listening and the sincere concern of a first-rate therapeutic relationship.

References

Apter, A. J., Boston, R. C., George, M., Norfleet, A. L., Tenhave, T., Coyne, J. C., et al. (2003). Modifiable barriers to adherence to inhaled steroids among adults with asthma: It's not just black and white. *Journal of Allergy and Clinical Immunology, 111,* 1219–1226.

Bartsch, A., Witt, E., Sahm, G., & Schneider, S. (1993). Correlates of objective patient compliance with removable appliance wear. *American Journal of Orthodontics & Dentofacial Orthopedics, 104,* 378–386.

Bayer, R., & Dupuis, L. (1995). Tuberculosis, public health, and civil liberties. *Annual Review* of *Public Health, 16,* 307–326.

Bender, B. G., Pedan, A., & Varasteh, L. T. (2006). Adherence and persistence with fluticasone propionate/salmeterol combination therapy. *Journal of Allergy and Clinical Immunology, 118,* 899–904.

Berg, J. S., Dischler, J., Wagner, D. J., Raia, J. J., & Palmer-Shevlin, N. (1993). Medication compliance: A healthcare problem. *Annals of Pharmacotherapy, 27,* S1–S24.

Besch, C. L. (1995). Compliance in clinical trials. *AIDS, 9,* 1–10.

Bosworth, H. B., Dudley, T., Olsen, M. K., Voils, C. I., Powers, B., Goldstein, M. K., et al. (2006). Racial differences in blood pressure control: Potential explanatory factors. *American Journal of Medicine, 119,* 70.e9–70.e15.

Britten, N. (1994) Patients' ideas about medicines: A qualitative study in a general practice population. *British Journal of General Practice, 44,* 465–468.

Brown, K. K., Rehmus, W. E., & Kimball, A. B. (2006). Determining the relative importance of patient motivations for nonadherence to topical corticosteroid therapy in psoriasis. *Journal of the American Academy of Dermatology, 55,* 607–613.

Cordero, L., Morehead, S., & Miller, R. (1993). Parental compliance with home apnea monitoring. *Journal of Perinatology, 13,* 448–452.

Coutts, J. A. P., Gibson, N. A., & Paton, J. Y. (1992). Measuring compliance with inhaled medication in asthma. *Archives of Disease in Childhood, 67,* 332–333.

Cramer, J. A., Mattson, R. H., Prevey, M. L., Scheyer, R. D., & Oullette, V. L. (1989). How often is medication taken as prescribed? A novel assessment technique. *Journal of the American Medical Association, 261,* 3273–3277.

Cramer, J., Vachon, L., Desforges, C., & Sussman, N. M. (1995). Dose frequency and dose interval compliance with multiple antilepileptic medications during a controlled clinical trial. *Epilepsia, 36,* 1111–1117.

Cromer, B. A., Steinberg, K., Gardner, L., Thornton, D., & Shannon, B. (1989). Psychosocial determinants of compliance in adolescents with iron deficiency. *American Journal of Diseases of Children, 143,* 55–58.

Davis, M. S. (1966). Variations in patients' compliance with doctors; orders: Analysis of congruence between survey responses and results of empirical investigations. *Journal of Medical Education, 41,* 1037–1048.

Diette, G. B., Wu, A. W., Skinner, E. A., Markson, L., Clark, R. D., McDonald, R. C., et al. (1999). Treatment patterns among adult patients with asthma: Factors associated with overuse of inhaled beta-agonists and underuse of inhaled corticosteroids. *Archives of Internal Medicine, 159,* 2697–2704.

DiMatteo, M. R. (2004a). Social support and patient adherence to medical treatment: A meta-analysis. *Health Psychology, 23,* 207–218.

DiMatteo, M. R. (2004b). Variations in patients' adherence to medical recommendations: A quantitative review of 50 years of research. *Medical Care, 42,* 200–209.

DiMatteo, M. R., Giordani, P. J., Lepper, H. S., & Croghan, T. W. (2002). Patient adherence and medical treatment outcomes: A meta-analysis. *Medical Care, 40,* 794–811.

DiMatteo, M. R., Sherbourne, C. D., Hays, R. D., Ordway, L., Kravitz, R. L., McGlynn, et al. (1993). Physicians' characteristics influence patients' adherence to medical treatment: Results from the medical outcomes study. *Health Psychology, 12,* 93–102.

Dolce, J., Crisp, C., Manzella, B., Richards, J. M., Harding, M., & Bailey, W. C. (1991). Medication adherence patterns in chronic obstructive pulmonary disease. *Chest, 99,* 837–841.

Dolder, C. R., Lacro, J. P., & Jeste, D. V. (2003). Adherence to antipsychotic and nonpsychiatric medications in middle-aged and older patients with psychotic disorders. *Psychosomatic Medicine, 65,* 156–162.

Donovan, J. L., & Blake, D. R. (1992). Patient non-compliance: Deviance or reasoned decision-making? *Social Science and Medicine, 34,* 507–513.

DuBard, M. B., Goldenberg, R. L., Copper, R. L., & Hauth, J. C. (1993). Are pill counts valid measures of compliance in clinical obstetric trials? *American Journal of Obstetrics and Gynecology, 169,* 1181–1182.

Dubbert, P. M., King, A., Rapp, S. R., Brief, D., Martin, J. E., & Lake, M. (1985). Riboflavin as a tracer of medication compliance. *Journal of Behavioral Medicine, 8,* 287–299.

Dunbar-Jacob, J. (1993). Contributions to patient adherence: Is it time to share the blame? *Health Psychology, 12,* 91–92.

Golin, C. E., Liu, H., Hays, R. D., Miller, L. G., Beck, C. K., Ickovics, J., et al. (2002). A prospective study of predictors of adherence to combination antiretroviral medication. *Journal of General Internal Medicine, 17,* 756–765.

Gordis, L. (1976). Methodologic issues in the measurement of patient compliance. In D. L. Sackett & R. B. Haynes (Eds.), *Compliance with therapeutic regimens* (pp. 51–66). Baltimore, MD: Johns Hopkins University Press.

Granger, B. B., Swedberg, K., Ekman, I., Granger, C. B., Olofsson, B., McMurray, J. J., et al. (2005). Adherence to candesartan and placebo and outcomes in chronic heart failure in the CHARM programme: Double-blind, randomised, controlled clinical trial. *Lancet, 366,* 2005–2011.

Grant, R. W., Singer, D. E., & Meigs, J. B. (2005). Medication adherence before an increase in antihypertensive therapy: A cohort study using pharmacy claims data. *Clinical Therapeutics, 27,* 773–781.

Gurwitz, J. H., Glynn, R. J., Monane, M., Everitt, D. E., Gilden, D., Smith, N., et al. (1993). Treatment for glaucoma: Adherence by the elderly. *American Journal of Public Health, 83,* 711–716.

Hamilton, G. A. (2003). Measuring adherence in a hypertension clinical trial. *European Journal of Cardiovascular Nursing, 2,* 219–228.

Hatton, M. Q. F., Allen, M. B., Vathenen, S. V., Feely, M. P., & Cooke, N. J. (1996). Compliance with oral corticosteroids during steroid trials in chronic airways obstruction. *Thorax, 51,* 323–324.

Heszen Klemens, I., & Lapinska, E. (1984). Doctor-patient interaction, patients' health behavior and effects of treatment. *Social Science and Medicine, 19,* 9–18.

Hilbrands, L. B., Hoitsma, A., & Koene, R. A. P. (1995). Medication compliance after renal transplantation. *Transplantation, 60,* 914–920.

Jayaweera, D. T., Kolber, M. A., Brill, M., Tanner, T., Campo, R., Rodriguez, A., et al. (2004). Effectiveness and tolerability of a once-daily amprenavir/ritonavir-containing highly active antiretroviral therapy regimen in antiretroviral-naive patients at risk for nonadherence: 48-week results after 24 weeks of directly observed therapy. *HIV Medicine, 5,* 364–370.

Kasl, S. V. (1975). Issues in patient adherence to health care regimens. *Journal of Human Stress, 1,* 5–17.

Koch, D. A., Giardina, P. J., Ryan, M., MacQueen, M., & Hilgartner, M. W. (1993). Behavioral contracting to improve adherence in patients with thalassemia. *Journal of Pediatric Nursing, 8,* 106–111.

Kraag, G. R., Gordon, D. A., Menard, H-A., Russell, A. S., & Kalish, G. H. (1994). Patient compliance with tenoxicam in family practice. *Clinical Therapy, 16,* 581–593.

Krishnan, J. A., Riekert, K. A., McCoy, J. V., Stewart, D. Y., Schmidt, S., Chanmugam, A., et al. (2004). Corticosteroid use after hospital discharge among high-risk adults with asthma. *American Journal of Respiratory and Critical Care Medicine, 170,* 1281–1285.

Laine, C., Newschaffer, C. J., Zhang, D., Cosler, L., Hauck, W. W., & Turner, B. J. (2000). Adherence to antiretroviral therapy by pregnant women infected with human immunodeficiency virus: A pharmacy claims-based analysis. *Obstetrics and Gynecology, 95,* 167–173.

Levine, A. J., Hinkin, C. H., Marion, S., Keuning, A., Castellon, S. A., Lam, M. M., et al. (2006). Adherence to antiretroviral medications in HIV: Differences in data collected via self-report and electronic monitoring. *Health Psychology, 25,* 329–335.

Liu, H., Golin, C. E., Miller, L. G., Hays, R. D., Beck, C. K., Sanandaji, S., et al. (2001). A comparison study of multiple measures of adherence to HIV protease inhibitors. *Annals of Internal Medicine, 134,* 968–977.

Liu, H., Kaplan, A. H., & Wenger, N. S. (2002). Measuring patient adherence. *Annals of Internal Medicine, 137,* 72–73.

Llabre, M. M., Weaver, K. E., Duran, R. E., Antoni, M. H., Pherson-Baker, S., & Schneiderman, N. (2006). A measurement model of medication adherence to highly active antiretroviral therapy and its relation to viral load in HIV-positive adults. *AIDS Patient Care and STDs, 20,* 701–711.

Lucas, G. M., Mullen, B. A., Weidle, P. J., Hader, S., McCaul, M. E., & Moore, R. D. (2006). Directly administered antiretroviral therapy in methadone clinics is associated with improved HIV treatment outcomes, compared with outcomes among concurrent comparison groups. *Clinical Infectious Diseases, 42,* 1628–1635.

Lucas, G. M., Weidle, P. J., Hader, S., & Moore, R. D. (2004). Directly administered antiretroviral therapy in an urban methadone maintenance clinic: A nonrandomized comparative study. *Clinical Infectious Diseases, 38* (Suppl. 5), 409–413.

Maenpaa, H., Manninen, V., & Heinonen, O. P. (1992). Compliance with medication in the Helsinki Heart Study. *European Journal of Clinical Pharmacology, 42,* 15–19.

Marceau, C., Lemiere, C., Berbiche, D., Perreault, S., & Blais, L. (2006). Persistence, adherence, and effectiveness of combination therapy among adult patients with asthma. *Journal Allergy Clinical Immunology, 118,* 574–581.

Maronde, R. F., Chan, L. S., Larsen, F. J., Strandberg, L. R., Laventurier, M. F., & Sullivan, S. R. (1989). Underutilization of antihypertensive drugs and associated hospitalization. *Medical Care, 27,* 1159–1166.

Mason, B. J., Matsuyama, J. R., & Jue, S. G. (1995). Assessment of sulfonylurea adherence and metabolic control. *Diabetes Educator, 21,* 52–57.

Matsui, D., Hermann, C., Klein, J., Berkovitch, M., Olivieri, N., & Koren, G. (1994). Critical comparison of novel and existing methods of compliance assessment during a clinical trial of an oral iron chelator. *Journal of Clinical Pharmacology, 34,* 944–949.

Mawhinney, H., Spector, S. L., Kinsman, R. A., Siegel, S. C., Rachelefsky, G. S., Katz, R. M., et al. (1991). Compliance in clinical trials of two nonbronchodilator, antiasthma medications. *Annals of Allergy, 66,* 294–299.

Melnikow, J., & Kiefe, C. (1994). Patient compliance and medical research: Issues in methodology. *Journal of General Internal Medicine, 9,* 96–105.

Miller, L. G., Liu, H., Hays, R. D., Golin, C. E., Beck, C. K., Asch, S. M., et al. (2002). How well do clinicians estimate patients' adherence to combination antiretroviral therapy? *Journal of General and Internal Medicine, 17,* 1–11.

Moss, A. R., Hahn, J. A., Perry, S., Charlebois, E. D., Guzman, D., Clark, R. A., et al. (2004). Adherence to highly active antiretroviral therapy in the homeless population in San Francisco: A prospective study. *Clinical Infectious Diseases, 39,* 1190–1198.

Nachega, J. B., Hislop, M., Dowdy, D. W., Lo, M., Omer, S. B., Regensberg, L., et al. (2006). Adherence to highly active antiretroviral therapy assessed by pharmacy claims predicts survival in HIV-infected South African adults. *Journal of Acquired Immune Deficiency Syndromes, 43,* 78–84.

Nides, M. A., Tashkin, D. P., Simmons, M. S., Wise, R. A., Li, V. C., & Rand, C. S. (1993). Improving inhaler adherence in a clinical trial through the use of the nebulizer chronology. *Chest, 104,* 501–507.

Parris, E. S., Lawrence, D. B., Mohn, L. A., & Long, L. B. (2005). Adherence to statin therapy and LDL cholesterol goal attainment by patients with diabetes and dyslipidemia. *Diabetes Care, 28,* 595–599.

Paulson, S. M., Krause, S., & Iber, R. (1977). Development and evaluation of a compliance test for patients taking disulfiram. *Johns Hopkins Medical Journal, 141,* 119–125.

Purcell, B. K., Dooley, D. P., Gray, P. J., Hill, K. J., & Oliverson, F. W. (2004). Experience with directly observed prophylaxis using erythromycin in military trainees exposed to pertussis. *Military Medicine, 169,* 417–420.

Rand, C., Bilderback, A., Schiller, K., Edelman, J. M., Hustad, C. M., & Zeiger, R. S. (2007). Adherence with montelukast or fluticasone in a long-term clinical trial: Results from the mild asthma montelukast versus inhaled corticosteroid trial. *Journal of Allergy and Clinical Immunology, 119,* 916–923.

Rand, C. S. (2000). "I took the medicine like you told me, doctor": Self-report of adherence with medical regimens. In A. A. Stone, J. S. Turkkan, C. A. Bachrach, J. B. Jobe, H. S. Kurtzman, & V. S. Cain (Eds.), *The science of self-report: Implications for research and practice* (pp. 257–276). Mahwah, NJ: Lawrence Earlbaum.

Rand, C. S. (2002). Adherence to asthma therapy in the preschool child. *Allergy, 57* (Suppl. 74), 48–57.

Rand, C. S., Nides, M., Cowles, M. K., Wise, R. A., & Connett, J. (1995). Long-term metered-dose inhaler adherence in a clinical trial. The Lung Health Study Research Group. *American Journal of Respiratory and Critical Care Medicine, 152,* 580–588.

Rand, C. S., & Sevick, M. A. (2000). Ethics in adherence promotion and monitoring. *Controlled Clinical Trials, 21,* 241S–247S.

Rand, C. S., & Wise, R. A. (1994). Measuring adherence to asthma medication regimens. *American Journal of Respiratory Critical Care & Medicine, 149,* S69–S76.

Rand, C. S., Wise, R. A., Nides, M., Simmons, M. S., Bleecker, E. R., Kusek, J. W., et al. (1992). MDI adherence in a clinical trial. *American Review of Respiratory Disorders, 146,* 1559–1564.

Riekert, K. A., & Rand, C. S. (2002). Electronic monitoring of medication adherence: When is high-tech best? *Journal of Clinical Psychology in Medical Settings, 9,* 25–34.

Rodewald, L. E., & Pichichero, M. E. (1993). Compliance with antibiotic therapy: A comparison of deuterium oxide tracer, urine bioassay, bottle weights, and parental reports. *Journal of Pediatrics, 123,* 143–147.

Ross, F. M. (1991). Patient compliance: Whose responsibility? *Social Science and Medicine, 32,* 89–94.

Sackett, D. L., & Haynes, R. B. (1976). *Compliance with therapeutic regimens.* Baltimore, MD: Johns Hopkins University Press.

Sale, J. E., Gignac, M., & Hawker, G. (2006). How "bad" does the pain have to be? A qualitative study examining adherence to pain medication in older adults with osteoarthritis. *Arthritis & Rheumatism, 55,* 272–278.

Schaub, A. F., Steiner, A., & Vetter, W. (1993). Compliance to treatment. Clinical and *Experimental Hypertension, 15,* 1121–1130.

Schectman, G., Hiatt, J., & Hartz, A. (1994). Telephone contacts do not improve adherence to niacin or bile acid sequestrant therapy. *Annals of Pharmacotherapy, 28,* 29–35.

Sherman, J., Hutson, A., Baumstein, S., & Hendeles, L. (2000). Telephoning the patient's pharmacy to assess adherence with asthma medications by measuring refill rate for prescriptions. *Journal of Pediatrics, 136,* 532–536.

Spitzer, W. O., Suissa, S., Ernst, P., Horwitz, R. I., Habbick, B., Cockcroft, D., et al. (1992). The use of B-agonists and the risk of death from asthma. *New England Journal of Medicine, 326,* 501–506.

Steele, D. J., Jackson, T. C., & Gutmann, M. C. (1990). Have you been taking your pill? The adherence-monitoring sequence in the medical interview. *Journal of Family Practice, 30,* 294–299.

Steele, R. G., Anderson, B., Rindel, B., Dreyer, M. L., Perrin, K., Christensen, R., et al. (2001). Adherence to antiretroviral therapy among HIV-positive children: Examination of the role of caregiver health beliefs. *AIDS Care, 13,* 617–629.

Stein, M. B., Cantrell, C. R., Sokol, M. C., Eaddy, M. T., & Shah, M. B. (2006). Antidepressant adherence and medical resource use among managed care patients with anxiety disorders. *Psychiatric Services, 57,* 673–680.

Steiner, J. F., Fihn, S. D., Blair, B., & Inui, T. S. (1991). Appropriate reductions in compliance among well-controlled hypertensive patients. *Journal of Clinical Epidemiology, 44,* 1361–1371.

Stempel, D. A., Stoloff, S. W., Carranza, R., Jr., Stanford, R. H., Ryskina, K. L., & Legorreta, A. P. (2005). Adherence to asthma controller medication regimens. *Respiratory Medicine, 99,* 1263–1267.

Tamblyn, R., Lavoie, G., Petrella, L., & Monette, J. (1995). The use of prescription claims databases in pharmacoepidemiological research: The accuracy and comprehensiveness of the prescription claims database in Quebec. *Journal of Clinical Epidemiology, 48,* 999–1009.

Urquhart, J. (1991). Patient compliance as an explanatory variable in four selected cardiovascular studies. In J. A. Cramer & B. Spilker (Eds.), *Patient compliance in medical practice and clinical trials* (pp. 301–322). New York: Raven.

Volmink, J., & Garner, P. (2000). Interventions for promoting adherence to tuberculosis management. *Cochran Database of Systematic Review,* CD000010.

Waitzkin, H. (1984). Doctor-patient communication. Clinical implications of social scientific research. *Journal of the American Medical Association, 252,* 2441–2446.

Wang, P. S., Benner, J. S., Glynn, R. J., Winkelmayer, W. C., Mogun, H., & Avorn, J. (2004). How well do patients report noncompliance with antihypertensive medications? A comparison of self-report versus filled prescriptions. *Pharmacoepidemiology and Drug Safety, 13,* 11–19.

Waterhouse, D. M., Calzone, K. A., Mele, C., & Brenner, D. E. (1993). Adherence to oral tamoxifen: A comparison of patient self report, pill counts, and microelectronic monitoring. *Journal of Clinical Oncology, 11,* 1189–1197.

Wysocki, T., Green, L., & Huxtable, K. (1989). Blood glucose monitoring by diabetic adolescents: Compliance and metabolic control. *Health Psychology, 8,* 267–284.

The Measurement of Physical Activity

17

Sara Wilcox and
Barbara E. Ainsworth

A growing body of work has focused on examining and improving the measurement of physical activity. In the past decade, several conferences and resources have focused on the assessment of physical activity with the goal of gaining insight into ways to increase precision within various measurement settings (Table 17.1). Within the health-related disciplines, there are at least four major reasons to measure physical activity: (1) to examine the role of physical activity as a risk or protective factor in the development of a particular disease such as cardiovascular disease or cancer, (2) to monitor changes in physical activity in a population over time (surveillance), (3) to examine the associations between physical activity and individual, social, and environmental factors for the purpose of informing interventions and identifying populations to target in interventions, and (4) to determine whether interventions at the individual and

17.1 Useful Resources for the Measurement of Physical Activity

Topic	Resource
Assessment of physical activity in specific populations and with specific methods	Proceedings of the October 1999 Cooper Institute Conference, *Measurement of Physical Activity.* Published in the June 2000 issue of *Research Quarterly for Exercise and Sport, 71,* Supplement to No. 2
Reproduction of commonly used self-report measures and reliability and validity references	Issue of *Medicine and Science in Sports and Exercise, 29*(6) (1997, Supplement)
Use of accelerometers in different settings and populations	Proceedings of the December 2004 conference *Objective Measurement of Physical Activity: Closing the Gaps in the Science of Accelerometery.* Published in *Medicine and Science in Sports and Exercise, 37*(11, Supplement) (November 2005)

population levels are effective. This chapter identifies definitions of terms used in physical activity assessment and reviews self-report and objective measures of physical activity. In each section, considerations that must be made when selecting measures for population subgroups (e.g., women, people of color, older adults, and children) are discussed where relevant.

Definitions

It is important to differentiate among physical activity, exercise, and energy expenditure. Physical activity is a complex behavior defined as any bodily movement produced by skeletal muscles that results in increased energy expenditure (Caspersen, Powell, & Christenson, 1985). This broad definition includes activities such as housework, yard work, child care, transportation, occupational activity, sport and exercise, and leisure-time activity. Exercise is a type of physical activity and is more narrowly defined as planned, structured, and repetitive bodily movements done to improve or maintain one or more components of physical fitness (Caspersen et al., 1985). Energy expenditure is the outcome of physical activity and is defined as the exchange of energy required to perform biological work. Components of total energy expenditure include basal metabolic rate (encompassing 50%–70% of total energy), the thermic effect of food (encompassing another 7%–10% of total energy), and physical activity (encompassing the remaining percentage of total energy) (Ravussin & Swinburn, 1992). Physical activity is the most variable component of total energy expenditure and makes up a greater proportion of energy expenditure in active than inactive individuals. This chapter focuses on the measurement of physical activity.

Physical activity can be measured using direct methods such motion detectors and by indirect methods such as questionnaires, records, and logs. Several dimensions of physical activity are typically measured, including frequency, duration, intensity, and type to assess the volume of activity performed and to estimate the energy expenditure if desired. Frequency is generally defined as the number of sessions or days per week or per month an activity is performed. Duration usually refers to the time (minutes or hours) spent in one bout of a specific activity. Intensity refers to the level of effort required to perform a specific activity and is often expressed in terms of metabolic equivalents (METs). METs are defined as the ratio of the energy cost of an activity divided by the energy cost of the resting metabolic rate (1 MET). One MET is roughly equivalent to expending 1 kcal per kilogram body weight per hour (1 kcal/kg/hr) (Taylor et al., 1978). Public health programs encourage participation in moderate intensity physical activity to reduce disease risks and enhance health. Moderate intensity physical activity is defined as three to six METs (Pate et al., 1995). Vigorous intensity physical activity is defined as more than six METs and is associated with improvement of cardiorespiratory fitness. Total physical activity is often reported as hours or minutes per week and is a function of the frequency, duration, and intensity of activity performed. As a weighted estimate of intensity, MET-hr/wk (or MET-min/wk) is computed by multiplying the appropriate weight metabolic equivalent value for each activity by the amount of time spent performing that specific activity in a given week (Ainsworth et al., 2000). Finally, comprehensive measures of physical activity also measure the type or mode of the activity performed (e.g., walking, vacuuming, jogging) to allow for understanding the context in which physical activity occurs.

Key Issues to Consider When Selecting a Measure

There are many issues to consider when choosing a physical activity measure. The measure should reflect the dimension(s) of greatest interest to the study or program. For example, if an intervention targets walking, walking should be a primary activity assessed in the measure. If, however, the intervention targets lifestyle activity (e.g., building more activity into one's daily routine), then a broader and more comprehensive assessment of physical activity is likely needed. Beyond the match between measure and purpose of the assessment, other issues to consider include reliability, validity, sensitivity to change, feasibility, reactivity, and potential sources of bias (Table 17.2).

Reliability indicates the degree to which a measure consistently produces the same results with repeated administration, or test-retest reliability. Interrater reliability, or the degree of agreement between two independent raters, is also relevant for interview-administered measures and direct observation of physical activity. It is important to remember that a measure can be reliable but not valid. That is, the measure might consistently yield the same score but not measure the underlying construct of physical activity. Validity indicates how well the measure assesses what it is purported to measure, typically referred to

17.2   Issues to Consider When Selecting a Physical Activity Measure

Measurement concerns	Definitions
Test-retest reliability	Degree to which a measure consistently produces the same results with repeated administration
Interrater reliability	Degree of agreement between two independent raters
Construct validity	How well the measure assesses what it is purported to measure
Criterion validity	Accuracy of a measure by comparing it with another measure which has been demonstrated to be valid
Convergent validity	How well two measures of the same construct correlate with each other
Sensitivity to change	Ability to detect a change when true behavior change occurs
Feasibility	Relates to the setting that measures will be used, the number of individuals measured, the cost of the measures, and the acceptability of the measures to the target population
Reactivity	Degree to which the simple act of measurement changes a person's behavior
Social desirability	The tendency for people to present themselves in an overly positive manner
Demand characteristics	The participant's tendency to respond in a manner consistent with what he/she perceives as the study hypotheses

as construct validity (Shadish, Cook, & Campbell, 2002). For example, an occupational questionnaire that accurately identifies the amount of physical activity performed in an occupational setting would have acceptable construct validity. Criterion-related validity is used to demonstrate the accuracy of a measure or procedure by comparing it with another measure or procedure that has been demonstrated to be valid. Assessing a measure's criterion-related validity is problematic for physical activity. Patterson (2000) notes that even objective measures, such as doubly labeled water, accelerometers, heart rate, and direct observation, are not likely true "gold standard measures" of physical activity as they singly do not assess the breadth of movement by type and intensity. Instead, she suggests that comparing a measure of interest to these more objective measures provides convergent validity, which is only one component of construct validity and reflects the degree that construct measures are related.

A measure's sensitivity to change is another important but sometimes overlooked issue to consider in the assessment of physical activity. A measure that is sensitive to change is one that detects a true change when it occurs. Sensitivity to change is most relevant in prospective and intervention (quasi-experimental and experimental) studies that rely on physical activity assessment tools to determine the effects of the intervention strategies on changing physical activity behaviors.

Feasibility issues often drive the selection of study measures. Some measures are more feasible than others depending on the setting in which they will be used, the number of individuals measured, the cost of the measures, and the acceptability of the measures to the target population. For example, expensive objective measures (i.e., accelerometers) are not very feasible for use in surveillance systems where large numbers of individuals are typically assessed via telephone. Some may feel the measures pose too much of a participant burden, are perceived as intrusive, or are too expensive to administer. It is interesting to note, however, that physical activity was recently measured with accelerometers in the National Health and Nutrition Examination Survey and found to be acceptable by the study participants (Troiano, 2005). Finally, potential sources of bias (often called threats to construct validity) (Shadish et al., 2002) must be considered when selecting a measure and interpreting study findings. Reactivity, social desirability, and demand characteristics are some of the most likely sources of bias in physical activity measurement. Reactivity refers to the idea that the simple act of measurement may change a person's behavior. For example, keeping a diary of activity or wearing a pedometer may cause a person to alter his activity level. Social desirability refers to the tendency for people to present themselves in an overly positive manner—for example, as more physically active than they actually are. Demand characteristics refer to participants' tendency to respond in a manner consistent with what they perceive as the study hypotheses. For example, participants may over report physical activity after an intervention if they know the purpose of the study is to increase physical activity. Social desirability and demand characteristic biases are of particular concern with self-report measures. For more details regarding these and other sources of bias, the reader is referred elsewhere (Shadish et al., 2002). Each of these issues is highlighted in the review of physical activity measurement approaches.

It is important to keep in mind that there is no "perfect" measure of physical activity. Typically, one must weigh the pros and cons relative to the issues just described. Wherever possible, it is advisable to use more than one method of measuring physical activity to help balance different sources of bias.

Types of Physical Activity Measures

Indirect Measures—Self-Report of Physical Activity

Self-report measures are the most frequently used method of assessing physical activity due in large part to their low cost and ease of use. Self-administered measures (e.g., paper-and-pencil questionnaires), interview-administered measures, and physical activity records and logs are described in this section.

Self- and Interview-Administered Self-Report Measures

A large number of self-report measures are available for use in general as well as specific populations, and they vary greatly in complexity and length, assessment time frame, domain of activity assessed, and expression of physical activity (e.g., unitless value, MET hrs/wk, minutes/week). Examples of self-report measures are presented in Table 17.3. Global measures tend to be very brief and typically ask participants to rate their physical activity level on a Likert-type scale. Participation in specific types of activities is not assessed, and often the participant is asked to respond relative to a "usual" or "typical" day. These measures tend to be used to measure physical activity when it is not the primary behavior of interest, for example, to control for physical activity in a study of dietary behavior.

Self-report recall measures can range from very short questionnaires or interviews that are used in surveillance studies to more lengthy questionnaires. Surveillance measures are typically used to categorize people into groups (e.g., percentage meeting physical activity recommendations) rather than to provide a precise estimate of physical activity. Longer, more comprehensive measures ask participants to report their participation in specific types of activities, as well as the frequency and duration of the activities. There is some variation in the time frame assessed in recall measures, although the time frame generally ranges from the preceding 24 hours to the previous month.

Finally, historical self-report questionnaires most commonly assess physical activity patterns over the past 12 months or one's lifetime. These measures are useful for assessing typical patterns of physical activity and for relating long-term physical activity or inactivity to various health outcomes.

Overall, when deciding on what time frame is most appropriate for the assessment of physical activity, it is important to consider how well the assessment method fits with the study purpose. In addition, the advantage of shorter time frames is that recall bias is likely to be reduced as people aren't required to think back over a long period of time, whereas the disadvantage is that the previous 24 hours or week may not be typical of the person's physical activity due to illness, a stressful life event, or other factors. Measures that assess longer time frames, such as the past year, are more likely to assess an individual's usual pattern of behavior but are more susceptible to recall errors.

Finally, self-report measures vary in the domains of physical activity they capture. Examples of domains included on many self-report questionnaires include leisure-time physical activity, sport, exercise, household activities, yard work, transportation-related activity, and child-care-related activities. Measures that contain domains related to the primary purpose of the study should be chosen.

Self- and Interview-Administered Self-Report Measures—Reliability, Validity, Sensitivity, Feasibility, and Bias

Self-report measures typically have fairly high test-retest reliability in adult samples (Sallis & Saelens, 2000). It is important to keep in mind that reliability correlations can be attenuated due to actual variability in physical activity levels over time. Validity of self-report measures is more difficult to assess because of the lack of appropriate criterion measures discussed earlier. When researchers compared objective measures such as doubly labeled water, accelerometers, and heart rate monitoring to commonly used measures, validity correlations were found to be lower than reliability correlations, ranging from r = .14 to .36, although the Seven-Day Physical Activity Recall (PAR) had higher correlations

17.3 Examples of Self-Report Physical Activity Measures for Adults

Measure	Reference	Number of items	Recall time frame	Domains assessed
Brief, global				
Lipid Research Clinics Physical Activity Questionnaire	Ainsworth, Jacobs, & Leon, 1993	4	Usual day	Occupational exercise
Stanford Usual Activity Questionnaire	Sallis et al., 1985	2	Usual activity unspecified & usual activity in the last 3 months	Moderate-intensity and vigorous-intensity activity
Recall questionnaires or interviews				
Baecke Questionnaire of Habitual Physical Activity	Baecke, Burema, & Frijters, 1982	16	Usual activity	Sport, leisure, occupational
Behavioral Risk Factor Surveillance System (BRFSS)	Centers for Disease Control, 2005	6	Usual week	Moderate-intensity and vigorous-intensity lifestyle physical activity
Community Healthy Activities Model Programs for Seniors (CHAMPS)	Stewart et al., 2001	42	Typical week in the past 4 weeks	Exercise, sport, leisure, occupational, transportation
Physical Activity Scale for the Elderly (interview- or self-administered)	Washburn et al., 1999; Washburn et al., 1993	10	Past 7 days	Leisure, household, occupational
Seven-Day Physical Activity Recall (interview-administered)	Blair et al., 1985	Not applicable (guided recall of activity in morning, afternoon, and evening in past 7 days)	Past 7 days	Exercise, leisure, occupational

(Continued)

17.3 Examples of Self-Report Physical Activity Measures for Adults (*Continued*)

Measure	Reference	Number of items	Recall time frame	Domains assessed
Historical questionnaires				
CARDIA Physical Activity History	Jacobs et al., 1989	60 (if all questions are answered yes)	Past 12 months	Leisure, occupational, household
Historical Leisure Activity Questionnaire	Kriska et al., 1990	List of 39 activities is read (plus "other") and for those done >10 times, participant reports on 4 periods in life	Lifetime	Exercise, sports
Lifetime Total Physical Activity Questionnaire	Friedenreich et al., 1998	Open-ended question for each domain	Lifetime	Exercise/sports, occupational, household
Minnesota Leisure-Time Physical Activity Questionnaire	Taylor et al., 1978	63	Past 12 months	Exercise, sports, recreation, yard, household

with accelerometers (range of r = .50 to .53) (Sallis & Saelens, 2000). Higher-intensity physical activities are more accurately reported than lower-intensity activities, likely because they are more memorable and time-limited than light- and moderate-intensity activities (Sallis et al., 1985; Sallis & Saelens, 2000).

Self-report measures are often selected because of their feasibility. They are inexpensive and generally easy for participants to complete, therefore presenting relatively low participant burden, and can be used in a wide variety of settings. Data regarding sensitivity of measures to change are often not reported to the extent that validity and reliability data are. The potential for bias is the most substantial concern with self-report measures. While reactivity is not a concern, social desirability biases and demand characteristics are among the most commonly voiced concerns with self-report measures. The reader is also referred to an excellent paper by Choi and Pak (2005), which outlines a number of additional biases in self-report measures and ways to minimize these biases.

Several approaches have been used to try to identify and minimize bias in questionnaire development. Durante and Ainsworth (1996) discuss a cognitive model that can be used to identify potential sources of bias in questionnaires.

They propose four stages of cognitive processing that influence how respondents answer questions: (1) comprehension, (2) retrieval, (3) decision making, and (4) response generation. Ambiguities in the question impact comprehension. For example, if respondents are left to define critical terms (e.g., "a city block," "moderate-intensity"), biases are likely in this first stage of comprehension. Challenges related to mental operations required in the decision-making stage (e.g., summing time walked over a one- to seven-day period) could produce errors in this stage. Further, errors in translating information from the decision-making stage to the response generation stage could result in errors. Several ways to reduce such sources of error have been recommended. First, questions are often subjected to cognitive testing. Respondents are asked, for example, to rephrase what they think the question means or to state how confident they are in the accuracy of their response. Another approach that enhances accuracy is to provide contextual cues and recall calendars. For example, in the Seven Day Physical Activity Recall (Sallis et al., 1985), participants are asked to think about the activities they did in a given day (e.g., when did they wake up? Did they work that day? Did they have class that day?) in order to give greater context to their day and thus enable them to report physical activity more accurately. Recall calendars (e.g., focused on educational and occupational activities and life events) are used in the Lifetime Total Physical Activity Questionnaire (Friedenreich, Courneya, & Bryant, 1998) to help serve as memory aids for the participant. Another approach to minimizing self-report errors has been used to attempt to reduce social desirability. The Community Healthy Activities Model Program for Seniors (CHAMPS) physical activity questionnaire (Stewart et al., 2001) asks about activities that are not physical in nature (e.g., visiting with friends, reading, working on a computer) in addition to physical activities. The rationale is that individuals will be more likely to truly respond negatively to items if there are some activities included to which they can respond positively. Finally, in the area of dietary assessment, some used a social desirability measure as a way to estimate bias and control for it in analyses (Hebert, Clemow, Pbert, Ockene, & Ockene, 1995). A similar approach could be used in physical activity assessment. Additional techniques to minimize reporting errors are discussed elsewhere (Choi & Pak, 2005; Durante & Ainsworth, 1996).

Self- and Interview-Administered Measures in Population Subgroups

There are several factors that must be considered when using self-report measures in children, older adults, women, and persons of color. Sallis and colleagues reviewed self-report measures used in the 1990s for children, adults, and older adults (Sallis & Saelens, 2000). Children, particularly those under the age of 9 years, are more limited in their cognitive functioning than adults, translating into less accurate recall of physical activity and an inability to accurately estimate time on self-report measures (Welk, Corbin, & Dale, 2000). Therefore, self-report measures are not recommended for children under the age of 9 years. In a review of self-report measures for children age 9 years and older (Sallis & Saelens, 2000), test-retest reliability correlations for self-report measures were generally acceptable (range: $r = .60$ to $.98$), but validity correlations were variable, ranging from $r = .07$ to $r = .88$ for self-administered surveys and from $r = .17$ to $r = .72$ for interview-administered measures. However, they noted that approximately half of the measures assessed had validity correlation coefficients of r = .50 or higher. In an effort to reduce cognitive demands, the Previous Day Physical Activity Recall (PDPAR) was developed for use with children and validated (Weston, Petosa, & Pate, 1997). Children are asked to recall the dominant activity engaged in during a series of 30-minute time increments and the intensity of the activity. A MET value is assigned to each activity corresponding to the activity type and intensity. Multiple days of recalls must be collected, as is the case in the 3-Day Physical Activity Recall (3DPAR) (Pate, Ross, Dowda, Trost, & Sirard, 2003).

Women and persons of color are less likely than men and non-Hispanic whites to participate in structured, vigorous-intensity physical activity. Instead, they are more likely to participate in activities that are less structured and of light- to moderate-intensity, such occupational, household, and family-care activities (Ainsworth, 2000b). Many self-report measures do not assess these types of activities, and thus the physical activity levels of women and ethnic minority adults are likely underestimated (Ainsworth, 2000a; Kriska, 2000; Mâsse et al., 1998). Indeed, Brownson and colleagues (Brownson et al., 2000) found that when a broader definition of physical activity was used that included occupational activity and housework, nearly three-fourths of women in the U.S. Women's Determinants Study were classified as regularly active. Ainsworth and colleagues (Ainsworth, Irwin, Addy, Whitt, & Stolarczyk, 1999) reported similar findings in that 63% to 70% of African American and Native American women over the age of 40 years were classified as regularly active when activities such as household chores, occupation activity, and child care were assessed. Related, most available questionnaires have not been critically evaluated as to the extent that they are culturally and gender sensitive (Mâsse et al., 1998). Terms such as "moderate intensity," "vigorous," "exercise," "leisure-time," and "physical activity" may not be interpreted the same way across study populations (Tortolero, Mâsse, Fulton, Torres, & Kohl, 1999). Furthermore, as was noted earlier, lower-intensity activities are recalled with poorer accuracy than higher-intensity activities, posing challenges for valid and reliable physical activity assessment in women and persons of color.

Mâsse and colleagues (Mâsse et al., 1998) outlined a number of recommendations for assessing physical activity in midlife, older, and minority women. These include being sensitive to the characteristics of the study population, accounting for various dimensions of physical activity performed, measuring moderate and intermittent activities as well as vigorous and continuous activities, and designing and administering surveys that are culturally inviting to the study population. In response to a number of these concerns and consistent with Mâsse and colleague's recommendations, Ainsworth and colleagues developed a self-report survey to assess physical activity among White, African American, and Native American women (Ainsworth et al., 1999). Survey items were generated based on detailed physical activity records kept by women that characterized types and patterns of physical activity in which they participated. The resulting questionnaire is one of the few developed specifically for ethnic minority women.

Finally, there are unique considerations in the measurement of physical activity in older adults. Some of the same challenges that affect the assessment of physical activity in women and persons of color apply to older adults. Although there is a great deal of diversity within the older population, low- and moderate-intensity physical activities are much more common than vigorous-intensity physical activities, potentially creating problems in accurate recall as well as in the appropriate inclusion of activities on surveys (Mâsse et al., 1998). Thus, prevalence studies likely underestimate physical activity participation among older adults because of the types of questions that are included in most self-report surveys. Another challenge in assessing physical activity in older adults relates to cognitive and sensory impairments. Cognitive impairments and age-related sensory declines in vision and hearing, which increase with age, may attenuate the accuracy of self-report measures. Thus, when considering which measure to use with an older population, the time frame and types of activities assessed are important considerations. Ideally, measures should ask about the past week or a usual week and should include household, yard, and caregiving activities. Older adults should be reminded to bring visual and hearing aids as needed, the interviewer should avoid speaking softly or in a high-pitched tone, and a larger font size (14 point) and matte rather than glossy paper should be used.

Several physical activity questionnaires have been developed specifically for older adults. Washburn (2000) reviewed four measures and reported adequate test-retest reliability correlations (range: $r = .42$ to .75) and validity correlations (range: $r = .42$ to .75). As noted by Washburn, validity studies were relatively rare and consisted of small samples. The four surveys were the Modified Baecke Questionnaire for Older Adults (Voorrips, Ravelli, Dongelmans, Deurenberg, & Van Staveren, 1991), the Zutphen Physical Activity Survey (Caspersen, Bloemberg, Saris, Merritt, & Kromhout, 1991), the Yale Physical Activity Survey (Dipietro, Caspersen, Ostfeld, & Nadel, 1993), and the Physical Activity Scale for the Elderly (Washburn, McAuley, Katula, Mihalko, & Boileau, 1999; Washburn, Smith, Jette, & Janney, 1993). Since that publication, Stewart and colleagues (Stewart et al., 2001) reported on the development of the Community Healthy Activities Model Program for Seniors (CHAMPS) physical activity questionnaire. This measure has comparably high reliability and validity correlations and has been shown to be sensitive to change in a number of intervention studies. Although the Zutphen Physical Activity measure only assesses leisure activity, the other measures assess broader domains, including household and occupational activity.

Physical Activity Records and Logs

Another type of self-report measure is a physical activity record or log. Physical activity records are typically detailed accounts of the types of activity in which participants engaged over the course of days or weeks. More detailed records might ask participants to report all activities in which they engaged, the duration of the activities, and perceived effort, whereas other, somewhat less detailed records might have participants record their activity at specified time intervals. This approach is similar to a food diary and can be completed as the person is going about her day. More detailed records can be used to validate other physical activity measures, since issues of recall bias are greatly minimized due to near-real-time recording (Ainsworth et al., 1999).

Physical activity logs are similar to records but are generally less burdensome. Typically, a checklist of activities and intensity levels is included for the participant to complete at specified time intervals (e.g., every 15 minutes). The logs are completed at the end of the day, and intensity values from the Compendium of Physical Activity (Ainsworth et al., 2000) are assigned to each activity. Examples of physical activity logs include the Bouchard Physical Activity Log (Bouchard et al., 1983) and the Ainsworth Physical Activity Log (LaMonte, Ainsworth, & Tudor-Locke, 2003). Finally, in the context of intervention studies, very simple logs are often used to record bouts of physical activity. For example, in a walking study, participants could record the total minutes they walked each day for exercise on a calendar and return this log to staff on a monthly basis.

Physical Activity Records and Logs—Reliability, Validity, Sensitivity, Feasibility, and Bias

The psychometric properties of physical activity records and logs have not been studied as extensively as self- and interview-administered self-report questionnaires. However, because these records or logs are typically completed during the course of the day or at the end of the day, it is assumed that the degree of recall bias is considerably less than with questionnaires, thus enhancing reliability and validity. As noted earlier, detailed physical activity records are sometimes used to validate self-report measures. When compared to accelerometer counts, physical activity records have relatively high validity correlations (Richardson, Leon, Jacobs, Ainsworth, & Serfass, 1995). When records are completed over short periods of time, participant burden is relatively low. Similarly, physical activity logs, especially brief ones, impose very little participant burden. However, detailed records kept over longer periods of time can pose more substantial participant burden and can require substantial research staff time to code behavior, enter data, and synthesize data. Thus, feasibility is dependent on the level of detail required and the length of the reporting period. While reactivity is of minimal concern with questionnaires as the mere act of completing them is unlikely to change behavior, reactivity is of greater concern with physical activity records and logs. That is, the act of recording activities could change actual behavior patterns. The effects of social desirability and demand pressures are more worrisome with physical activity questionnaires and logs than with objective measures but are of less concern than when self- and interview-administered questionnaires are used. However, these biases may still operate, as participants may overestimate duration or intensity due to social desirability and demand characteristic biases.

Direct Measures of Physical Activity

Accelerometers

Accelerometers are increasingly being used to measure physical activity as availability and improvements in technology continue. While the Caltrac (Muscle Dynamics, Torrence, CA) was the first accelerometer to be widely used in research, there are currently a number of accelerometers available for use, including Tritrac-R3D, RT3, Actigraph, Actical, ActiTrac, Actiwatch, BioTrainer, Tracmor, and SenseWear PRO_2. Accelerometers are small, battery-operated devices, typically worn at the hip (although arm and ankle placements are also used), that measure movement and velocity of movement. Most use piezoelectric sensors that detect movement in one to three planes. Accelerometers can be programmed to assess movement at different intervals or epochs (e.g., every minute) and store data for extended periods (up to 28 days of minute-by-minute recording). Data stored on the device are later downloaded, and regression equations based on laboratory calibration studies can be applied to classify physical activity into intensity categories using various cutpoints (Freedson, Melanson, & Sirard, 1998; Freedson, Pober, & Janz, 2005; Matthew, 2005).

Both uniaxial and triaxial accelerometers have been used to assess physical activity in various settings. Uniaxial accelerometers measure movement in one plane, typically the number and velocity of vertical movements. A commonly used uniaxial accelerometer is the Actigraph (formerly called the Computer Science Application or CSA; Actigraph, LLC, Fort Walton Beach, FL). Triaxial accelerometers measure movement in three dimensions. A commonly used triaxial accelerometer is the RT3 Triaxial Research Tracker (StayHealthy, Inc., Monrovia, CA). The Actical (Mini Mitter Co., Inc., Bend, OR) is an example of a newer triaxial accelerometer that is becoming widely used. It can record physical activity counts for up to 45 days (using minute-by-minute recording). In addition to the uniaxial and triaxial accelerometers, emerging technologies in accelerometers are described by Chen and Bassett (2005). These include accelerometers that take multiple measurements at different body segments, devices that combined accelerometry with other physiological measurements (e.g., heart rate, temperature), and shoe- and ankle-mounted accelerometers. Multisensor accelerometers such as the Intelligent Device for Energy Expenditure and Activity (IDEEA, MiniSun LLC, Fresno, CA) hold promise for enhancing prediction accuracy.

Reliability, Validity, Sensitivity, Feasibility, and Bias

Accelerometers are often selected because they remove the need for participant recall and thus eliminate self-report biases that limit reliability and validity. When compared to oxygen consumption and similar measures in controlled laboratory settings, accelerometers have high validity and reliability, particularly for dynamic activities such as walking and running, which are among the more common activities adults undertake (Matthew, 2005). Theoretically, triaxial accelerometers should be more accurate than uniaxial accelerometers because they should better characterize human movement and reflect movement in all geometric planes (e.g., forward, back, sideways, uphill, and downhill), but data reduction programs do not fully capitalize on this potential strength (Chen & Bassett, 2005), and validity coefficients have tended to be only marginally higher in triaxial models than in uniaxial models (Trost, McIver, & Pate, 2005). Accelerometers are not as valid for activities that require upper-body movement, strength training, water activities, or more complex activities. There is also evidence from validation studies. that accelerometers tend to underestimate energy expenditure, particularly for lifestyle activities, with triaxial accelerometers performing only slightly better than uniaxial accelerometers (Trost et al., 2005). In addition, while an appeal of accelerometers is that they measure both time and intensity, there are some instances where intensity is not properly assessed, such as walking or hiking on an incline.

With regard to feasibility, accelerometers typically impose only a modest participant burden. However, accuracy is threatened if the monitor is not worn properly, if the participant forgets to wear it or wears it for only part of a day, or if the monitor is not returned to the researcher. Thus, participant compliance is essential. Because of day-to-day variability in physical activity, it is recommended that the accelerometer be worn for 3 to 5 days in adults and 7 days in children to obtain adequate reliability coefficients (Trost et al., 2005). The cost of accelerometers ($300–$600) limits their feasibility in some contexts, such as population-based studies, and, because the monitor must be distributed and then collected some period of time later, its use is limited in some settings. Reactivity is a potential bias with the accelerometer because people may alter their behavior if they know it is being measured. However, the accelerometer does not provide feedback to the participant, thus minimizing this bias. An appeal of the accelerometer is that, because it eliminates the need for self-report, it is not subject to recall biases, social desirability, or demand characteristics.

Pedometers

The pedometer is another measure of physical activity that has grown in popularity in part because of its low cost and small size. Pedometers are worn at the waist and are triggered by the vertical accelerations of the hip that cause a horizontal spring-suspended level arm to move up and down, resulting in counted "steps." Pedometers are typically used to obtain a step count over a specified period, typically over the course of a day. They are used both as a measurement tool, particularly to assess walking, and as a self-monitoring and self-motivation tool in intervention studies. With regard to typical step counts one can expect, a systematic review of 32 empirical studies reported that 12,000–16,000 steps/day for 8–10-year-old children, 7,000–13,000 steps/day for relatively healthy, younger adults, 6,000–8,500 steps/day for healthy older adults, and 3,500–5,500 steps/day for individuals living with disabilities and chronic illnesses is typical (Tudor-Locke & Myers, 2001). Counts are lower in girls and women than in boys and men. The pedometer also has been used to assess population levels of physical activity (Tudor-Locke, 2002; Tudor-Locke et al., 2004). Tudor-Locke (2002) provides a comprehensive description of the use of pedometers for surveillance and research and in practice settings.

Reliability, Validity, Sensitivity, Feasibility, and Bias

In many settings the pedometer is a feasible alternative to the accelerometer because of its substantially lower cost ($20–$30). When walking is the primary activity of interest, a number of pedometers are available that are valid and reliable (Schneider, Crouter, & Bassett, 2004; Schneider, Crouter, Lukajic, & Bassett, 2003). Three days of measurement are considered necessary to obtain acceptable reliability coefficients with a pedometer (Tudor-Locke et al., 2005). The pedometer does not perform as well for very slow walking speeds and does not assess some types of physical activity, including upper-body exercises, strength training, and water activities. Placement and type of pedometer may be particularly important issues to attend to in obese individuals, especially when assessing very slow walking speeds (Crouter et al., 2005). Pedometers also provide no information regarding intensity of activity, duration of activity bouts, type of activity, or when the activity was performed.

As with the accelerometer, the participant burden imposed by the pedometer tends to be low, and participant compliance is important for accurate measurement. The participant must wear the pedometer correctly and consistently, record steps on a log at the end of the day, and zero it out every day. When it is used as a measurement tool, the pedometer does create a potential for reactivity. Because the participant gets feedback on number of steps taken, he can modify (increase) physical activity behavior as a result of assessment. One way to lessen reactivity is to have the participant wear the pedometer for a longer period of time than needed and to use only data acquired after several days of wearing. The novelty of the pedometer is likely to decrease after a few days of measurement. Also like the accelerometer, the pedometer eliminates recall biases. Assuming that the participant properly records his steps in a log, the biases imposed by social desirability and demand characteristic are minimal with pedometers.

Accelerometers and Pedometers in Population Subgroups

Because self-report measures have more limited reliability and validity in children, particularly young children, than in adults, accelerometers and pedometers are appealing. The reliability and validity of pedometers have not been examined extensively in children, but there is concern that children tend to react to the monitor and manipulate it and therefore reduce its validity (Ward, Saunders, & Pate, 2007). Nonetheless, Rowlands and colleagues reported a high correlation between pedometer and Tritrac accelerometer counts (r = .90) in a sample of children ages 8–10 years (Rowlands & Eston, 2005), and Eston and colleagues reported a high correlation (r = .78) between pedometer steps and oxygen uptake for treadmill walking and an even higher correlation with unregulated play activities (r = .92) (Eston, Rowlands, & Ingledew, 1998). Another study, however, found that pedometers did not fare well in a comparison with a direct observation system in younger children (Oliver, Schofield, Kolt, & Schluter, 2006).

Accelerometers, on the other hand, have been widely used in studies of children, and acceptable reliability and validity have been shown in both laboratory and field conditions (Trost et al., 2005; Welk et al., 2000). The Actigraph, Actical, and RT3 Triaxial Research Tracker have been studied most extensively. A key issue in assessing physical activity with children through accelerometers is that children tend to have more intermittent bursts of behavior. Thus, using time intervals or epochs of 1 minute, as is common in adults, is too long for children. Shorter time epochs should be used (e.g., 15 or 30 seconds). More days of monitoring (five to nine) are needed for children than for adults, and 7 days are recommended (Trost et al., 2005).

While the use of objective monitors in older adults is appealing as a way to avoid recall biases, few data are available regarding the reliability and validity of accelerometers in this population. There is some evidence, however, that pedometers underestimate steps taken by older adults with a slow walking speed and those with gait disorders, thus limiting their utility with frail individuals

(Cyarto, Myers, & Tudor-Locke, 2004). However, pedometers can be used with a high degree of reliability and validity with healthy older adult populations.

Direct Observation

The final direct approach to the measurement of physical activity is direct observation. Because of some of the limitations inherent in the measurement of physical activity in children via self-report measures, direct observation has been used almost exclusively in the context of assessing physical activity in children. Examples of observational systems include the Children's Activity Rating Scale (CARS) (Puhl, Greaves, Hoyt, & Baranowski, 1990), the System of Observing Play and Leisure Activity in Youth (SOPLAY) (McKenzie, Marshall, Sallis, & Conway, 2000), the System for Observing Fitness Instruction Time (SOFIT) (McKenzie, Sallis, & Nader, 1991), BEACHES (McKenzie et al., 1991), and the Observational System for Recording Physical Activity in Children-Preschool Version (OSRAC-P) (Brown et al., 2006). For example, SOPLAY is based on momentary time sampling and is used to obtain observational data on activity levels among children during play and leisure opportunities. During a scan, the physical activity of each child in the study is coded as sedentary, walking, or very active. Additional contextual information is also noted, including accessibility, usability, and availability of equipment. The type of activity in which the child is engaged is also recorded. For the activity measures, counts are tallied for sedentary, walking and very active behavior, and counts are transformed into estimates of energy expenditure. The system requires extensive training to ensure that observers reach acceptable criteria for reliable assessment.

Reliability, Validity, Sensitivity, Feasibility, and Bias

Observational systems have been shown to be reliable and valid and are often used to validate other measures. However, proper training and assessment are necessary to ensure adequate interrater reliability and to prevent coder drift over time. Ideally, multiple raters code behavior and interrater reliability is assessed, at least for a sample of observations. While this approach eliminates participant burden, it can be a time-intensive and thus expensive approach for the investigator. This approach is not feasible for population-based studies. In addition, the information learned is restricted to a narrow time window and to a limited setting or context (e.g., physical education class, playground). Direct observation can be very informative for understanding the contextual factors that influence physical activity and for quantifying physical activity in specific situations (e.g., physical education classes). It is a less useful method for estimating total physical activity.

Summary and Conclusions

A number of options exist for assessing physical activity in children and adults, but these options vary in their level of precision. Ideally, where possible, multiple measures (i.e., direct and indirect measures concurrently) should be used to adequately capture frequency, intensity, type, duration, and context of this complex behavior. All measurement methods have limitations to some degree in their reliability, validity, sensitivity, feasibility, reactivity, and potential sources of bias. Thus, these issues must be considered when selecting a measure for the specific study population. Indirect methods used to assess physical activity, such as self-report measures, are commonly used because of their low cost, low participant burden, ease of use, and limited reactivity. However, depending on the measure, reliability and validity can be limited due to recall and other self-report biases. Direct methods used to assess physical activity, such as objective monitoring devices (accelerometers and pedometers), are appealing because they eliminate recall biases and are generally reliable and valid, although some types of activity may not be captured and some types of activity (slow walking, lifestyle activities) are less accurately measured. In addition, the type of activity performed and the context in which it is performed are not recorded. Accelerometers are expensive, require high participant compliance, and require up to a week of wearing to gather reliable data, thus limiting their use in some settings. Pedometers are inexpensive but do not store data and thus require participant logging of steps. In addition, pedometers do not capture the dimensions of type, duration, or intensity of activity bouts. Finally, direct observation is an objective approach that is used to measure physical activity in children in specific settings such as physical education class or recess. This approach eliminates participant recall bias and participant burden and is considered high in validity and reliability, but substantial training of observers is required to obtain high interrater reliability. This approach can also be expensive in terms of staffing and data reduction.

While there is no perfect measure of physical activity, the study purpose, setting, and resources must be considered to identify the optimal method to assess physical activity. Prior to adopting a method to assess physical activity, investigators must carefully evaluate the method for its measurement properties and for its suitability for the study population.

References

Ainsworth, B. E. (2000a). Challenges in measuring physical activity in women. *Exercise and Sport Sciences Reviews, 28*(2), 93–96.

Ainsworth, B. E. (2000b). Issues in the assessment of physical activity in women. *Research Quarterly for Exercise and Sport, 71*(2 Suppl.), S37–S42.

Ainsworth, B. E., Haskell, W. L., Whitt, M. C., Irwin, M. L., Swartz, A. M., Strath, S. J., et al. (2000). Compendium of physical activities: An update of activity codes and MET intensities. *Medicine and Science in Sports and Exercise, 32*(9 Suppl.), S498–S504.

Ainsworth, B. E., Irwin, M. L., Addy, C. L., Whitt, M. C., & Stolarczyk, L. M. (1999). Moderate physical activity patterns of minority women: The Cross-Cultural Activity Participation Study. *Journal of Womens Health and Gender Based Medicine, 8*(6), 805–813.

Ainsworth, B. E., Jacobs, D. R., Jr., & Leon, A. S. (1993). Validity and reliability of self-reported physical activity status: The Lipid Research Clinics questionnaire. *Medicine and Science in Sports and Exercise, 25*(1), 92–98.

Baecke, J. A., Burema, J., & Frijters, J. E. (1982). A short questionnaire for the measurement of habitual physical activity in epidemiological studies. *American Journal of Clinical Nutrition, 36*(5), 936–942.

Blair, S. N., Haskell, W. L., Ho, P., Paffenbarger, R. S., Jr., Vranizan, K. M., Farquhar, J. W., et al. (1985). Assessment of habitual physical activity by a seven-day recall in a community survey and controlled experiments. *American Journal of Epidemiology, 122*(5), 794–804.

Bouchard, C., Tremblay, A., Leblanc, C., Lortie, G., Savard, R., & Theriault, G. (1983). A method to assess energy expenditure in children and adults. *American Journal of Clinical Nutrition, 37*(3), 461–467.

Brown, W. H., Pfeiffer, K. A., McLver, K. L., Dowda, M., Almeida, M. J., & Pate, R. R. (2006). Assessing preschool children's physical activity: The Observational System for Recording Physical Activity in children-preschool version. *Research Quarterly for Exercise and Sport, 77*(2), 167–176.

Brownson, R. C., Eyler, A. A., King, A. C., Brown, D. R., Shyu, Y. L., & Sallis, J. F. (2000). Patterns and correlates of physical activity among U.S. women 40 years and older. *American Journal of Public Health, 90*(2), 264–270.

Caspersen, C. J., Bloemberg, B. P., Saris, W. H., Merritt, R. K., & Kromhout, D. (1991). The prevalence of selected physical activities and their relation with coronary heart disease risk factors in elderly men: The Zutphen Study, 1985. *American Journal of Epidemiology, 133*(11), 1078–1092.

Caspersen, C. J., Powell, K. E., & Christenson, G. M. (1985). Physical activity, exercise, and physical fitness: Definitions and distinctions for health-related research. *Public Health Reports, 100*(2), 126–131.

Centers for Disease Control and Prevention. (2005). *Behavioral Risk Factor Surveillance System, 2005 Survey Questions.* Retrieved March 16, 2007, from http://www.cdc.gov/brfss/questionnaires/english.htm

Chen, K. Y., & Bassett, D. R., Jr. (2005). The technology of accelerometry-based activity monitors: Current and future. *Medicine and Science in Sports and Exercise, 37*(11 Suppl.), S490–S500.

Choi, B., & Pak, A. (2005). A catalog of biases in questionnaires. *Preventing Chronic Disease [serial online], 2*(1), 1–13.

Crouter, S. E., Schneider, P. L., & Bassett, D. R., Jr. (2005). Spring-levered versus piezo-electric pedometer accuracy in overweight and obese adults. *Medicine and Science in Sports and Exercise, 37*(10), 1673–1679.

Cyarto, E. V., Myers, A. M., & Tudor-Locke, C. (2004). Pedometer accuracy in nursing home and community-dwelling older adults. *Medicine and Science in Sports and Exercise, 36*(2), 205–209.

Dipietro, L., Caspersen, C. J., Ostfeld, A. M., & Nadel, E. R. (1993). A survey for assessing physical activity among older adults. *Medicine and Science in Sports and Exercise, 25*(5), 628–642.

Durante, R., & Ainsworth, B. E. (1996). The recall of physical activity: Using a cognitive model of the question-answering process. *Medicine and Science in Sports and Exercise, 28*(10), 1282–1291.

Eston, R. G., Rowlands, A. V., & Ingledew, D. K. (1998). Validity of heart rate, pedometry, and accelerometry for predicting the energy cost of children's activities. *Journal of Applied Physiology, 84*(1), 362–371.

Freedson, P., Pober, D., & Janz, K. F. (2005). Calibration of accelerometer output for children. *Medicine and Science in Sports and Exercise, 37*(11 Suppl.), S523–S530.

Freedson, P. S., Melanson, E., & Sirard, J. (1998). Calibration of the Computer Science and Applications, Inc. accelerometer. *Medicine and Science in Sports and Exercise, 30*(5), 777–781.

Friedenreich, C. M., Courneya, K. S., & Bryant, H. E. (1998). The lifetime total physical activity questionnaire: Development and reliability. *Medicine and Science in Sports and Exercise, 30*(2), 266–274.

Hebert, J. R., Clemow, L., Pbert, L., Ockene, I. S., & Ockene, J. K. (1995). Social desirability bias in dietary self-report may compromise the validity of dietary intake measures. *International Journal of Epidemiology, 24*(2), 389–398.

Jacobs, D. R., Jr., Hahn, L. P., Haskell, W. L., Pirie, P., & Sidney, S. (1989). Reliability and validity of a short physical activity history: CARDIA and the Minnesota Heart Health Program. *Journal of Cardiopulmonary Rehabilitation, 9*, 448–459.

Kriska, A. M. (2000). Ethnic and cultural issues in assessing physical activity. *Research Quarterly for Exercise and Sport, 71*(2 Suppl.), S47–S53.

Kriska, A. M., Knowler, W. C., LaPorte, R. E., Drash, A. L., Wing, R. R., Blair, S. N., et al. (1990). Development of questionnaire to examine relationship of physical activity and diabetes in Pima Indians. *Diabetes Care, 13*(4), 401–411.

Kriska, A. M., Sandler, R. B., Cauley, J. A., LaPorte, R. E., Hom, D. L., & Pambianco, G. (1988). The assessment of historical physical activity and its relation to adult bone parameters. *American Journal of Epidemiology, 127*(5), 1053–1063.

LaMonte, M., Ainsworth, B. E., & Tudor-Locke, C. (2003). Assessment of physical activity and energy expenditure. In R. E. Andersen (Ed.), *Obesity—etiology, assessment, treatment, and prevention* (pp. 111–140). Champaign, IL: Human Kinetics.

Mâsse, L. C., Ainsworth, B. E., Tortolero, S., Levin, S., Fulton, J. E., Henderson, K. A., et al. (1998). Measuring physical activity in midlife, older, and minority women: Issues from an expert panel. *Journal of Women's Health, 7*(1), 57–67.

Matthew, C. E. (2005). Calibration of accelerometer output for adults. *Medicine and Science in Sports and Exercise, 37*(11 Suppl.), S512–S522.

McKenzie, T. L., Marshall, S. J., Sallis, J. F., & Conway, T. L. (2000). Leisure-time physical activity in school environments: An observational study using SOPLAY. *Preventive Medicine, 30*(1), 70–77.

McKenzie, T. L., Sallis, J. F., & Nader, P. R. (1991). SOFIT: System for observing fitness instruction time. *Journal of Teaching Physical Education, 11,* 195–205.

McKenzie, T. L., Sallis, J. F., Nader, P. R., Patterson, T. L., Elder, J. P., Berry, C. C., et al. (1991). BEACHES: An observational system for assessing children's eating and physical activity behaviors and associated events. *Journal of Applied Behavioral Analysis, 24*(1), 141–151.

Oliver, M., Schofield, G. M., Kolt, G. S., & Schluter, P. J. (2006). Pedometer accuracy in physical activity assessment of preschool children. *Journal of Science and Medicine in Sport, 10*(5), 303–310.

Pate, R. R., Pratt, M., Blair, S. N., Haskell, W. L., Macera, C. A., Bouchard, C., et al. (1995). Physical activity and public health. A recommendation from the Centers for Disease Control and Prevention and the American College of Sports Medicine. *Journal of the American Medical Association, 273*(5), 402–407.

Pate, R. R., Ross, R., Dowda, M., Trost, S. G., & Sirard, J. (2003). Validation of a three-day physical activity recall instrument in female youth. *Pediatric Exercise Science, 15,* 257–265.

Patterson, P. (2000). Reliability, validity, and methodological response to the assessment of physical activity via self-report. *Research Quarterly for Exercise and Sport, 71*(2 Suppl), S15–S20.

Puhl, J., Greaves, K., Hoyt, M., & Baranowski, T. (1990). Children's Activity Rating Scale (CARS): Description and calibration. *Research Quarterly for Exercise and Sport, 61*(1), 26–36.

Ravussin, E., & Swinburn, B. A. (1992). Pathophysiology of obesity. *Lancet, 340*(8816), 404–408.

Richardson, M. T., Leon, A. S., Jacobs, D. R., Jr., Ainsworth, B. E., & Serfass, R. (1995). Ability of the Caltrac accelerometer to assess daily physical activity levels. *Journal of Cardiopulmonary Rehabilitation, 15*(2), 107–113.

Rowlands, A. V., & Eston, R. G. (2005). Comparison of accelerometer and pedometer measures of physical activity in boys and girls, ages 8–10 years. *Research Quarterly for Exercise and Sport, 76*(3), 251–257.

Sallis, J. F., Haskell, W. L., Wood, P. D., Fortmann, S. P., Rogers, T., Blair, S. N., et al. (1985). Physical activity assessment methodology in the Five-City Project. *American Journal of Epidemiology, 121*(1), 91–106.

Sallis, J. F., & Saelens, B. E. (2000). Assessment of physical activity by self-report: Status, limitations, and future directions. *Research Quarterly for Exercise and Sport, 71*(2 Suppl.), S1–S14.

Schneider, P. L., Crouter, S. E., & Bassett, D. R. (2004). Pedometer measures of free-living physical activity: Comparison of 13 models. *Medicine and Science in Sports and Exercise, 36*(2), 331–335.

Schneider, P. L., Crouter, S. E., Lukajic, O., & Bassett, D. R., Jr. (2003). Accuracy and reliability of 10 pedometers for measuring steps over a 400-m walk. *Medicine and Science in Sports and Exercise, 35*(10), 1779–1784.

Shadish, W. R., Cook, T. D., & Campbell, D. T. (2002). *Experimental and quasi-experimental designs for generalized causal inference.* Boston: Houghton Mifflin.

Stewart, A. L., Mills, K. M., King, A. C., Haskell, W. L., Gillis, D., & Ritter, P. L. (2001). CHAMPS Physical Activity Questionnaire for Older Adults: Outcomes for interventions. *Medicine and Science in Sports and Exercise, 33*(7), 1126–1141.

Taylor, H. L., Jacobs, D. R., Jr., Schucker, B., Knudsen, J., Leon, A. S., & Debacker, G. (1978). A questionnaire for the assessment of leisure time physical activities. *Journal of Chronic Disease, 31*(12), 741–755.

Tortolero, S. R., Mâsse, L. C., Fulton, J. E., Torres, I., & Kohl, H. W., III. (1999). Assessing physical activity among minority women: Focus group results. *Womens Health Issues, 9*(3), 135–142.

Troiano, R. P. (2005). A timely meeting: Objective measurement of physical activity. *Medicine and Science in Sports and Exercise, 37*(11 Suppl.), S487–S489.

Trost, S. G., McIver, K. L., & Pate, R. R. (2005). Conducting accelerometer-based activity assessments in field-based research. *Medicine and Science in Sports and Exercise, 37*(11 Suppl.), S531–S543.

Tudor-Locke, C. (2002). Taking steps toward increased physical activity: Using pedometers to measure and motivate. Retrieved April 24, 2007, from http://www.fitness.gov/pcpfsdigestjune2002.pdf

Tudor-Locke, C. E., Burkett, L., Reis, J. P., Ainsworth, B. E., Macera, C. A., & Wilson, D. K. (2005). How many days of pedometer monitoring predict weekly physical activity in adults? *Preventive Medicine, 40*(3), 293–298.

Tudor-Locke, C. E., Ham, S. A., Macera, C. A., Ainsworth, B. E., Kirtland, K. A., Reis, J. P., et al. (2004). Descriptive epidemiology of pedometer-determined physical activity. *Medicine and Science in Sports and Exercise, 36*(9), 1567–1573.

Tudor-Locke, C. E., & Myers, A. M. (2001). Methodological considerations for researchers and practitioners using pedometers to measure physical (ambulatory) activity. *Research Quarterly for Exercise and Sport, 72*(1), 1–12.

Voorrips, L. E., Ravelli, A. C., Dongelmans, P. C., Deurenberg, P., & Van Staveren, W. A. (1991). A physical activity questionnaire for the elderly. *Medicine and Science in Sports and Exercise, 23*(8), 974–979.

Ward, D. S., Saunders, R. P., & Pate, R. R. (2007). Measuring physical activity. In *Physical activity interventions in children and adolescents.* Champaign, IL: Human Kinetics.

Washburn, R. A. (2000). Assessment of physical activity in older adults. *Research Quarterly for Exercise and Sport, 71*(2 Suppl.), S79–S88.

Washburn, R. A., McAuley, E., Katula, J., Mihalko, S. L., & Boileau, R. A. (1999). The physical activity scale for the elderly (PASE): Evidence for validity. *Journal of Clinical Epidemiology, 52*(7), 643–651.

Washburn, R. A., Smith, K. W., Jette, A. M., & Janney, C. A. (1993). The Physical Activity Scale for the Elderly (PASE): Development and evaluation. *Journal of Clinical Epidemiology, 46*(2), 153–162.

Welk, G. J., Corbin, C. B., & Dale, D. (2000). Measurement issues in the assessment of physical activity in children. *Research Quarterly for Exercise and Sport, 71*(2 Suppl.), S59–S73.

Weston, A. T., Petosa, R., & Pate, R. R. (1997). Validity of an instrument for measurement of physical activity in youth. *Medicine and Science in Sports and Exercise, 29*(1), 138–143.

Changes in Substance Use Behavior

18

Donald M. Dougherty,
Michael A. Dawes,
and Sylvain Nouvion

This chapter describes a number of techniques and tools available for the measurement of substance use behaviors, changes in these behaviors, and risk and factors that predict changes in substance use behavior. Measurement of substance use behavior requires repeated use of multiple measures and informants to capture the patterns and changes in substance use that occur over time. The chapter includes definitions of substance use behavior and describes the developmental patterning of substance use behavior. Also included are sections and tables on questionnaires and biological measures that assess substance use behavior in adolescents and adults. We review risk and protective factors that are associated with the onset, progression, and continuation of substance use behavior and measures that assess these factors. Finally, we discuss challenges related to current methods of assessment and measurement, as well as future directions.

Substance Use Behavior

Substance use is the use of any substance that acts on the central nervous system in a manner other than prescribed and often features impaired control related to substance intake and difficulty in self-regulation of substance intake, despite negative outcomes (Martin, Fillmore, Chung, Easdon, & Miczek, 2006). Substance use disorders (abuse and dependence) are maladaptive patterns of substance use that include clinically significant impairment or distress, as manifested by occurrence of specific symptoms that have occurred within a year (American Psychiatric Association, 2000).

Substance use behaviors are pervasive among adolescents and young adults in the United States and present a significant burden to both the user and society. The National Survey on Drug Use and Health (Substance Abuse & Mental Health Services Administration, 2006) found that 19.7 million individuals over the age of 12 had used an illicit drug in the past month, representing approximately 8% of the population 12 years or older. Marijuana was the most widely used illicit substance, although "harder" drugs such as cocaine and other stimulants, including methamphetamine, were also prevalent.

An important developmental model of substance use is the "gateway" theory (Kandel, 1975), which describes sequential stages of *onset* of drug use (Kandel, Yamaguchi, & Klein, 2006). The first stage involves use of beer or wine; the user then progresses to use of hard liquor and cigarettes (stage 2), marijuana (stage 3), and, ultimately, other illicit drugs (stage 4). These transitions occur *across* classes of drugs, as progression from less severe drugs (e.g., marijuana) toward more severe drugs (e.g., cocaine, heroin). However, the gateway theory does not adequately explain the behaviors involved in the progression of substance use *within* classes (e.g., maintenance of use, increasing use). Although gateway effects may exist, a common factor (drug use propensity) may also predispose the initiation and continuation of drug use (Dawes et al., 2000; Morral, McCaffrey, & Paddock, 2002).

Theories explaining onset of substance use must be viewed in a broader context that includes transitions *within* stages. For example, the development of substance use disorders has been described as transitioning through five stages: (1) Initiation, (2) Continuation, (3) Maintenance and progression within a drug class, (4) Progression across drug classes, and (5) Regression, cessation, and relapse cycles (Clayton, 1992). Initiation is the phase when a nonuser begins to use a particular substance. Continuation is the transition of drug use just beyond initiation, when first exposure leads to increased use. Maintenance of use includes persistence of both moderate and excessive usage. Progression within a drug class refers to increased consumption of the substance, as well as progression in route of administration of the substance (e.g., from snorting cocaine to smoking it). Progression across drug classes is the transition from use of one substance to polysubstance use. Finally, regression, cessation, and relapse cycles are transitions from use to nonuse and back to use.

Assessment of Substance Use Behavior

Substance Use Severity

Substance use behaviors are more accurately measured along a continuum of severity of involvement: experimental use, early abuse, abuse, dependence, and recovery. Experimental use coincides with the initiation and continuation stages and involves minimal, often recreational, use. Early abuse is present early in the maintenance stage and involves more established use, with adverse consequences beginning to emerge. Abuse occurs later in the maintenance stage and involves regular use over an extended period with several adverse consequences. Dependence is present toward the end of the continuum and involves repeated use, severe consequences, signs of tolerance, and schedule accommodation for drug seeking (Winters, Latimer, & Stinchfeld, 2001). Abstinence is cessation of use after a period of abuse or dependence. The optimal assessment of substance use involvement should assess changes severity and consequences of substance use over time (Clark & Winters, 2002).

Measurement and Validity

In order to accurately assess substance use behavior, it is essential to use sensitive, reliable, and valid methods of measurement. Available measures fall into two general categories: questionnaires and laboratory tests. Questionnaires include self-report and parent-report measures. Structured and semistructured interviews assess substance use severity, psychopathology, presence of risk and protective factors, and cognitive domains of substance use. Laboratory measures include testing blood samples, urine samples, breath samples, and other biological samples.

Clearly, questionnaires and interviews require the cooperation of the individual being assessed. Furthermore, the individual should demonstrate some degree of insight into the condition, willingness to accept the existence of problems, and motivation to seek assessment and treatment. Assessment can be hindered because substance-using individuals may have impairments in cognitive and decision-making abilities that can affect their willingness to address problems (Noam & Houlihan, 1990). For adolescents, assessments and corroborating parental reports require honesty and accurate insight, as well as objective reporting concerning their child and knowledge of their child's substance use behaviors. Often, parents cannot provide meaningful information concerning the substance use behaviors of their children (Winters et al., 2001). Self-report measures have received considerable scrutiny, with support both for and against validity (Winters et al., 2001). To increase validity, standardized instruments should include response bias scales and interviewing techniques that help the individual feel comfortable and therefore more likely to disclose substance use (Winters et al., 2001).

Comprehensive Assessment

Comprehensive assessment of the severity of current substance use is a multifaceted process that utilizes questionnaires, interviews, and laboratory measures. The first step, screening, should address multiple domains of functioning, using instruments with high reliability, validity, and predictive ability. The screening assessment should focus both on severity of use and the effects of use on everyday functioning across many domains (e.g., school, home). If indicated (i.e., signs of poor functioning across several domains due to substance use), further assessment should be undertaken by a trained professional.

The second step, diagnostic assessment, requires use of multiple measures and multiple informants. Structured or semistructured interviews and drug monitoring in urine samples provide information about the severity of substance abuse, psychiatric comorbidity, and medical and health status to determine what level of intervention and/or treatment is indicated (Substance Abuse and Mental Health Services Administration [SAMHSA], 1999). The purposes of the diagnostic assessment are to (1) identify if a substance use disorder and a psychiatric comorbidity exist, (2) determine those individuals in need of treatment, (3) determine to what extent the individual's environment affects substance use behavior, and (4) develop a plan for treatment (SAMHSA, 1999).

Questionnaire Measures

"Questionnaire measures" describe the tools (typically pen-and-paper measures) used to gather nonbiological information related to substance use behaviors. Measures used in adolescents and adults all differ, although some have been altered to be compatible with broader populations. In adolescents, a critical measurement issue is the necessity of corroborating information (e.g., from parents or teachers). Information gathered from adolescents and informants includes, but is not limited to, history of use, current patterns of use, presence of risk/protective factors, and cognitive beliefs concerning substance use (Winters et al., 2001).

Adolescent Measures—Screening Instruments

Screening instruments should be used to estimate where an individual stands on the continuum of severity of substance use. Generally, screening instruments provide a brief estimation of substance use severity and indications that further assessment is needed. Many screening tools are available for use in adolescents and are appropriate for different situations. Some cover items strictly related to substance use, while others provide a more multidimensional screening. Screening instruments include the Drug Use Screening Inventory—Revised (DUSI-R; Kirisci, Mezzich, & Tarter, 1995), the Problem Oriented Screening Instrument for Teenagers (POSIT; Rahdert, 1991), and screening instruments to assess adolescent alcohol and drug use in primary care (CRAFFT; Knight, Sherritt, Shrier, Harris, & Chang, 2002), alcohol use (Adolescent Alcohol Involvement Scale, AAIS; Mayer & Filstead, 1979), drug use and dependence (Adolescent Drug Involvement Scale, ADIS; Moberg & Hahn, 1991) and problems arising from alcohol use (Rutgers Alcohol Problem Index, RAPI; White & Labouvie, 1989). For a comparison of the properties of these adolescent screening measures, please see items 1 through 6 in Table 18.1.

18.1 Substance Use Screening Measures, Questionnaires, and Structured and Semistructured Interviews

Instrument/ Measure	Items: Administration Time	Age Range	Use	Key Features	Citation
1. *Drug Use Screening Inventory—Revised* (DUSI-R)	159 items: 20–40 minutes	Adolescent to adult	Evaluate suspected drug using individuals; quantify severity of consequences of drug use	Can be used in adolescents and adults; Lie Scale included; Spanish version available; self-administered	Tarter, 1990
2. *Problem Oriented Screening Instrument for Teenagers* (POSIT)	139 items: 20–30 minutes	12–19	Identify potential problems requiring further assessment in 10 areas	Assesses multiple domains; modified form for repeatability available; can be used by school, juvenile, and family court personnel; follow-up can be used as a measure of change; self-administered	Rahdert, 1991
3. *CRAFFT Substance Abuse Screening Test* (CRAFFT)	6 items: 5 minutes	Adolescents	Drug use screening in adolescents	Specific for adolescents; very brief; screens for drugs and alcohol; self- or interviewer-administered	Knight et al., 2002
4. *Adolescent Alcohol Involvement Scale* (AAIS)	14 items: 5 minutes	Adolescents	Brief standardized measure for detecting adolescents' use and misuse of alcohol	Assesses quantitative use and psychosocial consequences in three domains: psychological functioning, social relations and family living; self-administered	Mayer and Filstead, 1979

(Continued)

18.1 Substance Use Screening Measures, Questionnaires, and Structured and Semistructured Interviews (*Continued*)

Instrument/ Measure	Items: Administration Time	Age Range	Use	Key Features	Citation
5. *Adolescent Drug Involvement Scale* (ADIS)	12 items: 5 minutes	Adolescents	Distinguish heavier problematic users from less involved users	Used for both research and screening: drug involvement defined in terms of consequences, motivations, and sense of control: self-administered	Moberg and Hahn, 1991
6. *Rutgers Alcohol Problem Index* (RAPI)	23 items: 10 minutes	Adolescents	Screening tool for assessing adolescent problem drinking	Easily administered: no training required: usable in clinical and nonclinical samples: self-administered	White and Labouvie, 1989
7. *Diagnostic Interview for Children and Adolescents* (DICA)	416 items: 60–90 minutes	6–18	Semistructured interview assessing 19 DSM-IV disorders, including substance use disorders	Detailed substance abuse section: separate versions for children 6–12 and adolescents 13–18: computerized version available: interviewer-administered or self-administered on computer	Reich et al., 1982
8. *Diagnostic Interview Schedule for Children* (DISC-C)	358 "stem" questions: 70–120 minutes	6–17	Highly structured interview designed to assess DSM-IV psychiatric disorders, including substance use disorders	Separate parent and child versions: designed for epidemiological research: generates symptom counts and diagnoses: interviewer-administered	Shaffer et al., 1996
9. *Kiddie Schedule for Affective Disorders and Schizophrenia* (K-SADS)	300 items: 90–120 minutes	6–18	Semistructured interview covering a broad spectrum of child psychiatric diagnoses, including substance use disorders	Used primarily in research settings. not ordinary clinical settings: administered by a trained clinician	Endicott and Spitzer, 1978

10. *Modified Struc-* *tured Clinical* *Interview for the* *DSM-IV (mSCID)*	92 items: 45–60 minutes	Adolescents	Structured interview assessing age of substance use onset and frequency of use	Assess developmentally appropriate drug problems: should be administered to the adolescent and the parent: interviewer- administered	First et al. 1997; Martin et al. 1995
11. *Adolescent Diag-* *nostic Interview* *(ADI)*	213 items: 30–90 minutes	12–18	Structured interview assessing psychoac- tive substance use disorders	Screens for accompanying mental/behav- ioral problems: Based on DSM-III and IV criteria: Interviewer-administered	Winters and Henly, 1993
12. *Adolescent Self-* *Assessment Pro-* *file (ASAP)*	225 items: 25–50 minutes	Adolescents	Assessment of psycho- social adjustment and substance use involvement	May be used for, during, and after treatment to determine changes in perception of adolescents' psychosocial and substance use problems: self-administered	Leccese and Waldron, 1994
13. *Adolescent Drug* *Abuse Diagnosis* *(ADAD)*	150 items: 45–55 minutes	Adolescents	Structured interview assessing substance use and other life problems	Comprehensive evaluation yielding 10-point severity ratings in nine life problem areas: 83 items are used for measuring change: interviewer-administered	Leccese and Waldron, 1994
14. *Comprehensive* *Addiction Severity* *Index for Adoles-* *cents* (CASI-A)	10 modules: 45–90 minutes	Adolescents	Semistructured clinical interview for evaluat- ing adolescents in many domains, in- cluding substance use	Can be used in many provider settings and repeated at follow-up: assesses many domains; incorporates urine drug screen results; interviewer-administered	Meyers, 1991
15. *American Drug* *and Alcohol Survey* *(ADAS)*	55 items: 30–50 minutes	4th–12th grade	Self-report inventory of drug use and related behaviors	Administered at school: child (4th–6th grade) and adolescent (6th–12th grade) versions: provides information to help school dis- tricts understand extent of local substance use: self-administered	Conoley and Impara, 1995

(continued)

18.1 Substance Use Screening Measures, Questionnaires, and Structured and Semistructured Interviews (Continued)

Instrument/Measure	Items: Administration Time	Age Range	Use	Key Features	Citation
16. *Personal Experience Inventory* (PEI)	276 items: 60–90 minutes	12–18	Self-report inventory documenting onset, nature, degree, and duration of chemical involvement	Screening includes possible family problems, sexual abuse, physical abuse, eating disorder, and suicide potential; self-administered	Winters and Henly, 1989
17. *Alcohol Expectancy Questionnaire—Adolescent Version* (AEQ)	100 items: 10–15 minutes	12–19	Assess individual's expectancy of effects of alcohol use	Assists in identifying factors in the process of transition to, or persistence of, problem drinking; self-administered	Brown et al., 1987
18. *Problem Recognition Questionnaire* (PRQ)	25 items: 5 minutes	Adolescents over 16 years	Assess user's recognition of problem drug use and readiness for treatment	Evaluates degree of problem recognition and willingness to change; self-administered	Cady et al., 1996
19. *Stages of Change Readiness and Treatment Eagerness Scale* (SOCRATES)	19 items: 3 minutes	12–18	Assess readiness for change in alcohol abusers	Three scales: problem recognition, ambivalence, and taking steps; can assist clinicians in treatment plans; self-administered	Maisto et al., 2003
20. *CAGE Questionnaire* (CAGE)	4 items: 1 minute	Adolescents 16 or over; Adults	Screening for problem alcohol use	Single positive answer has 90% detection rate for alcohol use disorder; computerized version available; self-administered	Mayfield et al., 1974

21. *Drug Abuse Screening Test* (DAST)	28 items: 5 minutes	Adolescents Adults	Brief method for identifying individuals who are abusing psychoactive drugs	Shortened versions of 10 and 20 items available: identifies individuals needing further assessment: self-administered	Skinner, 1982
22. *Alcohol Use Disorders Identification Test* (AUDIT)	10 items: 2 minutes	Adults	Screen to identify persons whose alcohol consumption has become hazardous or harmful to their health	Optional Clinical Screening Procedure includes a blood test: self-administered	Allen et al. 1997
23. *Michigan Alcohol Screening Test* (MAST)	25 items: 8 minutes	Adolescents Adults	Provide rapid screening for lifetime alcohol-related problems	Shortened versions of 9, 10, and 13 items available: widely used measure for assessing alcohol abuse: self-administered	Allen and Columbus, 1995
24. *TWEAK* (TWEAK)	5 items: 1–2 minutes	Adult women	Screen for risk drinking during pregnancy	Specific to pregnant women: self-administered	Russell et al. 1991
25. *Structured Clinical Interview for the DSM-IV* (SCID)	4 abuse items, 9 dependence items: 10–45 minutes	Adults	Structured interview to diagnose DSM-IV substance use disorders for all major drugs of abuse	Very commonly utilized: interviewer-administered	Spitzer et al. 1987
26. *Timeline Follow-Back* (TLFB)	30–360 items: 10–30 minutes	Adolescents Adults	Obtains estimates of daily drinking up to the past 12 months	Evaluated in clinical and non-clinical populations: allows several dimensions of drinking to be examined: variability, pattern, and extent: interviewer-administered	Sobell and Sobell, 1992

(continued)

18.1 Substance Use Screening Measures, Questionnaires, and Structured and Semistructured Interviews (Continued)

Instrument/ Measure	Items; Administration Time	Age Range	Use	Key Features	Citation
27. Addiction Severity Index (ASI)	200 items: 50–60 minutes	Adults	Semistructured interview providing an overview of problems related to substance use	Assesses problems in medical status, employment, drug and alcohol use, legal/family/social status, and psychiatric status; interviewer-administered	McLellan et al., 1992
28. Drinker Inventory of Consequences (DrInC)	50 items; 10 minutes	Adults	Measure adverse consequences of alcohol abuse in five areas	Areas assessed: interpersonal, physical, social, impulsive, and intrapersonal; can be used for treatment planning and evaluation; self-administered	Miller et al., 1995
29. Alcohol Expectancy Questionnaire—Adult Version (AEQ)	120 items (90 scored); 10–15 minutes	Adults	Assess domain of alcohol reinforcement expectancies on six subscales	Six subscales: positive global changes, sexual enhancement, social and physical pleasure, assertiveness, relaxation/tension reduction, and arousal/interpersonal power; self-administered	Brown et al., 1987

Adolescent Measures—Psychiatric Interviews/Instruments Assessing Substance Use Disorders

Similarly, there are a number of structured and semistructured psychiatric interviews available for assessing substance use in adolescents. These include the Diagnostic Interview for Children and Adolescents (DICA; Reich, Herjanic, Welner, & Gandhy, 1982), the Diagnostic Interview Schedule for Children (DISC-C; Shaffer, Fisher, & Dulcan, 1996), the Kiddie Schedule for Affective Disorders and Schizophrenia (K-SADS; Endicott & Spitzer, 1978), the modified Structured Clinical Interview for the DSM-IV (mSCID; First, Spitzer, & Gibbon, 1997; Martin, Kaczynski, Maisto, Bukstein, & Moss, 1995; Spitzer, Williams, & Gibbon, 1987), the Adolescent Diagnostic Interview (ADI; Winters & Henly, 1993), the Adolescent Self-Assessment Profile (ASAP; Leccese & Waldron, 1994) and the Adolescent Drug Abuse Diagnosis (ADAD; Leccese & Waldron, 1994). As with the screening instruments, these interviews branch into other areas of functioning to help determine not only whether substance use is present but also the extent of the impact of substance use in the lives of adolescents. (See items 7 through 13 in Table 18.1 for specific information regarding these interviews.)

Additional Interviews Available

The Comprehensive Addiction Severity Index for Adolescents (CASI-A; Meyers, 1991) addresses many domains and incorporates urine drug screen results and assessor observations. The American Drug and Alcohol Survey (ADAS; Conoley & Impara, 1995) is administered to youth while at school and is used by school districts to gauge substance use among students in an effort to create awareness of use and to develop effective prevention strategies. The Personal Experience Inventory (PEI; Winters and Henly, 1989) assesses use of all substances and problems associated with substance use. (See items 14 through 16 in Table 18.1 for details.)

Adolescent Measures—Substance Use Expectancy and Behavior Change Readiness

The following measures are useful in determining the expected effects of substance use (e.g., expectation of positive outcomes of use) and the ability to self-report problem drug use. Additionally, the following provide measures of the user's readiness to change substance-using behaviors. The Alcohol Expectancy Questionnaire—Adolescent Version (AEQ; Brown, Christiansen, & Goldman, 1987) assesses an individual's expectancy of effects of alcohol use and can be used in adolescent and adult populations. The Problem Recognition Questionnaire (PRQ; Cady, Winters, Jordan, & Solheim, 1996) assesses the user's recognition of problem drug use and their readiness for treatment, and the Stages of Change Readiness and Treatment Eagerness Scale (SOCRATES; Maisto, Chung, Cornelius, & Martin, 2003) assesses two factors: taking steps and recognition. Please see items 17 through 19 in Table 18.1 for information regarding these measures.

Summary of Adolescent Measures: Stability and Changes in Substance Use Behaviors

Screening Measures

The POSIT has been used as a repeated measure to screen for substance abuse and related problems. In a sample of adolescents 12–16 years olds, the POSIT was administered twice, 30 weeks apart. Results indicated that scores on the substance use component of the POSIT were not statistically different after 30 weeks (Tuttle, Campbell-Heider, & David, 2006). In another study (Dembo, Schmeidler, Borden, Turner, Sue, & Manning, 1996), the POSIT was found to be a useful tool to determine which youths were in need of intervention and treatment services. Finally, Knight, Goodman, Pulerwitz, and DuRant (2001) demonstrated that the substance use/abuse scales of the POSIT have favorable test-retest reliability when administered to teenage patients a week apart.

Diagnostic Interviews

The modified SCID has been used in a longitudinal study following participants from the age of 10–12 up to 25 (Cornelius, Clark, Reynolds, Kirisci, & Tarter, 2006). Participants completed the SCID at age of intake, and at ages 14, 16, 19, 22, and 25 years, demonstrating the ability to use this diagnostic instrument repeatedly and to detect stability and change in substance use behavior. Tarter, Vanyukov, Kirisci, Reynolds, and Clark (2006), using some of the same cohort as the Cornelius et al. (2006) study, administered the modified SCID to participants at ages 12–14, 16, 19, and 22. Together, these studies support the predictive validity of the modified SCID and the ability of this measure to assess transitions in substance use behavior during adolescence and young adulthood.

Substance Abuse and Expectancy Changes

The Alcohol Expectancy Questionnaire-Adolescent Version (AEQ-A) has been administered to a group of 924 seventh graders at three time points over a 2-year period (Natvig Aas, Leigh, Anderssen, & Jakobsen, 1998). The authors reported that among those adolescents who were drinkers at the start of the study, there were expectations of positive social effects for drinking across the 2-year period.

Adult Measures—Screening Instruments

Screening instruments available for adult populations include the CAGE Questionnaire (CAGE; Mayfield, McLeod, & Hall, 1974), the Drug Abuse Screening Test (DAST; Skinner, 1982), and screening instruments used to assess harmful alcohol use (Alcohol Use Disorders Identification Test, AUDIT; Allen, Litten, & Fertig, 1997), lifetime alcohol use (Michigan Alcohol Screening Test, MAST; Allen & Columbus, 1995), and alcohol use during pregnancy (TWEAK; Russell, Czarnecki, & Cowan, 1991). (See items 20 through 24 of Table 18.1 for a comparison of these screening tools.)

Adult Measures—Psychiatric Interviews/Instruments Assessing Substance Use Disorders

The Structured Clinical Interview for the DSM-IV (SCID; First et al., 1997; Martin et al., 1995; Spitzer et al., 1987) is one of the most commonly used structured interviews to assess substance use disorders (Item 25, Table 18.1). It provides psychiatric diagnoses from the Diagnostic and Statistical Manual, Fourth Edition (DSM-IV; APA, 2000). The Timeline Follow-Back (Item 26, Table 18.1) (TLFB; Sobell & Sobell, 1992) reconstructs the individual's type, quantity, and frequency of substance use during the past 3 months up to the last year (Brandon, Copeland, & Saper, 1995). The Addiction Severity Index (Item 27, Table 18.1) (ASI; McLellan, Kushner, & Metzger, 1992) is a structured interview designed to assess problems in seven areas that frequently influence substance use disorders. The Drinker Inventory of Consequences (Item 28, Table 18.1) (DrInC; Miller, Tonigan, & Longabaugh, 1995) measures recent and lifetime negative consequences related to alcohol use.

Adult Measures—Measures of Substance Use Expectancy and Behavior Change Readiness

The Alcohol Expectancy Questionnaire—Adult Version (Item 29, Table 18.1) (AEQ; Brown et al., 1987) consists of 90 scored items regarding an individual's expectancy of effects of alcohol use and has been used in adolescent and adult populations.

Laboratory Measures—Urine Samples for Drug Testing

Laboratory measures of biological specimens provide complementary methods to self-report methodology for the determination of recent substance use. The presence of drugs, their metabolites, or both is most commonly determined from urine tests, which can be performed rapidly and inexpensively. A disadvantage of urine testing for recent substance use is that drug metabolites vary in detection times, and this can lead to inaccurate results. For example, metabolites of marijuana may be detectable in urine for several weeks in a chronic user, regardless of whether the user has abstained for several days, in which case a positive test for current use would be incorrect (Cone, 1997). Furthermore, detection can vary by other factors, including dose, frequency of administration, and metabolism (Cone, 1997). (For an overview of laboratory methods for drug screening, see Table 18.2.)

It is critical that laboratory measures of drug use be both precise and accurate because results can have a negative impact on those individuals being tested, especially if the result is a false positive. A valid method must be able to detect the drug and/or its metabolites (Gorodetzky, 1972). Valid laboratory assessment of drug use is ensured by first using a screening measure, which when positive should be followed by a more specific analytical method (Goldberger & Jenkins, 1999). Techniques to detect drugs in urine fall into two categories: immunological and chromatographic. Immunological tests include radioimmunoassay, enzyme immunoassay, fluorescence polarization immunoassay, and

18.2   Laboratory Measures of Substance Use

Test	Time frame	Drugs tested	Key features	Citation
Urine Samples—Enzyme Immunoassay	Mostly recent use (12–96 hours); Longer for chronic marijuana use	Amphetamines: Benzodiazepines: Cocaine: GHB: LSD: MDMA: Marijuana: Opiates	Fast: simple: sensitive: inexpensive: on-site testing: covers most common substances of abuse: semiquantitative	Verstraete. 2004
Urine Samples—Chromatography/Mass Spectroscopy	Mostly recent use (12–96 hours); Longer for chronic marijuana use	Amphetamines: Benzodiazepines: Cocaine: GHB: LSD: MDMA: Marijuana: Opiates	Commonly used to confirm presumptive samples; can detect quantities down to 0.1–5 ng/ml	Verstraete. 2004
Breath Samples	Recent use (minutes to hours)	Alcohol	Fast: noninvasive: inexpensive: high sensitivity and specificity	
Blood/Serum/Plasma Samples	Recent use (5–48 hours): Chronic use for alcohol	Alcohol: Amphetamines: Benzodiazepines: Cocaine: GHB MDMA: Marijuana: Opiates	Chronic alcohol use determined by increase in mean corpuscular volume and increased liver enzymes	Verstraete. 2004: Kolodziej et al., 2002
Saliva Samples	Recent use (5–50 hours)	Alcohol: Amphetamines: Benzodiazepines: Cocaine: GHB: MDMA: Marijuana: Opiates	Noninvasive: inexpensive	Verstraete. 2004

Sweat Samples	Recent and chronic use (minutes to 1 week or longer)	Amphetamines; Cocaine; MDMA; Marijuana; Opiates	Hampered by contamination and large variability	Kintz et al., 2000; Samyn and van Haeren, 2000; Samyn et al., 2002
Hair Samples	Chronic use (months)	Amphetamines; Cocaine; MDMA; Opiates	Noninvasive; low potential for sample manipulation	Cone, 1997; Musshoff and Madea, 2007
Emerging Biomarkers— Alcohol	Recent and chronic use	Alcohol	Biomarkers: ethyl glucuronide; phosphatidyl ethanol; fatty acid ethyl esters; sialic acid index of plasma apolipoprotein J	Wurst et al. 2005
Quantitative Urine Test Marijuana	Recent and chronic use	Marijuana	Biomarkers: THC/Creatinine ratio; 11-nor-9-carboxy-Δ 9-tetrahydrocannabinal	Huestis and Cone, 1998
Quantitative Urine Test Benzoylecgonine	Recent use	Cocaine	Urine Benzoylecgonine	Delucchi et al., 1997

particle immunoassay. Chromatographic tests include thin-layer chromatography, high-performance liquid chromatography, and gas chromatography.

Immunoassay techniques are based on competitive binding of both a labeled and an unlabeled antigen to a specific antibody. In the most commonly used technique (enzyme immunoassay), the competition occurs between the unlabeled drug and the drug covalently bound to a specific enzyme. When the drug binds to the antibody, enzyme activity is decreased, but when the unlabeled drug displaces the drug-labeled enzyme, the free enzyme catalyzes a reaction that can be used to quantify drug presence in the sample (Goldberger & Jenkins, 1999). Advantages of the immunoassay techniques include speed, sensitivity, availability for all common substances of abuse, simplicity, qualitative and semiquantitative results, and the ability to test onsite (eliminating the need for expensive equipment and skilled operators). Disadvantages (mainly for radioimmunoassay methods) include a short shelf life and the extra safety precautions required with the use of radioisotopes.

Chromatographic and mass spectroscopy techniques are often used by laboratories to confirm a positive test. Chromatographic techniques separate liquid solutions into component parts through interaction with mobile and stationary phases (Bowers, Ullman, & Burtis, 1994). In gas chromatography, liquid extracts are vaporized and the remaining solid components are resuspended in a buffered solution and then transferred to a column in which components become separated. Components are identified and quantified by a detector as they elute from the column. Detection is by mass spectroscopy, which can detect quantities as small as 0.1–5 ng/ml (Bowers et al., 1994).

Laboratory Measures—Recent Drug Use

Alternate methods to test for substance use include analysis of samples of breath, blood, saliva, sweat, and hair (see Table 18.2). Breath samples are used primarily to detect alcohol use and have high sensitivity and specificity. Breath testing is rapid, noninvasive, and inexpensive. The primary disadvantage is that breath sampling has a narrow window of assessment (i.e., minutes to hours). Blood samples detect recent heavy drug use or consequences of chronic alcohol use. Chronic alcohol use may be determined by an increase in red blood cell mean corpuscular volume (MCV) and increased levels of glycoprotein carbohydrate-deficient transferrin (CDT), γ-glutamyl transferase (GGT), or other liver enzymes, which can indicate hepatic disease such as hepatitis or cirrhosis (Kolodziej, Greenfield, & Weiss, 2002). Saliva testing is noninvasive and cost-effective.

Laboratory Measures—Chronic Drug Use

Testing of sweat provides information on both current and cumulative drug use, with detection times of minutes to 1 week or longer (see Table 18.2). Sweat testing is hampered by possible environmental contamination and large variability among subjects. Hair testing provides an additional long-term measure of drug use, with a detection time of months. Hair testing is noninvasive and has a low potential for manipulation by the individual being tested, although it cannot measure current drug use (Cone, 1997).

Laboratory Measures—Emerging Biomarkers

Sensitive and specific biomarkers for alcohol and other drug use are needed for assessment and treatment of substance use disorders. Recently, several potential biomarkers of alcohol consumption have been identified. These include direct ethanol metabolites, such as ethyl glucuronide (EtG), phosphatidyl ethanol (PEth), fatty acid ethyl esters (FAEEs), and sialic acid index of plasma apolipoprotein J (SIJ) (Wurst et al., 2005). Overall, PEth appears to be the best candidate for a stand-alone marker for ethanol consumption.

Quantitative Urine Measures to Detect Changes in Drug Use

The use of quantitative urine tests to detect changes in drug use is an area of active research. One example is the use of the THC/Creatinine Ratio. Abstinence from cannabis use can be verified by daily quantitative (e.g., continuous outcome measure) urine tests. To detect changes in cannabis use or relapse, gas chromatographic-mass spectroscopic levels of 11-nor-9-carboxy-Δ 9-tetrahydrocannabinal (THCCOOH), the primary cannabis metabolite, are normalized to urine creatinine concentration to obtain a metabolite-creatinine ratio (THC/Cr). The recommended standard to confirm abstinence from recent cannabis use is a THC/Cr ratio greater than 50% from the previous visit to indicate recent cannabis use, and changes of <50% indicate abstinence (Huestis & Cone, 1998). Quantitative urine screening (THC/Cr) is the benchmark for monitoring abstinence in cannabis withdrawal studies. A second example of a quantitative urine test is the determination of the concentration of benzoylecgonine, a major metabolite of cocaine, in studies of cocaine treatment. Findings from placebo-control trials of fluoxetine as an adjunct to treatment cocaine abuse have shown that urine benzylecgonine level is related to self-reports of recent drug use and is independent of anxiety, and depression (Delucchi, Jones, & Batki, 1997). Together, these findings suggest that quantitative urine tests can be used for monitoring abstinence from cannabis use and cocaine use in clinical research studies.

Multiple Repeated Measures of Substance Use Behaviors

In addition to screening and diagnostic assessment of psychiatric and substance use disorders, a thorough history should include assessment of developmental, family, social, and environmental factors. During the assessment, it may also be necessary to use some of the laboratory measures described earlier, to determine the recency of substance use. Particularly for the assessment of adolescents, corroborating information from multiple informants increases accuracy. The assessment should then be used as a guide for a biopsychosocial formulation of a treatment plan for the particular individual. For treatment or prospective follow-up, substance use behaviors should be monitored regularly via the laboratory measures and self-report measures described earlier.

In addition to measuring and monitoring substance use behaviors during treatment and/or follow-up, it is beneficial to determine what risk and protective factors for substance use are present. Assessment of risk and protective factors can provide invaluable information to help predict the developmental course and/or treatment course of substance use and related disorders.

Biopsychosocial Risk and Protective Factors

As with all neurobehavioral disorders, a multifactorial model of inheritance (Falconer, 1965; Lander & Schork, 1994) provides a broad enough theoretical framework to encompass specific gene-gene and gene-environment interactions that predict stages of substance use involvement. From this model, characterization of the clinical phenotype (e.g., clinical characteristics, severity, family history, age of onset), along with specific risk and protective factors, are likely to be particularly useful in identifying groups of individuals at risk for developing substance use disorders (Falconer, 1965; Lander & Schork, 1994). Risk factors for substance use increase the probability of use, while protective factors decrease the probability of use. Specific genetic and environmental risk factors may predispose an individual to behaviors leading to substance use, abuse, and dependence. For example, children of substance-using parents, school dropouts, delinquent youth, and youth with mental health problems are all at high risk for the development of substance use disorders by young adulthood. Among college students, high-risk drinking and related consequences appears to be problematic within fraternities and sororities, as well as among student athletes (Turrisi, Mallett, Mastroleo, & Larimer, 2006). Throughout adulthood, the physical and social consequences of chronic alcohol and drug use can become severe, especially for individuals with risk factors such as poor health and pain (Christensen, Low, & Anstey, 2006). Risk status for drug use and related problems among adolescents and young adults can be screened using the DUSI-R, POSIT, ADI, ASAP and ADAD, whereas for adults, measures such as the ASI are recommended (see Table 18.1 for details). The incidence of drug use initiation generally increases to the age of 18 years, whereupon a rapid decline in the onset of drug use occurs throughout young adulthood (Kandel & Logan, 1984; Yamaguchi & Kandel, 1984a; Yamaguchi & Kandel, 1984b). However, the prevalence of substance abuse and related problems can continue throughout adulthood and lead to increased impairment in older adults who are heavy users (Christensen et al., 2006).

Measurement Issues for Assessment of Risk

For research purposes, it is necessary to demonstrate interrater reliability throughout each study that assesses changes in risk, since interrater indices evaluate both the instruments and the performance of the raters themselves. Reliability should be assessed by the scoring of recorded interviews by several raters, joint interviews, and use of test-retest methodology. One measure of interrater agreement is the kappa statistic, which corrects for chance agreement (Shrout, Spitzer, & Fleiss, 1987). Interrater agreement should be checked periodically, to prevent rater drift (Sanson-Fisher & Martin, 1981).

Research participants may also provide inconsistent or discrepant information, requiring use of multiple sources of information to establish the best estimate for psychiatric diagnoses and other measures of risk. The best estimate method uses multiple sources of information to establish diagnoses, based on all available information, by expert clinicians (Leckman, Sholomskas, Thompson,

Belanger, & Weissmain, 1982). Use of best-estimate methods helps to establish accurate diagnoses and minimizes the chance of missed diagnoses (Kosten & Rounsaville, 1992).

Domains

Three general domains encompass the majority of factors that predict substance use behavior throughout the life span: (1) genetic, (2) individual characteristics, and (3) social-environmental (Bry, McKeon, & Pandina, 1982; Hawkins & Catalano, 1989; Labouvie, Pandina, White, & Johnson, 1986; Newcomb, Maddahian, & Bentler, 1986). Before discussing specific factors in these domains, some general principles should be noted. First, risk factors are either present or not, and presence of a risk factor increases likelihood of drug use. Second, the presence of a protective factor does not guarantee abstinence. Third, as the number of risk factors increase, the likelihood of drug use increases. Fourth, risk and protective factors can be categorical or dimensional constructs. Finally, preventive interventions aim to decrease the likelihood of developing a disorder but do not necessarily eliminate all risk factors (Clayton, 1992).

Genetic Factors

Substance use disorders, like other neuropsychiatric disorders, are complex and multifactorially inherited (Falconer, 1965; Lander & Schork, 1994). Evidence for multifactorial inheritance is supported by both animal and human studies (Cadoret, O'Gorman, Troughton, & Heywood, 1986; Falconer, 1965; Lander & Schork, 1994; Li, Lumeg, McBride, & Murphy, 1987). Twin studies have demonstrated that identical (i.e., monozygotic) twins are more likely to be concordant for alcoholism than fraternal (i.e., dyzygotic) twins (Cloninger, Bohman, & Sigvardsson, 1981; Hrubec & Omenn, 1981). Some (Goodwin, Schulsinger, Hermansen, Guze, & Winokur, 1973) but not all (Clifford, Fulker, Gurling, & Murray, 1981) adoption studies have demonstrated that children of alcoholics (especially boys), when reared apart from biological parents, are more likely to develop alcohol problems than children of nonalcoholic parents. Children of alcoholic parents (Hill & Hruska, 1992) and of polysubstance-dependent fathers also appear to be at increased risk for substance use involvement (Cadoret, 1992). Linkage-based genome scans now provide converging evidence that specific chromosomal regions contain common allelic variants that confer human vulnerability to addiction across multiple classes of drugs (Uhl, 2004, 2006).

Individual Characteristics

A number of personal characteristics may predispose an individual to substance use. For example, sensation seeking (a need for varied, novel, and complex sensations and experiences, Zuckerman, 1979; Cloninger, 1987), impulsivity, and deficits in information processing have been associated with alcohol and drug use. Males are at greater risk to develop substance use (Coffey, Lynskey, Wolfe, & Patton, 2000; Kosterman, Hawkins, Guo, Catalano, & Abbott, 2000; Von Sydow, Lieb, Pfister, Hofler, Sonntag, & Wittchen, 2001), although girls with an early onset of puberty have greater alcohol and substance use than those with typical or late-onset puberty (Lanza & Collins, 2002). A particularly robust predictor of substance use is antisocial behavior. For instance, conduct problems (Coffey et al., 2000), deviance (Wills, Vaccaro, McNamara, & Hirky, 1996), rebelliousness (Hawkins, Catalano, & Miller, 1992), delinquency (Flory, Lynam, Milich, Leukefeld, & Clayton, 2004), and violence (Van den Bree & Pickworth, 2005) have all been associated with substance use development, particularly if present before middle adolescence; such individuals are more likely to escalate from use to abuse by young adulthood (Dishion & Loeber, 1985). For those individuals who continue to use drugs throughout adulthood, chronic alcohol and drug use can produce severe consequences and additional risk factors for continued drug use, such as poor health and pain (Christensen et al., 2006). All of these individual factors may play a role in the development of substance use initiation and progression through the stages of use, and it is very likely that these factors interact with social and environmental domains to produce substance use and substance use disorders.

Social and Environmental Factors

Family, peer, and dyadic relationships are strongly related to social environment (Dishion, Capaldi, & Yoerger, 1999), and reciprocal influences among social and environmental factors occur throughout childhood and adolescence (Stice & Barrera, 1995; Stice, Barrera, & Chassin, 1993). Parental influence in the initiation of drug use is more powerful in boys in early adolescence (Moss, Clark, & Kirisci, 1997), and parental influence continues to be a major risk factor for both genders throughout adolescence (Kandel, 1985). Dishion, Patterson, Stoolmiller, & Skinner (1991) and Patterson, Reid, & Dishion (1992) have shown that family influences precede the choice of, and direct the child toward, deviant peer groups.

The influence of the family structure has been studied as a risk factor for the initiation of substance use. For example, Kellam, Simon, & Ensminger (1983) found that the two-parent stable family is no longer the norm and that adolescents' solitude after the divorce of parents predicts drug use more in boys than in girls. In contrast, remarriage of the custodial parent is more related to drug use in girls than boys (Needle, Su, & Doherty, 1990). Additional familial risk factors for the development of substance use include the availability of alcohol or drugs in the home and the use of drugs or alcohol by parents or older siblings (Baumrind, 1983; Brook, Kessler, & Cohen, 1999); sexual or physical abuse (Dembo, Dertke, La Voie, Borders, Washburn, & Schmeidler, 1987), lack of closeness to parents (Kandel, 1982); and poor role modeling by parents or older siblings (Kaminer, 1994).

Peer affiliation is a key social factor in predicting the initiation and progression of substance abuse in adolescents and young adults (Swadi, 1999). Strong peer influence, peer pressure, and peer affiliation all predict more severe behavioral undercontrol and substance use (Fergusson, Linskey, Howard, 1995; Kandel, Kessler, & Margulies, 1978; Krohn, Lizotte, Thornberry, Smith, & McDowell, 1996; Swadi, 1999). Fergusson and colleagues (1995) found that hazardous alcohol use is best predicted by the extent of affiliation with substance-using peers. Best friends' smoking behavior consistently predicts adolescent smoking progression (Wang, Fitzhungh, Eddy, Fu, & Turner, 1997). Deviant peer influence strongly predicts marijuana use (Kandel et al., 1975). Krohn and colleagues (1996) have shown reciprocal causal effects between adolescent and peer drug use, with the influence of peer drug use on progression of adolescent drug use increasing over time. Peer encouragement to use drugs predicts escalated alcohol, cigarette, and marijuana use (Duncan, Tildesley, Duncan, & Hops, 1995). Other social risk factors for substance use related to school include low grades, poor school performance, and dropping out (Clayton, 1992; Mensch & Kandel, 1988). Among college students, high-risk drinking and related consequences are especially prevalent within fraternities and sororities, as well as among student athletes (Turrisi et al., 2006). For college students in these environments, there appears to be strongly ingrained traditions to drink and low concern about the consequences of drinking (Turrisi et al., 2006).

Measures of Social and Environmental Factors

Two instruments of particular use in assessing the social environment are the ADAD and ASAP. Both thoroughly assess social and family factors, and both can be administered repeatedly to gauge changes in family dynamics and substance use involvement over time. To assess peer relations and peer substance use during adolescence and young adulthood, the DUSI-R is a good screening instrument. For more thorough assessment of peer environment during adolescence, the DICA covers school and peer functioning more extensively. School performance can be assessed using the ASAP, ADAD, or CASI-A. For adults, the ASI provides measures of employment and legal, family, and social functioning. Additional details on measures of social and environmental factors are in Table 18.1.

Conclusions

Problems With Current Diagnostic Nosology

In the United States, substance use disorders are diagnosed by DSM-IV-TR criteria. Unfortunately, there is controversy because of the lack of clarity and questions about the developmental appropriateness of the specific DSM criteria for diagnosing substance use disorders in adolescents (Harrison, Fulkerson, & Beebe, 1998; Martin et al., 1995; Pollock & Martin, 1999). For example, defining any amount of substance use as a substance use disorder in adolescents limits the usefulness of the term, because the classification is too inclusive (Harrison et al., 1998). The categorical nature of the DSM-IV-TR can lead to diagnostic uncertainty for the case of substance-using adolescents. For example, an adolescent may meet one or two dependence criteria while meeting no abuse criteria, which would leave the adolescent being undiagnosed according to DSM-IV-TR, despite the presence of dependence criteria and impairment. These adolescents who do not fit neatly into the current DSM criteria are termed "diagnostic orphans" and have included up to 30% of adolescents in some studies (Winters, Latimer, & Stinchfeld, 2001). Clearly, this is an issue for concern that remains to be resolved. This example is another illustration of our previous recommendation that it is often useful to include a multidimensional assessment for psychiatric diagnoses and other risk factors, especially in the case of adolescents. Finally, it is also important to remember that "experimentation" with substances during adolescence and young adulthood may be a normative aspect of development, and the developmental outcomes may not necessarily be a substance use disorder. Many adolescents experiment with early "gateway" drugs, but most do not progress by young adulthood to use of more severe substances (Winters et al., 2001).

Future Directions

The measurement of substance use behavior and of changes in substance use behavior requires appropriate screening and comprehensive assessment. The specific screening and assessment tools depend on the purpose of the evaluation. Future studies on measurement of substance use behavior will need to determine which diagnostic criteria apply, especially for adolescent populations. Additional research will be needed to determine the most effective use and combinations of genotyping and biomarkers to further refine the behavioral phenotypes that define substance use behavior. Future longitudinal studies should include assessment using multiple measures of behavioral undercontrol, psychiatric comorbidity, substance use severity, and the severity, timing, and duration of environmental stressors. Future work in adolescent and young-adult populations should more effectively define and assess the social and environmental processes that increase or decrease the risk of substance use initiation and progression to substance use disorders. For adults with chronic use, prospective studies should examine the consequences and risk factors of continued use, examining how poor health and pain contribute to continued drug use.

References

Allen, J., & Columbus, M. (1995). *Assessing alcohol problems: A guide for clinicians and researchers.* Rockville, MD: National Institute on Alcohol Abuse and Alcoholism.

Allen, J., Litten, R., & Fertig, J. (1997). A review of research on the Alcohol Use Disorders Identification Test (AUDIT). *Alcoholism Clinical and Experimental Research, 21,* 613–619.

American Psychiatric Association. (2000). *Diagnostic and statistical manual of mental disorders, 4th Edition, Text Revision.* Washington, DC: American Psychiatric Association.

Baumrind, D. (1983). Specious causal attributions in the social sciences: The reformulated stepping-stone theory of heroin use as exemplar. *Journal of Personality and Social Psychology, 45,* 1289–1298.

Bowers, L. D., Ullman, M. D., & Burtis, C. A. (1994). Chromatography. In C. A. Burtis & E. R. Ashwood (Eds.), *Tietz textbook of clinical chemistry* (2nd ed.). Philadelphia: Saunders.

Brandon, T. H., Copeland, A. L., & Saper, Z. L. (1995). Programmed therapeutic messages as a smoking treatment adjunct: Reducing the impact of negative affect. *Health Psychology, 14,* 41–47.

Brook, J. S., Kessler, R. C., & Cohen, P. (1999). The onset of marijuana use from preadolescence and early adolescence to young adulthood. *Development and Psychopathology, 11,* 901–914.

Brown, S. A., Christiansen, B. A., & Goldman, M. S. (1987). The Alcohol Expectancies Questionnaire: An instrument for the assessment of adolescent and adult alcohol expectancies. *Journal of Studies on Alcohol, 48,* 483–491.

Brown, S. A., Myers, M. G., Lippke, L., Tapert, S. F., Stewart, D. G., & Vik, P. W. (1998). Psychometric evaluation of the Customary Drinking and Drug Use Record (CDDR): A measure of adolescent alcohol and drug involvement. *Journal of Studies on Alcohol, 59,* 427–438.

Bry, B. H., McKeon, P., & Pandina, R. J. (1982). Extent of drug use as a function of the number of risk factors. *Journal of Abnormal Psychology, 91,* 273–279.

Cadoret, R. J. (1992). Genetic and environmental factors in initiation of drug use and the transition to abuse. In M. Glantz & R. Pickens (Eds.), *Vulnerability to drug abuse* (pp. 99–113). Washington, DC: American Psychological Association.

Cadoret, R. J., O'Gorman, T., Troughton, E., & Heywood, E. (1986). An adoption study of genetic and environmental factors in drug abuse. *Archives of General Psychiatry, 43,* 1131–1136.

Cady, M., Winters, K. C., Jordan, D., & Solheim, K. (1996). Motivation to change as a predictor of treatment outcomes for adolescent substance abusers. *Journal of Child and Adolescent Substance Abuse, 5,* 73–91.

Christensen, H., Low, L. F., & Anstey, K. J. (2006). Prevalence, risk factors and treatment of substance abuse in older adults. *Current Opinion in Psychiatry, 19,* 587–592.

Clark, D. B., & Winters, K. C. (2002) Measuring risks and outcomes in substance use disorders prevention research. *Journal of Consulting and Clinical Psychology, 70,* 1207–1223.

Clayton, R. R. (1992). Transitions in drug use: Risk and protective factors. In M. Glantz & R. Pickens (Eds.), *Vulnerability to drug abuse* (pp. 15–51). Washington, DC: American Psychological Association.

Clifford, C. A., Fulker, D. W., Gurling, H. M. D., & Murray, R. M. (1981). *Preliminary findings from a twin study of alcohol use. Twin Research 3 Part C: Epidemiological and Clinical Studies.* New York: Alan R. Liss.

Cloninger, C. R. (1987). Neurogenetic adaptive mechanisms in alcoholism. *Science, 236,* 410–415.

Cloninger, C. R., Bohman, M., & Sigvardsson, S. (1981). Inheritance of alcohol abuse: Cross fostering analysis of adopted men. *Archives of General Psychiatry, 38,* 861–868.

Cocco, K. M., & Carey, K. B. (1998). Psychometric properties of the drug abuse screening test in psychiatric outpatients. *Psychological Assessment, 10,* 408–414.

Coffey, C., Lynskey, M., Wolfe, R., & Patton, G. C. (2000). Initiation and progression of cannabis use in a population-based Australian adolescent longitudinal study. *Addiction, 95,* 1679–1690.

Cone, E. J. (1997). New developments in biological measures of drug prevalence. In L. Harrison & A. Hughes (Eds.), *The validity of self-reported drug use: Improving the accuracy of survey estimates* (pp. 108–129). NIDA Research Monograph 167, NIH Publ. No. 97-4147. Rockville, MD: U.S. Department of Health and Human Services.

Conoley, J. C., & Impara, J. C. (1995). *Mental measurements yearbook* (12th ed). Lincoln, NE: Buros Institute of Mental Measurements

Cornelius, J. R., Clark, D. B., Reynolds, M., Kirisci, L., & Tarter, R. (2006). Early age of first sexual intercourse and affiliation with deviant peers predict development of SUD: A prospective longitudinal study. *Addictive Behaviors, 32,* 850–854.

Dawes, M. A., Antelman, S. M., Vanyukov, M. M., Giancola, P., Tarter, R. E., Susman, E. J., et al. (2000). Developmental sources of variation in liability to adolescent substance use disorders. *Drug and Alcohol Dependence, 61,* 3–14.

Delucchi, K. L., Jones, R. T., & Batki, S. L. (1997). Measurement properties of quantitative urine benzoylecgonine in clinical trials research. *Addiction, 92,* 297–302.

Dembo, R., Dertke, M., La Voie, L., Borders, S., Washburn, M., & Schmeidler, J. (1987). Physical abuse, sexual victimization and illicit drug use: A structural analysis among high risk adolescents. *Journal of Adolescence, 10,* 13–34.

Dembo, R., Schmeidler, J., Borden, P., Turner, G., Sue, C. C., & Manning, D. (1996). Examination of the reliability of the Problem Oriented Screening Instrument for Teenagers (POSIT) among arrested youths entering a juvenile assessment center. *Substance Use and Misuse, 31,* 785–824.

Dishion, T. J., Capaldi, D. M., & Yoerger, K. (1999). Middle childhood antecedents to progressions in male adolescent substance use: An ecological analysis of risk and protection. *Journal of Adolescent Research, 14,* 175–205.

Dishion, T. J., & Loeber, R. (1985). Adolescent marijuana and alcohol use: The role of parents and peers revisited. *American Journal of Drug and Alcohol Abuse, 11,* 11–25.

Dishion, T. J., Patterson, G. R., Stoolmiller, M., & Skinner, M. L. (1991). Family, school, and behavioral antecedents to early adolescent involvement with antisocial peers. *Developmental Psychology, 27,* 172–180.

Duncan, T. E., Tildesley, E., Duncan, S. C., & Hops, H. (1995). The consistency of family and peer influences on the development of substance use in adolescence. *Addiction, 90,* 1647–1660.

Endicott, J., & Spitzer, R. L. (1978). A diagnostic interview: The schedule for affective disorder and schizophrenia. *Archives of General Psychiatry, 35,* 837–844.

Falconer, D. S. (1965). The inheritance of liability to certain diseases, estimated from the incidence among relatives. *Annals of Human Genetics 29,* 51–76.

Fergusson, D. M., Linskey, M. T., & Howard, L. J. (1995). The role of peer affiliations, social, family, and individual factors in continuities in cigarette smoking between childhood and adolescence. *Addiction 90,* 647–659.

First, M., Spitzer, R., & Gibbon, M. (1997). *Structured clinical interview for DSM-IV Axis I Disorders—Patient Version 2.0 (SCID-I/P).* New York: New York State Psychiatric Institute.

Fisher, P., Shaffer, D., Piacentini, J. C., Lapkin, J., Kafantaris, V., Leonard, H., et al. (1993). Sensitivity of the Diagnostic Interview Schedule for Children (2nd ed.) (DISC 2.1) for specific diagnoses of children and adolescents. *Journal of the American Academy of Child and Adolescent Psychiatry, 32,* 666–673.

Flory, K., Lynam, D., Milich, R., Leukefeld, C., & Clayton, R. (2004). Early adolescent through young adult alcohol and marijuana use trajectories: Early predictors, young adult outcomes, and predictive utility. *Development and Psychopathology, 16,* 193–213.

Goldberger, B. A., & Jenkins, A. J. (1999). Drug toxicology. In P. J. Ott, R. E. Tarter, & R. T. Ammerman (Eds.), *Sourcebook on substance abuse* (pp. 185–196). Needham Heights, MA: Allyn & Bacon.

Goodwin, D. W., Schulsinger, F., Hermansen, L., Guze, S. B., & Winokur, G. (1973). Alcohol problems in adoptees raised apart from alcoholic biological parents. *Archives of General Psychiatry, 28,* 238–242.

Gorodetzky, C. W. (1972). *Validity of urine tests in monitoring drug abuse.* Report of the Thirty-Fourth Annual Scientific Meeting Committee on Problems of Drug Dependence, Ann Arbor, MI.

Harrison, P. A., Fulkerson, J. A., & Beebe, T. J. (1998). DSM-IV substance use disorder criteria for adolescents: A critical examination based on a statewide school survey. *American Journal of Psychiatry, 155,* 486–492.

Hawkins, J. D., & Catalano, R. F. (1989). *Risk and protective factors for alcohol and other drug problems: Implications for substance abuse prevention.* Unpublished manuscript.

Hawkins, J. D., Catalano, R. F., & Miller, J. Y. (1992). Risk and protective factors for alcohol and other drug problems in adolescence and early adulthood: Implications for substance abuse prevention. *Psychological Bulletin, 112,* 64–105.

Heustis, M. A., & Cone, E. J. (1998). Differentiating new marijuana use from residual drug excretion in occasional marijuana users. *Journal of Analytical Toxicology, 22,* 445–454.

Hill, S. Y., & Hruska, D. R. (1992). Childhood psychopathology in families with multigenerational alcoholism. *Journal of the American Academy of Child and Adolescent Psychiatry, 31,* 1024–1030.

Hrubec, Z., & Omenn, G. (1981). Evidence of genetic predisposition to alcoholic cirrhosis and psychosis: Twin concordance for alcoholism and its biological end-points by zygosity among male veterans. *Alcoholism: Clinical and Experimental Research, 5,* 207–235.

Kaminer, Y. (1994). *Adolescent substance abuse: A comprehensive guide to theory and practice.* New York: Plenum Medical Book Company.

Kandel, D. B. (1975). Stages in adolescent involvement in drug use. *Science, 190,* 912–914.

Kandel, D. B. (1982). Epidemiological and psychosocial perspectives on adolescent drug use. *Journal of the American Academy of Child Psychiatry, 21,* 328–347.

Kandel, D. B. (1985). On process of peer influences in adolescent drug use: A developmental perspective. *Advances in Alcohol and Substance Abuse, 4,* 139–163.

Kandel, D. B., Kessler, R. C., & Margulies, R. Z. (1978). Antecedents of adolescent initiation into stages of drug use: A developmental analysis. *Journal of Youth and Adolescence, 7,* 13–40.

Kandel, D. B., & Logan, J. A. (1984). Patterns of drug use from adolescence to young adulthood: I. Periods of risk for initiation, continued use, and discontinuation. *American Journal of Public Health, 74,* 660–666.

Kandel, D. B., Yamaguchi, K., & Klein, L. C. (2006). Testing the gateway hypothesis. *Addiction, 101,* 470–476.

Kellam, S. G., Simon, M. B., & Ensminger, M. E. (1983). Antecedent of teenage drug use and psychological well-being: A ten-year community wide prospective study. In D. Ricks & B. S. Dohrenwend (Eds.), *Origins of psychopathology: Research and public policy* (pp. 17–42). Cambridge, MA: Cambridge University Press.

Kintz, P., Cirimele, V., & Ludes, B. (2000). Detection of cannabis in oral fluid (saliva) and forehead wipes (sweat) from impaired drivers. *Journal of Analytical Toxicology, 24,* 557–561.

Kirisci, L., Mezzich, A., & Tarter, R. (1995). Norms and sensitivity of the adolescent version of the Drug Use Screening Inventory. *Addictive Behaviors, 20,* 149–157.

Knight, J. R., Goodman, E., Pulerwitz, T., & DuRant, R. H. (2001). Reliability of the problem oriented screening instrument for teenagers (POSIT) in adolescent medical practice. *Journal of Adolescent Health, 29,* 125–130.

Knight, J. R., Sherritt, L., Shrier, L A., Harris, S. K., & Chang, G. (2002). Validity of the CRAFFT substance abuse screening test among adolescent clinic patients. *Archives of Pediatrics & Adolescent Medicine, 156,* 607–614.

Kolodziej, M. E., Greenfield, S. F., & Weiss, R. D. (2002). Outcome measurement in substance use disorders. In W. W. Ishak, T. Burt, & L. I. Sederer (Eds.), *Outcome measurement in psychiatry: a critical review* (pp. 207–220). Washington, DC: American Psychiatric Publishing.

Kosten, T. A., & Ronsaville, B. J. (1992). Sensitivity of psychiatric diagnosis based on the best estimate procedure. *American Journal of Psychiatry, 149,* 1225–1227.

Kosterman, R., Hawkins, J. D., Guo, J., Catalano, R. F., & Abbott, R. D. (2000). The dynamics of alcohol and marijuana initiation: Patterns and predictors of first use in adolescence. *American Journal of Public Health, 90,* 360–366.

Krohn, M. D., Lizotte, A. J., Thornberry, T. P., Smith, C., & McDowell, D. (1996). Reciprocal causal relationships among drug use, peers, and beliefs: A five-wave panel model. *Journal of Drug Issues, 26,* 405–428.

Labouvie, E. W., Pandina, R. J., White, H. R., & Johnson, V. (1986). *Risk factors of adolescent drug use: A cross-sequential study.* Unpublished manuscript.

Lander, E. S., & Schork, N. J. (1994). Genetic dissection of complex traits. *Science, 265,* 2037–2048.

Lanza, S. T., & Collins, L. M. (2002). Pubertal timing and the onset of substance use in females during early adolescence. *Prevention Science, 3,* 69–82.

Latimer, W. W., Winters, K. C., & Stinchfield, R. D. (1997). Screening for drug abuse among adolescents in clinical and correctional settings using the Problem-Oriented Screening Instrument for Teenagers. *American Journal of Drug and Alcohol Abuse, 23,* 79–98.

Leccese, W. W., & Waldron, H. B. (1994). Assessing adolescent substance use: A critique of current measurement instruments. *Journal of Substance Abuse Treatment, 11,* 553–563.

Leckman, J. F., Sholomskas, D., Thompson, W. D., Belanger, A., & Weissmain, M. M. (1982). Best estimate of lifetime psychiatric diagnosis: A methodological study. *Archives of General Psychiatry, 39,* 879–883.

Li, T. Y., Lumeg, L., McBride, W. J., & Murphy, J. M. (1987). Rodent lines selected factors affecting alcohol consumption. *Alcoholism, 11,* 91–96.

Maisto, S. A., Chung, T. A., Cornelius, J. R., & Martin, C. S. (2003). Factor structure of the SOCRATES in a clinical sample of adolescents. *Psychology of Addictive Behaviors, 17,* 98–107.

Martin, C. S., Fillmore, M. T, Chung, T., Easdon, C. M., & Miczek, K. A. (2006). Multidisciplinary perspectives on impaired control over substance use. *Alcoholism: Clinical and Experimental Research, 30,* 265–271.

Martin, C. S., Kaczynski, N. A., Maisto, S. A., Bukstein, O. M., & Moss, H. B. (1995). Patterns of DSM-IV alcohol abuse and dependence symptoms in adolescent drinkers. *Journal of Studies and Alcohol, 56,* 672–680.

Martin, C. S., Kaczynski, N. A., Maisto, S. A., & Tarter, R. E. (1996). Polydrug use in adolescent drinkers with and without DSM-IV alcohol abuse and dependence. *Alcoholism, Clinical and Experimental Research, 20,* 1099–1108.

Martin, C., Pollock, N. K., Buckstein, O. M., & Lynch, K. G. (2000). Inter-rater reliability of the SCID alcohol use disorders section among adolescents. *Drug and Alcohol Dependence, 59,* 173–176.

Mayer, J., & Filstead, W. J. (1979). The adolescent alcohol involvement scale: An instrument for measuring adolescent use and misuse of alcohol. *Journal of Studies on Alcohol, 40,* 291–300.

Mayfield, D., McLeod, G., & Hall, P. (1974). The CAGE questionnaire: Validation of a new alcoholism screening instrument. *American Journal of Psychiatry, 131,* 1121–1123.

McLellan, A. T., Kushner, H., & Metzger, D. (1992). The fifth edition of the addiction severity index. *Journal of Substance Abuse Treatment, 9,* 199–213.

Mensch, B. S., & Kandel, D. B. (1988). Dropping out of high school and drug involvement. *Sociology of Education, 61*, 95–113.

Meyers, K. (1991). *Comprehensive Addiction Severity Index for Adolescents.* Philadelphia: University of Pennsylvania VA Medical Center.

Miller, W. R., Tonigan, J. S., & Longabaugh, R. (1995). *The Drinker Inventory of Consequences (DrInC): An instrument for assessing adverse consequences of alcohol abuse. Test Manual (NIAAA Project MATCH Monograph Series, Vol. 4).* NIH Publ. No. 95-3911. Washington, DC: U.S. Government Printing Office

Moberg, D. P., & Hahn, L., (1991). The adolescent drug involvement scale. *Journal of Adolescent Chemical Dependency, 2,* 75–88.

Morral, A. R., McCaffrey, D. F., & Paddock, S. M. (2002). Reassessing the marijuana gateway effect. *Addiction, 97,* 1493–1504.

Moss, H. B., Clark, D., & Kirisci, L., (1997). Timing of paternal substance use disorder cessation and the effects on problem behaviors in sons. *American Journal on Addictions, 6,* 30–37.

Musshoff, F., & Madea, B. (2007). New trends in hair analysis and scientific demands on validation and technical notes. *Forensic Science International, 165,* 204–215.

Natvig Aas, H., Leigh, B. C., Anderssen, N., & Jakobsen, R. (1998). Two-year longitudinal study of alcohol expectancies and drinking among Norwegian adolescents. *Addiction, 93,* 373–384.

Needle, R. H., Su, S., & Doherty, W. J. (1990). Divorce, remarriage, and adolescent substance use: A prospective longitudinal study. *Journal of Marriage and the Family, 52,* 157–169.

Newcomb, M. D., Maddahian, E., & Bentler, P. M. (1986). Risk factors for drug use among adolescents: Concurrent and longitudinal analyses. *American Journal of Public Health, 76,* 625–630.

Noam, G. G., & Houlihan, J. (1990). Developmental dimensions of DSM-III diagnoses in adolescent psychiatric patients. *American Journal of Orthopsychiatry, 60,* 371–378.

Orvaschel, H. (1985). Psychiatric interviews suitable for use in research with children and adolescents. *Psychopharmacology Bulletin, 21,* 737–745.

Patterson, G. R., Reid, J. B., & Dishion, T. J. (1992). *Antisocial boys.* Eugene, OR: Castilia.

Pollock, N. K., & Martin, C. S. (1999). Diagnostic orphans: Adolescents with alcohol symptom who do not qualify for DSM-IV abuse or dependence diagnoses. *American Journal of Psychiatry, 156,* 897–901.

Rahdert, E. (1991). *The Adolescent Assessment/Referral System Manual.* DHHS Pub. No. (ADM) 91-1735. Rockville, MD: U.S. Department of Health and Human Services, Alcohol, Drug Abuse and Mental Health Administration, National Institute on Drug Abuse.

Reich, W., Herjanic, B., Welner, Z., & Gandhy, P. R. (1982). Development of a structured psychiatric interview for children: Assessment on diagnosis comparing child and parent interviews. *Journal of Abnormal Child Psychology, 10,* 325–336.

Russell, M., Czarnecki, D., & Cowan, R. (1991). Measurements of maternal alcohol use as predictors of development in early childhood. *Alcoholism Clinical and Experimental Research, 15,* 991–1000.

Samyn, N., De Boeck, G., & Verstraete, A. G. (2002). The use of oral fluid and sweat wipes for the detection of drugs of abuse in drivers. *Journal of Forensic Science, 47,* 1380–1387.

Samyn, N., & van Haeren, C. (2000). On-site testing of saliva and sweat with Drugwipe and determination of concentrations of drugs of abuse in saliva, plasma and urine of suspected users. *International Journal of Legal Medicine, 113,* 150–154.

Sanson-Fisher, R. W., & Martin, C. (1981). Standardized interviews in psychiatry: Issues of reliability. *British Journal of Psychiatry, 139,* 138–143.

Shaffer, D., Fisher, P., & Dulcan M. (1996). The NIMH Diagnostic Interview Schedule for Children (DISC 2.3): Description, acceptability, prevalence, and performance in the MECA study. *Journal of the American Academy of Child and Adolescent Psychiatry, 335,* 865–877.

Shrout, P. E., Spitzer, R. L., & Fleiss, J. L. (1987). Quantification of agreement in psychiatric diagnosis revisited. *Archives of General Psychiatry, 44,* 172–177.

Skinner, H. A. (1982). The drug abuse screening test. *Addictive Behaviors, 7,* 363–371.

Sobell, L. C., & Sobell, M. B. (1992). Timeline follow-back: A technique for assessing self-reported alcohol consumption. In R. Litten & J. Allen, (Eds.), *Measuring alcohol consumption* (pp. 41–72). New York: Humana.

Spitzer, R. L., Endicott, J., & Robins, E. (1978). Research diagnostic criteria. *Archives of General Psychiatry, 35,* 773–782.

Spitzer, R., Williams, J., & Gibbon, B. (1987). *Instructions manual for the Structured Clinical Interview for the DSM-III-R.* New York: New York State Psychiatric Institute.

Stice, E., & Barrera, M. (1995). A longitudinal examination of the reciprocal relations between perceived parenting and adolescents' substance use and externalizing behaviors. *Developmental Psychology 31,* 322–334.

Stice, E., Barrera, M., & Chassin, L. (1993). Relation of parental support and control to adolescents' externalizing symptomatology and substance use: A longitudinal examination of curvilinear effects. *Journal of Abnormal Child Psychology, 21,* 609–629.

Substance Abuse and Mental Health Services Administration. (1999). *Screening and assessing adolescents for substance use disorders.* Center for Substance Abuse Treatment, Department of Health and Human Services Publication No. SMA 99–3282. Rockville, MD: Department of Health and Human Services.

Substance Abuse and Mental Health Services Administration. (2006). *Results from the 2005 National Survey on Drug Use and Health: National findings.* Office of Applied Studies, NSDUH Series H-30, DHHS Publication No. SMA 06-4194. Rockville, MD: Department of Health and Human Services.

Swadi, H. (1999). Individual risk factors for adolescent substance use. *Drug and Alcohol Dependence 55,* 209–224.

Tarter, R. (1990). Evaluation and treatment of adolescent substance abuse: A decision tree method. *American Journal of Drug and Alcohol Abuse, 16,* 1–46.

Tarter, R. E., Vanyukov, M., Kirisci, L., Reynolds, M., & Clark, D. B. (2006). Predictors of marijuana use in adolescents before and after licit drug use: Examination of the gateway hypothesis. *American Journal of Psychiatry, 163,* 2134–2140.

Turrisi, R., Mallett, K. A., Mastroleo, N. R., & Larimer, M. E. (2006). Heavy drinking in college students: Who is at risk and what is being done about it? *Journal of General Psychology, 133,* 401–420.

Tuttle, J., Campbell-Heider, N., & David, T. M. (2006). Positive adolescent life skills training for high-risk teens: Results of a group intervention study. *Journal of Pediatric Health Care, 20,* 184–191

Uhl, G. R. (2004). Molecular genetics of substance abuse vulnerability: Remarkable recent convergence of genome scan results. *Annals of the New York Academy of Sciences, 1025,* 1–13.

Uhl, G. R. (2006). Molecular genetics of addiction vulnerability. *NeuroRx, 3,* 295–301.

Van den Bree, M., & Pickworth, W. B. (2005). Risk factors predicting changes in marijuana involvement in teenagers. *Archives of General Psychiatry, 62,* 311–319.

Verstraete, A. G. (2004). Detection times of drugs of abuse in blood, urine, and oral fluid. *Therapeutic Drug Monitoring, 26,* 200–205.

Von Sydow, K., Lieb, R., Pfister, H., Hofler, M., Sonntag, H., & Wittchen, H. U. (2001). The natural course of cannabis use, abuse and dependence over four years: A longitudinal community study of adolescents and young adults. *Drug and Alcohol Dependence, 64,* 347–361.

Wang, M. Q., Fitzhugh, E. C., Eddy, J. M., Fu, Q., & Turner, L. (1997). Social influences on adolescents' smoking progress: A longitudinal analysis. *American Journal of Health Behavior, 21,* 111–117.

White, H. R., & Labouvie, E. W. (1989). Towards the assessment of adolescent problem drinking. *Journal of Studies on Alcohol, 50,* 30–37.

Williams, J. B., Gibbon, M., First, M. B., & Spitzer, R. L. (1992). The Structured Clinical Interview for DSM-III (SCID). II. Multisite test-retest reliability. *Archives of General Psychiatry, 49,* 630–636.

Wills, T. A., Vaccaro, D., McNamara, G., & Hirky, A. E. (1996). Escalated substance use: A longitudinal grouping analysis from early to middle adolescence. *Journal of Abnormal Psychology, 105,* 166–180.

Winters, K. C., & Henly, G. A. (1989). *Personal Experience Inventory and manual.* Los Angeles: Western Psychological Services.

Winters, K. C., & Henly, G. A. (1993). *Adolescent Diagnostic Interview schedule and manual.* Los Angeles: Western Psychological Services.

Winters, K. C., Latimer, W. W., & Stinchfeld, R. (2001). Assessing adolescent substance use. In E. F. Wagner & H. B. Waldron (Eds.), *Innovations in adolescent substance abuse interventions* (pp. 1–29). Oxford: Elsevier Science.

Wurst, F. M., Alling, C., Aradottir, S., Pragst, F., Allen, J. P., Weinmann, W., et al. (2005). Emerging biomarkers: New directions and clinical applications. *Alcoholism: Clinical and Experimental Research, 29,* 465–473.

Yamaguchi, K., & Kandel, D. B. (1984a). Patterns of drug use from adolescence to young adult-hood: II. Sequences of progression. *American Journal of Public Health, 74,* 668–672.

Yamaguchi, K., & Kandel, D. B. (1984b). Patterns of drug use from adolescence to young adult-hood: III. Predictors of progression. *American Journal of Public Health, 74,* 673–681.

Zuckerman, M. (1979). *Sensation seeking: Beyond the optimal level of arousal.* Hillsdale, NJ: Erlbaum.

Statistical Issues in Measuring Adherence: Methods for Incomplete Longitudinal Data

19

Mark R. Conaway,
W. Jack Rejeski, and
Michael E. Miller

In randomized controlled trials (RCTs) of drug therapy or other behavior change interventions, an inevitable methodological conundrum is nonadherence to treatment (Meichenbaum & Turk, 1987). From a design and data analytic perspective, there are three distinct issues that surface around the topic of nonadherence. First, how can one design behavior change interventions to better promote adherence? Second, given that nonadherence to treatment is an inevitable feature of behavioral interventions, how does one proceed with analysis of adherence data, when those who are not adherent are often those with missing data? And, third, what can be done to promote the collection of data related to

The Lifestyle Interventions and Independence for Elders Pilot (LIFE-P) Study was funded by a grant from the National Institute of Health/ National Institute on Aging (U01 AG22376) and supported in part by the Intramural Research Program, National Institute on Aging, NIH. Michael Miller received support from this grant.

treatment adherence? Although some of our own research has been directed at designing theoretically driven interventions that directly address the promotion of adherence to treatment in RCTs (Rejeski et al., 2003), the primary goal of this chapter is to examine various statistical approaches to handling missing adherence data. In addition, because the collection of adherence data is an issue that is distinct from promoting adherence itself, consideration is given to methodological factors that can enhance data acquisition.

Measuring and Analyzing Adherence

An analysis of patient adherence can be crucial to understanding the results of an intervention study or for planning a subsequent study. For example, not long ago, journal publications ignored dropouts, masking the potential negative effects that interventions may have had on specific subgroups. In our research with physical activity programming for older adults who have arthritis (Rejeski, Brawley, Ettinger, Morgan, & Thompson, 1997), we found that that it was not necessary for participants to exercise at the level that we originally set (40 minutes of continuous work each session) to derive benefit from treatment. In fact, those who were the most compliant did not benefit at all! In our future research on arthritis, this finding led us to promote multiple bouts of activity that were shorter in duration. This example illustrates the benefits of doing adherence analyses. There are also a number of well-cited examples of studies in which attention to dropout is a key part of the inference. Molenberghs and Kenward (2007) cite three trials for treating depression in which there is a substantial amount of dropout and in which failure to account for this during analyses could lead to inappropriate conclusions from the trial.

In investigations of pharmaceutical compounds, adherence may be measured in terms of actual pill counts, whereas, for behavioral studies trials that involve dietary or physical activity interventions, self-reported data may be essential for quantifying adherence. For example, dietary studies often rely on 24-hour food recalls or food frequency questionnaires administered at set intervals to validate the degree to which participants complied with intervention objectives (Crumb-Johnson, Smith-Bands, Hatcher, & Hagan, 1993; Van Horn, Dolecek, Grandits, & Skweres, 1997). Physical activity interventions may be measured by attendance at scheduled educational or activity intervention clinic sessions or by self-reported physical activity as was done in the Activity Counseling Trial (Blair et al., 1998). This illustrates that adherence can be measured either objectively or subjectively and can be assessed continuously or at set intervals. It is important to keep in mind that success in collection of subjective measures of adherence such as the self-report of physical activity can be influenced by social desirability, particularly when these data are collected by interventionists. When this type of adherence data is collected at set intervals by staff members who are blind to treatment assignment to reduce the influence of social desirability, then recall bias may be an issue of concern.

To obtain valid inferences from incomplete data, the mechanism (probability model) producing the missing observations must be considered when choosing an analysis technique. Different analysis techniques operate under different assumptions about the missing-data mechanism. The focus of this chapter is on methods for analyzing adherence data to obtain valid inference regarding adherence during follow-up when it is possible that missing adherence information may be related to patient characteristics or even the unobserved level of adherence. We have attempted to limit technical details and to concentrate on concepts related to what assumptions are made by various analytical methods so that analysts can make informed decisions when performing analyses of adherence data.

Two examples will serve to illustrate the methods. The first example is the Lifestyle Interventions and Independence for Elders (LIFE) pilot study, reported in Rejeski et al. (2005) and Pahor et al. (2006). A sample of 424 sedentary persons from four clinical sites were randomized to either a physical activity intervention or a successful-aging educational intervention. The primary outcome, measured at 6 and 12 months post-randomization, was the incidence of major mobility disability, defined as the inability to walk 400 meters within 15 minutes. The objectives of this pilot trial included obtaining data to be used in the sample-size calculations for a subsequent trial but also to assess adherence to the physical activity intervention as measured by self-report home exercise logs and the CHAMPS physical activity measure (Stewart et al., 2001).

A second example is the Leading the Way in Exercise and Diet (LEAD) study (Demark-Wahnefried et al., 2006). The goal of this study was to assess the effect of a 6-month home-based diet and exercise intervention on physical function in breast or prostate cancer survivors age 65 and older. A total of 182 subjects were randomized to either a diet and exercise intervention arm or a control arm that received general health information. The primary outcome of this trial is physical function as measured by the SF-36 Physical Function Subscale, augmented with four questions from Satariano, Ragheb, Branch, and Swanson (1990) at 6 and 12 months postrandomization. As in the previous example, physical activity was measured with the CHAMPS instrument.

In each of these examples, patient adherence to the intervention protocol is a key component of the evaluation of the trial. In the LIFE pilot study, an evaluation of adherence has implications for the design of the subsequent trial, both in terms of the sample size calculations and in terms of structuring the intervention protocol. The subjects in the LEAD study who were given the diet and activity intervention showed an improvement in physical function over those given the education-only intervention, but this difference was not statistically significant. By examining patient adherence to the protocol, researchers might be able to discover whether the next study would need a different type of intervention or whether the same intervention, with improved patient adherence, might be shown to be effective.

We note that other authors (Angrist, Imbens, & Rubin, 1996; Fischer-Lapp & Goetghebeur, 1999; Frangakis & Rubin, 1999, 2002) consider methods to account for nonadherence in analyzing the primary outcome variable. For example, these methods could be used in the LEAD study to compare the post-baseline physical function between the two arms, adjusting for patient adherence to the intervention protocol in the diet and exercise group, as well as for patients in the intervention group who adopt off-study diet and exercise changes (so-called drop-ins). Our focus is on methods for analyzing the adherence data alone, without regard to the outcome, in order to understand the level of adherence to the intervention.

Analyses of patient adherence are frequently complicated by subject dropout or missing data. Statistical methods for analyzing incomplete data are needed to obtain valid estimates of the degree of adherence. Extensive discussion of methods for incomplete data are given by a number of authors, such as Schafer and Graham (2002), Fitzmaurice, Laird, and Ware (2004), Little (1995), Hedeker and Gibbons (2006), and Molenberghs and Kenward (2007).

For adherence data, the analyses are made more challenging by the fact that rates of dropout or missing data may be related to subject characteristics or to the underlying unobserved degree of adherence. For example, subjects who are not adhering to the intervention protocol could be more likely to miss regular assessments or to not turn in the self-reported adherence information. This chapter begins with a discussion of "missing-data mechanisms," which give a formal framework for assumptions about how the probability of missing responses is related to subject characteristics or the underlying degree of adherence. This is followed by an overview of general classes of statistical methods for analyzing incomplete data, with a particular application to measuring adherence. The general classes include (1) analysis of only the observed data, often called the "complete-case" analysis, (2) imputation methods, (3) weighting, and (4) likelihood-based and Bayesian methods.

Missing-Data Mechanisms

Most discussions of missing data follow the terminology of Rubin (1976). The terminology distinguishes among studies where the data are "missing completely at random (MCAR)," those where the data are "missing at random (MAR)," and those where data are "missing not at random (MNAR)." The distinctions are important for a number of technical reasons, as described by Rubin (1976), but also for the practical reason that the type of mechanism determines which analysis method is appropriate. More detailed and mathematically precise discussions of this terminology are given later in this chapter, but we begin with a less technical discussion of why these cases are distinguished from one another and why data that are MCAR or MAR present much less of a challenge than data that are MNAR.

Roughly speaking, the difficulty with missing data is that the set of observed outcomes may no longer constitute a representative sample from the population. In principle, if it were known how the observed cases deviated from a representative sample, one could adjust the analyses in a way that could overcome the biases induced by having a nonrepresentative sample. To illustrate, suppose an investigator planned to take a random sample of 100 subjects from a population. Of the 100 subjects, outcomes are missing on 30 subjects for reasons unrelated to the outcome of interest or any characteristics of the subjects (MCAR). The remaining 70 subjects would still constitute a random sample from the population, and standard methods could be used on data from the 70 subjects.

Suppose, instead, that study participants who score below 25% adherence on a certain measure during follow-up have a high probability of not returning to provide adherence data at the next scheduled visit; whereas those who score above 25% always return. Further, assume that adherence information is collected on all participants at this prior visit. This is a simple illustration of a case where data are MAR because if we stratify on the basis of those that fall above and below 25% adherence at the antecedent visit, then for those with prior adherence <25%, "missingness" can be considered a random process with a specific probability of observing the follow-up measurement. Knowing the association between the probability of missing and the prior adherence measure would allow the researcher to adjust the results in the nonrepresentative sample to reduce bias.

Finally, suppose that, during follow-up, the research team is unable to obtain adherence measurements when participants have poor adherence. Further assume that there are no known covariates or prior observations collected that would permit formation of strata within which "missingness" is a result of chance alone. This would be considered a MNAR missing-data situation. Here, it is less clear how we should adjust the results in the sample to get accurate estimates for the population.

In order to be more precise about different forms of nonresponse, Rubin (1976) provides mathematical definition of the concepts. We will illustrate these definitions in the context of the LIFE and LEAD study examples mentioned earlier. Let $A = (A_0, A_6, A_{12})$ denote the measures of adherence from a subject at baseline (time 0) and at 6 and 12 months post-baseline. The values for (A_0, A_6, A_{12}) may be observed or unobserved, and we use indicators $R = (R_0, R_6, R_{12})$ to denote whether the adherence data at each time point for a particular subject is missing or observed. We assign $R_t = 1$ if the adherence data at time t is observed and $R_t = 0$ if the adherence data at time t is missing, for t = 0, 6, 12. Rubin (1976) partitions the adherence variables A into the missing and observed parts, $A = (A_{obs}, A_{mis})$. For example, if the adherence for a subject is observed at times 0 and 6 months but missing at 12 months, we have $A_{obs} = (A_0, A_6)$, $A_{mis} = (A_{12})$ and $R = (1, 1, 0)$.

Rubin's (1976) terminology classifies how the probability distribution of the set of missing data indicators, R, given the adherence variables A, depends on the missing and observed components of A. If the probability that the adherence is missing depends only on the observed components, $P(R \mid A_{obs}, A_{mis}) = P(R \mid A_{obs})$, Rubin (1976) denoted this as "missing at random," usually abbreviated "MAR." A special case of this, called "missing completely at random" (MCAR), occurs when the distribution of R does not depend on either A_{obs} or A_{mis}. If the distribution of R depends on A_{mis} alone or both A_{mis} and A_{obs}, then the mechanism is termed "missing not at random (MNAR)."

The terminology can be confusing, mainly, we believe, because the technical definition of the phrase "missing at random" does not coincide with how most people would interpret the phrase if used in a nontechnical context. In our experience, the term "missing at random" is taken to mean "missing completely at random." Since the majority of statistical methods for incomplete data are derived for the MAR case, they are applicable more generally than most practitioners would initially suppose.

For example, suppose that in a study like the LEAD or LIFE trials, with assessments at 0, 6, and 12 months following randomization, the data are missing only because of patient attrition. A fraction of subjects may fail to complete the study but are fully observed up to the last time they are observed. Table 19.1 contains an illustration of this pattern, often called "monotone missing data." In this pattern, a subject observed at 12 months is known to have been

19.1 A Monotone-Nonresponse Pattern			
Number of subjects	Baseline	6 months	12 months
n1	Observed	Observed	Observed
n2	Observed	Observed	Missing
n3	Observed	Missing	Missing

observed at both the baseline and the 6-month assessment; subjects observed at the 6-month assessment are known to be observed at baseline.

The corresponding R vectors for the n1 subjects are (1, 1, 1), for the n2 subjects the R vector is (1, 1, 0) and for the n3 subjects the R vector is (1, 0, 0). If the probability of missing does not depend on adherence at all, the mechanism is MCAR. If the probability that an adherence measure is missing at time t depends only on the degree of adherence at the last observed time, then the missing data mechanism is MAR. If the probability that an adherence measure is missing at time t depends on the adherence value at time t, then the mechanism is MNAR.

The discussion in the previous paragraph leaves out the important case where the probability of missing depends on covariates, such as patient characteristics or the intervention to which the patient is assigned. For the following description, we assume that covariates are always fully observed and not subject to missing values. When the probability of missing depends only on the covariates, Fitzmaurice, Laird, and Ware (2004) and Little (2005) use the term "covariate-dependent missingness" and note some subtle distinctions between this and MCAR. In this situation, by including important covariates in a model, one can obtain valid inference using estimation techniques that do not rely on maximum likelihood, such as generalized estimating equations (GEE) (Liang & Zeger, 1986). Data are said to be MAR if the probability of missing data depends on observed adherence and/or on covariates. Standard mixed-effects regression techniques based on maximum likelihood or Bayesian estimation or multiple imputation-based analyses can be used to obtain valid inference for MAR data. This again illustrates the generality of statistical methods derived under the assumption of MAR; the probability of missing can depend on observed adherence values and patient characteristics but still be "missing at random."

While the MCAR, MAR, and MNAR terminology is most commonly used to describe missing-data mechanisms, maximum likelihood and Bayesian methods for analyzing data containing missing outcomes tend to be described in terms of being applicable under assumptions of "ignorable" and " nonignorable" nonresponse mechanisms (Little & Rubin, 1987). In many cases, although not all, ignorable nonresponse mechanisms correspond to MCAR and MAR and nonignorable mechanisms correspond to NMAR cases. The importance of the distinction between ignorable and nonignorable mechanisms is that, for maximum likelihood methods, the same inference about the adherence measures is obtained under any ignorable model for nonresponse. For example, the probability of missing might depend on a patient's age, on gender, or on both age and gender. As long as the nonresponse model is ignorable in each of these cases, it does not matter which one of these models is "correct"; identical inference about the adherence parameters would be obtained. The technical details are given in Little and Rubin (1987).

Standard maximum likelihood analyses estimation techniques like those provided in PROC MIXED of SAS (SAS 9.1, Cary, NC) allow for valid inference of ignorable nonresponse if both the model for the mean and the covariance between repeated adherence measurements are correctly specified. In contrast, when the model for the nonresponse mechanism is not ignorable (i.e., the data are MNAR), one must make explicit assumptions and specify a model for nonresponse. Here, estimation can also be carried out through the use of maximum-likelihood techniques; however, these algorithms must incorporate these assumptions about the missing-data mechanism.

Methods for Analyzing Longitudinal Adherence Data

Complete-Case and Available-Case Methods

One of the most common methods of analyzing data subject to dropout or missing data is to do "complete-case analysis" in which only the subset of subjects observed on all measures is included. In the example displayed in Table 19.1, analysis would be based on the n1 subjects observed at all times. A similar method is termed " available-case" analysis by Schafer and Graham (2002) and uses different sets of subjects in different analyses depending on whether or not adherence is observed. For example, a summary of the change from baseline at 6 months would use data from n1 + n2 subjects; a summary of the change from baseline to 12 months would use data from n1 subjects. The main advantage of these methods is simplicity (i.e., standard least squares or maximum likelihood estimation can be used), but the methods can be highly biased when the data are not MCAR. Even when the data are MCAR, estimates from these procedures can be inefficient. As a result of these statistical properties, these methods have largely been discarded in the statistical literature.

Imputation Methods

There are many procedures for "imputing" or "filling in" missing observations in order to complete the dataset. One of the advantages of the various imputation methods is simplicity, in that once the data have been imputed, standard analysis methods can then be applied to the completed dataset. Imputation methods can be broadly classified as "single" or "multiple" imputation procedures. In single imputation, a single value is generated for each missing observation to complete the dataset. Once the dataset is completed, standard analyses are applied.

Methods for single imputation include "carried forward" analyses, as well as mean and regression imputation. Little and Rubin (1987) describe a number of other imputation procedures not discussed here, including "hot deck" and "cold deck" imputation procedures.

For longitudinal data, one of the most popular methods is "last-value-carried-forward" (LVCF). In LVCF, the last observed value is filled in for all subsequent time points for which the data are missing. For example, a subject observed to have values A0 and A6 for the baseline and 6-month follow-up but who is missing the 12-month observation would be assigned the A6 value at the 12-month follow-up. A subject missing both the 6- and 12-month follow-ups would be assigned the value A0 for the 6- and 12-month follow-ups. A number of authors have investigated the statistical properties of this procedure, including Shao and Zhong (2003). Fitzmaurice and colleagues. (2004, p. 393) and Molenberghs and Kenward (2007, p. 47) discuss the use of LVCF and describe how there are very few situations where the strong assumption that all observations following dropout remain constant is valid. They do not recommend the use of this procedure.

Other imputation procedures include "mean" imputation and "regression" imputation. To illustrate these methods, consider a subject in the LIFE or LEAD trials who is observed on the baseline and 6-month follow-up but for whom adherence data are missing for the 12-month follow-up. In regression imputation, the fully observed cases would be used to develop a regression model for predicting 12-month data from the baseline and 6-month adherence. "Mean" imputation is a special case where only an intercept is fit within the regression equation; thus, the missing 12-month values are replaced by the average of the observed 12-month adherence outcomes. To obtain proper inference, an element of randomness is often added to this procedure.

In multiple imputation, several values are generated for each missing value and standard analyses applied to each of the completed datasets. The final analysis accounts for the variability of the estimates within each completed dataset, as well as the variability across the completed datasets. Rubin (1987) gives an extensive treatment of procedures for multiple imputation. He argues that "proper" multiple imputation procedures should also account for the variability in the estimation of the parameters and provides a Bayesian solution for doing this.

Rubin (1987) also discusses multiple imputation methods when the data are MNAR. He notes that there are differences in the distribution of outcomes between a subject who completes the study, and one who drops out, even if the subjects have identical values on the outcomes observed up to the point of drop-out. The data do not provide a way of estimating this difference directly, and the conclusions can be sensitive to the assumptions used in modeling how the probability of dropout is related to missing outcomes. Rubin (1987) suggests some simple models for creating imputed values for MNAR cases from imputed values created under the assumption of MAR. One such model is to multiply the imputed value under MAR by a fixed factor, f, to obtain Y (imputed under MNAR) = f * Y (imputed under MAR). Rubin cautions on the use of these models, noting that the results can be sensitive to assumptions that cannot be verified directly.

Weighting

Weighting has long been used in the analysis of sample surveys to account for nonresponse or missing data. For analyzing missing data or dropouts in longitudinal data studies, the basic idea is to estimate the probability of remaining in the study and to weight the observed responses inversely proportional to this probability. For example, if we estimate that a subject has a 20% chance of remaining in the study, this person's responses are assigned weight 5. The probability can depend on subject characteristics or previously observed responses. Consequently, weighting provides a method that can be used in many different situations and in cases where the full likelihood is not completely specified, such as in generalized estimating equation (GEE) methods. Thus, through proper weighting of a GEE procedure, it is possible to extend this approach to handle data that are MAR. Examples of the use of weighting as a technique for analyzing incomplete data include Robins, Rotnitzky, and Scarfstein (1998) and Miller, Ten Have, Reboussin, Lohman, and Rejeski (2001).

Likelihood-Based Methods

Little and Rubin (1987) describe likelihood-based methods using the joint distribution of the adherence measures, A, and the missing data indicators, R. It is assumed that this joint distribution depends on a set of parameters θ, and estimates of θ can be obtained by maximum-likelihood or Bayesian methods. The methods are broad enough in scope that they can handle missing data mechanisms that are MCAR, MA R, or MNAR.

Two broad classes of models that have been developed to handle data that are MNAR include "pattern-mixture models" and "selection models" (Little & Rubin, 1987). "Pattern-mixture models" postulate assumptions about the distribution of adherence measures given particular patterns of the missing data indicators and the distribution of the missing data indicators without regard to adherence. Different nonresponse mechanisms can be modeled by specifying how the distribution of adherence depends on the pattern of observed or unobserved values. To illustrate, a pattern-mixture model in the LIFE study could state the assumptions that (1) mean adherence at each follow-up time is greater among those who complete the study than among those who dropped out, and (2) the probability of dropout is different at the 6-month and 12-month assessment times. Selection models specify (1) how the probability of nonresponse depends on the underlying adherence and (2) how adherence changes over the follow-up period. To illustrate a selection model for the LIFE study, one could assume that (1) the probability of nonresponse at the 6-month or 12-month assessments differs between those with high levels of adherence and those with low levels of adherence, and (2) adherence changes linearly over the follow-up period.

One specific type of selection model is termed a shared-parameter model (e.g., Ten Have, Kunselman, Pulkstenis, & Landis, 1998). This model specifies a mixed-effects model for the longitudinal adherence data and links this model to a model for the missing-data process by sharing a random effect between the two models. In its simplest form, the shared random effect allows the probability of missing response to be dependent on a random trend that characterizes the participant's adherence through time.

Each model has advantages in terms of interpretation. The pattern-mixture model provides an estimate of how the adherence variables differ across different patterns of nonresponse. On the other hand, the selection model explicitly states assumptions about the level of adherence over the follow-up period, which would be the quantity of interest if there were no missing data. Little (1995) provides an overview of the two types of models.

In either case, estimates of the parameters can be obtained by maximum-likelihood or Bayesian methods. It can be computationally difficult to maximize the likelihood directly, and methods based on procedures such as the EM algorithm (Dempster, Laird, & Rubin, 1977) have been suggested as a way of obtaining maximum-likelihood estimates.

Example From the Life Study

The LIFE pilot study randomized 213 participants to a comprehensive physical activity intervention with participants followed from between 12 and 18 months. The intervention had three defined phases: adoption (initial 8 weeks), transition (subsequent 15 weeks), and maintenance (week 24 through close-out). During maintenance, adherence to recommended levels of physical activity was measured using self-report home-based activity logs, which were collected monthly. These logs measured the number of times a participant was physically active and the number of minutes that the participant walked during the month. Exercise logs were received from 72% of the 213 participants during the maintenance period. The number of logs received in each month, the mean minutes of exercise per month, and the number of participants who turned in their last exercise log during each month are contained in Table 19.2.

We focus our analysis on those 154 participants who turned in at least one log during this time period, recognizing that those who never turned in a home-exercise log quite possibly had lower activity levels than those who returned at least one log. We explored whether having missing logs at subsequent months was related to the previously reported level of physical activity. We found that the odds of turning in future logs increased by 8.3% (p = 0.006) for each additional hour of reported physical activity. Thus, missing responses at subsequent visits were related to the observed responses at previous visits. Note that this relationship would violate the assumption of MCAR, where the probability of response cannot depend on previously observed responses.

To explore the longitudinal trend in physical activity, we fit a linear trend using three different longitudinal data analysis methods: GEE, a mixed-effects model, and a shared-parameter model. Because of skewness in the minutes/month outcome variable, a log transformation of the recorded minutes ($\log(\min + 1)$)

19.2	LIFE Home–Based Physical Activity Logs Collected During Maintenance		
Month	N	Mean (min/mo)	Last measurement
6	111	483	8
7	123	537	5
8	122	564	5
9	120	580	8
10	117	534	16
11	103	586	29
12	83	587	83

was applied prior to analysis. Thus, those recording 0 minutes received a value of 0 in the transformed distribution. The adherence model fit within GEE was:

$$A_i = \mu + \beta^* \, month_i + \varepsilon_i$$

with an unstructured covariance matrix. For the mixed-effects analysis, this adherence model was augmented with random intercept and slope terms (v)

$$A_i = \mu + \beta^* \, month_i + v_1 + v_2 \, month_i + \varepsilon_i.$$

An unstructured covariance matrix was used for the random-effects parameters. Finally, the shared-parameter model contained the random effects specified in the adherence model described earlier within both a model for adherence and a model for dropout. The dropout model took the form

$$\log(-\log(1 - P(D_i = j \mid D_i \geq j))) = \alpha_1 v_1 + \alpha_2 v_2$$

where D_i is an indicator variable that identifies if a participant discontinued handing in physical activity logs at time j. The left side of the equation represents the complementary log-log transformation, which is widely used to model binary observations. If α_1 and α_2 are zero, then the shared-parameter model reduces to the mixed-effects model.

The GEE approach provides inference under an assumption that the missing data are MCAR. The mixed-effects model provides inference under an assumption of MAR. The shared-parameter model operates under one specific alternative to MAR, namely that the missing data mechanism can be explained by a person-specific random trajectory that is shared between the model for adherence and that for dropout.

Results from these three approaches are presented in Table 19.3 and Figure 19.1. All methods indicate an increasing level of physical activity with increased follow-up; however, the slope relating the month of follow-up to adherence levels becomes nonsignificant ($p = 0.13$) when methods that account for MAR (mixed-effects) or NMAR (shared-parameter model) nonresponse are used. The estimates of α_1 ($p = 0.08$) and α_2 ($p = 0.85$) were not significantly different from zero in the dropout portion of the shared-parameter model, thus resulting in the similarity between estimates from this and the mixed-effects model. All three results permit an interpretation that the amount of physical activity was at least constant through the maintenance phase of the intervention. Had analyses

19.3	Estimated Intercepts and Slopes for Log Minutes of Physical Activity	
Method	Intercept	Slope
GEE	5.29	0.072 ($p = 0.033$)
Mixed-effects	5.23	0.043 ($p = 0.134$)
Shared-parameter	5.23	0.046 ($p = 0.137$)

19.1

Plot of actual and predicted values at each month of follow-up.

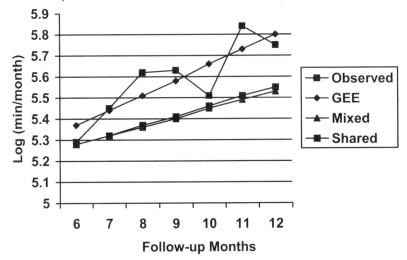

only been performed using the GEE approach, we might have concluded that activity levels increased.

In summary, our analyses showing that future missing data were dependent on previous observations led us to be suspicious of the MCAR assumption. The results from the mixed-effects analyses confirmed that different conclusions were obtained using an analysis technique applicable to data with MAR "missingness." Because it is very difficult to determine whether data may be NMAR, we explored the sensitivity of the conclusions to one form of NMAR and found that the conclusions were unchanged. By exploring the sensitivity of conclusions to different NMAR assumptions, one can have added confidence in the robustness of conclusions.

Avoiding Missing Data and Subject Dropout

The past 20–30 years have seen a rapid growth in the development of statistical methods for analyzing incomplete data, as well as a greater understanding of the statistical properties of older methods such as complete-case, available-case, and LVCF methods. While it is recognized that no statistical method is as good as having the actual data, a certain amount of missing data in clinical studies typically is unavoidable, as subjects either miss scheduled visits or drop out of the study. In addition, the collection of information on adherence to interventions is often complicated by the fact that participants are required to complete daily or weekly logs in order to track behavior in a continuous manner. In light of these challenges, investigators should take specific steps to retain participants in RCTs despite level of adherence to treatment and to devise strategies to facilitate data completeness when collecting data on a continuous schedule.

One of the strategies that has been advocated for reducing dropout is the use of pre-randomization screening for adherence. This screen can consist of a "placebo run-in" phase in which subjects are given a placebo and are monitored for compliance with the regimen. Subjects who do not comply are deemed ineligible for the trial. The perceived advantage of using the placebo run-in is statistical power. It is generally recognized that "noncompliers" tend to shrink the observed difference between treatment groups and consequently reduce power. By eliminating noncompliers, it is hoped that the statistical power is preserved. On the other hand, the use of these designs may reduce the generalizability of the findings.

The use of placebo run-ins is controversial. Senn (1997) raises objections on the basis of both ethical and statistical grounds. In a commentary on this article, Ramsey (1997) agreed that the statistical arguments supporting these designs are weak but notes that there are advantages to having pre-treatment information on subjects. For this reason, Ramsey (1997) argues that placebo run-ins should not be abandoned entirely. Pablos-Mendez, Barr, and Shea (1998) discuss placebo and active treatment run-ins as part of the design and conclude that these can either "dilute or enhance" the clinical applicability of a study, depending on the patient population to whom the results are applied. In a letter, Glynn, Buring, and Hennekens (1998) challenge these conclusions, arguing that the article overstates the generalizability of studies that remove subjects after the run-in period.

The retention of participants in RCTs for scheduled visits despite level of adherence is an area that has received particular attention at our own institutions. In general, the following steps are recommended. First, upon entry to a study, it is important to inform participants that the intervention and assessment visits represent distinct commitments. Thus, even if they are unable to participate in the intervention as intended, the hope is that they will still complete all assessment visits. We emphasize that their commitment to testing is critical to ensuring the scientific validity of study results. We ask participants to sign a form indicating that they understand the distinction between the intervention and assessment visits and agree to be contacted for assessments irrespective of their involvement in the intervention. Second, each time participants attend scheduled assessment visits, they are reimbursed for gas and given some small incentive as an appreciation for their attendance, and their names are placed in a lottery drawing that occurs at the end of each assessment cycle. Winners are announced by way of a newsletter that follows each cycle of assessment visits. We also provide feedback on several key variables that have significance for participants' health, such as levels of cholesterol and blood glucose. Third, assessment staff members are not involved in the interventions and never discuss participants' progress or level of participation in the intervention. At each assessment visit, staff members reinforce the importance of assessments visits to participants and thank them for their participation. And, fourth, we anticipate that participants who are ill around the time of assessments, those who have expressed a dislike for certain assessments, or those who are known dropout risks are less likely to attend assessment visits. Thus, assessment staff members are taught how to listen in a compassionate manner to participants concerns, to underscore the fact that partial data collection is extremely valuable even if participants cannot or do not want to complete specific assessments, and to be flexible with scheduling. Elapsed time from the target date for specific assessment visits can be recorded and adjusted for during analyses.

In addition to completion of scheduled assessments, evaluation of adherence can require that patients self-monitor and record behavior on a continued basis. For example, in weight loss interventions, it is informative to have patients track caloric intake along with minutes of physical activity. There are a number of strategies that can be useful when collecting this information. First, patients need to be educated on the need for and the value of such data. For example, it is well known that self-monitoring is a key strategy for successful behavior change. Hence, making this an integral part of treatment as opposed to apologizing to patients for having to collect such data dramatically influences patients' willingness to do so. We also recommend using these data to provide systematic feedback to patients so that their utility is emphasized. Second, it makes sense to reduce the burden of collecting these data as much as possible. Thus, while daily monitoring makes sense in the early phases of a trial, we have found that it is more tolerable to eventually switch to a schedule in which patients are asked to report data from 1 week of each month, ensuring that the week of recording is a typical week for each patient. And, third, when there are breaks in the intervention due to illness, caregiving, or other responsibilities, it is important to document nonadherence. This process is facilitated by normalizing gaps in treatment and renegotiating goals during transition periods.

As mentioned, it is impossible to have complete data related to adherence and to prevent every instance of early termination by patients in RCTs; however, we do find that an unwillingness to report on adherence and eventual dropping out often result from participants feeling that that they failed to meet the expectations of interventionists. A key to successful data acquisition and retention is to consistently communicate to patients that goals and expectations related to both treatment and assessment are established collaboratively. In addition, success can be defined in many different ways. For example, participants may not meet intervention goals, yet improve their health status. Also, we have had participants in weight loss trials who fail to lose weight but feel that they benefited from group interactions and education on how to eat healthy. It is important to identify and underscore progress of participants in intervention research even if the outcomes are unrelated to study objectives, since retention and the collection of adherence data are as important to the success of a trial as maximizing adherence.

Summary

In this chapter, we have reviewed some of the methods that could be used to analyze incomplete adherence data. When the probability of response depends on the unobserved outcome, the missing-data process is nonignorable, and using complete-case, available-case, or LVCF method can lead to biased estimates. Most model-based approaches for analyzing incomplete data can be summarized as a process whereby the analyst makes assumptions about the distribution of the missing data in an attempt to obtain unbiased estimates based on functions of the observed data. Unbiased estimates can be obtained if correct assumptions regarding the missing data process are made and incorporated into the analysis. To select an optimal statistical approach, the analyst must consider the underlying process that may have led to the missing observations, possibly using external data or expert knowledge from behavioral interventionists. In the face of uncertainty about the underlying missing data mechanism, we suggest that sensitivity analyses accompany most analyses of adherence data containing missing observations. When results from these analyses are similar, regardless of the nonresponse mechanism that is assumed, then the analyst can take comfort in knowing that conclusions made in the face of missing observations are robust to many assumptions regarding the missing-data process. When confronted by missing data, it is our view that the words of McCullough and Nelder (1999) that pertain in general to statistical models are quite applicable. They stated:

> *Modelling in science remains, partly at least, an art. Some principles do exist, however, to guide the modeler. A first, though at first sight, not a very helpful principle, is that all models are wrong; some, though are more useful than others and we should seek those. At the same time we must recognize that eternal truth is not within our grasp. (p. 8)*

References

Angrist, J., Imbens, G., & Rubin, D. (1996). "Identification of causal effects using instrumental variables." *Journal of the American Statistical Association*, 91, 444–455.

Blair, S. N., Applegate, W. B., Dunn, A. L., Ettinger, W. H., Haskell, W. L., King, A. C., et al. (1998). Simons-Morton DG for the Activity Counseling Trial Research Group. Activity Counseling Trial (ACT): Rationale, design, and methods. *Medicine & Science in Sports & Exercise, 30*(7), 1097–1106.

Block, G. (1982). A review of validations of dietary assessment methods. *American Journal of Epidemiology, 115*, 492–505.

Burke, L. E., Dunbar-Jacob, J. M., & Hill, M. N. (1997). Compliance with cardiovascular disease prevention strategies: A review of the research. *Annals of Behavioral Medicine 19*, 239–263.

Crumb-Johnson, R., Smith-Banes, M., Hatcher, L., & Hagan, D. W. (1993). Assessment of differences between compliers and noncompliers in outpatient research diet studies. *Journal of the American Dietetic Association, 93*(9), 1041–1042.

Demark-Wahnefried, W., Clipp, E. C., Morey, M. C., Pieper, C. F., Sloane, R., Snyder, D. C., et al. (2006). Lifestyle intervention development study to improve physical function in older adults with cancer: Outcomes from Project LEAD. *Journal of Clinical Oncology, 24*(21), 3465–3473.

Dempster, A., Laird, N., & Rubin, D. (1977). Maximum likelihood from incomplete data via the EM algorithm. *Journal of the Royal Statistical Society, Series B, 39*, 1–38.

Fischer-Lapp, K., & Goetghebeur, E. (1999). Practical properties of some structural mean analyses of the effect of compliance in randomized trials. *Randomized Controlled Trial Controlled Clinical Trials, 20*, 531–546.

Fitzmaurice, G., Laird, N., & Ware, J. (2004). *Applied longitudinal analysis*. Hoboken, NJ: Wiley.

Frangakis, C. E., & Rubin, D. B. (1999). Addressing complications of intention-to-treat analysis in the combined presence of all-or-none treatment-noncompliance and subsequent missing outcomes. *Biometrika, 86*, 365–379.

Frangakis, C., & Rubin, D. (2002). Principal stratification in causal inference. *Biometrics, 58*, 30–36.

Glynn, R., Buring, J., & Hennekens, C. (1998). Concerns about run-ins in randomized clinical trials. *Journal of the American Medical Association, 279*(19), 1526.

Hedeker, D., & Gibbons, R. (2006). *Longitudinal data analysis.* Hoboker, NJ: Wiley and Sons.

Huang, L., Chen, M.-H., & Ibrahim, J. (2005). Bayesian analysis for generalized linear models with nonignorably missing covariates. *Biometrics, 61,* 767–780.

Liang, K.-Y., & Zeger, S. L. (1986). Longitudinal data analysis using generalized linear models. *Biometrika, 73,* 13–22.

Little, R. J. (1992). Regression with missing X's—a review. *Journal of the American Statistical Association, 87,* 1227–1237.

Little, R. J. A. (1995). Modeling the drop-out mechanism in repeated-measures studies. *Journal of the American Statistical Association, 90,* 1112–1121.

Little, R. J., & Rubin, D. (1987). *Statistical analysis with missing data.* New York: John Wiley and Sons.

McCullough, P., & Nelder, J. A. (1989). *Generalized linear models* (2nd ed.). Boca Raton, FL: Chapman & Hall/CRC.

Meichenbaum, D., & Turk, D. C. (1987). *Facilitating treatment adherence: A practitioner's guidebook.* New York: Plenum.

Miller, M. E., Ten Have, T. R., Reboussin, B. A., Lohman, K., & Rejeski, W. J. (2001). A marginal model for analyzing discrete outcomes from longitudinal surveys with outcomes subject to multiple cause non-response. *Journal of the American Statistical Association, 96,* 844–857.

Molenberghs, G., & Kenward, M. G. (2007). *Missing data in clinical studies.* New York: John Wiley and Sons.

Pablos-Mendez, A., Barr, R., & Shea, S. (1998). Run-in periods in randomized trials: Implications for the application of results to clinical practice. *Journal of the American Medical Association, 279,* 222–225.

Pahor, M., Blair, S. N., Espeland, M., Fielding, R., Gill, T. M., Guralnik, J. M., et al. (2006). Effects of a physical activity intervention on measures of physical performance: Results of the Lifestyle Interventions and Independence for Elders Pilot (LIFE-P) Study. *The Journals of Gerontology Series A: Biological Sciences and Medical Sciences, 61*(11), 1157–1165.

Ramsey, L. (1997). Commentary: Placebo run-ins have some value. *British Medical Journal, 314,* 1193.

Rejeski, W. J., Brawley, L. R., Ambrosius, W., Brubaker P. H., Focht, B. C., Foy, C. G., et al. (2003). Older adults with chronic disease: The benefits of group mediated counseling in the promotion of physically active lifestyles. *Health Psychology, 22*(4), 414–423.

Rejeski, W. J., Brawley, L. R., Ettinger, W., Morgan, T., & Thompson, C. (1997). Compliance to therapy in older participants with knee osteoarthritis: Implications for treating disability. *Medicine and Science in Sports and Exercise, 29*(8), 977–985.

Rejeski, W. J., Fielding, R. A., Blair, S. N., Guralnik, J. M., Gill, T. M., Hadley, E. C., et al. (2005). The lifestyle interventions and independence for elders (LIFE) pilot study: Design and methods. *Contemporary Clinical Trials, 26,* 141–154.

Robins, J., Rotnitzky, A., & Scharfstein, D. (1998). Semiparametric regression for repeated outcomes with non-ignorable non-response. *Journal of the American Statistical Association, 93,* 1321–1339.

Rubin, D. (1976) Inference and Missing Data. *Biometrika, 63,* 581–592.

Rubin, D. (1987). *Multiple imputation for nonresponse in surveys.* New York: John Wiley and Sons.

SAS 9.1. The SAS Institute, Inc., Cary, NC.

Satariano, W., Ragheb, N., Branch, L. G., & Swanson, G. M. (1990) Difficulties in physical functioning reported by middle-aged and elderly women with breast cancer: Case-control comparison. *Journal of Gerontology, 45,* M3–M11.

Schafer, J., & Graham, J. (2002). Missing data: Our view of the state of the art. *Psychological Methods, 7,* 147–177.

Senn, S. (1997). Are placebo run-ins justified? *British Medical Journal, 314,* 1191–1192.

Shao, J., & Zhong, B. (2003). Last observation carry-forward and last observation analysis. *Statistics in Medicine, 22,* 2439–2441.

Stewart, A., Mills, K., King, A., Haskell, W., Gillis, D., & Ritter, P. (2001). CHAMPS physical activity questionnaire for older adults: Outcomes for interventions. *Medicine & Science in Sports & Exercise, 33*(7), 1126–1141.

Stubbendick, A. L., & Ibrahim, J. G. (2003). Maximum likelihood methods for nonignorable missing responses and covariates in random effects models. *Biometrics, 59,* 1140–1150.

Ten Have, T. R., Kunselman, A. R., Pulkstenis, E. P., & Landis, J. R. (1998). Mixed effects logistic regression models for longitudinal binary response data with informative drop-out. *Biometrics, 54,* 367–383.

Van Horn, L., Dolecek, T. A., Grandits, G. A., & Skweres, L. (1997). Adherence to dietary recommendations in the special intervention group in the Multiple Risk Factor Intervention Trial. *American Journal of Clinical Nutrition, 65*(1 Suppl.), 289S–304S.

Obstacles and Predictors of Lifestyle Change and Adherence

Section 4

Sally A. Shumaker
Editor

A number of complex factors influence whether people are able to change and maintain healthier behavior patterns. In Section IV authors explore these factors from the biological through the psychological, social, and policy levels of analysis. A significant change in this section from the prior edition of this book resides in the increased attention by all of the authors to the multiple and interrelated determinants of health behaviors. Together, these chapters provide critical insights into the relationships among various levels of influence on adherence and the challenges faced by individuals and health providers in trying to promote healthier lifestyles within a context that often thwarts such efforts.

In the first chapter, "Predictors of Patient Adherence: Patient Characteristics," Dunbar-Jacob, Gemmell, and Schlenk review a set of predictors of adherence that are specific to the individual. These authors provide an updated and detailed review of the studies that have looked at the degree to which psychological characteristics and cognitive and motivational factors influence adherence. In addition, they explore how the prior adherent behavior of an individual—either to a similar health regimen or to a new regimen—is predictive of future adherence. There is a long history of data on the influence of adverse side effects of medications on adherence. In this chapter, these data are updated and additional information is provided on the effects of symptoms benefits and adherence. Finally, the authors explore the world of health literacy—a major issue in the population today and one that often goes unacknowledged and thereby not addressed in the health provider–patient interaction.

In "Biopsychological Obstacles to Adoption and Maintenance of a Healthy Lifestyle," Grunberg and Klein retain the important and unique contribution to this field of their previous chapter (Grunberg & Klein, 1998) by fully exploring the biological aspects of health behavior including the absence or misinterpretation of biological cues, and physical and behavioral limitations. In addition, however, they expand on this biology-based perspective by considering the degree to which biological variables that influence healthy behaviors are, in turn, influenced by psychological and social factors. By applying this more systems-oriented analysis and considering the biopsychosocial aspects of adherence, Grunberg and Klein build an important bridge to understanding the interconnected influence of variables from the biological to the social that impact adherence, health behavior change, and maintenance.

Using adolescent tobacco exposure as the focus of the health behavior concern, Holub, Altman, and Jackson explore in "Adolescent Tobacco Use and the Social Context" the complex world embodied within the broad social context in this updated version of their previous chapter (Altman & Jackson, 1998). As noted by the authors, tobacco use remains the most preventable cause of morbidity and mortality in the United States despite significant strides made in the reduction of its use among adults and adolescents. However, recent trends in adolescent smoking behavior are of particular concern. Although there was a decline in smoking in the 1990s among adolescents, the trajectory of this decline began to slow in the 21st century. The authors tackle the challenge of understanding this persistent health concern by applying an ecological approach to the question. As noted by the authors, adolescent tobacco use is a complex behavior rooted in biological, social, environmental, historical, and cultural contexts. Their systems approach to this issue is similar to that considered by Grunberg and Klein—although the current authors focus more attention on the cultural and health policy aspects of the system.

In "Psychosocial Barriers to Adherence and Lifestyle Change," Williams, DiMatteo, and Haskard note that despite decades of research on patient adherence, questions continue about its causes and treatment. Approaching the issue from a systems perspective, with a focus on psychological and social factors, these authors explore what is known today about the complex factors that determine the ability and willingness of individuals to adhere to medical regimens and adopt and maintain health behaviors. In particular, they consider adherence as an ongoing process and describe the steps that individuals take throughout this process while considering the role of various psychosocial factors that contribute to a person's success or failure along the way.

In the final chapter in this section, "Changing Clinical Behavior: Implementing Guidelines to Improve Primary Care Practice," Dugan, Dodd, and Ellis consider the health provider, rather than the patient, and present a critical analysis of the world of evidence-based medicine and its relationship to adherence and health behaviors. The authors discuss the degree to which health care providers "adhere" to best practices as the health provider represents one of the key influences on the health behaviors of the general population. As noted by the authors, this area of research has grown substantially since the prior chapter on this topic (Dugan & Cohen, 1998), and these authors take full advantage of this growing field of inquiry by reviewing the complex, and sometimes dysfunctional, health care system in which clinical behavior occurs. Again, taking a systems approach and considering the components of that system (e.g., provider, practice setting, state or region, health maintenance organization, insurance providers, medical profession, and the United States) these authors consider why it is challenging for physicians to follow best practices and review the results of several interventions designed to improve primary care practices.

Predictors of Patient Adherence: Patient Characteristics

20

Jacqueline Dunbar-Jacob,
Leigh A. Gemmell,
and Elizabeth A.
Schlenk

With nonadherence rates ranging from 20% to 80% in practice and research settings, considerable health care resources are utilized in either remediating nonadherence or in addressing the consequences of inadequately treated diseases or risk factors. In the clinical research arena, further resources may be expended in the recruitment and management of additional participants to compensate for the loss of power due to dropouts or poor adherers. Resources might be better utilized at the outset of treatment or subject recruitment if individuals likely to have difficulty adhering could be identified. And, indeed, investigations have been undertaken directed toward the prediction of adherence.

A number of studies examined factors under the control of the provider that are likely to lead to nonadherence, such as prescription of multiple and/or complex regimens, lack of consistency in care providers, care provider behavior toward patients, adequacy of instructions, and convenience. Other sets of predictors are those that are more specific to the person than to the regimen, provider, or clinical setting. It is this latter set of factors that is addressed in this review. That is, what characteristics of the individual are likely to influence subsequent adherence to a health care regimen? We examine a number of areas, including psychological characteristics, cognitive-motivational factors, behavior itself, somatic and cognitive factors, and health literacy.

Psychological Characteristics as Predictors of Adherence

Several studies examined *personality traits* as predictors of adherence, and many use the Five Factor model of personality. For example, Stilley, Sereika, Muldoon, Ryan, and Dunbar-Jacob (2004) found that conscientiousness predicted medication adherence to cholesterol-lowering medications, but that neuroticism, extroversion, openness, and agreeableness did not. Extroversion predicted exercise adherence in an intervention group of cancer survivors but not in the control group (Courneya, Friedenreich, Sela, Quinney, & Rhodes, 2002). Neuroticism, conscientiousness, openness, and agreeableness did not predict adherence to exercise in either group. Finally, Hershberger, Robertson, and Markert (1999) found that appointment keeping was correlated with the personality factors of well-being, socialization, and communality in a sample of men in cardiac rehabilitation. The literature is too scant to permit us to draw any conclusions about the role of personality factors in adherence. However, the literature that exists suggests that different behaviors may be influenced by different factors.

Mood has also been examined as potential predictor of adherence. Overall, it appears that *depression* is often associated with poorer adherence. For example, measures of depression or depressive symptoms were related to poorer adherence to antihypertensive medications (Morris, Li, Kroenke, Bruner-England, Young, & Murray, 2006; Siegel, Lopez, & Meier, 2007), antiretroviral medications (Gordillo, del Amo, Soriano, & Gonzalez-Lahoz, 1999; Reynolds et al., 2004), cholesterol-lowering medications (Stilley et al., 2004), and medical appointment keeping (Mackin & Arean, 2007). Other studies have found that measures of depression or depressive symptoms are not related to adherence (Schweitzer, Head, & Dwyer, 2007; Shemesh et al., 2004). In these studies, depression or depressive symptoms were either measured through self-report questionnaires (Morris et al., 2006; Reynolds et al., 2004; Stilley et al., 2004; Gordillo et al., 1999; Schweitzer et al., 2007; Shemesh et al., 2004; Mackin & Arean, 2007) or by reviews of participants' medical records (Siegel et al., 2007). Adherence was assessed a number of different ways in these studies, including self-report questionnaires (Gordillo et al., 1999; Schweitzer et al., 2007; Morris et al., 2006; Reynolds et al., 2004), electronic monitoring (Stilley et al., 2004), pharmacy refill databases (Morris et al., 2006; Siegel et al., 2007), pill counts (Gordillo et al., 1999), missed appointments (Mackin & Arean, 2007) and biological data (Shemesh et al., 2004). No consistent patterns of associations between depressive symptoms and adherence emerged on the basis of the measurement methods used.

The Medical Outcomes Study reported that emotional distress over one's health predicted adherence (DiMatteo et al., 1993). Similarly, Dobkin, Sita, and Sewitch (2006) found that lower psychological distress was associated with better medication adherence in women with fibromyalgia. Naar-King and colleagues (2006) found that psychological distress predicted better self-reported adherence to HIV medication in youths.

Data are mixed regarding whether or not *anxiety* is related to adherence. Higher levels of anxiety were related to poorer adherence to taking cholesterol-lowering drugs (Stilley et al., 2004), overuse of medications among patients with asthma (Mawhinney et al., 1993), and poorer adherence to smoking and alcohol cessation guidelines in patients with chronic heart failure (Schweitzer et al., 2007). Lower levels of anxiety predicted greater exercise behavior among older adults (Emery, Hauck, & Blumenthal, 1992). In contrast to these findings, anxiety did not predict adherence to prenatal class attendance among primagravidas (Michie, Marteau, & Kidd, 1990), exercise adherence among healthy women (Welsh, Labbe, & Delaney, 1991), or older adults' adherence to medical appointment attendance (Mackin & Arean, 2007). One study found that the presence of anxiety symptoms was associated with *better* adherence to antiretroviral medications (Ingersoll, 2004). Thus, the relationship of anxiety to adherence is complex and not easily predicted. This suggests that efforts to raise anxiety in an attempt to raise adherence are unlikely to be successful, at best, and may lower adherence.

Investigators have also studied *coping styles* as potential predictors of adherence. Avoidant coping predicted better adherence to prenatal class attendance (Michie et al., 1990) and adherence in the Medical Outcomes Study as well (Sherbourne, Hays, Ordway, DiMatteo, & Kravitz, 1992). Instrumental coping was related to better medication adherence in women with fibromyalgia (Dobkin et al., 2006). Weaver et al. (2005) found that avoidance-oriented coping was related to poorer medication adherence to antiretroviral medications, but greater approach-oriented coping was not significantly associated with adherence. Finally, Heckman, Catz, Heckman, Miller, and Kalichman (2004) found that active coping with HIV-related stressors was associated with better adherence to antiretroviral therapy.

Hostility has been examined also in the context of adherence. Lee et al. (1992) found that participants who reported greater hostility skipped more doses of medication, although they did not report any greater difficulty in remembering to take medications. In contrast, Irvine et al. (1999) found that hostility was not associated with medication adherence in survivors of acute myocardial infarctions. Asthma patients who reported anger and irritation about their disease were more likely to attend an asthma education program (Yoon, McKenzie, Miles, & Bauman, 1991). Welsh et al. (1991) found that *Type A* and *Type H* (hard-driving) behavior was related to attendance in an exercise program designed for healthy women.

Other characteristics related to personality style have been examined, but limited evidence is available. For example, *self-motivation* is considered a possible characteristic that might influence adherence. Typically, however, self-motivation is inferred, not directly measured. Welsh et al. (1991) reported that self-motivation was not associated with exercise program attendance, but it was associated with exercise frequency. *Optimism* has also been associated with adherence to follow-up recommendations following detection of a suspicious skin lesion (Friedman, Webb, Bruce, Weinberg, & Cooper, 1995) and to adherence to attending a cardiac rehabilitation program (Glazer, Emery, Frid, & Banyasz, 2002).

Summary

The question arises as to why psychological states might predict adherence. It may be that psychological states directly influence adherence or that certain psychological states mediate the relationship between motivation and behavior. Certain psychological states may also be barriers to adherence. Although many studies have examined the relationships between psychological states and adherence, no clear patterns emerge.

Cognitive-Motivational Predictors of Adherence

Investigators have also examined beliefs and other cognitions as potential predictors of patient adherence, and it is in this area that much of the research on patient characteristics as an influence on adherence has focused. The principal models include health beliefs, intentions, self-efficacy, and stages of change.

The *Health Belief Model* is a cognitive-motivational model that states that recommended health actions will be taken if individuals believe that they are susceptible to the illness (perceived susceptibility), the consequences of the illness or of noncompliance are serious (perceived severity), the recommended action is beneficial or efficacious in reducing risk or severity (perceived benefits), and the barriers or costs of action do not exceed the benefits (perceived barriers). In addition to these beliefs, general health motivation is, at times, included in the model. General health motivation consists of both positive factors (e.g., engaging in healthy behaviors) and negative factors (e.g., worry or concern over health).

Perceived susceptibility has been the most commonly studied component of the Health Belief Model in studies examining predictors of patient adherence, but studies over the past 20 years have not supported its utility as a predictor of adherence. Perceived susceptibility did not predict adolescents' adherence to dental appointments (West, DuRant, & Pendergrast, 1993), follow-up appointment keeping in adults and children with otitis media (Jones, Jones, & Katz, 1989), medical follow-up for suspicious lesions in a skin cancer detection program (Friedman et al., 1995), participation in fecal occult blood testing among adults (Myers et al., 1994; Sandler, DeVellis, Blalock, & Holland, 1989), or mammography utilization in a community sample (Bastani, Marcus, Maxwell, Das, & Yan, 1994).

Perceived severity is a second component of the Health Belief Model. Lower ratings of perceived severity were related to poorer adherence to malaria medications in participants in a travel medicine clinic (Farquharson, Noble, Barker, & Behrens, 2004). Perceived severity has also been associated with appointment keeping among children and adults with otitis media (Jones et al., 1989) and participation in colorectal cancer screening in an HMO population (Myers et al., 1994). Perceived severity did not predict dental follow-up for adolescents (West et al., 1993) or medication adherence in chronically ill adults (Lorenc & Branthwaite, 1993).

Perceived benefits or efficacy of health behaviors as a modifier of disease is a third component of the Health Belief Model. A positive relationship has been demonstrated between perceived benefits and adherence to malaria medication (Farquharson et al., 2004), in myocardial infarction (MI) patients (Miller, Wikoff, McMahon, Garrett, & Ringel, 1988), as well as colorectal cancer (Myers et al., 1994), and mammography screening (Bastani et al., 1994). Perceived benefits did not predict follow-up appointment keeping in adults and children with otitis media (Jones et al., 1989) and medication adherence among adults with chronic conditions (Lorenc & Branthwaite, 1993).

Perceived barriers to health behavior are a fourth component of the Health Belief Model. There are mixed findings in studies that examine the relationship between perceived barriers and patient adherence. Perceived barriers have been predictive of medication adherence in adults with chronic conditions (Lorenc & Branthwaite, 1993) and mammography utilization (Bastani et al., 1994). Participants who perceived fewer barriers to obtaining mammography screenings were more likely to obtain repeated screenings (Russell, Champion, & Skinner, 2006) and adults in an anticoagulation clinic who obtained higher scores on measures of perceived barriers were less likely to refill their medication (Orensky & Holdford, 2005). In contrast, researchers found that perceived barriers were not associated with adolescents' appointment keeping for dental follow-up (West et al., 1993).

The predictive ability of health beliefs may vary among populations and behaviors. The number of studies in each of the areas mentioned is small, but those that have been undertaken suggest that an important direction in the study of health beliefs is an examination of the interaction of specific beliefs with types of health behaviors. A complicating factor in evaluating the effects of health beliefs on adherence is the time at which the assessment of health beliefs is undertaken in relation to diagnosis. Health beliefs may be modified with experience with a particular regimen (Beck, 1981). The ability of health beliefs to predict behavior may be related to whether or not individuals have experienced the behavior and adjusted their beliefs accordingly.

Several studies examined the associations between *behavioral intentions* and adherence. Courneya et al. (2004) examined intention to exercise as a predictor of behavior in a randomized-controlled trial of an exercise intervention for colorectal cancer survivors. They found that intentions predicted exercise behavior in the control group, but not in the treatment group. Blanchard et al. (2003) also found that intention predicted exercise adherence in patients attending a cardiac rehabilitation program. Other studies have also found a relationship between intentions and behavior (e.g., Myers et al., 1994). No association was found between intentions during hospitalization and adherence to activity, stress management, medication, or diet prescriptions 2 years later in post-MI patients (Miller, Wikoff, Garrett, McMahon, & Smith, 1990), suggesting that any relationship between intentions and behavior does not persist over the course of treatment.

A second theoretical model, *Self-Efficacy Theory* (Bandura, 1977), postulates that individuals will engage in or persist with a behavior to the extent that they believe themselves capable of carrying out that behavior (efficacy expectancy) and to the extent that they believe that the behavior will lead to a desired outcome (outcome expectancy). Overall, studies that examine the relationship between efficacy expectancy and self-efficacy support the notion that higher self-efficacy is associated with better adherence to HIV medications (Safren et al., 2001), and lower self-efficacy is associated with poorer adherence to HIV medications among younger, but not among older, participants (Barclay et al., 2007). Self-efficacy was also related to medication adherence in patients with rheumatoid arthritis (Brus, van de Laar, Taal, Rasker, & Wiegman, 1999) and multiple sclerosis (Fraser, Hadjimichael, & Vollmer, 2003; Fraser, Morgante, Hadjimichael, & Vollmer, 2004). In addition to being associated with medication adherence, self-efficacy has been found to be related to adherence to health behaviors including exercise regimen (McAuley, Courneya, Rudolph, & Lox, 1994) and preventive screening recommendations (Friedman et al., 1995; Myers et al., 1994). Conversely, self-efficacy was not related to exercise adherence in HIV-positive participants enrolled in an exercise intervention study (Pavone, Burnett, LaPerriere, & Perna, 1998). Finally, self-efficacy has been found to be related to adherence to diabetes self-management (Kavanagh, Gooley, & Wilson, 1993; Glasgow et al., 1989).

Few investigators have examined outcome expectancy either alone or in conjunction with self-efficacy. McCaul, Glasgow, and Schafer (1987) found that both self-efficacy and outcome expectancies were the strongest predictors of adherence for both the concurrent and prospective analyses in their study of patients with insulin-dependent diabetes mellitus. These findings held up among both adults and adolescents and across regimen: glucose monitoring, insulin administration, diet, and exercise. Researchers have also examined efficacy and outcome expectancies as determinants of adherence to exercise (Desharnais, Boullon, & Godin, 1986), medication-taking for rheumatoid arthritis (Dunbar-Jacob et al., 1993), and a cholesterol-lowering diet (Burke, Dunbar-Jacob, Sereika, & Rohay, 1996). Dunbar-Jacob et al. (1993) found that outcome expectancy was related to self-reported medication-taking but not to electronic monitoring of medication-taking. At least one study noted that self-efficacy is a stronger predictor of adherence than outcome expectancy. Desharnais et al. (1986) reported that at the outset of an exercise program, participants who became dropouts displayed lower self-efficacy related to attendance, even while expressing positive outcome expectancy.

A fourth cognitive-motivational meta-theoretical model, the *Transtheoretical Model* (DiClemente et al., 1991; Prochaska & DiClemente, 1983; Prochaska, DiClemente, & Norcross, 1992) addresses intentional behavior change. This model states that individuals move through five stages of change—precontemplation, contemplation, preparation, action, and maintenance—as they attempt to modify their behavior. This model states that progression through these stages is often nonlinear; rather, people tend to recycle through these stages. In general, people in the action and maintenance stages of change have the best adherence. Heapy et al. (2005) examined the relationship between stage of change and adherence in patients with chronic pain and found that the stage of change predicted adherence to coping skills practice. While this theory is promising, empirical reports to date tend to address clinical outcomes rather than adherence to treatment regimens. Also, the current literature tends to focus on the effects of stage-based interventions on adherence, not necessarily the relationship between the specific stage-of-change variables and adherence.

Summary

Cognitive-motivational models contribute to our understanding of patient adherence to health care regimens. Each proposes a slightly different schema for understanding the relationship between motivational cognitions and subsequent behavior. In most cases, studies find that these models account for a small proportion of the variance observed in adherence behavior. Further, studies in the health belief area suggest that the effect of beliefs on behavior may vary with the health behavior, as well as with the timing of the assessment of beliefs. Intentions and self-efficacy seem particularly promising as predictors of adherence. Aspects of health beliefs may also have a role, particularly perceived barriers, benefits, and severity. Both self-efficacy and health beliefs appear to be influenced by experience. As self-efficacy and health beliefs appear to change in the direction of the behavior change, however, one wonders if behavior itself is predictive of future behavior.

Health Behaviors as Predictors of Subsequent Adherence

Health behavior as a predictor of subsequent adherence can be examined along two dimensions. The first is whether adherence to a specific behavior predicts adherence to that same behavior in the future. The second is whether adherence to a specific behavior or set of behaviors predicts adherence to a different health behavior.

If individuals adhere to a health care regimen at one time, they may be more likely to do so at a later time. Indeed, the few studies that have examined the effect of adherence to a specific regimen on subsequent adherence to the same regimen do support such a hypothesis. This has been particularly evident with screening behaviors. Lechner, de Vries, and Offermans (1997) found that participants who had had breast cancer screening in the past were most likely to seek future screening. Previous mammography has been shown to be the best predictor of participation in mammography screening (Bastani et al., 1994), and the best predictor of follow-up on suspicious skin lesions was frequency of skin self-examination (Friedman et al., 1995). Interestingly, Myers et al. (1994) found that while past colorectal screening was predictive of screening in univariate analyses, in regression analyses past screening predicted intentions only and not actual screening, although intentions and screening behaviors were correlated. Studies of an adolescent population found that those who have visited dentists in the past were most likely to utilize preventive practices (West et al., 1993).

Several studies support the idea that past adherence is a predictor of subsequent adherence. For example, Ascher-Svanum, Zhu, Faries, Lacro, and Dolder (2006) found that past nonadherence to antipsychotic medications predicted future nonadherence in a sample of patients with schizophrenia. In the Lipid Research Clinics Coronary Primary Prevention Trial, a 10-year study of the cholesterol hypothesis, adherence to the study medication during the first month postrandomization accounted for 34.5% of the variance in adherence in the first year and approximately 24% in the seventh year (Dunbar & Knoke, 1986). Dubanoski (1988) also found that first-month adherence to tuberculosis preventive therapy was the strongest predictor of adherence at 6 months. Kribbs and colleagues (1993) found that adherence to nasal continuous positive airway pressure in the first month predicted usage at 3 months among patients with sleep apnea. The Medical Outcomes Study also reported that baseline adherence was associated with adherence 2 years later (DiMatteo et al., 1993). The ability of initial adherence to predict subsequent adherence over a 3-month to 7-year duration suggests certain stability to adherence based upon a pattern established early within a specific regimen. This growing body of evidence suggests interesting and valuable directions for the continued study of adherence to health regimens, in efforts to both understand and promote adherence.

Health behaviors other than early adherence to an intervention do not necessarily predict subsequent adherence to a specific regimen. For example, past exercise behaviors did not predict adherence to an exercise intervention for participants randomized to an exercise intervention group, but it did predict adherence in the control group (Courneya et al., 2002). This suggests that intervention may interrupt the early patterns. These studies suggest that behavior can predict behavior. The more similar the initial behavior is to the behavior to be predicted, the greater the ability to predict. However, there does not appear to be a set of behaviors that would allow prediction of individuals' adherence to a specific health regimen; that is, investigators could not predict that a health-oriented individual, as defined by the practice of a set of health behaviors, would necessarily adhere to a regimen solely on the basis of that earlier behavior. The studies do suggest that a history of adherence to a specific regimen predicts subsequent adherence to that regimen. Further study of the ability of behavior to predict subsequent adherence would be of interest and would be most useful in the selection of participants for clinical research efforts where maximal adherence to protocol regimen is desired.

Somatic and Cognitive Factors as Predictors of Adherence

Several studies examined aversive effects, as well as relief of symptoms due to treatment, as predictors of adherence. For example, physical discomfort during running predicted dropping out of a marathon training program (Heiby, Onorato, & Sato, 1985). Indeed, the amount of running done by the dropouts was a function of the number of injuries experienced. Other researchers similarly reported that adverse side effects, especially their number, nature, and perceived intensity, were inversely related to adherence in adolescents receiving iron supplements (Cromer, Steinberg, Gardner, Thornton, & Shannon, 1989) and in women prescribed ethinylestradiol (Kruse, Eggert-Kruse, Rampmaier, Runnebaum, & Weber, 1993). Ascher-Svanum et al. (2006) found that people with schizophrenia who were nonadherent to antipsychotic medication were more likely to report averse effects from the medication. Ickovics et al. (2006)

found that individuals living with HIV and on a highly active antiretroviral therapy regimen who reported fewer adverse events were more likely to adhere to treatment.

Adherence to self-management procedures for adults with chronic disease was related to fewer disease-related symptoms (Kravitz et al., 1993). Similarly, patients with chronic obstructive pulmonary disease who reported less shortness of breath were more likely to adhere to meter-dose inhaler regiments (Rand, Nides, Cowles, Wise, & Connett, 1995), and those with more severe dyspnea were more adherent to nebulizer therapy (Turner, Wright, Mendella, & Anthonisen, 1995). Two randomized clinical trials found that symptoms were not predictive of adherence (Jones et al., 1989; Yoon et al., 1991). The severity of disease among asthma patients did not affect their rate of attendance at an asthma education program after discharge from the hospital (Yoon et al., 1991). Duration and intensity of otitis media symptoms did not predict follow-up appointment keeping in adults and children presenting to an emergency department (Jones et al., 1989). Where an effect was found, fewer symptoms were associated with better adherence. The nature of the studies does not permit a clarification of the direction of the effect (e.g., whether fewer symptoms predict adherence or whether adherence leads to fewer symptoms).

Health Literacy as a Predictor of Adherence

Ratzan and Parker (2000) define health literacy as "the degree to which individuals have the capacity to obtain, process, and understand basic health information and services needed to make appropriate health decisions" (as cited in Institute of Medicine, 2004, p. 32). In 2003, the U.S. Department of Education conducted a National Assessment of Adult Literacy (NAAL), which included measures of health literacy. A separate report on the health literacy data suggested that higher levels of health literacy are associated with better overall self-reported health (Kutner, Greenberg, Jin, & Carlson, 2006), and, given this relationship, several researchers are beginning to examine the relationships between health literacy and patient adherence.

Several studies have examined the associations between health literacy and adherence and have obtained mixed results. Poor literacy was associated with poor adherence to HIV medications (Wolf et al., 2007), fewer medication refills in patients with glaucoma (Muir et al., 2006), and nonadherence to preoperative medications in patients who were preparing to undergo ambulatory surgery (Chew, Bradley, Flum, Cornia, & Koepsell, 2004). Although the majority of studies found that lower health literacy was related to poorer adherence, Paasche-Orlow et al. (2006) found that lower literacy was associated with better adherence to antiretroviral medications in HIV-positive participants.

Some researchers have not found an association between health literacy and patient adherence. Gazmararian et al. (2006) found that health literacy was not associated with medication refill adherence after controlling for several demographic variables and regimen complexity. Fang, Machtinger, Wang, and Schillinger (2006) also found that health literacy was not a predictor of adherence to warfarin therapy in patients attending an anticoagulation clinic. Data on health literacy and adherence are relatively recent, and, although there is some evidence to support a relationship, there are insufficient data to determine the nature, strength, or consistency of the relationship.

Summary

A variety of factors specific to the individual predict adherence. Among these are psychological characteristics; cognitive-motivational factors drawn from theories and models regarding health beliefs, intentions and behavior, self-efficacy, and stages of change; health behaviors; somatic and cognitive factors; and health literacy. Although each of these areas has something to contribute to our understanding of predictors of adherence, the power tends to be modest at best for any single factor. The most promising of these are self-efficacy, intentions, and prior adherence behavior. Not to be lost, however, is the role of depressive symptoms and emotional distress, perceptions about the illness or its consequences, and the experience or perceived experience of somatic complaints. Of more recent interest is the potential influence of health literacy in predicting adherence to treatment. Few of the areas have a sufficient number of studies to allow us to draw firm conclusions, but, as noted, the role of psychological and motivational factors are promising in our effort to understand adherence. Many questions still arise in the area of predictions of adherence. How do these individual factors function in different populations and health care settings, and how does the type of prescribed behavior influence adherence? Also, how do these multiple factors interact, if at all, to lead to adherence or nonadherence? None of the studies examined the influence of multiple factors. Although more is becoming known about individual factors that predict adherence, the relatively modest associations obtained in the research to date suggest that there is still much to be learned.

References

Ascher-Svanum, H., Zhu, B., Faries, D., Lacro, J. P., & Dolder, C. R. (2006). A prospective study of risk factors for nonadherence with antipsychotic medication in the treatment of schizophrenia. *Journal of Clinical Psychiatry, 67,* 1114–1123.

Bandura, A. (1977). Self-efficacy: Toward a unifying theory of behavioral change. *Psychological Review, 84,* 191–215.

Barclay, T. R., Hinkin, C. H., Castellon, S. A., Mason, K. I., Reinhard, M. J., Marion, S. D., et al. (2007). Age-associated predictors of medication adherence in HIV-positive adults: Health beliefs, self-efficacy, and neurocognitive status. *Health Psychology, 26,* 40–49.

Bastani, R., Marcus, A. C., Maxwell, A. E., Das, I. P., & Yan, K. X. (1994). Evaluation of an intervention to increase screening in Los Angeles. *Preventive Medicine, 23,* 83–90.

Beck, K. H. (1981). Driving while under the influence of alcohol: Relationship to attitudes and beliefs in a college population. *American Journal of Drug and Alcohol Abuse, 8,* 377–386.

Blanchard, C. M., Courneya, K. S., Rodgers, W. M., Fraser, S. N., Murray, T. C., Daub, B., et al. (2003). Is the theory of planned behavior a useful framework for understanding exercise adherence during phase II cardiac rehabilitation? *Journal of Cardiopulmonary Rehabilitation, 23,* 29–39.

Brus, H., van de Laar, M., Taal, E., Rasker, J., & Wiegman, O. (1999). Determinants of compliance with medication in patients with rheumatoid arthritis: The importance of self-efficacy expectations. *Patient Education and Counseling, 36,* 57–64.

Burke, L. E., Dunbar-Jacob, J., Serika, S., & Rohay, J. (1996). Outcome expectations vs. self-efficacy as predictive of dietary adherence in cardiac rehabilitation patients. (Abstract). Paper presented at the 4th International Congress of Behavioral Medicine. *Annals of Behavioral Medicine, 18*(Suppl.), S088.

Chew, L. D., Bradley, K. A., Flum, D. R., Cornia, P. B., & Koepsell, T. D. (2004). The impact of low health literacy on surgical practice. *American Journal of Surgery, 188,* 250–253.

Courneya, K. S., Friedenreich, C. M., Quinney, H. A., Fields, A. L., Jones, L. W. & Fairey, A. S. (2004). Predictors of adherence and contamination in a randomized controlled trial of exercise in colorectal cancer survivors. *Psychooncology, 13,* 857–866.

Courneya, K. S., Friedenreich, C. M., Sela, R. A., Quinney, H. A., & Rhodes, R. E. (2002). Correlates of adherence and contamination in a randomized controlled trial of exercise in cancer survivors: An application of the theory of planned behavior and the five factor model of personality. *Annals of Behavioral Medicine, 24,* 257–268.

Cromer, B. A., Steinberg, K., Gardner, L., Thornton, D., & Shannon, B. (1989). Psychosocial determinants of compliance in adolescents with iron deficiency. *American Journal of Diseases in Children, 143,* 55–58.

Desharnais, R., Boullon, J., & Godin, G. (1986). Self-efficacy and outcome expectations as determinants of exercise adherence. *Psychological Reports, 59,* 1155–1159.

DiClemente, C. C., Prochaska, J. O., Fairhurst, S. K., Velicer, W. F., Velasquez, M., & Rossi, J. S. (1991). The process of smoking cessation: An analysis of precontemplation, contemplation, and preparation stages of change. *Journal of Consulting and Clinical Psychology, 58,* 295–304.

DiMatteo, M. R., Sherbourne, C. D., Hays, R. D., Ordway, L., Kravitz, R. L., McGlynn, E. A., et al. (1993). Physicians' characteristics influence patients' adherence to medical treatment: Results from the Medical Outcomes Study. *Health Psychology, 12,* 93–102.

Dobkin, P. L., Sita, A., & Sewitch, M. J. (2006). Predictors of adherence to treatment in women with fibromyalgia. *Clinical Journal of Pain, 22,* 286–294.

Dubanoski, J. P. (1988). Preventive health behavior: A model of adherence prediction. *Dissertation Abstracts International, 48*(10-B), 3152.

Dunbar, J., & Knoke, J. (1986, March). *Prediction of medication adherence at one year and seven years: Behavioral and psychological factors.* Paper presented at the Society for Clinical Trials Annual Conference, Montreal, Canada.

Dunbar-Jacob, J., Serika, S., Burke, L. E., Kwoh, C. K., McCall, M., Locke, C., et al. (1993). Perceived treatment efficacy: Assessment in rheumatoid arthritis (Abstract). Paper presented at the 14th annual Scientific Sessions, Society of Behavioral Medicine. *Annals of Behavioral Medicine, 14*(Suppl.), S147.

Emery, C. F., Hauck, E. R., & Blumenthal, J. A. (1992). Exercise adherence or maintenance among older adults: 1-year follow-up study. *Psychology and Aging, 7,* 466–470.

Fang, M. C., Machtinger, E. L., Wang, F., & Schillinger, D. (2006). Health literacy and anticoagulation-related outcomes among patients taking warfarin. *Journal of General Internal Medicine, 21,* 1525–1497.

Farquharson, L., Noble, L. M., Barker, C., & Behrens, R. H. (2004). Health beliefs and communication in the travel clinic consultation as predictors of adherence to malaria chemoprophylaxis. *British Journal of Health Psychology, 9,* 210–217.

Fraser, C., Hadjimichael, O., & Vollmer, T. (2003). Predictors of adherence to glatiramer acetate therapy in individuals with self-reported progressive forms of multiple sclerosis. *Journal of Neuroscience Nursing, 35,* 163–170.

Fraser, C., Morgante, L., Hadjimichael, O., & Vollmer, T. (2004). A prospective study of adherence to glatiramer acetate in individuals with multiple sclerosis. *Journal of Neuroscience Nursing, 36,* 120–129.

Friedman, L. C., Webb, J. A., Bruce, S., Weinberg, A. D., & Cooper, H. P. (1995). Skin cancer prevention and early detection intentions and behavior. *American Journal of Preventive Medicine, 11,* 59–65.

Gazmararian, J. A., Kripalani, S., Miller, M. J., Echt, K. V., Ren, J., & Rask, K. (2006). Factors associated with medication refill adherence in cardiovascular-related diseases: A focus on health literacy. *Journal of General Internal Medicine, 21,* 1215–1221.

Glasgow, R. E., Toobert, D. J., Riddle, M., Donnelly, J., Mitchell, D. L., & Clader, D. (1989). Diabetes-specific social learning variables and self-care behaviors among persons with type II diabetes. *Health Psychology, 8,* 285–303.

Glazer, K. M., Emery, C. F., Frid, D. J., & Banyasz, R. E. (2002). Psychological predictors of adherence and outcomes among patients in cardiac rehabilitation. *Journal of Cardiopulmonary Rehabilitation, 22,* 40–46.

Gordillo, V., del Amo, J., Soriano, V., & Gonzalez-Lahoz, J. (1999). Sociodemographic and psychological variables influencing adherence to antiretroviral therapy. *AIDS, 13,* 1763–1769.

Heapy, A., Otis, J., Marcus, K. S., Frantsve, L. M., Janke, E. A., Shulman, M., et al. (2005). In-
tersession coping skill practice mediates the relationship between readiness for self-
management treatment and goal accomplishment. *Pain, 118,* 360–368.

Heckman, B. D., Catz, S. L., Heckman, T. G., Miller, J. G., & Kalichman, S. C. (2004). Adherence to
antiretroviral therapy in rural persons living with HIV disease in the United States. *AIDS
Care, 16,* 219–230.

Heiby, E. M., Onorato, V. A., & Sato, R. A. (1985, August). *A cognitive-behavioral model of adherence to health-related exercise.* Poster session presented at the American Psychological
Association 93rd Annual Convention, Los Angeles, CA.

Hershberger, P. J., Robertson, K. B. & Markert, R. J. (1999). Personality and appointment-
keeping adherence in cardiac rehabilitation. *Journal of Cardiopulmonary Rehabilitation,
19,* 106–111.

Ickovics, J. R., Cameron, A., Zackin, R., Bassett, R., Chesney, M., Johnson, V., et al. (2006). Consequences and determinants of adherence to antiretroviral medication: Results from Adult
AIDS Clinical Trials Group protocol 370. *Antiviral Therapy, 7,* 185–193.

Ingersoll, K. (2004). The impact of psychiatric symptoms, drug use, and medication regimen on
non-adherence to HIV treatment. *AIDS Care, 16,* 199–211.

Institute of Medicine. (2004). *Health literacy: A prescription to end confusion.* Washington, DC:
Institute of Medicine, Board on Neuroscience and Behavioral Health, Committee on
Health Literacy.

Irvine, J., Baker, B., Smith, J., Jandciu, S., Paquette, M., Cairns, J., et al. (1999). Poor adherence
to placebo to amiodarone therapy predicts mortality: Results from the CAMIAT study.
Psychosomatic Medicine, 61, 566–575.

Jones, S. L., Jones, P. K., & Katz, J. (1989). A nursing intervention to increase compliance in otitis
media patients. *Applied Nursing Research, 29,* 68–73.

Kavanagh, D. J., Gooley, S., & Wilson, P. H. (1993). Prediction of adherence and control in diabetes. *Journal of Behavioral Medicine, 16,* 509–522.

Kravitz, R. L., Hays, R. D., Sherbourne, C. D., DiMatteo, M. R., Rogers, W. H., Ordway, L., et al.
(1993). Recall of recommendations and adherence to advice among patients with chronic
medical conditions. *Archives of Internal Medicine, 153,* 1869–1878.

Kribbs, N. B., Pack, A. I., Kline, L. R., Smith, P. L., Schwartz, A. R., Schubert, N. M., et al. (1993).
Objective measurement of patterns of nasal CPAP use by patients with obstructive sleep
apnea. *American Review of Respiratory Disorders, 147,* 887–895.

Kruse, W., Eggert-Kruse, W., Rampmaier, J., Runnebaum, B., & Weber, E. (1993). Compliance
and adverse drug reactions: A prospective study with ethinylestradiol using continuous
compliance monitoring. *Clinical Investigator, 71,* 483–487.

Kutner, M., Greenberg, E., Jin, Y., & Paulsen, C. (2006). *The health literacy of America's adults:
Results from the 2003 National Assessment of Adult Literacy (NCES 2006-483).* U.S. Department of Education. Washington, DC: National Center for Education Statistics.

Lechner, L., de Vries, H., & Offermans, N. (1997). Participation in a breast cancer screening
program: Influence of past behavior and determinants on future screening participation.
Preventive Medicine, 26, 473–482.

Lee, D., DeLeon, C. F. M., Jenkins, C. D., Croog, S. H., Levine, S., & Sudilovsky, A. (1992). Relation
of hostility to medication adherence, symptom complaints, and blood pressure reduction
in a clinical field trial of antihypertensive medication. *Journal of Psychosomatic Research,
36,* 181–190.

Lorenc, L., & Branthwaite, A. (1993). Are older adults less compliant with prescribed medication than younger adults? *British Journal of Clinical Psychology, 32,* 485–492.

Mackin, R. S., & Arean, P. A. (2007). Cognitive and psychiatric predictors of medical treatment
adherence among older adults in primary care clinics. *International Journal of Geriatric
Psychiatry, 22,* 55–60.

Mawhinney, H., Spector, S. L., Heitjan, D., Kinsman, R. A., Dirks, J. F., & Pines, I. (1993). As-
needed medication use in asthma usage patterns and patient characteristics. *Journal of
Asthma, 30,* 61–71.

McAuley, E., Courneya, K. S., Rudolph, D. L., & Lox, C. L. (1994). Enhancing exercise adherence
in middle-aged males and females. *Preventive Medicine, 23,* 498–506.

McCaul, K. D., Glasgow, R. E., & Schafer, L. C. (1987). Diabetes regimen behaviors: Predicting
adherence. *Medical Care, 25,* 868–881.

Michie, S., Marteau, T. M., & Kidd, J. (1990). Cognitive predictors of attendance at antenatal classes. *British Journal of Clinical Psychology, 29,* 193–199.

Miller, P., Wikoff, R., Garrett, M. J., McMahon, M., & Smith, T. (1990). Regimen compliance two years after myocardial infarction. *Nursing Research, 30,* 333–336.

Miller, P., Wikoff, R., McMahon, M., Garrett, M. J., & Ringel, K. (1988). Influence of a nursing intervention on regimen adherence and societal adjustments post-myocardial infarction. *Nursing Research, 37,* 297–302.

Morris, A. B., Li, J., Kroenke, K., Bruner-England, T. E., Young, J. M., & Murray, M. D. (2006). Factors associated with drug adherence and blood pressure in patients with hypertension. *Pharmacotherapy, 26,* 483–492.

Muir, K. W., Santiago-Turla, C., Stinnett, S. S., Herndon, L. W., Allingham, R. R., Challa, P., et al. (2006). Health literacy and adherence to glaucoma therapy. *Opthalmology, 142,* 223–226.

Myers, R. E., Ross, E., Jepson, C., Wolf, T., Balshem, A., Millner, L., et al. (1994). Modeling adherence to colorectal cancer screening. *Preventive Medicine, 23,* 142–151.

Naar-King, S., Templin, T., Wright, K., Frey, M., Parsons, J. T., & Lam, P. (2006). Psychosocial factors and medication adherence in HIV-positive youth. *AIDS Patient Care STDS, 20,* 44–47.

Orensky, I. A., & Holdford, D. A. (2005). Predictors of noncompliance with warfarin therapy in an outpatient anticoagulation clinic. *Pharmacotherapy, 25,* 1801–1808.

Paasche-Orlow, M. K., Cheng, D. M., Palepu, A., Meli, S., Faber, V., & Samet, J. H. (2006). Health literacy, antiretroviral adherence and HIV-RNA suppression: A longitudinal perspective. *Journal of General Internal Medicine, 21,* 835–840.

Pavone, R. M., Burnett, K. F., LaPerriere, A., & Perna, F. M. (1998). Social cognitive and physical health determinants of exercise adherence for HIV-1 seropositive, early symptomatic men and women. *International Journal of Behavioral Medicine, 5,* 245–258.

Prochaska, J. O., & DiClemente, C. C. (1983). Stages and processes of self-change in smoking: Toward an integrative model of change. *Journal of Consulting and Clinical Psychology, 5,* 390–395.

Prochaska, J. O., DiClemente, C. C., & Norcross, J. C. (1992). In search of how people change. *American Psychologist, 47,* 1102–1114.

Rand, C. S., Nides, M., Cowles, M. K., Wise, R. A., & Connett, J. (1995). Long-term metered-dose inhaler adherence in a clinical trial. *American Journal of Respiratory and Critical Care Medicine, 152,* 580–588.

Ratzan, S. C., & Parker, R. M. (2000). Introduction. In C. R. Selden, M. Zorn, S. C. Ratzan, & R. M. Parker (Eds.), *National Library of Medicine current bibliographies in medicine: Health literacy.* NLM Pub. No. CBM 2000-1. Bethesda, MD: National Institutes of Health, U.S. Department of Health and Human Services.

Reynolds, N. R., Testa, M. A., Marc, L. G., Chesney, M. A., Neidig, J. L., Smith, S. R., et al. (2004). Factors influencing medication adherence beliefs and self-efficacy in persons naïve to antiretroviral therapy: A multicenter, cross-sectional study. *AIDS and Behavior, 8,* 141–150.

Russell, K. M., Champion, V. L., & Skinner, C. S. (2006). Psychosocial factors related to repeat mammography screening over 5 years in African American women. *Cancer Nursing, 29,* 236–243.

Safren, S. A., Otto, M. W., Worth, J. L., Salomon, E., Johnson, W., Mayer, K., et al. (2001). Two strategies to increase adherence to HIV antiretroviral medication: Life-steps and medication monitoring. *Behavior, Research, and Therapy, 39,* 1151–1162.

Sandler, R. S., DeVellis, B. M., Blalock, S. J., & Holland, K. L. (1989). Participation of high-risk subjects in colon cancer screening. *Cancer, 63,* 2211–2215.

Schweitzer, R. D., Head, K., & Dwyer, J. W. (2007). Psychological factors and treatment adherence behavior in patients with chronic heart failure. *Journal of Cardiovascular Nursing, 22,* 76–83.

Shemesh, E., Yehuda, R., Milo, O., Dinur, I., Rudnick, A., Vered, Z., et al. (2004). Posttraumatic stress, nonadherence, and adverse outcome in survivors of a myocardial infarction. *Psychosomatic Medicine, 66,* 521–526.

Sherbourne, C. D., Hays, R. D., Ordway, L., DiMatteo, M. R., & Kravitz, R. L. (1992). Antecedents of adherence to medical recommendations: Results from the Medical Outcomes Study. *Journal of Behavioral Medicine, 15,* 447–468.

Siegel, D., Lopez, J., & Meier, J. (2007). Antihypertensive medication adherence in the department of veteran affairs. *American Journal of Medicine, 120,* 26–32.

Stilley, C. S., Sereika, S., Muldoon, M. F., Ryan, C. M., & Dunbar-Jacob, J. (2004). Psychological and cognitive function: Predictors of adherence with cholesterol lowering treatment. *Annals of Behavioral Medicine, 27,* 117–124.

Turner, J., Wright, E., Mendella, L., & Anthonisen, N. (1995). Predictors of patient adherence to long-term home nebulizer therapy for COPD. IPPB Study Group. *Chest, 108,* 394–400.

Weaver, K. E., Llabre, M. M., Duran, R. E., Antoni, M. H., Ironson, G., Penedo, F. J., et al. (2005). A stress and coping model of medication adherence and viral load in HIV-positive men and women on highly active antiretroviral therapy (HAART). *Health Psychology, 24,* 385–392.

Welsh, M. C., Labbe, E. E., & Delaney, D. (1991). Cognitive strategies and personality variables in adherence to exercise. *Psychological Reports, 68,* 1327–1335.

West, K. P., DuRant, R. H., & Pendergrast, R. (1993). An experimental test of adolescents' compliance with dental appointments. *Journal of Adolescent Medicine, 14,* 384–389.

Wolf, M. S., Davis, T. C., Osborn, C. Y., Skripkauskas, S., Bennett, C. L., & Makoul, G. (2007). Literacy, self-efficacy, and HIV medication adherence. *Patient Education and Counseling, 65,* 253–260.

Yoon, R., McKenzie, D. K., Miles, D. A., & Bauman, A. (1991). Characteristics of attenders and non-attenders at an asthma education programme. *Thorax, 46,* 886–890.

Biopsychological Obstacles to Adoption and Maintenance of a Healthy Lifestyle

21

Neil E. Grunberg and
Laura Cousino Klein

Decades of research have made clear what we should do (e.g., eat in moderation; eat fruits, vegetables, and grains; exercise regularly; nurture social support; take our medicines) and what we should not do (e.g., not smoke cigarettes; not consume alcohol or other drugs in excess; not eat high-fat foods in excess; not experience too much chronic stress) to enjoy good health. Although we know what to do, it is often difficult to adopt and to maintain a healthy lifestyle

The views contained herein are the private ones of the authors and do not reflect those of the Uniformed Services University of the Health Sciences, the Department of Defense, or The Pennsylvania State University. Correspondence concerning this chapter should be addressed to Dr. Neil E. Grunberg, Department of Medical and Clinical Psychology, The Uniformed Services University of the Health Sciences, 4301 Jones Bridge Road, Bethesda, MD 20814–4799. Electronic mail may be sent to ngrunberg@usuhs.mil.

because of economic, social, psychological, and biological obstacles. This chapter discusses the biopsychological obstacles to adoption and maintenance of a healthy lifestyle.

Biological obstacles relevant to a healthy lifestyle received little attention before the 1990s. Grunberg and Lord (1990) first highlighted this category of variables and offered a framework to categorize biological barriers to the adoption and maintenance of health-promoting behaviors. Since then, the broad topic of compliance with health-related behaviors has received increased attention and has become a part of some medical and health care curricula. A computer literature search of *PubMed* for "compliance" or "adherence" lists more than 5,000 titles in 2007 alone, and, of these many reports, hundreds now consider biologically relevant aspects of compliance across many different scientific disciplines and domains. This chapter updates our previous report on this topic (Grunberg & Klein, 1998a) in light of recent scientific advances across many health-related disciplines, including psychology, medicine, and biobehavioral health.

Much of the information we discussed in 1998 regarding biological variables and compliance remains true today and is reiterated in this chapter. One of the marked and purposeful changes that we have made in this chapter is the revision of the title from "biological" to "biopsychological" obstacles. Another purposeful semantic change is from "health-promoting behaviors" to "healthy lifestyle." These changes reflect our opinion that (1) the biological variables that dissuade individuals from complying with medical and health-promoting behaviors are influenced by psychological factors and vice versa, and (2) health and the obstacles to maintaining health are affected by how individuals go about living their daily lives. Another important change in this revised chapter is the expansion of the types of biopsychological obstacles and a recategorization of these variables across several biopsychological domains, including physical, behavioral, cognitive, and motivational limitations. This expansion acknowledges the contributions of each of these domains to a healthy lifestyle, and it is our hope that readers will conceptualize practical and research issues with all four of these domains in mind. A final update is the change from strictly addressing "adherence" and "compliance" to the inclusion of "adoption" and "maintenance" because we believe that it is important to emphasize the collaborative role that patients should have with their health care provider to establish and to practice a healthy lifestyle.

As with our previous chapter, we continue to believe that marked technological advances in the biological and behavioral sciences, substantial expansion of interdisciplinary and multidisciplinary consideration of health issues, and incorporation of multilevel analyses in behavior and health work together to sustain a renewed mind-body monism. Advances in behavioral and cognitive neuroscience, genetics, molecular biology, and behavioral science all point to the effects of the mind on the body and the body on the mind. In the context of the present chapter and the present volume, biological variables are part of the biopsychological and environmental milieu that affects adoption and maintenance of healthy lifestyles and compliance and adherence to healthful behaviors and treatments.

Types of Biological Obstacles

The biological obstacles that affect adoption and maintenance of a healthy lifestyle can be organized across eight domains: (1) absence or misinterpretation of biological cues; (2) physical and behavioral limitations; (3) cognitive limitations; (4) motivational limitations; (5) interference of healthful behaviors with quality of life; (6) unpleasant side effects of treatments to enhance a healthy lifestyle; (7) common biopsychological obstacles; and (8) individual differences. Each major category is addressed in order.

Absence or Misinterpretation of Biological Cues

An important factor that may affect adoption and maintenance of a healthy lifestyle but that receives limited research attention is the patient's failure to experience or correctly interpret symptoms of underlying disorders. Basically, patients may feel fine and conclude that they are fine. As a result, they believe that they do not need bed rest, medications, restricted activities, or dietary changes. Premature discontinuation of therapy can be dangerous. For example, a patient typically feels better (e.g., no fever, weakness, pain, cough) before a course of antibiotic treatment is finished. If the antibiotic regimen is not completed, then drug-resistant strains of microorganisms can multiply and create a more serious health risk to the individual and to the general public. This serious scenario is playing out today in the development of drug-resistant and extensively drug resistant (XDR) strains of tuberculosis. Symptomless diseases such as hypertension or type II diabetes also require treatments (e.g., medication, regular medical tests and checkups, dietary changes, exercise) with physical effects that will not be felt by the patient. Preventive treatment for asthma with daily regimens of nonsteroidal (e.g., cromolyn sodium or Intal®) and leukotriene receptor antagonists (e.g., montelukast or Singulair®), along with peak flow meter evaluation, is not directly or immediately felt by the patient, and prevention efficacy is measured by decreased number of asthma attacks weeks later. In addition, misinterpretation of symptoms (e.g., "I get headaches whenever my blood pressure is high" or "I feel anxious right before I have an asthma attack") may lead to inappropriate self-dosing or inappropriate abstinence (e.g., "I don't have a headache, so I don't need to take my pills" or "My chest doesn't feel tight, so I don't need to use my inhaler").

A variant of this misinterpretation obstacle to promotion of a healthy lifestyle occurs when people feel fine and, therefore, believe that they do not need to do anything special to promote or improve health. For example, when people feel fine, they may assume that it is unnecessary to exercise, be careful about cholesterol intake, quit smoking, or avoid excess sun exposure.

Adoption and maintenance of a healthy lifestyle also are reduced when a given healthful behavior has no noticeable positive effects that are obvious to the individual. For example: "I've been exercising for weeks, but I don't feel any better (in fact, I feel worse because my muscles and back hurt); I've given up smoking for 3 months now, but I don't feel better (in fact, I've gained weight); I take my pills regularly, but I don't feel any different—I bet the doctor gave me sugar pills because he thinks I'm not sick or to stop me from bugging him; I've been getting allergy shots twice a week for over a year and I still sneeze around cats." These experiences and lack of awareness of bodily states, therapeutic effects, or preventive effects should be addressed and explained to patients.

Patient expectations about treatments and illnesses can be wrong. It is these expectations, however, that affect the confidence in a given healthful behavior, the credibility of a health care provider, and the likelihood that patients will adhere to and comply with healthy behaviors.

Physical and Behavioral Limitations

Another category of biological obstacles to adoption and maintenance of a healthy lifestyle involves problems or deficiencies in physical and behaviorally based abilities of patients. Impairment of a sensory system, such as hearing or vision, can interfere with the ability to gather or interpret information from the health care provider. These impairments also may make a patient more reluctant to ask questions of the health care provider. For example, impaired vision interferes with the processing of written instructions about prescribed health behaviors, and impaired hearing can make it difficult to understand oral instructions from the health care provider. Difficulties in visual acuity, myopia, and hyperopia all can act to make objectively clearly written instructions inaccessible to patients. Color deficiencies in an individual patient also can interfere with that patient's ability to adhere to medication regimens that require taking different colored pills on different days or at different times of the day.

Physical barriers to adoption and maintenance of a healthy lifestyle also include a variety of allergies and physical handicaps. For example, food allergies may interfere with nutrition or the ability to adopt a healthy diet (e.g., celiac disease or a gluten allergy prohibits consumption of wheat products), drug allergies may prevent the administration of effective pharmacologic agents, and contact dermatologic reactions may interfere with the use of some medications and some medicinal soaps and may prevent safe-sex practices. Respiratory allergic responses, such as extrinsic asthma or allergic rhinitis, can inhibit an individual from performing exercise activities, eating certain foods, and complying with immunotherapy (e.g., allergy shots).

Further, individuals with physical and hidden disabilities such as orthopedic, neuromuscular, cardiovascular, and pulmonary disorders (e.g., injury, muscular dystrophy, multiple sclerosis, cerebral palsy, amputation, heart disease, pulmonary disease) must rely on assistive devices such as wheelchairs, crutches, canes, prosthetic devices (artificial limbs), and oxygen to obtain mobility. These disabilities and physical challenges may require specialized attention to develop an individualized health adoption and maintenance plan across psychological and physical domains.

Cognitive Limitations

There are biologically based cognitive impairments that interfere with adoption and maintenance of a healthy lifestyle. These impairments include mental retardation, senile dementias, Alzheimer's Disease, Traumatic Brain Injury, acute illness-induced cognitive impairments, HIV-induced cognitive impairments, AIDS dementia, drug-induced dementias, and attentional disorders. As we enjoy the benefits of modern medicine and live well into our 80s, the likelihood that people will experience various cognitive limitations and the proportion of people so affected increases because of unhealthy aging, chronic diseases, and, for some people, reduced daily intellectual challenges. The aging demographics of today's society means that more people will (1) need help to maintain healthy lifestyles, (2) need continued medical attention, and (3) have some difficulty understanding that they need help, how and where to get this help, and how to put sound health-promoting advice into practice. An increasing source of cognitive limitations is the result of traumatic brain injuries (Wood & Rutterford, 2006). Traumatic brain injuries result from automotive accidents, falls, athletic collisions, and exposure to improvised explosive devices (IEDs). These injuries often have deleterious cognitive effects, including effects on executive function, organization skills, and memory. In the clinical realm, we need to screen for cognitive limitations to optimize the likelihood that people can understand what they need to do to engage in healthy lifestyles.

Motivational Limitations

It is relevant to consider how motivation may affect the adoption and maintenance of healthy lifestyles. Knowledge about nutrition, weight, exercise, long-term health, and the positive effects of taking various medications have little or no value for people who are apathetic or do not care about their current or long-term health status. Misunderstanding the importance of developing healthy lifestyles can undermine attempts by health care professionals and significant others to encourage the adoption and maintenance of a healthy lifestyle. Biopsychological conditions (fatigue, pain, depression, anxiety) can weaken motivations to practice a healthy lifestyle. Motivations are separate from behaviors and cognitions, which is an important distinction to make in order to understand how to increase motivations relevant to positive goals and to decrease motivations that interfere with positive goals.

Interestingly, the study of motivation was central to the discipline of psychology in the late 19th and early 20th centuries but was replaced in the mid-20th century with a focus on behavior per se. In the mid- to late 20th century, cognition slipped back in to psychology, but motivation still was largely set aside. In the late 20th century, behavior and cognition came together as cognitive-behavioral therapy, a surprising "marriage" for scholars and practitioners who had long considered these two approaches to be opposing and mutually exclusive. In the late 20th century and early 21st century, motivation has made a small comeback as a topic of study and construct for therapeutic intervention. Further, brain imaging studies have sought to determine which areas of the brain are active with particular emotions and motivations related to health, such as drug addiction, pain, and depression (Bär et al., 2007; Peyron, Laurent, & García-Larrea, 2000; Yücel et al., 2007). However, we believe that motivation remains a sleeping giant that must be awakened in the present biopsychological era of study and practice. With regard to healthy lifestyles, motivation is the engine that drives the relevant behaviors and cognitions and, therefore, deserves center stage for study.

Interference of Healthful Behaviors With Quality of Life

Restrictive diets designed to improve cardiovascular function (e.g., low-cholesterol diets), decrease the likelihood of cancer or diabetes (e.g., high-fiber or low-glycemic diet), or to help lose weight (e.g., diet with few sweet, high-caloric foods) promote health (Grunberg, 1987) but often are not enjoyable and may cause discomfort in some individuals who suffer from diet-related diseases such as celiac disease (i.e., gluten intolerance), lactose intolerance, or irritable bowel syndrome. Daily rituals (e.g., morning coffee, high-fat or high-cholesterol breakfast) may have biological actions to which we adapt, come to need, and enjoy. Undoubtedly, we miss such daily pleasures when they become unavailable. Perhaps the enjoyment associated with specific foods, such as salty or sweet foods, involves biologically driven hedonic preferences to consume food-stuffs needed by the body (Cabanac, 1971; Richter, 1943; Young, 1936, 1955). In this context, it is interesting to note that cigarette smokers prefer and consume more sweets after cessation of smoking (Grunberg, 1985, 1986a). Anecdotal reports indicate that similar phenomena accompany abstinence from habitual use of alcohol or narcotics. It has been hypothesized that the enjoyment derived from eating specific foods taps similar biological processes involved in the self-administration of some drugs of dependence (Grunberg & Baum, 1985; Grunberg & Klein, 1998b). Specifically, the unpleasantness associated with withdrawal from habitual drug use can be attenuated by the consumption of sweets and carbohydrates (Grunberg, 1986b; Grunberg & Baum, 1985). Whether or not this hypothesis linking drugs of dependence to food preferences is correct, it is clear that consumption of specific foods is enjoyable, that restricted diets are not, and that people often cheat on their diets.

In addition to eating, people enjoy drinking, smoking, and using "recreational" drugs. Consumption of alcohol, nicotine, marijuana, cocaine, Ecstasy, amphetamines, and other psychoactive drugs is reportedly enjoyable. These drugs have various effects and become desired by the users. Even when the health messages for these substances are well known (e.g., cigarette smoking is responsible for 400,000 deaths annually in the United States; driving while intoxicated can be lethal), individuals are motivated by the pleasurable effects of psychoactive drugs or by the discomfort of abstinence or withdrawal and, therefore, continue to self-administer rather than adopt more healthful behaviors.

Cigarette smoking is the single most preventable cause of premature death and illness (Centers for Disease Control and Prevention, 1993, 2006; U.S. Department of Health & Human Services, 1988). The health message is clear: do not smoke. Quitting smoking, however, is far more difficult than this simple health message leads us to believe. Use of tobacco products is an addictive behavior that involves powerful psychological and biological reinforcers. Consequently, asking habitual smokers to abstain from smoking requires the cessation of self-administration of an addictive pharmacological agent, namely nicotine. Smoking cessation results in irritability, anxiety, sleep disturbances, difficulty concentrating, and body weight gains (Grunberg & Bowen, 1985; Shiffman, 1979). These biologically based abstinence effects are powerful obstacles to adopting and maintaining a healthy lifestyle. In addition, abstinence means that the ex-smoker no longer will receive the effects of nicotine that are considered positive, such as decreased body weight, focused attention, and stress modulation.

Other abused substances, including alcohol, opiates, and sympathomimetics (e.g., cocaine, methamphetamine), similarly have biological effects that are reinforcing and abstinence effects that are unpleasant. Therefore, abstinence from use and abuse of these substances is hindered by biological obstacles, and it is important that health care providers and significant others become aware of the consequences of abstinence.

Moreover, some substances (e.g., alcohol, some tranquilizers), when used in excess, reduce motivation or competence to comply with instructions involving other healthful behaviors. Prodding, coercion, scare tactics, and hinting are minimally effective in changing a dazed, addicted individual into someone who exercises, eats right, and takes medications on the appropriate dosing schedule.

Safe-sex practices are another example of healthy behaviors that interfere with biologically based enjoyment. Sexual intercourse with condoms and abstinence from sexual intercourse are recommended to decrease the likelihood of transmission of HIV and sexually transmitted diseases (STDs). Safe-sex practices, however, may decrease or prevent sensuality and pleasures of sexual intimacy. They also take time and planning, which can interfere with intimate, arousing moments.

Medication schedules also can interfere with biologically based enjoyable behaviors. Some medications require administration during the night or during a sleep period. Other medications require administration either an hour before or 2 hours after a meal. These modifications or inconveniences pit the health-promoting behavior against a biologically necessary state. In addition to medication dosing schedules, some drugs are associated with behavioral restrictions that many people find enjoyable or necessary. For example, medications that are accompanied by the instruction "Do not operate a motor vehicle or other large equipment" can be a nuisance that interferes with pleasures and conveniences, or this instruction can interfere with one's livelihood. Instructions to avoid strenuous activities (e.g., physical activity, exercise, lifting, sexual activity) can interfere with jobs, hobbies, and general enjoyment. The development of long-acting drugs to enhance patient adherence are coming into the forefront of preventive medicine. For example, there have been tremendous advances in medications to treat osteoporosis, ranging from sodium alendronate (Fosamax®) and risedronate (Actonel®), taken once a week, to ibandronate (Boniva®), taken once a month, to the newly available bisphosphonate zoledronic acid (Reclast®), administered as a single, 15-minute, intravenous infusion once a year. Medications that are taken less frequently may help improve adoption and maintenance of a healthy lifestyle by minimizing the impact on quality of life.

In all of these cases, the interference of healthful behaviors with enjoyable behaviors is not insurmountable. However, the incompatible relationship of these behaviors and the intensity of the pleasures that are lost must be addressed by the health care provider and cannot be ignored. For example, most people agree that safe-sex practices are important. However, the decreased pleasure and inconveniences associated with abstinence or condom use may offset concerns about STDs or AIDS, especially when the likelihood

of contracting these infections is viewed as being minimal. In order to optimize adherence to healthful behaviors, the balance between biological and
psychological aspects of the healthful behaviors, with their impact on quality
of life, needs to be addressed.

Unpleasant Side Effects of Treatments to Enhance a Healthy Lifestyle

When a healthful behavior is physically unpleasant or painful or causes discomfort, people are less likely to adhere to the healthful behavior. This category
includes unpleasant biological side effects of nonmedicinal treatments; prescription medications; over-the-counter (OTC) medications; drug interactions
with alcohol; and drug-drug interactions.

Nonmedicinal Treatments

Rehabilitation medicine has expanded dramatically in the United States over
the past 25 years, and the role of physical and alternative therapies in medical treatment has earned respect. Unfortunately, physical therapy has a variety
of effects that can be considered to be unpleasant biological effects (or psy-
chobiological actions) that deter compliance. For example, an individual who
was rear-ended in rush hour traffic and suffered whiplash and minor apparent
bruises now receives muscle relaxants, analgesics, and several months to several years of physical therapy. This therapy may include traction, muscular and
neural electrical stimulation, heat and cold packs, specific exercise routines,
deep-muscle manipulation, muscular ultrasound, stretching exercises, and spinal disc manipulation. Although this therapeutic adjunct to pharmacotherapy
is valuable and effective, it may hurt and has effects that can be characterized
as biopsychological obstacles that may deter patients from compliance. Specifically, physical therapy can result in: headaches, numbness, nausea, muscle
aches, muscle fatigue, pain, sleep disturbances, and a cascade of other physical
discomforts, as physical therapy and manipulation has a domino effect on other,
presumably uninjured, parts of the body. As with other aspects of compliance,
predictability, identification of the cause of problems, understanding of the time
course or duration of discomfort, and communication among the health care
team of physicians, other health care specialists, and patients all are likely to
encourage maintenance of the behaviors that will help to restore or to optimize
health.

In addition to physical therapy, there are other nonmedical treatments that
result in discomfort and may act as biopsychological obstacles to compliance
with a particular treatment or lifestyle change. For example, surgeries that are
not required for survival are, indeed, unpleasant and frightening episodes that
we all would prefer to avoid. Even when we become convinced that the benefits
of surgery outweigh the risks, we also become aware of the impact of surgery
on our comfort and regular routines. When we know someone who has gone
through a similar experience and who reports being bedridden for weeks or
who reports the resultant pain and discomfort, we often can come up with reasons to put off that procedure just a bit longer. Communication from health
care providers that is credible in reporting the unpleasant side effects, yet that

presents a convincing rationale for the benefits of the procedure can go a long way to surmount the biopsychological obstacles. Perhaps health care providers who are faced with such obstacles that obstruct the best treatment procedures should consider the value of adopting a convincing and concerned advocacy position, rather than an authoritarian posture or a seemingly disinterested style. Moreover, the involvement of supportive significant others may help people to make sound decisions that will optimize long-term health.

Even rather innocuous changes, such as exercise and healthful dietary changes, may result in discomfort for individuals and, thereby, act as biopsychological obstacles. In these cases, anything that can be done to make the healthful behaviors accessible, positive, and rewarding would help. Enhancement of motivation is likely to help with compliance, particularly when the consequences may be uncomfortable.

Prescription Medications

Pharmaceutical houses certainly aim to develop and market drugs with the widest possible therapeutic range and the fewest and weakest unpleasant side effects. Unfortunately, many therapeutically effective and lifesaving drugs have unpleasant biopsychological effects that deter people from taking their medicine. These side effects range from mildly irritating to almost debilitating.

Unpleasant biopsychological effects of drugs that could interfere with adherence to drug-taking therapies become clear when one consults the *Physicians' Desk Reference* (2007) or reference books about pharmacotherapeutics (e.g., Brunton, Lazo, & Parker, 2006; Julien, 2005; Katzung, 2007; Melmon, Morrelli, Hoffman, & Nierenberg, 1992). There are many unpleasant side effects associated with a variety of drugs. For example, tricyclic antidepressants can cause hallucinations, disorientation, delusions, anxiety, restlessness, numbness and tingling in the extremities, lack of coordination, muscle spasms or tremors, seizures, confusion, convulsions, dry mouth, blurred vision, constipation, inability to urinate, rash, itching, sensitivity to bright light or sunlight, retention of fluids, fever, allergy, nausea, vomiting, loss of appetite, stomach upset, diarrhea, sleep disturbances, panic, black coloration of the tongue, yellowing of the eyes or skin, perspiration, frequent urination, dizziness, weakness, headache, and loss of hair. No wonder that a patient might not comply with this medication regimen.

Lifesaving antineoplastic drugs can cause many unpleasant side effects that can interfere with a patient's willingness to undergo cancer chemotherapy, including nausea and vomiting, peripheral neuropathies, cerebral blindness, loss of taste and hearing, and seizures (e.g., cisplatin or Platinol®); leukopenia, anemia, anorexia, nausea, vomiting, and diarrhea (e.g., cyclophosphamide or Cytoxan®); pain, scarring, diarrhea, anorexia, nausea, vomiting, and contact dermatitis (e.g., fluorouracil or Efudex®); or hepatotoxicity, cirrhosis, fetal death, anemia, leukopenia, thrombocytopenia, diarrhea, ulcerative stomatitis, nausea, vomiting and anorexia (e.g., methotrexate, formerly Amethopterin®). No wonder a patient might fail to completely follow a regimen of even a lifesaving drug.

Drugs taken to improve cardiovascular function can manifest a variety of unpleasant effects. For example, digitalis can cause abdominal discomfort, pain, and headaches; hydralazine can cause headaches, angina, myalgia, or chest pain;

methyldopa can cause diarrhea, blurred vision, dizziness, impaired concentration, and nightmares; propranolol can cause insomnia or sexual impairment; and metoprolol can cause fatigue and dizziness. These side effects can become obstacles to adherence to prescribed pharmaceutical regimens, especially in individuals whose condition is asymptomatic (e.g., hypertension).

Anti-HIV medications, such as nucleoside reverse transcriptase inhibitors (e.g., Truvada® [emtricitabine and tenofovir disoproxil fumarate]) and synthetic nucleoside analogues (e.g., Retrovir® [azidothymidine, AZT], Hivid® [zalcitabine, ddC], Videx® [didanosine, ddI], Zerit® [stavudine, d4T], and Epivir® [lamivudine, 3TC]), slow the progression of HIV disease but do not cure AIDS. Long-term use of several of these drugs can result in debilitating peripheral neuropathies, severe pain, and general toxicity (Berger et al., 1993; Border & Arcane, 1990; Cherry et al., 2006; Dubinsky, Arcane, Dalakas, & Border, 1989; Merigan Skowron, & ddC Study Group, 1990; Nolan & Mallal, 2004; Simpson, 2002; Youle, Osio, & ALCAR Study Group, 2007).

Over-the-Counter (OTC) Medications

The over-the-counter (OTC) pharmacopeia is becoming more and more impressive every day. This development helps keep prices down and makes medications more available but often makes the medicines seem like nonmedicines and the condition seem like a nonmedical condition. These medications, including bronchodilators, cough suppressants, antihistamines, painkillers, sleep aids, mild sympathomimetics, and treatments for yeast and fungal infections, can mask biological symptoms that otherwise would motivate individuals to seek medical attention. This desirable effect of treatment, therefore, can have the paradoxical effect of deterring patients from seeking and adopting health-promoting actions. Conversely, these medications, in some cases, can have side effects (e.g., gastrointestinal irritation, dermatologic irritation, sleep disturbances, tachycardia) that can be categorized as biological or biopsychological obstacles to compliance.

Drug Interactions With Alcohol

In addition to nonprescription medications, alcohol must be considered as a nonprescription drug that can interact with other drugs and medications to cause untoward side effects. It is noteworthy that negative interactions can occur with the use, not necessarily abuse, of alcohol. For example, many drugs that otherwise have a wide therapeutic range with few side effects cause serious problems when taken along with alcohol. Alcohol with antianginal drugs (e.g., nitroglycerin) results in hypertension, dizziness, and syncope; alcohol with anticoagulants (e.g., Coumadin®, dicumarol, Panwarfin®) alters the anticoagulant action depending on whether there is acute or chronic alcohol ingestion. Alcohol with antidiabetic drugs (e.g., Glucophage® [metformin], Prandin® [repaglinide], Orinase® [tolbutamide]) results in unpredictable blood sugar, disulfiram-like reactions, and angina pectoris; alcohol with antihypertensives has an additive hypotensive effect; alcohol with antitubercular drugs (e.g., Isoniazid, rifampin) decreases the therapeutic response and increases the likelihood of hepatotoxicity; alcohol with salicylates (e.g., aspirin) leads to gastrointestinal bleeding. Alcohol plus some antibiotics (e.g., cephalosporins, furazolidone) produces disulfiram-like reactions. Alcohol self-administration with benzodiazepines can contribute to adverse side effects such as vomiting and nausea.

Drug-Drug Interactions

Drug-drug interactions (involving substances besides alcohol) can be dangerous or unpleasant. Administration of OTC nonsteroidal anti-inflammatory drugs (NSAIDs) like ibuprofen (Advil®) with concomitant administration of certain antineoplastics (e.g., methotrexate) can cause unexpected, sometimes fatal, bone marrow suppression and gastrointestinal toxicity. Even simple antacids can potentiate the effects of anticholinergics; inhibit the actions of anticoagulants; and potentiate the effects of antihistamines, antimalarials, and bronchodilators (e.g., albuterol or Proventil®, beclomethasone dipropionate or Vanceril®). Nicotine (other than that derived from tobacco products) now is a prescription and OTC medication that can interact with other drugs. Nicotine is the active pharmacological agent in several smoking cessation aids (e.g., nicotine polacrilex gum, nicotine patch, nicotine nasal spray, nicotine lozenge) and is being tested as a medical agent for the treatment of several disorders (e.g., Parkinson's Disease, Gilles de la Tourette's Syndrome, Attention Deficit Disorder With and Without Hyperactivity, Parkinson's Disease, Alzheimer's Disease). Nicotine is a powerful sympathomimetic that affects catecholamines, indoleamines (including serotonin), sex hormones, pro-opiomelanocorticotropin hormones (including the endogenous opioid peptides), insulin, and other neurochemicals and hormones. There can be drug-drug interactions between nicotine and other medications that can result in uncomfortable effects and affect compliance.

There are many other undesirable side effects of drugs. This list is meant to provide an illustrative rather than a comprehensive review of biological and biopsychological effects that are unpleasant enough to become obstacles to compliance and adherence, particularly when weighed against the salience to the individual of the benefits of the given drugs.

Common Biopsychological Obstacles

This chapter purposely focuses on biopsychological obstacles to healthy lifestyle that may not be obvious and that, in our opinion, receive too little research, clinical, and public health attention. A discussion of biopsychological obstacles to a healthy lifestyle also must emphasize the most common health-relevant behaviors that involve biopsychological mechanisms: tobacco use and eating.

Despite the well-documented and well-publicized health hazards of tobacco use, roughly 20% of American adults continue to smoke tobacco cigarettes and even more use other tobacco products. It is clear that tobacco use involves biopsychological mechanisms, including nicotine addiction and reinforcement of behaviors, cognitions, and situations associated with tobacco use (Chaudhri et al., 2006; USDHHS, 1988; Wonnacott, Sidhpura, & Balfour, 2005). Tobacco use remains the single most important preventable cause of death and illness in the United States, but another behavior-related epidemic is close on its heels: obesity and excessive body weight. Today, almost 2/3 of Americans are obese or overweight, and the health risks of these conditions are staggering. Some experts argue that we live in a "toxic food environment" (Bray & Champagne, 2005; Lustig, 2006) of high-caloric fast foods that encourage our excessive eating. Other experts argue that we use our cars too much, sit at computers and watch television too much, and do not exercise enough or engage in enough physical activity of other sorts. It is clear that we must control eating and increase activity if we are to tackle the growing problem of obesity. Although U.S. citizens today enjoy a better life expectancy than prior generations, they rank much lower than citizens of many other countries in life expectancy, despite a government that spends more money per person on health care than any other country in the world.

In the context of common biopsychological obstacles to healthy lifestyle, consideration of tobacco and eating should be broadened. Specifically, the study, prevention, and treatment of tobacco use also are relevant to the study, prevention, and treatment of other substance abuse (including alcohol, opiates, amphetamines, and so on). The study, prevention, and treatment of eating must include conditions of eating disorders (including anorexia nervosa, bulimia nervosa, and eating disorders not otherwise specified).

There is one other important topic that we categorize as a common biopsychological obstacle to healthy lifestyle: sleep hygiene and sleep disruption. We spend roughly 1/3 of our lives sleeping, yet this behavior has received too little research attention with regard to its impact on health. There has been a marked increase in the study of sleep and health recently, including dramatic data regarding the inverse relationship between hours of sleep on one hand and obesity, type II diabetes and a wide range of physical and mental health conditions on the other (Jennings, Muldoon, Hall, Buysse, & Manuck, 2007; Knutson, Ryden, Mander, & Van Cauter, 2006; Knutson, Spiegel, Penev, & Van Cauter, 2007). Sleep is a crucial topic of study in the context of biopsychological variables that affect healthy behavior.

Individual Differences

Genetics

Since 1990, there has been an explosion in knowledge about genetics and an increased emphasis on the importance of genetic contributions to health conditions. This development is relevant to the present topic in several ways. First, there are likely to be biologically based individual differences in susceptibility to each of the effects that we delineate throughout this chapter. For example, certain individuals are more likely to experience a given side effect of particular medications or in response to a behavioral treatment. Second, there are likely to be marked biologically based differences in the likelihood of developing pathophysiologic conditions, psychopathologic conditions, and biobehavioral conditions that can become obstacles to compliance. For example, certain individuals are more likely to develop obesity, senile dementias, mood disorders, or substance abuse. These biologically based differences in the likelihood of developing a particular condition can differentially contribute to the role of the condition as a biopsychological obstacle to compliance. Third, there are likely to be genetically based differences in the moderation or mediation of a given set of variables (e.g., a given medication, dietary regimen, or physical activity) on the development of an adverse side effect, not simply because of individual differences in effect but because of individual differences in interaction. Fourth, there are ethical dilemmas that emerge as genetic mapping may allow prediction of probabilistic development of particular pathophysiologic conditions (e.g., cardiovascular disease, stroke, lung cancer, breast cancer, chronic obstructive lung disease, diabetes); biobehavioral conditions (e.g., obesity, anorexia nervosa, substance abuse, sleep disorders, AIDS); and psychopathologic conditions (e.g., depression, anxiety, obsessive-compulsive disorder, schizophrenia). For example, should we know what we are at risk of getting as a way to help us prevent the unwanted condition and to enhance our compliance with preventive measures and treatments? Or, does such knowledge give us excuses for developing these conditions and, thereby, act to deter compliance? At this point, this information may sound like science fiction, but the rate of information acquisition makes it all worthy of serious consideration.

We suspect that, within our lifetimes, we each will use our own genomic information to help determine the optimal pharmaceuticals that we each should take. We wonder if, within our lifetimes, we each will use our own genomic information to help determine the best strategies (i.e., behaviors, cognitions, and motivations) to optimize our healthy lifestyles.

Age and Gender

Most of the information relevant to this chapter is based on research, epidemiological data, and clinical reports focused on adults, both men and women. Age, of course, is relevant to biology, motivations, behaviors, cognitions, social interactions, and so on. In addition, women live longer than men. Therefore, it is reasonable to speculate that age and gender are relevant to the biopsychological obstacles to adoptions and maintenance of a healthy lifestyle. We know that appetites and taste preferences differ in children, middle-aged adults, and elderly adults and between men and women. We also know that physical ailments, recovery from injury, experiences of pain, and sleep patterns differ according to age and gender. We know that most if not all of the topics discussed in this chapter are affected by age and gender. We do not, however, have a clear and complete understanding of this information or how to use what knowledge we have to tailor enhancement of a healthy lifestyle to each age and gender group.

Ethnic, Cultural, and Socioeconomic Variables

Perhaps the most important topics that need increased attention are ethnic and cultural variables that affect healthy lifestyles. The health disparities that currently exist based on ethnic, cultural, and socioeconomic variables are truly disturbing (Seeman & Crimmins, 2001). Some of these disparities are understandable, such as lack of money to pay for health care and lack of transportation to travel to health care professionals. However, these logistical issues do not account for the extreme disparities that exist (Crimmins, Kim, Alley, Karlamangla, & Seeman, 2007).

Conclusions

Biopsychological obstacles are important and must be considered if we are to make headway in increasing the adoption and maintenance of behaviors that can lead to a healthy lifestyle and an improved quality of life. Over the past 20 years, there has been an impressive increase in knowledge about biopsychological obstacles that affect health. In this chapter, we categorize these obstacles in ways to help focus understanding, research, and therapeutic intervention. In light of the increased attention to these topics in the research, clinical, and public health literatures, we are optimistic that biopsychological obstacles can be surmounted. We hope to encourage increased research, clinical, and public health attention to these topics.

References

Bär, K. J., Wagner, G., Koschke, M., Boettger, S., Boettger, M. K., Schlösser, R., et al. (2007). Increased prefrontal activation during pain perception in major depression. *Biological Psychiatry, 62*, 1281–1287.

Berger, A. R., Arezzo, J. C., Schaumberg, H. H., Skowron, G., Merigan, T., Bozette, S., et al. (1993). 2′,3′-dideoxycytidine (ddC) toxic neuropathy: A study of 52 patients. *Neurology, 43*, 358–362.

Border, S., & Arcane, R. (1990). Dideoxycytidine: Current clinical experience and future prospects. *American Journal of Medicine, 88*(5B), 31S–33S.

Bray, G. A., & Champagne, C. M. (2005). Beyond energy balance: There is more to obesity than kilocalories. *Journal of the American Dietetic Association, 105*(Suppl.), S17–23.

Brunton, L. L., Lazo, J. S., & Parker, K. L. (Eds.). (2006). *Goodman and Gilman's: The pharmacological basics of therapeutics* (11th ed.). New York: McGraw-Hill.

Cabanac, M. (1971). Physiological role of pleasure. *Science, 173*, 1103–1107.

Centers for Disease Control and Prevention. (1993). Cigarette smoking-attributable mortality and years of potential life lost—United States, 1990. *Morbidity and Mortality Weekly Report [serial online], 42*, 645–649 [cited June 6, 2007]. Retrieved from http://www.cdc.gov/mmwr/preview/mmwrhtml/00021441.htm

Centers for Disease Control and Prevention. (2006, September). *Fact sheet: Cigarette smoking-related disease and mortality*. Retrieved June 6, 2007, from http://www.cdc.gov/tobacco/data_statistics/Factsheets/cig_smoking_mort.htm

Chaudhri, N., Caggiula, A. R., Donny, E. C., Palmatier, M. I., Liu, X., & Sved, A. F. (2006). Complex interactions between nicotine and nonpharmacological stimuli reveal multiple roles for nicotine in reinforcement. *Psychopharmacology, 184*, 353–366.

Cherry, C. L., Skolasky, R. L., Lal, L., Creighton, J., Hauer, P., Raman, S. P., et al. (2006). Antiretroviral use and other risks for HIV-associated neuropathies in an international cohort. *Neurology, 66*, 867–873.

Crimmins, E. M., Kim, J. K., Alley, D. E., Karlamangla, A., & Seeman, T. (2007). Hispanic paradox in biological risk profiles. *American Journal of Public Health, 97*, 1305–1310.

Dubinsky, R. M., Arcane, R., Dalakas, M., & Border, S. (1989). Reversible axonal neuropathy from the treatment of AIDS and related disorders with 2′,3′-dideoxycytidine (ddC). *Muscle & Nerve, 12*, 856–860.

Grunberg, N. E. (1985). Nicotine, cigarette smoking, and body weight. *British Journal of Addiction, 80*, 369–377.

Grunberg, N. E. (1986a). Behavioral and biological factors in the relationship between tobacco use and body weight. In E. S. Katkin & S. B. Manuck (Eds.), *Advances in behavioral medicine* (vol. 2, pp. 97–129). Greenwich, CT: JAI Press.

Grunberg, N. E. (1986b). Nicotine as a psychoactive drug: Appetite regulation. *Psychopharmacology Bulletin, 22*(3), 875–881.

Grunberg, N. E. (1987). Behavioral factors in preventive medicine and health promotion. In W. Gordon, A. Herd, & A. Baum (Eds.), *Perspectives on behavioral medicine* (vol. 3, pp. 1–41). New York: Academic Press.

Grunberg, N. E., & Baum, A. (1985). Biological commonalities of stress and substance abuse. In S. Shiffman & T. A. Wills (Eds.), *Coping and substance abuse* (pp. 25–62). New York: Academic Press.

Grunberg, N. E., & Bowen, D. J. (1985). Coping with the sequelae of smoking cessation. *Journal of Cardiopulmonary Rehabilitation, 5,* 285–289.

Grunberg, N. E., & Klein, L. C. (1998a). Biological obstacles to adoption and maintenance of health-promoting behaviors. In S. A. Shumaker, E. Schron, J. Ockene, & W. L. McBee (Eds.), *The handbook of health behavior changes* (2nd ed., pp. 269–282). New York: Springer Publishing Company.

Grunberg, N. E., & Klein, L. C. (1998b). The relevance of stress and eating to the study of gender and drugs. In C. L. Wetherington & A. B. Roman (Eds.), *Drug addiction research and the health of women* (pp. 173–186). NIH Publication No. 98-4290. Rockville, MD: National Institute on Drug Abuse.

Grunberg, N. E., & Lord, D. (1990). Biological barriers to adoption and maintenance of health-promoting behaviors. In S. A. Shumaker, E. B. Schron, & J. K. Ockene (Eds.), *The handbook of health behavior change* (pp. 221–230). New York: Springer Publishing Company.

Jennings, J. R., Muldoon, M. F., Hall, M., Buysse, D. J., & Manuck, S. B. (2007). Self-reported sleep quality is associated with the metabolic syndrome. *Sleep, 30,* 219–223.

Julien, R. M. (2005). *A primer of drug action* (10th ed.). New York: Worth.

Katzung, B. G. (2007). *Basic and clinical pharmacology* (10th ed.). New York: McGraw-Hill.

Knutson, K. L., Ryden, A. M., Mander, B. A., & Van Cauter, E. (2006). Role of sleep duration and quality in the risk and severity of type 2 diabetes mellitus. *Archives of Internal Medicine, 166,* 1768–1774.

Knutson, K. L., Spiegel, K., Penev, P., & Van Cauter, E. (2007). The metabolic consequences of sleep deprivation. *Sleep Medicine Reviews, 11,* 163–178.

Lustig, R. H. (2006). The "skinny" on childhood obesity: How our Western environment starves kids' brains. *Pediatric Annals, 35,* 898–902.

Melmon, K. L., Morrelli, H. F., Hoffman, B. B., & Nierenberg, D. W. (Eds.). (1992). *Melmon and Morrelli's clinical pharmacology: Basic principles in therapeutics* (3rd ed.). New York: McGraw-Hill.

Merigan, T. C., Skowron, G., & ddC Study Group of the AIDS Clinical Trials Group of the National Institute of Allergy and Infectious Diseases. (1990). Safety and tolerance of dideoxycytosine as a single agent. *American Journal of Medicine, 88*(5B), 11S–15S.

Nolan, D., & Mallal, S. (2004). Complications associated with NRTI therapy: Update on clinical features, and possible pathogenic mechanisms. *Antiviral Therapy, 9,* 849–863.

Peyron, R., Laurent, B., & García-Larrea, L. (2000). Functional imaging of brain responses to pain. A review and meta-analysis (2000). *Neurophysiologie Clinique, 30,* 263–288.

Physicians' Desk Reference. (61st ed.). (2007). Montvale, NJ: Medical Economics Data.

Richter, C. P. (1943). Total self regulatory functions in animals and human beings. *Harvey Lecture Series, 38,* 63–103.

Seeman, T. E., & Crimmins, E. (2001). Social environment effects on health and aging: Integrating epidemiologic and demographic approaches and perspectives. *Annals of the New York Academy of Sciences, 954,* 88–117.

Shiffman, S. M. (1979). The tobacco withdrawal syndrome. In N. A. Krasnegor (Ed.), *NIDA research monograph 23: Cigarette smoking as a dependence process* (pp. 158–184). Rockville, MD: U.S. Department of Health, Education, & Welfare, Alcohol, Drug Abuse and Mental Health Administration.

Simpson, D. M. (2002). Selected peripheral neuropathies associated with human immunodeficiency virus infection and antiretroviral therapy. *Journal of Neurovirology, 8*(Suppl.), 33–41.

U.S. Department of Health and Human Services. (1988). *The health consequences of smoking: Nicotine addiction. A report of the Surgeon General.* DHHS Pub. No. (CDC)88-8406. Washington, DC: U.S. Government Printing Office.

Wonnacott, S., Sidhpura, N., & Balfour, D. J. (2005). Nicotine: From molecular mechanisms to behaviour. *Current Opinions in Pharmacology, 5,* 53–59.

Wood, R. L., & Rutterford, N. A. (2006). Demographic and cognitive predictors of long-term psychosocial outcome following traumatic brain injury. *Journal of the International Neuropsychological Society, 12,* 350–358.

Youle, M., Osio, M., & ALCAR Study Group. (2007). A double-blind, parallel-group, placebo-controlled, multicentre study of acetyl L-carnitine in the symptomatic treatment of antiretroviral toxic neuropathy in patients with HIV-1 infection. *HIV Medicine, 8,* 241–250.

Young, P. T. (1936). *Motivation of behavior.* New York: Wiley.

Young, P. T. (1955). The role of hedonic processes in motivation. In M. R. Jones (Ed.), *Nebraska symposium on motivation* (pp. 193–238). Lincoln: University of Nebraska Press.

Yücel, M., Lubman, D. I., Harrison, B. J., Fornito, A., Allen, N. B., Wellard, R. M., et al. (2007). A combined spectroscopic and functional MRI investigation of the dorsal anterior cingulate region in opiate addiction. *Molecular Psychiatry, 12,* 691–702.

Adolescent Tobacco Use and the Social Context

22

Christina K. Holub,
David G. Altman,
and Christine
Jackson

The slowing decline of adolescent smoking rates continues to prompt the need for the development of even more robust prevention programs (Eaton et al., 2006). In the United States, a primary public health response to adolescent tobacco use has been school-based prevention programs. Data from evaluations of these programs suggest that their effects have been generally modest in the short term and uncertain in the long term (Glynn, 1989; Rooney & Murray, 1996; Thomas & Perera, 2006; U.S. Department of Health and Human Services, 1994). A notable exception is a 6-year longitudinal evaluation of a school-based program in 56 schools that presented the first encouraging news about the long-term efficacy of a model school-based intervention. In this study, the investigators found that smoking rates were 15%–25% lower in the intervention group (Botvin, Baker, Dusenbury, Botvin, & Diaz, 1995). Unfortunately, such high-quality programs have limited national dissemination. More commonly, schools around the country routinely implement untested or ineffective programs.

In a review of school-based programs, only modest evidence for a positive long-term impact was found (Thomas & Perera, 2006). In this review, among all interventions marked as high quality, only one scored high on both intervention quality and methodological rigor of the evaluation (the Hutchinson Smoking Prevention Project, or HSPP) (Peterson, Kealey, Mann, Marek, & Sarason, 2000). This large trial was well implemented and sufficiently powered and followed participants for 2 years after they left school. The study did not find evidence that the intervention influenced smoking prevalence, either immediately after leaving school or at the follow-up. Thomas and Perera (2006) examined the results of successful interventions pooled with interventions that were not successful (e.g., HSPP), and the end result was a beneficial, but not significant, effect on smoking behavior in the short and long terms.

The discrepancies between pro-health concepts taught in school-based prevention programs and the pro-smoking messages that youth observe and experience firsthand in their communities contribute to adolescent tobacco use. Preventing adolescent tobacco use is not simply a matter of equipping individuals with peer-pressure resistance skills. Teaching resistance skills is an important component of a comprehensive intervention, but neglecting factors that engender peer norms is a strategic error and is an example of focusing on a mediating rather than an antecedent cause of the problem. The Master Settlement Agreement of 1998 provided an opportunity to target many of these factors by funding the development of comprehensive tobacco control programs. However, allocation of funds used for adolescent prevention programs has been modest at best (Jones, Austin, Beach, & Altman, 2007). Given the predominant focus of interventions currently employed, it is not surprising that adolescent tobacco use continues to be a problem.

An Ecological Approach to Tobacco Control

Adolescent tobacco use is a complex behavior, rooted in biological, social, environmental, historical, and cultural contexts. In this chapter, we focus on how environmental, policy, and interpersonal factors influence tobacco use and offer suggestions for preventing adolescent tobacco use. Our approach is influenced by ecological and systems theories. These theories view behavior as a function of the surrounding context. Articulation of an ecological approach has been provided by others writing in diverse disciplines (Binder, Stokols, & Catalano, 1975; Bronfenbrenner, 1977; Ennett et al., 2006; Kelly, 1966, 1971; McLeroy, Bibeau, Steckler, & Glanz, 1988; Rappaport, 1977; Stokols, 1992). At its most basic level, ecological theory posits that individuals and settings are mutually influential, that this influence occurs in subsystems at multiple levels of analysis, and that influence changes over time and settings. Ecological theory is thus guided by the principle that the whole is more than the sum of its parts and that behavior and environment are viewed as interdependent rather than independent (Wicker, 1979). Furthermore, an ecological perspective considers different levels of analysis like the layers of an onion, each system nested within another, with each system constrained both by the system it surrounds and the system that surrounds it (Wicker, 1979). Central to this chapter are the implications for applying a social ecological perspective to design and implement tobacco control interventions. An interventionist committed to the ecological model would search for points of leverage at multiple levels of analysis in the sociocultural context and would use multiple approaches to change the behaviors.

Few studies of health behavior specify the sequence or causal linkages by which individuals influence, and are influenced by, the larger social context (Chuang, Ennett, Bauman, & Foshee, 2005; Ennett et al., 2006; Winett, King, & Altman, 1989). The ultimate goal of all interventions directed at tobacco-related behavior, regardless of the level of analysis, is to improve the health status of individuals, since individuals, not systems or environments, experience illness and health. The focus of macro-level interventions (e.g., increasing the tax on cigarettes) can also influence the actions that individuals take (e.g., not purchasing cigarettes). Similarly, a goal of many micro-level interventions (e.g., teaching worksite employees how to quit smoking) can influence actions taken at higher levels of analysis (e.g., implementation of a worksite smoking policy). There are interactional and synergistic connections among levels of analysis. The means by which individuals are reached and influenced, however, can vary as a function of the level at which one intervenes. In more cases than not, there is a reciprocity of influence between levels of analysis (Winett et al., 1989).

Cross-Disciplinary Research

In an effort to understand and intervene in adolescent tobacco use in multiple contexts, collecting and analyzing data at different levels of analysis are often required. This can be achieved through working with other fields or disciplines collaboratively (Maton, Perkins, & Saergert, 2006). Indeed, for future progress to be made on adolescent tobacco use, cross-disciplinary approaches will be needed. Within cross-disciplinary research, integrative research that spans across multiple disciplines can be viewed in three distinct forms: multidisciplinary research, interdisciplinary research, and transdisciplinary research (Stokols, 2006).

Multidisciplinary research occurs when researchers work independently from each other, concentrating on their field, to address a particular topic. Interdisciplinary research entails more communication and coordination among researchers, though the researchers remain committed to their discipline's perspectives and methods. On the other hand, transdisciplinary research is a process by which researchers work collaboratively to develop an integrative conceptual framework that incorporates, from the different disciplines, concepts, theories, and methods to address a shared research topic (Stokols, 2006). Recent developments in cross-disciplinary research have largely focused on the latter two forms.

Interdisciplinary research can present several challenges, including the fact that researchers often have different perspectives on design, measures, and the best analytic framework for addressing multiple levels of analysis; simply bringing together collaborators from multiple disciplines and community partners itself offers a challenge. Maton, Perkins, and Saegert (2006) identify several factors that contribute to successful interdisciplinary research. Successful interdisciplinary research teams have good leadership (shared mission and vision), good relationships among researchers (respect, commitment, and openness), and research questions that either are high-profile public issues or are problem focused, rather than theory focused. Individuals within successful teams are usually passionate, committed, willing to invest time for collaboration, and able to constructively negotiate conflicts or disagreements. External factors that facilitate successful interdisciplinary research include supportive organizational contexts, consistent external funding, and physical proximity of the team (Maton et al., 2006).

Transdisciplinary research has been offered as a solution to some of the challenges that interdisciplinary research has faced (Smith, 2006). Transdisciplinary research collaborations aim to produce shared and integrated conceptual formations (Stokols, 2006). In fact, several federal agencies and private organizations, including the National Institutes of Health and the Robert Wood Johnson Foundation, have invested in establishing transdisciplinary research that focuses on different societal problems, such as substance use, obesity, and smoking. The success of these collaborations will depend on the extent to which they promote the development of common, shared conceptual frameworks that integrate and extend concepts, theories, and methods from different fields (Stokols, 2006).

The Environmental Context of Tobacco Use Policy

Tobacco control policies not only work independently to reduce smoking by youth but can also interact with other social resources, including community, peer, and family influences. Policy can act to remove individual choice in smoking behavior, such as by prohibiting smoking in certain areas. In addition, the awareness of such policies can serve as a source of education on the harmful effects of tobacco use and can even influence the stigmatization of smoking in general. In particular, cigarette prices, youth access laws, clean air laws, and the Master Settlement are factors that have reduced the rates of smoking among the young.

Prices

Much of the research on tobacco control policies has centered on increasing cigarette prices through excise taxes. Over 40 years, a tax increase of $1.00 has the potential to reduce the smoking rate by 30% and the number of premature deaths by 17% (Levy, Cummings, & Hyland, 2000). Higher cigarette prices can have indirect and direct effects on cigarette availability and on the decision to smoke (Liang, Chaloupka, Nichter, & Clayton, 2003). Price increases can affect smoking initiation and experimentation, as well as cessation (Tauras, 2004). Although increases in cigarette prices affect all smokers, adolescents are more sensitive to price, especially established adolescent smokers (Chaloupka, 1999; Liang & Chaloupka, 2002; Warner, 1986). Young men are more sensitive to price changes than are young women, regardless of race. However, young Black men are more price sensitive than young White men;

a 10% increase in price results in a 16.5% decrease in smoking prevalence among young Black men but only an 8.6% decrease among young White men (Chaloupka & Pacula, 1999).

Higher cigarette prices can affect other contextual factors, in particular, the availability of tobacco from social sources (Jones, Sharp, Husten, & Crossett, 2002). When the cost is high and obtaining cigarettes is more difficult, peers are less willing to share them (Chaloupka, 2003). Also, when prices are high, families may make it more difficult for adolescents to take cigarettes, and they experience a reduction in general smoking, as well (Chaloupka, 2003). Thus, increasing the price of cigarettes on tobacco is an effective tobacco control intervention.

Youth Access Laws

Youth access laws are newer than other tobacco control policies and include minimum-age laws, bans on self-service displays, and license revocation for vendors who continue to violate these laws (Liang et al., 2003; Woollery, Asma, & Sharp, 2000). In 1992, Congress mandated that every state and territory must legally prohibit the sale of tobacco to minors by 1994 (U.S. Department of Health and Human Services, 1995). This federal law also mandates random, unannounced checks every year. Unfortunately, many states are not in full compliance with these laws (DiFranza, 2005; DiFranza & Rigotti, 1999).

If enforcement of tobacco sales laws is done right, it can have a major impact on adolescent tobacco use (DiFranza, 2000, 2005). If the enforcement is effective, access and availability are curtailed, leading to a reduction in smoking. There have also been discussions and recommendations to increase the legal minimum age for smoking to 21 (Ahmad, 2005). As with higher cigarette prices, there are direct (e.g., limited access) and indirect (e.g., reduction in smoking by peers) influences on adolescents' likelihood of smoking. As is the case for intervening across several contexts, combining youth access laws with increased taxation and other policies aimed at reducing adolescent smoking is likely to be most effective.

Clean Air Laws

There are health risks associated with exposure to secondhand smoke or environmental smoke, especially for nonsmokers and children. The vast majority of the states (49 plus the District of Columbia) has consequently adopted clean indoor air policies. These laws typically prohibit smoking in schools, public transportation, shopping malls, retail stores, workplaces, restaurants, and bars (Liang, Chaloupka, Nichter, & Clayton, 2003). Clean air laws have not been in place long enough to yield conclusive results, though there is some early evidence of their effectiveness (Abrams et al., 2006). In addition, some data have shown that clean air laws account for a small percentage of the success of tobacco control policies (Levy, Hyland, Hibgee, Remer, & Compton, 2007; Levy, Ross, Powell, Bauer, & Lee, 2007). Clean air laws likely operate through more indirect influences, such as by stigmatizing and changing social norms of smoking. Thus, changes due to clean air laws may occur at a slower pace, and, therefore, the effects of clean air laws will take longer to observe.

Master Settlement Agreement

In November 1998, attorneys general for 46 states, the District of Columbia, and five U.S. territories signed the Master Settlement Agreement (MSA) with the major tobacco companies (National Association of Attorneys General, 1998). The MSA required tobacco companies to pay more than $200 billion over the next 25 years in response to pending lawsuits by states for health care costs from tobacco-related illnesses. In addition, the settlement included restrictions on marketing and advertising tobacco to youth. Funds were also made available to support a national antismoking campaign targeted at youth.

While the MSA was intended to incentivize states to use funds for preventing and reducing tobacco use, especially among youth, allocation of funds for this purpose has been limited. In 2000 and 2001, 43% of the funding was allocated to general health care and only 9% to actual tobacco-related measures (Pollack & Jacobson, 2003). In North Carolina, in the period 2000–2004 the percentage of funds that went to youth tobacco use prevention and cessation programs was only 9.6%. When diverted funds and payments to tobacco quota owners and growers are included, this drops down to 2.3% (Jones, Austin, Beach, & Altman, 2007). The Centers for Disease Control and Prevention (CDC) developed tobacco control program guidelines, which require about 20%–25% of the state's settlement funds. Unfortunately, only four states (Arkansas, Delaware, Maine, and Mississippi) are at the minimum levels set forth in the guidelines. The sale of cigarettes decreased in states that spent more money on comprehensive tobacco control programs (Farrelly, Pechacek, & Chaloupka, 2003). If states had spent the CDC's minimum recommended funding between 1999 and 2000, it is estimated that the prevalence of smoking among the young would have been between 3.3% and 13.5% lower than what was observed (Taurus et al., 2004).

Despite these obstacles, the MSA has led to several public health achievements. First, there have been major changes in social norms by youth. The "Truth Campaign," a product of the American Legacy Foundation funded by the MSA, changed adolescents' beliefs and attitudes towards the tobacco industry (Hersey et al., 2005a). There are also fewer environmental visual cues such as billboards and sporting event sponsorships. Paraphernalia designed to attract youths' attention to smoking and cartoon figures, such as Joe Camel, are practically nonexistent. The removal of such cues to smoking and the encouragement of antismoking attitudes are large steps in the right direction. Nationally, tobacco control efforts have succeeded in changing public policy, influencing public attitudes and social norms, and encouraging discourse on tobacco use (Pollack & Jacobson, 2003). Policies can increase public awareness of the effects of secondhand smoke and thereby motivate families and parents to be more involved in antismoking socialization (Chaloupka, 2003).

Marketing

Expenditures

Tobacco company marketing expenditures increased rapidly in the past few decades, climbing from about $261 million in 1964, to $491 million in 1975, to more than $9 billion by the year 2000. During the mid-1990s, expenditures increased by almost $1 billion each year. In 2003, the amount spent on cigarette advertising and promotion exceeded $15 billion dollars. This represents a 35.0% increase from 2001 ($11.2 billion) and a 21.5% increase from 2002 ($12.5 billion) (Federal Trade Commission, 2005).

Effects on Adolescents

There is some evidence of an association between attention and participation in promotional campaigns and susceptibility to tobacco use (Altman, Levine, Coeytaux, Slade, & Jaffe, 1996). Altman and colleagues found that when an adolescent was aware of tobacco promotions, the predicted odds that that adolescent was a tobacco user or was susceptible to tobacco use were two times greater than those for an adolescent who was unaware of promotions. When an adolescent was aware of promotions, had an adolescent friend who owned a promotional item, had received tobacco, and had participated directly in a tobacco promotional campaign, the odds of becoming a smoker increased to about 22 (Altman et al., 1996). Pierce and colleagues (2005) found that curiosity and susceptibility to smoking were independently associated with smoking initiation; adolescents reporting curiosity about smoking were more likely to become susceptible to tobacco use, a factor that has often been viewed by advertising theorists as an intermediate goal to encouragement. Similarly, candy cigarette use in youth has been found to be associated with increased risk of smoking as adults (Klein, Thomas, & Sutter, 2007).

After a thorough review of the evidence, the FDA concluded that there was substantial quantitative and qualitative evidence supporting a causal relationship between tobacco product marketing and adolescent tobacco use. Likewise, the FDA suggested that there was strong evidence supporting the efficacy of antismoking media campaigns (Food and Drug Administration, 1995). While, in 2000, the U.S. Supreme Court ruled that the FDA does not have the legal authority to regulate tobacco, other studies have continued to demonstrate the link between marketing and adolescent smoking (cf. Wakefield, Flay, Nichter, & Giovino, 2003).

Evaluations of established antismoking media campaigns in California, Massachusetts, and Florida have shown that the campaigns do reduce smoking in adults and adolescents (Hersey et al., 2005b; Institute of Medicine and National Research Council, 2000; Sly, Heald, & Ray, 2001). California was the first U.S. state to have an ongoing comprehensive tobacco control program. Evaluations of the campaign demonstrated that children in grades 4–12 who participated had an increase in recall of the media campaign, more unfavorable attitudes toward smoking, a decrease in intention to smoke, and a decline in 30-day smoking prevalence (Popham, Potter, & Hedrick, 1994). Similarly, evaluations of antismoking campaigns in Massachusetts, which had the highest level of per capita funding in 1993, and of the "Truth" Campaign, launched in Florida in 1998, showed that both led to high recall of antismoking advertising and subsequent reduction in adolescent smoking (Harris, Connolly, Brooks, & Davis, 1996; Sly et al., 2001). Other evidence has shown that the impact of antismoking campaigns on adolescent smoking can be seen when funding for such efforts is cut. In 2003, when Minnesota's successful campaign was defunded, trends in measures of susceptibility to smoking, attitudes toward smoking, and intentions to smoke changed in the same direction that would increase risk for smoking, showing that discontinuing successful campaigns can have a negative impact (Sly et al., 2001). Overall, as a result of the MSA, significant tobacco product marketing aimed at youth has been curtailed.

Media Practices Affecting Modeling of Smoking

The portrayal of tobacco use in the mass media may play a role in the way that adolescents perceive social norms about use. In a sample of the top 20 highest-grossing films from 1990–1996, an average of 5 minutes per film involved a tobacco-related incident, of which only 43 seconds involved an antismoking message (Stockwell & Glantz, 1997). Movie stars may have the potential to be seen as role models because their behavior on screen and in real life is highly visible; it has been shown that having a favorite movie star who smokes increases teens' susceptibility to becoming smokers themselves (Distefan, Gilpin, & Sargent, 1999). In an experimental study assessing how on-screen smoking might influence young viewers (Pechmann & Shih, 1999), researchers compared the responses of 9th-graders to movies with and without smoking scenes. Movies with smoking scenes positively aroused the young viewers, enhanced the perception of a smoker's social stature, and increased their intent to smoke. Interestingly, if the young viewers were shown an antismoking advertisement before seeing the movie, these effects were nullified (Pechmann & Shih, 1999). While tobacco use is less frequent on television than in movies, there is evidence that depictions of smoking increased during the 1990s (Hazan & Glantz, 1995). Tobacco use also is recounted in music videos and lyrics. One study found tobacco use mentioned in 12% of country music videos and in 26% of videos on MTV (Durant, Romes, Rich, & Allred, 1997). The promotion of cigarettes in movies, on television, and in videos is planned and strategic, rather than coincidental. While the effects of these exposures on actual tobacco use behavior are difficult to assess, they contribute, in conjunction with other advertising and promotional strategies, to the idea that tobacco use is desirable.

Access to Cigarettes by Minors

Although most states have laws regulating tobacco sales to minors, these laws are rarely enforced (Food and Drug Administration, 1995; Inspector General, 1995; USDHHS, 1990, 1994, 1995), and minors have little trouble obtaining tobacco. A national survey representative of students attending school found that more than 76% of 8th-graders and 90% of 10th-graders believed that it would be "fairly easy" or "very easy" for them to obtain tobacco (Johnston, 1995). While over-the-counter access to cigarettes has been increasingly difficult for adolescents in recent years, there is some evidence that shoplifting and "bumming" cigarettes can be other sources for minors, especially among early adolescents (Cismoski & Sheridan, 1994; DiFranza, Eddy, Brown, & Ryan, 1995). Local laws restricting youth access to tobacco, including minimum-age laws and verification requirements, have been successful in the short term; long-term effects are still inconclusive (Chen & Forster, 2006). However, some researchers would argue that youth access interventions are simply not working (Craig & Boris, 2007; Fitchenburg & Glanz, 2002).

Access to cigarettes is a critical determinant of whether people (particularly children and adolescents) experiment with or maintain tobacco use. Since few smokers begin smoking after high school (Johnston, O'Malley, & Bachman, 1994), some begin even before high school (Johnston, O'Malley, Bachman, & Schulenberg, 2006), and the majority of adult smokers began to smoke at an early age, efforts to prevent the adoption of smoking must focus on preventing children and adolescents from becoming addicted. Limiting access to tobacco can contribute to prevention, but poor enforcement and advances in technology may be undermining recent achievements in tobacco control policies, including youth access laws.

Tobacco and the Internet

Stronger regulation and enforcement directed at those who sell cigarettes to minors and the imposition of consequences for such activities have made youth access to over-the-counter sources more difficult. One unintended consequence of this achievement is that youth may be more likely to use the Internet to obtain tobacco. When data on internet use in U.S. households were first collected in 1997, 18% of households reported having access (U.S. Census Bureau, 2004). Access more than doubled, to 41.5%, in 2000 and increased again to more than 50% in 2001. In 2001, approximately 65% of youth ages 10–14 and 68% of those ages 15–17 reported having access in the home.

The number of domestic Internet cigarette vendors has increased rapidly, from 88 in 2000 to more than 300 in 2005 (Ribisl, Kim, & Williams, 2001, 2007). In 2005, a total of 664 sites were identified, including those with domestic, international, and unknown vendor locations. The nature of the Internet makes it difficult to regulate and enforce youth access to tobacco. This is even more complex for vendors located in tribal lands and countries outside the United States (Ribisl et al., 2007). More than 75% of Internet cigarette vendors are estimated to advertise tax-free cigarettes (U.S. General Accounting Office, 2002). The sale of cheaper cigarettes is attractive to price-sensitive smokers, which includes adolescents and those who reside in high-excise-tax states (Ribisl et al., 2007; Turner, Mermelstein, & Flay, 2004). The availability of cheaper cigarettes may curtail the normal progression of price-sensitive smokers toward quitting or reducing tobacco use.

Adolescents are more responsive to price than are adults (Turner et al., 2004), which further reinforces the concern about youth access to cigarettes online. Several studies found that adolescents are capable of searching for and placing orders with tobacco vendors (often in under 20 minutes) and that more than 90% of them purchase products (Jensen, Hickman, Landrine, & Klonoff, 2004; Ribisl, 2003). Ribisl (2003) found that only 11% of the vendors asked for a copy of the buyer's photo ID for age verification. Even when ID was not provided, half of vendors still fulfilled the order. In 2005, 6.5% of 9th-grade smokers reported having bought cigarettes online, with 5.2% having bought cigarettes online in the past 30 days. The number of cigarettes bought by youth online in the past 30 days more than doubled between 2001 and 2005 (Fix et al., 2006). While a small proportion of youth smokers are currently buying cigarettes online, those who do are more likely to report difficulty in obtaining cigarettes from commercial and social sources (Ribisl et al., 2007). This suggests that, as completing over-the-counter purchases becomes more difficult for minors, they will turn to online sources.

As part of an Institute of Medicine report, Ribisl and colleagues (2007) proposed a framework of multiple policy strategies and recommendations aimed at effectively regulating Internet cigarette sales to youth. The framework, Q.U.I.T. (Quarantine of Unhealthy Internet Trade), recommended regulating the supply of cigarettes to Internet vendors, blocking or seizing Web site domains of vendors that are noncompliant with tax laws and age verification, preventing the major payment-processing companies (e.g., VISA, MasterCard) from approving transactions, regulating delivery services, and educating consumers about tax requirements. Several of these strategies have begun to be implemented, with some positive effect. For example, several major credit cards have stopped approving Internet cigarette sales, and shipping companies such as UPS and DHL have ceased shipping cigarettes to consumers. These actions have started to reduce Internet cigarette sales, but more collaborative work is needed. While the number of youth smokers who buy cigarettes online is still relatively low, as for other consumer products, the Internet has become a major method for gaining access to products.

Family Socialization Processes

Tobacco use by children and adolescents may be influenced by socialization processes within the family. Parents can have both direct and indirect influences on tobacco use, for example by influencing adolescents' affiliation with peers who smoke (Simons-Morton, Chen, Abroms, & Haynie, 2004). Siblings can also have considerable influence on tobacco use, since those with siblings who smoke are more likely to smoke themselves. High levels of social connectedness between siblings further enhances the effect of a shared environment (Slomkowski, Rende, Novak, Lloyd-Richardson, & Niaura, 2005). Particularly important to consider are general parenting style and tobacco-specific parenting practices, both of which can predispose some children to engage in risk-taking behaviors.

Parenting style refers to the general child-rearing practices of parents. Developmental theorists have identified parental demandingness, responsiveness, and degree of warmth and acceptance as the key dimensions of parenting style (Baumrind, 1978; Roberts, 1986; Steinberg, Elmen, & Mounts, 1989). Each dimension is a composite of parenting behaviors; for example, demandingness refers to setting and enforcing clear standards of behavior; active monitoring and supervision of a child's activities; maintenance of structure and regimen in a child's life; and making demands for maturity consistent with the child's developmental phase. Parental responsiveness includes supporting a child's independence and individuality; relating to the actual child rather than to an idealized child; respecting a child's rights; and expecting the child to respect a parent's rights.

The authoritative parenting style, defined by both high levels of demands and high levels of responsiveness and warmth, has been associated with reduced tobacco use among children and adolescents. Adolescents whose parents are more authoritative are less likely to smoke than are adolescents whose parents are less authoritative (Chassin et al., 2005; Pierce, Distefan, Jackson,

White, & Gilpin, 2002). In addition, parents with authoritative parenting styles are more likely to have children who see them as influential authority figures regarding substance use (Jackson, 2002). Chassin and colleagues (2005) found that adolescents in homes with authoritative parents reported having significantly more tobacco-specific discussions than did those in homes with authoritarian parents (high on demandingness, low on acceptance).

A parent's role in socialization related to tobacco can take several forms. Parents' own tobacco use is an important predictor of their children's use (Foster et al., 2007; Murray, Kiryluk, & Swan, 1985; Nolte, Smith, & O'Rourke, 1983; Peterson et al., 2006). Children of parents who smoke may be receiving cues that unintentionally encourage them to smoke. Parents are encouraged to quit smoking while their children are young. However, research has shown that children of parents who practice antismoking socialization (e.g., by communicating strong antismoking messages, establishing household smoking bans, perceiving that they can influence their child not to smoke) can impact children's smoking behavior, despite the parent's own smoking (Conley, 2005; Harakeh, Scholte, de Vries, & Engel, 2005; Jackson & Dickinson, 2006; Turner et al., 2004). Through these and other socializing mechanisms, parents influence their children's perceptions of the prevalence, social acceptability, and personal and social consequences of tobacco use.

Parenting style and tobacco-specific parenting practices not only are associated with smoking initiation but also have implications for regular smoking among adolescents and for the persistence of smoking into adulthood (Turner et al., 2004). As such, it is important to intervene in tobacco use when children are young. Jackson and Dickinson (2004) found that small increases in the number of cigarettes consumed when children were young translated to a significantly higher likelihood of current, established, and daily smoking in adolescence. While some parents may be proactive in socializing their children against tobacco use, it is likely that the majority of parents view tobacco use as a problem of adolescence and thus remain passive during the children's early years. Importantly, a passive orientation is not devoid of a socializing effect. Baumrind, for example, posits that children often interpret parent passivity as tacit approval or lack of disapproval (Baumrind & Moselle, 1985). Thus, parents who do not actively challenge the many prosmoking influences to which their children are exposed may effectively allow these other social influences to take effect.

Summary

A theme of this chapter is that tobacco-related behavior and the settings in which such behavior occurs are interdependent. Recognizing this point will help tobacco control researchers and advocates focus both on the settings in which tobacco use is most encouraged and salient and on the individual tobacco-related behaviors that occur in these settings. The physical and policy environments are central influences on the beliefs and behaviors of individuals. It can be difficult, however, to develop interventions that effectively target the multiple levels of influence on specific tobacco-related knowledge, attitudes, and behaviors. Similarly, assessing the interrelationships and potential synergistic effects among these levels of influence is difficult. The critical issue is how behavior is influenced by, and influences, multiple levels of analysis in a complex web of place and time. To address the need for multilevel analysis will require methodological advances. While the tools for measuring the social context of health phenomena are perhaps less developed than the tools for measuring psychosocial constructs, their development is essential if we are to develop an adequate understanding of contextual effects on health-related behaviors. Collaboration among social and health scientists in a search for complementary theories, concepts, and methodologies can assist in this endeavor.

Overall, few studies with a focus on the policy context of adolescent smoking incorporate micro-level factors such as community, family, and peer influences. Research that aims to examine multiple contexts, as well as their interaction, from a transdisciplinary perspective is needed. This would help to improve our understanding of the complex interaction of various influences on adolescent smoking, which would in turn help to inform the formulation of more effective policies and new prevention methods to reduce smoking among youth.

References

Abrams, S. M., Mahoney, M. C., Hyland, A., Cummings, M., Davis, W., & Song, L. (2006). Early evidence of the effectiveness of clean indoor air legislation in New York State. *American Journal of Public Health, 96,* 296–298.

Ahmad, S. (2005). Closing the youth access gap: The projected health benefits and cost savings of a national policy to raise the legal smoking age to 21 in the United States. *Health Policy, 75,* 74–84.

Altman, D. G., Levine, D. W., Coeytaux, R., Slade, J., & Jaffe, R. (1996). Tobacco promotion and susceptibility to tobacco use among adolescents aged 12 through 17 years in a nationally representative sample. *American Journal of Public Health, 86*(11), 1590–1593.

Andersen, M. R., Leroux, B. G., Marek, P. M., Peterson, A. V., Kealey K. A., & Sarason, I. G. (2002). Mothers' attitudes and concerns about their children smoking: Do they influence kids? *Preventive Medicine, 34,* 198–206.

Barker, D. (1994). Changes in the cigarette brand preferences of adolescent smokers—United States, 1989–1993. *Morbidity and Mortality Weekly Report, 43*(32), 577–581.

Bauman, K. E., Foshee, V., Ennett, S. T., Hicks, K., & Pemberton, M. (2001). Family matters: A family-directed program designed to prevent adolescent tobacco and alcohol use. *Health Promotion Practice, 2,* 81–96.

Baumrind, D. (1978). Parental disciplinary patterns and social competence in children. *Youth & Society, 9*(3), 239–275.

Baumrind, D., & Moselle, K. A. (1985). A developmental perspective on adolescent drug abuse. *Advances in Alcohol and Substance Abuse, 4,* 41–67.

Binder, A., Stokols, D., & Catalano, R. (1975). Social ecology: An emerging multidiscipline. *Journal of Environmental Education, 7,* 32–43.

Botvin, G. J., Baker, E., Dusenbury, L., Botvin, E. M., & Diaz, T. (1995). Long-term follow-up results of a randomized drug abuse prevention trial in a white middle-class population. *Journal of the American Medical Association, 273*(14), 1106–1112.

Bricker, J. B., Leroux, B. G., Andersen, M. R., Rajan, K. B., & Peterson, A. V. (2005). Parental smoking cessation and children's smoking: Mediation by antismoking actions. *Nicotine & Tobacco Research, 7,* 501–509.

Bronfenbrenner, U. (1977). Toward an experimental ecology of human development. *American Psychologist, 32*(7), 513–531.

Chaloupka, F. J. (1999). Macro-social influences: The effect of prices and tobacco control policies on the demand for tobacco products. *Nicotine & Tobacco Research, 1,* S105–S109.

Chaloupka, F. J. (2003). Contextual factors and youth tobacco use: Policy linkages. *Addiction, 98,* 147–149.

Chaloupka, F. J., & Pacula, R. L. (1999). Sex and race differences in young people's responsiveness to price and tobacco control policies. *Tobacco Control, 8,* 373–377.

Chapman, S., & Wong, W. L. (1990). *Tobacco control in the third world.* Penang: International Organisation of Consumers.

Chassin, L., Presson, C. C., Rose, J., Sherman, S. J., Davis, M. J., & Gonzalez, J. L. (2005). Parenting style and smoking-specific parenting practices as predictors of adolescent smoking onset. *Journal of Pediatric Psychology, 30,* 333–344.

Chen, V., & Forster, J. L. (2006). The long-term effect of local policies to restrict retail sale of tobacco to youth. *Nicotine & Tobacco Research, 8,* 371–377.

Chuang, Y. C., Ennett, S. T., Bauman, K. E., & Foshee, V. A. (2005). Neighborhood influences on adolescent cigarette and alcohol use: Mediating effects through parent and peer behaviors. *Journal of Health & Social Behavior, 46*(2), 187–204.

Cismoski, J., & Sheridan, M. (1994). Tobacco acquisition practices of adolescents in two Wisconsin communities. *Wisconsin Medical Journal, 93*(11), 585–591.

Clausen, J. A. (1968). Perspectives on childhood socialization. In J. A. Clausen (Ed.), *Socialization and society* (pp. 131–181). Boston: Little, Brown.

Conley, T. C., Siegel, M., Winickoff, J., Biener, L., & Rigotti, N. A. (2005). Household smoking bans and adolescents' perceived prevalence of smoking and social acceptability of smoking. *Preventive Medicine, 41,* 349–356.

Craig, M. J., & Boris, N. W. (2007). Youth tobacco access restrictions: Time to shift resources to other interventions? *Health Promotion and Practice, 8,* 22–27.

DiFranza, J. R. (2000). Youth access: The baby and the bath water. *Tobacco Control, 9,* 120–121.

DiFranza, J. R. (2005). Best practices for enforcing state laws prohibiting the sale of tobacco to minors. *Journal of Public Health Management & Practice, 11,* 559–565.

DiFranza, J. R., & Coleman, M. (2001). Sources of tobacco for youths in communities with strong enforcement of youth access laws. *Tobacco Control, 10,* 323–328.

DiFranza, J. R., Eddy, J. J., Brown, L. F., & Ryan, J. L. (1995). Tobacco acquisition and cigarette brand selection among youth. *Tobacco Control, 3,* 334–338.

DiFranza, J. R., & Rigotti, N. A. (1999). Impediments to the enforcement of youth access laws. *Tobacco Control, 8,* 152–155.

Distefan, J. M., Gilpin, E. A., & Sargent, J. D. (1999). Do movie stars encourage adolescents to start smoking? Evidence from California. *Preventive Medicine, 28,* 1–11.

Durant, R. H., Romes, E. S., Rich, M., & Allred, E. (1997). Tobacco and alcohol use behaviors portrayed in music videos: A content analysis. *American Journal of Public Health, 87,* 1131–1135.

Eaton, D. K., Kann, L., Kinchen, S., Ross, J., Hawkins, J., Harris, W. A., et al. (2006). Youth risk behavior surveillance—United States, 2005. *Morbidity and Mortality Weekly Report, 55* (SS-5), 1–112.

Ennett, S. T., Bauman, K. E., Hussong, A., Faris, R., Foshee, V. A., Cai, L., et al. (2006). The peer context of adolescent use: Findings from social network analysis. *Journal of Research on Adolescence, 16,* 159–186.

Ennett, S. T., Mauman, K. E., Pemberton, M., Foshee, V. A., Chuang, Y., King, T. S., et al. (2001). Mediation in a family-directed program for prevention of adolescent tobacco and alcohol use. *Preventive Medicine, 33,* 333–346.

Farrelly, M. C., Pechacek, T. F., & Chaloupka, F. J. (2003). The impact of tobacco control program expenditures on aggregate cigarette sales: 1981–2000. *Journal of Health Economics, 22*(5), 843–859.

Federal Trade Commission. (2005). *Cigarette Report for 2003.* Washington, DC: Federal Trade Commission.

Fichtenberg, C. M., & Glantz, S. A. (2002). Youth access interventions do not affect youth smoking. *Pediatrics, 109,* 1088–1092.

Fix, B. V., Zambon, M., Higbee, C., Cummings, K. M., Alford, T., & Hyland, A. (2006). Internet cigarette purchasing among 9th grade students in western New York: 2000–2001 vs. 2004–2005. *Preventive Medicine, 43,* 191–195.

Food and Drug Administration. (1995). Regulations restricting the sale and distribution of cigarettes and smokeless tobacco products to protect children and adolescents; proposed rule analysis regarding FDA's jurisdiction over nicotine-containing cigarettes and smokeless tobacco products. *Federal Register, 60*(155), 21 CFR Part 801. U.S. Department of Health and Human Services, Food and Drug Administration.

Foster, S. E., Jones, D. J., Olson, A. L., Forehand, R., Gaffney, C. A., Zens, M. S., et al. (2007). Family socialization of adolescent's self-reported cigarette use: The role of parents' history of regular smoking and parenting style. *Journal of Pediatric Psychology, 32,* 481–493.

Glynn, T. J. (1989). Essential elements of school-based smoking prevention programs. *Journal of School Health, 59,* 181–188.

Harakeh, Z., Scholte, R. H., de Vries, H., & Engels, R. C. (2005). Parental rules and communication: their association with adolescent smoking. *Addiction, 100,* 862–870.

Harris, J., Connolly, G., Brooks, D., & Davis, B. (1996). Cigarette smoking before and after an excise tax increase and an antismoking campaign—Massachusetts, 1990–1996. *Morbidity and Mortality Weekly Report, 45,* 966–970.

Hazan, A. R., & Glantz, S. A. (1995). Current trends in tobacco use in prime-time fictional television. *American Journal of Public Health, 85,* 116–117.

Hersey, J. C., Niederdeppe, J., Evans, W. D., Nonnemaker, J., Blahut, S., Holden, D., et al. (2005b). The theory of "truth": How counterindustry campaigns affect smoking behavior among teens. *Health Psychology, 24,* 22–31.

Hersey, J. C., Niederdeppe, J., Ng, S. W., Mowery, P., Farrelly, M., & Messeri, P. (2005a). How state counter-industry campaigns help prime perceptions of tobacco industry practices to promote reduction in youth smoking. *Tobacco Control, 14,* 377–383.

Inspector General. (1995). *State oversight of tobacco sales to minors.* Washington, DC: U.S. Department of Health & Human Services. Office of Inspector General.

Institute of Medicine and National Research Council. (2000). *State programs can reduce tobacco use.* Washington DC: National Academy of Sciences, National Cancer Policy Board, Institute of Medicine, National Research Council and Board on Health Promotion and Disease Prevention.

Jackson, C. (2002). Perceived legitimacy of parental authority and tobacco and alcohol use during early adolescence. *Journal of Adolescent Health, 31,* 425–432.

Jackson, C., & Dickinson, D. (2004). Cigarette consumption during childhood and persistence of smoking through adolescence. *Archives of Pediatric and Adolescent Medicine, 158,* 1050–1056.

Jackson, C., & Dickinson, D. (2006). Enabling parents who smoke to prevent their children from initiating smoking. *Archives of Pediatric and Adolescent Medicine, 160,* 56–62.

Jensen, J. A., Hickman, N. J., Landrine, H., & Klonoff, E. A. (2004). Availability of tobacco to youth via the Internet. *Journal of the American Medical Association, 291*(15), 1837.

Johnston, L. D. (1995). *Smoking rates climb among American teen-agers, who find smoking increasingly acceptable and seriously underestimate the risks.* Ann Arbor: University of Michigan News and Information Service.

Johnston, L. D., O'Malley, P. M., & Bachman, J. G. (1994). *National survey results on drug use from the monitoring the future study, 1975–1992: Vol. 1, Secondary school students.* Washington, DC: U.S. Department of Health and Human Services, Public Health Service, National Institutes of Health, National Institute on Drug Abuse.

Johnston, L. D., O'Malley, P. M., Bachman, J. G., & Schulenberg, J. E. (2006). *Monitoring the future national results on adolescent drug use: Overview of key findings, 2005.* National Institutes of Health, Bethesda, MD: National Institute of Drug Abuse.

Jones, A. S., Austin, W. D., Beach, R. H., & Altman, D. G. (2007). Funding of North Carolina tobacco control programs through the Master Settlement Agreement. *American Journal of Public Health, 97,* 36–43.

Jones, S. E., Sharp, D. J., Husten, C. G., & Crossett, L. S. (2002). Cigarette acquisition and proof of age among U.S. high school students who smoke. *Tobacco Control, 11,* 20–25.

Kelly, J. G. (1966). Ecological constraints on mental health services. *American Psychologist, 21,* 535–539.

Kelly, J. G. (1971). Qualities for the community psychologist. *American Psychologist, 26,* 897–903.

Klein, J. D., Thomas, R. K., & Sutter, E. J. (2007). History of childhood candy cigarette use is associated with tobacco smoking by adults. *Preventive Medicine, 45,* 26–30.

Laniado-Laborin, R., Woodruff, S. I., Candelaria, J. I., & Sallis, J. F. (2002). Parental prompting and smoking among Latino youth. *Ethnicity & Disease, 12,* 508–516.

Levy, D. T., Cummings, K. M., & Hyland, A. (2000). Increasing taxes as a strategy to reduce cigarette use and deaths: Results of a simulation model. *Preventive Medicine, 31,* 279–286.

Levy, D. T., Hyland, A., Higbee, C., Remer, L., & Compton, C. (2007). The role of public policies in reducing smoking prevalence in California: Results from the California Tobacco Policy Simulation Model. *Health Policy, 82,* 167–185.

Levy, D. T., Ross, H., Powell, L., Bauer, J. E., & Lee, H. R. (2007). The role of public policies in reducing smoking prevalence and deaths caused by smoking in Arizona: Results from the Arizona tobacco policy simulation model. *Journal of Public Health Management and Practice, 13,* 59–67.

Liang, L., & Chaloupka, F. J. (2002). Differential effects of cigarette price on youth smoking intensity. *Nicotine and Tobacco Research, 4,* 109–114.

Liang, L., Chaloupka, F. J., Nichter, M., & Clayton, R. (2003). Prices, policies, and youth smoking, May 2001. *Addiction, 98,* 105–122.

Mackay, J. M. (1994). The fight against tobacco in developing countries. *Tubercle and Lung Disease, 75,* 8–24.

Mackay, J. M. (2004). The tobacco industry in Asia: Revelations in the corporate documents. *Tobacco Control, 13*(Suppl.2), ii1–3.

Maton, K. I., Perkins, D. D., Altman, D. G., Gutierrez, L., Kelly, J. G., Rappaport, J., et al. (2006). *American Journal of Community Psychology, 38,* 1–7.

Maton, K. I., Perkins, D. D., & Saegert, S. (2006). Community psychology at the crossroads: Prospects for interdisciplinary research. *American Journal of Community Psychology, 38,* 9–21.

McLeroy, K. R., Bibeau, D., Steckler, A., & Glanz, K. (1988). An ecological perspective on health promotion programs. *Health Education Quarterly, 15*(4), 351–377.

Murray, M., Kiryluk, S., & Swan, A. V. (1985). Relation between parents' and children's smoking behaviour and attitudes. *Journal of Epidemiology and Community Health, 39,* 169–174.

Naett, C. (1994). The tobacco industry and Eastern Europe: International trade fair and symposium, Moscow, 21–24. *Tobacco Control, 3*(2), 163–165.

National Association of Attorneys General. (1998). *Tobacco Master Settlement Agreement.* Retrieved December 12, 2007, from www.naag.org/upload/1109185724_1032468605_cigmsa.pdf

Nichter, M., & Project Quit Tobacco International Group. (2006). Introducing tobacco cessation in developing countries: An overview of Project Quit Tobacco International. *Tobacco Control, 15*(Suppl. 1), i12–i17.

Niemeyer, D., Miner, K. R., Carlson, L. M., Baer, K., & Shorty, L. (2004). The 1998 Master Settlement Agreement: A public health opportunity realized—or lost? *Health Promotion Practice, 5,* 21–32.

Nolte, A. E., Smith, B. J., & O'Rourke, T. (1983). The relative importance of parental attitudes and behavior upon youth smoking behavior. *Journal of School Health, 53*(4), 264–271.

O'Callaghan, F. V., O'Callaghan, M., Najman, J. M., Williams, G. M., Bor, W., & Alati, R. (2006). Prediction of adolescent smoking from family and social risk factors at 5 years, and maternal smoking in pregnancy at 5 and 14 years. *Addiction, 101,* 282–290.

Pechmann, C., & Shih, C. F. (1999). Smoking scenes in movies and antismoking advertisements before movies: effects on youth. *Journal of Marketing, 63,* 1–13.

Peterson, A. V., Kealey, K. A., Mann, S. L., Marek, P. M., & Sarason, I. G. (2000). Hutchinson Smoking Prevention Project: Long-term randomized trial in school-based tobacco use prevention—results on smoking. *Journal of the National Cancer Institute, 92,* 1979–1991.

Peterson, A. V., Leroux, B. G., Bricker, J., Kealey, K. A., Marek, P. M., Sarason, I. G., et al. (2006). Nine-year prediction of adolescent smoking by number of smoking parents. *Addictive Behaviors, 31,* 788–801.

Pierce, J. P., Distefan, J. M., Jackson, C., White, M. M., & Gilpin, E. A. (2002). Does tobacco marketing undermine the influence of recommended parenting in discouraging adolescents from smoking? *American Journal of Preventive Medicine, 23,* 73–81.

Pierce, J. P., Distefan, J. M., Kaplan, R. M., & Gilpin, E. A. (2005). The role of curiosity in smoking initiation. *Addictive Behavior, 30,* 685–696.

Pollack, H. A., & Jacobson, P. D. (2003). Political economy of youth smoking regulation. *Addiction, 98,* 123–138.

Popham, W. J., Potter, L. D., & Hedrick, M. A. (1994). Effectiveness of the California 1990–91 tobacco education media campaign. *American Journal of Preventive Medicine, 10,* 319–326.

Rappaport, J. (1977). *Community psychology: Values, research, and action.* New York: Holt, Rinehart, and Winston.

Ribisl, K. M. (2003). The potential of the internet as a medium to encourage and discourage youth tobacco use. *Tobacco Control, 12*(1), i48–i59.

Ribisl, K. M., Kim, A. E., & Williams, R. S. (2001). Web sites selling cigarettes: How many are there in the U.S.A. and what are their sales practices? *Tobacco Control, 10,* 352–359.

Ribisl, K. M., Kim, A. E., & Williams, R. S. (2007). Sales and marketing of cigarettes on the Internet: Emerging threats to tobacco control and promising policy solutions. In R. J. Bonnie, K. Strattan, & R. B. Wallace (Eds.), *Ending the tobacco problem: A blueprint for the nation* (Appendix M, pp. 653–678). Washington, DC: Institute of Medicine.

Roberts, W. L. (1986). Nonlinear models of development: An example from the socialization of competence. *Child Development, 57,* 1166–1178.

Rooney, B. L., & Murray, D. M. (1996). A meta-analysis of smoking prevention programs after adjustment for errors in the unit of analysis. *Health Education Quarterly, 23*(1), 48–64.

Simons-Morton, B., Chen, R., Abroms, L., & Haynie, D. L. (2004). Latent growth curve analysis of peer and parental influences on smoking progression among early adolescents. *Health Psychology, 23,* 612–621.

Slomkowski, C., Rende, R., Novak, S., Lloyd-Richardson, E., & Niaura, R. (2005). Sibling effects on smoking in adolescence: Evidence for social influence from a genetically informative design. *Addiction, 100,* 430–438.

Sly, D. F., Heald, G. R., & Ray, S. (2001). The Florida "Truth" anti-tobacco media evaluation: Design, first year results and implications for planning future media evaluations. *Tobacco Control, 10,* 9–15.

Smith, J. (2006). At a crossroad: Standing still and moving forward. *American Journal of Community Psychology, 38,* 23–25.

Steinberg, L., Elmen, J. D., & Mounts, N. S. (1989). Authoritative parenting, psychosocial maturity, and academic success among adolescents. *Child Development, 60,* 1424–1436.

Stockwell, T. F., & Glantz, S. A. (1997). Tobacco use is increasing in popular films. *Tobacco Control, 6,* 282–284.

Stokols, D. (1992). Establishing and maintaining healthy environments: Toward a social ecology of health promotion. *American Psychologist, 47*(1), 6–22.

Stokols, D. (2006). Toward a science of transdisciplinary action research. *American Journal of Community Psychology, 38,* 63–77.

Tauras, J. A. (2004). Public policy and smoking cessation among young adults in the United States. *Health Policy, 68,* 321–332.

Thomas, R., & Perera, R. (2006). School-based programmes for preventing smoking. *Cochrane Database of Systematic Reviews, 3,* CD001293.

Turner, L., Mermelstein, R., & Flay, B. (2004). Individual and contextual influences on adolescent smoking. *Annals of New York Academy of Science, 1021,* 175–197.

U.S. Census Bureau. (2004). *Current Population Survey, September 2001.* Retrieved December 12, 2007, from http://www.census.gov/main/www/cen2000.html

U.S. Department of Health and Human Services (USDHHS). (1990). *Smoking and health, a national status report: A report to Congress/Department of Health and Human Services* (2nd ed.). Vol. DHHS (CDC) 87–8396. Rockville, MD: U.S. Department of Health and Human Services.

U.S. Department of Health and Human Services (USDHHS). (1994). *Preventing tobacco use among young: A report of the Surgeon General.* Atlanta: Public Health Service, Centers for Disease Control and Prevention, Office on Smoking and Health.

U.S. Department of Health and Human Services (USDHHS). (1995). *State oversight of tobacco sales to minors* 1. Rockville, MD: U.S. Department of Health and Human Services, Office of Inspector General.

U.S. General Accounting Office. (2002). *Internet cigarette sales: Giving ATF investigative authority may improve reporting and enforcement.* Washington, DC: Author.

Vincent, T. A., & Trickett, E. J. (1983). Preventive interventions and the human context: Ecological approaches to environmental assessment and change. In R. D. Felner (Ed.), *Preventive psychology: Theory, research and practice* (pp. 67–86). New York: Pergamon Press.

Wakefield, M., Flay, B., Nichter, M., & Giovino, G. (2003). Role of the media in influencing trajectories of youth smoking. *Addiction, 98*(S1), 79–103.

Warner, K. E. (1986). *Selling smoke: Cigarette advertising and public health.* Washington, DC: American Public Health Association.

Warner, K. E., Butler, J., Cummings, K. M., D'Onofrio, C., Davis, R. M., Flay, B., et al. (1992). Report of the tobacco policy research study group on tobacco marketing and promotion. *Tobacco Control, 1*(Suppl.), S19–S23.

Wicker, A. W. (1979). *An introduction to ecological psychology.* Monterey, CA: Brooks-Cole.

Winett, R. A., King, A. C., & Altman, D. G. (1989). *Health psychology and public health.* New York: Pergamon Press.

Woollery, T., Asma, S., & Sharp, D. (2000). Clean indoor air and youth access restrictions. In P. Jha & F. J. Chaloupka (Eds.), *Tobacco control in developing countries.* Oxford: Oxford University Press.

Psychosocial Barriers to Adherence and Lifestyle Change

23

Summer L. Williams,
M. Robin DiMatteo,
and Kelly B. Haskard

Despite the implications for patients' well-being and the danger of poor health outcomes, nonadherence to treatment and lifestyle recommendations continues to persist. Why do many patients ignore health advice in the face of disease progression, worsening symptoms, and the waste of precious health care dollars? How can the seemingly irrational act of patient nonadherence persist?

Despite decades of research on patient adherence, there remain many unanswered questions about its causes and treatment. Adhering to even a relatively

Acknowledgments: This work was supported by a Robert Wood Johnson Foundation Investigator Award in Health Policy Research, by a grant from the National Institute on Aging 5R03AG27552-02, and by the Committee on Research of the U.C. Riverside Academic Senate. The views expressed in this chapter are those of the authors alone and do not imply endorsement by the funding sources.

445

simple medication regimen can be intimidating, and major lifestyle changes can be daunting as patients face challenges to the management of their daily lives and routines. While some barriers to adhering are practical and relatively straightforward, such as having limited funds to purchase expensive medication, other barriers are more nuanced and complex, involving psychological and social impediments to action.

Patient adherence generally refers to the degree of success a patient has in carrying out prevention or treatment recommendations offered by a health professional (e.g., a nurse or physician) (DiMatteo & DiNicola, 1982). Research suggests that failure to adhere is a widespread problem; between 25% and 40% of patients are nonadherent, depending upon the length and complexity of medical recommendations (DiMatteo, 2004a; DiMatteo, 1994a; Dishman & Buckworth, 1997).

Psychosocial Factors Affecting Patient Adherence

Decades of research on patient adherence have identified myriad correlates. Nearly every psychological, social, interpersonal, and contextual element of patients' lives has been found to bear some relationship to their ability to follow health lifestyle and/or medical treatment recommendations. These correlates tend to fall into three general categories that provide a simple template for organizing and analyzing research findings, and for guiding clinical care. Simply put, in order to adhere, patients need to *know* what they must do to care for themselves, *want* to take those actions, and be *able* to take the necessary steps toward adherence. Thus, cognitive, motivational, and resource-based factors influence adherence. Improving adherence requires the patient's knowledge and understanding of the medical recommendations, the desire and motivation to adhere, and the ability and resources to carry out the required behaviors (DiMatteo & DiNicola, 1982).

Instrumental Communication in Adherence

Knowledge and understanding of the health care regimen requires effective cognitive functioning and planning. Patients forget much of what is told to them in their medical visits; the anxiety and novelty of the medical situation can interfere with their retention of information. Often, patients do not initially understand their medical directives, and as they attempt to adhere their confusion may increase (Kravitz et al., 1993; Ley & Spelman, 1965). Patients' health literacy may initially determine their comprehension of what they are told, and the quality of communication in the physician-patient interaction can serve as a prominent and essential element in determining whether or not the patient can adhere to the medical recommendations offered. Good rapport and a trusting physician-patient relationship can determine whether patients ask essential questions and voice preferences that are likely to guide their health behaviors.

Knowledge and Understanding

The medical visit exchange requires knowledge and understanding of the process of medical care, including the initiation and management of recommended treatments. It is vital, for example, that patients understand various aspects of the medical regimen, including dosage instructions, timing, and other treatment characteristics. When medical regimens and dosing schedules are complex and require habit and lifestyle changes, nonadherence can be as high as 70% (Chesney, 2000; Li, Brown, Ampil, Burton, Yu, & McDonald, 2000). Adherence to exercise, for example, can be as low as 19% (Kravitz et al., 1993).

Language barriers are associated with decreased patient adherence. Further, even when patients understand the *language* of their medical instructions, it can be difficult for them to comprehend the complexity of that information and precisely what is necessary for proper adherence (Williams et al., 1995). Likewise, a patient's beliefs about health and about treatment can influence how they adhere. Research has shown that patients on lifetime daily doses of medication such as antihypertensive treatments often believe that their medication need be taken only when they are symptomatic (Anarella, Roohan, Balistreri, & Gesten, 2004).

Studies indicate that patient satisfaction and adherence to regimen plans are related to the quality of information given and the patient's ability to comprehend it (Falvo & Tippy, 1988; Jolly, Scott, Feied, & Sanford, 1993; Krishal & Baraff, 1993). When patients are of low income, with little education, and have limited access to follow-up care, adherence may be in serious jeopardy. In the emergency department of an urban hospital, where patients were at risk for low adherence because of their limited understanding of treatment, one study found that cartoon illustrations effectively taught patients to properly care for themselves after release from the emergency department (Delp & Jones, 1996). Engaging and easily understood health information may be essential in the provision of information to patients toward the goal of adherence.

Cognitive Functioning, Planning, and Remembering

Planning and implementing the medical regimen can be a complex process requiring careful explanation, as well as scheduling, and tailoring the regimen to the patient's individual needs and circumstances. In a study of adherence to inhaled steroid use among asthmatic patients, direct clinician-to-patient feedback (i.e., constructive, positive discussion about the patient's adherence and problems adhering and information on techniques and strategies to improve adherence), significantly improved patients' adherence to their treatment (Onyirimba et al., 2003).

Recalling crucial information from a medical visit can be challenging, but it is essential that patients return home with a regimen plan they fully understand and have the ability to follow. Confusion about medication often leads to nonadherence, and patient distraction is a common cognitive factor that jeopardizes adherence. After leaving their provider's offices, patients may be able to recall only about 50% of the information given to them about their regimen (Ong, de Haes, Hoos, & Lammes, 1995). One reason may be that providers often speak in medical jargon and use technical medical language with which patients are unfamiliar, threatening patients' ability to understand and retain critical information (Jackson, 1992). Particularly when physicians operate under time limitations, they may fail to fully explain regimen details to their patients. Failure to ask patients to plan and rehearse the regimen in the presence of the physician can reduce the chances of patient adherence

(Stanton, 1987). Research has suggested the value of adherence-enhancing strategies such as additional treatment education and the use of adherence aids (e.g., medication lists, dosette boxes) (George, Kong, Thoman, & Stewart, 2005).

Patient Involvement

During the medical interaction, physicians may fail to take into account the patient's perspective on illness and thus fail to incorporate patients' explanations and concerns when reviewing presenting symptoms. Research has found that patients specifically mention their main concerns to their physicians in only 24% of all encounters (Korsch & Negrete, 1972). When patients are encouraged by their physicians to share their concerns and when physicians engage in active listening, use focused questions, follow up on patient cues, and engage patients in their interpretations of their conditions, patients tend to be more satisfied and reveal more adherence-relevant information to their providers (Lang, Floyd, Beine, & Buck, 2002).

Health Literacy

Limited literacy skills and poor understanding of spoken and written health information may be the larger and more problematic context in which nonadherence occurs, however (Davis et al., 1996, 1998; Williams et al., 1995). The concept of health literacy has gained considerable research attention in recent years and has broad effects on patients' adherence to treatment, as well as on healthy lifestyle practices. Health literacy can involve health knowledge and information about the body, disease, health risks, and the organization and functioning of the health care system, medical vocabulary, basic health concepts, and many other medically related issues; it is strongly related to overall literacy and can influence what happens with patients before they arrive at the medical visit. Health literacy affects the use of preventive measures such as screening and immunizations (Holloway et al., 2003; Lerman et al., 1992) and offers a context in which patients can interpret their symptoms and identify their need for medical treatment.

Health literacy can affect patient adherence at several points in the process of care, including visit preparation. It also touches on patient's skills and efficacy in identifying the details of precipitating events and symptoms and their reporting of actions they have taken to manage the condition. Health literacy affects patients' awareness of strategies available for risk avoidance and reduction, medical decision making, and participation in care, and it is essential for patient communication with the physician. Health literacy also influences how patients access health care information (e.g., through printed materials, Internet resources, or information and communication-technology resources) and media health issues to which patients attend (Eysenbach & Kohler, 2002; Query & Wright, 2003; Walters, Wright, & Shegog, 2006). Culturally competent health care contexts are also centrally important to adherence. Race, ethnicity, and language can affect the physician-patient relationship; minority patients who are not proficient in English are less likely to engender empathic communication from their physicians, are less likely to have good rapport with their physicians, and are less likely to receive adequate health information and to be encouraged to ask questions and be more active in their care (Ferguson & Candib, 2002).

Low health literacy is likely to affect adherence in multiple ways before, during, and after the medical visit (Kalichman, Ramachandran, & Catz, 1999) and has been linked to poor physician-patient communication, depression, and the quality of patients' conversations with their physicians (Schillinger et al., 2003; Kalichman et al., 1999). Low levels of health literacy can exacerbate chronic disease by leading to poor management or failure to use preventive health measures (DiMatteo, 1994a; DiMatteo & DiNicola, 1982; Dunbar-Jacob & Sereika, 2001; Health Literacy, 2004; Shumaker, Schron, & Ockene, 1998). Patients who are low in health literacy may be less likely to understand the risks and benefits of their treatments, putting them at greater risk for nonadherence (Paasche-Orlow et al., 2005). Among asthma patients, inadequate health literacy and limited knowledge of self-management skills has been associated with having less knowledge of asthma and medications, as well as with less appropriate use of metered-dosed inhalers (MDI) by patients (Paasche-Orlow et al., 2005). With complex regimens, such as those required for HIV patients, those with low health literacy were at greater risk for nonadherence to combination antiretroviral (ARV) therapies (Kalichman et al., 1999). Such patients also tend to have greater difficulty in the management of their illness and in implementing physician directives about care. Adherence to preoperative surgery recommendations, while generally poor in the elderly population, is an even greater problem for patients with low levels of health literacy, who have greater difficulty deciphering instructions from their physicians and understanding information given to them in printed pamphlets (Chew, Bradley, Flum, Cornia, & Koepsell, 2004). The potential difficulties presented by nonadherence to preoperative instructions can include increased morbidity, delays in surgery, surgery cancellations, and even increased risk or operative mortality (Chew et al., 2004).

Research suggests that adherence to disease management strategies partially depends on patients' confidence in their ability to exercise management options. Low health literacy threatens essential aspects of patients' relationship to their illness, and, without the skills and efficacy to gather essential management information (e.g., by asking questions and communicating clearly with health care providers), patients may remain unaware of the strategies available to them for improved adherence. Inadequate access to medical information or to the health care system may lead patients to have difficulty following recommended instructions (e.g., follow-up appointments, visits to specialists) and to feelings of discouragement.

Physician Communication and Empathy

Effective communication in provider-patient interaction requires that a physician demonstrate empathy, understanding of patients' feelings, trust, and rapport with patients. If a provider attends to biomedical issues alone, neglecting patients' emotional needs, the therapeutic relationship may fail, threatening the interpersonal elements necessary for healing and positive outcomes. Trust, open communication between provider and patient, and interpersonal rapport have been associated with patients' greater willingness to seek care and better adherence to treatment recommendations (Trachtenberg, Dugan, & Hall, 2005). Early research on adherence identified the physician-patient interaction as an essential element in care and found that adherence was enhanced both when patients were able to release tension in their interaction and when their questions received a response from the physician (Davis, 1968). Physician-patient rapport is essential to motivating patients to adhere (Jahng, Martin, Golin, & DiMatteo, 2005). Research findings demonstrate that patient satisfaction with physicians' *affective concern* is more important than patient satisfaction with physicians' technical competence in determining patients' commitment to treatment plans (Segall & Burnett, 1980). A provider's collaborative communication style influences treatment outcomes, including patient adherence, by enhancing the patient's knowledge of the medical regimen and by encouraging patients' commitment to and confidence in the regimen and their ability to follow it (Bultman & Svarstad, 2000).

Several interpersonal behaviors, both verbal and nonverbal, on the part of the physician have been found to foster patient outcomes such as recall of medical information and adherence to prescribed treatment (DiMatteo, 1994a). Verbal behaviors such as direct expressions of empathy, reassurance, support, patient-centered questioning, humor, psychosocial talk, health education and information-sharing, friendliness, and summarizing and clarifying the interaction have been associated with both patient satisfaction and adherence (Beck, Daughtridge, & Sloane, 2002). Likewise, nonverbal behaviors such as nodding the head, leaning forward, using a direct body orientation, uncrossing the arms and legs, placing the arms in a symmetrical position, and engaging in a limited amount of mutual gaze have been associated with patient satisfaction and adherence (Beck et al, 2002).

Adherence is greatest when patients feel that their expectations for the visit are being met and when providers elicit and respect patients' concerns and provide responsive information and feedback concerning the condition, diagnosis, method for treatment, and plan for adherence. Strategies for improved provider-patient communication may include ensuring that patients' health concerns are being addressed, taking patients' concerns seriously, asking questions of the patient and engaging in active listening, and determining the potential barriers that might impede the patient's knowledge and acceptance of the importance of the regimen. By taking steps toward improved patient health literacy and better provider-patient communication built on trust, respect, honesty, and integrity, health care providers can contribute directly to patients' adherence to their recommendations.

Motivational Elements in Adherence

Patients' motivations to adhere to lifestyle change and therapeutic regimens depend upon their health beliefs, perceptions, motivations, expectations about medical care and the health care system, and cultural values. Is the patient positive and optimistic or negative about treatment or recommended health behaviors? Does the patient believe that he can follow recommendations and fit those recommendations in with his lifestyle? And, is the patient willing to commit to behavioral changes and adopt new health behaviors and practices? Addressing these issues with patients and exploring their thoughts and beliefs about care may be essential to promoting patient adherence.

Patients' Perceptions: Health Beliefs, Attitudes, and Expectations

Patients' subjective health perceptions reflect their feelings, attitudes, and beliefs about their health status and about health care; such factors can influence patients' health decisions and participation in health behavior change (Olfson, Gilbert, Weissman, Blacklow, & Broadhead, 1995; Sewitch, Leffondre, & Dobkin, 2004; Sherbourne, Hays, Ordway, DiMatteo, & Kravitz, 1992). Patients' beliefs about their condition can strongly influence their behavior, and providers must thoughtfully and thoroughly listen to patients' concerns if they are to have an influence on their beliefs (Becker & Maiman, 1980). In posttransplant care, for example, patients may develop a false sense of security due to improved immunosuppressive drugs. Unrealistic beliefs in the power of a medication to cure, rather than simply manage, a condition such as renal transplant may interfere with patients' rigorous adherence to their posttransplant regimen (Rodriguez, Diaz, Colon, & Santiago-Delpin, 1991).

Beliefs about medication, particularly about side effects, can also be robust predictors of patient adherence; lower adherence is reported among patients who believe that their medication causes problematic side effects (Horne & Weinman, 1999). Between 30% and 83% of patients who begin antidepressant medication discontinue treatment prematurely, often because of incorrect beliefs about the value and the dangers of antidepressant medication (Aikens, Nease, Nau, Klinkman, & Schwenk, 2005). Patients' beliefs in treatment efficacy can also influence adherence. In a sample of Mexican-American women receiving dialysis treatment, adherence was related to the perceived efficacy of the regimen required of them. Those who believed, because they experienced no ill effects, that their nutritional and fluid restrictions made no difference in their outcome were much less likely to adhere than were those who believed in the regimen's efficacy (Tijerina, 2006).

Patients' perceptions of and experiences with the health system can also influence their adherence to treatment and medical recommendations. In one study of ethnically diverse, economically disadvantaged patients with rheumatoid arthritis and systemic lupus, nonadherence to treatment was correlated with patients' difficulties navigating the health care system and obtaining public funding (Garcia Popa-Lisseanu et al., 2005).

Physicians' understanding of their patients' health perceptions can have a positive impact on many health outcomes, particularly adherence (Chesney, Brown, Poe, & Gary, 1983; Starfield, Wray, Hess, Gross, Birk, & D'Lugoff, 1981; Stewart, McWhinney, & Buck, 1979). Physicians who seek to understand the health beliefs of their patients (such as those with HIV, who face the challenges of taking antiretroviral medications) and who educate their patients on the benefits of antiretroviral therapy can help improve their adherence (Schneider, Kaplan, Greenfield, Li, & Wilson, 2004). Strategies to improve adherence are most likely to be successful if they include attempts to modify patients' beliefs and perceptions regarding medication effectiveness and to address patients' concerns and fears about the risk of side effects (Garcia Popa-Lisseanu et al., 2005).

Patients' Cultural Background

Patients' unique social contexts, ethnicity, and cultural backgrounds are central factors that affect their adherence (Freimuth & Quinn, 2004). In a study of colorectal cancer screening, for example, researchers found that subjective norms, emotional support from family and friends, perceived behavioral control (over colorectal cancer screening), and perceived benefit of screening for colorectal cancer served to mediate the pathway from patients' contextual environment to adherence (Freimuth & Quinn, 2004).

Patients' cultural beliefs are often intricately tied to their health beliefs and illness perceptions; both personal and cultural beliefs influence medication taking and lifestyle changes (Gould, 1999; Rudd, 1993). Among elderly patients (over the age of 65 years), adherence can be less than optimal, often because of personal and cultural beliefs (Chia, Schlenk, & Dunbar-Jacob, 2006). African American older adults have been found to express more negative opinions or suspicions about their physician's recommendations than nonminority patients, and their distrust was found to relate to ethnic disparities in quality of care (Siegel, Karus, & Schrimshaw, 2000).

The Illness Behavior Model attempts to better understand the connections among patients' culture, health behaviors, and adherence (McHugh & Vallis, 1985). This model views an individual's response to illness as resulting from the dynamic interaction of factors clustering around four major dimensions: physiological, affective, cognitive, and phenomenological. These dimensions are shaped by the individual's ethnocultural context, within which day-to-day circumstances influence the individual's beliefs, norms, and experience of illness.

Central to adherence and health behavior change are the patient's motivation to follow medical recommendations, the belief that they are worth adhering to, and confidence in the ability to follow them. Overall, patients' health beliefs, attitudes, cognitions, health perceptions, expectations, and motivations can determine their success or failure with the regimen. Management of these elements of the patient's response to health care recommendations is a central task of the physician-patient relationship; thus, it is critical that health professionals listen to what their patients reveal about their motivations and establish treatment goals together with and individualized to their patient's needs and circumstances.

The Necessity of Resources

Resources, both practical and emotional, can strongly influence patient adherence to treatment; patients' socioeconomic status, education, and income can strongly influence their ability to follow through with health recommendations. Economically vulnerable patients, such as those at the poverty level, tend to be considerably less adherent than are patients with financial resources (Tijerina, 2006), and individuals in socially vulnerable subpopulations, such as the elderly, tend to be at increased risk of nonadherence (Balkrishnan, 1998). Limitations in emotional resources and the experience of stress, anxiety, depression, anger, guilt, and withdrawal can also impair a patient's ability to follow through with health behavior changes or to maintain necessary health behaviors (DiMatteo, Lepper, & Croghan, 2000). Social resources can also affect adherence. The degree and type of social support available to a patient is largely associated with the patient's ability to adhere. Without both practical and emotional support for following recommended guidelines for treatment, patients often have difficulty managing their illnesses (DiMatteo, 2004b).

Distressed Psychological States

Depression

Depression can thwart adequate adherence and improvements in health behavior for a number of reasons. Depression involves hopelessness and pessimism, making any positive action seem futile and undermining positive expectations about treatment efficacy (DiMatteo et al., 1993). Depression is also associated with social isolation and withdrawal from friends and family, limiting access to the social support that is essential to patient adherence (DiMatteo, 1994b; DiMatteo & DiNicola, 1982). Depression may also be associated with decreased cognitive functioning and diminished ability to concentrate, plan, and remember to follow through with recommendations and new health behaviors (Carson, Butcher, & Mineka, 2002). Mental health problems, particularly depression, are common among patients with serious diseases such as HIV and cancer and painful conditions such as arthritis, and can contribute to poor adherence (Morrison et al., 2002; Taal, Rasker, Seydel, & Wiegman, 1993; Tucker et al., 2004; Turner et al., 2001).

Despite the important role played by psychological problems in threatening patient adherence, physicians often fail to recognize or refer patients for psychological services or treatment (Badger et al., 1994; Higgins, 1994; Mechanic, 1992). Many physicians view psychological problems as common and as normal concomitants of illness (Peyrot et al., 2005; Thompson et al., 2000). Patients' mental health needs to be considered, however, and interventions are essential to address this important barrier to adherence.

Anxiety and Stress

The relationship of anxiety and stress to adherence is variable across a number of studies, and the exact relationship is not yet fully understood (DiMatteo et al., 2000). Anxiety can range from panic to obsessive-compulsive behaviors and generalized anxiety about health; anxiety is often comorbid with depression, and its unique effects are difficult to determine (Mineka, Watson, & Clark, 1998). Nonetheless, both disorders tap into negative affect such as distress, anger, fear, worry, and guilt (Watson et al., 1995), which can negatively affect the practice of health behaviors and adherence to medical recommendations (Ng & Jeffery, 2003). Worry often characterizes the experience of many ill patients, who fear that their illness will progress and prevent them from living their lives as they wish. Many also worry about their inability to work and to carry out family responsibilities while ill, about their financial futures, and about the effect of illness on their appearance (Peyrot et al., 2005). Psychological distress can influence patients' perceptions of support and contribute to negative social interactions, further reducing the practical and emotional social support available to them (Alferi, Carver, Antoni, Weiss, & Duran, 2001; Coyne, 1976).

Social Support

Social support benefits health by acting as a buffer against stress, influencing health behaviors and affective states (Cohen, 1988), and allowing individuals to take more positive action toward adherence (Wallston, Alagna, & DeVellis,

1983). Support from friends and family can encourage an individual to be optimistic, have increased self-esteem, less depression and pessimism, better sick-role behavior, and increased functional and emotional support during difficult times (Shumaker & Hill, 1991). Social support can also influence an individual's ability to adjust to and live with illness (Hegelson & Cohen, 1996), including adhering to treatment (DiMatteo, 2004b).

Social support comes in many forms, such as functional and tangible support, emotional support, and informational support. Functional social support (e.g., physical resources, information) has been shown to have stronger effects on adherence than structural social support (e.g., number of family members), suggesting that it is the *quality* of the relationships that the individual has with others rather than the number of friends and family (DiMatteo, 2004b). The value of social support for adherence may partially depend upon the type and severity of the individual's illness and the complexity of the treatment regimen (Martin, Davis, Baron, Suls, & Blanchard, 1994; Penninx et al., 1998). Patients who underwent coronary artery bypass surgery and who had significant emotional support demonstrated better emotional status (evidenced less anxiety and depression) and adhered better to recommended lifestyle changes and medication regimens than similar patients without such support (Kulik & Mahler, 1993).

The social control hypothesis theorizes that the presence of close others may facilitate adherence through the internalization of norms conducive to good health and the experience of sanctions for deviating from those norms (Lewis & Rook, 1999). Nonsupportive social networks, on the other hand, can actually work against patient adherence and positive health behavior change by robbing the patient of the time and energy to effectively manage an illness or engage in a healthier lifestyle (Kaplan & Hartwell, 1987; Revicki & May, 1985). Meta-analysis shows that, overall, the following social support variables are positively associated with higher levels of patient adherence: practical support, emotional support, unidimensional social support, family cohesiveness, being married, and living with someone (DiMatteo, 2004b). Low social support has been found to be related to biological and physiological variables such as increased prostate-specific antigen levels (Stone, Mezzacappa, Donatone, & Gonder, 1999), and patients with poor social support are less likely to adhere to their ARV medication regimens (HIV), although many do not recognize that their social support can play a role in their adherence (Catz, Kelly, Bogart, Benotsch, & McAuliffe, 2000; Gifford et al., 2000; Gordillo, del Amo, Soriano, & Gonzalez-Lahoz, 1999).

Social support can improve patient adherence by enhancing cognitive functioning, self-efficacy, intrinsic motivation, sense of personal control, confidence, self-esteem, mood, and by reducing emotional conflict, interpersonal strain, distress, and depression (DiMatteo, 2004b). Strong social ties can help a great deal in combating the psychosocial difficulties that threaten adherence to treatment.

Patient Adjustment to Illness

Psychosocial adjustment to illness can strongly influence the adherence process. Research shows that up to 30% of women with breast cancer fail to complete necessary chemotherapy following mastectomy, often as a result of psychological distress (Gilbar & De-Nour, 1989). Those who drop out or fail to follow through with treatment tend to have greater difficulty adjusting psychologically to their illnesses and adapting to the changes in functioning brought about by the illness in various areas of their lives. Cancer patients undergoing chemotherapy often must deal with many sources of stress arising from threats to bodily comfort, changes in self-perception, emotional variability, changes in social roles, threats to future plans, and day-to-day life hassles (Gilbar & De-Nour, 1989). Patients with cancer often deal with identity losses resulting from changed body image, heightened awareness of death, and family stressors such as family conflict; those with more stressors are more likely to be nonadherent (Tijerina, 2006).

Socioeconomic Status, Education, and Income

A patient's socioeconomic status (SES), education level, and income can strongly influence adherence. Lifestyle change may be difficult, or impossible, in the context of significant social and economic vulnerability. Factors such as lack of transportation and child care, unfamiliarity with the medical care system, and lack of or inadequate medical insurance coverage can threaten adherence, adding to the growing concern that economic disparities exist in the U.S. health care system. Patients with lower incomes, less education, and lower socioeconomic status are likely to face greater challenges to the achievement of good health behavior than those with higher incomes and socioeconomic status.

Lack of resources can constitute a significant impediment to behavior change despite the best of intentions from patients (DiMatteo & Martin, 2002). Economic vulnerability can lead to discontent, and even depression, and can contribute to limitations in adherence (Brand, Smith, & Brand, 1977). Low levels of education are often associated with poor adherence, and research on diabetics has found that low levels of education are associated with poor glycemic control (Lloyd, Wing, Orchard, & Becker, 1993). Cancer patients of lower socioeconomic status have lower rates of adherence to their chemotherapy medical regimens than those of higher socioeconomic status, likely because they possess fewer coping resources and are more vulnerable to the effects of illness on their lives (Lebovits et al., 1990). Research has shown that low socioeconomic status (SES) and low income strongly influence disease screening activities, as well as interactions with health care providers, especially among women patients. Women of lower SES continue to be less likely to receive adequate screening for breast cancer than those of high SES (O'Malley, Forrest, & Mandelblatt, 2002). Screening rates tend to rise, however, when physicians discuss mammography screening in a primary-care setting with low SES women and are enthusiastic about the screening (Friedman, Puryear, Moore, & Green, 2005).

Subpopulations

Patients who face limited resources in their later years often have difficulty adhering to medical regimens and lifestyle changes. Many older adults experience reductions in their income and health care insurance as they enter retirement, introducing significant challenges and limitations in the quality of health care coverage they receive (Chen & Landefeld, 2007). Despite government health care programs for older adults (Medicare), elderly adults often must pay for many of their medical expenses out-of-pocket, jeopardizing the use of preventive services and putting them at risk for poor management and control of disease (Sudano & Baker, 2006). Older patients often have more chronic conditions than others and as a result may receive prescriptions for a greater number of medications. Other changes that accompany aging also may negatively affect patient adherence (Balkrishnan, 1998). Elderly patients tend to be less likely to ask questions and be actively involved in their care, often leave the medical visit with questions unanswered, and are unclear about what they are supposed to do to care for themselves (Breemhaar, Visser, & Kleijnen, 1990; DiMatteo, Hays, & Sherbourne, 1992). To be effective in communicating and treating elderly patients, physicians must take factors that affect their elderly patient's adherence into account.

A patient's race, ethnicity, language, and income status all pose challenges to proper adherence. Many studies have documented these disparities in health care and their effects on patient adherence. Effective physician-patient communication is essential to adherence success, yet studies have shown that minority patients rate their medical visits as less participatory than do White patients (Cooper-Patrick et al., 1999). Minority patients also report less positive perceptions of their physicians and have less trust in their physicians than do White patients (Doescher, Saver, Franks, & Fiscella, 2000). Many poor and underserved women experience a lack of continuity and quality in their care and thus can develop distrust of the medical interaction and in their physicians (LaVeist, Keith, & Gutierrez, 1995). Trust is essential, however, and is significantly related to treatment continuity and to adherence (Safran et al., 1998; Thom, Ribisl, Stewart, & Luke, 1999).

A variety of patient psychosocial variables can interfere with the ability to adhere to a medical regimen, even if the patient understands what to do and is motivated. Helping patients overcome barriers has the potential to greatly increase the likelihood that they will follow through with medical recommendations and lifestyle changes.

Summary and Conclusion

Each of the psychosocial variables discussed in this chapter plays an important role in shaping patients' knowledge and understanding of their illness and medical treatment, in shaping their beliefs in the efficacy of the prescribed regimen, in motivating them to follow through with recommended health behaviors, and in shaping their ability to carry out the behaviors required to adhere effectively to treatment. Health care professionals and providers have at their disposal a variety of means to enhance patients' knowledge and understanding of, and beliefs in, treatment, as well as to improve the provider-patient relationship and to deal effectively with the barriers faced by a diverse population of patients. By examining and carefully attending to the steps involved in adherence to medical recommendations, providers can begin to untangle the web of psychosocial factors that may impede a patient's adherence to medical recommendations and health behavior change and thereby ultimately help to improve patients' health care outcomes.

References

Aikens, J. E., Nease, D. E., Jr., Nau, D. P., Klinkman, M. S., & Schwenk, T. L. (2005). Adherence to maintenance-phase antidepressant medication as a function of patient beliefs about medication. *Annals of Family Medicine, 3*(1), 23–30.

Alferi, S. M., Carver, C. S., Antoni, M. H., Weiss, S., & Duran, R. E. (2001). An exploratory study of social support, distress, and life disruption among low-income Hispanic women under treatment for early stage breast cancer. *Health Psychology, 20*(1), 41–46.

Anarella, J., Roohan, P., Balistreri, E., & Gesten, F. (2004). A survey of Medicaid recipients with asthma: perceptions of self-management, access, and care. *Chest, 125*(4), 1359–1367.

Badger, L. W., DeGruy, F. V., Hartman, J., Plant, M. A., Lepper, J., Anderson, R., et al. (1994). Patient presentation, interview, consent, and the detection of depression by primary care physicians. *Psychosomatic Medicine, 56,* 128–135.

Balkrishnan, R. (1998). Predictors of medication adherence in the elderly. *Clinical Therapeutics, 20*(4), 764–771.

Beck, R. S., Daughtridge, R., & Sloane, P. D. (2002). Physician-patient communication in the primary care office: A systematic review. *Journal of the American Board of Family Practice, 15*(1), 25–38.

Becker, M. H., & Maiman, L. A. (1980). Strategies for enhancing patient compliance. *Journal of Community Health, 6*(2), 113–135.

Brand, F. N., Smith, R. T., & Brand, P. A. (1977). Effect of economic barriers to medical care on patients' noncompliance. *Public Health Reports, 92*(1), 72–78.

Breemhaar, B., Visser, A. P., & Kleijnen, J. G. (1990). Perceptions and behaviour among elderly hospital patients: Description and explanation of age differences in satisfaction, knowledge, emotions and behaviour. *Social Science and Medicine, 31*(12), 1377–1385.

Bultman, D. C., & Svarstad, B. L. (2000). Effects of physician communication style on client medication beliefs and adherence with antidepressant treatment. *Patient Education and Counseling, 40*(2), 173–185.

California Health Literacy Initiative. (2000). *Healthy people 2010. U.S. Department of Health and Human Services. Understanding and improving health: Objectives for improving health* (2nd ed.). Washington, DC: Government Printing Office.

Carson, R. C., Butcher, J. N., & Mineka, S. (2002). *Fundamentals of abnormal psychology and modern life.* Boston: Allyn & Bacon.

Catz, S. L., Kelly, J. A., Bogart, L. M., Benotsch, E. G., & McAuliffe, T. L. (2000). Patterns, correlates, and barriers to medication adherence among persons prescribed new treatments for HIV disease. *Health Psychology, 19*(2), 124–133.

Chen, H., & Landefeld, S. C. (2007). The hidden poor: Care of the elderly. In W. M. King (Ed.), *Medical management of vulnerable and underserved patients* (pp. 199–209). New York: McGraw-Hill.

Chesney, A. P., Brown, K. A., Poe, C. W., & Gary, H. E., Jr. (1983). Physician-patient agreement on symptoms as a predictor of retention in outpatient care. *Hospital and Community Psychiatry, 34*(8), 737–739.

Chesney, M. A. (2000). Factors affecting adherence to antiretroviral therapy. *Clinical Infectious Diseases, 30*(Suppl.2), S171–176.

Chew, L. D., Bradley, K. A., Flum, D. R., Cornia, P. B., & Koepsell, T. D. (2004). The impact of low health literacy on surgical practice. *American Journal of Surgery, 188*(3), 250–253.

Chia, L. R., Schlenk, E. A., & Dunbar-Jacob, J. (2006). Effect of personal and cultural beliefs on medication adherence in the elderly. *Drugs and Aging, 23*(3), 191–202.

Cohen, S. (1988). Psychosocial models of the role of social support in the etiology of physical disease. *Health Psychology, 7*(3), 269–297.

Cooper-Patrick, L., Gallo, J. J., Gonzales, J. J., Vu, H. T., Powe, N. R., Nelson, C., et al. (1999). Race, gender, and partnership in the patient-physician relationship. *Journal of the American Medical Association, 282*(6), 583–589.

Coyne, J. C. (1976). Depression and the response of others. *Journal of Abnormal Psychology, 85*(2), 186–193.

Davis, M. S. (1968). Variations in patients' compliance with doctors' advice: An empirical analysis of patterns of communication. *American Journal of Public Health, 58*(2), 274–288.

Davis, T. C., Bocchini, J. A., Jr., Fredrickson, D., Arnold, C., Mayeaux, E. J., Murphy, P. W., et al. (1996). Parent comprehension of polio vaccine information pamphlets. *Pediatrics, 97*(6 Pt. 1), 804–810.

Davis, T. C., Fredrickson, D. D., Arnold, C., Murphy, P. W., Herbst, M., & Bocchini, J. A. (1998). A polio immunization pamphlet with increased appeal and simplified language does not improve comprehension to an acceptable level. *Patient Education and Counseling, 33*(1), 25–37.

Delp, C., & Jones, J. (1996). Communicating information to patients: The use of cartoon illustrations to improve comprehension of instructions. *Academic Emergency Medicine, 3*(3), 264–270.

DiMatteo, M. R. (1994a). Enhancing patient adherence to medical recommendations. *Journal of the American Medical Association, 271*(1), 79–83.

DiMatteo, M. R. (1994b). The physician-patient relationship: Effects on the quality of health care. *Clinical Obstetrics and Gynecology, 37*(1), 149–161.

DiMatteo, M. R. (2004a). Social support and patient adherence to medical treatment: A meta-analysis. *Health Psychology, 23*(2), 207–218.

DiMatteo, M. R. (2004b). Variations in patients' adherence to medical recommendations: A quantitative review of 50 years of research. *Medical Care, 42*(3), 200–209.

DiMatteo, M. R., & DiNicola, D. D. (1982). *Achieving patient compliance: The psychology of the medical practitioner's role.* New York: Pergamon Press.

DiMatteo, M. R., Hays, R. D., Gritz, E. R., Bastani, R., Crane, L., Elashoff, R., et al. (1993). Patient adherence to cancer control regimens: Scale development and initial validation. *Psychological Assessment, 5*(1), 102–112.

DiMatteo, M. R., Hays, R. D., & Sherbourne, C. D. (1992). Adherence to cancer regimens: Implications for treating the older patient. *Oncology (Williston Park), 6*(2 Suppl.), 50–57.

DiMatteo, M. R., Lepper, H. S., & Croghan, T. W. (2000). Depression is a risk factor for noncompliance with medical treatment: Meta-analysis of the effects of anxiety and depression on patient adherence. *Archives of Internal Medicine, 160*(14), 2101–2107.

DiMatteo, M. R., & Martin, L. R. (2002). *Health psychology.* Boston: Allyn & Bacon.

Dishman, R. K., & Buckworth, J. (1997). Adherence to physical activity. In W. P. Morgan (Ed.), *Physical activity and mental health.* Washington, DC: Taylor & Francis.

Doescher, M. P., Saver, B. G., Franks, P., & Fiscella, K. (2000). Racial and ethnic disparities in perceptions of physician style and trust. *Archives of Family Medicine, 9*(10), 1156–1163.

Dunbar-Jacob, J., & Sereika, S. M. (2001). Conceptual and methodological problems. In L. E. Burke & I. S. Ockene (Eds.), *Compliance in healthcare and research* (pp. 93–104). Armonk, NY: Futura.

Eysenbach, G., & Kohler, C. (2002). How do consumers search for and appraise health information on the world wide web? Qualitative study using focus groups, usability tests, and in-depth interviews. *British Medical Journal, 324*(7337), 573–577.

Falvo, D., & Tippy, P. (1988). Communicating information to patients. Patient satisfaction and adherence as associated with resident skill. *Journal of Family Practice, 26*(6), 643–647.

Ferguson, W. J., & Candib, L. M. (2002). Culture, language, and the doctor-patient relationship. *Family Medicine, 34*(5), 353–361.

Finney Rutten, L. J., & Iannotti, R. J. (2003). Health beliefs, salience of breast cancer family history, and involvement with breast cancer issues: Adherence to annual mammography screening recommendations. *Cancer Detection and Prevention, 27*(5), 353–359.

Freimuth, V. S., & Quinn, S. C. (2004). The contributions of health communication to eliminating health disparities. *American Journal of Public Health, 94*(12), 2053–2055.

Friedman, L. C., Puryear, L. J., Moore, A., & Greene, C. E. (2005). Breast and colorectal cancer screening among low-income women with psychiatric disorders. *Psychooncology, 14*(9), 786–91.

Garcia Popa-Lisseanu, M. G., Greisinger, A., Richardson, M., O'Malley, K. J., Janssen, N. M., Marcus, D. M., et al. (2005). Determinants of treatment adherence in ethnically diverse, economically disadvantaged patients with rheumatic disease. *Journal of Rheumatology, 32*(5), 913–919.

George, J., Kong, D. C., Thoman, R., & Stewart, K. (2005). Factors associated with medication nonadherence in patients with COPD. *Chest, 128*(5), 3198–3204.

Gifford, A. L., Bormann, J. E., Shively, M. J., Wright, B. C., Richman, D. D., & Bozzette, S. A. (2000). Predictors of self-reported adherence and plasma HIV concentrations in patients on multidrug antiretroviral regimens. *Journal of the Acquired Immune Deficiency Syndrome, 23*(5), 386–395.

Gilbar, O., & De-Nour, A. K. (1989). Adjustment to illness and dropout of chemotherapy. *Journal of Psychosomatic Research, 33*(1), 1–5.

Gordillo, V., del Amo, J., Soriano, V., & Gonzalez-Lahoz, J. (1999). Sociodemographic and psychological variables influencing adherence to antiretroviral therapy. *AIDS, 13*(13), 1763–1769.

Gould, O. N. (1999). Cognition and socio-affective factors in medication adherence. In D. C. Park, R. W. Morrell, & K. Shifren (Eds.), *Processing of medical information in aging patients: Cognitive and human factors perspectives.* Hillsdale, NJ: Erlbaum.

Health Literacy. (2004). *A prescription to end the confusion.* Washington, DC: Institute of Medicine.

Helgeson, V. S., & Cohen, S. (1996). Social support and adjustment to cancer: Reconciling descriptive, correlational, and intervention research. *Health Psychology, 15*(2), 135–148.

Higgins, E. S. (1994). A review of unrecognized mental illness in primary care. Prevalence, natural history, and efforts to change the course. *Archives of Family Medicine, 3*(10), 908–917.

Holloway, R. M., Wilkinson, C., Peters, T. J., Russell, I., Cohen, D., Hale, J., et al. (2003). Cluster-randomised trial of risk communication to enhance informed uptake of cervical screening. *British Journal of General Practice, 53*(493), 620–625.

Horne, R., & Weinman, J. (1999). Patients' beliefs about prescribed medicines and their role in adherence to treatment in chronic physical illness. *Journal of Psychosomatic Research, 47*(6), 555–567.

Jackson, L. D. (1992). Information complexity and medical communication: The effects of technical language and amount of information in a medical message. *Health Communication, 4,* 197–210.

Jahng, K. H., Martin, L. R., Golin, C. E., & DiMatteo, M. R. (2005). Preferences for medical collaboration: patient-physician congruence and patient outcomes. *Patient Education and Counseling, 57*(3), 308–314.

Jolly, B. T., Scott, J. L., Feied, C. F., & Sanford, S. M. (1993). Functional illiteracy among emergency department patients: A preliminary study. *Annals of Emergency Medicine, 22*(3), 573–578.

Kalichman, S. C., Ramachandran, B., & Catz, S. (1999). Adherence to combination antiretroviral therapies in HIV patients of low health literacy. *Journal of General Internal Medicine, 14*(5), 267–273.

Kaplan, R. M., & Hartwell, S. L. (1987). Differential effects of social support and social network on physiological and social outcomes in men and women with type II diabetes mellitus. *Health Psychology, 6*(5), 387–398.

Korsch, B. M., & Negrete, V. F. (1972). Doctor-patient communication. *Scientific American, 227*(2), 66–74.

Kravitz, R. L., Hays, R. D., Sherbourne, C. D., DiMatteo, M. R., Rogers, W. H., Ordway, L., et al. (1993). Recall of recommendations and adherence to advice among patients with chronic medical conditions. *Archives of Internal Medicine, 153*(16), 1869–1878.

Krishel, S., & Baraff, L. J. (1993). Effect of emergency department information on patient satisfaction. *Annals of Emergency Medicine, 22*(3), 568–572.

Kulik, J. A., & Mahler, H. I. (1993). Emotional support as a moderator of adjustment and compliance after coronary artery bypass surgery: A longitudinal study. *Journal of Behavioral Medicine, 16*(1), 45–63.

Lang, F., Floyd, M. R., Beine, K. L., & Buck, P. (2002). Sequenced questioning to elicit the patient's perspective on illness: Effects on information disclosure, patient satisfaction, and time expenditure. *Family Medicine, 34*(5), 325–330.

LaVeist, T. A., Keith, V. M., & Gutierrez, M. L. (1995). Black/white differences in prenatal care utilization: An assessment of predisposing and enabling factors. *Health Services Research, 30*(1), 43–58.

Lebovits, A. H., Strain, J. J., Schleifer, S. J., Tanaka, J. S., Bhardwaj, S., & Messe, M. R. (1990). Patient noncompliance with self-administered chemotherapy. *Cancer, 65*(1), 17–22.

Lerman, C., Hanjani, P., Caputo, C., Miller, S., Delmoor, E., Nolte, S., et al. (1992). Telephone counseling improves adherence to colposcopy among lower-income minority women. *Journal of Clinical Oncology, 10*(2), 330–333.

Lewis, M. A., & Rook, K. S. (1999). Social control in personal relationships: Impact on health behaviors and psychological distress. *Health Psychology, 18*(1), 63–71.

Ley, P., & Spelman, M. S. (1965). Communications in an out-patient setting. *British Journal of Social and Clinical Psychology, 4*(2), 114–116.

Li, B. D., Brown, W. A., Ampil, F. L., Burton, G. V., Yu, H., & McDonald, J. C. (2000). Patient compliance is critical for equivalent clinical outcomes for breast cancer treated by breast-conservation therapy. *Annals of Surgery, 231*(6), 883–889.

Lloyd, C. E., Wing, R. R., Orchard, T. J., & Becker, D. J. (1993). Psychosocial correlates of glycemic control: The Pittsburgh Epidemiology of Diabetes Complications (EDC) Study. *Diabetes Research and Clinical Practice, 21*(2–3), 187–195.

Martin, R., Davis, G. M., Baron, R. S., Suls, J., & Blanchard, E. B. (1994). Specificity in social support: perceptions of helpful and unhelpful provider behaviors among irritable bowel syndrome, headache, and cancer patients. *Health Psychology, 13*(5), 432–439.

McHugh, S., & Vallis, T. M. (1985). *Illness behavior: Operationalization of the biopsychosocial model.* New York: Plenum Press.

Mechanic, D. (1992). Health and illness behavior and patient-practitioner relationships. *Social Science and Medicine, 34*(12), 1345–1350.

Mickey, R. M., Vezina, J. L., Worden, J. K., & Warner, S. L. (1997). Breast screening behavior and interactions with health care providers among lower income women. *Medical Care, 35*(12), 1204–1211.

Mineka, S., Watson, D., & Clark, L. A. (1998). Comorbidity of anxiety and unipolar mood disorders. *Annual Review of Psychology, 49,* 377–412.

Morrison, M. F., Petitto, J. M., Ten Have, T., Gettes, D. R., Chiappini, M. S., Weber, A. L., et al. (2002). Depressive and anxiety disorders in women with HIV infection. *American Journal of Psychiatry, 159*(5), 789–796.

Ng, D. M., & Jeffery, R. W. (2003). Relationships between perceived stress and health behaviors in a sample of working adults. *Health Psychology, 22*(6), 638–642.

Olfson, M., Gilbert, T., Weissman, M., Blacklow, R. S., & Broadhead, W. E. (1995). Recognition of emotional distress in physically healthy primary care patients who perceive poor physical health. *General Hospital Psychiatry, 17*(3), 173–180.

O'Malley, A. S., Forrest, C. B., & Mandelblatt, J. (2002). Adherence of low-income women to cancer screening recommendations. *Journal of General Internal Medicine,* 17(2), 144–154.

Ong, L. M., de Haes, J. C., Hoos, A. M., & Lammes, F. B. (1995). Doctor-patient communication: A review of the literature. *Social Science and Medicine, 40*(7), 903–918.

Onyirimba, F., Apter, A., Reisine, S., Litt, M., McCusker, C., Connors, M., et al. (2003). Direct clinician-to-patient feedback discussion of inhaled steroid use: Its effect on adherence. *Annals of Allergy Asthma and Immunology, 90*(4), 411–415.

Paasche-Orlow, M. K., Riekert, K. A., Bilderback, A., Chanmugam, A., Hill, P., Rand, C. S., et al. (2005). Tailored education may reduce health literacy disparities in asthma self-management. *American Journal of Respiratory and Critical Care Medicine, 172*(8), 980–986.

Penninx, B. W., van Tilburg, T., Boeke, A. J., Deeg, D. J., Kriegsman, D. M., & van Eijk, J. T. (1998). Effects of social support and personal coping resources on depressive symptoms: different for various chronic diseases? *Health Psychology, 17*(6), 551–558.

Peyrot, M., Rubin, R. R., Lauritzen, T., Snoek, F. J., Matthews, D. R., & Skovlund, S. E. (2005). Psychosocial problems and barriers to improved diabetes management: results of the Cross-National Diabetes Attitudes, Wishes and Needs (DAWN) Study. *Diabetic Medicine, 22*(10), 1379–1385.

Query, J. L., Jr., & Wright, K. (2003). Assessing communication competence in an online study: toward informing subsequent interventions among older adults with cancer, their lay caregivers, and peers. *Health Communication, 15*(2), 203–218.

Revieki, D. A., & May, H. J. (1985). Occupational stress, social support, and depression. *Health Psychology, 4,* 61–77.

Rodriguez, A., Diaz, M., Colon, A., & Santiago-Delpin, E. A. (1991). Psychosocial profile of non-compliant transplant patients. *Transplant Proceedings, 23*(2), 1807–1809.

Rudd, P. (1993). The measurement of compliance: Medication taking. In A. Krasnegor, L. Epstein, & S. B. Johnson (Eds.), *Developmental aspects of health compliance behavior.* Hillsdale, NJ: Erlbaum.

Safran, D. G., Taira, D. A., Rogers, W. H., Kosinski, M., Ware, J. E., & Tarlov, A. R. (1998). Linking primary care performance to outcomes of care. *Journal of Family Practice, 47*(3), 213–220.

Schillinger, D., Piette, J., Grumbach, K., Wang, F., Wilson, C., Daher, C., et al. (2003). Closing the loop: Physician communication with diabetic patients who have low health literacy. *Archives of Internal Medicine, 163*(1), 83–90.

Schneider, J., Kaplan, S. H., Greenfield, S., Li, W., & Wilson, I. B. (2004). Better physician-patient relationships are associated with higher reported adherence to antiretroviral therapy in patients with HIV infection. *Journal of General Internal Medicine, 19*(11), 1096–1103.

Segall, A., & Burnett, M. (1980). Patient evaluation of physician role performance. *Social Science and Medicine, 14A*(4), 269–278.

Sewitch, M. J., Leffondre, K., & Dobkin, P. L. (2004). Clustering patients according to health perceptions: Relationships to psychosocial characteristics and medication nonadherence. *Journal of Psychosomatic Research, 56*(3), 323–332.

Sherbourne, C. D., Hays, R. D., Ordway, L., DiMatteo, M. R., & Kravitz, R. L. (1992). Antecedents of adherence to medical recommendations: Results from the Medical Outcomes Study. *Journal of Behavioral Medicine, 15*(5), 447–468.

Shumaker, S. A., & Hill, D. R. (1991). Gender differences in social support and physical health. *Health Psychology, 10*(2), 102–111.

Shumaker, S. A., Schron, E. B., & Ockene, J. K. (1998). *The handbook of health behavior change* (2nd ed.). New York: Springer Publishing Company.

Siegel, K., Karus, D., & Schrimshaw, E. W. (2000). Racial differences in attitudes toward protease inhibitors among older HIV-infected men. *AIDS Care, 12*(4), 423–434.

Stanton, A. L. (1987). Determinants of adherence to medical regimens by hypertensive patients. *Journal of Behavioral Medicine, 10*(4), 377–394.

Starfield, B., Wray, C., Hess, K., Gross, R., Birk, P. S., & D'Lugoff, B. C. (1981). The influence of patient-practitioner agreement on outcome of care. *American Journal of Public Health, 71*(2), 127–131.

Stewart, M. A., McWhinney, I. R., & Buck, C. W. (1979). The doctor/patient relationship and its effect upon outcome. *Journal of the Royal College of General Practitioners, 29*(199), 77–81.

Stone, A. A., Mezzacappa, E. S., Donatone, B. A., & Gonder, M. (1999). Psychosocial stress and social support are associated with prostate-specific antigen levels in men: Results from a community screening program. *Health Psychology, 18*(5), 482–486.

Sudano, J. J., & Baker, D. W. (2006). Explaining U.S. racial/ethnic disparities in health declines and mortality in late middle age: The roles of socioeconomic status, health behaviors, and health insurance. *Social Science and Medicine, 62*(4), 909–922.

Taal, E., Rasker, J. J., Seydel, E. R., & Wiegman, O. (1993). Health status, adherence with health recommendations, self-efficacy and social support in patients with rheumatoid arthritis. *Patient Education and Counseling, 20*(2–3), 63–76.

Thom, D. H., Ribisl, K. M., Stewart, A. L., & Luke, D. A. (1999). Further validation and reliability testing of the Trust in Physician Scale. The Stanford Trust Study Physicians. *Medical Care, 37*(5), 510–517.

Thompson, C., Kinmonth, A. L., Stevens, L., Peveler, R. C., Stevens, A., Ostler, K. J., et al. (2000). Effects of a clinical-practice guideline and practice-based education on detection and outcome of depression in primary care: Hampshire Depression Project randomised controlled trial. *Lancet, 355*(9199), 185–191.

Tijerina, M. S. (2006). Psychosocial factors influencing Mexican-American women's adherence with hemodialysis treatment. *Social Work in Health Care, 43*(1), 57–74.

Trachtenberg, F., Dugan, E., & Hall, M. A. (2005). How patients' trust relates to their involvement in medical care. *Journal of Family Practice, 54*(4), 344–352.

Tucker, J. S., Orlando, M., Burnam, M. A., Sherbourne, C. D., Kung, F. Y., & Gifford, A. L. (2004). Psychosocial mediators of antiretroviral nonadherence in HIV-positive adults with substance use and mental health problems. *Health Psychology, 23*(4), 363–370.

Turner, B. J., Fleishman, J. A., Wenger, N., London, A. S., Burnam, M. A., Shapiro, M. F., et al. (2001). Effects of drug abuse and mental disorders on use and type of antiretroviral therapy in HIV-infected persons. *Journal of General Internal Medicine, 16*(9), 625–633.

Wallston, B. S., Alagna, S. W., & DeVellis, R. F. (1983). Social support and physical health. *Health Psychology, 2,* 367–391.

Walters, S. T., Wright, J. A., & Shegog, R. (2006). A review of computer and Internet-based interventions for smoking behavior. *Addictive Behaviors, 31,* 264–277.

Watson, D., Clark, L. A., Weber, K., Assenheimer, J. S., Strauss, M. E., & McCormick, R. A. (1995). Testing a tripartite model: I. Evaluating the convergent and discriminant validity of anxiety and depression symptom scales. *Journal of Abnormal Psychology, 104,* 3–14.

Williams, M. V., Parker, R. M., Baker, D. W., Parikh, N. S., Pitkin, K., Coates, W. C., et al. (1995). Inadequate functional health literacy among patients at two public hospitals. *Journal of the American Medical Association, 274*(21), 1677–1682.

Changing Clinical Behavior: Implementing Guidelines to Improve Primary Care Practice

24

Elizabeth Dugan,
Katherine Dodd, and
Shellie Ellis

Modifying any human behavior is not easy, and changing the behavior of health care providers presents an even greater challenge because of the many factors that influence clinical practice. Theories of behavior change, a number of them elegantly explained elsewhere in this book, tend to note the importance of two concepts: self-efficacy and the readiness for change. However, interventions to improve clinical behavior require more than targeting a provider's readiness to change or fostering a strong belief that the desired change is possible. Clinical behavior occurs within a complex, and sometimes remarkably dysfunctional, health care system—and each component of the system (e.g., a provider, a practice setting, a state or region, a health maintenance organization, insurance providers, the medical profession, the federal government) exerts forces that may impede or facilitate desired behavior change.

Yet, clinical practice guidelines—the blueprint for desired improvements in clinical behavior—continue to be developed at an impressive rate. There are more than 2,000 guidelines available at the National Guideline Clearinghouse (www.guideline.gov), which is maintained by the Agency for Healthcare Research and Quality (AHRQ) and is, by far, the best-regulated repository of guidelines. AHRQ defines clinical guidelines as systematically developed statements to help patients and providers make decisions about appropriate health care. Guidelines usually contain recommendations about prevention, screening, diagnosing, treating, and living with diseases and conditions. Clinical practice guidelines are valuable because they summarize the vast scientific evidence surrounding a clinical issue and provide guidance as to the best practices for that specific issue. Thus, they are a great help to practitioners who do not have the time, expertise, or interest to carefully evaluate all of the latest research findings about a disease.

It is encouraging to note that the field has grown substantially since the previous edition of this volume. Recognition of the long trajectory of translating research findings into clinical practice—estimated at 17 years (Antman, Lau, Kupelnick, Mosteller, & Chalmers, 1992; Kumar, 1992)—has spurred efforts to address this unacceptable lag. For example, there is now a journal *(Implementation Science)* that focuses on the "scientific study of methods to promote the uptake of research findings into routine healthcare in both clinical and policy contexts" (Eccles & Mittman, 2006). Canada has formed the Improved Clinical Effectiveness Through Behavioral Research Group, which is supported by the Canadian Institutes of Health Research and the Ontario Ministry of Health (ICEBeRG, 2006). In the United States guideline research funding opportunities, such as those funded by the National Institutes of Health, have increased. Finally, theoretical constructs on which to base this research are steadily emerging (Newton et al., 2007; Sladek, Phillips, & Bond, 2006), as is the development of more accurate measures (Hakkennes & Green, 2006). Yet, even with the promising growth in the field, many researchers and clinicians still struggle when trying to improve primary care practices. Despite the development of theory and methods to smooth implementation of effective interventions, there is still often a large gap between the desired and the delivered quality of care.

A systematic review of 235 studies designed to improve practices illustrates the problem. Overall, the interventions showed a very modest impact—in fact, the absolute improvements in care ranged from only 6% to 14.1% (Grimshaw et al., 2006a). Moreover, there are even fewer studies that look beyond the documentation of changes in the processes of care to improvement in patient outcomes, and these demonstrate only modest impact.

Why Is It Hard to Change Clinical Behavior?

Unfortunately, there is often a gap between the best practice as outlined in a clinical practice guideline and what actually happens in everyday clinical practice (McGlynn et al., 2003). Those of us involved in medical education recognize that much of what we teach to medical students and residents is out of date in just a few years because of the rapid development of new medications, medical devices, and procedures. We stress the importance of lifelong learning to our students because they will need to be proactive in order to maintain excellent clinical skills. Guidelines are important learning tools. Yet, there are barriers to their use. The sheer number of guidelines available to study is one barrier. For example, there are guidelines focused on a range of important issues, such as hypertension, diabetes, incontinence, smoking cessation, or depression. Primary-care practice is demanding, and the time pressures are significant. There isn't time to read all the guidelines, and they are not all of the same quality, so the process of how to select the best guideline is unclear.

Another barrier to guideline implementation is the difficulty of objectively assessing one's own clinical performance. Remember that clinical behavior change requires effort. If there is no perceived problem, why would anyone invest the effort to change? Providers may believe they are delivering outstanding care (when they are not), and thus may not be motivated to make any sort of change. Quality reporting (e.g., monitoring of administrative data by health plans to determine if a quality-of-care indicator—like cancer screening mammography—is performed) provides some objective, but limited, information about provider performance.

Individual provider-level factors play a role in clinical behavior change. Cabana et al. (1999) noted six barriers to clinical behavior change: lack of awareness; lack of familiarity; disagreement with the guideline; disbelief that the guideline will result in the intended outcome; lack of self-efficacy to perform the behavior; and practice inertia. Some providers are not ready or prepared to make a change in their clinical behavior.

Similarly, there are patient factors that can impede guideline implementation. For example, patients may be resistant to a change. To illustrate, consider the case of Dr. Kidd, who decided, after attending a seminar, to improve screening for domestic violence in her general internal medicine primary-care practice. To prepare for the change she read up on the topic, became familiar with local resources, and had one of her staff add programmed alerts to her computerized medical record system to remind her to routinely integrate screening questions into the history section of every patient interview. Yet, by the end of the quarter, she noted that a surprisingly large number of patients in her rural Colorado practice were upset about being asked about a stigmatized condition. The patients resisted her *new and improved* clinical behavior. As a result of the patients' reactions, Dr. Kidd reevaluated the situation and decided to drop the domestic-violence screening questions and abandoned her efforts to implement the clinical practice guideline.

Not only do patient and provider factors conspire to impede clinical behavior change, but aspects of the practice setting, such as resources (materials, staff, hours of operation) may also interfere (Gravel, Legare, & Graham, 2006). At the system level, the reimbursement policies of health insurers are potential barriers to clinical improvement. To illustrate, let's consider Dr. Kidd again. She read an alarming article in the *Journal of the American Medical Association* about very high rates of medication errors and serious adverse drug events in older adults. Dr. Kidd wants to talk with all her older patients at every visit about *all* the medications (e.g., prescription, over-the-counter, herbs) they are taking. But she also wants her practice to remain financially solvent and has found that primary-care visits for her older patients tend to take longer than those for her younger patients, because of differences in the average number of chronic conditions that have to be addressed and the numbers of medications prescribed. Yet, insurance reimbursement rates generally do not reflect this reality and pose a barrier to her achieving a potentially life-saving clinical improvement goal. Thus, making this change in clinical behavior will cost her both time and money.

What Interventions Facilitate Clinical Behavior Change?

The best interventions usually focus on more than one component in the system and are described later in this chapter. But multilevel and multimethod interventions are expensive, resource intensive, and difficult to implement. As a result, most clinical behavior change strategies have focused on the individual provider. Typical interventions targeting providers aim to increase knowledge and motivation for change. Printed materials or the recommendation of a respected local opinion leader may be disseminated to providers to facilitate clinical behavior change. Interventions aimed at the systems level include administrative policies, care plans, treatment protocols, provision of free samples, and audit and feedback.

Education Materials and Continuing Medical Education

Continuing medical education (CME) and the distribution of educational materials are the most widely used interventions, despite evidence suggesting only modest effects on clinical behavior (Sohn, Ismail, & Tellez, 2004). They are widely used because of familiarity and ease of implementation. While passive educational strategies hold little promise, active educational interventions do show moderate benefit (O'Brien, 2007). The most effective educational strategies use multiple interventions, two-way communications, printed and graphic materials delivered in person, and locally respected health personnel as educators (Cauffman et al., 2002; Griffin et al., 2004).

Soumerai reviewed a number of educational interventions and identified the characteristics of those activities most likely to influence behavior. Ignoring design limitations of the studies reviewed, the researchers found that educational materials alone showed no significant effect, while participatory guideline development did lead to significant changes. Three other strategies—educational materials along with drug sample distribution; one-on-one education; and group education—all showed mixed results (Soumerai & Avorn, 1987; Soumerai, McLaughlin, & Avorn, 1989; Soumerai et al., 1993a, 1993b).

Time constraints may pose a barrier to physicians' participation in educational activities. However, one method to overcome this barrier is to present educational materials within the context of already scheduled events. For example, successful dissemination of new knowledge may occur with the integration of educational seminars within the context of grand rounds or monthly departmental meetings.

Conferences and Seminars

Continuing medical education may be provided via conferences and seminars; however, it can be difficult to recruit physicians to attend because of scheduling conflicts (Cabana et al., 2004). Physician recruitment necessitates personal and multiple contacts and careful planning of seminar location, time, and content.

Industry-sponsored luxury conferences can be powerful agents of change (Orlowski & Wateska, 1992). In a natural experiment, two new drugs were introduced via all-expenses paid symposia for MDs at the Cleveland Clinic. Drug A, an intravenous antibiotic, was launched at a California luxury beach resort over 4 days. Drug B, an intravenous cardiovascular agent, was introduced during a 5-day Caribbean island resort conference. Although 85% of physicians asked before the symposia predicted that the trips would have absolutely no impact on their prescribing patterns (only 5% thought that they might), time trend data show that prescribing of Drug A *doubled* and prescribing of Drug B more than *tripled* after the trips (Orlowski & Wateska, 1992). Even though conferences are a passive strategy of information transmission, if conducted in a luxury setting they seem to be extraordinarily effective in changing behavior.

Advertising

Studies of intensive marketing campaigns conducted by pharmaceutical companies show they can be effective in changing practice, even when the care provided may be contrary to evidence (Avorn, Chen, & Hartley, 1982). Following heavy advertising of the analgesic propoxyphene, Avorn et al. surveyed physicians' opinions on whether it was better than aspirin. Eighty percent of doctors said that the drug was better or the same as aspirin, when in fact the drug was no better, possibly worse, and more expensive than aspirin.

Opinion Leaders

Opinion leaders and local consensus exert influence on clinical behavior. Promotion of a particular intervention, method, or process by opinion leaders often leads to adoption by medical associations, hospitals, and providers. Opinion leaders are a major source of information diffusion. In fact, medical innovations introduced by opinion leaders are quickly adopted by physicians as the diffusion process is expedited. Clinicians often rely on local sources of information to seek knowledge about an issue they are uncertain about (Buller, Young, Fisher, & Maloy, 2007). Specific opinion leaders are more appropriate for a particular issue than are others (Grimshaw et al., 2006b).

Medical professional societies serve as natural opinion leaders and have become involved in promoting behavior change, both in developing guidelines and in encouraging their adoption. Genuine interest in improving health outcomes and eagerness to maintain autonomy in monitoring and directing practice pattern changes have prompted professional societies to embark on quasi-experimental research to impact practice. Examples include the American College of Cardiology's Guidelines Applied in Practice and the American Heart Association's "Get With the Guidelines" modules for stroke, coronary artery disease, and heart failure.

Academic Detailing

The pharmaceutical industry invests billions of dollars per year on "detailing," an estimated $8,000 to $13,000 per year for each physician (Wazana, 2000).

Given the for-profit nature of the industry, this approach must be effective to justify the investment. "Academic detailing" was developed in response to the "detailing" of health care providers that pharmaceutical sales representatives perform. Harvard's Jerry Avorn and colleagues (1982) recognized that successful pharmaceutical salespersons were usually attractive, articulate, and engaging professionals who provide user-friendly information and, often, lunch, all the while seeking to promote the sales of their company's drugs. Avorn believed and has proven that a noncommercial approach can change clinical behavior, too. Academic detailing is an "unsales" approach—where unbiased, commercial-free information about optimal care is provided to a clinician to improve care. Educational interventions are delivered by clinician-educators (generally physicians or pharmacists) who are experts in the field and specially trained in communication strategies. These experts visit the practice site and provide tailored information and encouragement to targeted clinicians. Academic detailers explore the provider's current knowledge and motivation, define clear educational and behavioral objects, and support the provider in making the desired change. For example, in a randomized controlled trial of 435 physicians with patterns of overprescribing three ineffective, harmful, and expensive drugs—propoxyphene, cerebral vasodilators, and cephalexin—academic detailing caused a 25% decrease in the troublesome prescribing (Avorn et al., 1982).

Detailing interventions seem most effective if physicians are targeted for intervention on the basis of need (e.g., prescribing data, opinion leaders); credible messengers and data sources are used; person-to-person interactions occur; key messages are repeated and reinforced over time; behavioral alternatives are discouraged; and brief, graphic educational materials are used (Soumerai & Avorn, 1990).

Audit and Feedback (Practice Reports)

The National Institute for Clinical Excellence (NICE) defines audit and feedback as a quality improvement practice aimed at improving patient care and outcomes through systematic review of care against specific criteria and the implementation of change. A five-step process is used to initiate and sustain the audit process. These steps include (1) preparing for the audit, (2) selecting criteria, (3) measuring the level of performance, (4) making improvements, and (5) sustaining improvement. In preparing for an audit, an organization should secure stakeholders' involvement, determine the purpose and goal of the audit, and identify what resources will be necessary to carry out the audit process. Selection, process, and outcome criteria must be chosen on the basis of their measurability, their relations to important aspects of care, and whether they are evidence based. Clear and concise definitions should be developed to adequately measure performance levels. For example, key elements that need defining are the user group, the professionals involved, and the time period over which criteria will be applied. External relationships and utilization of other supporting interventions should be considered when making improvements. Identifying potential barriers and implementing change will also help to make successful improvements. Once improvements have been made, they must be sustained by continuous monitoring and evaluation, development of an organizational framework, and leadership.

Audit and feedback as a method to improve clinical behavior have had mixed results. Feedback of aggregate data alone has not produced consistent results, but feedback strategies that target specific patients or provide worksheets, additional clinical services, or other tools have produced mixed results. In a systematic review of 118 studies, adjusted change among audit and feedback strategies ranged from a 10% drop in performance as measured against a control to a 70% improvement (Jamtvedt, Young, Kristoffersen, O'Brien, & Oxman, 2006).

The variation in effectiveness may be a result of the specific behaviors targeted or the person conducting the feedback. Further research is necessary to determine how and in what environments audit and feedback works best. The strategies shown most effective in the Jamfvedt and colleagues review (2006) were those where baseline compliance to guidelines was low and the intensity of the interventions was high. Several qualitative studies have explored characteristics of effective feedback strategies. Radford and colleagues noted that the *perceived accuracy* of the feedback and the source of data (internal vs. external) conferred validity on the data. Further, timeliness of effective reports was based on the *frequency of reporting* performance feedback. The impact of the feedback was heightened if the physician was compared to like providers (e.g., same specialty and same type of practice setting). Finally, the usefulness varied by who received the data and in what forum, who provided the data, and how the data were formatted (Bradley et al., 2001). Another study of high- and low-performing facilities' use of clinical audit data for feedback purposes suggested that high-performing sites provided timely, individualized, nonpunitive feedback to providers, while low-performing sites showed more variability in timeliness and punitive action and relied more heavily on standardized, facility level reports (Hysong, Best, & Pugh, 2006).

Incentives and Financial Rewards (Pay for Performance)

Pay for performance embraces the idea that providers should be rewarded for outstanding quality-of-care performance. It is reasonable to believe that financial incentives will have a positive impact on clinicians' behavior. A common type of financial reward is value-based purchasing. Value-based purchasing is a system in which employers and other purchasers collect and analyze data related to the costs and quality of various competing providers and health plans (Rowe, 2006). In this system, the best-performing plans and health care providers are rewarded with greater volume of enrollees or patients. The degree to which health care providers respond to value-based purchasing initiatives is greatly influenced by the extent to which a clinical practice is dependent upon the purchasing entity making the payments. Approximately 40% of managed care organizations offer financial incentives to affect practice patterns, a much lower rate of utilization than that for other behavior change strategies (Soumerai et al., 1989). Currently, most incentives are less than 10% of a provider's salary.

More recent policy initiatives have layered financial incentives with accountability for good patient outcomes at a systems level. Medicare's Pay for Performance initiative is one example. Under pay-for-performance pilot programs, hospitals scoring in the top 10% received a 2% bonus payment in addition to their standard Diagnosis-Related Group payment. The next highest-scoring 10% received a 1% bonus, and hospitals that did not meet threshold score were subject to *reductions* in payment. Evaluation of the pilot program indicated that the pay-for-performance demonstration initiative had a significant impact on the rate and magnitude of performance improvement at one hospital (Grossbart, 2006), and early indicators suggest the 10 large, multispecialty group practices participating in the 3-year trial are making strides in identifying Medicare patients with chronic, high-cost conditions and closing the gaps in their care (Klein, 2006).

Public Reporting of Quality-of-Care Indicators

Report cards have been developed to measure and compare health plans (e.g., Healthcare Effectiveness Data and Information Set, Consumer Assessment of Healthcare Providers and Systems) and the Leapfrog Group, a consortium of employer payers, has designated minimum criteria for health care quality and requires public reporting of these indices. In some instances the risk adjustment methodologies are inadequate and sometimes not even reported. However, to date, the release of information to the public does not appear to have had an effect on patients' decisions to select particular physicians as their provider (Rosenthal, Fernandopulle, Song, & Landon, 2004).

Organizational Interventions

A review of organizational interventions showed inconsistent effects. But, on the basis of the weak designs of the studies, Wensing, Wollersheim, and Grol (2006) suggest that revision of professional roles and computer systems changed provider behavior and that implementation of multidisciplinary teams, integrated care services, and computer systems impacted patient outcomes. However, they concluded that the benefits of quality management strategies remained uncertain.

Administrative Policies

At the systems level, incentives and disincentives have been used to influence provider behavior. Almost all managed care organizations report using formularies, and approximately 90% use drug utilization review, to direct specific prescribing practices (Soumerai et al., 1989). Formulary approaches can reduce medication use and costs. However, the impact on total health care costs and health outcomes has received little attention. Other administrative policies such as mandatory switching, coverage limits, and use of prior authorization can increase prescribing of preferred drugs, although a small percentage of patients do switch back to the original therapy, and forced switching may result in a temporary increase in office visits (Soumerai et al., 1989).

One tenet of system strategies is to make it easy to do the right thing and difficult to do the wrong thing. Prior authorization, in which the practice is not reimbursed for care that has not been authorized by the payer in advance, is one such barrier and has been implemented in 80% of managed care organizations (Soumerai et al., 1989).

Care Plans, Protocols, Pathways

Other organizational plans and policies may reduce variation by standardization. Care pathways may help clinicians select and make adjustments to appropriate medications quickly, reduce risk of errors, and have a positive impact on outcomes.

Care protocols document required actions that should be taken in a specific circumstance. Clinical pathways are patient-focused tools that describe the time frame and sequencing of routine, predictable, multidisciplinary care patterns and the patient outcomes expected from them. They are most successful in situations in which care is provided for a high volume of patients with similar needs (e.g., hip fracture patients have similar hospital courses following surgery, so rehabilitation services can be standardized by day postsurgery).

One successful approach is the Guidelines Applied in Practice (GAP) program (Mehta et al., 2002). GAP used standard orders, pocket guidelines cards, clinical pathways, patient information forms, and patient discharge forms to improve care of acute myocardial infarction patients and showed small, but significantly increased trends in health care providers' adherence to prescribing beta blockers, aspirin, and cholesterol lowering medications, and reductions in time to acute care therapies (Mehta et al., 2002).

Drug Samples

Distributing drug samples is one approach to encourage specific prescribing patterns. The pharmaceutical industry spends an estimated $8 billion per year in the United States on drug samples. Not surprisingly, the use of generic drugs has been shown to be negatively influenced by the presence of brand samples in a primary care clinic (Miller, 2005). In a survey of physicians who used drug samples, 91% stated the sample given was not their preferred drug, but 69% of them would not switch the patient to their preferred drug once the patient's hypertension was controlled (Chew et al., 2000).

Reminders

Many interventions are built upon the simple concept of reminding physicians of guidelines, preventative tests due, and other processes of care to be followed. Several systems have been utilized, including chart-attached reminders, nurse-prepared checklists, and computer prompts. A review of reminder interventions looked at nine comparisons between physicians who received reminders and those with no intervention and showed absolute increases in preventive services varying from 5% to 24% (Hulscher, Wensing, van Der, & Grol, 2001). In a review of cluster randomized trials of various reminder strategies, Grimshaw et al. (2006b) found a median absolute improvement of 14.1% among physicians who received reminders, but the researchers doubt that these effects can be replicated outside a rigorous trial setting. Computerized reminder systems are becoming more common. However, it seems that paper-based reminders are a more effective reminder strategy (Dexheimer, Sanders, Rosenbloom, & Aronsky, 2005).

Decision Support Tools (Point-of-Care Calculators, Care Protocols)

In a landmark article, McDonald (1976) suggested that humans were limited in data-processing capacity and that computers held the promise of helping clinicians to reduce errors and improve patient care. More than two decades later, in *To Err Is Human* (2000) and *Crossing the Quality Chasm* (2001), the Institute of Medicine declared that information technology is a cornerstone of efforts to improve patient safety. Two health information technologies are essential to improving patient safety: electronic medical records (EMR) and computerized physician order entry (CPOE). These technologies narrow variation from evidence-based practice and prevent medical errors (Berwick, 2003). A cadre of national organizations, including the Institute of Medicine, the Leapfrog Group, and the Agency for Healthcare Research and Quality (AHRQ), have endorsed CPOE as an intervention that may dramatically improve patient safety (Institute of Medicine, 2000, 2001). There have also been legislative initiatives at both the state and the federal levels to promote implementation of information technology in hospitals (Institute of Medicine, 2000).

Use of computer-based clinical decision support systems (CDSSs) are thought to improve adherence to guideline recommendations; improve patient outcomes; reduce inappropriate variation in clinical practice; reduce errors and oversights; and decrease costs of care. CPOE may significantly improve patient care and safety by eliminating illegible orders and reducing transcription errors (Mekhjian et al., 2002). CPOE provides a platform for diagnosis-specific order sets and corollary orders, which enhance compliance with evidence-based guidelines and improve medication monitoring (Overhage, Tierney, Zhou, & McDonald, 1997). CPOE facilitates the use of reminders to enhance adherence to preventive-care routines or protocols (Dexter et al., 2001). The approach constrains choices such as selection of medications, both improving medication selection and dosage and reducing time to therapeutic level (Teich et al., 2000). It reduces medication errors and facilitates allergy identification, leading to substantial reductions in potential adverse drug events (Bates et al., 1998; Teich et al., 1999).

A key to the effectiveness of CPOE is the linkage to computerized clinical decision support systems (CDSS). In medication management, for example, CDSS can provide computerized rules and algorithms to "alert" physicians to the presence of potentially unsafe drug-drug interactions, the need to adjust drug dosage, and contraindications to specific drugs based on the presence of a medication allergy or comorbidity (Wang, Shabot, Duncan, Polaschek, & Jones, 2002). As with other implementation strategies, the evidence base has not caught up with the enthusiasm.

Although clinical decision support (CDS) tools may positively affect the cost, quality, and safety of health care delivery, studies find a rather low acceptance rate among clinicians. It takes an investment of time to use CDS effectively, and time constraints are a reason why more physicians do not use them. Even if a physician is inclined to use CDS, the effects of the system's support may not be optimal, as many physicians can override or ignore the messages the system provides. Physicians who do effectively use CDS, however, claim that it helps them take better care of their patients and reminds them of important activities or appointments. Physicians using handheld decision support tools in a critical care setting have decreased their patient's length of stay and their prescribing of antibiotics (Sintchenko, Iredell, Gilbert, & Coiera, 2005).

Patient Activation Tools

The pharmaceutical industry has capitalized on direct-to-consumer advertising to promote the sale of target drugs. Several academic interventions have also capitalized on the physician-patient interaction to promote guideline adherence. These patient activation approaches engage the patient as a catalyst to remind the care provider of guideline protocols. Other strategies have employed posters in the exam room describing appropriate care and engage patients in their own care by providing care records or test results such as written blood pressure results with notes regarding threshold values and encouragement to discuss abnormal results with the physician (Ellis et al., 2007). Evidence suggests that such interventions can alter the interaction between patients and practitioners (Griffin et al., 2004).

Multifaceted Interventions

A review of the impact of multifaceted interventions found 14 comparisons between groups that received multifaceted interventions and controls that received no intervention that showed an absolute change in the performance of preventive services of between negative 3% and positive 64% in the group that received multifaceted interventions; 6 comparisons between groups that received multifaceted interventions and groups that received group education produced absolute changes ranging from negative 31% to 28% in the first group (Hulscher et al., 2001). Grimshaw, Eccles, & Tetroe (2004a) found that multifaceted interventions were no more effective than single interventions and also found no relationship between the number of components and the effects of multifaceted interventions (Grimshaw et al., 2006a). In response, more rigorous studies have been designed to test the incremental effects of patient-specific reminders delivered at the point of care with brief treatment guidelines endorsed by local opinion leaders (McAlister et al., 2006) and other mixed-methods approaches (Johnson et al., 2006).

Tailored Interventions

Tailored interventions are designed to be flexible enough to allow providers to select aspects of the intervention that will "fit" in their setting. This flexibility recognizes that no one size fits all and that if providers are able to choose aspects of the intervention, they are more likely to be influenced by it. Tailored interventions have been effective in research studies using nonexperimental designs (Bonds, Ellis, Weeks, Palla, & Lichstein, 2006) and experimental designs (Eccles et al., 2006).

Why Does It Matter?

Unfortunately, there is often a chasm between the gold standard of care as outlined in clinical practice guidelines and the care that is actually delivered on a day-to-day basis. The practice of medicine usually involves a dynamic relationship between a health care provider and a patient. Thus, a patient who is cared for by a physician using best practices is going to have every advantage in achieving adherence over a patient who is not seen by a high-performing clinician. The physician's behavior has clear implications for the patient's health behavior and outcomes. If that weren't reason enough to learn about the challenges of guideline implementation, the fact that the health care landscape is constantly changing provides another compelling reason. As advances in techniques, diagnostic equipment, and medications emerge at rapid rates, clinical behavior will have to change in response if clinical excellence is to be realized. In this chapter, we highlighted the challenges in changing clinical behavior in primary care practice. We emphasized the importance of thinking about clinical behavior change as occurring in a context and of developing systems to support the desired behavior change. The approaches and models that seem to work best have been noted, as have notable failures. Future research in this area should consider whether it is important to disentangle the effects of multilevel and multimethod interventions and how such effects could be isolated and measured.

References

Antman, E. M., Lau, J., Kupelnick, B., Mosteller, F., & Chalmers, T. C. (1992). A comparison of results of meta-analyses of randomized control trials and recommendations of clinical experts. Treatments for myocardial infarction. *Journal of the American Medical Association, 268,* 240–248.

Avorn, J., Chen, M., & Hartley, R. (1982). Scientific versus commercial sources of influence on the prescribing behavior of physicians. *American Journal of Medicine, 73,* 4–8.

Barr, V. J., Robinson, S., Marin-Link, B., Underhill, L., Dotts, A., Ravensdale, D., et al. (2003). The expanded Chronic Care Model: An integration of concepts and strategies from population health promotion and the Chronic Care Model. *Hospital Quarterly, 7,* 73–82.

Bates, D. W., Leape, L. L., Cullen, D. J., Laird, N., Petersen, L. A., Teich, J. M., et al. (1998). Effect of computerized physician order entry and a team intervention on prevention of serious medication errors. *Journal of the American Medical Association, 280,* 1311–1316.

Bates, D. W., Teich, J. M., Lee, J., Seger, D., Kuperman, G. J., Ma'Luf, N., et al. (1999). The impact of computerized physician order entry on medication error prevention. *Journal of the American Medical Informatics Association, 6,* 313–321.

Berwick, D. M. (2003). Errors today and errors tomorrow. *New England Journal of Medicine, 348,* 2570–2572.

Bloom, B. S. (2005). Effects of continuing medical education on improving physician clinical care and patient health: a review of systematic reviews. *International Journal of Technology Assessment in Health Care, 21,* 380–385.

Bonds, D. E., Ellis, S. D., Weeks, E., Palla, S. L., & Lichstein, P. (2006). A practice-centered intervention to increase screening for domestic violence in primary care practices. *BMC Family Practice, 7,* 63.

Bradley, E. H., Holmboe, E. S., Mattera, J. A., Roumanis, S. A., Radford, M. J., & Krumholz, H. M. (2001). A qualitative study of increasing beta-blocker use after myocardial infarction: Why do some hospitals succeed? *Journal of the American Medical Association, 285,* 2604–2611.

Buller, D. B., Young, W. F., Fisher, K. H., & Maloy, J. A. (2007). The effect of endorsement by local opinion leaders and testimonials from teachers on the dissemination of a Web-based smoking prevention program. *Health Education Research, 22,* 609–618.

Cabana, M. D., Brown, R., Clark, N. M., White, D. F., Lyons, J., Lang, S. W., et al. (2004). Improving physician attendance at educational seminars sponsored by Managed Care Organizations. *Managed Care, 13,* 49–56.

Cabana, M. D., Rand, C. S., Powe, N. R., Wu, A. W., Wilson, M. H., Abboud, P. A., et al. (1999). Why don't physicians follow clinical practice guidelines? A framework for improvement. *Journal of the American Medical Association, 282,* 1458–1465.

Cauffman, J. G., Forsyth, R. A., Clark, V. A., Foster, J. P., Martin, K. J., Lapsys, F. X., et al. (2002). Randomized controlled trials of continuing medical education: What makes them most effective? *Journal of Continuing Education in the Health Professions, 22,* 214–221.

Chew, L. D., O'Young, T. S., Hazlet, T. K., Bradley, K. A., Maynard, C., & Lessler, D. S. (2000). A physician survey of the effect of drug sample availability on physicians' behavior. *Journal of General Internal Medicine, 15,* 478–483.

Choudhry, N. K., Fletcher, R. H., & Soumerai, S. B. (2005). Systematic review: The relationship between clinical experience and quality of health care. *Annals of Internal Medicine, 142,* 260–273.

Dexheimer, J. W., Sanders, D. L., Rosenbloom, S. T., & Aronsky, D. (2005). Prompting clinicians: A systematic review of preventive care reminders. *AMIA Annual Symposium Proceedings,* 938.

Dexter, P. R., Perkins, S., Overhage, J. M., Maharry, K., Kohler, R. B., & McDonald, C. J. (2001). A computerized reminder system to increase the use of preventive care for hospitalized patients. *New England Journal of Medicine, 345,* 965–970.

Eccles, M. P., Foy, R., Bamford, C. H., Hughes, J. C., Johnston, M., Whitty, P. M., et al. (2006). A trial platform to develop a tailored theory-based intervention to improve professional practice in the disclosure of a diagnosis of dementia: Study protocol [ISRCTN15871014]. *Implementation Science, 1,* 7.

Eccles, M. P., & Mittman, B. (2006). Welcome to Implementation Science. *Implementation Science, 1,* 1–3.

Ellis, S. D., Bertoni, A. G., Bonds, D. E., Clinch, C. R., Balasubramanyam, A., Blackwell, C., et al. (2007). Value of recruitment strategies used in a primary care practice-based trial. *Contemporary Clinical Trials, 28,* 258–267.

Gravel, K., Legare, F., & Graham, I. D. (2006). Barriers and facilitators to implementing shared decision-making in clinical practice: A systematic review of health professionals' perceptions. *Implementation Science, 1,* 16.

Griffin, S. J., Kinmonth, A. L., Veltman, M. W., Gillard, S., Grant, J., & Stewart, M. (2004). Effect on health-related outcomes of interventions to alter the interaction between patients and practitioners: a systematic review of trials. *Annals of Family Medicine, 2,* 595–608.

Grimshaw, J., Eccles, M., & Tetroe, J. (2004a). Implementing clinical guidelines: Current evidence and future implications. *Journal of Continuing Education in the Health Professions, 24*(Suppl. 1), S31–S37.

Grimshaw, J., Eccles, M., Thomas, R., Maclennan, G., Ramsay, C., Fraser, C., et al. (2006a). Toward evidence-based quality improvement. Evidence (and its limitations) of the effectiveness of guideline dissemination and implementation strategies 1966–1998. *Journal of General Internal Medicine, 21*(Suppl. 2), S14–S20.

Grimshaw, J. M., Eccles, M. P., Greener, J., Maclennan, G., Ibbotson, T., Kahan, J. P., et al. (2006b). Is the involvement of opinion leaders in the implementation of research findings a feasible strategy? *Implementation Science, 1,* 3.

Grossbart, S. R. (2006). What's the return? Assessing the effect of "pay-for-performance" initiatives on the quality of care delivery. *Medical Care Research and Review, 63,* 29S–48S.

Hakkennes, S., & Green, S. (2006). Measures for assessing practice change in medical practitioners. *Implementation Science, 1,* 29.

Hulscher, M. E., Wensing, M., van Der, W. T., & Grol, R. (2001). Interventions to implement prevention in primary care. *Cochrane Database of Systematic Reviews,* CD000362.

Hysong, S. J., Best, R. G., & Pugh, J. A. (2006). Audit and feedback and clinical practice guideline adherence: Making feedback actionable. *Implementation Science, 1,* 9.

ICEBeRG. (2006). Designing theoretically informed implementation interventions. *Implementation Science, 1,* 4.

Institute of Medicine. (2000). *To err is human: Building a safer health system.* Washington, DC: National Academies Press.

Institute of Medicine. (2001). *Crossing the quality chasm: A new health system for the 21st century.* Washington, DC: National Academies Press.

Jamtvedt, G., Young, J. M., Kristoffersen, D. T., O'Brien, M. A., & Oxman, A. D. (2006). Audit and feedback: Effects on professional practice and health care outcomes. *Cochrane Database of Systematic Reviews,* CD000259.

Johnson, D. W., Craig, W., Brant, R., Mitton, C., Svenson, L., & Klassen, T. P. (2006). A cluster randomized controlled trial comparing three methods of disseminating practice guidelines for children with croup [ISRCTN73394937]. *Implementation Science, 1,* 10.

Johnston, M. E., Langton, K. B., Haynes, R. B., & Mathieu, A. (1994). Effects of computer-based clinical decision support systems on clinician performance and patient outcome. A critical appraisal of research. *Annals of Internal Medicine, 120,* 135–142.

Kaushal, R., Shojania, K. G., & Bates, D. W. (2003). Effects of computerized physician order entry and clinical decision support systems on medication safety: A systematic review. *Archives of Internal Medicine, 163,* 1409–1416.

Klein, C. J. (2006). Linking competency-based assessment to successful clinical practice. *Journal of Nursing Education, 45,* 379–383.

Kumar, P. D. (1992). Publication lag intervals—a reason for authors' apathy? *Journal of the Association of Physicians of India, 40,* 623–624.

Leclere, J., Ollivier, L., Ruszniewski, M., & Neuenschwander, S. (2006). Improving overall patient care during imaging studies: The radiologist's CREDO and PERLES. *Journal of Radiology, 87,* 1831–1836.

McAlister, F. A., Fradette, M., Graham, M., Majumdar, S. R., Ghali, W. A., Williams, R., et al. (2006). A randomized trial to assess the impact of opinion leader endorsed evidence summaries on the use of secondary prevention strategies in patients with coronary artery disease: The ESP-CAD trial protocol [NCT00175240]. *Implementation Science, 1,* 11.

McDonald, C. J. (1976). Protocol-based computer reminders, the quality of care and the non-perfectability of man. *New England Journal of Medicine, 295,* 1351–1355.

McGlynn, E. A., Asch, S. M., Adams, J., Keesey, J., Hicks, J., DeCristofaro, A., et al. (2003). The quality of health care delivered to adults in the United States. *New England Journal of Medicine, 348,* 2635–2645.

Mehta, R. H., Montoye, C. K., Gallogly, M., Baker, P., Blount, A., Faul, J., et al. (2002). Improving quality of care for acute myocardial infarction: The Guidelines Applied in Practice (GAP) Initiative. *Journal of the American Medical Association, 287,* 1269–1276.

Mekhjian, H. S., Kumar, R. R., Kuehn, L., Bentley, T. D., Teater, P., Thomas, A., et al. (2002). Immediate benefits realized following implementation of physician order entry at an academic medical center. *Journal of the American Medical Informatics Association, 9,* 529–539.

Miller, D. (2005). *The impact of drug samples on prescribing by primary care physicians.* Unpublished.

Newton, M. S., Estabrooks, C. A., Norton, P., Birdsell, J. M., Adewale, A. J., & Thornley, R. (2007). Health researchers in Alberta: An exploratory comparison of defining characteristics and knowledge translation activities. *Implementation Science, 2,* 1.

O'Brien, S. M., Shahian, D. M., DeLong, E. R., Normand, S. L., Edwards, F. H., Ferraris, V. A., et al. (2007). Quality measurement in adult cardiac surgery: Part 2—Statistical considerations in composite measure scoring and provider rating. *Annals of Thoracic Surgery, 83,* S13–S26.

Orlowski, J. P., & Wateska, L. (1992). The effects of pharmaceutical firm enticements on physician prescribing patterns. There's no such thing as a free lunch. *Chest, 102,* 270–273.

Overhage, J. M., Tierney, W. M., Zhou, X. H., & McDonald, C. J. (1997). A randomized trial of "corollary orders" to prevent errors of omission. *Journal of the American Medical Informatics Association, 4,* 364–375.

Ramnarayan, P., Winrow, A., Coren, M., Nanduri, V., Buchdahl, R., Jacobs, B., et al. (2006). Diagnostic omission errors in acute paediatric practice: Impact of a reminder system on decision-making. *BMC Medical Informatics and Decision Making, 6,* 37.

Rosenthal, M. B., Fernandopulle, R., Song, H. R., & Landon, B. (2004). Paying for quality: Providers' incentives for quality improvement. *Health Affairs (Millwood), 23,* 127–141.

Rowe, J. W. (2006). Pay-for-performance and accountability: Related themes in improving health care. *Annals of Internal Medicine, 145,* 695–699.

Shaw, B., Cheater, F., Baker, R., Gillies, C., Hearnshaw, H., Flottorp, S., et al. (2005). Tailored interventions to overcome identified barriers to change: Effects on professional practice and health care outcomes. *Cochrane Database of Systematic Reviews,* CD005470.

Sintchenko, V., Iredell, J. R., Gilbert, G. L., & Coiera, E. (2005). Handheld computer-based decision support reduces patient length of stay and antibiotic prescribing in critical care. *Journal of the American Medical Informatics Association, 12,* 398–402.

Sladek, R. M., Phillips, P. A., & Bond, M. J. (2006). Implementation science: A role for parallel dual processing models of reasoning? *Implementation Science, 1,* 12.

Sohn, W., Ismail, A. I., & Tellez, M. (2004). Efficacy of educational interventions targeting primary care providers' practice behaviors: An overview of published systematic reviews. *Journal of Public Health Dentistry, 64,* 164–172.

Soumerai, S. B., & Avorn, J. (1987). Changing prescribing practices through individual continuing education. *Journal of the American Medical Association, 257,* 487.

Soumerai, S. B., & Avorn, J. (1990). Principles of educational outreach ("academic detailing") to improve clinical decision making. *Journal of the American Medical Association, 263,* 549–556.

Soumerai, S. B., Avorn, J., Taylor, W. C., Wessels, M., Maher, D., & Hawley, S. L. (1993a). Improving choice of prescribed antibiotics through concurrent reminders in an educational order form. *Medical Care, 31,* 552–558.

Soumerai, S. B., McLaughlin, T. J., & Avorn, J. (1989). Improving drug prescribing in primary care: A critical analysis of the experimental literature. *Milbank Quarterly, 67,* 268–317.

Soumerai, S. B., Salem-Schatz, S., Avorn, J., Casteris, C. S., Ross-Degnan, D., & Popovsky, M. A. (1993b). A controlled trial of educational outreach to improve blood transfusion practice. *Journal of the American Medical Association, 270,* 961–966.

Stetler, C. B., Legro, M. W., Rycroft-Malone, J., Bowman, C., Curran, G., Guihan, M., et al. (2006). Role of "external facilitation" in implementation of research findings: A qualitative evaluation of facilitation experiences in the Veterans Health Administration. *Implementation Science, 1,* 23.

Teich, J. M., Glaser, J. P., Beckley, R. F., Aranow, M., Bates, D. W., Kuperman, G. J., et al. (1999). The Brigham integrated computing system (BICS): Advanced clinical systems in an academic hospital environment. *International Journal of Medical Informatics, 54,* 197–208.

Teich, J. M., Merchia, P. R., Schmiz, J. L., Kuperman, G. J., Spurr, C. D., & Bates, D. W. (2000). Effects of computerized physician order entry on prescribing practices. *Archives of Internal Medicine, 160,* 2741–2747.

Wang, J. K., Shabot, M. M., Duncan, R. G., Polaschek, J. X., & Jones, D. T. (2002). A clinical rules taxonomy for the implementation of a computerized physician order entry (CPOE) system. *Proceedings of the AMIA Symposium,* 860–863.

Wazana, A. (2000). Physicians and the pharmaceutical industry: Is a gift ever just a gift? *Journal of the American Medical Association, 283,* 373–380.

Wensing, M., Wollersheim, H., & Grol, R. (2006). Organizational interventions to implement improvements in patient care: A structured review of reviews. *Implementation Science, 1,* 2.

Worrall, G., Chaulk, P., & Freake, D. (1997). The effects of clinical practice guidelines on patient outcomes in primary care: A systematic review. *Canadian Medical Association Journal, 156,* 1705–1712.

Lifestyle Change and Adherence Issues Within Specific Populations

Section 5

Sally A. Shumaker
Editor

There are many factors discussed throughout the current volume that influence lifestyle changes and adherence that are common across groups. However, there are also factors that are specific within groups. Such population strata variables include economic status, education, gender, ethnicity and race, rural versus urban, access to care, and age. Each of these strata contain characteristics that differentially explain a group's receptiveness and ability to initiate healthy lifestyle changes as well as the group's ability to maintain new behaviors over time. To maximize the effectiveness of strategies designed to initiate and maintain healthy behaviors it is important for behavioral scientists and health care providers to be sensitive to both within- and between-group differences. And, as noted throughout this volume, it is critical to go beyond these two levels of analysis and consider health behaviors within the broader and complex social system. In the previous edition, we explored the role of adherence and health behavior among three specific population groups: the young, adolescents with chronic diseases, and the elderly. In this edition, in addition to significantly updating each of the previous chapters, we added chapters on older adults with cognitive impairments and health disparities and minority health.

In "Lifestyle Interventions for the Young," Ievers-Landis and Witherspoon present a compelling argument for developing healthy behaviors as early as possible in a person's development, as such behaviors influence both current and future health. Further, the behaviors instilled in childhood (whether healthy or unhealthy) are most likely to be sustained throughout the lifetime. This latter point is underscored by the difficulty with which health behavior changes (e.g., increased physical activity, smoking cessation, and a healthy diet) are initiated and sustained in adulthood. In considering healthy lifestyles in the young, Ievers-Landis and Witherspoon address two age groups: preschool and middle childhood (i.e., ages 3–12). Noting that the success of healthy lifestyle interventions is dependent on the developmental stage of the child, the authors discuss where such interventions are likely to be most successful at different age groups and present different approaches by age and situation— considering the family and home environment, the classroom, the built environment, and the primary care physician's clinic. The authors conclude with a critical review of interventions that have been developed to enhance healthy behaviors in children and discuss the relative merit of each program.

Murdaugh and Insel provide an update on the chapter in the previous volume (Murdaugh, 1998) in "Problems With Adherence in the Elderly." The elderly represent the fastest growing portion of the population in the United States, and an increasing number of aging adults are living into their 80s and further. And, for many older adults, the behaviors required to improve their health run counter to lifelong habits that are well-established and resistant to change. Further exacerbating this situation is the fact that chronic illnesses increase with age, and often older adults are faced with multiple comorbidities that require complex behavioral and pharmacological interventions. In this chapter, Murdaugh and Insel begin with a description of the types of nonadherence that occur in the aging population. They provide an in-depth review of the complex nature of nonadherence and the multiple factors that influence it among older adults (e.g., ability, desire, physical and emotional health, the social environment, and pharmacokinetics). Although they focus primarily on adherence to prescribed medication regimens for chronic conditions, these authors note that many of the factors that promote nonadherence and adherence are applicable to other types of regimens or lifestyle changes in which adherence is an issue. Recognizing the heterogeneity of the elderly population, these authors go on to consider methods to assess an elder's capacity to adhere. They conclude the chapter with a critical analysis of potential strategies for enhancing optimal adherence among the elderly.

Resnick, Galik, Nahm, Shaughnessy, and Michael discuss the complex challenges involved in "Optimizing Adherence in Older Adults With Cognitive Impairment." The prevalence of dementia and mild cognitive impairment increases dramatically over age 65. About 5%–8% of people over age 65 suffer from dementia. Currently, it is estimated that 4.5 million Americans suffer from Alzheimer's disease, and because of increases in life expectancy it is projected that by 2050 approximately 13.2 million Americans will be affected by the disease. When less dramatic declines in cognitive functioning are considered, the rates of elderly with some cognitive impairment are significantly higher. Health-promoting behaviors are the same for adults with cognitive impairment (CI) as the general population. Further, adults with CI benefit from successfully achieving health behavior changes (e.g., increased physical activity). However, cognitive impairment presents a unique set of challenges within the context of adherence and sustained health-behavior changes. In this chapter, Resnick and colleagues provide a detailed review of the evidence supporting the value of health-behavior change interventions among older adults with cognitive impairment. In addition, they discuss the factors that predict poor or good adherence in this cohort. In the final section of the chapter, the authors discuss the value of applying a social-ecological model to interventions designed to enhance health behaviors among cognitively impaired adults. They provide several excellent examples of specific intervention programs and critically assess the relative value of each. This chapter represents a unique and valuable resource to the health professional working with the cognitively impaired—whether within an institutionalized population or living at home. The authors provide a sense of efficacy and hope for improving the outcomes for this growing population.

In "Adherence Issues Among Adolescents With Chronic Diseases" Rapoff and Smith provide an excellent update on the chapter from the previous volume (Rapoff, 1998) in which this critical issue was addressed. The authors begin by defining adherence versus compliance—a critical distinction for any population and particularly sensitive during adolescence when individuals are testing their independent status. Rapoff and Smith also distinguish between volitional and nonvolitional nonadherence—further clarifying the importance of choice, knowledge, and independence among adolescents. They note that although chronic diseases are present in a relatively small percentage of the adolescent population in the United States, the consequences of such conditions are major with respect to the quality of life of the teen and the significant medical and psychosocial implications. In addition, chronic diseases among adolescents carry a disproportionate economic burden. Further, although rates are relatively low, with increased obesity, sedentary lifestyles, and diabetes among young adults, the rate of chronic disease in adolescents is increasing. Also, adolescents are at particularly high risk for nonadherence to medical and healthy lifestyle interventions. In this chapter the authors review the degree to which nonadherence is a problem among teens, and its consequences. In addition, they critically review potential strategies for improving adherence.

A major issue in today's health arena revolves around ethnic and racial diversity and its relationship to health disparities. In their chapter, "Health Disparities and Minority Health," Whitt-Glover, Beech, Bell, Jackson, Loftin-Bell, and Mount tackle this important and complex issue—and relate it to healthy lifestyle behaviors and adherence. The authors set the stage for their analysis by providing two critical historical pieces that lay the groundwork for the remainder of the chapter and underscore the importance of context in understanding how minority status influences health behaviors and change. They first provide a history of the concept of *minority,* and its changing use, meaning, and application over time in the United States. In addition, they consider the implications of these changes for how minorities are viewed historically and how this influences data collection and ultimately our understanding of the health status of various groups. The next section is an analysis of the term *health disparities*—again noting the variability with which the term has been used over time and how it is currently applied to a range of health behaviors and conditions. With this grounding established along with the implied caveats in place, the authors then move on to a review of the literature on the prevalence of a selected group of lifestyle and clinical behaviors, and adherence rates and their predictors, among minorities. The chapter concludes with suggested strategies for enhancing adherence among minority groups—within a social-ecological model. The authors consider strategies at the individual and community levels of analysis and discuss the degree to which various interventions have been successfully adapted to the intended culture.

Lifestyle Interventions for the Young

25

Carolyn E.
Ievers-Landis and
Dawn Witherspoon

In this chapter we provide an overview of the rationale for lifestyle interventions in the young (early and middle childhood) and brief descriptions of recent examples of the wide range of such interventions. Lifestyle interventions influence both the current and future health status of children, even into their older years (e.g., the prevention of osteoporosis) (Ievers-Landis et al., 2003, 2005). Health behavior change interventions may be most cost-efficient and effective when delivered early in an individual's life. We begin this chapter by providing an overview of the need for delivering lifestyle interventions to the young. The variety of these interventions and the choices researchers make during the design and implementation phases of research are highlighted throughout the remainder of the chapter. Lifestyle interventions can be designed for a number of health-related targets and goals, and some of the most common and novel ones are described. In addition, the relationship of the design and implementation of lifestyle interventions to age and developmental stage is considered. Finally, the range of approaches selected to implement interventions are presented, as well as the types of intervention strategies used.

Research shows that intervening with children to promote healthy lifestyles is vitally important. When children are taught appropriate health behaviors early, these behaviors are more likely to become habitual and continue into adulthood (O'Brien & Bush, 1997; Taylor, 1999). Intervening with a population before it has developed habitually unhealthy behaviors is an added benefit of the timing of such interventions. The health behaviors of children are strongly influenced by early experiences and socialization, especially from parents as both positive and negative role models. Parents' eating behaviors, for example, may play a role in the development and maintenance of childhood obesity. In one study researchers found that children ages 3–6 years had more difficulty adjusting their eating in response to increases in the caloric density of the diet if their parents reported higher dietary disinhibition (e.g., eating large amounts of food without regard for hunger or fullness cues) (Johnson & Birch, 1994). In contrast, parents may model healthy behaviors for their children that become automatic, like wearing seatbelts (Damashek & Peterson, 2002).

Efforts to promote health in children often focus on educational opportunities to prevent poor health behaviors from developing (Turrisi et al., 2004). Early interactions align with "teachable moments," that is, moments when a child is cognitively ready to learn about a health behavior and has not yet developed a poor health habit in that area. Children benefit from intervention programs designed specifically for their level of cognitive development. As early as preschool, children can develop responsibility for some of their own health behaviors, such as crossing the street safely and wearing seat belts (O'Brien & Bush, 1997; Taylor, 1999).

Another reason to promote appropriate health behaviors in the young is that precautions taken either before or during adolescence may be more likely to prevent some diseases in later adulthood rather than waiting to improve health behaviors until initial symptoms arise (Chavarro, Peterson, Sobol, Wiecha, & Gortmaker, 2005; Cummings, Kelsey, Nevitt, & O'Dowd, 1985). Chronic conditions that arise in adulthood may be directly linked to childhood health habits. Examples include osteoporosis and skin cancer (Davis, Cokkinides, Weinstock, Connell, & Wingo, 2002; Ievers-Landis et al., 2005).

A number of lifestyle behaviors are identified as the leading causes of morbidity and mortality in the United States (Mokdad, Marks, Stroup, & Gerberding, 2000). The most prevalent among these are physical inactivity, unhealthy dietary patterns and behaviors that contribute to unintentional injury, and all of these are linked to behaviors that can be established in childhood and adolescence. (Other important behaviors linked to morbidity and mortality are substance abuse and unsafe sexual behaviors—both of which are covered in other chapters in this book.)

Child Age Range

Early Childhood

Some interventions are best suited for children in the "preschool" age range (3–6). These interventions usually include parental involvement (e.g., Fitzgibbon et al., 2004) and may be wholly directed to changing the parents' beliefs, attitudes and behaviors in order to benefit the children's health (e.g., Sääkslahti et al., 2004). Beginning interventions at this time is important as food preferences and physical activity habits are set relatively early in life (Sullivan & Birch, 1990; Trost, Sirard, Dowda, Pfeiffer, & Pate, 2003), and both are important for future health behaviors (Sherry, 2005). Also, early intervention can affect the timing of adiposity rebound, which is the second rise in body mass index (BMI) that occurs between 3 and 7 years of age. Early age at adiposity rebound is known to be a risk factor for later obesity (Cole, 2004; Trost et al., 2003). Additionally, children who are overweight between the ages of 3 and 5 are 7.9 times more likely to be obese as adults than their normal-weight peers (Whitaker, Wright, Pepe, Seidel, & Dietz, 1997). As children become older and remain overweight, their risk of remaining obese into adulthood dramatically increases.

Middle Childhood

Interventions aimed at middle childhood (6–12 years of age) usually involve a much larger component directed to the child than do interventions for younger children. These interventions often use creative strategies, such as multimedia games (Cullen, Watson, Baranowski, Baranowski, & Zakeri, 2005) or creative physical activities such as jump roping (Ievers-Landis et al., 2005), which are inappropriate for younger children and less appealing to the majority of older adolescents. Children in this middle age group are at the concrete-thinking stage of cognitive development and benefit from direct information and practice in performing healthy behaviors (O'Brien & Bush, 1997). In many cases, adding the participation of parents to the intervention leads to greater long-term success in changing the child's health behaviors because parents and caregivers are still primarily responsible for most of the child's choices and actions, and the parents continue to function as important role models.

Reasons to intervene to promote healthy lifestyles during middle childhood are quite similar to those for preschool-age children. However, many more lifestyle interventions are aimed at children in this age group than at preschool-age children. The reason is that some of the physical factors that lead to chronic diseases in adulthood begin during middle childhood. For instance, peak bone mass, which is a predictor of later osteoporosis, is built and enlarged during middle childhood and early adolescence (Cummings et al., 1985). Another reason is that it is easier to work with older children as they are able to complete self-report questionnaires and provide fairly reliable responses regarding their own perceptions and feelings (e.g., self-efficacy, social support). To date, researchers have been unable to develop valid methods to reliably assess young children's internal thought processes. Older children are also more accessible, as the majority of them attend schools in which intervention programs can be implemented, whereas a smaller proportion of younger children regularly attend preschool.

Intervention Approaches

Classroom

The school environment is used increasingly to implement interventions for improving the health of children. One advantage of designing interventions for children in the school setting is that most of the targeted population can be reached (Taylor, 1999). This is especially true for younger children and preadolescents, who have lower rates of skipping school than older adolescents. Schools also have a natural intervention setting—the classroom. Classes provide structured settings of approximately 1-hour duration, and this characteristic is adaptable to interventions (Taylor, 1999). Additionally, schools are already involved in promoting the health of students. Local and state laws typically require public schools to obtain records of required immunizations and physicals before children begin classes, and school nurses provide information to students and parents regarding recommendations for preventing the spread of acute illnesses. Also, Head Start programs usually have a health component that promotes preventive healthy behaviors in a preschool setting.

Parents/Family

As the primary caregivers of children, parents play a significant role in the development of a child's health behaviors, beliefs and practices. Parents' lifestyle behaviors such as dietary intake and physical activity levels correspond to their children's behaviors (Cullen et al., 2001). For example, the amount of time parents allow their children to spend outdoors is positively related to children's physical activity behavior (Ferreira et al., 2006). Conversely, children can develop unhealthy behaviors that are similar to their parents' and other family members' (Cullen et al., 2001). Parental obesity has been found to be one of the strongest factors in predicting whether children will be overweight from birth to 9.5 years (Agras, Hammer, McNicholas, & Kraemer, 2004). In addition to a genetic influence, parents influence their children's weight by their practices during mealtimes, which may play a role in the development of childhood overweight. The less parents monitor children's food selections, the greater the children's consumption of nonnutritious foods and the higher the caloric content of their meals (Klesges, Eck, Hanson, Haddock, & Klesges, 1990). If children grow up in homes in which healthy behaviors are infrequently practiced, then other interventions (i.e., through school or clinic) may be less effective (Winett et al., 1992). Family-based behavioral interventions or the inclusion of a parent component in another type of intervention (e.g., school-based) may exert influence both directly on the child and through the family by educating parents regarding the health recommendations for their children.

Environment

The built environment can be important in efforts to improve the lifestyle be-haviors of children. The built environment is defined as consisting of neighbor-hoods, roads, buildings, food sources, and recreational facilities in which people live, work, are educated, eat, and play (Sallis & Glanz, 2006). Environmental influences on food choices and physical activities such as aspects of the home and school are associated with children's lifestyle behaviors. For example, the physical activity–related policies in schools significantly influence children's engagement in physical activity (Ferreira et al., 2006). Environmental aspects of the local neighborhood, such as parents' perceptions that the neighborhood has heavy traffic and no lights or safe crossings or that children need to cross sev-eral roads to reach play areas, are related to a decreased likelihood of children walking or cycling at least three times per week, depending on the child's age and gender (Timperio, Crawford, Telford, & Salmon, 2004). Social ecological models support the hypothesis that behaviors are influenced by both the social and physical environments, as well as by intrapersonal factors (Sallis & Owen, 1999). The focus of interventions drawn from a social ecological model is on the implementation of structural changes in the environment rather than on individual-level approaches (Matson-Koffman, Brownstein, Neiner, & Greaney, 2005). Examples include increasing the availability of low-fat foods (e.g., through school policies aimed at reducing fat in school lunches) and implementing reg-ulations requiring sidewalks within a community.

Clinic/Primary Care

Health behavior change interventions that are delivered by physicians or other medical staff in the clinic are usually perceived as credible by the targeted per-son. Physicians also are able to monitor children's health and to check their health status against national norms (e.g., BMI) over time (Wald et al., 2005). The one-on-one setting promotes discussion about the individual child's health needs (Taylor, 1999), and parents may be more willing to voice their concerns about their child's health to a trusted family pediatrician than to an unfamil-iar behavioral interventionist. In many cases, the family doctor will also have knowledge about the child's family's medical history and health behavior (e.g., history of cancer, diabetes, obesity, or smoking). Another advantage is that par-ents may be more likely to follow a pediatrician's recommendations for health change. Some innovative physician practices are attempting to integrate "health coaches" to better motivate patients to make health behavior changes (Adelman & Graybill, 2005). One drawback to implementing health behavior change inter-ventions through a physician's office is that only one child is helped at a time. Also, depending on the age of the child and the frequency of medical visits, the follow-ups may be too few and far between.

Intervention Strategies

The types of interventions used with children vary and may include a combi-nation of behavioral, educational, and environmental components. Behavioral interventions may include such strategies as self-monitoring via charting, goal setting, and the earning of rewards for appropriate gains. Educational interventions are based on the belief that children and parents will change their health behaviors if they are given adequate information about desirable health behaviors. Environmental interventions use strategies that involve changing the physical surroundings and social, economic or organizational systems to promote individual behavior change.

Interventions to Improve Lifestyle Behaviors in the General Population

Two of the most common causes of disease, disability, and premature death in the United States are the health risk behaviors of consumption of an unhealthy diet and physical inactivity (Mokdad et al., 2000). Therefore, a general purpose of lifestyle interventions for the young, regardless of risk status, is to promote the adoption of healthy lifestyle behaviors for reducing the risk of diseases such as type 2 diabetes mellitus, cardiovascular disease, hyperlipidemia, and certain types of cancer that may occur in childhood or later in adulthood. These interventions target dietary intake, physical activity, sedentary behavior, or a combination of these.

As an example of a dietary change intervention, a school-based program targeted fruit, 100% juice, and vegetable (FJV) consumption changes by meal among fourth graders participating in "Squire's Quest!," a 10-session individualized multimedia game (Cullen et al., 2005). The game involves many meal- and environment-specific behavioral change techniques and is based on social cognitive theory (Bandura, 1986). At each session, students set goals to make at home the recipe prepared in the virtual kitchen and to eat an FJV serving at a specified meal and snack at home and at school. A total of 26 elementary schools were randomly assigned to treatment or control groups. Results were that students in the intervention group consumed one more serving FJV per day, with significantly more servings of fruits and 100% fruit juice at snacks and more vegetables at lunch than did children in the control condition schools. Conclusions were that while multimedia games with meal- and environment-targeted goal setting may improve dietary habits within the school setting, additional research is needed to generalize these improvements to meals eaten outside school.

As an example of a lifestyle-intervention targeting physical activity, 30 preadolescent girls from two after school programs were randomized to a Pilates intervention or control group (Jago, Jonker, Missaghian, & Baranowski, 2006). The Pilates classes were provided free for an hour per day, 5 days a week, for 1 month. Mean attendance was 75%. Findings were significant time by group interactions for BMI percentile, with small changes in BMI percentiles for the intervention group. Another intervention targeted the physical activities of 228 children over a 3-year period, from ages 3 to 7 years (Sääkslahti et al., 2004). Parents in the intervention group attended annual hour-long meetings to discuss the importance of physical activity for children. Twice yearly they were provided with printed education materials and activity posters. In addition, they were given a board game that involved practicing many different fundamental motor skills. Children in the intervention group spent significantly more time playing outside, and engagement in high-activity play increased with age in the intervention group but not for the controls.

Interventions for the Prevention or Treatment of Childhood Obesity

Other lifestyle interventions for the young are specifically designed for the prevention and treatment of childhood overweight. The prevalence of childhood overweight is growing at an alarming rate and is linked to serious short- and long-term morbidity (Freedman, Dietz, Srinivasan, & Berenson, 1999; Strauss, 1999; Williams et al., 2002). Unfortunately, young children are not immune from the growing trend, and even preschool-age children are evidencing increasing rates of becoming overweight (Mei, Scanlon, Grummer-Strawn, Freedman, Yip, & Trowbridge, 1998; Ogden et al., 1997). In an overview of obesity prevention, Baranowski and colleagues (2000) noted that increased activity and improved diet are beneficial for everyone regardless of their risk for obesity. Testing broad, population-based prevention programs may be reasonable to reduce adiposity for the overweight, to potentially lower the overall incidence of obesity, and to improve protective behaviors against chronic disease among all children who are targets of the programs. Targeting interventions to children who are already overweight or obese is valuable because it directs a program at those most likely to benefit. Much progress has been made in the treatment of childhood obesity (Epstein, Myers, Raynor, & Saelens, 1998), and reviews suggest that behavioral treatments of childhood obesity targeting lifestyle behaviors are considered to be empirically validated treatments (Jelalian & Saelens, 1999).

Prevention of Childhood Obesity

An obesity prevention program specifically targeting preschoolers is "Hip-Hop to Health, Jr." (Fitzgibbon et al., 2004; Stolley et al., 2003). This is a well-designed 5-year randomized clinical trial of a dietary and physical activity intervention targeting 3- to 5-year-old minority children enrolled in Head Start. Children in the intervention arm participated in a 14-week healthy eating and physical activity program (40 minutes at three times per week) that involved a 20-minute lesson with colorful handheld puppets and 20 minutes of physical activity. Parents of children in the intervention arm received weekly newsletters with information on healthy eating and physical activity that included a homework assignment, and they received a $5 coupon for each assignment they turned in. The controls received a 14-week program on general health with a similar parent newsletter. Results for 197 intervention and 212 control children were that the intervention group had significantly smaller increases in BMI than did controls at 1- and 2-year follow-ups (approximately .54 kg/m^2). No significant differences were found for parent-reported food intake/physical activity except that the percentage of calories from saturated fat was higher in controls at 1-year follow-up. The sample included primarily African American children, and approximately 1/3 of the children were overweight or obese. Relative effects of the intervention were similar for children who were of normal weight and those who were either overweight or obese (i.e., at or above the 85th percentile of BMI) at baseline.

Treatment of Childhood Obesity

Interventions targeted at high-risk groups, such as children who are obese or who have one or more obese parents, are an alternative approach to prevention (Baranowski et al., 2000). In one study of 63 8–12-year-old obese children, various methods for reducing sedentary behavior were compared. Epstein and colleagues (Epstein, Paluch, Kilanowski, & Raynor, 2004) evaluated family-based behavioral treatment that included either reinforcement or stimulus control of sedentary behavior. In the reinforced group, positive reinforcement was contingent on reducing targeted sedentary behaviors; in the stimulus control group, positive reinforcement was contingent on recording targeted sedentary behaviors. The treatment program for both groups included 16 weekly meetings, followed by four follow-up meetings during a 6-month period. Families received workbooks for weight self-monitoring, information on the *Traffic Light Diet* and behavior change techniques, and suggestions for maintenance of behavior change. Findings were significant, with equivalent improvements in lifestyle behaviors noted for both groups. Children who substituted physical activity for sedentary behaviors had significantly greater BMI z-score changes at 6- and 12-month follow-ups.

The primary care setting has been a recently expanding area for intervening to prevent or treat childhood obesity. In a pilot study by Wald et al. (2005), an intervention was tested in two diverse primary care settings where physicians were trained in using brief motivational strategies to help parents make health behavior changes related to nutrition and physical activity for their overweight or obese children. The intervention was successful at increasing physicians' willingness to engage in discussions about nutrition and weight status with parents of their high-risk child patients. The practice of measuring and charting the children's BMI-for-age percentiles was easily integrated into current practice.

Interventions for Risk Reduction for Specific Future Health Conditions

Osteoporosis

Prevention of osteoporosis provides an opportunity to test behavioral interventions for improving healthy lifestyle behaviors among children (Ievers-Landis et al., 2003). Although commonly associated with postmenopausal women and the elderly, osteoporosis has been linked to bone development during childhood and adolescence (Cummings et al., 1985). Peak bone mass is one of the major predictors of the risk of fracture in osteoporosis, and approximately 40% of the skeletal structure is built and enlarged during late childhood and early adolescence (Cummings et al., 1985). Females are particularly at risk for development of osteoporosis. The risk of developing osteoporosis can be reduced by the adoption of healthy lifestyle behaviors (e.g., increasing dietary calcium [Ca] intake and weight-bearing physical activity [WBPA]) (Teegarden, Lyle, Prouiz, Johnston, & Weaver, 1999).

A randomized controlled trial of a behavioral-educational intervention for the primary prevention of osteoporosis was conducted for 247 preadolescent girls via their Girl Scout troops (Ievers-Landis et al., 2005). Troops were randomly assigned to two intervention groups, girls only or girls with their mothers, or to a healthy lifestyles control group. The program, *Know Bones About It,* involved skills training in enhancement of dietary Ca intake and WBPA using self-monitoring, feedback on goal attainment, social persuasion, problem-solving training, role modeling, and practice of the desired behaviors (e.g., jumping rope and eating Ca-rich snacks). Sessions for the group that included mothers were the same as those for the girls-only group but included two interactive sessions led by a psychologist who focused on maternal role modeling, creating a healthy environment, and positive reinforcement. Among girls who met the recommended levels of Ca at baseline, those in the intervention groups were significantly more likely to maintain or improve their intake at follow-up visits than were girls in the control group. No significant group differences were found for changes in WBPA.

Risk Reduction for Skin Cancer

The American Academy of Dermatology reports that almost one in six people will develop some type of skin cancer in his or her lifetime, and other reports show 25% of people under the age of 40 will develop melanoma (Ahmedin, Thomas, Murray, & Thun, 2002; Turrisi et al., 2004). The majority of the reported cases of skin cancer are now believed to be the result of the use of tanning equipment and salons, inadequate sun protection (misuse or lack of sun block) and excessive intentional sun bathing (Hall, May, Lew, Koh, & Nadel, 1997; Thompson, Jolley, & Marks, 1993; Turrisi et al., 2004). Interventions aimed at reducing unsafe sun behaviors have addressed individuals' beliefs about sun safe behaviors and sun risk through educational programs (Turrisi et al., 2004). Hypotheses are that beliefs about risks posed by exposure to the sun will influence intentional sun-related behaviors (tanning and sunbathing) and consequences (Clarke, Williams, & Arthey, 1997; Turrisi et al., 2004).

An intervention study by Turrisi et al. (2004) was designed to prevent skin cancer in children and young adolescents by using parents as the primary change agents. Four hundred and sixty nine children were divided into intervention and control groups. Parents in the intervention group were given a handbook that provided background information on the incidence of skin cancer and consequences of UV exposure. The handbook included intervention materials that instructed parents on how to initiate conversations about skin cancer, including discussions of high-risk and positive "sun-safe" behaviors. Other materials included teaching children assertiveness skills and techniques for dealing with peer pressure. Evaluation of the intervention outcomes found significant differences between treatment and control groups; participants in the treatment group became sunburned less often and had less severe burns than did those in the control group. The groups also differed significantly in terms of sunbathing tendencies and attitudes and beliefs about sunbathing, tanning, appearance, and skin cancer risk.

Risk Reduction for Other Types of Cancer

Risk reduction efforts for other types of cancers related to lifestyle behaviors should begin in childhood and continue throughout all stages of life (Uauy & Solomons, 2005). Even among young children, being overweight is linked to potentially increased cancer risk (Berkey, Gardner, Frazier, & Colditz, 2000; Freedson, Melanson, & Sirard, 1998; Strauss, 1999). By age 6, children who are overweight show hormonal changes that are risk factors for cancer in adults who are obese (Gascon et al., 2004). Girls who are overweight and inactive in preadolescence may experience early menarche, a risk factor for breast cancer (Chavarro et al., 2005). Physical activity and body size and composition are well-recognized strong predictors of the initiation of menses (Berkey et al., 2000). If the trend toward a greater incidence of childhood overweight continues, we can expect an increase in the incidence of certain types of cancer as these children become adults. Obesity in adulthood is a proven risk factor for cancers of the colon, female breast, endometrium, kidney, esophagus, and liver (Bugianesi, 2005; Key, Allen, Spencer, & Travis, 2002; Key et al., 2004). Cancer risk reduction beginning with young children is also vital because food preferences and physical activity habits are set relatively early in life (Birch et al, 2001), and both may be important for prevention of cancer (Key et al., 2002, 2004). Fruit and vegetables may reduce the adult risk for cancers of the oral cavity, esophagus, stomach, and colon, and physical activity reduces risk for colorectal and possibly breast cancer (Key et al., 2004).

Although not yet a common focus, interventions are being designed to address the link between lifestyle behaviors in childhood and future cancer risk. For example, recently published results from a school-based obesity prevention program demonstrated that a one-unit increase in baseline BMI was associated with a 7% increased risk of early menarche. Attending a school assigned to intervention status was associated with a decreased risk of experiencing early menarche during the 19-month study period (Chavarro et al., 2005). Other interventions with children that focus on healthy lifestyles or prevention and treatment of obesity may have an impact on later cancer incidence. Specific mediators in addition to weight status, hormonal changes and time of menarche related to health behaviors may predict future cancer risk for children and should be explored. Examining animal models may lead to the identification of other mediators to be examined, though the time factor in determining whether risk reduction interventions will be effective in reducing cancer incidence makes this area quite challenging.

Interventions to Reduce Accidents or Unintentional Injury

A majority of children and adolescents are at risk for death due to preventable accidents or unintentional injuries. According to the Centers for Disease Control statistics (Centers for Disease Control, 2004), accidents or unintentional injuries were the leading cause of death for this population. Children are at a greater risk for morbidity and mortality due to unintentional injuries than are adults. In Westernized countries, unintentional injuries have replaced infectious disease as the major cause of death in childhood (Bockholdt & Schneider, 2003). The strongest predictors of injury are male gender, inadequate supervision, and an impulsive temperament (Brehaut, Miller, Raina, & McGrail, 2003).

Every year about 1 million people die and about 10 million are seriously injured on the roads across the globe (Murray & Lopez, 1996). The World Health Organization (WHO) has reported that for children, adolescence and young adults ages 3–35 years, road traffic crashes are now the leading cause of disablement and death. Children are particularly vulnerable, and pedestrian injuries account for most of the childhood road deaths each year (Duperrex, Bunn, & Roberts, 2002; Murray & Lopez, 1996; Rivara, 1990). To reduce and possibly prevent pedestrian injuries, educational measures to teach children how to cope with traffic are considered to be an important part of any intervention (Duperrex et al., 2002). Duperrex et al. (2002) reviewed current randomized controlled trials on pedestrian road-crossing behavior. Their aim was to identify the effectiveness of safety education interventions for pedestrians in improving knowledge and behavior as a means for preventing pedestrian-related motor vehicle accidents. Their findings were mixed, partly because of the multiple risk factors for child pedestrian injuries. They found that behaviorally oriented interventions might be best able to address these issues.

One such intervention designed by Barton, Schwebel, and Morrongiello (2006) tested a skill-based training intervention for increasing safe road-crossing behaviors in children. The intervention targeted multiple basic pedestrian skills, such as waiting for safe traffic gaps and looking right and left before crossing. The intervention components were designed to be delivered in a single brief session (less than 15 minutes) and could be taught by parents. The intervention was delivered to 85 children ages 5–8 and utilized a pre-post design. Results of the study indicate that children behaved more safely following training. Specifically, children attended more to traffic patterns, waited longer before crossing the street and waited for larger gaps between vehicles prior to crossing. The study also found that girls and older children engaged in safer pedestrian behaviors than did boys and younger children.

Future Directions

Sleep Enhancement Interventions

Sleep is often overlooked in discussions of lifestyle behaviors, but children's sleep habits are as important as diet and activity levels for their present and future health (Ievers-Landis & Redline, 2007). As a prime example, insufficient sleep is one potentially vital factor that has been neglected in interventions to prevent or reduce childhood overweight; lack of sleep is emerging as a novel risk factor for overweight in both children and adults. A review by D. B. Allison and colleagues (Keith et al., 2006) of novel risk factors for the obesity epidemic recently identified a number of environmental and sociocultural factors that have changed since 1970 with the substantial increase of obesity. In addition to environmental changes that focus on food marketing practices and institution-driven reductions in physical activity, this group identified at least 10 additional explanations, including sleep debt. Longitudinal data suggest a causative role for short sleep in the preschool period for the later development of childhood overweight (Agras et al., 2004). In a prospective study of 150 children, hours of sleep reported annually for children ages 3 to 5 were negatively related with overweight status at 9.5 years of age (Agras et al., 2004). Children who were to become overweight were reported to sleep 30 minutes less on average in a

24-hour period than those who remained normal weight. Several large cross-sectional studies of childhood obesity have reported strong associations between obesity and short sleep duration, including among children as young as 5 (Locard et al., 1992; Sekine et al., 2002; Von Kries, Toschke, Wurmser, Sauerwald, & Koletzko, 2002). Short sleep duration has emerged as a stronger predictor of childhood overweight than parent education, parent BMI, children's birth weight, snacking habits, and sedentary behavior. An urgent need exists for the development, validation, and dissemination of sleep enhancement interventions for children of all ages.

Primary Care Practice for Supporting Healthy Behaviors

Many of the issues in this chapter may be addressed by prevention counseling practices of primary care pediatricians. Further efforts are needed to improve the ability of pediatricians to effectively deliver educational materials, individualized advice and recommendations of resources for further reading (e.g., specially created Internet portals) or for local classes and memberships (e.g., referral to a dietitian, recommendation to join a gym) to parents. As examples, currently primary care pediatricians may not be adequately addressing osteoporosis and obesity prevention. According to a survey of 187 primary care pediatricians, knowledge of the U.S. recommended daily allowance for Ca in children and adolescents was limited, with only 23.7% and 32.3% correctly identifying the recommended values for children and adolescents, respectively (Fleming & Patrick, 2002). Additionally, fewer than half reported that they counseled patients to reduce osteoporosis risk because other issues took priority or they lacked the sufficient time to bring up such issues. A survey of 1,066 physicians regarding their attitudes and practices related to treatment of childhood overweight in primary care settings found that only 26.6% of physicians discussed weight with children age 12 and younger who were mildly overweight, while 95.5% discussed weight with children who were morbidly overweight (Jelalian, Boergers, Alday, & Frank, 2003). Physicians may benefit by obtaining ongoing education about lifestyle behavior (e.g., obtaining specialized training by attending workshops) and by reading brief information sheets about the prevention of future health conditions such as osteoporosis and skin cancer (Fleming & Patrick, 2002).

Another area of growth could be via the inclusion of motivational interviewing (MI) techniques into the primary care setting. MI is designed to increase intrinsic motivation in patients by exploring and resolving areas of ambivalence (Miller & Rollnick, 2002). MI is a patient-centered directive therapy that is based on the five guiding principles of showing empathy, being aware of ambivalence, understanding resistance to change, avoiding arguments, and supporting self-efficacy (Miller & Rollnick, 2002). In a study by Adelman and Graybill (2005), the use of MI-consistent strategies by a "health coach" in primary care settings led 48% of the adult patients studied to initiate health behavior change in their physical activity or eating habits. Exploring the use of MI-consistent strategies delivered by a health coach in pediatric offices to work with both parents and with older children regarding their ambivalence about behavior change is an area for further exploration.

Summary

Lifestyle interventions for the young include a wide range of approaches and settings, including the classroom, with parents and family in the home, and environmental, clinic-based, and primary care settings. Strategies to change behaviors often take into account a combination of behavioral, educational, and environmental factors. Although many of these interventions focus on improving children's dietary intake and activity levels, the stated purposes of the interventions vary from general prevention of later health conditions regardless of risk status to specific goals for treatment of childhood obesity or prevention of osteoporosis, various cancers and accidents or unintentional injuries. In the future, researchers are encouraged to consider the addition of sleep as a vital lifestyle behavior because of the consistent finding of a strong relationship between insufficient sleep and childhood obesity. Also, efforts for greater involvement of pediatricians are strongly encouraged to strengthen existing pilot work and to build on successful programs with adult patients, such as the use of MI-consistent strategies using a "health coach."

References

Adelman, A. M., & Graybill, M. (2005). Integrating a health coach into primary care: Reflections from the Penn State ambulatory research network. *Annals of Family Medicine, 3*(2), S33–S35.

Agras, W. S., Hammer, L. D., McNicholas, F., & Kraemer, H. C. (2004). Risk factors for Childhood overweight: A prospective study from birth to 9.5 years. *Journal of Pediatrics, 145,* 20–25.

Ahmedin, J., Thomas, A., Murray, T., & Thun, M. (2002). Cancer statistics, 2002. *CA: A Cancer Journal for Clinicians, 52,* 23–45.

Bandura, A. (1986). *Social foundations for thought and action: A social cognitive theory.* Englewood Cliffs, NJ: Prentice-Hall.

Baranowski, T., Mendlein, J., Resnicow, K., Frank, E., Cullen, K. W., & Baranowski, J. (2000). Physical activity and nutrition in children and youth: An overview of obesity prevention. *Preventive Medicine, 31,* S1–S10.

Barton, B. K., Schwebel, D. C., & Morrongiello, B. A. (2006). Brief report: Increasing children's safe pedestrian behaviors through simple skills training. *Journal of Pediatric Psychology, 32,* 475–480.

Berkey, C. S., Gardner, J. D., Frazier, A. L., & Colditz, G. A. (2000). Relation of childhood diet and body size to menarche and adolescent growth in girls. *American Journal of Epidemiology, 152,* 446–452.

Birch, L. L., Fisher, J. O., Grimm-Thomas, K., Markey, C. N., Sawyer, R., & Johnson, S. L. (2001). Confirmatory factor analysis of the Child Feeding Questionnaire: A measure of parental attitudes, beliefs and practices about child feeding and obesity proneness. *Appetite, 36,* 201–210.

Bockholdt, B., & Schneider, V., (2003). The injury pattern to children involved in lethal traffic accidents in Berlin. *Legal Medicine, 5*(Suppl. 11), 390–392.

Brehaut, J. C., Miller, A., Raina, P., & McGrail, K. M. (2003). Childhood behavior disorders and injuries among children and youth: A population-based study. *Pediatrics, 111,* 262–269.

Bugianesi, E. (2005). Review article: Steatosis, the metabolic syndrome and cancer. *Ailmentary Pharmacology & Therapeutics, 22*(Suppl. 2), 40–43.

Centers for Disease Control. (2004). *Unintentional injuries, violence, and the health of young people.* Retrieved June 17, 2008, from http://www.cdc.gov/healthyyouth/injury/facts.htm

Chavarro, J. E., Peterson, K. E., Sobol, A. M., Wiecha, J. L., & Gortmaker, S. L. (2005). Effects of a school-based obesity prevention intervention on menarche. *Cancer Causes and Control, 16,* 1245–1252.

Clarke, V. A., Williams, T., & Arthey, S. (1997). Skin type and optimistic bias in relation to the sun protection and suntanning behaviors of young adults. *Journal of Behavioral Medicine, 20,* 207–222.

Cole, T. J. (2004). Children grow and horses race: Is the adiposity rebound a critical period for later obesity? *BMC Pediatrics, 4,* 6.

Cullen, K., Baranowski, T., Rittenberry, L., Cosart, C., Hebert, D., & de Moor, C. (2001). Child-reported family and peer influences on fruit, juice, and vegetable consumption: Reliability and validity of measures. *Health Education Research, 16,* 187–200.

Cullen, K. W., Watson, K., Baranowski, T., Baranowski, J. H., & Zakeri, I. (2005). Squire's quest: Intervention changes occurred at lunch and snack meals. *Appetite, 45,* 148–151.

Cummings, S. R., Kelsey, J. L., Nevitt, M. C., & O'Dowd, K. J. (1985). Epidemiology of osteoporosis and osteoporosis fractures. *Epidemiologic Reviews, 7,* 178–208.

Damashek, A., & Peterson, L. (2002). Unintentional injury prevention efforts for young children: Levels, methods, types, and targets. *Journal of Developmental and Behavioral Pediatrics, 23,* 443–455.

Davis, K. J., Cokkinides, V. E., Weinstock, M. A., O'Connell, M. C., & Wingo, P. A. (2002). Summer sunburn and sun exposure among U.S. youth ages 11 to 18: National prevalence and associated factors. *Pediatrics, 110,* 27–35.

Duperrex, O., Bunn, F., & Roberts, I. (2002). Safety education of pedestrians for injury prevention: A systematic review of randomized controlled trials. *British Medical Journal, 324,* 1129.

Ekelund, U., Ong, K., Linne, Y., Neovius, M., Brage, S., Dunger, D. B., et al. (2006). Upward weight percentile crossing in infancy and early childhood independently predicts fat mass in young adults: The Stockholm Weight Development Study (SWEDES). *American Journal of Clinical Nutrition, 83,* 324–330.

Epstein, L. H., Myers, M. D., Raynor, H. A., & Saelens, B. E. (1998). Treatment of pediatric obesity. *Pediatrics, 101,* 554–570.

Epstein, L. H., Paluch, R. A., Kilanowski, C. K., & Raynor, H. A. (2004). The effect of reinforcement or stimulus control to reduce sedentary behavior in the treatment of pediatric obesity. *Health Psychology, 23,* 371–380.

Ferreira, E., van der Horst, K., Wendel-Vos, W., Kremer, S., van Lenthe, F. J., & Brug, J. (2006). Environmental correlates of physical activity in youth—a review and update. *Obesity Reviews, 8,* 129–154.

Fitzgibbon, M. L., Stolley, M. R., Schiffer, L., Van Horn, L., Kaufer Christoffel, D., & Dyer, A. (2004). Two-year follow-up results for Hip-Hop to Health, Jr.: A randomized controlled trial for overweight prevention in preschool minority children. *Journal of Pediatrics, 146,* 618–625.

Fleming, R., & Patrick, K. (2002). Osteoporosis prevention: Pediatricians' knowledge, attitudes and counseling practices. *Preventive Medicine, 34,* 411–421.

Freedman, D., Dietz, W., Srinivasan, S., & Berenson, G. (1999). The relation of overweight to cardiovascular risk factors among children and adolescents: The Bogalusa Heart Study. *Pediatrics, 103,* 1175–1182.

Freedson, P. S., Melanson, E., & Sirard, J. (1998). Calibration of the computer science and applications, Inc. accelerometer. *Medicine and Science in Sports and Exercise, 30,* 777–781.

Gascon, F., Valle, M., Martos, R., Zafra, M., Morales, R., & Castano, M. A. (2004). Childhood obesity and hormonal abnormalities associated with cancer risk. *European Journal of Cancer Prevention, 13,* 193–197.

Hall, H. I., May, D. S., Lew, R. A., Koh, H. K., & Nadel, M. (1997). Sun protection behaviors of the U.S. white population. *Preventive Medicine, 26,* 401–407.

Ievers-Landis, C. E., Burant, B., Drotar, D., Morgan, L., Trapl, E. S., Colabianchi, N., et al. (2005). A randomized controlled trial for the primary prevention of osteoporosis among preadolescent Girl Scouts: One-year outcomes of a behavioral program. *Journal of Pediatric Psychology, 30,* 155–165.

Ievers-Landis, C. E., Burant, C., Drotar, D., Morgan, L., Trapl, E. S., & Kwoh, C. K. (2003). Social support, knowledge, and self-efficacy as correlates of osteoporosis preventive behaviors among preadolescent females. *Journal of Pediatric Psychology, 28,* 335–345.

Ievers-Landis, C. E., & Redline, S. (2007). Pediatric sleep apnea: Implications of the epidemic of childhood overweight. *American Journal of Respiratory and Critical Care Medicine, 175,* 436–441.

Jago, R., Jonker, M. L., Missaghian, M., & Baranowski, T. (2006). Effect of 4 weeks of Pilates on the body composition of young girls. *Preventive Medicine, 42,* 177–180.

Jelalian, E., Boergers, J., Alday, C. S., & Frank, R. (2003). Survey of physician attitudes and practices related to pediatric obesity. *Clinical Pediatrics, 42,* 235–245.

Jelalian, E., & Saelens, B. E. (1999). Empirically supported treatments in pediatric psychology: Pediatric obesity. *Journal of Pediatric Psychology, 24,* 223–248.

Johnson, S. L., & Birch, L. L. (1994). Parents' and children's adiposity and eating style. *Pediatrics, 94,* 653–661.

Keith, S.W., Redden, D. T., Katzmarzyk, P. T., Boggiano, M. M., Hanlon, E. C., Benca, R. M., et al. (2006). Putative contributors to the secular increase in obesity: Exploring the roads less traveled. *International Journal of Obesity, 30,* 1585–1594.

Key, T. J., Allen, N. E., Spencer, E. A., & Travis, R. C. (2002). The effect of diet on risk of cancer. *Lancet, 360,* 861–868.

Key, T. J., Schatzkin, A., Willett, W. C., Allen, N. E., Spencer, E. A., & Travis, R. C. (2004). Diet, nutrition and the prevention of cancer. *Public Health Nutrition, 7,* 187–200.

Klesges, R. C., Eck, L. H., Hanson, C. L., Haddock, C. K., & Klesges, L. M. (1990). Effects of obesity, social interactions, and physical environment on physical activity in preschoolers. *Health Psychology, 9,* 435–449.

Locard, E., Mamelle, N., Billette, A., Miginiac, M., Munoz, F., & Rey, S. (1992). Risk factors of obesity in a five-year-old population. Parental versus environmental factors. *International Journal of Obesity Related Metabolic Disorders, 16,* 721–729.

Matson-Koffman, D. M., Brownstein, J. N., Neiner, J. A., & Greaney, M. L. (2005). A site-specific literature review of policy and environmental interventions that promote physical activity and nutrition for cardiovascular health: What works? *American Journal of Health Promotion, 19*(3), 167–193.

Mei, Z., Scanlon, K., Grummer-Strawn, L., Freedman, D., Yip, R., & Trowbridge, F. (1998). Increasing prevalence of overweight among U.S. low-income preschool children: The Centers for Disease Control and Prevention pediatric nutrition surveillance, 1983 to 1995. *Pediatrics, 101*(1), E12.

Miller, W. R., & Rollnick, S. (2002). *Motivational interviewing: Preparing people for change* (2nd ed.). New York: Guilford Press.

Mokdad, A. H., Marks, J. S., Stroup, D. F., & Gerberding, J. L. (2000). Actual causes of death in the United States. *Journal of the American Medical Association, 291,* 1238–1245.

Murray, C. J., & Lopez, A. D. (1996). *Global health statistics: A compendium of incidence, prevalence and mortality estimates for over 200 conditions.* Geneva: World Health Organization.

O'Brien, R. W., & Bush, P. J. (1997). Health behavior in children. In David S. Gochman (Ed.), *Handbook of health behavior research III: Demography, development, and diversity.* New York: Plenum Press.

Ogden, C. L., Flegal, K. M., Carroll, M. D., & Johnson, C. L. (2002). Prevalence and trends in overweight among U.S. children and adolescents, 1999–2000. *Journal of the American Medical Association, 288,* 1728–1732.

Ogden, C. L., Troiano, R., Briefel, R., Kuczmarski, R., Flegal, K., & Johnson, C. (1997). Prevalence of overweight among preschool children in the United States, 1971 through 1994. *Pediatrics, 99,* 4, E1.

Rivara, F. P. (1990). Child pedestrian injuries in the United States. Current status of the problem, potential interventions, and future research needs. *American Journal of Diseases of Children, 144,* 692–696.

Sääkslahti, A., Numminen, P., Varstala, V., Helenius, H., Tammi, A., Viikari, J., et al. (2004). Physical activity as a preventive measure for coronary heart disease risk factors in early childhood. *Scandinavian Journal of Medicine & Science in Sports, 14,* 143–149.

Sallis, J. F., & Glanz, D. (2006). The role of built environments in physical activity, eating, and obesity in childhood. *Future Child, 16*(1), 89–108.

Sallis, J. F., & Owen, N. (1999). *Physical activity and behavioral medicine.* Thousand Oaks, CA: Sage.

Sekine, M., Yamagami, T., Handa, K., Saito, T., Nanri, S., Kawaminami, K., et al. (2002). A dose-response relationship between short sleeping hours and childhood obesity: Results of the Toyama Birth Cohort Study. *Child Care Health and Development, 28,* 163–170.

Sherry, B. (2005). Food behaviors and other strategies to prevent and treat pediatric overweight. *International Journal of Obesity, 29,* S116–S126.

Stolley, M. R., Fitzgibbon, M. L., Dyer, A., Van Horn, L., KauferChristoffel, K., & Schiffer, L. (2003). Hip-hop to Health, Jr., an obesity prevention program for minority preschool children: Baseline characteristics of participants. *Preventive Medicine, 36,* 320–329.

Strauss, R. (1999). Childhood obesity. *Current Problems in Pediatrics, 29,* 1–29.

Sullivan, S. A., & Birch, L. L. (1990). Pass the sugar, pass the salt: Experiences dictates preferences. *Developmental Psychology, 26,* 546–555.

Taylor, S. E. (1999). *Health psychology* (4th ed.). Boston: McGraw-Hill.

Teegarden, D., Lyle, R. M., Proulx, W. R., Johnston, C. C., & Weaver, C. M. (1999). Previous milk consumption is associated with greater bone density in young women. *The American Journal of Clinical Nutrition, 69,* 1014–1017.

Thompson, S. C., Jolley, D., & Marks, R. (1993). Reduction of solar keratoses by regular sunscreen use. *New England Journal of Medicine, 329,* 1147–1151.

Timperio, A., Crawford, D., Telford, A., & Salmon, J. (2004). Perceptions about the local neighborhood and walking and cycling among children. *Preventive Medicine, 38,* 39–47.

Trost, S. G., Sirard, J. R., Dowda, M., Pfeiffer, K. A., & Pate, R. R. (2003). Physical activity in overweight and non-overweight preschool children. *International Journal of Obesity, 27,* 834–839.

Turrisi, R., Hillhouse, J., Heavin, S., Robinson, J., Adams, M., & Berry, J. (2004). Examination of the short-term efficacy of a parent-based intervention to prevent skin cancer. *Journal of Behavioral Medicine, 27,* 393–412.

Uauy, R., & Solomons, N. (2005). Diet, nutrition, and the life-course approach to cancer prevention. *Journal of Nutrition, 135,* 29345S–2945S.

Von Kries, R., Toschke, A. M., Wurmser, H., Sauerwald, T., & Koletzko, B. (2002). Reduced risk for overweight and obesity in 5- and 6-yr-old children by duration of sleep—a cross-sectional study. *International Journal of Obesity and Related Metabolic Disorders, 26,* 710–716.

Wald, E. R., Ewing, L., Cluss, P., Goldstrohm, S., Cipriani, L., & Colborn, K. (2005). Establishing a family-based intervention for overweight children in pediatric practice. *Annals of Family Medicine, 3*(2), S45–S47.

Whitaker, R. C., Wright, J. A., Pepe, M. S., Seidel, K. D., & Dietz, W. H. (1997). Predicting obesity in young adulthood from childhood and parental obesity. *New England Journal of Medicine, 337,* 869–73.

Williams, C. L., Hayman, L. L., Daniels, S. R., Robinson, T. N., Steinberger, J., Pardon, S., et al. (2002). Cardiovascular health in childhood. *Circulation, 106,* 143–160.

Winett, R. A., Anderson, E. S., Moore, J. F., Sikkema, K. J., Hook, R. J., & Webster, D. A. (1992). Family/media approach to HIV prevention: Results with a home-based, parent-teen video program. *Health Psychology, 11,* 203–206.

Problems With Adherence in the Elderly

26

Carolyn L. Murdaugh
and Kathleen Insel

The aging population in the United States is one of the major public health challenges in the 21st century. Two factors, longevity and aging baby boomers, will influence the growth of Americans 65 years or older during the next 25 years (Centers for Disease Control and Prevention [CDC] and Merck Company Foundation [MCF], 2007). Baby boomers, those born between 1946 and 1964, represent nearly one-third of the population and will begin turning age 65 in 2011; by 2020, all of the baby boomers will be age 65 or older. As a result, older Americans are expected to make up 20% of the total population (U.S. Bureau of the Census, 2000).

Improved medical care and prevention efforts have contributed to dramatic increases in life expectancy. Persons born in 1900 could expect a life expectancy of 47 years, whereas those born in 2001 can expect to live 77 years (CDC & MCF,

2007). As a result of longer life spans, major shifts have occurred in the leading causes of death. Infectious and acute diseases have been replaced by chronic and degenerative diseases. The three leading causes of death in persons 65 years and older are heart disease, cancer, and stroke. It is estimated that 80% of older Americans have a minimum of one chronic disease, and 50% have at least two (National Center for Health Statistics [NCHS], 2006). More than two-thirds of health care costs are currently spent treating chronic illness conditions in older adults, with 95% of the health care expenditures for the three major chronic diseases. By 2030, it is expected that health care expenditures will increase by 25%, without taking inflation into account, because of the demographic shift to an elderly population.

The expanding aging population and its accompanying increased burden of chronic diseases have created new challenges to ensure that the added years are quality ones. A major challenge is management of medical regimens (CDC & MCF, 2007). Almost half of all older Americans are treated for hypertension or arthritis. Other chronic conditions requiring treatment include heart disease, cancer, stroke, and diabetes. At some point, all chronic conditions require adherence to complex medication regimens or other types of treatments to effectively manage the disease and postpone disability and death. However, adherence rates to long-term regimens average 50%, regardless of the illness, regimen, or adherence criteria (World Health Organization [WHO], 2003). Nonadherence is most common with chronic conditions, in long-term therapy, and in preventive efforts (WHO, 2003). Thus, adherence is and will persist as a major health care issue in the elderly.

This chapter discusses the multiple factors that contribute to nonadherence to medical regimens in the elderly. First, types of nonadherence are described. Factors that influence one's ability or desire to adhere, such as quality of patient-provider relationships, regimen complexity, presence of adverse side effects, personal and cultural beliefs, health literacy, physical changes, cognitive alterations, depression, and adequacy of social and financial resources, are then summarized. Methods to assess an older person's capacity to adhere are described, and the chapter concludes with a review of strategies to increase adherence in the elderly. Adherence to prescribed medication regimens for chronic conditions is the focus of the chapter. However, many of the factors that promote nonadherence, as well as the strategies to promote adherence, are applicable to other types of regimens or lifestyle changes in which adherence is an issue.

Types of Nonadherence

Persons 65 and older are the largest consumers of pharmaceutical agents. Although the elderly comprise only 13% of the population, they use more than 34% of all prescription medications and approximately 30% of nonprescription drugs (Haynes et al., 2005). An average of 11 prescriptions is filled each year by elderly persons living in the community. The elderly also purchase and consume seven times the number of over-the-counter medications purchased by younger persons (Anderson, Ory, Cohen, & McBride, 2000). The commonly used over-the-counter drugs are analgesics, laxatives, antihistamines, and sympathomimetics.

Medication costs are second only to nursing home costs in out-of-pocket expenses in this age group. Health care costs are also incurred because of the large number of hospitalizations for drug-related illnesses. More than 200,000 elderly are admitted to hospitals annually because of adverse drug reactions, or they may have prolonged hospital stays because of an adverse drug reaction during hospitalization (Esposito, 1995).

Medication adherence in the elderly has been estimated to be as low as 40% and as high as 75% (Haynes et al., 2005). Medication nonadherence places an elderly person at risk for debilitating health problems, increased hospitalization, and death. Approximately 11% of hospitalizations in persons over the age of 65 have been attributed to medication nonadherence (Vik, Maxwell, & Hogan, 2004). Increased physician outpatient and emergency room visits, hospitalizations, and nursing home admissions place the cost of nonadherence at $13 to $22 billion per year. Nonadherence is not a dichotomized behavior, as medication use is complex. Persons may not adhere intentionally or unintentionally. Or nonadherence may result from taking an incorrect dosage of medication or taking medications at an incorrect time or sequence.

Intentional and Nonintentional Nonadherence

Intentional and nonintentional medication overuse and underuse are two types of nonadherence to medication regimens in the elderly (Atkins & Fallowfield, 2006; Brookhart et al., 2007). Intentional nonadherence occurs when a patient makes a specific decision not to take the medication as prescribed. Intentional nonadherence may be due to (1) lack of information about the pros and cons of treatment, (2) lack of immediate benefit from the medication, and/or (3) negative beliefs about the value of the medication (Atkins & Fallowfield, 2006). Intentional underuse may occur when elders deny the diagnosis of an illness. Intentional underuse also occurs when the patient does not believe the medication is needed or does not want to be overmedicated. Medication "hoarding," or saving medication for a future problem, is another example of intentional underuse and is often related to the high costs of drugs. Intentional underuse may result from a lack of financial resources to pay for prescriptions, as some prescriptions are never filled. Uncomfortable side effects of medications may also result in intentional underuse or even termination of the medication. For example, diuretics are often considered a hindrance to activities and may be taken only in response to symptoms, instead of as prescribed. Medication regimens that are disruptive to the person's daily activities or routines result in intentional underuse. For example, doses may be skipped or eliminated if they interfere with social or lifestyle activities. Intentional overuse is often attributed to the belief that the prescribed dose is ineffective or that "more is better" to relieve symptoms or promote recovery.

Drug holidays, another form of intentional nonadherence, refer to interruptions in medication use lasting more than 3 days (Brookhart et al., 2007). Drug holidays have been observed when medications have been electronically monitored in controlled settings. Long, unexplained drug holidays have been commonly reported among users of osteoporosis medications, as women stop and restart medications (Brookhart et al., 2007). Women are more likely to restart if the drug holiday is less than 120 days. Cyclic nonadherence points to the complexity and need to evaluate both intentional and nonintentional nonadherence simultaneously to better understand medication taking.

Unintentional nonadherence may be due to forgetting or misunderstanding instructions. Forgetfulness may result in unintentional overuse if the patient does not remember taking a medication and takes a second dose. Forgetfulness is the most common reason for unintentional underuse of medications. The inability to perform simple tasks that depend on adequate functional performance, such as the ability to open a medication bottle or cut pills, may also result in unintentional underuse.

Nonadherence may also occur when medications are not taken at the correct time or in the correct sequence. Patients have reported modifying doses and dosing regimens to accommodate their daily activities and commitments. For example, a medication prescribed twice a day may be taken only once daily, or a medication prescribed every 6 hours may be taken every 4 hours. Timing errors may result in what the health care provider perceives as treatment failure or precipitate unnecessary or inappropriate treatment changes.

Factors That Promote Nonadherence in the Elderly

Multiple factors contribute to the problem of nonadherence in elderly persons. First, patient-provider relationships are a key factor. Second, the complexity of the medical regimen may promote nonadherence, as may adverse side effects of the medications. Physical changes that occur with aging, such as declining functional performance and visual and hearing alterations, as well as cognitive changes, may have an effect on adherence (Lehane & McCarthy, 2007).

Emotional health, specifically depression, is also considered a factor in nonadherence in older persons. The lack of resources, including social networks and social support (presence of companions or friends, living arrangements) and financial resources, also promotes nonadherence. Personal and cultural beliefs and health literacy have also been documented to contribute to nonadherence. Each of these factors is described in detail to provide an understanding of their potential role in the problem of nonadherence in the elderly.

Patient-Provider Relationships

The relationship between patients and health care providers has long been associated with adherence, presumably because good relationships are associated with improved communication (Honda & Kagawa-Singer, 2006; Madigan, Majumdar, & Johnson, 2005). The behavior and attitudes of health care professionals, as well as the amount of time spent with patients in a supportive environment, can have either positive or negative effects on adherence (Tarn et al., 2006). Providers may lack the expertise to assess adherence appropriately, or they may not have the time to discuss adherence. Closed-ended questions, requiring just a yes or no response from the patient, do not provide opportunities for discussion (Bokhour, Berlowitz, Long, & Kressin, 2006). If patients are not satisfied that their questions are being answered or if their expectations for the encounter have not been met, they are more likely to be nonadherent (Burge et al., 2005). Although patients expect their health care providers to be their primary information resource, they report that they often feel inferior or do not understand the provider's medical jargon or think they are given too little information for it to be helpful (Gordon, Smith, & Dhillion, 2007).

Complexity of Drug Regimen

Regimen complexity is routinely cited as a reason for nonadherence (Dunbar-Jacobs, Erlen, Schlenk, et al., 2000; McNabb, Nicolau, Stoner, & Ross, 2003), although some reports also indicate that complexity may not influence medication adherence (Shalansky, 2002, Burge et al., 2005). Polypharmacy regimens report adherence rates 10% to 20% lower than monotherapy regimens (Larson, Vaccherei, Anderson, Montanaro, & Berbman, 2000; Melekian, White, Vanderplas, Dezeii, & Change, 2002). Patients with type two diabetes have been shown to have adherence rates of 79% with once daily dosing compared to 38% for three times daily. In addition, medications were taken at the correct prescribed time in 77% of cases for once daily dosing compared to 5% for three times a day dosing (Rubin, 2005).

The presence of more than one chronic illness in many elderly patients results in the administration of a large number of medications. More than one specialist may be consulted, resulting in multiple prescribers and prescriptions. Thus, polypharmacy is commonplace. Excessive and often inappropriate prescribing is not uncommon. Reasons for this have been documented and include the failure to make an accurate diagnosis due to inadequate clinical assessment before issuing the initial prescription; the influence of the pharmaceutical industry, which promotes prescribing; overenergetic treatment, which leads to incremental prescribing; patient or family demands; failure to conduct careful medication histories; inadequate review of patient records, resulting in a failure to discontinue drugs; and lack of continuity of care between acute and outpatient facilities (Walley & Scott, 1995). Having a larger number of drugs associated with a more complex administration schedule is also a deterrent to adherence. Multiple dosing schedules, rather than a single dose or twice-daily doses, may interfere with leisure activities or sleep and are more likely to be forgotten by the elderly. In addition, the consumption of multiple drugs may result in unpleasant drug-drug interactions in which one drug may either interfere with or enhance the action of another, or one drug may change the manner in which the body handles a second drug (Yee & Williams, 2002). Changes in drug regimens or switches from brand names to generic drugs are also confusing to the elderly and may result in nonadherence (Sorenson, Stokes, Purdue, Woodward, & Roberts, 2005).

Adverse Side Effects

Drug-Age Pharmokinetics

Because of age-related changes that occur in the body, older persons respond differently from younger people to medication. Pharmokinetic alterations include changes in absorption, distribution, metabolism, and elimination. Absorption of drugs by passive diffusion is not affected by aging. However, alterations in gastric motility and blood flow can influence drug absorption. Distribution or transportation of drugs throughout the body may be altered by age-related changes, including decreased lean body mass, increased body fat, and decreased total body water. Thus, dosages of water-soluble drugs, including digoxin, propranolol, and cimetidine, need to be altered, as well as those for drugs that are distributed into adipose tissue. In addition, fat-soluble drugs such as barbiturates and phenothiazines produce prolonged actions or adverse effects due to the large amounts that may be stored in fat.

The major site for drug metabolism is in the liver. Hepatic mass and hepatic blood flow decrease with age. The decreased blood flow means a decreased extraction (first pass) of the drug by the liver, which produces an increase in serum drug levels and strengthens the clinical effects of certain drugs, such as propanalol, verapamil, and some opiates.

The kidney is the major organ of drug excretion. Renal blood flow and perfusion decrease with age. Therefore, dosages must be reduced for drugs that are dependent on renal blood for excretion, such as digoxin, lithium, and antibiotics. In addition to the effects of aging, common chronic illnesses, such as congestive heart failure, cirrhosis, nutritional deficiencies, hypertension, and kidney diseases, may impair absorption, metabolism, and excretion.

Adverse Effects

Significant adverse side effects and toxicity may occur if the physician does not understand age-related changes in pharmokinetics when prescribing pharmacologic therapies and prescribes incorrect doses. Deleterious effects or perceived lack of benefits result in nonadherence, as well as increased health care costs due to hospitalizations.

Adverse side effects are thought to be the most common reason for nonadherence. Adverse side effects increase the risk of nonadherence, as they are often more troublesome than the disease itself, as in the case of hypertension, which is usually asymptomatic. In addition, many side effects make it difficult for an elderly person to continue the treatment regimen because of the annoying nature of the symptoms, such as confusion, sedation, dizziness, diuresis, appetite and mood changes, constipation, sleep disturbances, and problems with gait instability and physical performance. Antihypertensive agents, the most commonly prescribed medication in the elderly, may cause psychiatric symptoms (Siegel, Lopez, & Meier, 2007). Any of these side effects may cause deterioration in both physical health and quality of life. Although adverse side effects may be serious and long lasting, they are rarely addressed in office visits, as it has been documented that fewer than 25% of patients mention side effects to their health care providers (Rubin, 2005). Many elderly do not report side effects because they do not consider the side effects to be abnormal, or they may not know what to do if side effects occur. In addition, they may be embarrassed to report symptoms, such as forgetfulness or confusion, because they believe they will be labeled demented.

Lack of Information and Inadequate Instructions

Lack of knowledge of medications and their side effects is a major factor in nonadherence; the problem is twofold. Physicians and other health care professionals often do not provide adequate information, and many elderly are hesitant to ask for information. Many older persons believe they do not receive adequate information about their prescriptions from their health care providers (Gordon et al, 2007). It is estimated that as many as 50% of patients leave physicians' offices without understanding their medical regimens. When explanations are provided, they are couched in medical terminology that is foreign to most people, including elderly patients. Persons are less likely to follow a prescribed regimen when the instructions are not clear and understandable. Elderly patients do not want to be viewed as what they perceive to be a "problem patient," so they do not acknowledge their lack of understanding. Hearing and visual difficulties, as well as increased forgetfulness and decreased attention span, also interfere with an elderly person's ability to understand and remember instructions. Persons adhere to regimens they understand and believe in and have the ability to follow. Patients vary in the type and level of information needed, so tailoring information and instructions is key to promoting medication adherence.

Personal and Cultural Beliefs

The personal and cultural health beliefs of older adults may influence adherence both positively and negatively. Older adults have higher reported adherence when they believe that the prescribed medication is essential for their health and that they will derive benefits from taking it and when they have few concerns about side effects (Chia, Schlenk, & Dunbar-Jacobs, 2006). Patients must believe in the value of the regimen and also believe that they have the ability to overcome barriers to adherence.

The health care environment in which older persons receive treatment must not be in conflict with their cultural beliefs if they are to adhere to treatment for chronic diseases (Hughes, 2004). If patients' views of illness and treatment are not consistent with the views of the health care provider, they are less likely to accept the prescribed therapy. All cultures have explanatory models of health, and many are not congruent with the traditional biomedical model (Schraufnagal, Wagner, Miranda, & Roy-Bryne, 2006). Strong ties with family and friends reinforce patients' cultural beliefs, often resulting in a reluctance to seek treatment and a tendency not to adhere to treatment regiments. For example, older persons who believe that natural products and home remedies will be more effective than conventional therapies are more likely to take home remedies than their prescribed medications.

Persons who hold fatalistic beliefs or accept an external locus of control are also more likely to exhibit poor adherence. Both types of beliefs have been associated with decreased access to care and low adherence, as these persons believe they have little control over their own health and are often more passive in health care encounters (Schraufnagal et al., 2006).

Health Literacy

It is estimated that 48% of the adult population in the United States lack the literacy proficiency needed to understand and act on health information (Institute of Medicine [IOM], 2004). Health literacy, defined as the degree to which the patient has the capacity to obtain, process, and understand health information and services needed to make appropriate health decisions, goes unrecognized by health care providers, who rarely verify patients' recall and comprehension of their treatment regimens (Schillinger, Grumbach, & Piette, 2002; Selden, Zorn, Ratzan, & Parker, 2000). Limited health literacy predicts less successful self-care and worse health outcomes, as studies show that patients with lower health literacy are less likely to understand verbal or written instructions for self-care, including medication regimens (Kripalani et al., 2007). Patients with low health literacy may not be able to read or understand medication labels, leading to nonintentional nonadherence. There are economic consequences to limited health literacy; these individuals are more inefficient in their use of health care services and incur greater health care costs than people with greater health literacy (Howard, Gazmararian, & Parker, 2005). In persons with limited health literacy skills, nonadherence and other adverse health outcomes are associated with limited chronic disease knowledge, poor self-management skills, and failure to use appropriate preventive services (Wolf, Gazmararian, & Baker, 2007).

Functional Performance Changes

Functional performance declines in the elderly. More than poor posture results from decreases in strength and flexibility. Loss of strength and flexibility compounds problems in walking or performing activities of daily living (Lewis, 2002). However, decreases in strength may go unnoticed for long periods because normal daily activities do not require great strength. Strength, flexibility, and balance ensure adequate gait or mobility. Bilateral standing balance is necessary to free the upper extremities for activities, while unilateral balance is essential for stepping over obstacles and climbing stairs. Changes in gait that occur in aging include slowed walking speed, flexion in the thoracic spinal area, a loss of the lordic curve in the lumbar spine, a forward head position, short shuffling steps, and a loss of normal arm movement. Functional performance is essential to accomplish everyday activities such as bathing, dressing, toileting, shopping, preparing meals, using transportation, and performing simple psychomotor skills. Functional performance is important in taking medications, as older persons may experience problems in manipulating packaging, especially child-resistant containers and blister packs. Any changes that result in a deterioration in functional performance and the capacity to maintain independence affect one's ability to perform activities necessary to adhere to certain treatments regimens.

Visual Changes

Visual changes occur with aging; reduced vision is the most common sensory problem in the aged, and at least 90% of persons over age 60 need vision correction (Heath, 1992a). The major visual impairment in the elderly, presbyopia, is caused by a loss of elasticity and increased density of the lens. The ciliary muscles that hold the lens also lose their ability to accommodate rapidly, resulting in the need for bifocal lenses. Age-related ocular changes include altered depth perception, increased light threshold, arcus senility, increased eyelid laxity, and decreased tear production. Cataracts are the most common ocular disease in the elderly. Two other major ocular diseases affecting the elderly are glaucoma and macular degeneration. All three of these diseases result in visual impairments, and glaucoma and macular degeneration can result in blindness. In addition, chronic diseases, such as diabetes mellitus, cause eye changes that may result in blindness. Visual problems often go undetected until late in the disease process, because these changes may be associated with aging and overlooked. Visual deficits create nonadherence due to patients' difficulties in reading and following written instructions, as patients cannot adhere if they are unable to read the instructions.

Hearing Changes

Hearing loss, or presbycusis, is the most underreported and unrecognized sensory impairment in geriatric medicine (Heath, 1992b). Elderly persons with hearing problems may wait 5 years or more before seeking medical assistance. Hearing loss results in a decreased perception of higher frequency tones, as well as auditory signal distortion, which may result in inappropriate responses. Such responses are often misinterpreted, and elderly people who experience this problem may withdraw in frustration. Withdrawal from conversations, inappropriate responses, inattentiveness, and difficulty following directions are often interpreted as confusion or cognitive decline in the elderly instead of being seen as a potentially correctable hearing problem. Because hearing loss is usually not diagnosed and managed appropriately, elderly people who do not hear or who misinterpret medical information or who are reluctant to ask questions because they are concerned they will not hear the response may be more likely to be nonadherent to medical regimens.

Cognitive Alterations

Age effects on adherence are thought to be mediated through cognitive function (Hutchinson, Jones, West, & Wei, 2006). Older age is associated with changes in cognitive abilities, including declines in memory, judgment, perception, attention and concentration, perceptual speed, spatial manipulation, and reasoning (Anstey & Low, 2004; Schonknecht, Pantel, Kruse, & Schroder, 2005). The ability to recall and plan medication regimens may be sufficiently reduced in patients with mild cognitive impairments to result in medication errors. Age-associated cognitive decline has been shown to have a prevalence rate of 20% to 27% in elderly populations and 13% in the 60–64-year-old population (Schonknecht et al., 2005). Most cognitive deficits remain subtle over a long period, and silent or unrecognized dementia has been reported to be as high as 52% among persons with early cognitive deterioration (Ross et al., 1997). Early signs of cognitive impairment are often ignored or diagnosed as "normal" aging, hearing loss, or depression, and the impairment may remain undetected until the advanced stages.

Age differences have been noted in the comprehension of medical information. Understanding medical information requires several cognitive and noncognitive processes. Information must be presented, learned, and remembered at the appropriate time. Older adults have more difficulty attending to information and inhibiting irrelevant information or stimuli (Salthouse, 2003). Many older adults experience changes in memory at a stage in life when there is an increasing need to follow complex medication regimens (Craik, 1999; Craik & Salthouse, 2007).

Executive function and working memory are cognitive processes that are particularly susceptible to the effects of aging. These two cognitive processes are not automatic. Executive function is involved in maintaining attention to a task, switching tasks, planning, organizing, making decisions, and sequencing goal-directed behavior (Fuster, 1997). Each of these executive-function tasks is involved in behaviors associated with medication taking. Working memory has also been shown to decline among older adults. Working memory is described as the capacity for online processing, which is the holding of information while manipulating it. Holding information about the medication while listening to further instructions may be more difficult for older adults. Changes in executive function and working memory in one's later years have been shown to be associated with adherence among older adults living in the community and taking at least one prescribed medication (Insel, Morrow, Brewer, & Figueredo, 2006).

Cognitive abilities are considered to be the most important resource for maintaining everyday functioning. Thus, cognitive changes, namely memory loss, become issues when an elderly person is unable to recall and use the information necessary to perform everyday activities, including the ability to remember information needed to plan and follow treatment regimens.

Emotional Health: Depression

Depression is one of the major predictors of nonadherence (DiMatteo, Lepper, & Croghan, 2000). The incidence of depression among individuals with chronic disease is significant. Losses associated with aging, such as death of a spouse or friends, moving from one's home, and termination of a career, are also thought to contribute to depression. Older adults as a group are more active and healthier in retirement than in prior years; however, role transitions contain both opportunities and challenges. Signs of depression should be noted, as they can influence motivation to adhere to treatment regimens.

Depression may produce physical, psychological, and cognitive symptoms (Teri & Wagner, 1992). Physical symptoms include sleep disturbances, appetite or weight changes, fatigue, and loss of libido. Emotional aspects include a pervasive dysphoric mood, feelings of worthlessness, suicidal thoughts, and loss of self-esteem. Cognitive symptoms may include difficulty with memory and concentration and confusion. As with other changes in the elderly, depressive symptoms are often considered predictable complaints of chronic illnesses and ignored.

Several aspects of depression are thought to have negative effects on adherence. These include a pessimistic attitude about the effectiveness of the treatment; changes in memory, attention, and cognition; decreased desire for self-care; lack of motivation, isolation, and even possible intentional self-harm (Wang et al., 2002). Depression has been reported to have a negative effect on adherence to medications in multiple chronic diseases, including coronary artery disease, HIV disease, asthma, renal transplantation, and hypertension (Wang et al, 2002). These findings point to a need to screen for depressive symptoms and to monitor adherence, as elderly depressed patients are particularly vulnerable to nonadherence because of multiple chronic illnesses and, consequently, multiple medications regimens (Schraufnagel et al., 2006).

Resources: Social Network and Social Support

Social networks and supports are well-documented links to the health and well-being of older persons (Antonucci, 1990). Social networks provide access to support and other needed resources. The major types of social support are emotional, informational, and instrumental or tangible support. Supportive contacts and relationships may positively affect health by allowing for earlier recognition of the adverse effects of medications, increasing the likelihood that the person will seek medical care, and providing assistance needed to sustain treatment regimens. The lack of social and community relationships has been associated with poor adherence (Tucker et al., 2004). Estimates indicate that between 25% and 35% of persons over age 65 live alone. Elderly persons who live alone, especially elderly women, are also more likely to have lower incomes than those who live with other people. Both of these factors contribute to the difficulties encountered by elderly persons in adhering to a treatment regimen.

Resources: Financial

One of the major challenges created by an increased life span and the growing burden of chronic illnesses is health care costs (CDC & MCF, 2007). The cost of providing health care for a person over age 65 is three to five times higher than the cost of caring for a person younger than age 65. Between 1980 and 2002, Medicare spending grew from $33.9 billion to $252 billion. This increase is a result, in part, of the increased numbers of persons over age 65.

The high costs of prescriptions and medical supplies are barriers to adherence for persons with low or fixed incomes. Many elderly cannot afford to pay for all of the medications prescribed and make their own decisions about which ones to omit. Persons on fixed incomes usually have limited funds available after paying for food, housing, and other medical care, resulting in unfilled drug prescriptions or intentional dose skipping, dosage reductions, such as cutting pills in half, or drug hoarding.

Assessment of the Capacity to Adhere

The first step in facilitating adherence in the elderly is to assess the person's capacity to follow a regimen, as physical, cognitive, and social environmental barriers place older persons at risk for nonadherence. Such an approach needs to occur before a medication or treatment regimen begins, not after a program has been implemented. Assessment enables the health care provider to evaluate the elderly person's understanding, as well as capacity to follow a treatment program. Comprehension is a key component in decision making, as elderly persons must understand information in order to make appropriate decisions. Adherence is not likely if they do not comprehend the instructions. Since impaired mental status is a major risk factor for nonadherence, assessment of cognitive status is essential. Tests, such as the Mini-Mental Status Examination, are simple to administer and will alert the health care professional to potential problems. In addition, a cognitive assessment will assist in planning strategies to promote adherence in these patients.

Physical functioning also needs to be observed when assessing the capacity of elders to adhere. For example, the ability to perform self-care and the instrumental activities of daily living provides information on elderly persons' ability to care for themselves. Hearing and visual difficulties also need to be assessed, as they may interfere with comprehension and implementation of the treatment regimen.

Assessment of cognitive functioning, as well as physical functioning, prior to initiating a regimen is achieved through open communication with a health care professional. The time allotted to an initial detailed assessment will pay off over time. Short, reliable, and valid questionnaires that are easy to administer are available to assess cognitive functioning, self-care, and the ability to perform the instrumental activities of daily living. It must be kept in mind that many factors influence compliance other than the ability to initiate and follow a regimen. However, an initial thorough assessment provides a major step in reducing potential barriers to adherence.

Strategies to Increase Adherence in the Elderly

In spite of many studies of adherence and the identification of factors that predict variability in adherence, there is still not enough evidence to support any one type of strategy or intervention (Higgins & Regan, 2004; Patel & David, 2004). The many factors that predict nonadherence point to the need for tailored interventions that incorporate multiple strategies. Successful interventions are complex and need to include tailored educational strategies appropriate for the person, as well as behavior strategies with external cognitive supports. Patients must be active participants in their care, and health care providers must acknowledge the complexity of the problem and be supported by multidisciplinary teams.

Adherence to the current medication regimen should be evaluated following assessment of the elderly person's capacity to follow the prescribed therapy. A detailed medication history is necessary prior to implementing an educational program so that strategies to increase adherence can be tailored to the person's individual needs. As stated earlier, communication between the elderly person and the health care professional, using the appropriate language, is a major factor in improving adherence. Therefore, the health care provider must understand the elements of effective communication that promote adherence, as well as the principles of health literacy. Since forgetting is a major problem in adherence in the elderly, educational and behavioral strategies that promote remembering to take medications should be initiated. Last, a multidisciplinary approach is central to promoting adherence in the elderly.

Medication History Assessment

Initially, a detailed medication history should be taken to obtain information about the use of current prescription and over-the-counter medications, prior prescription and over-the-counter medications, and home remedies. Social drug use, including alcohol, tobacco, and caffeine intake, should also be ascertained, as these may interfere with or alter the absorption of prescribed drugs.

A successful strategy is to request that the person bring in all prescription, over-the-counter, borrowed, and outdated medications in the home to the initial visit. This "brown bag assessment" will provide a picture of the person's medication habits (Bergman-Evans, 2006). Next, the elderly person should be queried about the medications. Questions need to be asked to obtain information about dosages and schedules, side effects and other problems when taking the medications, and knowledge about the drugs and disease being treated. Questions should be open ended and asked in a supportive, nonpunitive manner in language understandable to the patient. A supportive atmosphere will facilitate honest answers about adherence issues without fear of reprisal.

Medication Regimen Analysis

Potential adherence issues may be addressed through an ongoing review of the medication regimen, while focusing on the patient, as well as the disease. First, prescription instructions should be given in detail, avoiding directions such as "take as directed" or "take as needed," as these may not be understood. Easily administered dosage forms that consider such problems as difficulty in swallowing pills are preferable. The physician should undertake a careful review to simplify the regimen as much as possible, as the elderly should take as few drugs as necessary. Drugs that can be administered in a single or twice-daily dose should be prescribed whenever possible. The idea of a "polypill," in which one combination pill contains multiple medications, has generated interest in the literature as a way to increase adherence, as only one pill daily would be required (Wald & Law, 2003). The prescriber should time the dosage so that the schedule does not conflict with the person's daily activities. Therapeutic endpoints for prescribed drugs should be established, and medications that are no longer needed should be discontinued as soon as possible. In general, dispensing pharmacies should avoid safety caps, as many elderly are unable to open medications with these caps. Ongoing attention through regular visits and consistent assessment of all aspects of the medication regimen decreases the potential for adverse side effects and increases the likelihood of adherence. Physicians and other health care providers who prescribe need to be educated, in addition to educating the elderly.

Effective Communication

Timing of communication episodes, quality of the encounter, and involvement of a supportive other have been shown to promote constructive communication between health care professionals and elderly persons. Effective communication enables health care providers to furnish essential information in a meaningful manner, as well as to elicit the elderly person's concerns and questions about the medication regimen. Effective communication also enables the health care provider to learn about any personal and cultural beliefs that may interfere with the person's adherence to the prescribed regimen.

Timing

Scheduled ongoing contacts with a consistent health care provider, rather than "as needed" visits, are necessary to prevent or reduce side effects and polypharmacy and to monitor cognitive and physical changes which may interfere with adherence (Patel & David, 2004). Follow-up visits are critical after a hospital or other health care facility discharge, the death of a spouse, a change in living arrangements, or a decline in cognitive or physical functioning, as any transition increases the elder's risk for nonadherence, as well as other potentially debilitating consequences.

Quality of Encounter

The quality of the patient–health care provider relationship has a significant bearing on satisfaction with care, which in turn influences an elderly person's motivation to adhere to a prescribed regimen. The health care provider-patient interaction may be the most important ingredient in whether behavior change occurs, as research has shown that it influences the patient's care seeking and active participation in the treatment regimen (Schilder et al., 2001). Empathic listening and genuine interest in the person convey respect, instill trust, and decrease communication barriers. Sensitivity to cognitive, physical, and social environmental barriers enables health care providers to plan and implement realistic regimens with supports essential for success. The quality of the encounter is enriched when sufficient time is spent with the person to allow the health care provider to offer individualized information, assess the patient's response to current medications, answer questions, address concerns, and provide encouragement and support. A quality encounter occurs when health literacy barriers of the patient are assessed and addressed. Patients with limited literacy have less general knowledge of their disease and its treatment. The provider may need to administer scales that measure literacy in health care settings early in the encounter to know the knowledge and language level to use with the particular person. For example, the Rapid Estimate of Adult Literacy in Medicine (REALM) is a health word recognition test in which patients are asked to read aloud medical terms (Davis, Kennen, Gazararian, & Williams, 2004). Education, at a level and in a language that are understood, is critical to promote comprehension of the disease and prescribed treatments.

Involvement of a Supportive Other

Inclusion of the spouse or another family member or friend is a major factor in facilitating management of the elderly person's chronic-illness treatment regimen, especially in the presence of declining cognitive or physical functioning. Household members can contribute information about the person and his living environments that is crucial to understanding potential adherence issues. A supportive other may also administer the medications or ensure that the person is taking the medication. Illness is a family affair, as everyone in the household is affected. Therefore, active participation by another person facilitates adherence to medication and other treatments that may be prescribed. In addition, side effects or other problems are likely to be observed and reported earlier when there is a supportive other monitoring the functioning of the patient, decreasing the need for hospitalization. Supportive others need to be present during provider-patient communications about the medication regimens and during all educational activities.

Educational Strategies

Educational strategies have traditionally been the mainstay of efforts to improve adherence to medication and other treatment regimens and have achieved varying levels of success for persons of all ages (Haynes et al, 2005). Educational strategies are based on the premise that providing patients with information about their disease and its treatment is a necessary first step. In other words, elderly persons must first understand their illness and its consequences and comprehend the benefits of the prescribed regimen before they are able to make the lifestyle adjustments needed to implement a regimen. Multiple educational strategies are more effective than a single strategy. For example, a combination of verbal and written information is more beneficial than written information alone. Multiple strategies that take into account verbal, visual, and auditory channels are particularly effective to reinforce information in the elderly. Strategies to facilitate comprehension include simplifying language, organizing information to match patients' expectations, and including pictorials that reinforce verbal and written instructions. Medical and technical terminology should be avoided when possible, and the provider must be careful not to present too much information in one session, as a reduced attention span may result in the elderly person's remembering only some or none of the information. A stepwise approach, in which information is presented in small increments, enables the elderly person to believe that adherence is both beneficial and possible. Individualized educational sessions that are flexible are more effective than structured group approaches. Tailoring the educational process is critical to adjust for varying levels of involvement, difficulties with comprehension, and changes in beliefs and attitudes. Other educational strategies include active involvement of the elderly as much as possible in the teaching-learning process. Active involvement enables the health care provider to evaluate how much the person understands of the information being provided and gives the elderly person opportunities to ask questions and practice new skills, such as insulin injections or urine checks. The "show and tell" technique is an effective teaching strategy. First, the medication is shown to the patient. The patient is then told what the medication is for, how is it to be taken and what types of problems, if any, might be experienced. Attention to design and packaging information, which takes into account visual and physical functional problems and health literacy levels, is also critical to promote adherence.

Behavioral Strategies

Behavioral strategies are based on the premise that behavior is learned and can be modified. Behavioral strategies include such things as reminders and the use of self-monitoring tools or other aids to increase adherence. Behavioral strategies are effective, as they address the problem of declining cognitive and physical functioning in the elderly. Research indicates that instructions aimed at the process (medication taking) are more effective than instructions aimed at the health behavior goal (Theunissen, de Ridder, Bensing, & Rutten, 2003). Reminders may be as simple as a chart, special medication containers such as a daily dispenser or weekly medication tray, or a special calendar or mealtime dispensing pack. These organizers help the patient identify whether the medication has been taken, eliminating confusion at a later time. Color-coded bottles have also been used. Special packaging simplifies the medication regimen by organizing the medications. The packaging can also serve as a mechanism to monitor adherence. Telephone or mail prompts to refill prescriptions are also helpful in promoting adherence.

Additional strategies to address declining memory have been implemented with varying levels of success. Interventions that support remembering to take medications and monitor completion of medication taking are important (Insel & Coe, 2005). Cues within the environment that are specific to the patient's home and routines are frequently used as reminders. Elderly persons can be taught to establish a routine for taking the medication. For example, taking medications everyday can be associated with drinking morning coffee or juice, meal times, or certain television programs. Or patients may devise their own cues. Research indicates that linking an intended action (medication taking) with an event improves adherence (Einstein, McDaniel, Manzi, Cochran, & Baker, 2000). Reminders from a significant other are valuable complements to environmental cues.

The formation of implementation intentions has also been found to be effective in promoting adherence (Liu & Park, 2004; Milne, Orbell, & Sheeran, 2002). Implementation intentions refer to planning when and where medication taking will occur, rather than just planning to take the medicine. For example, adherence is more likely to occur if patients plan the time and location for taking the medication and associate the taking of the medication with certain activities, rather than having a general plan for taking the medications. Forming implementation intentions is also associated with success in beginning and adhering to other types of treatment regimens, such as physical activity.

Multidisciplinary Approach

A team approach, in which the expertise of physicians, pharmacists, and registered nurses is incorporated, is essential for comprehensive care and successful adherence (Yam et al., 2006). Each provider contributes special expertise that is complementary, rather than competitive. For example, physicians are responsible for diagnosing and prescribing medications. Physicians also monitor patients for adverse side effects and provide education. Pharmacists fill prescriptions and review drugs for potential drug-drug interactions. They conduct drug reviews to reduce the cost of medications, as well as reduce the number of medicines prescribed. Pharmacists dispense information and may provide education as well. The responsibilities of registered nurses vary with their role. Nurse practitioners may prescribe medications, educate, and monitor for adverse side effects. Nurses in institutional-care settings administer medications and monitor patients for effectiveness and adverse side effects. In addition, nurses provide information about the medication regimen and teach skills that may be needed to administer medications, such as insulin injections. In the community setting, nurses make home visits to monitor the elderly for side effects and other issues that may influence adherence to the medication regimen. Ongoing communication among all health care providers is essential to optimize care and promote adherence.

Summary

The number of persons over the age of 65 is increasing faster than that for any other segment of the population and has become the largest consumer of health care services. The increase in life span and the increased burden of chronic illnesses in the elderly necessitate lifelong, complex medication and treatment programs that may produce unpleasant and uncomfortable side effects. Problems with adherence result from multiple issues, including health care provider factors, patient factors, and regimen factors. Thus, improving adherence in the elderly is complex. Health care providers need to begin with an assessment of factors that influence an elderly person's capacity to adhere. Potential causes of nonadherence, including the complexity of the regimen, the presence of adverse side effects, a lack of understanding, lack of health literacy, and personal and cultural beliefs should be explored by the prescriber in order to facilitate the choice of strategies to increase adherence. Consistent, effective communication between the elderly person and the health care provider is paramount. While educational and behavioral strategies may promote adherence, no one strategy is completely effective. Ongoing research is critical, as the problem of nonadherence in the elderly is considered a silent epidemic that is expected to increase as the elderly population continues to grow.

References

Anderson, R. T., Ory, M., Cohen, S., & McBride, J. (2000). Issues of aging and adherence to health interventions. *Controlled Clinical Trials, 21,* 171S–183S.

Anstey, K. J., & Low, L. (2004). Normal cognitive changes in aging. *Australian + Family Physician, 33*(10), 782–787.

Antonucci, T. C. (1990). Social supports and social relationships. In R. H. Binstock & L. K. George (Eds.), *Handbook of aging and the social sciences* (3rd ed., pp. 205–226). San Diego: Academic Press.

Atkins, L., & Fallowfield, L. (2006). Intentional and nonintentional non-adherence to medication amongst breast cancer patients. *European Journal of Cancer, 42,* 2271–2276.

Bergman-Evans, B. (2006). Aides to improving medication adherence in older adults. *Geriatric Nursing, 27*(3), 174–182.

Bokhour, B. G., Berlowitz, D. R., Long, J. A., & Kressin, N. R. (2006). How do providers assess antihypertensive medication adherence in medical encounters? *Journal of General Internal Medicine, 21*(6), 577–583.

Brookhart, M. A., Avorn, J., Katz, J. A., Finkerstein, J. S., Arnold, M., Potinski, M., et al. (2007). Gaps in treatment among users of osteoporosis medications: The dynamics of noncompliance. *American Journal of Medicine, 120,* 251–256.

Burge, S., While, D., Bajorek, E., Bazaldua, O., Trevino, J., Albright, T., et al. (2005). Correlates of medication knowledge and adherence: Findings from the residency research network of south Texas. *Family Medicine, 37*(10), 712–718.

Centers for Disease Control and Prevention and the Merck Company Foundation. (2007). *The state of aging and health in America.* Whitehouse Station, NJ: Merck Company Foundation.

Chia, L., Schlenk, E. A., & Dunbar-Jacobs, J. (2006). Effect of personal and cultural beliefs on medication adherence in the elderly. *Drugs and Aging, 23*(3), 191–202.

Craik, F. I. (1999). Age-related changes in human memory. In D. C. Park & N. Schwarz (Eds.), *Cognitive aging: A primer* (pp. 75–92), London, UK: Psychology Press.

Craik, F. I. M., & Salthouse, T. A. (2007). *The handbook of aging and cognition* (3rd ed.). London, UK: Psychology Press.

Davis, T. C., Kennen, E. M., Gazmararian, J. A., & Williams, M. V. (2004). Literacy testing in health care research. In J. G. Schwartzberg, J. B. VanGees, & C. C. Wang (Eds.), *Understanding health literacy: Implications for medicine, public health* (pp. 157–179). Chicago: AMA Press.

DiMatteo, M. R., Lepper, H. S., & Croghan, T. W. (2000). Depression is a risk factor for noncompliance with medical treatment: Meta-analysis of the effects of anxiety and depression inpatient adherence. *Archives of Internal Medicine, 160,* 2101–2107.

Dunbar-Jacobs, J., Erlen, J. A., Schlenk, E. A., Ryan, C. M., Sereika, S. M., & Doswell, W. M. (2000). Adherence in chronic disease. *Annual Review of Nursing Research, 18,* 48–90.

Einstein, G. O., McDaniel, M. A., Manzi, M., Cochran, B., & Baker, M. (2000). Prospective memory and aging: Forgetting intentions over short delays. *Psychology & Aging, 15*(4), 671–683.

Eposito, L. (1995). The effects of medication education on adherence to medication regimens in an elderly population. *Journal of Advanced Nursing, 21,* 935–943.

Fuster, J. M. (1997). *The prefrontal cortex anatomy, physiology, and neuropsychology of the frontal lobe* (3rd ed.). Philadelphia: Lippincott-Raven.

Gordon, K., Smith, F., & Dhillion, S. (2007). Effective chronic disease management: Patients' perspectives on medication-related problems. *Patient Education and Counseling, 65,* 407–415.

Haynes, R. B., Yao, X., Degani, A., Kripalani, S., Garg, A., & McDonald, H. P. (2005). Interventions to enhance medication adherence. *Cochrane Database of Systematic Reviews, 10*(4) CD000011.

Heath, J. M. (1992a). Vision. In R. J. Ham & P. D. Sloane (Eds.), *Primary care geriatrics* (2nd ed., pp. 482–489). St. Louis: Mosby Year Book.

Heath, J. M. (1992b). Hearing. In R. J. Ham & P. D. Sloane (Eds.), *Primary care geriatrics* (2nd ed., pp. 490–497). St. Louis: Mosby Year Book.

Higgins, N., & Regan, C. (2004). A systematic review of the effectiveness of interventions to help older people adhere to education regimens. *Age & Aging, 33,* 224–229.

Honda, K., & Kagawa-Singer, M. (2006). Cognitive mediators linking social support networks to colorectal cancer screening adherence. *Journal of Behavioral Medicine, 29*(5), 449–460.

Howard, D. H., Gazmararian, J., & Parker, R. M. (2005). The impact of low health literacy on the medical costs of Medicare managed care enrollees. *American Journal of Medicine, 118,* 371–377.

Hughes, C. M. (2004). Medication non-adherence in the elderly: How big is the problem? *Drugs and Aging, 21*(12), 793–811.

Hutchinson, L. C., Jones, S., West, D. S., & Wei, J. Y. (2006). Assessment of medication management by community-living elderly persons with two standardized assessment tools: A cross-sectional study. *American Journal of Geriatric Pharmacotherapy, 4*(2), 144–153.

Insel, K., Morrow, D., Brewer, B., & Figueredo, A. (2006). Executive function, working memory, and medication adherence among older adults. *Journals of Gerontology Series B: Psychological Sciences & Social Sciences, 61*(2), 102–107.

Insel, K. C., & Cole, L. (2005). Individualizing memory strategies to improve medication adherence. *Applied Nursing Research, 18,* 199–204.

Institute of Medicine. (2004). *Health literacy: A prescription to end confusion.* Washington, DC: National Academies Press.

Kripalani, S., Robertson, R., Love-Ghaffari, M. H., Henderson, L. E., Praska, J., Strawder, A., et al. (2007). Development of an illustrated medication schedule as a low-literacy patient education tool. *Patient Education and Counseling, 66*(3), 368–377.

Larson, J., Vaccherei, A., Anderson, M., Montanaro, N., & Bergman, I. J. (2000). Lack of adherence to lipid lowering drug treatment: A comparison of utilization patterns in defined populations in Funent, Denmark, and Bologna, Italy. *British Journal of Clinical Pharmacology, 49,* 463–471.

Lehane, E., & McCarthy, G. (2007). Intentional and unintentional medication nonadherence: A comprehensive framework for clinical research and practice: A discussion paper. *International Journal of Nursing Studies, 44*(8), 1468–1477.

Lewis, C. B. (2002). Musculoskeletal changes with age: Clinical implications. In C. B. Lewis (Ed.), *Aging: The health care challenge* (3rd ed.) (pp. 147–176). Philadelphia: F. A. Davis.

Liu, L. L., & Park, D. C. (2004). Aging and medical adherence: The use of automatic processes to achieve effortful things. *Psychology & Aging, 19*(2), 318–325.

Madigan, S. L., Majumdar, S. R., & Johnson, J. A. (2005). Understanding the complex associations between patient-provider relationships, self-care behaviors, and health-related quality of life in type 2 diabetes: A structural equation modeling approach. *Quality of Life Research, 14*(6), 1489–1500.

McNabb, J. J., Nicolau, D. P., Stoner, J. A., & Ross, J. (2003). Patterns of adherence to antiretroviral medications: The value of electronic monitoring. *AIDS, 17*(12), 1763–1767.

Melekian, C., White, R. J., Vanderplas, A., Dezeii, C. M., & Change, E. (2002). Adherence to oral antidiabetic therapy in a managed care organization: A comparison of monotherapy, combination therapy, and fixed dose combination therapy. *Clinical Therapeutics, 24,* 460–467.

Milne, S., Orbell, S., & Sheeran, P. (2002). Combining motivational and volitional interventions to promote exercise participation: Protection motivation theory and implementation intentions. *British Journal of Health Psychology, 7*(2), 163–184.

National Center for Health Statistics. (2006). *Health, United States with chart books for trends in the health of Americans.* Washington, DC: U.S. Government Printing Office.

Patel, M., & David, A. S. (2004). Medication adherence: Predictive factors and enhancement strategies. *Psychiatry, 3*(10), 41–44.

Ross, W., Abbot, R., Petrovich, H., Masaki, K., Murdaugh, C., & White, C. (1997). Silent dementia: Frequency and characteristics in elderly Japanese-American men: The Honolulu-Asia Study. *Journal of the American Medical Association, 277*(10), 800–805.

Rubin, R. R. (2005). Adherence to pharmacologic therapy in patients with type 2 diabetes mellitus. *American Journal of Medicine, 118*(5A), 27S–34S.

Salthouse, T. A. (2003). Interrelation of aging, knowledge and cognitive performance. In U. M. Staudinger & U. Lindenberger (Eds.), *Understanding human development: Dialogue with lifespan psychology* (pp. 435–489). Dordrecht: Kluwer Academic Publishers.

Schilder, A. J., Kennedy, C., Goldstone, I. L., Ogden, R. D., Hogg, R. S., & O'Shaughnessy, M. V. (2001). "Being dealt with as a whole person." Careseeking and adherence: The benefits of culturally competent care. *Social Science and Medicine, 52,* 643–659.

Schillinger, D., Grumbach, K. & Piette, J. (2002). Association of health literacy with diabetes outcomes. *Journal of the American Medical Association, 288,* 475–482.

Schonknecht, P., Pantel, J., Kruse, A. & Schroder, J. (2005). Prevalence and natural course of aging-associated cognitive decline in a population-based sample of young-old adults. *American Journal of Psychiatry, 162*(11), 2071–2077.

Schraufnagal, T. J., Wagner, A. W., Miranda, J., & Roy-Bryne, P. P. (2006). Treating minority patients with depression and anxiety: What does the evidence tell us? *General Hospital Psychiatry, 28,* 27–36.

Seldon, C. R., Zorn, M., Ratzman, S., & Parke, R. M. (2000), *Current bibliographies in medicine: Health literacy.* Bethesda, MD: National Library of Medicine.

Shalansky, S. J. (2002). Effect of number of medications on cardiovascular therapy adherence. *Annals of Pharmacology, 36,* 1532–1538.

Siegel, D., Lopez, J., & Meier, J. (2007). Antihypertensive medication adherence in the Department of Veterans Affairs. *American Journal of Medicine, 120,* 26–32.

Sorenson, L., Stokes, J. A., Purdue, D., Woodward, M., & Roberts, M. S. (2005). Medication management at home: Medication-related risk factors associated with poor health outcomes. *Age and Aging, 34,* 626–632.

Tarn, D. M., Heritage, J., Paternite, D. A., Hays, R. D., Kravitz, R. L., & Wenger, N. S. (2006). Physician communication when prescribing new medications. *Archives of Internal Medicine, 25,* 1855–1862.

Teri, L., & Wagner, A. (1992). Alzheimer's disease and depression. *Journal of Consulting and Clinical Psychology, 60,* 379–391.

Theunissen, N. C., de Ridder, D. T., Bensing, J. M., & Rutten, G. E. (2003). Manipulation of patient-provider interaction: Discussing illness representations or action plans concerning adherence. *Patient Education & Counseling, 51*(3), 247–258.

Tucker, J. S., Orlando, M., Barnum, M. A., Sherbourne, C. D., King, F. Y., & Gifford, A. L. (2004). Psychosocial mediators of antiretroviral nonadherence in HIV-positive adults with substance abuse and mental health problems. *Topics in HIV Medicine, 8,* 21–30.

U.S. Bureau of the Census. (2000). *Population division.* Retrieved April 12, 2007, from www.census.gov/population

Vik, A., Maxwell, C. J., & Hogan, D. B. (2004). Measurement, correlates and health outcomes of medication adherence among seniors. *Annals of Pharmacotherapy, 38,* 303–312.

Wald, M. J., & Law, M. R. (2003). A strategy to reduce cardiovascular disease by 80%. *British Medical Journal, 326,* 1419–1424.

Wally, T., & Scott, A. K. (1995). Prescribing in the elderly. *Postgraduate Medical Journal, 71,* 466–471.

Wang, P. S., Bohn, R. L., Knight, E., Glynn, R. J., Magun, H., & Avorn, J. (2002). Noncompliance with antihypertensive medications: The impact of depressive symptoms and psychosocial factors. *Journal of General Internal Medicine, 17,* 504–511.

Wolf, M. S., Gazmararian, J. A., & Baker, D. W. (2007). Health literacy and health risk behaviors among older adults. *American Journal of Preventive Medicine, 32*(1), 19–24.

World Health Organization. (2003). *Adherence to long term therapies—Evidence for action.* Geneva: WHO Publications.

Yam, F. K., Akers, W., Ferraris, V. A., Smith, K., Ramaiah, C., Camp, P., et al. (2006). Interventions to improve guideline compliance following coronary artery bypass grafting. *Surgery, 140,* 541–552.

Yee, B. W. K., & Williams, B. J. (2002). Medication management and appropriate substance use in the elderly. In C. B. Lewis (Ed.), *Aging: The health care challenge* (3rd ed., pp. 325–363). Philadelphia: F. A. Davis.

Optimizing Adherence in Older Adults With Cognitive Impairment

27

Barbara Resnick,
Elizabeth Galik,
Eun Shim Nahm,
Marianne
Shaughnessy, and
Kathleen Michael

Dementia has been defined as a global decline in cognitive functioning that occurs in the absence of delirium and is severe enough that it affects social and occupational functioning. The prevalence of dementia increases dramatically in people over the age of 65. Among people 65 years old and older, 50–80 per 1,000 (5% to 8%) have dementia (Rabins, Lyketsos, & Steele, 2006). The prevalence of dementia is highest at 350–400 per 1,000 (35%–40%) among individuals who are 85 years old or older (Rabins et al., 2006). Currently, it is estimated that 4.5 million Americans have Alzheimer's disease, and, because of increases in life expectancy, it is projected that approximately 13.2 million Americans will be affected by Alzheimer's disease in the year 2050.

Optimizing Health Through Adherence to Healthy Behaviors

Health promotion is the science and art of helping people change their life-styles to move toward a state of optimal health, defined as a balance of physical, emotional, social, spiritual, and intellectual health (Green & Kreuter, 2001). The purpose of health promotion and disease prevention is to reduce the poten-tial years of life lost to premature mortality and to ensure better quality of re-maining life among those with cognitive impairment (CI). Adherence to specific health promotion activities among these individuals is therefore critical and has been noted to improve clinical outcomes particularly with regard to mental health and quality of life (Markle-Reid et al., 2006).

Health promotion activities include the use of immunizations to prevent the occurrence of acute problems such as influenza and pneumonia, risk factor reduction through lifestyle modifications such as smoking cessation or regular physical activity, and the prophylactic use of medication to prevent cardiovascu-lar disease or musculoskeletal disorders. In addition, health promotion includes screening to facilitate the early identification of disease so that treatment can be initiated and unnecessary pain and discomfort avoided.

There are multiple guidelines for health promotion activities available for health care providers, as well as patient-specific information to help older in-dividuals decide what type of health promotion activities they want to engage in. These guidelines are no different for those who have CI. The decisions about whether to adhere to these guidelines are, however, complicated by the cogni-tive status of these individuals and about decisions related to their length and quality of life. Decisions about health promotion activities for individuals with CI are generally made by the power of attorney (POA) for health care once it has been deemed that the individual is incompetent (Raik, Miller, & Fins, 2004).

Prevalence of Nonadherence

Compliance with recommended immunization guidelines for older adults has improved (Daniels, Nguyen, Gildengorin, & Pérez-Stable, 2004), although the goal set in *Healthy People 2010* of 95% adherence to immunization has not been met. To facilitate compliance, the federal government in 2002 approved stand-ing orders for annual influenza vaccinations and pneumococcal pneumonia vaccination for older adults in institutional settings and home health agencies for all Medicare and Medicaid beneficiaries. With regard to smoking cessation, despite the fact that older adults are less likely to get counseled for smoking cessation, they have the same quit rates as younger individuals. Annually, it is reported that 70% of older smokers want to quit, and 46% make some attempt each year at quitting (Hyland, Rezaishiraz, Bauer, Giovino, & Cummings, 2005). While there is some support to indicate that quitting smoking even after age 65 can increase years of life (Houston et al., 2005), it may be more important to focus on the potential improvement in quality of life with smoking cessation such as safety issues related to fires and improvement in cardiovascular function and memory (Reitz, Luchsinger, Tang, & Mayeux, 2005).

Moderate alcohol intake is believed to be health promoting (Byles, Young, Furuya, & Parkinson, 2006). Unfortunately, however, 5.6% of people 65 years of age or older engage in binge drinking, 1.6% engage in heavy alcohol use, and .5% are known to be alcohol dependent (Office of Applied Studies, 2000). Although older adults with CI do not drink more than other older individuals (Reid, Boutros, O'Connor, Cadariu, & Concato, 2002), alcohol has the potential to be beneficial or harmful to health and quality of life.

Physical activity is an important aspect of health promotion among CI older adults as physical activity may help them maintain function and optimize quality of life, even at relatively low levels of physical activity or exercise intensity (defined as activities that use a metabolic energy equivalent of <4.0) (Roddy et al., 2005). For older adults living in nursing homes, at least half of whom are likely to have moderate to severe CI (Magaziner, Zimmerman, Fox, & Burns, 1998; Rosenblatt et al., 2004), lack of physical activity exacerbates functional impairment (Luukinen et al., 2006). A recent study of 21,670 nursing home residents examined the change in physical function in adults with moderate and severe CI with no comorbid illness over a 6-month time period (Carpenter, Hastie, Morris, Fries, & Ankri, 2006). Overall physical function of residents with moderate CI worsened significantly by 1.78 points (95% CI; 1.67 to 1.91) on the Minimum Data Set Activities of Daily Living (MDS-ADL) with dependence on staff being highest for functions related to personal hygiene, dressing, and toileting (Carpenter et al., 2006). Overall physical function of residents with severe CI also worsened significantly by 1.70 points on the MDS-ADL (95% CI; 1.59 to 1.83) over the 6-month time period, with dependence on staff being highest in activities related to eating (Carpenter et al., 2006). Each ADL item, such as bed mobility, transfer, locomotion, dressing, eating, toileting, and personal hygiene, showed a significant worsening at both 3 and 6 months for both groups of cognitively impaired residents (Carpenter et al., 2006).

Evaluating food intake in older adults is particularly important as inadequate intake can result in weight loss and loss of muscle mass, which may result in decreased strength and power, decreased walking speed and impaired balance, and a decline in activity (Bourre, 2006). Most micronutrients (vitamins and trace elements) have been directly evaluated in the setting of cerebral functioning. For instance, to produce energy, the use of glucose by nervous tissue implies the presence of vitamin B1, and this vitamin modulates cognitive performance, especially in the elderly. Vitamin B9 preserves brain during its development and memory during aging. Vitamins B6 and B12, among others, are directly involved in the synthesis of some neurotransmitters. Vitamin B12 delays the onset of signs of dementia (and blood abnormalities), provided it is administered in a precise clinical timing window, before the onset of the first symptoms. The Modified Food Pyramid can be used to guide individuals toward adequate nutritional intake.

There is no evidence to support differences in micronutrient status among those with or without dementia. Although the association is not always strong, there is evidence to suggest a relationship between body weight and CI such that those with CI are more likely to have body mass indexes (BMI) higher or lower than normal. CI was also more frequently detected in subjects with metabolic syndrome (MetS) than in subjects without MetS (7.2 vs. 2.8%; $p < 0.001$) (Vanhanen et al., 2006). Specifically, it was noted that Alzheimer's disease was associated with obesity (odds ratio [OR] 9.5, 95% confidence interval [CI] 2.4–37.3, p = 0.001), being underweight (OR 5.4, CI 0.9–33.7, p = 0.07) and abdominal obesity (OR 2.5, CI 1.1–5.7, p = 0.027), after adjusting for age, sex, and living location (e.g., institution versus community) (Razay, Vreugdenhil, & Wilcock, 2006). Women who developed dementia between ages 79 and 88 years were overweight, with a higher average BMI at age 70 years (27.7 vs. 25.7; P = .007), 75 years (27.9 vs. 25.0; P < .001), and 79 years (26.9 vs. 25.1; P = .02) than was found among non-demented women. A higher degree of overweight was observed in women who developed AD at 70 years (29.3; P = .009), 75 years (29.6; P < .001), and 79 years (28.2; P = .003) than in nondemented women. For every 1.0 increase in BMI at age 70 years, AD risk increased by 36%.

The impact of screening or not screening for cancer among older adults has not been well studied among older adults with cognitive impairment. There is some evidence, however, that these individuals are less likely to adhere to screening; researchers found that individuals with CI tend to be diagnosed with breast cancer at later stages than individuals without evidence of CI. Patients with CI were not diagnosed until tumors were larger and the likelihood of lymph node involvement had increased. Likewise, with colon cancer, patients with CI were twice as likely to have colon cancer reported after death (i.e., autopsy or death certificate) (adjusted odds ratio [AOR] = 2.31, 95% confidence interval [CI] = 1.79–3.00) (Gorin, Heck, Albert, & Hershman, 2005).

Impact of Nonadherence

Lack of adherence to health-promoting activities such as maintenance of optimal weight and dietary intake, particularly of micronutrients; adherence to physical activity recommendations; cancer screening; smoking cessation; and moderate use of alcohol may have a significant impact on the quality of life of older adults with CI and their ability to function at their highest cognitive and physical level. Optimal dietary intake and maintaining an ideal body weight may help to ensure the highest level of cognitive ability and physical activity in individuals with CI and thereby improve health (Zizzi et al., 2006). With regard to alcohol intake, CI is noted to be higher for those who exceed one wine-equivalent liter among men and 0.5 liter among women, daily. Nonadherence to moderate alcohol intake may exacerbate cognitive function and cardiovascular disease and increase the risk of accidents (Hollingworth et al., 2006; Li et al., 2006; Wendel-Vos et al., 2004).

Analytic reviews provide strong evidence that participation in either nonspecific physical activity or specific aerobic or resistive exercise is associated with a variety of health improvements, such as decreased risk of coronary heart disease and stroke (Cornelissen & Fagard, 2005; Lee, Folsom, & Blair, 2003; Wendel-Vos et al., 2004); decreased progression of degenerative joint disease (Roddy, Zhang, & Doherty, 2005; Roddy et al., 2005); prevention of osteoporosis of the lumbar spine (Palombaro, 2005); decreased incidences of falls (Chang et al., 2004; Weatherall, 1994); increased gait speed if the activity is of sufficient intensity and dosage (Lopopolo, Greco, Sullivan, Craik, & Mangione, 2006); improved cognitive function in sedentary older adults (Colcombe et al., 2006) and in those with dementia (Heyn, Abreu, & Ottenbacher, 2004); a modest benefit in quality of life for frail older adults (Schechtman & Ory, 2001); and successful aging (Depp & Jeste, 2006). Given the strong support for adherence to physical activity guidelines for older adults, lack of adherence among older adults with CI can have multiple consequences, all of which are critical to quality of life rather than longevity. Moreover, the well-known association between CI and functional decline is exacerbated by inadequate amounts of time spent in physical activity.

In addition to clinical benefits associated with physical activity, the impact that lack of activity has on functional decline can have serious implications for the amount of care needed, increasing health risks associated with decreased mobility, the cost of providing care, and the quality of life for individuals with CI (Hill, Fillit, Thomas, & Chang, 2006; Vestergaard, Kronborg-Andersen, Korsholm, & Puggaard, 2006). Researchers conclude that in older adults with dementia, functional disability increases the cost of Medicare services by more than $399 per additional ADL disability per year. Functional decline is costly, and individuals with disabilities caused by disorders of the central nervous system, such as dementia, represent a group of ever increasing size (Thomas et al., 2002). Until CI can be prevented or cured, promoting the maintenance of functional abilities through physical activity in this population remains a priority in clinical practice and research (Rolland et al., 2007). Volicer and colleagues (2006), for example, were able to demonstrate that a continuous-activity program for nursing home residents with severe CI resulted in a significant decrease in behavioral symptoms and a decline in the use of psychotropic medications among the study participants. It appears that providing opportunities and motivating nursing home residents with CI to engage in meaningful activities is an important strategy for preventing agitated behaviors and ultimately improving residents' quality of life.

There continues to be a clinical and ethical debate about screening for cancer among older adults in general, and specifically for those with CI. This debate generally is based on the cost/benefit associated with screening to the individual and the health care system. The impact of nonadherence to screening has not been well studied.

Factors That Influence Adherence Among Older Adults With Cognitive Impairment

Memory

Given that older adults with moderate to severe CI may not be able to elucidate their wishes with regard to health-promoting behaviors or explain their rationale for nonadherence, it is possible to address only relationships between factors that are known to influence adherence by non-CI patients and these behaviors among those with CI. Underlying physical status, and the impact of this on function, can have a major influence on participation and adherence to health-promoting behaviors. In some cases, health care providers may assume that, in light of physical and functional decline, there is no benefit to health-promoting activities; they may believe that they won't make a difference in clinical outcomes or quality of life of the individual. Underlying physical status can also influence individuals' beliefs in their abilities to engage in healthy behaviors such as exercise or to be able to tolerate health promotion screenings such as mammography or bone densitometry.

Psychosocial Factors: Mood and Fear

The most commonly noted psychosocial factors influencing adherence to healthy behaviors, particularly physical activity guidelines, are fear of falling or exacerbating underlying problems (e.g., causing a decline in memory or increasing musculoskeletal pain) (Bruce, Devine, & Prince, 2002; Fletcher & Hirdes, 2004; Martin, Hart, Spector, Doyle, & Harari, 2005) and depressive symptoms (Tinetti, 2003; van Wijk et al., 2006). Fear of falling, for example, is commonly associated with a decline in physical activity (Bruce et al., 2002; Fletcher & Hirdes, 2004; Martin et al., 2005) and influences exercise behavior. Fear of the impact of screening in terms of diagnosis and/or treatment-related issues may inhibit older adults with CI and/or their decision makers from having the older individual with CI undergo screenings (Fowler, 2006; Tessaro, Mangone, Parkar, & Pawar, 2006).

Depression, which is prevalent among older adults with CI, can also impact individuals' willingness to engage in any type of health-promoting behaviors, such as exercise, eating, or even getting immunizations (Jensen, Decker, & Andersen, 2006).

Behavioral Symptoms

The motivational challenges that face those who attempt to engage older adults with CI is exacerbated for those elderly persons who exhibit complicating behavioral and psychiatric symptoms in the context of their dementia. The prevalence of agitated and/or aggressive behaviors among nursing home residents with dementia is often greater than 80% (Aalten et al., 2006). Functional dependence and impaired mobility have also been associated with problematic behavioral symptoms and depression among long-term-care residents with CI (Boustani et al., 2005; Gruber-Baldini, 2004). The presence of behavioral disturbance may also adversely affect the adherence of older adults with CI to interventions designed to maintain or improve functional abilities or overall health. For example, Rolland et al. (2007) found that the adherence of cognitively impaired nursing home residents to an exercise intervention that occurred two times a week for 1 year was low, with only 47.8% of the subjects participating in more than one-third of the exercise sessions. Verbal disagreement and behavioral disorders among the cognitively impaired participants accounted for 75% of the nonadherence to the exercise intervention.

Apathy

In addition to the frequency of problematic behavioral symptoms among cognitively impaired nursing home residents, this population is faced with the additional motivational challenge of apathy. Apathy is a neuropsychiatric symptom that results in a loss of motivation due to disturbance of intellect, emotion, or level of consciousness (Marin, 1991). It has been repeatedly demonstrated that cognitively impaired older adults are more likely than their cognitively intact counterparts to suffer from severe apathy (Buettner & Fitzsimmons, 2006), which is believed to affect 61%–88% of individuals with CI (Galynker, Roane, Miner, Feinberg, & Watts, 1995). While apathy does not seem to respond to medical interventions (Rabins, Lyketsos, & Steele, 2006), it has been demonstrated that caregiver behavioral approaches that assist with the motivation and initial cuing to engage in specific activities such as those related to physical activity are effective (Beck et al., 1997; Chang & Lin, 2005; Engelman, Altus, & Hosier, 2003; Teri et al., 2003; Volicer, Simard, Heartquist-Pupa, Medrek, & Riordan, 2006; Yu, Evans, & Sullivan-Marx, 2005). In addition, apathy can be decreased through the use of music (Holmes et al., 2006).

Social Support

Social support networks, including family, friends, peers, medical professionals, and nursing home staff, are important determinants of health-promoting behaviors (Resnick, Orwig, Magaziner, & Wynne, 2002). Repeatedly, motivation to perform functional activities and exercise has been found to be influenced by the social milieu of the care setting (Rose & Pruchno, 1999; Waters, 1994). The influence of any member of the social network of the older adult with CI can be positive or negative, depending on the person's philosophy and beliefs related to restorative care. There is a need to establish a system within the social network and a culture of care in which there are interactions that will motivate individuals with CI to engage in health-promoting activities and achieve realistic goals given their underlying disease.

Self-Efficacy and Outcome Expectations

Bandura (1977, 1997) described self-efficacy and outcome expectations as two of the central concepts within Social Cognitive Theory. Specifically, self-efficacy expectations are individuals' beliefs in their capabilities to perform a course of action to attain a desired outcome, and outcome expectations are the beliefs that a certain consequence will be produced by personal action. Efficacy expectations are dynamic and are both appraised and enhanced by four mechanisms (Bandura, 1997): (1) enactive mastery experience, or successful performance of the activity of interest; (2) verbal persuasion, or verbal encouragement given by a credible source that the individual is capable of performing the activity of interest; (3) vicarious experience, or seeing similar individuals perform a specific activity; and (4) physiological and affective states such as pain, fatigue, or anxiety associated with a given activity. Both self-efficacy and outcome expectations play an influential role in the performance of healthy activities (Collins, Lee, Albright, & King, 2004; Cress et al., 2005; King et al., 2000; Taylor-Piliae & Froelicher, 2005) and in the adoption and maintenance of exercise behavior (Conn, Burks, Pomeroy, Ulbrich, & Cochran, 2003; Dunstan et al., 2002; Litt, Kleppinger, & Judge, 2002; McAuley, Marquez, Jerome, Blissmer, & Katula, 2002; O'Connor, Rousseau, & Maki, 2004).

Outcome expectations are particularly relevant to older adults. These individuals may have high self-efficacy expectations for exercise, but if they do not believe in the outcomes associated with the behavior, for example, that screening for bowel cancer may identify early disease that is easily treated, then it is unlikely that they will be willing to undergo screening. Older adults with mild CI can evaluate their current self-efficacy and outcome expectations with regard to specific health behaviors, but those with moderate to severe cognitive changes may not be able to adequately articulate these beliefs. That is not to say, however, that self-efficacy-based interventions do not work with these individuals. Rather, we have multiple examples in which self-efficacy-based interventions have changed behavior among older individuals with CI (Resnick, 2004; Resnick, Allen, & Ruane, 2002; Resnick, Simpson, Galik, et al., 2006).

Innovative behavioral-care approaches with older adults with CI have utilized techniques based on components of self-efficacy theory, such as verbal encouragement, cueing, role modeling, positive reinforcement, and development of a routine to successfully motivate these individuals to perform health-promoting activities (Engelman et al., 2003; Lim, 2003; Teri et al., 2003). The theory of self-efficacy has also been applied to improving behavioral interactions between family caregivers and individuals with CI (DiBartolo, 2002; Gottlieb & Rooney, 2004).

Self-efficacy-based staff motivational systems such as behavioral supervision, observing and providing nursing assistants (NAs) with verbal feedback related to care activities (Chang & Lin, 2005; Field, 2004; Sacre, 2004; Teri et al., 2003), have been used successfully to implement interventions to improve adherence to healthy behaviors.

Resilience

In contrast to apathy, resilience is an individual's capacity to make a "psycho-social comeback in adversity" (Kadner, 1989) and is defined as the ability to achieve, retain, or regain a level of physical or emotional health after illness or loss (Felten & Hall, 2001). Resilient individuals tend to manifest adaptive behavior, especially with regard to social functioning, morale, and somatic health and are less likely to succumb to illness (Wagnild, 2003). Resilience, as a component of the individual's personality, develops and changes over time through ongoing experiences with the physical and social environment (Glantz & Johnson, 1999). Older women who have successfully recovered from orthopedic or other stressful events describe themselves as resilient and determined (Felten & Hall, 2001). Community-dwelling older adults who are resilient were noted to have better function, mood, and quality of life than those who were less resilient (Hardy, Concato, & Gill, 2004; Wagnild, 2003). Resilience is also noted to be related to self-efficacy and outcome expectations and a predictor of adherence to exercise in older women after hip fracture (Inguito & Resnick, 2007). Older adults with CI who are resilient may therefore be more likely to continue to engage in healthy behaviors.

Culture, the Environment, and Institutional Procedures

Environments that facilitate healthy behaviors such as physical activity can influence participation in these activities (Iwarsson & Isacsson, 1996; Iwarsson

& Slaug, 2001) and enable people to achieve their highest level of function and well-being (Humpel, Owen, & Leslie, 2002; Takano, Nakamura, & Watanabe, 2002). Unfortunately, many environments in which older adults with CI live are limited with regard to space for exercise. Accessible and safe walking paths are often not present, nor are heart-healthy food choices (i.e., low-cholesterol and low-fat meals) or finger foods for easy snacking available for those who need to increase their caloric content (Humpel et al., 2002; Takano et al., 2002). Altering the environment has been noted to impact behavior (Takano et al., 2002).

Policy

New practice guidelines associated with "Welcome to Medicare" (Centers for Disease Control and Prevention Behavioral Risk Factor Surveillance System) and Health Plan Employer Data and Information Set (HEDIS®) programs provide reimbursement and regulatory incentives for providers to take the time to discuss and encourage health-promotion activities such as physical activity. The availability of this opportunity should encourage providers and patients to partake of these services. It is not known, however, how extensively these guidelines are being utilized in practice or whether older adults with CI are excluded from these welcome visits because the health care provider assumes that health-promoting activities will not improve the CI patient's quality of life.

National policies have not been established related to physical activity. With regard to function, the Omnibus Budget Reconciliation Act (OBRA) of 1987 mandated that residents in nursing homes attain and maintain their highest level of function. Consequently, caregivers in nursing homes have attempted to develop and implement restorative-care programs to increase physical activity among older adults with CI. The impact and success of this policy has not been evaluated. Policy has been successful, however, in changing health behaviors in areas such as the use of seat belts, suggesting that policy can have an important impact on behavior (Salzberg & Moffat, 2004).

Use of a Social Ecological Model to Optimize Adherence

As described earlier, the reasons for poor adherence to health-promoting behaviors among older adults with CI are multifactorial and therefore best explained using a social ecological model (Sallis & Glanz, 2006; Sallis et al., 2006). Specifically, a social ecological model suggests that an individual's behavior is affected by a wide sphere of influences: intrapersonal, interpersonal, institutional/organizational/environment, and public policy. In addition to the intrapersonal factors previously addressed, such as psychological factors (e.g., mood and motivation), there are also nonmodifiable factors, including demographic variables such as age, gender, and race. While it is useful to acknowledge the presence of these factors, it is challenging to relate them directly to function, as there is a good deal of interindividual variability. Moreover, it is impossible to separate out the multiple comorbidities common in older individuals with CI. Appreciating the potential impact of these variables, however, can help guide interventions.

Interpersonal factors that influence participation in health-promotion activities are particularly important among older adults with CI whose engagement in these activities may be driven by the influence of a caregiver or by a power of attorney for health care. For example, social interactions can alter the underlying physical status of the individual with CI. Degenerative joint disease, for example, that imposes limitations in range of motion may have a smaller impact on functional limitation in dressing in individuals who are encouraged by a family member to dress themselves than in individuals who are dressed by a family member or whose family member insists that the NA dress the individual, not allowing the older individual optimal range and function.

Environment and organizational factors that optimize adherence to health-promoting behaviors can influence outcomes with regard to adherence to those behaviors (Crews, 2005; Iwarsson, 2005; Takano et al., 2002). Having visible exercise-related areas, walkable spaces, safe areas for exercise, and interesting walking destinations have been shown to improve physical activity among residents (Joseph, Szimring, Harris-Kojetin, & Kiefer, 2005). Simple and cost-efficient modifications can be made, such as improving lighting, displaying signs that specifically promote active living, and providing physical activity stations throughout the facility and outdoors. Policies and procedures within the organizational environment are also critical. For example, facility-based policies related to use of shared space areas, provision of care, and availability of services can influence participation in physical activities and function among residents. If outdoor space for walking is locked and made inaccessible, or if the underlying philosophy or culture within the facility is to provide care rather than to optimize function, perceptions and expectations among residents, staff, and families or their proxies can be affected, leading to decreased promotion of healthy activities such as exercise.

Public health policies can influence adherence to health-promoting activities for older adults with CI. Nursing homes serving Medicare and Medicaid patients have to provide immunizations against influenza and pneumococcal disease to all residents if they want to continue in the programs (Hinman, Urquhart, Strikas, & National Vaccine Advisory Committee, 2007). In some states, implementation of this policy has resulted in an increase in adherence to immunizations (Dunn, Misra, Habermann, & Griffin, 2003). Public policy related to physical activity has not been as well enforced, although increased recognition among caregivers and proxies for individuals with CI of the benefits of physical activity has led them to provide verbal encouragement to individuals with CI to engage in physical activity. The implications for reimbursement associated with screening as noted by Medicare have a significant impact on participation in screening activities. Reimbursement may be unavailable for some preventive interventions (e.g., hearing tests, over-the-counter medications, smoking-cessation products) and may be available within narrowly defined time frames for screenings such as colonoscopy (Dunn et al., 2003).

Although the components of the social ecological model were described separately, it is critical to recognize that these factors are interrelated in real-world settings. The intra-individual level of the model, for example, explains the functional changes that can occur within the individual. The interpersonal level influences the intra-individual level of the model through the theory of self-efficacy such that interactions with caregivers can help to engage older adults with CI in health-promoting behaviors. At the institutional or organizational and environmental level, interventions can be implemented to influence the impact of the environment on the individual and the interpersonal interactions that are ongoing. Last, enforcement of policy guidelines can significantly influence all other aspects of the model. Guidelines requiring walking paths in nursing homes, for example, could influence the environment, affect interpersonal activities that occur in those settings with family, and improve intrapersonal factors related to health status by increasing physical activity of persons with CI.

Special Challenges: Adherence in Select Populations

Older Adults Poststroke

Many older adult stroke survivors struggle with the sudden onset of neurological deficits that cause profound changes in their daily lives. Many continue to have persistent risk factors that put them at significant risk for a future stroke event. In a recent study of 364 community-dwelling stroke survivors, 99% of volunteers for an exercise study had at least one suboptimally controlled cardiovascular risk factor, and 91% had two or more concurrent risk factors that were being inadequately treated (Kopunek et al., 2007). Eighty percent of the participants had prehypertension or hypertension, 67% were overweight or obese, 60% had suboptimal LDL, 45% had impaired fasting glucose, 34% had low HDL, and 14% were current smokers, all the while reportedly receiving routine medical care (Kopunek et al., 2007). Every stroke survivor should be evaluated for risk of stroke at least annually and more often if multiple risk factors are present. Patients must be queried at every visit (in the home, at the practitioner's office, or at the hospital) regarding risk factors and educated regarding the importance of aggressive management and control.

Adherence to medication, diet, or exercise regimens designed to modify risk-factor profiles may seem an overwhelming task for many older stroke survivors. Rehabilitation may focus on the development of new adaptive and compensatory strategies to facilitate independence and function, imposing a steep learning curve to acquire and restore needed skills. The combination of sudden neurological and functional changes, along with age-related declines, can present significant challenges. Alterations in perception and motivation that result from damage to specific areas of the brain further confront the ability of individuals with stroke to perform health-promoting behaviors. Add to this clinical picture the possibility of stroke-related CI, and the challenges are compounded.

Assessment of older adults' understanding of their health status is a critical starting point for any intervention. The health care provider should ask stroke survivors to explain what they have been told about each medical problem. Using this information, an educational plan can be designed to improve understanding, provide feedback, and reinforce adherence to recommended regimens. Reliable sites on the Web, such as those supported by the National Institutes of Health or disease-specific foundations, are useful sources to download and print information for patients to take home to reinforce in-person teaching efforts. These educational tools have been adapted for stroke patients, who frequently have associated visual or hearing deficits. Font size and visual contrast must be adequate, and the language must be appropriate for the person's educational level.

With regard to medication management and adherence, the use of pillboxes may be valuable. Part of the assessment of health management should be an inquiry into whether finances influence the person's medication-taking practices. Medicare Part D has impacted most older adults and confused many recipients regarding the available benefits.

Patient education among those who have had a stroke is not sufficient to change behavior poststroke. Rather, adherence to medication, exercise, or treatment regimens is closely associated with changing their beliefs. As previously described, social cognitive theory indicates that specific efficacy expectations affect behavior, motivational level, thought patterns, and emotional reactions to any situation (Bandura, 1977). These beliefs are essential to the adoption and maintenance of self-care activities, such as engaging in physical activity after stroke (Robinson-Smith, Johnston, & Allen, 2000; Shaughnessy et al., 2005). Bolstering self-efficacy to make significant lifestyle modifications can be accomplished through (1) offering education and encouragement; (2) providing specific tasks to accomplish and directions on how to complete the task; (3) identifying and addressing barriers to compliance; and (4) cuing behaviors through role-modeling or self-modeling. Finally, education regarding expected benefits may provide further incentives and motivation to change behaviors. Helping an older adult stroke survivor to choose a healthier diet, lose weight, begin an exercise program, or adhere to a medication regimen requires time, care, and lots of encouragement in selecting goals and interventions for behavior modification and should be a routine part of medical and nursing assessment and surveillance.

In the course of a stroke, survivors have sustained some type of brain injury that may or may not affect their cognitive function. Depending on the location and extent of the stroke, patients may be independent in all matters regarding their own health care or dependent on others for many aspects of day-to-day living. As cognitive screening is part of a standardized neurological assessment for all stroke survivors, accommodations for cognitive deficits must be made accordingly, particularly for those with attention or memory dysfunction. Further, improvements in cognition may occur during the recovery process and require ongoing evaluation and adjustment of treatment plans. Alterations in cognition may signify other medical conditions that commonly occur with stroke, so astute recognition of change is important.

Older Adults With Moderate to Severe Cognitive Impairment

Older adults with moderate to severe CI do not have the underlying cognitive ability to consciously decide to adhere or not to adhere to health-promoting behaviors. Therefore, ethical decisions and decisions about the futility of interventions need to be considered by their caregivers (Resnick et al., 2005). Medical futility is described as evidence from the available data that a proposed therapy should not be performed because it will not improve the patient's medical condition (Bernat,

2005). The health-promotion plan of care for the older individual with moderate to severe CI must be established with the proxy. Once the goals are determined, then interventions can be implemented to optimize the individual's participation in the health-promotion goals. There is evidence that physical activity can be increased among individuals with CI, as well as increased participation in functional activities (Kuiack, Campbell, & Evans, 2003; Tappen, Roach, Applegate, & Stowell, 2000; Tsai, 2003). Consistently across all these studies, encouraging adherence to physical activity among older adults with moderate to severe CI optimized their participation in functional activities and walking programs.

To increase participation in eating, particularly eating independently, for older adults with moderate to severe CI, teaching interventions for caregivers have been implemented with some success (Chang & Lin, 2005). When caregivers allowed the study participants to control more of their own eating process, and when they provided verbal prompts and positive reinforcement for eating, there was improvement in independent eating. Other techniques that have been successfully utilized to engage older adults with moderate to severe CI in healthy behaviors include prompting the individual with simple one-step commands (Beck et al., 2003; Lim & Taylor, 2005).

In a recent study, Galik and Resnick (2007) specifically explored strategies that would successfully motivate nursing home residents with moderate to severe CI to engage in functional activities and exercise. This study used a qualitative design with a focus-group methodology. A total of 26 different codes were identified, which were reduced to the following four themes describing effective techniques for promoting participation in healthy behaviors: (1) communication techniques (13% of total codes); (2) caring (34% of total codes); (3) magnified sensory stimulation (19% of total codes); and (4) general innovative techniques (34% of total codes). Table 27.1 incorporates the findings from prior quantitative studies and this recent qualitative work and outlines the interventions that effectively improve adherence to healthy behaviors among older adults with moderate to severe CI.

Use of Technology to Optimize Adherence in Older Adults With Cognitive Impairment

As prevalence of dementia has become a significant public health problem among older adults (Rabins et al., 2006), researchers and professionals in various fields have been making efforts to develop innovative technologies to assist these individuals to maintain activities of daily living and overall well-being. A burgeoning scientific effort is to develop "cognitive prosthetics" or "cognitive orthoses" for cognitively impaired individuals (Center for Aging Services Technologies, 2004; Kuwahara, 2006; Wherton & Monk, 2006). The term "cognitive prosthetics" or "cognitive orthoses" is rooted in the terms for physical prostheses that augment various physical disabilities. Among different definitions (LoPresti & Kirsch, 2004; Lynch & George, 2002), Lynch (Lynch & George, 2002) defines a "cognitive prosthetic" as "any computer-based system that has been designed for a specific individual to accomplish one or more designated tasks related to activities of daily living, including work." Development of a cognitive prosthetic requires multidisciplinary collaboration in the areas of cognitive

27.1   Description of the Interventions to Facilitate Adherence in CI Older Adults

Mastery experiences	An effective way of creating a strong sense of efficacy is through mastery of experiences. Mastery involves the actual performance and successful completion of an activity.

- NAs will be encouraged to provide opportunities for cognitively impaired residents to do a functional task for themselves rather than simply doing it for residents (i.e., comb hair, wash face, put arm in shirt sleeve, drink with a no-spill cup, feed self with an adaptive utensil).
- NAs will be taught techniques to actively engage residents with moderate to severe cognitive impairment in restorative care activities by positively acknowledging any and all attempts of successful completion of goal activities.
- NAs will be encouraged to strive for a restorative care approach with every resident encounter.

Vicarious experience	Role modeling by Restorative Care Nurse to NAs.

- Demonstration of techniques to optimize functional performance of residents with moderate to severe cognitive impairment (i.e., simplify presentation of food so as not to overwhelm resident, physically model/demonstrate the functional behavior rather than using lengthy verbal directions).
- Demonstration of techniques to encourage participation (i.e., using music as a motivator, encouraging resident activities that are consistent with past life experience, such as folding clothes, packing a briefcase).
- Demonstration of exercise routine (i.e., range of motion, small-group activities with functional/physical activity focus).
- Teaching NAs how to pair cognitively impaired residents to motivate each other (i.e., pair a resident who can self-propel in her wheelchair with a resident who is more sedentary, pair a resident who is slightly more independent at mealtime with a resident who might benefit from the visual cues).
- Verbal encouragement, praise, and recognition of NAs for efforts to engage residents in restorative-care activities.

Self-modeling:

- Offer NAs an opportunity to return demonstrate or verbalize creative techniques learned to optimize physical function in residents with moderate to severe cognitive impairment.
- Encourage NAs to share resident's progress in restorative-care goals with family and significant others.

Verbal encouragement	*Education* regarding the philosophy of restorative care with the moderate to severely cognitively impaired during the Res-Care-CI in-service classes and during coaching/mentoring on the units.

- Review the benefits of restorative care for residents and NAs.
- Review Restorative Care Interventions with NAs in terms of ADLs (i.e., bathing [washing mitt, liquid soap, modeling action]; dressing [laying clothes out in order that they are to be put on]; feeding [adaptive utensils, no-spill cups, simplify food presentation]; continence [toileting schedule, running water as auditory cue]; communication [use of old photographs to start conversation; organization of activities around more energetic times of the day]).

27.1 Description of the Interventions to Facilittate Adherence in CI Older Adults (*Continued*)

- Offer caregiver tips on how to motivate cognitively impaired residents to participate in functional activities (i.e., use of humor, activities consistent with past life experiences).
- Discuss how to incorporate restorative care into daily routine.
- Discuss potential effects of cognitive impairment on mood, affect, and behavior of patient.
- Discuss the similarities and differences between restorative care and behavior management.

Encouragement, including initial goal identification with NA, resident, and family. During coaching and mentoring, the restorative care nurse will work with the NA, resident, and family to identify daily short-term goals for the resident. These goals will focus on performing a specific functional activity or exercise activity. A long-term goal will also be identified and will vary on the basis of what is relevant to the individual (i.e., being able to go on a trip or to a family outing).

- Goals are written on a special Goal Identification Form (Appendix).
- Completion of restorative-care activities and time spent in individual activities is documented by the NA on Documentation of Restorative Care Flow Sheet. Instruction on the use of the flow sheet is provided during the Res-Care-CI classes.
- Goals are graduated, from easy to more difficult.
- Goals are reviewed weekly with NA, resident, and/or family and revised as appropriate.

Physiological feedback

Teaching NAs to assess for and manage physiological feedback that may affect the participation of residents with moderate to severe cognitive impairment in restorative-care activities.

- Caregivers are taught to recognize symptoms such as aphasia, motor apraxia, agnosia, tremor, and increased tone/cogwheeling that may affect the individual's ability to participate in goal activities.
- Caregivers are instructed to assess residents on a daily basis to ascertain if they experience pain, anxiety, behavioral disturbance, fatigue, shortness of breath, or chest pain associated with functional activities or exercise that may make the individual not want to perform functional activities or exercise.

Interventions to decrease these unpleasant sensations will be initiated by NAs and include:

- *Management of Aphasia:*
  - Use simple words and phrases.
  - Anticipate a resident's verbal response delay. Teach NAs to wait for the resident to answer questions or respond.
  - Use physical gesturing and modeling with residents who have a difficult time understanding spoken language.
- *Management of Motor Apraxia:*
  - Teach NAs how to recognize symptoms of motor apraxia.
  - Reinforce and engage residents in physical activities and functional activities that reinforce repetitive and simple movements.

(Continued)

27.1 Description of the Interventions to Facilitate Adherence in CI Older Adults (*Continued*)

- Engage residents in functional activities that they performed every day.
- Simplify functional tasks (break down into steps) that are too difficult for residents to perform.
- Demonstrate or model the activity for the resident.
- Use adaptive clothing (Velcro, elastic-waist pants).
- Teach NAs the benefit of hand-over-hand activity for residents with severe motor apraxia.
- *Management of Agnosia:*
  - Encourage family members to bring in familiar objects for the resident's room.
  - Explain tasks/activities, provide verbal cues to prevent the resident from misinterpreting situations.
  - Attempt to provide activities that are consistent with the resident's previous personal routine.
- *Management of Tremor:* Discuss use of alternate clothing choices (i.e., pullovers rather than button-down shirts, loafers, elastic shoelaces). Weighted cups with lids, weighted utensils, or use of wrist weights. Use of electric razor instead of straight razor.
- *Management of Increased Tone/Cogwheeling:* Review with NA how to identify cogwheeling and reinforce that this is a neurological symptom and not the resident being resistive. Provide the resident with opportunities for range of motion (creative ways to engage cognitively impaired residents in ROM include reaching for item in closet or cupboard, sweeping, kicking a ball, folding and flying a paper airplane, folding clothes, tapping a balloon, pressing down on a "gas pedal").
- *Management of Pain:* Advocate for adequate pain relief (i.e., pain medications can be scheduled to be given prior to more physically active times; using complementary techniques to decrease pain as appropriate such as heat and ice; using relaxation techniques such as deep breathing and distraction to decrease pain. Also, will discuss role of range-of-motion exercises in muscle soreness and rigidity. Teach techniques for proper body alignment and positioning of residents (rolled towels, splints, specific positioning devices for bed and/or chair).
- *Management of Anxiety/Behavioral Disturbance:*
  - Teach NAs to approach resident with calm, unhurried, and pleasant attitude.
  - Use humor and smile as cognitively impaired residents are highly influenced by the emotional state of their caregivers.
  - Teach NAs to be alert to excessive levels of noise, temperature, and visual stimulation in the environment. A quieter, less stimulating environment may work better for residents who are easily overwhelmed.
  - Use more cueing and modeling and less direct hands-on care (as individuals with cognitive impairment may misinterpret a caregiver's touch).
  - Be patient and reapproach the resident at another time if he is anxious or uncooperative.
- *Management of Fatigue:* Educate nursing assistant to (1) schedule rest periods to augment restorative-care time; (2) be flexible with restorative-care activities so that the resident can rest first and then perform the activity.

27.1	**Description of the Interventions to Facilitate Adherence in CI Older Adults (*Continued*)**

■ *Management of Shortness of Breath (SOB):* If shortness of breath is a new symptom, increases suddenly, or increases significantly with activity or at rest, the NA is to halt the activity and to call and discuss situation with health care provider. Remind NA to provide rest time between steps in completion of any activity.

■ *Management of Chest Pain:* If chest pain is a new symptom or increases significantly with activity, then the activity is to be halted and the caregiver will be taught to notify the charge nurse, who can discuss with health care provider or access emergency services.

NAs are instructed to discuss the occurrence of any unpleasant sensations with the charge nurse and the investigator so that a plan of care can be developed to specifically focus on decreasing those sensations.

science, technology, human computer interaction design, and health care (Alm et al., 2004; LoPresti & Kirsch, 2004).

Cognitive impairment can be caused by various conditions and illnesses, such as motor vehicle accidents, stroke, or dementia. Although the fundamental principles of cognitive prosthesis can be applied to most conditions or illnesses, each condition may require assistance in different areas, such as long-term memory loss or short-term memory loss (LoPresti & Kirsch, 2004). In this chapter, we focus on supportive technologies for older adults suffering from dementia or Alzheimer's disease (AD).

For individuals with dementia and AD, cognitive decline mainly affects episodic memory (memories of personally experienced events) and executive functions (planning, sequencing, and control) (Graham, Emery, & Hodges, 2004; Wherton & Monk, 2006). Executive functions are necessary to carry out individuals' activities of daily living, and many cognitive assistive devices have been and continue to be developed to compensate for losses in these functions (Adlam & Orpwood, 2004; Center for Aging Services Technologies, 2004; Chen, Kam, Zhang, Liu, & Shue, 2005; LoPresti & Kirsch, 2004; Rowe, Lane, & Phipps, 2007). The Center for Aging Services Technologies (CAST), a program of the American Association of Homes and Services, has been a leading national force in developing such technologies. Developed in collaboration with government, academia, and industry, the CAST Web site includes a comprehensive list of evolving technologies and research efforts in the field (Center for Aging Services Technologies, 2004). Selected examples include monitoring technologies, smart homes, medicine management systems, and wander management systems.

Assistive technologies can help cognitively impaired individuals maintain activities of daily living by using several approaches, such as providing cues and instructions for specific functions, alarming individuals for imminent hazardous behaviors (e.g., imminent flooding from the sink, smoking detector) (Adlam & Orpwood, 2004; Chen et al., 2005), helping frail older adults manage medications (Quirk, 2006; AgeLab, 2006), and providing information about their whereabouts or directions (Associated Press, 2007; Global Action on Aging, 2005).

A prototype computerized device, the COACH, was developed to help individuals with dementia perform activities of daily living with less dependence on a caregiver. The COACH was developed using a personal computer and a single video camera to unobtrusively track a user during an activity (e.g., hand washing). When the program detects an error by the user, it provides prerecorded verbal prompts (cues), and if the user does not correct or stop the behavior, the computer calls for a caregiver (LoPresti & Kirsch, 2004). Another example is SmartHome (Adlam & Orpwood, 2004). The Bath Institute of Medical Engineering (BIME), in the United Kingdom, partnered with commercial and nonprofit organizations and developed smart-house systems for people with dementia. This home combines several unique existing technologies. The Bath and Basin Monitor is a system that prevents flooding from the bath or basin; the Night Light provides gentle lighting to residents at night using motion-detector technologies; the Time of Day voice reminder provides messaging through voice units distributed around the house; and the Cooker Monitor and Cooker Minder monitor the stove and turns it off if smoke or gas is detected.

A great deal of effort has been put into the area of medication management. An example of an innovative device includes a "smart" pillbox (the MD.2) from Interactive Medical Developments, L.C. (2007). Currently, the researcher Karen Marek is conducting a study to examine the effects of the MD.2 on frail older adults' health outcomes. This medication box, which is connected to the service center by phone, dispenses medications and reminds patients when it's time to take their medication. If older adults do not retrieve the medicine as scheduled, the machine beeps for 45 minutes, then calls the service center (Quirk, 2006).

In the AgeLab at the Massachusetts Institute of Technology (MIT) School of Engineering's Engineering Systems Division, a multidisciplinary team of researchers, business partners, and advocates for the aging are working on innovative technologies to improve older adults' well-being. One such technology is an "Electronic Pill Pet," which uses play and emotion to remind older adults to take their medications (AgeLab, 2006).

Often, Global Positioning System (GPS) systems are being used by caregivers to locate wondering Alzheimer patients (Associated Press, 2007). However, some other services use GPS technology to provide forgetful older adults with a sense of their whereabouts or to give them directions, as well as to help caregivers rescue these frail older adults in emergencies (Global Action on Aging, 2005). For instance, Secom Company in Japan runs a service that provides positional information on these individuals through GPS satellites and mobile phones (Global Action on Aging, 2005).

Considering the rapidly changing modern technologies and the growing number of older adults, research and business in the area of cognitive assistive technology will expand exponentially. In particular, in collaboration with academia and organizations for the aging, large industry corporation labs such as those at Intel (Intel Corporation, 2007) and IBM (SeniorNet, 2006), are making great efforts toward creating new technologies for older adults. There are, however, many other issues surrounding this area, such as ethical issues, safety, and cost-effectiveness. More research efforts must be undertaken to address these issues.

Examples of Innovative Behavior Change Programs for Older Adults With CI

The Res-Care Intervention: Optimizing Function and Physical Activity Restorative nursing care program focuses on the restoration and/or maintenance of physical function and helps older adults with CI to compensate for functional impairments so that they achieve and maintain the highest possible level of function (Resnick, 2004). This type of care attempts to maximize the ability of the resident, focuses on what the individual can do instead of what they can't do, optimizes independence, reduces the level of care required, and ultimately improves quality of life, self-image, and self-esteem. Health care providers working with older adults may be familiar with restorative care, have the skills to engage in this type of caregiving, and believe in the many benefits of engaging in restorative-care activities, but the resident may resist these activities. Unfortunately, older individuals with CI may not believe that they are capable of performing physical activities, may not see the benefit to participating in restorative-care activities, or may feel that caregivers should perform their personal care activities. Consequently, a major aspect of implementing a restorative-care program is to motivate older adults to engage in these activities.

The Res-Care Intervention is a two-tiered motivational intervention that involves teaching and motivating caregivers to engage in restorative-care activities with residents. Specifically, the caregivers are taught techniques, using a self-efficacy approach, to motivate residents to engage in appropriate functional activities and exercise. The first aspect of the Res-Care Intervention involves exposure to a 6-week educational series provided by two advanced-practice nurses. The educational series includes six different 30-minute sessions covering the philosophy of restorative care, a review of specific restorative-care skills, techniques to motivate residents to perform restorative-care activities, and practical ways to integrate restorative-care activities into daily care. In addition, the Res-Care Intervention includes the direction and oversight of a restorative-care nurse coordinator (RCC).

The RCC is ideally a registered nurse with experience in restorative care and rehabilitation nursing. The RCC does an initial evaluation of the resident and, on the basis of this evaluation, the resident, the RCC, and a nursing assistant (and/or family caregiver) who know the resident establish restorative-care goals. The goals are written on a goal form to communicate to all nursing assistants, nurses, and family or friends working with the resident what activities the resident should engage in. The goal form, for example, indicates if the resident should walk to the dining room or self-propel the wheelchair, eat independently after set-up, or participate in daily range-of-motion exercises.

In addition to the goal form, all participating residents have a poster that highlights the benefits of engaging in physical activity placed in their room. The RCC checks with the nursing assistants on a weekly basis to establish whether restorative-care activities are being completed, whether goals are achieved, and/or whether new goals are needed and informally provides verbal encouragement to residents to engage in restorative-care activities. Nursing assistants are encouraged to inform the RCC of challenges related to the implementation of restorative care, and, as appropriate, the RCC attempts to remove any barriers. Exercise activities are encouraged for all residents and built into their daily activities. Such things as walk-to-dine programs, daily exercise sessions that involve stretching and strengthening activities, and dance classes are encouraged. This type of program has been shown to be helpful in changing the philosophy of care in long-term care settings so that the focus is on the function of the resident and not on the completion of the task (Resnick, Allen, et al., 2002; Resnick & Simpson, 2003; Resnick, Simpson, Bercovitz, et al., 2006; Resnick, Simpson, Galik, et al., 2006).

The WALC Intervention

The WALC intervention (Resnick, 2002) is a self-efficacy-based intervention that incorporates all of the known sources of efficacy-enhancing information (Bandura, 1977, 1997) in an attempt to increase physical activity among older adults with mild CI. The intervention was developed for older adults with mild CI who live in the community or in a continuing-care retirement community setting. The "W" refers to participating in a walking program, and all study participants randomized to treatment were invited to join the Walking Group or to walk on their own for 30 minutes daily. The "A" within the WALC intervention refers to addressing potential pain, fear, and fatigue associated with exercise. The primary care health provider (PCP) asked the participant, initially weekly and monthly, about any unpleasant sensations they were experiencing in association with walking. Individualized interventions were implemented to decrease these unpleasant sensations. The "L" within the WALC intervention, also completed with the PCP, reviewed exercise benefits and established specific goals for each participant. Last, the "C" within the WALC intervention involved providing cues (visual cues such as a monthly calendar and the goal forms) for the participant to exercise. The WALC intervention can also be implemented in a group setting by providing education to the group and using group support and encouragement to help establish and achieve goals, and to provide ongoing verbal encouragement (Resnick, Vogel, & Luisi, 2006).

References

Aalten, P., van Valen, E., de Vugt, M. E., Lousberg, R., Jolles, J., & Verhey, F. R. (2006). Awareness and behavioral problems in dementia patients: A prospective study. *International Psychogeriatrics, 18*(1), 3–17.

Adlam, T. D., & Orpwood, R. D. (2004, September 7). *Taking the Gloucester Smart House from the laboratory to the living room. Work in progress bringing smart house technology for people with dementia to its intended users.* Paper presented at the 3rd International Workshop on Ubiquitous Computing for Pervasive Healthcare Applications, Nottingham, UK.

AgeLab, Massachusetts Institute of Technology. (2006). *Pill pet.* Retrieved March 1, 2007, from http://web.mit.edu/agelab/projects_wellness.shtml#1

Alm, N., Astell, A., Ellis, M., Dye, R., Gowans, G., & Campbell, J. (2004). A cognitive prosthesis and communication support for people with dementia. *Neuropsychological Rehabilitation, 14*(1/2), 117–134.

Associated Press. (2007). *GPS shoes make tracking kids, elderly easier.* Retrieved March 1, 2007, from http://www.foxnews.com/story/0,2933,251122,00.html

Bandura, A. (1977). Self-efficacy: Toward a unifying theory of behavioral change. *Psychological Review, 84,* 191–215.

Bandura, A. (1997). *Self-efficacy: The exercise of control.* New York: W. H. Freeman.

Beck, C., Heacock, P., Mercer, S. O., Walls, R. C., Rapp, C. G., & Vogelpohl, T. S. (1997). Improving dressing behavior in cognitively impaired nursing home residents. *Nursing Research, 46*(3), 126–132.

Beck, C. K., Vogelpohl, T. S., Rasin, J. H., Uriri, J. T., O'Sullivan, P., Walls, R. et al. (2002). Effects of behavioral interventions on disruptive behavior and affect in demented nursing home residents. *Nursing Research, 51*(4), 219–228.

Bernat, J. L. (2005). Medical futility: Definition, determination, and disputes in critical care. *Neurocritical Care, 2*(2), 198–205.

Bourre, J. M. (2006). Effects of nutrients (in food) on the structure and function of the nervous system: update on dietary requirements for brain. Part 2: Macronutrients. *Journal of Nutrition, Health and Aging, 10*(5), 389–399.

Boustani, M., Zimmerman, S., Williams, C. S., Gruber-Baldini, A. W. L., Reed, P., & Sloane, P. (2005). Characteristics associated with behavioral symptoms related to dementia in long-term care residents. *Gerontologist, 45,* 56–61.

Bruce, D. G., Devine, A., & Prince, R. L. (2002). Recreational physical activity levels in healthy older women: The importance of fear of falling. *Journal of the American Geriatric Society, 50,* 84–89.

Buettner, L., & Fitzsimmons, S. (2006). Mixed behaviors in dementia: The need for a paradigm shift. *Journal of Gerontological Nursing, 32*(7), 15–22.

Byles, J., Young, A., Furuya, H., & Parkinson, L. (2006). A drink to healthy aging: The association between older women's use of alcohol and their health-related quality of life. *Journal of the American Geriatric Society, 54*(9), 1341–1347.

Carpenter, G. I., Hastie, C. L., Morris, J. N., Fries, B.E., & Ankri, J. (2006). Measuring change in activities of daily living in nursing home residents with moderate to severe cognitive impairment. *Biomedical Central Geriatrics, 6,* 7.

Center for Aging Services Technologies. (2004). *CAST Clearinghouse.* Retrieved March 1, 2007, from http://www.agingtech.org/Browsemain.aspx

Centers for Disease Control and Prevention Behavioral Risk Factor Surveillance System. (2006). Retrieved April 17, 2008, from https://www.cdc.gov/brfss

Chang, C., & Lin, L. C. (2005). Effects of a feeding skills training programme on nursing assistants and dementia patients. *Journal of Clinical Nursing, 14*(10), 1185–1192.

Chang, J. T., Morton, S. C., Rubenstein, L. Z., Mojica, W. A., Maglione, M., Suttorp, M. J., et al. (2004). Interventions for the prevention of falls in older adults: Systematic review and meta-analysis of randomized clinical trials. *British Medical Journal, 328*(7441), 653–654.

Chen, J., Kam, A. H., Zhang, J., Liu, N., & Shue, L. (2005, May). *Bathroom activity monitoring based on sound.* Paper presented at the 3rd International Conference: Pervasive Computing, Munich, Germany.

Colcombe, S. J., Erickson, K. I., Scalf, P. E., Kim, J. S., Prakash, R., McAuley, E., et al. (2006). Aerobic exercise training increases brain volume in aging humans. *Journal of Gerontology Series A, Biological Sciences and Medical Sciences, 61*(11), 1166–1170.

Collins, R., Lee, R. E., Albright, C. L., & King, A.C. (2004). Ready to be physically active? The effects of a course preparing low-income multiethnic women to be more physically active. *Health Education and Behavior, 31*(1), 47–64.

Conn, V., Burks, K. J., Pomeroy, S. H., Ulbrich, S. L., & Cochran, J. E. (2003). Older women and exercise: Explanatory concepts. *Womens Health Issues, 13*(4), 158–166.

Cornelissen, V. A., & Fagard, R. H. (2005). Effect of resistance training on resting blood pressure: A meta-analysis of randomized controlled trials. *Journal of Hypertension, 23*(2), 251–259.

Cress, M., Buchner, D., Prochaska, T., Rimmer, J., Brown, M., Macera, C., et al. (2005). Best practices for physical activity programs and behavior counseling in older adult populations. *Journal of Aging and Physical Activity, 13*(1), 61–74.

Crews, D. (2005). Artificial environments and an aging population: Designing for age related functional losses. *Journal of Physiological Anthropology, 24*(1), 103–109.

Daniels, N. A., Nguyen, T. T., Gildengorin, G., & Pérez-Stable, E. J. (2004). Adult immunization in university-based primary care and specialty practices. *Journal of the American Geriatric Society, 52*(6), 1007–1012.

Depp, C. A., & Jeste, D. V. (2006). Definitions and predictors of successful aging: A comprehensive review of larger quantitative studies. *American Journal of Geriatric Psychiatry, 14*(1), 6–20.

DiBartolo, M. C. (2002). Exploring self-efficacy and hardiness in spousal caregivers of individuals with dementia. *Journal of Gerontological Nursing, 28*(4), 24–33.

Dunn, M. K., Misra, S., Habermann. R., & Griffin, M. R. (2003). Pneumococcal vaccination in nursing homes: Does policy change practice? *Journal of the American Medical Directors Association, 4*(3), 135–138.

Dunstan, D., Daly, R., Owen, N., Jolley, D., DeCourten, M., Shaw, J., & Zimmet, P. (2002). High intensity resistance training improves glycemic control in older patients with type-2 diabetes. *Diabetes Care, 25,* 1729–1736.

Engelman, K. K., Altus, D. E., & Hosier, M. C. (2003). Brief training to promote the use of less intrusive prompts by nursing assistants in a dementia care unit. *Journal of Applied Behavior Analysis, 36,* 129–132.

Felten, B., & Hall, J. (2001). Conceptualizing resilience in women older than 85: Overcoming adversity from illness of loss. *Journal of Gerontological Nursing, 27*(1), 46–54.

Field, C. (2004, February). The 'gift' of restorative nursing: Focusing on restorative care benefits both residents and staff at Cove's Edge Comprehensive Care Center. *Nursing Homes.* Retrieved July, 2008, from http://findarticles.com/p/articles/mi_m3830/is_2_53/ai_n60941 26?tag=artBody;coll

Fletcher, P., & Hirdes, J. P. (2004). Restriction in activity associated with fear of falling among community based seniors using home care services. *Age and Ageing, 33*(3), 273–279.

Fowler, B. A. (2006). Social processes used by African American women in making decisions about mammography screening. *Journal of Nursing Scholarship, 38*(3), 247–254.

Galik, E., & Resnick, B. (2007). Moving beyond behavior. *Topics in Geriatric Rehabilitation, 10*(2), 4–9.

Galynker, I. I., Roane, D. M., Miner, C., Feinberg, T., & Watts, B. (1995). Negative symptoms in patients with Alzheimer's disease. *American Journal of Geriatric Psychiatry, 3*(1), 52–59.

Glantz, M., & Johnson, J. (1999). *Resilience and development: Positive life adaptations.* New York: Kluwer Academic Press.

Global Action on Aging. (2005). *Targeting elderly needing help by GPS.* Retrieved March 1, 2007, from http://www.globalaging.org/elderrights/world/2005/gps.htm

Gorin, S. S., Heck, J. E., Albert, S., & Hershman, D. (2005). Treatment for breast cancer in patients with Alzheimer's disease. *Journal of the American Geriatric Society, 53*(11), 1897–1904.

Gottlieb, B. H., & Rooney, J. A. (2004). Coping effectiveness: Determinants and relevance to the mental health and affect of family caregivers of persons with dementia. *Aging Mental Health, 8,* 4364–4373.

Graham, N. L., Emery, T., & Hodges, J. R. (2004). Distinctive cognitive profiles in Alzheimer's disease and subcortical vascular dementia. *Journal of Neurology Neurosurgery and Psychiatry, 75,* 61–71.

Green L., & Kreuter, M. (2001). *Health promotion planning: An educational and environmental approach.* Mountain View, CA: Mayfield.

Gruber-Baldini, A. L., Boustani, M., Sloane, P., & Zimmerman, S. (2004). Behavioral symptoms in residential care/assisted living facilities: Prevalence, risk factors, and medication management. *Journal of the American Geriatrics Society, 52,* 1610–1617.

Hardy, S., Concato, J., & Gill, T. M. (2004). Resilience of community-dwelling older persons. *Journal of the American Geriatrics Society, 52*(2), 257–262.

Heyn, P., Abreu, B. C., & Ottenbacher, K. J. (2004). The effects of exercise training on elderly persons with cognitive impairment and dementia: A meta-analysis. *Archives of Physical Medicine and Rehabilitation, 85*(10), 1694–1704.

Hill, J., Fillit, H., Thomas, S. K., & Chang, S. (2006). Functional impairment, healthcare costs and the prevalence of institutionalization in patients with Alzheimer's disease and other dementias. *Pharmacoeconomics, 24,* 3265–3280.

Hinman, A. R., Urquhart, G. A., Strikas, R. A., & National Vaccine Advisory Committee. (2007). Immunization information systems: National vaccine advisory committee progress report, 2007. *Journal of Public Health Management and Practice, 13*(6), 553–558.

Hollingworth, W., Ebel, B. E., McCarty, C. A., Garrison, M. M., Christakis, D. A., & Rivara, F. P. (2006). Prevention of deaths from harmful drinking in the United States: The potential effects of tax increases and advertising bans on young drinkers. *Journal of Studies on Alcohol, 67*(2), 300–308.

Holmes, C. K. A., Dean, C., Hodkinson, S., & Hopkins, V. (2006). Keep music live: Music and the alleviation of apathy in dementia subjects. *International Psychogeriatrics, 18*(4), 623–630.

Houston, T. K., Allison, J. J., Person, S., Kovac, S., Williams, O. D., & Kiefe, C. I. (2005). Post-myocardial infarction smoking cessation counseling: Associations with immediate and late mortality in older Medicare patients. *American Journal of Medicine, 118*(3), 269–275.

Humpel, N., Owen, N., & Leslie, E. (2002). Environmental factors associated with adults' participation in physical activity: A review. *American Journal of Preventive Medicine, 22*(3), 188–199.

Hyland, A., Rezaishiraz, H., Bauer, J., Giovino, G. A., & Cummings, K. M. (2005). Characteristics of low-level smokers. *Nicotine and Tobacco Research, 7*(3), 461–468.

Inguito, P., & Resnick, B. (2007). Factors that influence long term adherence to exercise post hip fracture. *Journal of the American Geriatric Society, 47*(2), 120.

Intel Corporation. (2007). *Helping the elderly age gracefully at home.* Retrieved March 1, 2007, from http://www.intel.com/research/prohealth/cs-aging_in_place.htm

Interactive Medical Developments. (2007). MD.2 Personal Medication System. Retrieved March 1, 2007, from http://www.imd2.com/

Iwarsson, S. (2005). A long-term perspective on person-environment fit and ADL dependence among older Swedish adults. *Gerontologist, 45*(3), 327–336.

Iwarsson, S., & Isacsson, A. (1996). Housing standards, environmental barriers in the home, and subjective general apprehension of housing situation among the rural elderly. *Scandinavian Journal of Occupational Therapy, 3*, 52–61.

Iwarsson, S., & Slaug, B. (2001). *Housing enabler information.* Retrieved April 17, 2008, from http://www.housingenabler.com

Jensen, L. W., Decker, L., & Andersen, M. M. (2006). Depression and health-promoting lifestyles of persons with mental illnesses. *Issues in Mental Health Nursing, 27*(6), 617–624.

Joseph, A., Szimring, C., Harris-Kojetin, L., & Kiefer, K. (2005). Presence and visibility of outdoor and indoor physical activity features and participation in physical activity among older adults in retirement communities. In S. Rodiek & B. Schwarz (Eds.), *The role of the outdoors in residential environments for aging.* New York: Haworth Press.

Kadner, K. (1989). Resilience: Responding to adversity. *Journal of Psychosocial Nursing, 27*, 20–25.

King, A. C., Pruitt, L. A., Phillips, W., Oka, R., Rodenburg, A., & Haskell, W. L. (2000). Comparative effects of two physical activity programs on measured and perceived physical functioning and other health related quality of life outcomes in older adults. *Journal of Gerontology: Medical Sciences, 55*, M74–M83.

Kopunek, S. P., Michael, K. M., Shaughnessy, M., Resnick, B., Nahm, E. S., Whitall, J., et al. (2007). Cardiovascular risk in survivors of stroke. *American Journal of Preventive Medicine, 32*(5), 408–412.

Kuiack, S. L., Campbell, W. W., & Evans, W. J. (2003). Structured resistive training program improves muscle strength and power in elderly persons with dementia. *Activities, Adaptation and Aging, 28*(1), 35–47.

Kuwahara, N. (2006). *International workshop on cognitive prostheses and assisted communication.* Retrieved March 1, 2007, from http://www.irc.atr.jp/cpac2006/

Lee, C. D., Folsom, A. R., & Blair, S. N. (2003). Physical activity and stroke risk: A meta-analysis. *Stroke, 34*(10), 2475–2481.

Li, Y., Wang, J. G., Gao, P. J., Wang, G. L., Qian, Y. S., Zhu, D. L., et al. (2006). Interaction between body mass index and alcohol intake in relation to blood pressure in Han and She Chinese. *American Journal of Hypertension, 19*(5), 448–453.

Lim, K., & Taylor, L. (2005). Factors associated with physical activity among older people—a population-based study. *Preventive Medicine, 40*(1), 33–40.

Lim, Y. (2003). Nursing intervention for grooming of elders with mild cognitive impairments in Korea. *Geriatric Nursing, 24*(1), 11–15.

Litt, M., Kleppinger, A., & Judge, J. (2002). Initiation and maintenance of exercise behavior in older women: Predictors from the social learning model. *Journal of Behavioral Medicine, 25*(1), 83–97.

Lopopolo, R. B., Greco, M., Sullivan, D., Craik, R. L., & Mangione, K. K. (2006). Effect of therapeutic exercise on gait speed in community-dwelling elderly people: A meta-analysis. *Physical Therapy, 86*, 4520–4540.

LoPresti, E., & Kirsch, N. (2004). Assistive technology for cognitive rehabilitation: State of the art. *Neuropsychological Rehabilitation, 14*(1/2), 5–40.

Luukinen, H., Lehtola, S., Jokelainen, J., Vaananen-Sainio, R., Lotvonen, S., & Koistinen, P. (2006). Prevention of disability by exercise among the elderly: A population-based, randomized, controlled trial. *Scandinavian Journal of Primary Health Care, 24*(4), 199–205.

Lynch, S. M., & George, L. K. (2002). Interlocking trajectories of loss-related events and depressive symptoms among elders. *Journal of Gerontology, Series B Psychological Science and Social Sciences, 57*(2), S117–S125.

Magaziner, J., Zimmerman, S. I., Fox, K. M., & Burns, B. J. (1998). Dementia in United States nursing homes: Descriptive epidemiology and implications for long-term residential care. *Aging and Mental Health, 2*(1), 28–35.

Marin, R. S. (1991). Apathy: A neuropsychiatric syndrome. *Journal of Neuropsychiatry and Clinical Neurosciences, 3*(3), 243–254.

Markle-Reid, M., Weir, R., Browne, G., Roberts, J., Gafni, A., & Henderson, S. (2006). Health promotion for frail older home care clients. *Journal of Advanced Nursing, 54*(3), 381–395.

Martin, F. C., Hart, D., Spector, T., Doyle, D. V., & Harari, D. (2005). Fear of falling limiting activity in young-old women is associated with reduced functional mobility rather than psychological factors. *Age and Ageing, 34,* 281–287.

McAuley, E., Marquez, D. X., Jerome, G. J., Blissmer, B., & Katula, J. (2002). Physical activity and physique anxiety in older adults: Fitness, and efficacy influences. *Aging and Mental Health, 6*(3), 222–230.

O'Connor, B. P., Rousseau, F. L., & Maki, S. A. (2004). Physical exercise and experienced bodily changes: the emergence of benefits and limits on benefits. *International Journal of Aging and Human Development, 59*(3), 177–203.

Office of Applied Studies. (2000). *Summary of findings from the 1999 National Household Survey on Drug Abuse.* Rockville, MD: Substance Abuse and Mental Health Services Administration.

Omnibus Budget Reconciliation Act (OBRA). (1987). Nursing Home Reform Act. P.L. 100–203 § 1819 [42 USC § 1395i-3]. Requirements for and assuring quality of care in skilled nursing facilities.

Palombaro, K. M. (2005). Effects of walking-only interventions on bone mineral density at various skeletal sites: A meta-analysis. *Journal of Geriatric Physical Therapy, 28*(3), 102–107.

Quirk, K. (2006). *"Smart" pillbox could help seniors live at home longer.* Retrieved March 1, 2007, from http://www.uwm.edu/News/Features/06.05/Smart_Pillbox.html

Rabins, P., Lyketsos, C., & Steele, C. (2006). *Practical dementia care* (2nd ed.). New York: Oxford University Press.

Raik, B. L., Miller, F. G., & Fins, J. J. (2004). Screening and cognitive impairment: Ethics of forgoing mammography in older women. *Journal of the American Geriatric Society, 52*(3), 440–444.

Razay, G., Vreugdenhil, A., & Wilcock, G. (2006). Obesity, abdominal obesity and Alzheimer disease. *Dementia and Geriatric Cognitive Disorders, 22*(2), 173–176.

Reid, M. C., Boutros, N. N., O'Connor, P. G., Cadariu, A., & Concato, J. (2002). The health-related effects of alcohol use in older persons: A systematic review. *Substance Abuse, 23*(3), 149–164.

Reitz, C., Luchsinger, J., Tang, M. X., & Mayeux, R. (2005). Effect of smoking and time on cognitive function in the elderly without dementia. *Neurology, 65*(6), 870–875.

Resnick, B. (2002). Testing the impact of the WALC intervention on exercise adherence in older adults. *Journal of Gerontological Nursing, 28*(6), 32–40.

Resnick, B. (2004). *Restorative care nursing for older adults.* New York: Springer Publishing Company.

Resnick, B., Allen, P., & Ruane, K. (2002). Testing the effectiveness of a restorative care program. *Long-Term Care Interface, 3*(11), 25–30.

Resnick, B., Orwig, D., Magaziner, J., & Wynne, C. (2002). The effect of social support on exercise behavior in older adults. *Clinical Nursing Research, 11*(1), 52–70.

Resnick, B., Orwig, D., Wehren, L., Zimmerman, S., Simpson, M., & Magaziner, J. (2005). The Exercise Plus Program for older women post hip fracture: Participant perspectives. *Gerontologist, 45*(4), 539–544.

Resnick, B., & Simpson, M. (2003). Restorative care nursing activities: Pilot testing self efficacy and outcome expectation measures. *Geriatric Nursing, 24*(2), 83–87.

Resnick, B., Simpson, M., Bercovitz, A., Galik, E., Gruber-Baldini, A., Zimmerman, S., et al. (2006). Pilot testing of the restorative care program: Impact on residents. *Journal of Gerontological Nursing, 2,* 11–14.

Resnick, B., Simpson, M., Galik, E., Bercovitz, A., Gruber-Baldini, A., Zimmerman, S., et al. (2006). Making a difference: Nursing assistants perspectives of restorative care nursing. *Rehabilitation Nursing, 31*(2), 78–86.

Resnick, B., Vogel, A., & Luisi, D. (2006). Motivating minority older adults to exercise. *Cultural Diversity and Ethnic Minority Psychology, 3,* 17–21.

Robinson-Smith, G., Johnston, M. V., & Allen, J. (2000). Self-care, self-efficacy, quality of life, and depression after stroke. *Archives of Physical Medicine and Rehabilitation, 81*(4), 460–464.

Roddy, E., Zhang, W., & Doherty, M. (2005). Aerobic walking or strengthening exercise for osteoarthritis of the knee? A systematic review. *Annals of Rheumatic Disease, 64*(4), 544–548.

Roddy, E., Zhang, W., Doherty, M., Arden, N. K., Barlow, J., Birrell, F., et al. (2005). Evidence-based recommendations for the role of exercise in the management of osteoarthritis of the hip or knee—the MOVE consensus. *Rheumatology, 44*(1), 67–73.

Rolland, Y., Pillard, F., Klapouszczak, A., Reynish, E., Thomas, D., Andrieu, S., et al. (2007). Exercise program for nursing home residents with Alzheimer's disease: A 1-year randomized, controlled trial. *Journal of the American Geriatric Society, 55*(2), 158–165.

Rose, M., & Pruchno, R. (1999). Behavior sequences of long-term care residents and their social partners. *Journal of Gerontology, Series B, Psychological Science and Social Sciences, 54B*(2), S75–S83.

Rosenblatt, A., Samus, Q., Steele, C., Baker, A., Harper, M., Brandt, J., et al. (2004). The Maryland Assisted Living Study: Prevalence, recognition, and treatment of dementia and other psychiatric disorders in the assisted living population of central Maryland. *Journal of the American Geriatrics Society, 52,* 1618–1625.

Rowe, M., Lane, S., & Phipps, C. (2007). CareWatch. *Topics in Geriatric Rehabilitation, 23*(1), 3–8.

Sacre, S. (2004). The total restorative care concept. *Nursing Homes, 3,* 58.

Sallis, J., Cervero, R. B., Ascher, W., Henderson, K. A., Kraft, M. K., & Kerr, J. (2006). Ecological approach to creating active living communities. *Annual Review of Public Health, 27,* 297–322.

Sallis, J., & Glanz, K. (2006). The role of built environments in physical activity, eating, and obesity in childhood. *The Future of Children, 16*(1), 89–108.

Salzberg, P., & Moffat, J. M. (2004). Ninety-five percent: An evaluation of law, policy, and programs to promote seat belt use in Washington state. *Journal of Safety Research, 35*(2), 215–222.

Schechtman, K. B., & Ory, M. G. (2001). Frailty and injuries: Cooperative studies of intervention techniques: The effects of exercise on the quality of life of frail older adults: A preplanned meta-analysis of the FICSIT trial. *Annals of Behavioral Medicine, 23*(3), 186–197.

SeniorNet. (2006). *IBM and SeniorNet unlock the World Wide Web for millions more users.* Retrieved March 1, 2007, from http://www.seniornet.org/php/default.php?PageID=6583&Version=0&Font=0

Shaughnessy, M., Michael, K., Resnick, B., Nahm, E., Kopunek, S., & Orwig, D. (2005). Clinical trials and tribulations: Challenges to realizing intervention research. Symposium, Gerontological Society of America. *Gerontologist, 45*(11), 670.

Takano, T., Nakamura, K., & Watanabe, M. (2002). Urban residential environments and senior citizens' longevity in mega-city areas: The importance of walkable green spaces. *Journal of Epidemiology and Community Health, 56,* 913–918.

Tappen, R. M., Roach, K., Applegate, E. B., & Stowell, P. (2000). Effect of a combined walking and conversation intervention on functional mobility of nursing home residents with Alzheimer disease. *Alzheimer Disease and Associated Disorders, 14*(4), 196–201.

Taylor-Piliae, R., & Froelicher, E. (2005). Measurement properties of Tai Chi exercise self-efficacy among ethnic Chinese with coronary heart disease risk factors: A pilot study. *European Journal of Cardiovascular Nursing, 3*(4), 287–294.

Teri, L., Gibbons, L. E., McCurry, S. M., Logsdon, R. G., Buchner, D. M., Barlow, W. E., et al. (2003). Exercise plus behavioral management in patients with Alzheimer's disease: A randomized controlled trial. *Journal of the American Medical Association, 290*(15), 2015–2022.

Tessaro, I., Mangone, C., Parkar, I., & Pawar, V. (2006). Knowledge, barriers, and predictors of colorectal cancer screening in an Appalachian church population. *Preventing Chronic Disease 3*(4), A123.

Thomas, K., Muir, K. R., Doherty, M., Jones, A. C., O'Reilly, S. C., & Bassey, E. J. (2002). Home based exercise programme for knee pain and knee osteoarthritis: Randomized controlled trial. *British Medical Journal, 325*(7367), 752.

Thompson, J., Stopford, C. L., Snowden, J. S., & Neary, D. (2005). Qualitative neuropsychological performance characteristics in frontotemporal dementia and Alzheimer's disease. *Journal of Neurology Neurosurgery Psychiatry, 76*(7), 920–927.

Tinetti, M. E. (2003). Preventing falls in elderly persons. *New England Journal of Medicine, 348*(1), 42–49.

Tsai, P. (2003). Determinants of the white-coat effect in normotensives and never-treated mild hypertensives. *Clinical and Experimental Hypertension, 25*(7), 443–454.

Vanhanen, M., Koivisto, K., Moilanen, L., Helkala, E. L., Hanninen, T., Soininen, H., et al. (2006). Association of metabolic syndrome with Alzheimer disease: A population-based study. *Neurology, 67*(5), 843–847.

van Wijk, I., Algra, A., van de Port, I. G., Bevaart, B., & Lindeman, E. (2006). Change in mobility activity in the second year after stroke in a rehabilitation population: Who is at risk for decline? *Archives of Physical Medicine and Rehabilitation, 87*(1), 45–50.

Vestergaard, S., Kronborg-Andersen, C., Korsholm, L., & Puggaard, L. (2006). Exercise intervention of 65+-year-old men and women: Functional ability and health care costs. *Aging Clinical and Experimental Research, 18,* 3227–3234.

Volicer, L., Simard, J., Heartquist-Pupa, J., Medrek, R., & Riordan, M. (2006). Effects of continuous activity programming on behavioral symptoms of dementia. *Journal of the American Medical Directors Association, 7,* 426–431.

Wagnild, G. (2003). Resilience and successful aging. Comparison among low and high income older adults. *Journal of Gerontological Nursing, 29*(12), 42–49.

Waters, K. (1994). Getting dressed in the early morning: Styles of staff/patient interaction on rehabilitation hospital wards for elderly people. *Journal of Advanced Nursing, 19,* 239–247.

Weatherall, M. (1994). One year follow-up of patients with fracture of the proximal femur. *New Zealand Medical Journal, 107,* 308–309.

Wendel-Vos, G. C., Schuit, A. J., Feskens, E. J., Boshuizen, H. C., Verschuren, W. M., Saris, W. H., et al. (2004). Physical activity and stroke: A meta-analysis of observational data. *International Journal of Epidemiology, 33,* 4787–4798.

Wherton, J., & Monk, A. (2006, April 24–27). *Cognitive support for dementia.* Paper presented at the Association for Computing Machinery: Computer-Human Interaction2006 Workshop on Designing Technology for People with Cognitive Impairments, Montréal, Quebec, Canada.

Yu, F., Evans, L. K., & Sullivan-Marx, E. M. (2005). Functional outcomes for older people with cognitive impairment in a comprehensive outpatient rehabilitation facility. *Journal of the American Geriatrics Society, 53,* 1599–1606.

Zizzi, S., Goodrich, D., Wu, Y., Parker, L., Rye, S., Pawar, V., et al. (2006). Correlates of physical activity in a community sample of older adults in Appalachia. *Journal of Aging and Physical Activity, 14*(4), 423–438.

Adherence Issues Among Adolescents With Chronic Diseases

28

Michael A. Rapoff

The term "adherence" (rather than "compliance") reflects a more active role for patients in consenting to and following prescribed treatments (Lutfey & Wishner, 1999; Rapoff, 1999). The World Health Organization defines adherence as "the extent to which a person's behavior—taking medication, following a diet, or executing lifestyle changes—corresponds with agreed recommendations from a health care provider" (World Health Organization, 2003, pp. 3–4). This definition acknowledges that regimens for chronic conditions involve multiple behavioral components with varying levels of adherence to each component and that agreement to follow regimens has been secured from the patient. In pediatrics, agreement to follow prescribed regimens may need to be obtained from caretakers, as well as patients.

Another potentially useful distinction in the adherence literature is between inadvertent (nonvolitional) and volitional (or intentional) nonadherence (Adams, Dreyer, Dinakar, & Portnoy, 2004). Inadvertent nonadherence may involve patients forgetting to take a medication dose or being away from home without access to medications. Volitional nonadherence may involve a reasoned and purposeful decision by patients to omit a medication dose because they are asymptomatic or because taking medications interferes with their lifestyle. In the case of inadvertent nonadherence, one can help patients problem-solve about how to keep track of medication doses (such as using a pill-reminder case) and to have medications with them when away from home. In the case of volitional nonadherence, one needs to negotiate with adolescents and their families to obtain agreement on what they are willing to do to treat their disease without compromising their quality of life.

Although chronic physical illnesses affect a relatively small proportion of adolescents (Newacheck, 1989; Newacheck & Taylor, 1992), they carry the potential for causing significant medical and psychosocial morbidity and even increased mortality, while consuming a disproportionate amount of health care resources (Holden & Nitz, 1995). Nonadherence to medical treatment is considered a major contributor to increased morbidity, mortality, and health care utilization and costs (Jay, Litt, & DuRant, 1984; Rapoff, 1999). Adolescents are at risk for nonadherence to regimens for *asthma* (Jónasson, Carlsen, & Mowinckel, 2000; Kelloway, Wyatt, & Adlis, 1994; McQuaid, Kopel, Klein, & Fritz, 2003; Walders, Kopel, Koins-Mitchell, & McQuaid, 2005), *cancer* (Smith, Rosen, Trueworthy, & Lowman, 1979; Tebbi, Cummings, Zevon, Smith, Richards, & Mallon, 1986), *cystic fibrosis* (Gudas, Koocher, & Wypij, 1991; Patterson, 1985), *diabetes* (Anderson, Auslander, Jung, Miller, & Santiago, 1990; Anderson, Ho, Brackett, Finkelstein, & Laffel, 1997; Bond, Aiken, & Somerville, 1992; Holmes et al., 2006; Jacobson et al., 1987, 1990; Johnson et al., 1992; Kovacs, Goldston, Obrosky, & Iyengar, 1992; La Greca et al., 1990; Stewart et al., 2003), *heart* or *heart/lung disease posttransplantation* (Serrano-Ikkos, Lask, Whitehead, & Eisler, 1998), *HIV* (Williams et al., 2006), *juvenile rheumatoid arthritis* (Feldman et al., 2007), *renal disease* (Beck et al., 1980; Brownbridge & Fielding, 1994), and *renal disease posttransplantation* (Feinstein et al., 2005).

In addition to negotiating the normal developmental challenges, adolescents with chronic diseases have to cope with pain, fatigue, limitations in their daily activities, and demanding medical regimens. These regimens can be time consuming, intrusive, and of little immediate benefit (Rapoff, 1999). In this chapter, I review the prevalence, consequences, and predictors of adherence problems for adolescents with chronic diseases and strategies for improving adherence. Clinical and research implications are offered from a normative developmental framework to increase sensitivity to the reality that adolescents with chronic diseases, like other people their age, are best understood within this context.

Prevalence of Adherence Problems

The average nonadherence rate to medical regimens for chronic pediatric diseases is often cited to be about 50% (Rapoff, 1999). However, nonadherence rates vary across different diseases, types of regimens, and methods of defining and measuring adherence. There is also variability in adherence across persons and age groupings and within the same persons over time.

Table 28.1 summarizes nonadherence rates to various chronic disease regimens from 54 studies that included or reported exclusively on adolescents with chronic diseases. Several conclusions can be drawn from reviewing these studies: (1) there is wide variability in nonadherence rates across different diseases and types of regimens, with a tendency toward lower adherence to more complex and intrusive regimen components, such as dietary modifications in the treatment of cystic fibrosis (Passero, Remor, & Salomon, 1981) and dietary and blood glucose monitoring in the treatment of diabetes (Jacobson et al., 1987); (2) adherence to regimens for diabetes has been studied most frequently (26% of studies), followed by medications for asthma (20% of studies), medications post-transplantation (17%), medications for cancer (15%), and relatively few (<10%) for the remaining chronic diseases; (3) the majority of these studies (67%) assessed adherence to medications only; (4) many of these studies (41%) relied on less objective methods of assessing adherence, such as patient, parent, or health care provider ratings, but, encouragingly, 39% of studies used more objective methods, such as assays or electronic monitors; (5) varied and relatively arbitrary criteria have been used to classify patients in a dichotomous fashion (adherent or nonadherent) on the basis of cross-sectional and single assessments of adherence; and (6) adherence was higher to regimens for more imminently life-threatening conditions, such as insulin for diabetes and immunosuppressive medications for HIV.

Nonadherence Consequences

Potentially serious health consequences can result from adherence failures (Rapoff, 1999). Bauman et al. (2002) reported that those who were nonadherent to asthma regimens had increased morbidity, including higher hospitalizations, missed more school, had poorer overall functioning, and had more days with wheezing and restricted activities. The Diabetes Control and Complications Trial (DCCT) showed that maintaining excellent glycemic control through intensive therapy delays the onset and slows the progression of long-term complications of diabetes (such as blindness) and that this requires a high level of adherence to regimens for diabetes (DCCT Research Group, 1994). Nonadherence has been consistently linked to a lack of viral suppression in the treatment of HIV, which in turn results in compromised health status and disease progression (Steele & Grauer, 2003). Incomplete adherence to immunosuppressive drugs has been linked to heart, kidney, and liver transplant failures (Magee et al., 2004; Stuber, 1993). Ettenger et al. (1991) found that 64% (30/47) of adolescents were found to be nonadherent, with 15% rejecting their allograft and 26% experiencing graft dysfunction attributed to nonadherence. Jarzembowski et al. (2004) found that 5 years after renal transplantation, African Americans had a lower rate of graft survival (42%) than Whites (71%) and Hispanics (95%) and that nonadherence accounted for 71% of cases of graft loss among African Americans. These adherence-related transplant failures are particularly tragic given

28.1 Nonadherence Rates for Selected Chronic Disease Regimens (Studies That Include or Exclusively Report on Adolescents)

Reference	Sample	Regimen	Adherence measure	Results
			Asthma	
Bender et al., 2006	N = 5,504 5–96 years (N = 423. 13–20 years)	Inhaled steroid/ beta-agonist combination	Pharmacy refill data	Overall adherence = 22% of days covered by refills (16% for 13–10 year olds)
Celano et al., 1998	N = 55 6–17 years	Inhaled steroid	Canister weight	Mean adherence = 44%
Coutts et al., 1992	N = 14 9–16 years	Inhaled steroid	Nebulizer Chronolog	Underuse recorded on 55% of days and overuse on 2%
Eney & Goldstein. 1976	N = 43 3–16 years	Theophylline	Serum assay (therapeutic range = 10–20ug/ ml or higher)	88% of sample had subtherapeutic levels: median level = 2.65ug/ml: range = 0–15.4
Jónasson et al., 2000	N = 122 7–16 years	Inhaled steroid placebo (clinical trial)	Count of remaining doses in inhaler	Adherence lower for adolescents throughout the 27 months of the trial. Adherence to inhaled steroid dropped from 77% at 3 months to 49% at 27 months
Kelloway et al., 1994	N = 14 12–17 years (remainder of sample was 105 patients 18–65 years)	Theophylline inhaled steroid	Comparison of pharmacy claims to prescribed orders in medical charts	Theophylline adherence = 73% Inhaled steroid adherence = 30% (both figures lower for adolescents than for adults)
McQuaid et al., 2003	N = 106 8–16 years	Inhaled steroid	MDILog (electronic monitor)	Mean adherence = 48%

McQuaid et al., 2005	N = 53 (subsample of N = 115) 7–16 years	Inhaled steroid	MDILog	Mean adherence = 51%
Radius et al., 1978	N = 80 9 mos.–17 years (M = 7.7 yrs)	Theophylline	Serum Assay	34% had negative values
Simmons et al., 1997	N = 14 12–16 years	Inhaled beta-agonist (salmeterol) vs. placebo (clinical trial)	Nebulizer Chronolog	11 of 13 patients (85%) were >85% adherent to salmeterol; 7 of 13 (54%) were adherent to placebo
Walders et al., 2005	N = 75 8–16 years	Inhaled quick-relief (as needed) and longer-term controller (daily) medications	MDILog	Mean daily controller medications taken 46% of time; quick-relief medication use varied between 0 and 251 doses taken over 1 month

Cancer

Festa et al., 1992	N = 50 (2 samples with M = 15.6 yrs and M = 19.1 yrs)	Prednisone (N = 21) for ALL. Penicillin (N = 29) for postsplenectomy prophylaxis.	Serum assay for prednisone; urine assay for penicillin	52% nonadherent to prednisone; 48% nonadherent to penicillin

(continued)

28.1 Nonadherence Rates for Selected Chronic Disease Regimens (Studies That Include or Exclusively Report on Adolescents) (*continued*)

Reference	Sample	Regimen	Adherence measure	Results
			Cancer	
Kennard et al., 2004	N = 44 M = 15.3 years	Trimethoprim/ sulfamethoxa-zole	Serum assay	27% nonadherent
Lancaster et al., 1997	N = 496 5–18 years	6-Mercaptopu-rine	Blood assay	42% had subtherapeutic levels 2% had completely undetectable metabolites on one or more occasions
Lansky et al., 1983	N = 31 2.1–14.3 years (M = 7.2 yrs)	Prednisone	Urine assay (<18.7kgs/cr defined as sub-therapeutic)	42% had subtherapeutic levels (M = 19.88; range = 4.95–40.05)
Lau et al., 1998	N = 24 2.6–17 years	6-Mercaptopu-rine	MEMS (electronic monitor)	17% nonadherent (<80% of doses taken)
Phipps & De-Cuir-Whalley, 1990	N = 54 1mos.–20 years (M = 9 yrs)	Antibiotics as part of bone marrow trans-plant	Review of patient chart and notes from psy-chosocial team meetings	"Significant" adherence difficulties identified in 52% of sample
Smith et al., 1979	N = 52 8mos–17 years	Prednisone	Urine assay (<18.7kgs/cr defined as sub-therapeutic)	33% had subtherapeutic levels
Tebbi et al., 1986	N = 46 2.5–23 years (M = 6.85 yrs)	Prednisone	Patient and parent report (corroborated by serum assay). Nonadherence defined as any missed dose during preceding month.	Nonadherence rates, postdiagnoses, at 2 wks = 18.8%; at 20wks = 39.5%; at 50wks = 35%

Cystic fibrosis

Czajkowski & Koucher, 1986	N = 40 13–23 years	Chest physiotherapy, diet, medications, Recording daily input and output, and co-operating with medical tests (on inpatient unit).	Medical and nursing notes used to rate degree of adherence (rater not specified)	35% of sample identified as being nonadherent
Passero et al., 1981	N = 58 (no specific ages given)	Antibiotics, vitamins, chest physiotherapy, and diet	Patient report	Incomplete adherence for: antibiotics = 7%; vitamins = 10%; chest physiotherapy = 60%; diet = 80%

Diabetes

Anderson et al., 1997	N = 89 10–15 years	Blood glucose monitoring	Provider rating 3 to 4 months prior to clinic visit	39% of younger patients (10–12 years) monitored blood glucose four or more times daily; 10% of older patients (p < 0.007) did so
Hentinen & Kyngas, 1992	N = 47 15–17 years	Insulin; diet; glucose monitoring	Patient report (questionnaire) with patient responses used to categorize adherence as high, average, or low	Percent of patients categorized as having low adherence by regimen component: insulin = 3%; diet = 34%; glucose monitoring = 38%

(continued)

28.1 Nonadherence Rates for Selected Chronic Disease Regimens (Studies That Include or Exclusively Report on Adolescents) (continued)

Reference	Sample	Regimen	Adherence measure	Results
Diabetes				
Jacobson et al., 1987	N = 57 9–15 years (M = 12.8 yrs)	Diet: insulin usage: blood glucose moni-toring	Health care provider ratings on a 4-point scale (4 = excellent. 3 = good. 2 = fair. 1 = poor) for each regimen component and a composite index	First 9-mos interval mean adherence ratings by regimen: diet = 3.2; insulin usage = 3.3 blood glucose monitoring = 2.8 composite index = 3 Second 9-mos interval mean adherence ratings by regimen: diet = 2.9; insulin usage = 3; blood glucose monitoring = 2.5 and composite index = 2.7 (second 9-mos interval significantly lower than first) Adolescents had significantly lower adher-ence on diet, blood glucose monitoring, and the composite index than preadolescents
Jacobson et al., 1990	N = 61 9–16 years	Diet: insulin usage: blood glucose moni-toring	Health care provider ratings on a 4-point scale (4 = excellent. 3 = good. 2 = fair. 1 = poor). Composite index derived from regi-men components	Mean adherence ratings by year: Yr. 1 = 3.07: Yr. 2 = 2.83: Yr. 3 = 2.63: and Yr. 4 = 2.43
Kovacs et al., 1992	N = 95 8–13 years (M = 11.1 yrs)	Insulin use: glu-cose monitor-ing: diet	Diagnosis of medical nonadherence by clini-cians based on structured interviews with patients and parents	29.5% of sample were nonadherent Nonadherence emerged an average of 3.5 yrs after disease onset

Lorenz et al., 1985	N = 90 9–15 years (M = 12.8 yrs)	Diet	Observations (unobtrusively done in camp setting) Error rate calculated by summing additions and deletions to meal plan divided by the total number of exchanges	Mean error rate = .35 (standard deviation = .19)
Miller & Drotar, 2003	N = 82 11–17 years	Diabetes tasks (e.g., monitoring blood glucose)	Self-Care Inventory ratings of 14 tasks by parents (5-point scale, "never do it" to "always do as recommended without fail") and average number of blood glucose tests over the previous 2 weeks as recorded on glucose meter obtained from medical chart	Mean parent rating = 3.92 and patient rating = 3.93; mean number of glucose tests/day = 2.66
Miller & Drotar, 2007	N = 63 11–17 years	Diabetes tasks (e.g., monitoring blood glucose)	Self-Care Inventory ratings of 14 tasks by parents (5-point scale, "never do it" to "always do as recommended without fail") and provider rating of 9 aspects of care; average number of blood glucose tests over the previous 2 weeks as recorded on glucose meter obtained from medical chart	Mean rating by parent = 3.72 and by provider = 3.25; mean number of glucose tests/day = 2.77
Naar-King et al., 2006	N = 119 10–17 years	Diet, insulin injections, blood glucose monitoring, and exercise	Ratings by parents and patients (0–100%, assessing "what percent of time do you/your teen" complete each regimen component in past month)	Mean parent rating = 68.04; mean patient rating = 65.49

(continued)

28.1 Nonadherence Rates for Selected Chronic Disease Regimens (Studies That Include or Exclusively Report on Adolescents) (continued)

Reference	Sample	Regimen	Adherence measure	Results
Diabetes				
Schmidt et al., 1992	N = 69 4–18 years (M = 14.2 yrs)	Diet	Patient dietary records over a 3 day period. Registered dietitian tallied the number of food exchanges that deviated from prescribed meal plans	Mean daily deviation from prescribed food exchanges = 23.8% (patients added or deleted. on average. about one of four exchanges)
Stewart et al., 2003	N = 56 10–23 years	Insulin injection. diet. blood glucose testing. exercise. treating reactions, maintaining blood glucose levels, and remembering to do everything every day.	Patient rated each care behavior from 20 ("failure") to 100 ("an A+"); average computed across the 7 behaviors to create an adherence composite	Time 1 adherence composite mean = 65.64 vs. Time 2 (12–24 months after Time 1) mean = 67.94
Wiebe et al., 2005	N = 127 10–15 years	14 diabetes managements tasks	Self-Care Inventory patient-rated adherence to 14 tasks ("1 = never did it to 5 = always did as recommended without fail"): average ratings computed across tasks	Mean composite rating = 3.62
Wilson & Endres. 1986	N = 18 12–18 years	Blood glucose monitoring	Meters with memory (patients and parents unaware of memory capabilities)	30% of blood tests not performed over 6 wks. Mean = 40% of blood tests recorded by patient but not registered by meter. Mean = 18% of blood tests not recorded by patients were registered by meter

Study	N / Age	Adherence behavior	Measurement	Findings
Wing et al., 1986	N = 62 (M = 13.5 yrs)	Blood glucose monitoring	Observation of blood glucose monitoring technique by trained observers in clinic	48% estimated blood glucose within 20% of actual value: sterile technique poor: only 10% worked on a tissue or paper towel and none washed hands; 40% incorrectly timed test; 21% did not adequately wipe blood from testing strip
HIV/AIDS				
Dolezal et al., 2003	N = 48 Parent-youth dyads 7–14 years	Antiretroviral medications	Caregiver and youths ratings of adherence over past 2 days and previous week	In 46% of caregiver-youth dyads, at least one of the pair reported adherence problems in last 2 days and 44% reported missing doses in past week: level of agreement among dyads was low (e.g., 38% in disagreement about missed, partial, or off-schedule medications)
Van Dyke et al., 2002	N = 125 4 mos–17 years	Antiretroviral medications	Caregiver or youth ratings in past 3 days	70% reported full adherence: 25% reported missing some doses; 5% missed all doses
Williams et al., 2006	N = 2,088 8–14 years	Antiretroviral medications	Caregiver or youth ratings in past 3 days	84% reported full adherence: lower for 15–18-year-olds (76%) than for younger children (83%–89%)
Juvenile rheumatoid arthritis (JRA)				
Feldman et al., 2007	N = 175 2–18 years	Medications and exercise	Caregiver rated over past 3 months	Adherence at baseline, 3, 6, 9, and 12 months for medications was 86%, 92%, 90%, 92%, and 89%; for exercises 55%, 64%, 61%, 63%, and 54%

(continued)

28.1 Nonadherence Rates for Selected Chronic Disease Regimens (Studies That Include or Exclusively Report on Adolescents) (continued)

Reference	Sample	Regimen	Adherence measure	Results
Juvenile rheumatoid arthritis (JRA)				
Kvien & Reimers, 1983	N = 25 4–15 years	Salicylates or Naproxen	Pill count	95% adherent overall
Litt & Cuskey, 1981	N = 82 (M = 12 yrs)	Salicylates	Serum assay (<20mg/dl defined nonadherence)	45% of patients nonadherent; mean serum level = 21.3mg/dl
Litt et al., 1982	N = 38 (M = 14 yrs)	Salicylates	Serum assay (<20mg/dl defined nonadherence)	45% of patients nonadherent; mean serum level = 20.79mg/dl
Rapoff et al., 2005	N = 48 2.3–16.7 years	Nonsteroidal antiinflammatory drugs	MEMS (electronic monitor)	Monitored over 28 consecutive days: 48% nonadherent (<80% of doses taken): median levels showed full adherence on 70% of days, partial on 14%, and no adherence on 7%
Seizures				
Friedman et al., 1986	N = 25 9–17 years	Phenobarbital	Saliva assay (<3.0 ug/ml defined nonadherence)	21% of patients nonadherent Mean saliva level = 5.11 ug/ml
Hazzard et al., 1990	N = 35 9–16 years	Anticonvulsant medications	Serum assay (nonadherence defined as subtherapeutic levels for 3 separate assays obtained an average of 2.52 months apart)	56% of patients nonadherent

Transplantation

Study	Sample	Regimen	Measure	Findings
Beck et al., 1980	N = 21 3–20 years	Immunosuppressive drug, postrenal transplant	Pill counts	43% of patients were nonadherent (all were adolescents)
Blowey et al., 1997	N = 19 13–18 years	Immunosuppressive drug, postrenal transplant	MEMS (electronic monitor)	21% nonadherent (<80% of doses taken)
Feinstein et al., 2005	N = 79 1.7–23 years	Immunosuppressive drug, postrenal transplant	Patient report and plasma assay	16% were nonadherent (all but one of 13 were adolescents)
Gerson et al., 2004	N = 13 2–21 years	Immunosuppressive drug, post renal transplant	MEMS (electronic monitor) and assay	Mean adherence by MEMS = 80% (mean adherence by MEMS for patients classified by assay as probably nonadherent = 69% and 95% for those classified as probably adherent)
Kurtin et al., 1994	N = 23 10–19 years (M = 16 yrs)	Medications and diet	Nurse rated adherence on a 5-point scale ("very often" to "never"); nonadherence defined as those patients rated as "sometimes," "almost never," or "never" adherent	59% of patients rated as nonadherent
Penkower et al., 2003	N = 22 13–18 years	Immunosuppressive drug, postrenal transplant	Patient report (deemed nonadherent for failing to take medication ≥ 3 times a month)	13.6% nonadherent at baseline and 12 months later

(continued)

Reference	Sample	Regimen	Adherence measure	Results
			Transplantation	
Serrano-Ikkos et al., 1998	N = 53 Mean age = 10.2 years	Immunosuppressive drug, postheart or heart-lung transplant	Patient medication diaries and blood assays	70% had good adherence (completed 80% of diaries and blood levels in acceptable range), 21% had moderate adherence (unsatisfactory diary completion), and 9% had poor adherence (unsatisfactory drug levels)
Shemesh et al., 2004	N = 81 2–22 years	Immunosuppressive drug, postliver transplant	Physicians, nurses, caregivers, and patients ratings (1 = "I always take my medications" to 4 = "I rarely take my medications as prescribed"); blood assay	Ratings of 1 ("ideally adherent") were given to 61% of patients by physicians, to 52% by nurses, to 70% by caregivers, and to 70% by patients themselves; only assay levels were significantly correlated with rejection episodes
Tucker et al., 2002	N = 68 (26 African American and 42 European American) 6–21 years	Immunosuppressive drug, postrenal transplant	Patient and physician rating, pill counts, and blood assay (all scored on 5-point scale, with 1 = "very nonadherent" and 5 = "very adherent")	Among African American patients, mean rating by patient = 3.89, by physician = 4.06, by pill count = 3.91, and assay = 4.13; among European American patients, mean rating by patient = 4.37, by physician = 4.02, by pill count = 3.58, and assay = 4.44

that approximately 19% of adolescent heart transplant recipients die while on organ transplant lists, as do 12% of adolescent potential liver and 1% of adolescent potential kidney recipients (Stuber, 1993). Adherence failures have also been implicated in the reemergence of drug-resistant infectious diseases such as tuberculosis (Bloom & Murray, 1992; Gibbons, 1992). Drug-resistant microbes evolve when bacteria exposed to different and incomplete doses of antimicrobials develop defenses against these drugs. This is particularly critical because drug companies are not developing new types of antimicrobials (Gibbons, 1992). The potential development of drug-resistant microbes could be especially threatening to young people with compromised immunity, such as those with cancer and cystic fibrosis, who are vulnerable to opportunistic infections.

Variations in adherence can also negatively impact medical decisions and outcomes of clinical drug trials. Physicians, unaware of adherence problems, may incorrectly assume that poor therapeutic outcomes are due to inadequacies in the regimen and prescribe more potent medicines with more serious side effects (Rapoff, 1999). Nonadherence can also interfere with effectiveness trials of medications (Fletcher, Fletcher, & Wagner, 1988) or clinical trials that try to determine the effectiveness of drugs given under ordinary circumstances. The variability in drug absorption (within and across persons) commonly found in clinical trials may be partially due to variability in adherence (Haynes & Dantes, 1987).

The cost-effectiveness of medical care can also be adversely affected by nonadherence (Rapoff, 1999; Smith, 1985). Overall, noncompliance with medical regimens accounts for up to $100 billion in health care and productivity costs in the United States (National Pharmaceutical Council, 1994). The annual cost of hospitalizations due to medication nonadherence in the United States is about $13.35 billion, which represents 1.7% of all health care expenditures. Costs associated with loss of productivity and premature death due to medication nonadherence have been estimated at $4.21 billion to $26.71 billion per year (Cleemput, Kesteloot, & DeGeest, 2002). The costs associated with treating drug-resistant infections have been estimated to be between $100 million and $200 million a year in the United States (Gibbons, 1992). These potentially unnecessary expenses may add to the existing economic burden on families of chronically ill adolescents and society in general, in the form of increased insurance costs and taxes. Conversely, interventions that improve adherence may also reduce unnecessary health care costs (Cleemput et al., 2002; National Pharmaceutical Council, 1994). In a large retrospective cohort study of 137,277 patients under the age of 65 years with congestive heart failure, diabetes, hypercholesterolemia, or hypertension, disease-related and all-cause medical costs and hospitalization rates were significantly lower for patients with higher medication adherence (Sokol, McGuigan, Verbrugge, & Epstein, 2005).

These serious health and economic consequences of nonadherence illustrate the importance of identifying predictors of adherence, particularly those that can be modified to improve adherence to therapeutic regimens. These efforts have the potential of increasing treatment efficacy, reducing disease-related morbidity and mortality, reducing unnecessary health care costs, and improving the yield from clinical drug trials.

Predictors of Nonadherence

There are few extant theoretical models that have been proposed and tested that are relevant to the pediatric medical adherence literature, with the exception of variations on the Health Belief Model (HBM) (Rapoff, 1996). Most studies examine predictors of adherence through correlational or regression analyses or classify patients as adherent or nonadherent and test for significant between-group differences along factorial dimensions. Patient, family, disease, and regimen factors have been commonly studied as predictors of adherence. These types of studies can be helpful in identifying risk factors for adherence problems, even if a particular variable (e.g., age) cannot be altered to improve adherence. These empirically-derived factors can also assist researchers in formulating adherence theories that can then be tested and refined through experimentation (Rapoff, 1999). Studies relevant to each factor are reviewed followed by a discussion of the implications of these findings for improving adherence.

Patient/Family Factors

Demographics

A number of patient- and family-related demographic variables have been associated with adherence. As mentioned in the introduction, adolescents are at higher risk for nonadherence to regimens for asthma, cancer, cystic fibrosis, diabetes, heart or heart/lung disease posttransplantation, HIV, juvenile rheumatoid arthritis (JRA), renal disease, and renal disease posttransplantation. However, one study found that adolescents with asthma were more adherent than older patients (Bender, Pedan, & Varasteh, 2006), and another study found no significant differences in adherence to medications between preadolescents and adolescents with JRA (Litt & Cuskey, 1981).

The few studies that have examined patient gender effects have been less clear than those that have examined patient age. Males have been found to be less adherent to regimens for cystic fibrosis (Patterson, 1985), diabetes (Lorenz, Christensen, & Pichert, 1985; Naar-King et al., 2006), and after renal transplantation (Fennell, Tucker, & Pedersen, 2001). However, other studies found that males were more adherent to regimens for asthma (Bender et al., 2006) and diabetes (Johnson, Freund, Silverstein, Hansen, & Malone, 1990; Patino, Sanchez, Eidson, & Delamater, 2005; Stewart et al., 2003). Patients identifying as Hispanic or African American have been found to be less adherent than Caucasians to regimens for asthma (McQuaid, Kopel, Klein, & Fritz, 2003) and seizures (Snodgrass, Vedanarayanan, Parker, & Parks, 2001).

Parental and family demographics have also been studied as predictors of adherence. Lower socioeconomic status (SES), in general, and lower educational levels in parents, specifically, have been associated with nonadherence to regimens for asthma (Radius et al., 1978), cystic fibrosis (Patterson, 1985), diabetes (Bobrow, AvRuskin, & Siller, 1985), JRA (Rapoff et al., 2005), and renal disease (Brownbridge & Fielding, 1994). Adolescents whose parents are separated or divorced are less likely to be adherent to regimens for asthma (Radius et al.,

1978), heart or heart/lung disease requiring transplantation (Serrano-Ikkos et al., 1998), liver disease requiring transplantation (Lurie et al., 2000), and renal disease (Brownbridge & Fielding, 1994). In addition, patients in larger families and in families where the mother works outside the home are less likely to be adherent to regimens for cystic fibrosis (Patterson, 1985).

Knowledge/Health Beliefs

Patients who are less knowledgeable about their disease and treatment tend to be less adherent to regimens for cancer than those who are better informed (Tebbi et al., 1986), cystic fibrosis (Gudas et al., 1991), diabetes (La Greca et al., 1990), and renal disease after transplantation (Tucker et al., 2001). However, patient knowledge in one study was not associated with adherence to medications for renal disease (Beck et al., 1980). A different picture emerges when parents are knowledgeable about their child's disease and treatment. Parental knowledge of diabetes (La Greca et al., 1990) and sickle cell disease (Jensen et al., 2005) was significantly correlated with adherence for preadolescents but not adolescents.

Factors related to the HBM have been examined in several studies from parents' and patients' perspectives. The HBM posits four sets of variables that predict or explain adherence: (1) perceived susceptibility, (2) perceived severity, (3) perceived benefits, and (4) perceived barriers (Janz & Becker, 1984). In addition, the HBM emphasizes the importance of internal or external cues to action to prompt adherence.

Higher susceptibility or vulnerability and severity, as rated by mothers, has been associated with better adherence to medications for asthma (Radius et al., 1978) and, as rated by patients, for cancer (Tamaroff, Festa, Adesman, & Walco, 1992). In contrast, higher perceived threat or severity by adolescents has been associated with lower adherence to regimens for diabetes (Bond et al., 1992) and to lower adherence to chest physiotherapy for cystic fibrosis (Gudas et al., 1991). Higher levels of perceived benefits, as assessed by mothers, has been associated with better adherence to asthma medications (Radius et al., 1978) and (as assessed by patients) with diabetes regimens (Bobrow et al., 1985; Bond et al., 1992; McCaul, Glasgow, & Schafer, 1987). Among African American renal transplant patients, lower certainty that medications help to keep transplanted kidneys healthy was related to lower adherence (Tucker et al., 2001). Perceptions among parents and adolescents of higher barriers to adherence have been uniformly related to poorer adherence to regimens for asthma (Radius et al., 1978) and diabetes (Glasgow, McCaul, & Schafer, 1986; McCaul et al., 1987). The presence of relevant cues to action has been associated with better adherence to regimens for asthma (Slack & Brooks, 1995; Van Es et al., 1998), diabetes (Bond et al., 1992), and HIV (Williams et al., 2006). Interestingly, a study that included a high percent of African American adolescents found no support for HBM factors in the prediction of adherence (Patino et al., 2005).

Adjustment and Coping

Adolescent adjustment and coping variables have been frequently examined as correlates of adherence, with fairly consistent results. Higher self-esteem has been associated with better adherence to diabetes (Jacobson et al., 1987), JRA (Litt, Cuskey, & Rosenberg, 1982), and seizure (Friedman et al., 1986) regimens. Greater autonomy and personal independence have been related to higher adherence to regimens for JRA (Litt et al., 1982) and seizures (Friedman et al., 1986). Higher social functioning, better disease-specific adjustment, an internal locus of control, and higher self-efficacy have all been associated with higher adherence to diabetes regimens (Holmes et al., 2006; Jacobson et al., 1987). A sense of optimism has been associated with better adherence to regimens for cystic fibrosis (Gudas et al., 1991) and greater problem-solving skills predicted higher adherence to diabetes regimens (McCaul et al., 1987). Patient and parental satisfaction with care has been associated with better adherence to seizure medications (Hazzard, Hutchinson, & Krawiecki, 1990). Higher scores on standardized memory scales have been associated with higher adherence to regimens for diabetes (Holmes et al., 2006). Adolescents taking medication for attention deficit hyperactivity disorder or antipsychotic medications were more adherent to medications for HIV (Williams et al., 2006).

On the negative side of the ledger, behavioral problems have been related to lower adherence to regimens for asthma, cystic fibrosis, diabetes, and renal disease posttransplantation (Gerson, Furth, Neu, & Fivush, 2004; Greening, Stoppelbein, Konishi, Jordan, & Moll, 2007; Jacobson et al., 1987; Miller & Drotar, 2003; Modi & Quittner, 2006; Naar-King et al., 2006). Adolescents who have a psychiatric disorder are also less likely to be adherent to regimens for diabetes (Kovacs et al., 1992) and to medications after liver transplantation (Lurie et al., 2000). Repeating a grade in school has been associated with lower adherence to medications for HIV (Williams et al., 2006), and a history of dropping out of school has been associated with lower adherence to medications after liver transplantation (Lurie et al., 2000). Increased anxiety and depression have also been related to lower adherence to regimens for cancer (Kennard et al., 2004), diabetes (Naar-King et al., 2006), and renal disease (Brownbridge & Fielding, 1994). Denial has been associated with poor adherence to medications for asthma (Buston & Wood, 2000) and cancer (Tamaroff et al., 1992). Higher levels of anger predicted lower adherence to medications after renal transplantation (Penkower et al., 2003) Maladaptive decision making (hypervigilance) has been associated with lower adherence to regimens for diabetes (Miller & Drotar, 2007). A history of substance abuse and physical or sexual abuse has been associated with lower adherence to medications after liver transplantation (Lurie et al., 2000).

Several studies have examined family and parental adjustment and coping as correlates of adherence, with family environment variables studied most frequently. Greater family support, communication, expressiveness, harmony, integration, cohesion, organization, balance, and collaboration with health care providers have been associated with higher adherence to regimens for asthma (Gavin, Wamboldt, Sorokin, Levy, & Wamboldt, 1999; McQuaid et al., 2005), cystic fibrosis (Patterson, 1985), diabetes (Hauser et al., 1990; La Greca et al., 1995; Lewin et al., 2006; McCaul et al., 1987), JRA (Kyngäs, 2002), renal disease (Feinstein et al., 2005; Kurtin, Landgraf, & Abetz, 1994), and seizures (Friedman et al., 1986). In addition, mother-daughter interactions characterized by clear communication, empathy, and positive conflict resolution have been associated with higher adherence to diabetes regimens (Bobrow et al., 1985).

Somewhat surprisingly, paternal nagging has been associated with better adherence to diabetes regimens (Burroughs, Pontious, & Santiago, 1993). Though poorly studied, greater father involvement (both amount and helpfulness) has been related to higher adherence to regimens for asthma, cystic fibrosis, diabetes, inflammatory bowel disease, phenylketonuria, and spina bifida (Wysocki & Gavin, 2006). In contrast, reporting by mothers of lower levels of spousal support is associated with lower adherence to regimens for diabetes (Lewandowski & Drotar, 2007).

Family dysfunction (poor problem solving and communication, conflicts, and critical parenting) has been related to lower adherence to regimens for asthma (Weinstein & Faust, 1997), diabetes (Lewandowski & Drotar, 2007; Lewin et al., 2006; Miller & Drotar, 2007), HIV (Hammami et al., 2004), renal disease posttransplantation (Gerson et al., 2004), and sickle cell disease (Barakat, Smith-Whitley, & Ohene-Frempong, 2002). Somewhat surprisingly, higher marital satisfaction has been related to lower adherence to cystic fibrosis regimens (Geiss, Hobbs, Hammersley-Maercklein, Kramer, & Henley, 1992). Parental coping difficulties have been associated with poor adherence to JRA (Wynn & Eckel, 1986) and renal (Brownbridge & Fielding, 1994) regimens. Parental depression has been related to poor adherence to asthma and renal disease regimens (Brownbridge & Fielding, 1994). Parental anxiety has been related to lower adherence to seizure medications (Hazzard et al., 1990). Parental stress, passive parental coping styles, and maternal uninvolvement have been associated with lower adherence to regimens for diabetes, renal disease posttransplantation, and sickle cell disease (Barakat et al., 2002; Gerson et al., 2004; Wiebe et al., 2005). Also, those parents who placed more behavioral restrictions on their children tended to have children who were less adherent to their seizure medications (Hazzard et al., 1990).

Parental Monitoring

Lack of parental monitoring of adolescents' adherence to treatment-related activities has been implicated as a contributor to nonadherence. Family situations where there is ambiguity about who assumes primary responsibility for regimen tasks or where parental monitoring and supervision are low have been associated with lower adherence to regimens for asthma (Walders et al., 2000), cancer (Tebbi, Richards, Cummings, Zevon, & Mallon, 1988), diabetes (Anderson et al., 1990, 1997; Bobrow et al., 1985; Holmes et al., 2006; Ingersoll, Orr, Herrold, & Golden, 1986), and renal disease (Beck et al., 1980; Feinstein et al., 2005). In a sample of 12- to 21-year-olds with diabetes, parental supervision virtually ceased by the time children were 15 years of age (Ingersoll et al., 1986). Another study found that primary responsibility for taking immunosuppressive medications after liver transplantation shifted to children at about age 12 years (Shemesh et al., 2004). The lack of parental monitoring or involvement may explain why parental knowledge of diabetes is unrelated to adherence for adolescents but significantly correlated with adherence for preadolescents (La Greca et al., 1990) and why parental ratings of adherence for older adolescents are a poor predictor of metabolic control for that group but a significant predictor for younger adolescents (Burroughs et al., 1993).

Disease Factors

Duration

Longer disease duration has been associated with poorer adherence to regimens for diabetes (Bond et al., 1992; Patino et al., 2005), JRA (Litt & Cuskey, 1981), and renal disease (Brownbridge & Fielding, 1994). Also, longitudinal studies have found significant deterioration in adherence over time to diabetes regimens, with nonadherence emerging an average of 3.5 years after the onset of the disease (Jacobson et al., 1990; Kovacs et al., 1992).

Disease Course and Symptoms

Chronic diseases often fluctuate in terms of the presence and severity of symptoms. Adherence may be particularly difficult to sustain during periods when patients are relatively asymptomatic, such as with asthma (van Es et al., 1998) and JRA (Rapoff et al., 2005). However, studies involving adolescents with JRA (Feldman et al., 2007) and seizures (Hazzard et al., 1990) found that lower disease activity was associated with higher adherence.

Perceived Severity

Patients' perception of higher severity has been related to lower adherence (Gudas et al., 1991) while parents' perception of higher severity relates to higher adherence (Radius et al., 1978). However, patients' and parents' ratings of severity seem be more useful in predicting adherence than are severity ratings by health care providers (Rapoff, 1999).

Regimen Factors

Type and Complexity

Adherence tends to be lower with complex regimens such as chest physiotherapy for cystic fibrosis (Passero et al., 1981), dietary regimens for diabetes (Glasgow et al., 1986), medications for HIV (Van Dyke et al., 2002), exercise regimens for JRA (April et al., 2006; Feldman et al., 2007; Rapoff, Lindsley, & Christophersen, 1985), and medications after renal transplantation (Tucker et al., 2002). Lower rates of adherence have been reported for inhaled than for oral medications used in the treatment of asthma (Kelloway et al., 1994) and for pills than for liquid medications in the treatment of HIV (Van Dyke et al., 2002). Bad-tasting medications or the need to swallow larger pills has been cited as reasons for lower adherence to asthma medications (Celano, Geller, Phillips, & Ziman, 1998; Radius et al., 1978; Slack & Brooks, 1995; van Es et al., 1998) and medications after renal transplantation (Tucker et al., 2002). Morning doses are reported to be more difficult to remember to take than evening doses in the treatment of asthma (Jónasson et al., 2000; van Es et al., 1998). Patients who had had heart/lung transplantation were found to be less adherent to immunosuppressant medications than were those who had received heart transplantation only (Serrano-Ikkos et al., 1998). African American adolescents were less adherent to immunosuppressant medications after renal transplantation if they had not had dialysis prior to transplantation and if they had received a living-related organ donation (Fennell et al., 2001).

Costs

Treatment costs can be prohibitive for some families and result in nonadherence (Rapoff, 1999). A telephone survey of 138 patients with rheumatic diseases revealed that of those who had a physician visit and purchase of medication in the month before the survey, 40.7% of the parents reported difficulty paying physician-related charges and 25.3% had problems paying medication-related expenses (McCormick, Stemmler, & Athreya, 1986). Higher costs of medications have been related to lower adherence to medications for asthma (Bender et al., 2006), and lack of insurance has been associated with lower adherence to medications for seizures (Snodgrass et al., 2001).

Side Effects and Inconvenience

Having or avoiding side effects of medications has been cited as a reason for not taking medications for asthma (Buston & Wood, 2000; Slack & Brooks, 1995). The inconvenience or embarrassment of taking medications outside the home have been cited as reasons for nonadherence to medications in the treatment of asthma (Buston & Wood, 2000; Celano et al., 1998; Slack & Brooks, 1995).

Efficacy

Regimens that are perceived by parents and patients as more efficacious or beneficial are better adhered to (Bobrow et al., 1985; Bond et al., 1992; Feldman et al., 2007; McCaul et al., 1987; Radius et al., 1978). However, regimen efficacy (in terms of treatment outcome) is usually assumed to be partially determined by adherence. There is support for this connection, as higher adherence has been related to better metabolic control of diabetes (Burroughs et al., 1993; Johnson et al., 1992; Kovacs et al., 1992; Kuttner, Delameter, & Santiago, 1990). The relationship between efficacy and adherence is most likely bidirectional. A related issue is the delayed benefits of treatments even when patients are highly adherent (Rapoff, 1999). For example, an adequate trial of nonsteroidal anti-inflammatory medications in the treatment of JRA is considered to be at least 8 weeks (Lovell, Giannini, & Brewer, 1984).

Summary and Implications

The following adherence "risk profile" can be developed for adolescents with chronic diseases. They tend to come from families that are preoccupied with dysfunctional interaction patterns or, by contrast, with positive social and recreational activities outside the home that consume time, energy, and resources that could be directed to supervising and managing treatment regimens. Their families are also likely to be larger, in the lower socioeconomic strata, and from minority groups, and there is likely to be only one parent living in the home.

Their parents tend to be less educated, in general, or specifically about their children's disease and treatment. Also, their parents are prone to adjustment and coping difficulties and may place undue restrictions on their children's activities. Adolescents are also likely to have adjustment and coping difficulties and be less knowledgeable about their disease and treatment than more adherent peers. They are also likely to have primary responsibility for carrying out regimen tasks, with little or no direct supervision by their parents. Both the parents and the adolescents tend to hold beliefs that undermine adherence efforts; for example, they may perceive more costs than benefits from adhering to treatment regimens. These adolescents have also had to cope with their disease and treatment over a period of years, with fluctuations in the type and severity of symptoms associated with their disease. They have also been prescribed regimens that are often complex, intrusive, and costly, that produce negative side effects, and that are not immediately efficacious.

On the positive side, there are "resource" factors that can also be gleaned from these studies that point to specific ways patients can be helped to achieve better adherence. A positive family environment is critical for supporting adolescent adherence to chronic-disease regimens. This makes perfect sense from a normative developmental context. Despite the widespread notion that adolescent-parent relations are "stormy," most adolescents report being close to their parents, respect them, and rely on them for support (Coleman & Hendry, 1990; Crockett & Petersen, 1993). Part of this support by parents involves shared responsibility for treatment regimen tasks and monitoring. Again, this makes sense from a developmental perspective. Developing autonomy from parents is an important developmental task for adolescents, and close supervision by parents is not as feasible or, in some cases, desirable (Coleman & Hendry, 1990; Crockett & Petersen, 1993). For some adolescents, this decrease in parental supervision increases the likelihood of engaging in misconduct and health-risking behaviors (Crockett & Petersen, 1993). Thus, parents have to balance their adolescent's needs for autonomy with the need for supervision.

Adherence Improvement

Adherence improvement strategies can be broadly classified as educational, organizational, or behavioral (Rapoff, 1999). Educational strategies rely primarily on verbal and written instructions designed to inform patients and their parents about the illness, regimen tasks, the importance of adherence, and strategies for improving adherence. Organizational strategies target changes in the health care delivery system, such as increasing accessibility to health care services, simplifying regimens, and providing more intense supervision of patients by health care providers. Behavioral strategies refer to behavior change procedures, such as patient or parental monitoring, contracting, and token economy programs, designed to alter specific adherence behaviors. Most studies utilize these strategies in combination.

Table 28.2 provides details on adherence improvement studies, primarily conducted with chronically ill adolescents. Overall, there are strikingly few intervention studies. Nine of the 17 studies located were concerned with improving adherence to diabetes regimens, and no studies were located that were relevant to regimens for cancer, cystic fibrosis, renal disease, seizures, or posttransplantation. However, several conclusions can be drawn from these studies.

Educational strategies are rarely attempted in isolation but are usually combined with behavioral strategies (e.g., Pieper, Rapoff, Purviance, & Lindsley, 1989). This may occur because educational strategies have limited utility in improving adherence, in part, due to ceiling effects. That is, those patients selected for intervention studies were probably exposed to extensive educational efforts that had their impact on adherence prior to the patient's entry into the study (Rapoff & Barnard, 1991). Also, knowing about something (declarative knowledge) is quite different from knowing how to do something (procedural knowledge) or performing in accordance with expectations (Glaser & Bassok, 1989; Reese, 1989).

The primary organizational strategies used have been monitoring by a physician and simplification of regimens. Increased physician monitoring has improved adherence to asthma medications (Eney & Goldstein, 1976). Simplifying regimens, by reducing the number of medication doses, has improved adherence to medications for asthma (Tinkelman, Vanderpool, Carroll, Page, & Spangler, 1980) and JRA (Rapoff, Purviance, & Lindsley, 1988a).

By far the most frequently tested and effective strategies have been behaviorally based, including explicit training and feedback (Epstein, Figueroa, Farkas, & Beck, 1981), goal setting and contracting (Schafer, Glasgow, & McCaul, 1982), and reinforcement programs (Carney, Schechter, & Davis, 1983; Rapoff et al., 1988a, 1988b; Wysocki, Green, & Huxtable, 1989). Sometimes punishment procedures have been added when reinforcement contingencies have not been sufficient (Snyder, 1987). However, most of these studies have included small samples and have used fairly complicated interventions that are not likely to be feasible for routine use in subspecialty settings.

Several studies are noteworthy. One of the most intriguing studies reviewed in Table 28.2 is reported by Satin, La Greca, Zigo, and Skyler (1989), who employed a parent simulation component whereby parents simulated their children's diabetes regimens (gave themselves normal saline shots, followed the diet, checked blood glucose levels, and so on). This simulation, coupled with weekly support and educational sessions, resulted in improvements in metabolic control of patients' diabetes. Perhaps parents became more sensitized to adherence-related issues and were more attentive to and supportive of their children's efforts to adhere. Regimen simulation has been added as a component in behavioral family systems therapy for improving adherence to regimens for diabetes (Wysocki et al., 2006) and warrants replication with other chronic diseases. It might be interesting to extend these simulations to providers; they might enhance providers' sensitivity to adherence-related barriers and possible responses to these problems. Intensive home- and community-based family therapy ("multisystemic therapy") has been effective in increasing adherence to blood glucose testing in adolescents with diabetes (Ellis et al., 2005, 2007) and warrants further replications with other chronic conditions. Finally, the study by our group of JRA patients (Rapoff et al., 2002) was unique in that we focused on preventing the expected drop in adherence over time that has been documented for other chronic diseases by intervening with newly diagnosed patients. We were successful in that the experimental group showed maintenance

28.2 Adherence Intervention Studies Involving Adolescents With Chronic Diseases

Reference	Sample	Regimen/ measure	Procedures	Outcome
			Asthma	
Chan et al., 2007	N = 120 (6–17 yrs)	Inhaled steroids; pharmacy refill; symptom diaries completed	Random assignment to office-based (traditional in-person education and case management) or virtual group (received computers, Internet connections, in-home Internet-based education and case management via study Web site) over a 12-month period	No differences between groups on adherence to inhaled steroids; significantly greater diary completion in the virtual group (35.4%) than in the office-based group (20.8%); no differences between groups in ER visits, hospitalizations, unscheduled asthma-related clinic visits, pulmonary function, asthma knowledge scores, or quality of life
Eney & Goldstein, 1976	N = 90 (3–16 yrs)	Theophylline: serum/salivary assays	Random selection but not assignment to 2 groups: Gr 1 had no specific intervention; Gr 2 patients informed that drug ingestion was being monitored and physicians were more directive in discussing adherence	11% of patients in Gr 1 and 42% in Gr 2 had therapeutic drug levels
Tinkelman et al., 1980	N = 20 (11–18 yrs)	Theophylline: serum assay and pill counts	Random assignment to short-acting (q 6 hr) or sustained-release (q 12 hrs) theophylline; dosing instructions given for both preparations	Significantly higher adherence with sustained-release than with short-acting theophylline by pill counts; no significant difference in serum levels
			Diabetes	
Carney et al., 1983	N = 3 (10–14 yrs)	Blood glucose testing; patient records and used t	Multiple baseline-across-subjects with baseline followed by point system exchanged for money and special activities	All 3 patients showed improvement in % of tests performed, with 2 patients improving from <5% in baseline to 87% and 93%

	esting strips: Ghb levels		after treatment; gains were maintained at 4-mos follow-up: Ghb levels improved from baseline (10.1%, 15.2%, & 9.1%) to follow-up (9.4%, 11.7%, & 6.0%)
Ellis et al., 2005	N = 127 (10–17 yrs)	Insulin use, diet, and blood glucose testing by 24–recall interview; blood glucose by electronic monitor (glucometer)	Random assignment to standard care or multisystemic therapy (MST). MST is an intensive home- and community-based family therapy approach that includes a variety of interventions that can be selected, including cognitive-behavioral therapy, parent training, family therapy, support from school personnel and peers, and work with health care team (mean length of MST was 5.7 months)
			Significant improvement in the frequency of blood glucose testing (24-hr recall and glucometer) in the MST group over the standard-care group; no significant difference between groups on metabolic control, insulin or dietary adherence, or ER visits; youth in MST groups showed significant reductions in hospital admissions
Ellis et al., 2007	N = 127 (10–17 yrs)	Blood glucose testing; electronic monitor (glucometer)	Random assignment to standard care or multisystemic therapy (MST). MST is an intensive home- and community-based family therapy approach which includes a variety of interventions that can be selected including cognitive-behavioral therapy; parent training, family therapy, enlisting support from school personnel and peers, and working with health care team (mean length of MST was 5.7 months)
			Significant improvement in the frequency of blood glucose testing in the MST group over the standard-care group. Trend for youths receiving MST to show greater improvements in metabolic control; youths in the MST group from single-parent families showed a significant improvement in metabolic control No differences in primary caregiver support for diabetes; youth in two-parent families did report significantly greater increase in secondary caregiver support than did controls in two-parent families

(continued)

28.2   Adherence Intervention Studies Involving Adolescents With Chronic Diseases (*continued*)

Reference	Sample	Regimen/ measure	Procedures	Outcome
			Asthma	
Epstein et al., 1981	N = 17 (6–16 yrs)	Urine glucose testing: direct observation	Random assignment to practice condition (patients tested 20 prepared samples but were not informed of results) or feedback condition (patients tested samples and given feedback about accuracy)	Mean number of correct urine glucose estimations were significantly higher for feedback (7.2) than for practice (3.8) conditions posttraining
Satin et al., 1989	N = 32 (mean age = 14.6 yrs)	Insulin use: urine glucose testing; diet: exercise Parental ratings of self-care (1 = very careful to 5 = careless) Ghb levels Attitudes toward teenager with diabetes scales Family Environment Scale.	Random assignment to one of three groups: Gr 1–patients and parents met for 6 weekly sessions to discuss diabetes and management: Gr 2–identical to Gr 1 plus included a parent simulation of diabetes regimen: or Gr 3–control group	No significant differences between groups in self-care ratings: significant decrease in Ghb levels at 6-wk postintervention for Gr 2 compared to Gr 3: significant difference in attitudes towards teenager with diabetes (more positive) for Gr's 1 & 2

Study	Sample	Measures	Design/Intervention	Results
Schafer et al., 1982	N = 3 (16–18 yrs)	Urine glucose testing, insulin use, exercise; wearing diabetic information bracelet; blood glucose testing; assessed by patient self-monitoring records	Multiple baseline-across-behaviors design with baseline followed by goal setting and (if needed) contingency contracting conditions	Goal setting alone effective in improving adherence to wearing info, exercise, & urine testing for subject 1 & for urine testing and exercise for subject 2; goal setting plus contracting improved adherence to insulin use for subject 2; nothing effective for subject 3, who was experiencing severe family problems
Snyder, 1987	N = 1 (14 yrs)	Insulin use; urine glucose testing; diet patient self-monitoring records with independent checks by mother and school nurse	Quasi-experimental single-subject design. Following self-monitoring baseline, patient exposed to self-monitoring plus monetary incentives and then to an additional condition involving hospitalization contingent on hypo- or hyperglycemic episodes for 36 hrs in a private room with no TV, visitors, books, and minimal staff interaction. Behavioral contacting and communication/conflict resolution training also implemented for antisocial behavior and mother-child conflict	Mean number of diabetes self-care activities performed was 5.6 during self-monitoring baseline, 6.3 during self-monitoring + reinforcement, and 8.5 during self-monitoring + reinforcement + punishment; 1-mos follow-up showed maintenance of gains. Decreases in antisocial behavior and conflicts and increases in school attendance noted; however, anecdotal reports at 6-mos posttreatment indicated deterioration of gains, with patient hospitalized for drug abuse

(continued)

28.2 Adherence Intervention Studies Involving Adolescents With Chronic Diseases (*continued*)

Reference	Sample	Regimen/ measure	Procedures	Outcome
			Asthma	
Wysocki et al., 1989	N = 42 (mean age = 14 yrs)	Blood glucose testing; insulin use; diet; exercise; automated recording of blood glucose (reflectance meters). 24-hr recall patient and parent interviews. Ghb levels. Attitudes toward diabetes and diabetes adjustment scales	30 patients randomly assigned to meter-alone (MA) or meter-plus-contract (MC) groups; remaining 12 patients in conventional-therapy (CT) control group. MA Gr patients earned money for bringing meters to clinic; MC Gr patients earned money contingent on glucose testing frequency	By 8th week, MC Gr had significantly higher frequency of glucose testing; no differences in overall adherence, Ghb levels, or patient/parent attitudes and adjustment to diabetes

Wysocki et al., 2006	N = 92 (11–16 yrs)	Insulin use, blood glucose testing, diet, exercise, and managing hypoglycemia by structured interview	Random assignment to standard care (SC), educational support (ES: 12 multifamily meetings for diabetes education and support), or behavioral family systems therapy for diabetes (BFST-D: 12 sessions focusing on problem-solving, communication, cognitive restructuring, and family therapy). The BFST-D revised for this study to also include having families target two or more diabetes-related problems, go through behavioral contracting training, use self-monitoring of blood glucose data, and have parents simulate living with diabetes for 1 week	Main effect of group and the group X time interaction showed no significant differences on adherence. BFST-D did yield significant improvements (or fewer declines) for youth with higher baseline HbA1c levels when compared to the other groups
				Main effect of group and the group X time interaction showed no significant differences on metabolic control.
				Improvements in metabolic control were significantly greater for those with higher baseline HbA1c for the BFST-D and ES groups than for the SC group.
				Diabetes responsibility and conflict scores significantly improved for the BFST-D but not for the other groups.
				Parental-adolescent relationship scores (conflict, extreme belief, family structure) did not differ among the groups.

(continued)

28.2 Adherence Intervention Studies Involving Adolescents With Chronic Diseases (*continued*)

Reference	Sample	Regimen/ measure	Procedures	Outcome
			HIV	
Garvie et al., 2007	N = 23 (4–22 yrs)	Highly active anti- retroviral ther- apy (HAART) by pharmacy pill counts	Retrospective chart review of 23 patients clinically referred for pill-swallowing problems; modeling and shaping (starting with small pieces of candy and progress- ing to placebo pills the size of prescribed medications) used to teach pill swallow- ing	Adherence increased by a median of 9.8%; percentage of patients showing no evi- dence of immune suppression increased from 50% at baseline to 81.8% at ~6 months
			Rheumatic Diseases	
Pieper et al., 1989	N = 3 (11–18 yrs) 2 patients with Systemic Lupus Erythematosus & one with Der- matomyositis	Medications: pill counts	Multiple baseline-across-subjects: follow- ing baseline, patients and parents given instructions in clinic about medications, adherence, and monitoring/reinforcement strategies	Because over as well as underdosing oc- curred, patients classified as adherent if pill counts indicated 80–120% of doses were taken: mean % of pill counts in ac- ceptable range was baseline = 38%, 7%, and 33%: intervention = 89%, 67%, & 88%: 6- mos follow-up = 100% for all patients: and 12-mos follow-up = 67% for 2 patients

Rapoff et al. 1988a	N = 1 (14 yrs) with JRA	Medications; pill counts	Single-subject withdrawal design: following baseline, regimen simplified (q.i.d to t.i.d): token system in the home for 10 weeks, then withdrawn for 7 weeks, reinstated for 7 wks, and then maintenance phase for 8 wks (where token system reintroduced if adherence was <80% for 2 consecutive weeks): token system then completely withdrawn.	Mean adherence levels by condition were baseline = 44%: simplified regimen = 59%: token system = 100%: withdrawal of token system = 77%: token system reinstated = 99%: maintenance phase = 92%: and 9-mos follow-up = 97%: less disease activity evident during simplified regimen and token system phases
Rapoff et al. 1988b	N = 3 (3, 10, & 13 yrs) with JRA	Medications; pill counts	Multiple-baseline across subjects design. Following baseline, treatment introduced across participants in a time-staggered fashion and involved a single home visit where information was reviewed about type and purpose of medications prescribed. the importance of consistent adherence. how to prevent medication side effects, and monitoring of adherence and positive feedback	By visual inspection. adherence improved for the 10- and 3-yr-old participants from mean baseline levels of 38% and 54%. respectively. to 97% and 92%. respectively during intervention: at 4-mos follow-up. mean adherence levels were 56% and 89%. respectively: for these participants. Adherence increased only slightly for the 13-yr-old participant. averaging 44% at baseline and 49% during intervention: at 4-mos follow-up. adherence dropped to an average of 24%

(continued)

575

28.2 Adherence Intervention Studies Involving Adolescents With Chronic Diseases (*continued*)

Reference	Sample	Regimen/ measure	Procedures	Outcome
Rapoff et al., 2002	N = 34 (2–16 yrs) newly diagnosed patients with JRA	Medications: electronic monitor (MEMS)	Random assignment to education/behavioral intervention or education-only control group. Procedures for both groups introduced during 30-min clinic visit by the clinic nurse, following which the nurse phoned participants every 2 weeks for 2 month and then monthly for 10 months. Audiovisual programs and handouts used with both groups. Education group received information about types of JRA, signs and symptoms, and treatments; education/behavioral group received information identical to control group plus strategies for maintaining adherence, such as cueing, monitoring, positive reinforcement, and discipline	Over the 52-wk period of study, participants in the education/behavioral group showed significant better overall mean adherence than controls (77.7% vs. 56.9%); no significant differences between groups on measures of disease activity (active joint counts, morning stiffness, global disease severity, or functional limitations)

of adherence over a 52-week period (mean = 77.7% vs. 56.9% for controls), but there was no effect on disease activity, possibly due to "floor" effects (patients in both groups had low disease activity at baseline).

Clinical and Research Implications

On the basis of this and other reviews (Friedman & Litt, 1987; Jay et al., 1984; Meichenbaum & Turk, 1987; Rapoff, 1999; Rapoff & Barnard, 1991; Rapoff & Christophersen, 1982; Varni & Wallander, 1984), several clinical and research implications can be drawn.

Clinical Implications

Cooperative Alliance

Patients and their families are no longer satisfied (if they ever were) with a passive role in their health care. They want a greater role in making decisions regarding their health (Cassell, 1991). Chronic disease care needs to be a collaborative effort among adolescents, their parents, and providers. A first step in this approach is to set explicit and mutually agreed upon treatment goals. Patients and their families may be less inclined to follow treatment plans that fail to address their goals, which are usually related to functional concerns such as relating to peers, achieving academic success, and engaging in recreational and social activities. Greater involvement of adolescents in this clinical alliance also recognizes their need for autonomy and their increased cognitive sophistication (Coleman & Hendry, 1990; Crockett & Petersen, 1993).

Developmental Sensitivity

Providers who treat adolescents need to be sensitive to their developmental needs, challenges, and capacities. Among these are physical, cognitive, self-identity and esteem, and autonomy issues (see Crockett & Petersen, 1993, for an excellent review of individual and social factors that affect health promotion with adolescents). For example, we expect adolescents, in their transition to adulthood, to be more self-governed and responsible for their behavior. However, there needs to be a balance between giving adolescents opportunities to exercise their autonomy and minimizing risks to their health and well-being (Crockett & Petersen, 1993). The role of parental monitoring and support is critical in this process.

Parental Monitoring and Support

Clearly, parental involvement, in the form of appropriate monitoring, shared responsibility, and articulation and enforcement of reasonable limits, is critical to enhancing adherence to medical regimens and the competencies of adolescents, in general (Crockett & Petersen, 1993). An authoritative parenting style seems to be the most useful approach. This style has been characterized as a constellation of parent attributes that includes emotional support, high standards, appropriate granting of autonomy, and clear, bidirectional communication (Darling & Steinberg, 1993). As shown in this review, this type of parenting approach has been associated with better adherence to medical regimens for adolescents. The message for parents and health care providers seems clear: *be careful not to abruptly or completely discontinue monitoring and support* (Ingersoll et al., 1986; La Greca et al., 1995). Part of this support by providers is educational in nature.

Education

Most likely, educational strategies are *necessary but not sufficient* to maintain adherence to regimens for chronic diseases (Rapoff & Christophersen, 1982). However, they are necessary, and the content needs to be expanded to include not only disease and treatment information but specific instructions on how to maintain adherence and why consistent adherence is important (Rapoff, 1999). Educational methods also need to be expanded beyond verbal and written information giving to include modeling, behavioral rehearsal, and contingent performance feedback (e.g., Epstein et al., 1981). Educational content and methods need to capitalize on the developing ability of adolescents to engage in abstract thinking (Crockett & Petersen, 1993). In addition, education needs to be viewed as an ongoing process for patients and families. When patients are first diagnosed, they and their parents may be too anxious to adequately attend to and retain complex information required to master multicomponent chronic-disease regimens. Also, regimens are periodically altered, which necessitates educational updates or booster sessions.

Health Care Delivery

Providers may blame patients and their families for adherence problems while ignoring how they interact with patients and families to deliver health care (Dunbar-Jacob, 1993; Rapoff, 1999). Generally, consumer-friendly clinical settings need to be developed in order to enhance satisfaction with medical care and thereby promote adherence. This includes pleasant physical surroundings, prompt and accessible care, and a consistent provider (Rapoff, 1999). Also, providers need to take care how they prescribe regimens. Patients and their families have a finite amount of time, energy, and resources to devote to medical regimens, if they are to maintain some semblance of a normal family life (Patterson, 1985). Providers need to minimize the complexity, costs, and negative side effects of regimens. It is also incumbent on providers to prescribe regimens that are efficacious. Patients and families want their provider to be sensitive and caring, but not at the expense of competency.

Adherence Incentives

Ideally, patients are prescribed treatments that rapidly and pervasively control their disease symptoms. Thus, the natural reinforcer for adherence is that patients get and feel better. However, this rarely happens in the treatment of complex chronic diseases. This situation creates the necessity of using contrived reinforcers, such as token systems, to improve and maintain adherence until disease symptoms abate or remit. This review and others (Friedman & Litt, 1987; Jay et al., 1984; Meichenbaum & Turk, 1987; Rapoff, 1999; Rapoff & Barnard, 1991; Rapoff & Christophersen, 1982; Varni & Wallander, 1984) clearly show the effectiveness of behavioral procedures in improving adherence to chronic-disease regimens. But, positive reinforcement may not be sufficient in some cases (e.g., Snyder, 1987). Parents may need assistance in the use of appropriate discipline strategies, such as token fines (Rapoff, 1994). This may be particularly difficult for parents of chronically ill patients, as evidenced by studies that show that these parents (more than parents of healthy children) are more likely to excuse their children's misbehavior and fail to set limits (Ievers, Drotar, Dahms, Doershuk, & Stern, 1994; Walker, Garber, & Van Slyke, 1995). The importance of setting and enforcing reasonable limits can be explained to parents as vital to fostering self-discipline in their children. This is particularly important for adolescents with chronic diseases, who need a higher level of self-discipline than healthy adolescents, given the increased demands and challenges of living with a chronic illness.

At-Risk Patients and Families

In some cases, medical nonadherence can be symptomatic of, or exist concurrently with, patient or family dysfunction. For some adolescents, nonadherence may be part of a broader pattern of externalizing (e.g., oppositional and defiant disorder) or internalizing disorders (e.g., depression). There may also be parental or family problems. These types of problems may need to be addressed before or concurrent with efforts to manage medical nonadherence and are better addressed by mental health professionals who have extensive experience with adolescents in medical settings (Rapoff, 1999). Family- and community-based interventions may be needed to improve adherence among at-risk patients and their families (Ellis et al., 2005, 2007; Wysocki et al., 2006).

Research Implications

Assessment and Classification of Adherence Levels

All measures of adherence have advantages and disadvantages (Rapoff, 1999). Therefore, the use of multiple measures may yield a more complete assessment of adherence than the use of one indicator. The gold standard in adherence assessment might well be the combination of assays and electronic monitors for medications and direct observation for nonmedication regimens. Also, research is needed to establish what level of adherence is necessary for particular regimens to produce acceptable therapeutic outcomes (Rapoff & Christophersen, 1982). In general, this has not been done for pediatric chronic diseases.

Samples and Regimens

There is a need to expand adherence research to include patients with diseases other than diabetes and to nonmedication regimens. Also, adolescents from minority groups need to be included in adherence studies. As argued by Tucker and her colleagues (Tucker et al., 2002) a "difference model" research approach is needed when studying minority groups to identify culture-specific (within-group) factors in adherence rather than a "deficit model," which interprets differences between ethnic groups by using the behavior of the dominant ethnic group (Whites) as the norm (between-groups comparison). Given some of the common regimens (e.g., medications) and predictors of adherence, a noncategorical approach may be also useful to include patients with a variety of chronic diseases (cf. Stein & Jessop, 1989). This would be helpful given the relatively small samples of homogeneous patient groups that are available in most settings.

Correlations and Causation

As noted in this review, much of the literature on adherence is concerned with identifying predictors of adherence. However, many of these variables have limited utility because they are "marker" or "higher-level" variables (Haynes, 1992). A marker variable (such as age, gender, or SES) is one that is statistically associated with a parameter but does not have causal properties; it marks other variables that function as causal agents. For example, adolescent age has been associated with poorer adherence. What does this mean? Why are adolescents more likely to be nonadherent? The answers to these questions will help elucidate the potential underlying causal mechanisms. For example, adolescents may be less adherent because they are trying to be independent of parental influence or fit in with their peers.

Some of the correlational studies have investigated higher-level variables, which are molar or more inferential variables (such as family cohesion, autonomy needs, and negative self-concept). Higher-level variables are problematic because they subsume more multiple causal pathways than lower-level variables and are subject to greater measurement problems (Haynes, 1992). Thus, higher-level variables need to be disentangled and translated into lower, more utilitarian, levels. For example, what are the elements of cohesive families? What do such families look like in terms of how they interact, solve problems, and conduct their lives? The answers to these questions are likely to lead to specific and testable hypotheses regarding causal mechanisms (see Snyder, 1987, for an example of this approach utilizing Patterson's coercion theory).

Adherence Theories

With the exception of variants of the HBM, there are no explicit and comprehensive theories related to pediatric medical adherence. Theories are important because they influence methodological considerations, the data collected, and how researchers react to their data (Rapoff, 1996). Data on predictors of adherence can be combined to refute or support existing theories or to help formulate new theories, which can then be further refined through continued experimentation. For example, correlates of adherence reviewed in this chapter are supportive of the HBM and family systems models.

Controlled Studies

There is a clear need for prospective studies involving experimental manipulation of variables to improve adherence (Rapoff, 1999). This is the most stringent test of causal models. Single-subject designs may be particularly well suited for this endeavor because they accommodate small sample sizes and allow for repeated assessments of adherence over time (Barlow & Hersen, 1984; Powers, Piazza-Waggoner, Jones, Ferguson, Daines, & Acton, 2006; Rapoff, 1999). These designs are also flexible, allowing for changes in the treatment protocol depending on the patients' responses. Once effective strategies are isolated using single-subject designs, they can be tested in comparisons with each other or control conditions in conventional, between-group designs. This phase requires larger samples and argues for multicenter collaborative trials.

Cost-Effective Computer-Based Interventions

Adolescents have grown up with computers and are sophisticated users of CD-ROM games and the Internet. Interactive CD-ROM and Internet-based programs have been developed for children with asthma and cystic fibrosis (Chan et al., 2007; Davis, Quittner, Stack, & Yang, 2004; McPherson, Glazebrook, Forster, James, & Smyth, 2006), but they have not directly assessed or targeted adherence. These types of programs can be cost-effective, standardized, and tailored or flexible when needed, and are more accessible than direct contact interventions.

References

Adams, C. D., Dreyer, M. L., Dinakar, C., & Portnoy, J. M. (2004). Pediatric asthma: A look at adherence from the patient and family perspective. *Current Allergy & Asthma Reports, 4,* 425–432

Anderson, B. J., Auslander, W. F., Jung, K. C., Miller, J. P., & Santiago, J. V. (1990). Assessing family sharing of diabetes responsibilities. *Journal of Pediatric Psychology, 15,* 477–492.

Anderson, B., Ho, J., Brackett, J., Finkelstein, D., & Laffel, L. (1997). Parental involvement in diabetes management tasks: Relationships to blood glucose monitoring adherence and metabolic control in young adolescents with insulin-dependent diabetes mellitus. *Journal of Pediatrics, 130,* 257–265.

April, K. T., Feldman, D. E., Platt, R. W., & Duffy, C. M. (2006). Comparison between children with juvenile idiopathic arthritis and their parents concerning perceived treatment adherence. *Arthritis Care & Research, 55,* 558–563.

Barakat, L. P., Smith-Whitley, K., & Ohene-Frempong, K. (2002). Treatment adherence in children with sickle cell disease: Disease-related risk and psychosocial resistance factors. *Journal of Clinical Psychology in Medical Settings, 9,* 201–209.

Barlow, D. H., & Hersen, M. (1984). *Single case experimental designs: Strategies for studying behavior change* (2nd ed.). New York: Pergamon Press.

Bauman, L. J., Wright, E., Leickly, F. E., Crain, E., Kruszon-Moran, D., Wade, S. L., et al. (2002). Relationship of adherence to pediatric asthma morbidity among inner-city children. *Pediatrics, 110,* 1–7.

Beck, D. E., Fennell, R. S., Yost, R. L., Robinson, J. D., Geary, D., & Richards, G. A. (1980). Evaluation of an educational program on compliance with medication regimens in pediatric patients with renal transplants. *Journal of Pediatrics, 96,* 1094–1097.

Bender, B. G., Pedan, A., & Varasteh, L. T. (2006). Adherence and persistence with fluticasone propionate/salmeterol combination therapy. *Journal of Allergy & Clinical Immunology, 118,* 899–904.

Bloom, B. R., & Murray, C. J. L. (1992). Tuberculosis: Commentary on a reemergent killer. *Science, 257,* 1055–1064.

Blowey, D. L., Hébert, D., Arbus, G. S., Pool, R., Korus, M., & Koren, G. (1997). Compliance with cyclosporine in adolescent renal transplant recipients. *Pediatric Nephrology, 11,* 547–551.

Bobrow, E. S., AvRuskin, T. W., & Siller, J., (1985). Mother-daughter interaction and adherence to diabetes regimens. *Diabetes Care, 8,* 146–151.

Bond, G. G., Aiken, L. S., & Somerville, S. C. (1992). The health belief model and adolescents with insulin-dependent diabetes mellitus. *Health Psychology, 11,* 190–198.

Brownbridge, G., & Fielding, D. M. (1994). Psychosocial adjustment and adherence to dialysis treatment regimes. *Pediatric Nephrology, 8,* 744–749.

Burroughs, T. E., Pontious, S. L., & Santiago, J. V. (1993). The relationship among six psychosocial domains: Age, health care adherence, and metabolic control in adolescents with IDDM. *Diabetes Educator, 19,* 396–402.

Buston, K. M., & Wood, S. F. (2000). Non-compliance amongst adolescents with asthma: Listening to what they tell us about self-management. *Family Practice, 17,* 134–138.

Carney, R. M., Schechter, K., & Davis, T. (1983). Improving adherence to blood glucose testing in insulin-dependent diabetic children. *Behavior Therapy, 14,* 247–254.

Cassell, E. J. (1991). *The nature of suffering.* New York: Oxford University Press.

Celano, M., Geller, R. J., Phillips, K. M., & Ziman, R. (1998). Treatment adherence among low-income children with asthma. *Journal of Pediatric Psychology, 23,* 345–349.

Chan, D. S., Callahan, C. W., Hatch-Pigott, V. B., Lawless, A., Proffitt, H., Manning, N. E., et al. (2007). Internet-based home monitoring and education of children with asthma is comparable to ideal office-based care: Results of a 1-year asthma in-home monitoring trial. *Pediatrics, 119,* 569–578.

Cleemput, I., Kesteloot, K., & DeGeest, S. (2002). A review of the literature on the economics of noncompliance. Room for methodological improvement. *Health Policy, 59,* 65–94.

Coleman, J. C., & Hendry, L. (1990). *The nature of adolescence* (2nd ed.). New York: Routledge.

Coutts, J. A. P., Gibson, N. A., & Paton, J. Y. (1992). Measuring compliance with inhaled medication in asthma. *Archives of Diseases of Children, 67,* 332–333.

Crockett, L. J., & Petersen, A. C. (1993). Adolescent development: Health risks and opportunities for health promotion. In S. G. Millstein, A. C. Petersen, & E. O. Nightingale (Eds.), *Promoting the health of adolescents: New directions for the twenty-first century* (pp. 13–37). New York: Oxford University Press.

Czajkowski, D. R., & Koucher, G. P. (1987). Medical compliance and coping with cystic fibrosis. *Journal of Child Psychology and Psychiatry, 28,* 311–319.

Darling, N., & Steinberg, L. (1993). Parenting style as context: An integrative model. *Psychological Bulletin, 113,* 487–496.

Davis, M. A., Quittner, A. L., Stack, C. M., & Yang, M. C. K. (2004). Controlled evaluation of the STARBRIGHT CD-ROM program for children and adolescents with cystic fibrosis. *Journal of Pediatric Psychology, 29,* 259–267.

Diabetes Control and Complications Trial Research Group. (1994). Effect of intensive diabetes treatment on the development and progression of long term complications in adolescents with insulin-dependent diabetes mellitus: Diabetes Control and Complications Trial. *Journal of Pediatrics, 125,* 177–188.

DiMatteo, M. R., & DiNicola, D. D. (1982). *Achieving patient compliance: The psychology of the medical practitioner's role.* New York: Pergamon Press.

Dolezal, C., Mellins, C., Brackis-Cott, E., & Abrams, E. J. (2003). The reliability of reports of medical adherence from children with HIV and their adult caregivers. *Journal of Pediatric Psychology, 28,* 355–361.

Dunbar-Jacob, J. (1993). Contributions to patient adherence: Is it time to share the blame? *Health Psychology, 12,* 91–92.

Elliott, D. S. (1993). Health-enhancing and health-compromising lifestyles. In S. G. Millstein, A. C. Petersen, & E. O. Nightingale (Eds.), *Promoting the health of adolescents: New directions for the twenty-first century* (pp. 119–145). New York: Oxford University Press.

Ellis, D. A., Frey, M. A., Naar-King, S., Templin, T., Cunningham, P., & Cakan, N. (2005). Use of multisystemic therapy to improve regimen adherence among adolescents with type 1 diabetes in chronic poor metabolic control. *Diabetes Care, 28,* 1604–1610.

Ellis, D. A., Yopp, J., Templin, T., Naar-King, S., Frey, M. A., Cunningham, P. B., et al. (2007). Family mediators and moderators of treatment outcomes among youths with poorly controlled type 1 diabetes: Results from a randomized controlled trial. *Journal of Pediatric Psychology, 32,* 194–205.

Eney, R. D., & Goldstein, E. O. (1976). Compliance of chronic asthmatics with oral administration of theophylline as measured by serum and salivary levels. *Pediatrics, 57,* 513–517.

Epstein, L. H., Figueroa, J., Farkas, G. M., & Beck, S. (1981). The short-term effects of feedback on accuracy of urine glucose determinations in insulin dependent diabetic children. *Behavior Therapy, 12,* 560–564.

Ettenger, R. B., Rosenthal, J. T., Marik, J. L., Malekzadeh, M., Forsythe, S. B., Kamil, E. S., et al. (1991). Improved cadaveric renal transplant outcomes in children. *Pediatric Nephrology, 5,* 137–142.

Feinstein, S., Keich, R., Becker-Cohen, R., Rinat, C., Schwartz, S. B., & Frishberg, Y. (2005). Is noncompliance among adolescent renal transplant recipients inevitable? *Pediatrics, 115,* 969–973.

Feldman, D. E., De Civita, M., Dobkin, P. L., Malleson, P., Meshefedjian, G., & Duffy, C. (2007). Perceived adherence to prescribed treatment in juvenile idiopathic arthritis over a one-year period. *Arthritis Care & Research, 57,* 226–233.

Fennell, R. S., Tucker, C., & Pedersen, T. (2001). Demographic and medical predictors of medication compliance among ethnically different pediatric renal transplant patients. *Pediatric Transplantation, 5,* 343–348.

Festa, R. S., Tamaroff, M. H., Chasalow, F., & Lanzkowsky, P. (1992). Therapeutic adherence to oral medication regimens by adolescents with cancer. I. Laboratory assessment. *Journal of Pediatrics, 120,* 807–811.

Fletcher, R. H., Fletcher, S. W., & Wagner, E. H. (1988). *Clinical epidemiology: The essentials* (2nd ed.). Baltimore: Williams & Wilkins.

Friedman, I. M., & Litt, I. F. (1987). Adolescents' compliance with therapeutic regimens. *Journal of Adolescent Health Care, 8,* 52–67.

Friedman, I. M., Litt, I. F., King, D. R., Henson, R., Holtzman, D., Halverson, D., et al. (1986). Compliance with anticonvulsant therapy by epileptic youth. *Journal of Adolescent Health Care, 7,* 12–17.

Garvie, P. A., Lensing, S., & Rai, S. N. (2007). Efficacy of pill-swallowing training intervention to improve antiretroviral medication adherence in pediatric patients with HIV/AIDS. *Pediatrics, 119,* 893–899.

Gavin, L. A., Wamboldt, M. Z., Sorokin, N., Levy, S. Y., & Wamboldt, F. S. (1999). Treatment alliance and its association with family functioning, adherence, and medical outcome in adolescents with severe, chronic asthma. *Journal of Pediatric Psychology, 24,* 355–365.

Geiss, S. K., Hobbs, S. A., Hammersley-Maercklein, F., Kramer, J. C., & Henley, M. (1992). Psychosocial factors related to perceived compliance with cystic fibrosis treatment. *Journal of Clinical Psychology, 48,* 99–103.

Gerson, A. C., Furth, S. L., Neu, A. M., & Fivush, B. A. (2004). Assessing associations between medication adherence and potentially modifiable psychosocial variables in pediatric kidney transplant recipients and their families. *Pediatric Transplantation, 8,* 543–550.

Gibbons, A. (1992). Exploring new strategies to fight drug-resistant microbes. *Science, 257,* 1036–1038.

Glaser, R., & Bassok, M. (1989). Learning theory and the study of instruction. *Annual Review of Psychology, 40,* 631–666.

Glasgow, R. E., McCaul, K. D., & Schafer, L. C. (1986). Barriers to regimen adherence among persons with insulin-dependent diabetes. *Journal of Behavioral Medicine, 9,* 65–77.

Greening, L., Stoppelbein, L., Konishi, C., Jordan, S. S., & Moll, G. (2007). Child routines and youths' adherence to treatment for type 1 diabetes. *Journal of Pediatric Psychology, 32,* 437–447.

Gudas, L. J., Koocher, G. P., & Wypij, D. (1991). Perceptions of medical compliance in children and adolescents with cystic fibrosis. *Journal of Developmental and Behavioral Pediatrics, 12,* 236–242.

Hammami, N., Nöstlinger, C., Hoerée, T., Lefèvre, P., Jonckheer, T., & Kilsteren, P. (2004). Integrating adherence to highly active antiretroviral therapy into children's daily lives: A qualitative study. *Pediatrics, 114,* 591–597.

Hauser, S. T., Jacobson, A. M., Lavori, P., Wolfsdorf, J. I., Herskowitz, R. D., Milley, J. E., et al. (1990). Adherence among children and adolescents with insulin-dependent diabetes mellitus over a four-year longitudinal follow-up. II. Immediate and long-term linkages with the family milieu. *Journal of Pediatric Psychology, 15,* 527–541.

Haynes, R. B., & Dantes, R. (1987). Patient compliance and the conduct and interpretation of therapeutic trials. *Controlled Clinical Trials, 8,* 12–19.

Haynes, S. N. (1992). *Models of causality in psychopathology.* New York: Macmillian.

Hazzard, A., Hutchinson, S. J., & Krawiecki, N. (1990). Factors related to adherence to medication regimens in pediatric seizure patients. *Journal of Pediatric Psychology, 15,* 543–555.

Hentinen, M., & Kyngas, H. (1992). Compliance of young diabetics with health regimens. *Journal of Advanced Nursing, 17,* 530–536.

Holden, E. W., & Nitz, K. (1995). Epidemiology of adolescent health disorders. In J. L. Wallander & L. J. Siegel (Eds.), *Adolescent health problems: Behavioral perspectives* (pp. 7–21). New York: Guilford Press.

Holmes, C. S., Chen, R., Streisand, R., Marschall, D. E., Souter, S., Swift, E. E., et al. (2006). Predictors of youth diabetes care behaviors and metabolic control: A structural equation modeling approach. *Journal of Pediatric Psychology, 31,* 770–784.

Ievers, C. E., Drotar, D., Dahms, W. T., Doershuk, C. F., & Stern, R. S. (1994). Maternal child-rearing behavior in three groups: Cystic fibrosis, insulin-dependent diabetes mellitus, and healthy children. *Journal of Pediatric Psychology, 19,* 681–687.

Ingersoll, G. M., Orr, D. P., Herrold, A. J., & Golden, M. P. (1986). Cognitive maturity and self-management among adolescents with insulin-dependent diabetes mellitus. *Journal of Pediatrics, 108,* 620–623.

Jacobson, A. M., Hauser, S. T., Lavori, P., Wolfsdorf, J. I., Herskowitz, R. D., Milley, J. E., et al. (1990). Adherence among children and adolescents with insulin-dependent diabetes mellitus over a four-year longitudinal follow-up. I. The influence of patient coping and adjustment. *Journal of Pediatric Psychology, 15,* 511–526.

Jacobson, A. M., Hauser, S. T., Wolfsdorf, J. I., Houlihan, J., Milley, J. E., Herskowitz, R. D., et al. (1987). Psychologic predictors of compliance in children with recent onset of diabetes mellitus. *Journal of Pediatrics, 110,* 805–811.

Janz, N. K., & Becker, M. H. (1984). The health belief model: A decade later. *Health Education Quarterly, 11,* 1–47.

Jarzembowski, T., John, E., Panaro, F., Heiliczer, J., Kraft, K., Bogetti, D., et al. (2004). Impact of non-compliance on outcome after pediatric kidney transplantation: An analysis in racial subgroups. *Pediatric Transplantation, 8,* 367–371.

Jay, S., Litt, I. F., & Durant, R. H. (1984). Compliance with therapeutic regimens. *Journal of Adolescent Health Care, 5,* 124–136.

Jensen, S. A., Elkin, T. D., Hilker, K., Jordan, S., Iyer, R., & Smith, M. G. (2005). Caregiver knowledge and adherence in children with sickle cell disease: Knowing is not doing. *Journal of Clinical Psychology in Medical Settings, 12,* 333–348.

Johnson, S. B., Freund, A., Silverstein, J., Hansen, C. A., & Malone, J. (1990). Adherence-health status relationships in childhood diabetes. *Health Psychology, 9,* 606–631.

Johnson, S. B., Kelly, M., Henretta, J. C., Cunningham, W. R., Tomer, A., & Silverstein, J. H. (1992). A longitudinal analysis of adherence and health status in childhood diabetes. *Journal of Pediatric Psychology, 17,* 537–553.

Jónasson, G., Carlsen, K.-H., & Mowinckel, P. (2000). Asthma drug adherence in a long term clinical trial. *Archives of Disease in Childhood, 83,* 330–333.

Kelloway, J. S., Wyatt, R. A., & Adlis, S. A. (1994). Comparison of patients' compliance with prescribed oral and inhaled asthma medications. *Archives of Internal Medicine, 154,* 1349–1352.

Kennard, B. D., Stewart, S. M., Olvera, R., Bawdon, R. E., O hAilin, A., Lewis, C. P., et al. (2004). Nonadherence in adolescent oncology patients: Preliminary data on psychological risk factors and relationship to outcome. *Journal of Clinical Psychology in Medical Settings, 11,* 31–39.

Kovacs, M., Goldston, D., Obrosky, S., & Iyengar, S. (1992). Prevalence and predictors of pervasive noncompliance with medical treatment among youths with insulin-dependent diabetes mellitus. *Journal of American Academy of Child and Adolescent Psychiatry, 31,* 1112–1119.

Kurtin, P. S., Landgraf, J. M., & Abetz, L. (1994). Patient-based health status measurements in pediatric dialysis: Expanding the assessment of outcome. *American Journal of Kidney Diseases, 24,* 376–382.

Kuttner, M. J., Delamater, A. M., & Santiago, J. V. (1990). Learned helplessness in diabetic youths. *Journal of Pediatric Psychology, 15,* 581–594.

Kvien, T. K., & Reimers, S. (1983). Drug handling and patient compliance in an outpatient paediatric trial. *Journal of Clinical & Hospital Pharmacy, 8,* 251–257.

Kyngäs, H. (2002). Motivation as a crucial predictor of good compliance in adolescents with rheumatoid arthritis. *International Journal of Nursing Practice, 8,* 336–341.

La Greca, A. M., Auslander, W. F., Greco, P., Spetter, D., Fisher, E. B., & Santiago, J. V. (1995). I get by with a little help from my family and friends: Adolescents' support for diabetes care. *Journal of Pediatric Psychology, 20,* 449–476.

La Greca, A. M., Follansbee, D., & Skyler, J. S. (1990). Developmental and behavioral aspects of diabetes management in youngsters. *Children's Health Care, 19,* 132–139.

Lancaster, D., Lennard, L., & Lilleyman, J. S. (1997). Profile of non-compliance in lymphoblastic leukaemia. *Archives of Disease in Childhood, 76,* 365–366.

Lansky, S. B., Smith, S. D., Cairns, N. U., & Cairns, G. F. (1983). Psychological correlates of compliance. *American Journal of Pediatric Hematology/Oncology, 5,* 87–92.

Lau, R. C. W., Matsui, D., Greenberg, M., & Koren, G. (1998). Electronic measurement of compliance with mercaptopurine in pediatric patients with acute lymphoblastic leukemia. *Medical and Pediatric Oncology, 30,* 85–90.

Lewandowski, A., & Drotar, D. (2007). The relationship between parent-reported social support and adherence to medical treatment in families of adolescents with type 1 diabetes. *Journal of Pediatric Psychology, 32,* 427–436.

Lewin, A. B., Heidgerken, A. D., Geffken, G. R., Williams, L. B., Storch, E. A., Gelfand, K. M., et al. (2006). The relation between family factors and metabolic control: The role of diabetes adherence. *Journal of Pediatric Psychology, 31,* 174–183.

Litt, I. F., & Cuskey, W. R. (1981). Compliance with salicylate therapy in adolescents with juvenile rheumatoid arthritis. *American Journal of Diseases of Children, 135,* 434–436.

Litt, I. F., Cuskey, W. R., & Rosenberg, B. A. (1982). Role of self-esteem and autonomy in determining medication compliance among adolescents with juvenile rheumatoid arthritis. *Pediatrics, 69,* 15–17.

Lorenz, R. A., Christensen, N. K., & Pichert, J. W. (1985). Diet-related knowledge, skill, and adherence among children with insulin-dependent diabetes mellitus. *Pediatrics, 75,* 872–876.

Lovell, D. J., Giannini, E. H., & Brewer, E. J. (1984). Time course of response to nonsteroidal antiinflammatory drugs in juvenile rheumatoid arthritis. *Arthritis and Rheumatism, 27,* 1433–1437.

Lurie, S., Shemesh, E., Sheiner, P. A., Emre, S., Tindle, H. L., Melchionna, L., et al. (2000). Nonadherence in pediatric liver transplant recipients—an assessment of risk factors and natural history. *Pediatric Transplantation, 4,* 200–206.

Lutfey, K. E., & Wishner, W. J. (1999). Beyond "compliance" is "adherence." *Diabetes Care, 22,* 635–639.

Magee, J. C., Bucuvalas, J. C., Farmer, D. G., Harmon, W. E., Hulbert-Shearon, T. E., & Mendeloff, E. N. (2004). Pediatric transplantation. *American Journal of Transplantation, 4,* 54–71.

McCaul, K. D., Glasgow, R. E., & Schafer, L. C. (1987). Diabetes regimen behaviors: Predicting adherence. *Medical Care, 25,* 868–881.

McCormick, M. C., Stemmler, M. M., & Athreya, B. H. (1986). The impact of childhood rheumatic diseases on the family. *Arthritis and Rheumatism, 29,* 872–879.

McPherson, A. C., Glazebrook, C., Forster, D., James, C., & Smyth, A. (2006). A randomized, controlled trial of an interactive educational computer package for children with asthma. *Pediatrics, 117,* 1046–1054.

McQuaid, E. L., Kopel, S. J., Klein, R. B., & Fritz, G. K. (2003). Medication adherence in pediatric asthma: Reasoning, responsibility, and behavior. *Journal of Pediatric Psychology, 28,* 323–333.

McQuaid, E. L., Walders, N., Kopel, S. J., Fritz, G. K., & Klinnert, M. D. (2005). Pediatric asthma management in the family context: The family asthma management system scale. *Journal of Pediatric Psychology, 30,* 492–502.

Meichenbaum, D., & Turk, D. C. (1987). *Facilitating treatment adherence: A practitioner's guidebook.* New York: Plenum Press.

Miller, V. A., & Drotar, D. (2003). Discrepancies between mother and adolescent perceptions of diabetes-related decision-making autonomy and their relationship to diabetes-related conflict and adherence to treatment. *Journal of Pediatric Psychology, 28,* 265–274.

Miller, V. A., & Drotar, D. (2007). Decision-making competence and adherence to treatment in adolescents with diabetes. *Journal of Pediatric Psychology, 32,* 178–188.

Modi, A. C., & Quittner, A. L. (2006). Barriers to treatment adherence for children with cystic fibrosis and asthma: What gets in the way? *Journal of Pediatric Psychology, 31,* 846–858.

Naar-King, S., Idalski, A., Ellis, D., Frey, M., Templin, T., Cunningham, P. B., et al. (2006). Gender differences in adherence and metabolic control in urban youth with poorly controlled type 1 diabetes: The mediating role of mental health symptoms. *Journal of Pediatric Psychology, 31,* 793–802.

National Pharmaceutical Council. (1994). *Noncompliance with medications: An economic tragedy with important implications for health care reform.* Baltimore: National Pharmaceutical Council.

Newacheck, P. W. (1989). Adolescents with special health needs: Prevalence, severity, and access to health services. *Pediatrics, 85,* 872–881.

Newacheck, P. W., & Taylor, W. R. (1992). Childhood chronic illness: Prevalence, severity, and impact. *American Journal of Public Health, 82,* 364–371.

Passero, M. A., Remor, B., & Salomon, J. (1981). Patient-reported compliance with cystic fibrosis therapy. *Clinical Pediatrics, 20,* 264–268.

Patino, A. M., Sanchez, J., Eidson, M., & Delamater, A. M. (2005). Health beliefs and regimen adherence in minority adolescents with type 1 diabetes. *Journal of Pediatric Psychology, 30,* 503–512.

Patterson, J. M. (1985). Critical factors affecting family compliance with home treatment for children with cystic fibrosis. *Family Relations, 34,* 79–89.

Penkower, L., Dew, M. A., Ellis, D., Sereika, S. M., Kitutu, J. M. M., & Shapiro, R. (2003). Psychological distress and adherence to the medical regimen among adolescent renal transplant recipients. *American Journal of Transplantation, 3,* 1418–1425.

Phipps, S., & DeCuir-Whalley, S. (1990). Adherence issues in pediatric bone marrow transplantation. *Journal of Pediatric Psychology, 15,* 459–475.

Pieper, K. B., Rapoff, M. A., Purviance, M. R., & Lindsley, C. B. (1989). Improving compliance with prednisone therapy in pediatric patients with rheumatic disease. *Arthritis Care and Research, 2,* 132–135.

Powers, S. W., Piazza-Waggoner, C., Jones, J. S., Ferguson, K. S., Daines, C., & Acton, J. D. (2006). Examining clinical trial results with single-subject analysis: An example involving behavioral and nutrition treatment for young children with cystic fibrosis. *Journal of Pediatric Psychology, 31,* 574–581.

Radius, S. M., Becker, M. H., Rosenstock, I. M., Drachman, R. H., Schuberth, K. C., & Teets, K. C. (1978). Factors influencing mother's compliance with a medication regimen for asthmatic children. *Journal of Asthma Research, 15,* 133–149.

Rapoff, M. A. (1989). Compliance with treatment regimens for pediatric rheumatic diseases. *Arthritis Care and Research, 2,* S40–S47.

Rapoff, M. A. (1994). *Helping children follow their medical treatment program: Guidelines for parents of children with rheumatic diseases.* Available from Michael Rapoff, PhD, University of Kansas Medical Center, Department of Pediatrics, 3901 Rainbow Blvd., Kansas City, KS 66160–7330.

Rapoff, M. A. (1996). Why comply? Theories in pediatric medical adherence research. *Progress Notes: Newsletter of the Society of Pediatric Psychology, 20*(2–3), 6.

Rapoff, M. A. (1999). *Adherence to pediatric medical regimens.* New York: Kluwer/Plenum.

Rapoff, M. A., & Barnard, M. U. (1991). Compliance with pediatric medical regimens. In J. A. Cramer & B. Spilker (Eds.), *Patient compliance in medical practice and clinical trials* (pp. 73–98). New York: Raven Press.

Rapoff, M. A., Belmont, J. M., Lindsley, C. B., & Olson, N. Y. (2005). Electronically monitored adherence to medications by newly diagnosed patients with juvenile rheumatoid arthritis. *Arthritis Care & Research, 53,* 905–910.

Rapoff, M. A., Belmont, J., Lindsley, C. B., Olson, N. Y., & Padur, J. (2002). Prevention of nonadherence to non-steroidal anti-inflammatory medications for newly diagnosed patients with juvenile rheumatoid arthritis. *Health Psychology, 21,* 620–623.

Rapoff, M. A., & Christophersen, E. R. (1982). Compliance of pediatric patients with medical regimens: A review and evaluation. In R. B. Stuart (Ed.), *Adherence, compliance and generalization in behavioral medicine* (pp. 79–124). New York: Brunner/Mazel.

Rapoff, M. A., Lindsley, C. B., & Christophersen, E. R. (1985). Parent perceptions of problems experienced by their children in complying with treatments for juvenile rheumatoid arthritis. *Archives of Physical Medicine and Rehabilitation, 66,* 427–429.

Rapoff, M. A., Purviance, M. R., & Lindsley, C. B. (1988a). Improving medication compliance for juvenile rheumatoid arthritis and its effect on clinical outcome: A single subject analysis. *Arthritis Care and Research, 1,* 1–5.

Rapoff, M. A., Purviance, M. R., & Lindsley, C. B. (1988b). Educational and behavioral strategies for improving medication compliance in juvenile rheumatoid arthritis. *Archives of Physical Medicine and Rehabilitation, 69,* 439–441.

Reese, H. W. (1989). Rules and rule-governance: Cognitive and behavioristic views. In S. C. Hayes (Ed.), *Rule-governed behavior: Cognition, contingencies, and instructional control* (pp. 3–84). New York: Plenum Press.

Satin, W., La Greca, A. M., Zigo, M. A., & Skyler, J. S. (1989). Diabetes in adolescence: Effects of a multifamily group intervention and parent simulation of diabetes. *Journal of Pediatric Psychology, 14,* 259–275.

Schafer, L. C., Glasgow, R. E., & McCaul, K. D. (1982). Increasing the adherence of diabetic adolescents. *Journal of Behavioral Medicine, 5,* 353–362.

Schmidt, L. E., Klover, R. V., Arfken, C. L., Delamater, A. M., & Hobson, D. (1992). Compliance with dietary prescriptions in children and adolescents with insulin-dependent diabetes mellitus. *Journal of the American Dietetic Association, 92,* 567–570.

Serrano-Ikkos, E., Lask, B., Whitehead, B., & Eisler, I. (1998). Incomplete adherence after pediatric heart and heart-lung transplantation. *Journal of Heart & Lung Transplantation, 17,* 1177–1183.

Shemesh, E., Shneider, B. L., Savitzky, J. K., Arnott, L., Gondolesi, G. E., Krieger, N. R., et al. (2004). Medication adherence in pediatric and adolescent liver transplant recipients. *Pediatrics, 113,* 825–832.

Simmons, F. E. R., Gerstner, T. V., & Cheang, M. S. (1997). Tolerance to bronchoprotective effect of salmeterol in adolescents with exercise-induced asthma using concurrent inhaled glucocorticoid treatment. *Pediatrics, 99,* 655–659.

Slack, M. K., & Brooks, A. J. (1995). Medication management issues for adolescents with asthma. *American Journal of Health-System Pharmacy, 52,* 1417–1421.

Smith, M. (1985). The cost of noncompliance and the capacity of improved compliance to reduce health care expenditures. In *Improving medication compliance: Proceedings of a symposium.* Washington, DC: National Pharmaceutical Council.

Smith, S. D., Rosen, D., Trueworthy, R. C., & Lowman, J. T. (1979). A reliable method for evaluation drug compliance in children with cancer. *Cancer, 43,* 169–173.

Snodgrasss, S. R., Vedanarayanan, V. V., Parker, C. C., & Parks, B. R. (2001). Pediatric patients with undetectable anticonvulsant blood levels: Comparison with compliant patients. *Journal of Child Neurology, 16,* 164–168.

Snyder, J. (1987). Behavioral analysis and treatment of poor diabetic self-care and antisocial behavior: A single-subject experimental study. *Behavior Therapy, 18,* 251–263.

Sokol, M., McGuigan, K. A., Verbrugge, R. R., & Epstein, R. S. (2005). Impact of medication adherence on hospitalization risk and healthcare cost. *Medical Care, 43,* 521–530.

Steele, R. G., & Grauer, D. (2003). Adherence to antiretroviral therapy for pediatric HIV infection: Review of the literature and recommendations for research. *Clinical Child & Family Psychology Review, 6,* 17–30.

Stein, R. E. K., & Jessop, D. J. (1989). What diagnosis does not tell: The case for a noncategorical approach to chronic illness in childhood. *Social Science and Medicine, 29,* 769–778.

Stewart, S. M., Lee, P. W. H., Waller, D., Hughes, C. W., Low, L. C. K., Kennard, B. D., et al. (2003). A follow-up study of adherence and glycemic control among Hong Kong youths with diabetes. *Journal of Pediatric Psychology, 28,* 67–79.

Stuber, M. (1993). Psychiatric aspects of organ transplantation in children and adolescents. *Organ Transplantation in Children and Adolescents, 34,* 379–387.

Tamaroff, M. H., Festa, R. S., Adesman, A. R., & Walco, G. A., (1992). Therapeutic adherence to oral medication regimens by adolescents with cancer. II. Clinical and psychologic correlates, *Journal of Pediatrics, 120,* 812–817.

Tebbi, C. K., Cummings, K. M., Zevon, M., Smith, L., Richards, J., & Mallon, J. (1986). Compliance of pediatric and adolescent cancer patients. *Cancer, 58,* 1179–1184.

Tebbi, C. K., Richards, M. E., Cummings, K. M., Zevon, M. A., & Mallon, J. (1988). The role of parent-adolescent concordance in compliance with cancer chemotherapy. *Adolescence, 23,* 599–611.

Tinkelman, D. G., Vanderpool, G. E., Carroll, M. S., Page, E. G., & Spangler, D. L. (1980). Compliance differences following administration of theophylline at six- and twelve-hour intervals. *Annals of Allergy, 44,* 283–286.

Tucker, C. M., Fennell, R. S., Pedersen, T., Higley, B. P., Wallack, C. E., & Peterson, S. (2002). Associations with medication adherence among ethnically different pediatric patients with renal transplants. *Pediatric Nephrology, 17,* 251–256.

Tucker, C. M., Petersen, S., Herman, K. C., Fennell, R. S., Bowling, B., Pedersen, T., et al. (2001). Self-regulation predictors of medication adherence among ethnically different pediatric patients with renal transplants. *Journal of Pediatric Psychology, 26,* 455–464.

Van Dyke, R. B., Lee, S., Johnson, G. M., Wiznia, A., Mohan, K., Stanley, K., et al. (2002). Reported adherence as a determinant of response to highly active antiretroviral therapy in children who have human immunodeficiency virus infection. *Pediatrics, 109,* 1–7.

Van Es, S. M., le Coq, E. M., Brouwer, A. I., Mesters, I., Nagelkerke, A. F., & Colland, V. T. (1998). Adherence-related behavior in adolescents with asthma: Results from focus group interviews. *Journal of Asthma, 35,* 637–646.

Varni, J. W., & Wallander, J. L. (1984). Adherence to health-related regimens in pediatric chronic disorders. *Clinical Psychology Review, 4,* 585–596.

Walders, N., Drotar, D., & Kercsmar, C. (2000). The allocation of family responsibility for asthma management tasks in African-American adolescents. *Journal of Asthma, 37,* 89–99.

Walders, N., Kopel, S. J., Koins-Mitchell, D., & McQuaid, E. L. (2005). Patterns of quick-relief and long-term controller medication use in pediatric asthma. *Journal of Pediatrics, 146,* 177–182.

Walker, L. S., Garber, J., & Van Slyke, D. A. (1995). Do parents excuse the misbehavior of children with physical or emotional symptoms? An investigation of the pediatric sick role. *Journal of Pediatric Psychology, 20,* 329–345.

Weinstein, A. G., & Faust, D. (1997). Maintaining theophylline compliance/adherence in severely asthmatic children: The role of psychologic functioning of the child and family. *Annals of Allergy, Asthma & Immunology, 79,* 311–318.

Wiebe, D. J., Berg, C. A., Korbel, C., Palmer, D. L., Beveridge, R. M., Upchurch, R., et al. (2005). Children's appraisals of maternal involvement in coping with diabetes: Enhancing our understanding of adherence, metabolic control, and quality of life across adolescence. *Journal of Pediatric Psychology, 30,* 167–178.

Williams, P. L., Storm, D., Montepiedra, G., Nichols, S., Kammerer, B., Sirois, P. A., et al. (2006). Predictors of adherence to antiretroviral medications in children and adolescents with HIV infection. *Pediatrics, 118,* 1745–1757.

Wilson, D. P., & Endres, R. K. (1986). Compliance with blood glucose monitoring in children with type I diabetes mellitus. *Journal of Pediatrics, 108,* 1022–1024.

Wing, R. R., Koeske, R., New, A., Lamparski, D., & Becker, D. (1986). Behavioral skills in self-monitoring of blood glucose: Relationship to accuracy. *Diabetes Care, 9,* 330–333.

World Health Organization. (2003). *Adherence to long-term therapies: Evidence for action.* Geneva, Switzerland.

Wynn, K. S., & Eckel, E. M. (1986). Juvenile rheumatoid arthritis and home physical therapy program compliance. *Physical & Occupational Therapy in Pediatrics, 6,* 55–63.

Wysocki, T., & Gavin, L. (2006). Paternal involvement in the management of pediatric chronic diseases: Associations with adherence, quality of life, and health status. *Journal of Pediatric Psychology, 31,* 501–511.

Wysocki, T., Green, L., & Huxtable, K. (1989). Blood glucose monitoring by diabetic adolescents: Compliance and metabolic control. *Health Psychology, 8,* 267–284.

Wysocki, T., Harris, M. A., Buckloh, L. M., Mertlich, D., Lochrie, A. S., Taylor, A., et al. (2006). Effects of behavioral family systems therapy for diabetes on adolescents' family relationships, treatment adherence, and metabolic control. *Journal of Pediatric Psychology, 31,* 928–938.

Health Disparities and Minority Health

29

Melicia C.
Whitt-Glover,
Bettina M. Beech,
Ronny A. Bell,
Sharon A. Jackson,
Kismet A. Loftin-Bell,
and David L. Mount

In 2005, the total U.S. population was 288,378,137 and was composed of a large proportion of racial and ethnic minorities (~26%), including ~35 million Blacks/African Americans (12.1%), ~12.5 million Asians (4.3%), ~2.4 million American Indian and Alaska Natives (0.8%), nearly 400,000 Native Hawaiians and other Pacific Islanders (0.1%), and ~42 million Hispanics/Latinos (14.5%) (U.S. Census Bureau, 2005). Although racial and ethnic minorities make up only 26% of the U.S. population, they share a disproportionate burden of chronic disease. In 2004, 4 of the 10 leading causes of death among racial and ethnic minorities, as well as among the general population, were chronic diseases directly related to modifiable risk factors associated with lifestyle and clinical behaviors (National Center for Health Statistics, 2006). These chronic diseases were heart disease, cancer (specifically colon and breast cancer), diabetes, and stroke. For each of these health outcomes and their related risk factors, morbidity and mortality rates are also higher among racial and ethnic minorities than for non-Hispanic Whites.

The increased morbidity and mortality rates for chronic diseases among racial and ethnic minorities is associated with lower adherence to recommendations for healthy lifestyle and clinical behaviors. This may be related to reduced access to adequate health care (Hargraves, Cunningham, & Hughes, 2001; Hargraves & Hadley, 2003); lower participation in early and regular screening for disease (Bazargan, Bazargan, Farooq, & Baker, 2004; Wells & Roetzheim, 2007); and reduced access to resources associated with healthier lifestyles (e.g., parks, sources for healthy foods) (Gordon-Larsen, Nelson, Page, & Popkin, 2006; Taylor, Floyd, Whitt-Glover, & Brooks, 2007) among racial and ethnic minority groups, which leads to an increased burden on the health care system. Despite major advances in public health, medicine, economic prosperity, and wealth, disparities in morbidity and mortality rates for certain chronic diseases persisted into the current century and increased for some health outcomes (e.g., diabetes). Thus, addressing and reducing morbidity and mortality rates among minorities, particularly those health outcomes with modifiable risk factors, is a major public health priority. Such efforts will be integral to achieving the two overarching goals set forth in *Healthy People 2010*—increase the years of healthy life, and eliminate health disparities among different groups within the overall population (U.S. Department of Health and Human Services, 2000).

No consensus definition exists for the term "health disparity" or for the related terms "health inequality" and "health inequity." Generally, each of these terms refers to health-associated differences among groups. However, the terms "health inequity" and "health disparity" carry the additional connotation of health-associated differences that are judged to be ethically unfair and unjust. Definitions for the term "health disparity" have been proposed by various organizations and agencies. The National Institutes of Health (NIH) defines health disparities as "differences in the incidence, prevalence, mortality, and burden of diseases and other adverse health conditions that exist among specific population groups in the United States" (U.S. Department of Health and Human Services, 2002). Health disparities are measured by comparing the health of one group (usually defined as the reference group) to that of different groups. Health disparities reveal important information about the health of a population that is not as evident using population-wide health measures. Disparities indicate that certain groups of individuals are experiencing worse health or are at greater risk of poor health than are other groups in a population. Assessing the underlying causes of disparities can help provide policymakers, health care providers and educators, public health officials, and the lay public with important information related to how the distribution of efforts and resources is used to reduce or eliminate disparities.

In this chapter, we discuss adherence issues related to lifestyle and clinical behaviors among racial and ethnic minority groups. We highlight the prevalence of selected recommended lifestyle and clinical behaviors among racial and ethnic minorities, discuss factors associated with adherence and nonadherence to these recommended behaviors, and review several strategies for increasing adherence to recommended lifestyle and clinical behaviors among racial and ethnic minorities.

Prevalence of Selected Lifestyle and Clinical Behaviors Among Minority Populations

Lifestyle Behaviors

While some variation exists across studies and population subgroups, racial and ethnic minorities generally fare worse than non-Hispanic Whites in their rates of healthy lifestyle behaviors for primary and secondary disease prevention. Factors that may affect variations across these groups include age, gender, geographic region, socioeconomic status, and country of origin (for Hispanics and Asian Americans) or tribal affiliation (for American Indians).

Data from the National Health Interview Survey (Adams & Schoenborn, 2006) indicate that rates of physical inactivity and obesity are highest for African Americans and American Indians, with notably high rates for African American women. Rates of physical inactivity among African American women have declined significantly in recent years; the rate of physical inactivity among African American women was 45.7% in 1994 and 33.9% in 2004, but these rates remain higher than those of other racial and ethnic groups of women (Centers for Disease Control and Prevention, 2005). Rates of cigarette smoking are highest among American Indians, with nearly one-third of adults classified as current smokers. However, data from other sources indicate significant variation across tribes and regions in smoking rates and in the number of cigarettes consumed among current smokers (Denny, Holtzman, & Cobb, 2003; Levin, Welch, Bell, & Casper, 2002; Welty et al., 1995). Consumption of at least five alcoholic drinks in 1 day in the preceding year is highest for Native Hawaiians and other Pacific Islanders, non-Hispanic Whites, and American Indians and lowest for Asian Americans and African Americans (Adams & Schoenborn, 2006).

Racial and ethnic variations exist with regard to many of the nutritional factors associated with chronic diseases. Data from the Multi-Ethnic Cohort study showed that, among five ethnic groups, African Americans had the highest energy density from their diet and Japanese Americans had the lowest, which may partially explain the wide variations in body mass index in these populations (Howarth, Murphy, Wilkens, Hankin, & Kolonel, 2006). The 2000 National Health Interview Survey showed that intake of calories from fat was higher among both African American men and women than among Hispanic, non-Hispanic White, and other non-Hispanic men and women (Thompson et al., 2005). However, Hispanic men and women had higher levels of intake of fruits and vegetables and dietary fiber than did members of other racial and ethnic groups.

High rates of sexually transmitted diseases among many ethnic minority groups, particularly African Americans, largely reflect these groups' unsafe sexual practices. Data from the 2002 National Survey of Family Growth showed that African American young adults had higher rates of increased risk for HIV transmission than Hispanic and non-Hispanic White young adults (Anderson, Mosher, & Chandra, 2006). The differences were most pronounced among those who had lower levels of formal education. Nearly one-third of African American young adults with less than a high school education were at increased risk of HIV transmission, whereas approximately 15% of Hispanics and Whites had high risks of transmission. These rates dramatically decline to approximately 14% for African American college graduates, but there is no appreciable change with differences in education level for Hispanics and Whites (Anderson et al., 2006).

Clinical Behaviors

A number of clinical practices are recommended for prevention or management of acute and chronic illnesses and for general well-being (U.S. Preventive Services Task Force, 1989). Despite our wealth of knowledge about the importance of these practices in maintaining overall health and well-being, disparities continue to exist among racial and ethnic groups in the receipt of many of these services. Many of these disparities exist even after researchers control for socioeconomic status and access to health care providers.

Regular screening for some of the major forms of cancer, including breast and colon cancer, is important for early detection and effective treatment of these conditions (Maciosek, Solberg, Coffield, Edwards, & Goodman, 2006). Unfortunately, racial and ethnic minority women are less likely than White women to receive adequate mammography screening, and African American women in particular are more likely to have advanced tumors on diagnosis than are women from all other racial and ethnic minority groups (Smith-Bindman et al., 2006). Similarly, racial and ethnic minorities are less likely to receive colorectal cancer screening than are non-Hispanic Whites. Data from the 2000 National Health Interview Survey showed that Hispanics were 29% less likely and African Americans were 18% less likely to be adherent to colorectal cancer screening guidelines, defined as a sigmoidoscopy or proctoscopy test within the past 5 years, colonoscopy test within the past 10 years, or home fetal occult blood test within the last year (James, Greiner, Ellerbeck, Feng, & Ahluwalia, 2006).

One of the more sizable racial and ethnic disparities exists in the receipt of influenza and pneumococcal vaccinations, which African Americans are significantly less likely to obtain than members of other groups in the population (Egede & Zheng, 2003; Winston, Wortley, & Lees, 2006). Data from the 2000–2001 National Health Interview Survey showed that rates of pneumococcal vaccination among African American and Hispanic adults >65 years of age were nearly 50% lower than those for non-Hispanic Whites and nearly 25% lower for influenza vaccinations. This disparity exists even in uniformed health care settings such as the Veterans Administration health care system (Straits-Troster et al., 2006), and in high-risk populations such as those with diabetes (Brown et al., 2005).

Adherence and Nonadherence to Selected Lifestyle and Clinical Behaviors Among Minorities

Despite clinical recommendations for lifestyle and clinical behaviors related to improved health, the data presented in the previous section suggest that adherence to these recommendations is lower among racial and ethnic minorities than among non-Hispanic whites. Demographic characteristics such as age, education, income, and acculturation have a major impact on adherence to lifestyle behavior and clinical recommendations. Increasing age, education, and income are associated with increased adherence to recommendations for breast and cervical cancer screening and knowledge about cancer screening (Bazargan et al., 2004; Breitkopf, Pearson, & Breitkopf, 2005; Halbert et al., 2006; Jennings-Dozier & Lawrence, 2000; Juon, Kim, Shankar, & Han, 2004; Leong-Wu & Fernandez, 2006; Rosenberg, Wise, Palmer, Horton, & Adams-Campbell, 2005; Russell, Champion, & Skinner, 2006). Increasing age has also been associated with lower levels of participation in healthy lifestyle behaviors such as participating in physical activity and following dietary recommendations (Berrigan, Troiano, McNeel, DiSogra, & Ballard-Barbash, 2006; Weir et al., 2000). Data suggest that those more likely to adhere to dietary recommendations include those with higher levels of education, Hispanics older than 31 years, Hispanic women, and unacculturated Hispanics (Hulme et al., 2003). Those least likely to adhere to dietary recommendations include Korean Americans (Kim, Ahn, Chon, Bowen, & Khan, 2005). Being single or not living with a partner has been associated with adherence to safe sexual practices, including using a female condom and being tested for HIV (Sly et al., 1997) and engaging in increased levels of physical activity (Weir et al., 2000).

Acculturation impacts adherence to certain lifestyle health behaviors. Among Asian Americans, speaking fluent English and the number of years in the United States is associated with adherence to recommendations for mammography screening (Juon et al., 2004; Leong-Wu & Fernandez, 2006). The evidence for Hispanic women is less clear. A study of cervical cancer screening showed that better ability to speak English was associated with lower likelihood of screening among underserved Hispanic women (Bazargan et al., 2004). A separate study found that Hispanic women who reported adherence to Pap smear screening recommendations were more likely to have been born in the mainland United States and to speak English at home than were those who were nonadherent (Jennings-Dozier & Lawrence, 2000). Lower adherence to recommendations for self-monitoring of blood glucose levels among Hispanics and Asian and Pacific Islanders was associated with difficulties communicating in English or preferring a language other than English (Karter, Ferrara, Darbinian, Ackerson, & Selby, 2000). Adherence to general healthy behaviors among Hispanics has been associated with acculturation (increased acculturation is related to increased adherence) (Hulme et al., 2003).

Many factors that are specific to the patient can impact adherence to recommendations for clinical and lifestyle behaviors. Among the most important factors is the perception of barriers. Data suggest that individuals, regardless of racial and ethnic minority status, who perceive fewer barriers and have greater self-efficacy are more likely to adhere to recommendations for clinical behaviors. For example, Black women who had had five mammograms in the past 5 years perceived a lower mean number of barriers (e.g., inconvenience, time involved, forgetfulness, worry about finding cancer, embarrassment, pain, costs, and worry about radiation) than did the rest of the study group (Russell et al., 2006). In addition, this subgroup had the highest self-efficacy (confidence in ability to get a mammogram, including knowing the process, having the needed resources, talking with staff about concerns, and getting a mammogram even if worried or did not know what to expect) (Russell et al., 2006). Black women who had no child care responsibilities were more likely to undergo mammography on a regular basis (Rosenberg et al., 2005). Perceiving fewer barriers was also associated with adherence to flexible sigmoidoscopy for colorectal cancer screening (Brenes & Paskett, 2000). Research has shown that knowledge about the purpose of screening tests, screening guidelines, and protocols for what to do about abnormal findings is associated with increased cancer screening rates (Breitkopf et al., 2005; Juon et al., 2004; Russell et al., 2006).

Adherence to recommendations for lifestyle behaviors may be hampered by patient perceptions such as feeling that recommendations are unrealistic, the goals are unattainable, recommendations do not fit their lifestyles, or recommendations are unclear or not specific enough (e.g., a recommendation to "get more exercise" is not as clear as a recommendation to walk five or more days per week for at least 30 minutes at a time at an intensity level that increases your heart rate and breathing) (Dailey, Schwartz, Binienda, Moorman, & Neale, 2006). Patients may also feel that they do not have the tools necessary to implement the recommended lifestyle changes (e.g., patients may feel the need for special kitchen equipment for healthy cooking). Potential barriers that apply to all groups but may be more prevalent among racial and ethnic minority communities include a lack of social support or positive community norms and role models; lack of access (e.g., to safe and affordable means to be physically active or to healthy food options); multiple role obligations, including caregiving responsibilities; a higher priority on caregiving than on self-care; busy schedules and limited time for discretionary physical activity; perceived lack of energy; attitudes that predispose to resting rather than being physically active as a way of restoring health balance; a significant number of problematic life events and other sources of stress; health problems such as knee pain, foot problems, or extreme obesity that directly increase the difficulty of and lower self-efficacy for exercise; role expectations or identities (e.g., being a grandmother) that may be perceived as making certain types of activities socially inappropriate; limited understanding of or belief in the positive benefits (short term or long term) of changing lifestyle behaviors; some negative perceptions of the effects of changing lifestyle behaviors (e.g., exercising raises blood pressure, makes one sweaty, may require the use of public showers, ruins hair, boredom); and general attitudes of distrust with respect to messages perceived as coming from outside of the Black community (Airhihenbuwa, Kumanyika, Agurs, & Lowe, 1995; Baranowski et al., 1990; Broman, 1995; Dattilo, Dattilo, Samdahl, & Kleiber, 1994; Eyler et al., 2002; Fisher, Auslander, Sussman, Owens, & Jackson-Thompson, 1992; King et al., 2000; Lewis et al., 1993; Mayo, 1992; Yancey, 1999). Additional research points to factors associated with increased levels of physical activity, including family centeredness (e.g., among African Americans); a preference for exercising with friends and family members and for certain types of active recreation (e.g., participation in sports, exercising and dancing in general and particularly when music can be selected that is culturally relevant and appropriate); having a relatively positive body image even if obese (e.g., potentially less self-consciousness about exercising); and positive expectations about the effects of increased participation in physical activity (feeling better, sleeping better, increased sense of well-being, decreased anxiety and ability to manage stress, better cognitive ability, alleviation of some health problems such as lower extremity edema, facilitating weight loss, and improving appearance [e.g., "toning"]) (Airhihenbuwa et al., 1995; Eyler et al., 2002; Klesges, Klesges, Swenson, & Pheley, 1985; Kumanyika & Charleston, 1992; Lasco et al., 1989; Mayo, 1992; Sullivan & Carter, 1985).

Even if individuals have knowledge related to clinical behaviors, lack of access to health care may pose a problem for screening adherence. Data suggest that health insurance coverage is strongly associated with adherence to recommendations for cancer-screening mammography among Black and Asian American women (Jennings-Dozier & Lawrence, 2000; Leong-Wu & Fernandez, 2006; Rosenberg et al., 2005). Underserved Hispanic and Black women who reported having no medical coverage, those who reported lack of continuity of care, and those who reported a lower level of use of public services and benefits were less likely to report having a Pap smear within a 12-month period (Bazargan et al., 2004). Although not specific to racial and ethnic minority groups, out-of-pocket costs (e.g., for testing supplies, medical appointments) have been shown to be associated with lower adherence to recommendations for care seeking and disease self-management and treatment (Karter et al., 2000). Even those who are employed but who do not have health insurance report lower adherence to recommendations for cancer screening than those who have health insurance (Juon et al., 2004).

Engaging in health-related behaviors other than the one targeted has been associated with improved adherence to cancer screening. Among Black women, having a Pap smear within the 2 years before baseline and practicing breast self-exam was significantly associated with regular mammography use (Rosenberg et al., 2005). Black women who reported taking a multivitamin or female hormone supplements and those who did not smoke were more likely to be regular mammography users (Rosenberg et al., 2005). Abstinence from cigarettes and alcohol was associated with shorter time to cessation of use of drugs among injection drug users (Shah, Galai, Celentano, Vlahov, & Strathdee, 2006).

Engaging in risky health behaviors may also impact adherence to recommendations for lifestyle or clinical behaviors. A study among inner-city minority patients with type 2 diabetes mellitus showed that drinking alcohol was associated with poorer adherence to prescribed dietary recommendations and attendance at outpatient follow-up visits (Johnson, Bazargan, & Bing, 2000). Use of illicit drugs or abuse of other substances (e.g., cigarette smoking) has been shown to be associated with nonadherence to disease treatment protocols (e.g., hemodialysis treatments among hemodialysis patients) (Unruh, Evans, Fink, Powe, & Meyer, 2005). Those least likely to adhere to dietary recommendations include individuals who consume moderate to high amounts of alcohol (Johnson, Bazargan, & Bing, 2000).

Presence of a health outcome or known family history of disease is associated with increased screening for disease. Among Black women, those with fibrocystic breast disease or a family history of breast cancer are more likely to be regular mammography users (Rosenberg et al., 2005). Asian American women with a family history of breast cancer were twice as likely to have ever obtained a mammogram (Leong-Wu & Fernandez, 2006). Underserved Black and Hispanic women who reported a better level of perceived health status were less likely to receive a Pap smear in the 12 months prior to interview (Bazargan et al., 2004).

Providers' advice regarding clinical behaviors can also play an important role in individuals' adherence to recommendations. Research suggests that provider recommendation is associated with increased odds of cancer screening among minority groups members (Brenes & Paskett, 2000; Juon et al., 2004;

Russell et al., 2006). Among underserved Hispanic and Black women, those who reported that no health practitioners had ever recommended a Pap smear were less likely to have received a Pap smear in the 12 months before interviews (Bazargan et al., 2004). Despite the knowledge of their importance for patient health, physicians do not always offer advice or recommendations related to patients' health behaviors. According to Dailey et al. (2006), physicians reported barriers to their offering recommendations that included lack of patient education; lack of time; perceived unrealistic guideline goals (Dailey et al., 2006); inadequate knowledge about the factors on which to counsel (e.g., inadequate knowledge of diet and physical activity recommendations); personal attitudes; and lack of confidence about their lifestyle counseling skills. Physicians are also influenced by their perceptions of patient barriers, patients' willingness and ability to change lifestyle behaviors or to adhere to clinical recommendations, and a belief that patients will be noncompliant ("Barriers to guideline adherence. Based on a presentation by Michael Cabana, MD," 1998). Reported physician barriers to counseling on the JNC-VI guidelines for high blood pressure included lack of awareness, lack of agreement with the guidelines, lack of self-efficacy that they can effectively counsel on the guidelines, lack of outcome expectancy, and lack of a cuing mechanism or reminders to initiate counseling ("Barriers to guideline adherence. Based on a presentation by Michael Cabana, MD," 1998).

Many patients present to physicians with multiple comorbidities or health issues, and another barrier to provider counseling is having too many problems on which to focus (Dailey et al., 2006). This can sometimes result in a provider electing to treat one condition at a time, rather than treating all conditions together. Providers' perceptions of the patient's knowledge of the condition also influences counseling behavior (i.e., physicians who perceive more patient knowledge of a condition may be more likely to provide counseling as they feel more confident with patients who are educated because they feel their job is easier) (Dailey et al., 2006).

Nested within issues related to adherence to lifestyle behavior recommendations is the limited minority health care workforce in place to address the dynamic needs of the U.S. minority population (Sullivan Commission, 2003). The percentage of African Americans (11.5% to 20.5%) and Latinos and Hispanics (10.5% to 15.4%) who earn college degrees has increased. However, access to graduate-level education in the health professions for these groups has not increased accordingly (Reede, 2003). Following the civil rights movement in the late 1960s, a slight increase in minority medical school enrollment was observed in 1974; however, this was slowed by the decision by the U.S. Supreme Court in the 1978 case of *Regents of the University of California v. Bakke*, which deemed unlawful special admission programs (e.g., active recruitment of specified percentages of students from certain minority groups) implemented by the medical school at the University of California at Davis. Secondary to federal mandates, affirmative-action initiatives, and other programs to offset the adverse impact of discrimination, another wave of increased minority enrollment in medical schools occurred between 1982 and 1995, with enrollment spiking anywhere from 8.4% to 12.4% (Reede, 2003; Saha, Taggart, Komaromy, & Bindman, 2000). Since 1995, several states with relatively large minority constituencies have eliminated race, ethnicity, and gender as factors in the medical school admission process. American Indian, Hispanic and Latino, and African American doctorate-level health care providers are underrepresented relative to their proportion of the general population. In 2000, 1.6% of medical students and 5.5% of medical school faculty were from these groups, although these traditionally underserved groups collectively represent greater than 25% of the population in the United States (Reede, 2003; Saha et al., 2000). This trend is potentially problematic given the research suggesting that minorities prefer receiving care from race-concordant providers (Cooper et al., 2003; LaVeist & Carroll, 2002; LaVeist & Nuru-Jeter, 2002). The Sullivan Commission on Diversity report provides 37 recommendations to address the lack of diversity in the health professions, a challenge that represents one historical phase of the differential legacy of health and health care in North America (Sullivan Commission, 2003). It is plausible to conclude that the growing interest in cultural competency is an acknowledgment of the low availability of minority doctoral-level providers, although no such suggestion has been made in the literature.

Strategies for Improving Adherence to Lifestyle and Clinical Behaviors Among Minority Populations

Improving adherence to lifestyle interventions among racial and ethnic minority populations is particularly critical given the disproportionate burden of chronic disease experienced by populations of color in the United States. Illness and health behavior occur within a cultural context. Many racial and ethnic minority populations are characterized by having a collectivist culture, that is, one in which individuals characterize themselves in relation to others and identify as part of a network of interconnected people. In contrast, in an individualist culture, people distinguish themselves from others and identify as autonomous (Lewis et al., 2002). Although the material presented in this section is organizationally divided into individual and community-level strategies to improve lifestyle adherence among minority populations, this material should be considered within a collectivist context.

Individual-Level Strategies

The need to tailor behavioral intervention strategies to subgroups defined by demographic, health, and psychosocial characteristics and particularly to align such strategies with the cultural and ethnic milieu of the target population has been recognized in recent years (Harris-Davis & Haughton, 2000; Resnicow, Baranowski, Ahluwalia, & Braithwaite, 1999; Taylor, Baranowski, & Young, 1998). The challenges are to identify the relevant tailoring variables and then to operationalize these in the design of intervention strategies. Many variables relevant to the design of obesity-related interventions in African Americans have been deemed effective (Airhihenbuwa et al., 1995; Flynn & Fitzgibbon, 1998). For example, Airhihenbuwa et al. (1995) reported that among African Americans, rest was considered more important to one's health than exercise; in addition, their work activities were considered an important form of exercise.

Motivational interviewing (MI) is a second individual-level strategy that has shown preliminary efficacy in improving adherence to lifestyle interventions.

Originally used in alcohol treatment, MI is a client-centered counseling style for eliciting behavior change by helping clients resolve ambivalence (Rollnick & Miller, 1995). MI differs in several ways from traditional health education and social marketing. Rather than attempt to persuade clients, in MI, the counselor enables clients to write their own "advertisement for change." Rather than "pushing" information or persuasive messages to the client, in MI the counselor elicits the client's subjective pros and cons for change and helps create discrepancies between the person's current health behavior and his core values and life goals. The goal is to elicit change generated by the client. The use of MI has evolved from its initial use in the addiction field (Rollnick, Heather, Gold, & Hall, 1992) to a broader use in health promotion and disease prevention, including diet and weight control (Berg-Smith et al., 1999; Mhurchu, Margetts, & Speller, 1998; Resnicow et al., 2000; Smith, Heckemeyer, Kratt, & Mason, 1997), smoking (Colby et al., 1998; Lawendowski, 1998; Velasquez et al., 2000), physical activity (Harland et al., 1999), preventive screening (Rakowski et al., 1992; Taplin et al., 2000), HIV prevention (Carey et al., 1997) and diabetes management (Stott, Rollnick, Rees, & Pill, 1995). MI has been shown to be effective in addressing multiple risk behaviors, supporting smoking cessation, weight loss, dietary change, and elimination of substance abuse among various minority population groups. For example, coupled with behavioral counseling and case management, motivational interviewing has been shown to be effective in helping Hispanic intravenous drug users to reduce drug use and HIV-risk (Robles et al., 2004).

Community-Level Strategies

Culturally relevant conceptual models and frameworks are needed for the development and implementation of effective behavioral strategies to enhance adherence to lifestyle interventions. The PEN-3 conceptual framework is such a framework. Originally developed for use in African countries and since adapted for use with African Americans in the United States (Airhihenbuwa, 1995; Airhihenbuwa & Webster, 2004), the PEN-3 model was designed as a culturally relevant framework for the development of health education strategies and programs. It consists of three interrelated and interdependent dimensions of health (cultural identity, relationships and expectations, and cultural empowerment). As shown in Figure 29.1, each dimension has three components, which form the PEN acronym.

The first dimension of the framework, cultural identity, assists in defining the target audience (person, extended family, and neighborhood). The second dimension of the PEN-3 framework is relationships and expectations. This dimension focuses on determining, through interviews, focus groups, or surveys, the factors that influence the person, family, and/or community actions (perceptions, enablers, and nurturers). Perceptions include the knowledge, attitudes, and beliefs that may contribute to or hinder engagement in a particular health behavior. Enablers are community or structural factors such as availability of resources, accessibility, referrals, skills, and types of services. Nurturers are the reinforcing factors that the target audience receives from their social networks. A third and unique component of the model is cultural empowerment. This component is crucial in the development of culturally relevant interventions and instruments to assess the target health behavior of ethnic minority cultures. Its components are positive, existential, and negative. The "positive"

PEN-3 conceptual framework.

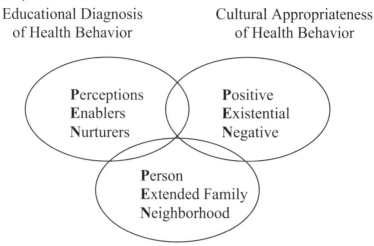

Educational Diagnosis
of Health Behavior

Cultural Appropriateness
of Health Behavior

Perceptions
Enablers
Nurturers

Positive
Existential
Negative

Person
Extended Family
Neighborhood

component refers to perceptions, enablers, and nurturers that lead the target audience to engage in the health behavior. The "existential" component refers to practices that have no harmful health consequences and should not be changed but incorporated in the intervention or instrument. The "negative" component refers to perceptions, enablers, and nurturers that prevent the target audience from engaging in the health behavior or that lead them to engage in a harmful behavior (e.g., smoking). This framework has been effective in the development of effective strategies for smoking cessation (Beech & Scarinci, 2003); obesity prevention (Airhihenbuwa, Kumanyika, TenHave, & Morssink, 2000), and physical activity (Airhihenbuwa et al., 1995) interventions for African Americans.

Culturally Adapted vs. Nonadapted Strategies

In the previous sections, we mentioned that adherence to healthy lifestyle behaviors has been and continues to be an issue, particularly for those who are low income, of racial and ethnic minorities, older, less educated, un- or underinsured, and living in rural areas (Beswick et al., 2005; Vellozzi, Romans, & Rothenberg, 1996). However, by acknowledging the issue of adherence among racial and ethnic minority populations, many researchers have sought to develop alternative strategies, including more culturally appropriate or culturally sensitive strategies. For the purposes of this discussion, culturally adapted strategies are defined as interventions that are specific to a particular culture — activities, language, and cultural norms that are aptly identified by a particular racial or ethnic group (e.g., gospel aerobics). Nonadapted strategies include interventions that do not relate to a specific culture, that is, interventions that can be implemented across the board with limited modifications for particular populations.

While many interventions have been developed to increase health among minority populations, there is limited research available that specifically relates to interventions to increase adherence to healthy behaviors and medication up-take in these groups. To make the distinction, many interventions have been developed to address the concern of health disparities among minority popula-tions; however, even after the primary causes of the disparity, such as access, have been addressed, issues of compliance remain. Furthermore, most of the available research focuses on identifying the barriers to adherence to medically recommended health behaviors and broadly focuses on the general population. However, the current research does overlap in basic concepts, while providing insight and overarching themes of culturally adapted and nonadapted strate-gies for improving adherence.

Interventions for addressing disparities in health often have been designed around specific cultures (i.e., African American, Latino/Hispanic). These in-terventions incorporate strategies that include developing healthy recipes of traditional foods or using culturally related music (e.g., gospel or hip hop) in aerobics classes or utilizing locations of trust within specific communities (e.g., churches or other places of worship), which, it has been suggested, increase adherence. For instance, a program in Arkansas titled "Witnessing in the Delta" put into practice the act of "witnessing," which is often part of African American church experience, by utilizing role models to discuss their personal experience with breast cancer with a small group of women in a church setting (Vellozzi et al., 1996). This intervention was successful not only in reaching low-income African American women who believed that they were not at risk for breast cancer but also in increasing the frequency with which the women performed breast self-examinations and obtained mammograms (Erwin, Spatz, & Turturro, 1992). A study aimed at improving metabolic control among Puerto Ricans with type 2 diabetes incorporated a *telenovela*, a popular Spanish-styled soap opera often watched by both genders, that included health messages related to the maintenance of diabetes (Rosal et al., 2005). Throughout the reading of the *tele-novela*, discussions focused on key health issues. The final assessments showed statistically significant differences in glycated hemoglobin levels between the intervention and control groups, in addition to a trend toward increased physi-cal activity in the intervention group. Other types of culturally adapted strate-gies include faith-based efforts (Vellozzi et al., 1996), use of lay health advisers (Vellozzi et al., 1996), and development of race-concordant services (Paschal, Lewis, Martin, Shipp, & Simpson, 2006). There are some strategies that are both culturally adapted and traditional. These strategies include television and radio campaigns and use of other forms of media (Vellozzi et al., 1996). These strat-egies contain elements that are both culturally adapted, such as language or style, and nonadapted, but the basic idea can be used across cultures.

Nonadapted strategies include making modifications to the management systems, such as sending patient tracking or reminder letters or postcards to providers and consumers, and the use of community-based outreach. An inter-vention aimed at increasing breast cancer screening among Hispanic Amer-ican women used both patient and physician reminders about the need for screening and led to a 13% increase in the number of women being screened (Zapka et al., 1993). A study aimed at low-income African American women used a variety of unadapted strategies, including a "Women's Fest," educational brochures, mass media, monthly classes, birthday cards with the study logo, targeted mailings, and one-on-one sessions in women's homes (Paskett et al.,

1999) and increased the percentage of women reported having a mammogram in the intervention city from 31% at baseline to 56%. Interestingly, a review of research on adherence to HIV and general medication regimens indicated that persons who had more complex medication regimens were more likely to adhere to the medical instruction (Burge et al., 2005; Fogarty et al., 2002). Other nonadapted strategies include integration of preventive services at primary health care sites (e.g., provider reminder systems [Vellozzi et al., 1996]), provider and consumer education [Beswick et al., 2005; Vellozzi et al., 1996], use of nurses and nurse practitioners), mobile mammography units and mobile clinics, community-based outreach (e.g., education delivered at community sites, consumer incentives, door-to-door recruitment), personalized communications (e.g., direct mailings, telephone reminders) (Vellozzi et al., 1996) and behavioral tools (e.g., providing pill boxes, role-playing medication schedule adjustments, teaching self-monitoring skills) (Fogarty et al., 2002).

In conclusion, a variety of interventions are available to increase adherence among racial and ethnic minority populations. While much of the research has not specifically focused on adherence or uptake of interventions, it does provide insight into additional methods for improving adherence. One review of the literature indicated that a combination of strategies should be used because not all strategies work for all target populations (Vellozzi et al., 1996). Determining the most effective will depend upon the types of strategies, the number of strategies, and the target population. Continued work is needed to determine the most effective strategies to increase adherence of health behaviors among minority populations.

Summary

Lifestyle and clinical behaviors that can lead to poor health are more prevalent among racial and ethnic minority communities, and many of these behaviors result in increased morbidity and mortality rates in these communities. Factors related to adherence and nonadherence grow out of both lifestyle and clinical behaviors. While many of these factors are not unique to racial and ethnic minority communities, these factors are often more common among racial and ethnic minorities (e.g., perceived barriers to behavior change, poor access to health care, difficulty communicating in English), which can lead to poor health-related behaviors and poor health. Several strategies to improve adherence to recommendations for healthy lifestyle behaviors have been identified. Some of these strategies take culture into account; however, many successful strategies do not necessarily rely on culture. Rather, they require targeted strategies for increasing awareness of recommendations for health-related behaviors, increasing access to resources necessary to engage in healthy behaviors, and potential changes in management systems that encourage participation in healthy behaviors. Strategies grounded in conceptual models and frameworks with appropriate cultural adaptations may have more promise for success; however, additional work is needed to identify the most successful strategies for increasing adherence to healthy lifestyle behaviors among racial and ethnic minority groups, which should lead to the elimination of health disparities.

References

Adams, P. F., & Schoenborn, C. A. (2006). Health behaviors of adults: United States, 2002–04. *Vital Health Statistics, 10*(230), 1–140.

Airhihenbuwa, C. O. (1995). *Health and culture: Beyond the Western paradigm*. Thousand Oaks, CA: Sage.

Airhihenbuwa, C. O., Kumanyika, S., Agurs, T. D., & Lowe, A. (1995). Perceptions and beliefs about exercise, rest, and health among African-Americans. *American Journal of Health Promotion, 9*(6), 426–429.

Airhihenbuwa, C. O., Kumanyika, S. K., TenHave, T. R., & Morssink, C. B. (2000). Cultural identity and health lifestyles among African Americans: A new direction for health intervention research? *Ethnicity and Disease, 10*(2), 148–164.

Airhihenbuwa, C. O., & Webster, J. D. (2004). Culture and African contexts of HIV/AIDS prevention, care and support. *Sahara Journal, 1*(4), 4–13.

Anderson, J. E., Mosher, W. D., & Chandra, A. (2006). Measuring HIV risk in the U.S. population aged 15–44: Results from Cycle 6 of the National Survey of Family Growth. *Advance Data, (377)*, 1–27.

Baranowski, T., Simons-Morton, B., Hooks, P., Henske, J., Tiernan, K., Dunn, J. K., et al. (1990). A center-based program for exercise change among black-American families. *Health Education Quarterly, 17*(2), 179–196.

Barriers to guideline adherence. Based on a presentation by Michael Cabana, MD. (1998). *American Journal of Managed Care, 4*(12 Suppl.), S741–S744; discussion S745–S748.

Bazargan, M., Bazargan, S. H., Farooq, M., & Baker, R. S. (2004). Correlates of cervical cancer screening among underserved Hispanic and African-American women. *Preventive Medicine, 39*(3), 465–473.

Beech, B. M., & Scarinci, I. C. (2003). Smoking attitudes and practices among low-income African-Americans: Qualitative assessment of contributing factors. *American Journal of Health Promotion, 17*(4), 240–248.

Berg-Smith, S. M., Stevens, V. J., Brown, K. M., Van Horn, L., Gernhofer, N., Peters, E., et al. (1999). A brief motivational intervention to improve dietary adherence in adolescents. The Dietary Intervention Study in Children (DISC) Research Group. *Health Education Research, 14*(3), 399–410.

Berrigan, D., Troiano, R. P., McNeel, T., DiSogra, C., & Ballard-Barbash, R. (2006). Active transportation increases adherence to activity recommendations. *American Journal of Preventive Medicine, 31*(3), 210–216.

Beswick, A. D., Rees, K., West, R. R., Taylor, F. C., Burke, M., Griebsch, I., et al. (2005). Improving uptake and adherence in cardiac rehabilitation: Literature review. *Journal of Advanced Nursing, 49*, 538–555.

Breitkopf, C. R., Pearson, H. C., & Breitkopf, D. M. (2005). Poor knowledge regarding the Pap test among low-income women undergoing routine screening. *Perspectives on Sexual and Reproductive Health, 37*(2), 78–84.

Brenes, G. A., & Paskett, E. D. (2000). Predictors of stage of adoption for colorectal cancer screening. *Preventive Medicine, 31*(4), 410–416.

Broman, C. L. (1995). Leisure-time physical activity in an African-American population. *Journal of Behavioral Medicine, 18*(4), 341–353.

Brown, A. F., Gregg, E. W., Stevens, M. R., Karter, A. J., Weinberger, M., Safford, M. M., et al. (2005). Race, ethnicity, socioeconomic position, and quality of care for adults with diabetes enrolled in managed care: The Translating Research Into Action for Diabetes (TRIAD) study. *Diabetes Care, 28*(12), 2864–2870.

Burge, S., White, D., Bajorek, E., Bazaldua, O., Trevino, J., Albright, H., et al. (2005). Correlates of medication knowledge and adherence: Findings from the Residency Research Network of South Texas. *Family Medicine, 37*(10), 712–718.

Carey, M. P., Maisto, S. A., Kalichman, S. C., Forsyth, A. D., Wright, E. M., & Johnson, B. T. (1997). Enhancing motivation to reduce the risk of HIV infection for economically disadvantaged urban women. *Journal of Consulting and Clinical Psychology, 65*(4), 531–541.

Centers for Disease Control and Prevention. (2005). Trends in leisure-time physical inactivity by age, sex, and race/ethnicity—United States, 1994–2004. *Morbidity and Mortality Weekly Report, 54*(39), 991–994.

Colby, S. M., Monti, P. M., Barnett, N. P., Rohsenow, D. J., Weissman, K., Spirito, A., et al. (1998). Brief motivational interviewing in a hospital setting for adolescent smoking: A preliminary study. *Journal of Consulting and Clinical Psychology, 66*(3), 574–578.

Cooper, L. A., Roter, D. L., Johnson, R. L., Ford, D. E., Steinwachs, D. M., & Powe, N. R. (2003). Patient-centered communication, ratings of care, and concordance of patient and physician race. *Annals of Internal Medicine, 139*(11), 907–915.

Dailey, R., Schwartz, K. L., Binienda, J., Moorman, J., & Neale, A. V. (2006). Challenges in making therapeutic lifestyle changes among hypercholesterolemic African-American patients and their physicians. *Journal of the National Medical Association, 98*(12), 1895–1903.

Dattilo, J., Dattilo, A. M., Samdahl, D. M., & Kleiber, D. A. (1994). Leisure orientations and self-esteem in women with low incomes who are overweight. *Journal of Leisure Research, 26*(1), 21–38.

Denny, C. H., Holtzman, D., & Cobb, N. (2003). Surveillance for health behaviors of American Indians and Alaska Natives. Findings from the Behavioral Risk Factor Surveillance System, 1997–2000. *MMWR Surveillance Summary, 52*(7), 1–13.

Egede, L. E., & Zheng, D. (2003). Racial/ethnic differences in influenza vaccination coverage in high-risk adults. *American Journal of Public Health, 93*(12), 2074–2078.

Erwin, D., Spatz, T., & Turturro, C. (1992). Development of an African American role model intervention to increase breast self-examination and mammography. *Journal of Cancer Education, 7*(4), 311–319.

Eyler, A. E., Wilcox, S., Matson-Koffman, D., Evenson, K. R., Sanderson, B., Thompson, J., et al. (2002). Correlates of physical activity among women from diverse racial/ethnic groups. *Journal of Womens Health and Gender Based Medicine, 11*(3), 239–253.

Fisher, E. B., Jr., Auslander, W., Sussman, L., Owens, N., & Jackson-Thompson, J. (1992). Community organization and health promotion in minority neighborhoods. *Ethnicity and Disease, 2*(3), 252–272.

Flynn, K. J., & Fitzgibbon, M. (1998). Body images and obesity risk among black females: A review of the literature. *Annals of Behavioral Medicine, 20*(1), 13–24.

Fogarty, L., Roter, D., Larson, S., Burke, J., Gillespie, J., & Levy, R. (2002). Patient adherence to HIV medication regimens: A review of published and abstract reports. *Patient Education and Counseling, 46*(2), 93–108.

Gordon-Larsen, P., Nelson, M. C., Page, P., & Popkin, B. M. (2006). Inequality in the built environment underlies key health disparities in physical activity and obesity. *Pediatrics, 117*(2), 417–424.

Halbert, C. H., Kessler, L., Wileyto, E. P., Weathers, B., Stopfer, J., Domchek, S., et al. (2006). Breast cancer screening behaviors among African American women with a strong family history of breast cancer. *Preventive Medicine, 43*(5), 385–388.

Hargraves, J. L., Cunningham, P. J., & Hughes, R. G. (2001). Racial and ethnic differences in access to medical care in managed care plans. *Health Services Research, 36*(5), 853–868.

Hargraves, J. L., & Hadley, J. (2003). The contribution of insurance coverage and community resources to reducing racial/ethnic disparities in access to care. *Health Services Research, 38*(3), 809–829.

Harland, J., White, M., Drinkwater, C., Chinn, D., Farr, L., & Howel, D. (1999). The Newcastle exercise project: A randomised controlled trial of methods to promote physical activity in primary care. *British Medical Journal, 319*(7213), 828–832.

Harris-Davis, E., & Haughton, B. (2000). Model for multicultural nutrition counseling competencies. *Journal of the American Dietetic Association, 100*(10), 1178–1185.

Howarth, N. C., Murphy, S. P., Wilkens, L. R., Hankin, J. H., & Kolonel, L. N. (2006). Dietary energy density is associated with overweight status among 5 ethnic groups in the multiethnic cohort study. *Journal of Nutrition, 136*(8), 2243–2248.

Hulme, P. A., Walker, S. N., Effle, K. J., Jorgensen, L., McGowan, M. G., Nelson, J. D., et al. (2003). Health-promoting lifestyle behaviors of Spanish-speaking Hispanic adults. *Journal of Transcultural Nursing, 14*, 244–254.

James, T. M., Greiner, K. A., Ellerbeck, E. F., Feng, C., & Ahluwalia, J. S. (2006). Disparities in colorectal cancer screening: A guideline-based analysis of adherence. *Ethnicity and Disease, 16*(1), 228–233.

Jennings-Dozier, K., & Lawrence, D. (2000). Sociodemographic predictors of adherence to annual cervical cancer screening in minority women. *Cancer Nursing, 23*(5), 350–356; quiz, 357–358.

Johnson, K. H., Bazargan, M., & Bing, E. G. (2000). Alcohol consumption and compliance among inner-city minority patients with type 2 diabetes mellitus. *Archives of Family Medicine, 9,* 964–970.

Juon, H. S., Kim, M., Shankar, S., & Han, W. (2004). Predictors of adherence to screening mammography among Korean American women. *Preventive Medicine, 39*(3), 474–481.

Karter, A. J., Ferrara, A., Darbinian, J. A., Ackerson, L. M., & Selby, J. V. (2000). Self-monitoring of blood glucose: Language and financial barriers in a managed care population with diabetes. *Diabetes Care, 23*(4), 477–483.

Kim, M. J., Ahn, Y.-H., Chon, C., Bowen, P., & Khan, S. (2005). Health disparities in lifestyle choices among hypertensive Korean Americans, non-Hispanic Whites, and Blacks. *Biological Research for Nursing, 7,* 67–74.

King, A. C., Castro, C., Wilcox, S., Eyler, A. A., Sallis, J. F., & Brownson, R. C. (2000). Personal and environmental factors associated with physical inactivity among different racial-ethnic groups of U.S. middle-aged and older-aged women. *Health Psychology, 19*(4), 354–364.

Klesges, R. C., Klesges, L. M., Swenson, A. M., & Pheley, A. M. (1985). A validation of two motion sensors in the prediction of child and adult physical activity levels. *American Journal of Epidemiology, 122*(3), 400–410.

Kumanyika, S. K., & Charleston, J. B. (1992). Lose weight and win: A church-based weight loss program for blood pressure control among black women. *Patient Education and Counseling, 19*(1), 19–32.

Lasco, R. A., Curry, R. H., Dickson, V. J., Powers, J., Menes, S., & Merritt, R. K. (1989). Participation rates, weight loss, and blood pressure changes among obese women in a nutrition-exercise program. *Public Health Reports, 104*(6), 640–646.

LaVeist, T. A., & Carroll, T. (2002). Race of physician and satisfaction with care among African-American patients. *Journal of the National Medical Association, 94*(11), 937–943.

LaVeist, T. A., & Nuru-Jeter, A. (2002). Is doctor-patient race concordance associated with greater satisfaction with care? *Journal of Health and Social Behavior, 43*(3), 296–306.

Lawendowski, L. A. (1998). A motivational intervention for adolescent smokers. *Preventive Medicine, 27*(5 Pt. 3), A39–A46.

Leong-Wu, C. A., & Fernandez, M. E. (2006). Correlates of breast cancer screening among Asian Americans enrolled in ENCOREplus. *Journal of Immigrant and Minority Health, 8*(3), 235–243.

Levin, S., Welch, V. L., Bell, R. A., & Casper, M. L. (2002). Geographic variation in cardiovascular disease risk factors among American Indians and comparisons with the corresponding state populations. *Ethnicity and Health, 7*(1), 57–67.

Lewis, C. E., Raczynski, J. M., Heath, G. W., Levinson, R., Hilyer, J. C., Jr., & Cutter, G. R. (1993). Promoting physical activity in low-income African-American communities: The PARR project. *Ethnicity and Disease, 3*(2), 106–118.

Maciosek, M. V., Solberg, L. I., Coffield, A. B., Edwards, N. M., & Goodman, M. J. (2006). Colorectal cancer screening: Health impact and cost effectiveness. *American Journal of Preventive Medicine, 31*(1), 80–89.

Mayo, K. (1992). Physical activity practices among American Black working women. *Qualitative Health Research, 2*(3), 318–333.

Mhurchu, C. N., Margetts, B. M., & Speller, V. (1998). Randomized clinical trial comparing the effectiveness of two dietary interventions for patients with hyperlipidaemia. *Clinical Science (Lond), 95*(4), 479–487.

National Center for Health Statistics. (2006). *Health, United States, 2006, With Chartbook on Trends in the Health of Americans.* Hyattsville, MD: Author.

Paschal, A. M., Lewis, R. K., Martin, A., Shipp, D. D., & Simpson, D. S. (2006). Evaluating the impact of a hypertension program for African Americans. *Journal of the National Medical Association, 98*(4), 607–615.

Paskett, E. D., Tatum, C. M., D'Agostino, R., Jr., Rushing, J., Velez, R., Michielutte, R., et al. (1999). Community-based interventions to improve breast and cervical cancer screening: Results of the Forsyth County Cancer Screening (FoCaS) Project. *Cancer Epidemiology, Biomarkers and Prevention, 8,* 453–459.

Racial/ethnic disparities in influenza and pneumococcal vaccination levels among persons aged > or = 65 years—United States, 1989–2001. (2003). *Morbidity and Mortality Weekly Report, 52*(40), 958–962.

Rakowski, W., Dube, C. E., Marcus, B. H., Prochaska, J. O., Velicer, W. F., & Abrams, D. B. (1992). Assessing elements of women's decisions about mammography. *Health Psychology, 11*(2), 111–118.

Reede, J. Y. (2003). A recurring theme: The need for minority physicians. *Health Affairs (Millwood), 22*(4), 91–93.

Resnicow, K., Baranowski, T., Ahluwalia, J. S., & Braithwaite, R. L. (1999). Cultural sensitivity in public health: Defined and demystified. *Ethnicity and Disease, 9*(1), 10–21.

Resnicow, K., Yaroch, A. L., Davis, A., Wang, D. T., Carter, S., Slaughter, L., et al. (2000). GO GIRLS!: Results from a nutrition and physical activity program for low-income, overweight African American adolescent females. *Health Education and Behavior, 27*(5), 616–631.

Robles, R. R., Reyes, J. C., Colon, H. M., Sahai, H., Marrero, C. A., Matos, T. D., et al. (2004). Effects of combined counseling and case management to reduce HIV risk behaviors among Hispanic drug injectors in Puerto Rico: A randomized controlled study. *Journal of Substance Abuse Treatment, 27*(2), 145–152.

Rollnick, S., Heather, N., Gold, R., & Hall, W. (1992). Development of a short "readiness to change" questionnaire for use in brief, opportunistic interventions among excessive drinkers. *British Journal of Addiction, 87*(5), 743–754.

Rollnick, S., & Miller, W. R. (1995). What is motivational interviewing? *Behavioural & Cognitive Psychotherapy, 23,* 325–334.

Rosal, M. C., Olendzki, B., Reed, G. W., Gumieniak, O., Scavron, J., & Ockene, I. (2005). Diabetes self-management among low-income Spanish-speaking patients: A pilot study. *Annals of Behavioral Medicine, 29,* 225–235.

Rosenberg, L., Wise, L. A., Palmer, J. R., Horton, N. J., & Adams-Campbell, L. L. (2005). A multilevel study of socioeconomic predictors of regular mammography use among African-American women. *Cancer Epidemiology, Biomarkers and Prevention, 14*(11 Pt .1), 2628–2633.

Russell, K. M., Champion, V. L., & Skinner, C. S. (2006). Psychosocial factors related to repeat mammography screening over 5 years in African American women. *Cancer Nursing, 29*(3), 236–243.

Saha, S., Taggart, S. H., Komaromy, M., & Bindman, A. B. (2000). Do patients choose physicians of their own race? *Health Affairs (Millwood), 19*(4), 76–83.

Shah, N. G., Galai, N., Celentano, D. D., Vlahov, D., & Strathdee, S. A. (2006). Longitudinal predictors of injection cessation and subsequent relapse among a cohort of injection drug users in Baltimore, MD, 1988–2000. *Drug & Alcohol Dependence, 83*(2), 147–156.

Sly, D. F., Quadagno, D., Harrison, D. F., Eberstein, I. W., Riehman, K., & Bailey, M. (1997). Factors associated with use of the female condom. *Family Planning Perspectives, 29*(4), 181–184.

Smith-Bindman, R., Miglioretti, D. L., Lurie, N., Abraham, L., Barbash, R. B., Strzelczyk, J., et al. (2006). Does utilization of screening mammography explain racial and ethnic differences in breast cancer? *Annals of Internal Medicine, 144*(8), 541–553.

Smith, D. E., Heckemeyer, C. M., Kratt, P. P., & Mason, D. A. (1997). Motivational interviewing to improve adherence to a behavioral weight-control program for older obese women with NIDDM. A pilot study. *Diabetes Care, 20*(1), 52–54.

Stott, N. C., Rollnick, S., Rees, M. R., & Pill, R. M. (1995). Innovation in clinical method: diabetes care and negotiating skills. *Family Practice, 12*(4), 413–418.

Straits-Troster, K. A., Kahwati, L. C., Kinsinger, L. S., Orelien, J., Burdick, M. B., & Yevich, S. J. (2006). Racial/ethnic differences in influenza vaccination in the Veterans Affairs Healthcare System. *American Journal of Preventive Medicine, 31*(5), 375–382.

Sullivan Commission. (2003). *Missing persons in the health professions: A report of the Sullivan Commission on Diversity in the Healthcare Workforce.* Retrieved October 26, 2005, from http://admissions.duhs.duke.edu/sullivancommission/documents/Sullivan_Final_Report_000.pdf

Sullivan, J., & Carter, J. P. (1985). A nutrition-physical fitness intervention program for low-income black parents. *Journal of the National Medical Association, 77*(1), 39–43.

Taplin, S. H., Barlow, W. E., Ludman, E., MacLehos, R., Meyer, D. M., Seger, D., et al. (2000). Testing reminder and motivational telephone calls to increase screening mammography: A randomized study. *Journal of the National Cancer Institute, 92*(3), 233–242.

Taylor, W. C., Baranowski, T., & Young, D. R. (1998). Physical activity interventions in low-income, ethnic minority, and populations with disability. *American Journal of Preventive Medicine, 15*(4), 334–343.

Taylor, W. C., Floyd, M. F., Whitt-Glover, M. C., & Brooks, J. (2007). Environmental justice: A framework for collaboration between the public health and parks and recreation fields to study disparities in physical activity. *Journal of Physical Activity & Health, 4*(Suppl. 1), S1–S14.

Thompson, F. E., Midthune, D., Subar, A. F., McNeel, T., Berrigan, D., & Kipnis, V. (2005). Dietary intake estimates in the National Health Interview Survey, 2000: Methodology, results, and interpretation. *Journal of the American Dietetic Association, 105*(3), 352–363; quiz, 487.

U.S. Census Bureau. (2005). *2005 American community survey: Data profile highlights.* Retrieved March 10, 2007, from http://factfinder.census.gov/home/saff/aff_acs2005_quickguide.pdf

U.S. Department of Health and Human Services. (2000). *Healthy People 2010.* Washington, DC: U.S. Government Printing Office.

U.S. Department of Health and Human Services. (2002). *Strategic research plan and budget to reduce and ultimately eliminate health disparities: Vol. 1: Fiscal Years 2002–2006.* Retrieved from http://obssr.od.nih.gov/Content/Sttrategic_Planning/Health_Disparities/Health Disp.htm

U.S. Preventive Services Task Force. (1989). *Guide to clinical preventive services* (2nd ed.) Retrieved from http://odphp.osophs.dhhs.gov/pubs/guidecps/

Unruh, M. L., Evans, I. V., Fink, N. E., Powe, N. R., & Meyer, K. B. (2005). Skipped treatments, markers of nutritional nonadherence, and survival among incident hemodialysis patients. *American Journal of Kidney Diseases, 46*(6), 1107–1116.

Velasquez, M. M., Hecht, J., Quinn, V. P., Emmons, K. M., DiClemente, C. C., & Dolan-Mullen, P. (2000). Application of motivational interviewing to prenatal smoking cessation: Training and implementation issues. *Tobacco Control, 9*(Suppl.3), III36–III40.

Vellozzi, C. J., Romans, M., & Rothenberg, R. B. (1996). Delivering breast and cervical cancer screening services to underserved women: Part I. Literature review and telephone survey. *Women's Health Issues, 6*(2), 65–73.

Weir, M. R., Maibach, E. W., Bakris, G. L., Black, H. R., Chawla, P., Messerli, F. H., et al. (2000). Implications of a health lifestyle and medication analysis for improving hypertension control. *Archives of Internal Medicine, 160,* 481–490.

Wells, K. J., & Roetzheim, R. G. (2007). Health disparities in receipt of screening mammography in Latinas: A critical review of recent literature. *Cancer Control, 14*(4), 369–379.

Welty, T. K., Lee, E. T., Yeh, J., Cowan, L. D., Go, O., Fabsitz, R. R., et al. (1995). Cardiovascular disease risk factors among American Indians. The Strong Heart Study. *American Journal of Epidemiology, 142*(3), 269–287.

Winston, C. A., Wortley, P. M., & Lees, K. A. (2006). Factors associated with vaccination of Medicare beneficiaries in five U.S. communities: Results from the racial and ethnic adult disparities in immunization initiative survey, 2003. *Journal of the American Geriatric Society, 54*(2), 303–310.

Yancey, A. K. (1999). Facilitating health promotion in communities of color. *Cancer Research Therapy & Control, 8,* 133–122.

Zapka, J. G., Harris, D. R., Hosmer, D., Costanza, M. E., Mas, E., & Barth, R. (1993). Effect of a community health center intervention on breast cancer screening among Hispanic American women. *Health Services Research, 28*(2), 223–235.

Lifestyle Change and Adherence Issues Among Patients With Chronic Diseases

Section 6

Kristin A. Riekert
Editor

As the population ages and medical care innovations advance, more and more people will be living with a chronic illness that requires daily adherence to an often complicated regimen. Section VI highlights the difficulties of maintaining positive health behavior and adherence when one is living with a chronic health condition.

Chronic Obstructive Pulmonary Disease (chapter 30) and Heart Disease (chapter 34) are consistently among the top causes of mortality worldwide. As described in these chapters, rehabilitation services and multidisciplinary care, which include intensive medical management as well as diet, exercise, or other risk-reduction counseling, are the standard of care for patients with these conditions in the United States. While randomized trials of multidisciplinary care have shown that such care has the potential to improve health outcomes, there has been remarkably little attention to either the influence of adherence to medication or lifestyle recommendations on health outcomes or whether the inclusion of counseling on these topics improves adherence.

Two chapter focus on the effect of cognitive decline on adherence to a diabetes regimen. Mount (chapter 35) describes the association between diabetes and dementia, the effect of cognitive deficits on adherence, and how specific cognitive deficits can affect patient care and self-management of type 2 diabetes. In contrast, Coker (chapter 31) focuses on cognitive and functional declines commonly seen among older adults with diabetes and how these may affect adherence, when and how to involve a caregiver in diabetes management and, importantly, the educational and support needs of the new caregiver, as well as the person with diabetes.

Cancer and HIV are diseases whose diagnosis was once viewed as an inevitable death sentence, but, with medical advances, they have now evolved into chronic long-term illnesses that require long-term regimen adherence and lifestyle changes to maintain quality of life. As Peterman, Victorson, and Cella (chapter 32) highlight, however, there has been remarkable little research on rates of nonadherence to treatment, and even less is known about interventions to support adherence to cancer regimens. Similarly, as Rhodes and colleagues (chapter 33) discuss, HIV affects many people already marginalized by society, and regimen adherence has implications not only for the patient's well-being but also for public health. For these reasons, it is all the more important to understand the factors that affect lifelong HIV regimen adherence and design interventions not only to improve adherence in the short-term but to sustain it for the long term.

Common to all chapters in this section is the call to move beyond merely assessing the prevalence of nonadherence toward studies that advance our knowledge of which intervention strategies are efficacious in improving adherence.

Adherence for Patients With Chronic Obstructive Pulmonary Disease

30

Robert M. Kaplan

Chronic Obstructive Pulmonary Disease (COPD) is a chronic medical condition associated with airflow obstruction due to chronic bronchitis or emphysema or a combination of the two. Emphysema is characterized by abnormal permanent enlargement of the air spaces resulting from destruction of the walls of the alveoli. Alveoli are clusters of air spaces at the ends of the airways in the lung. As the alveolar walls break down, individual alveoli collapse, and the

Portions of this text previously appeared in: "Co-Management of Chronic Obstructive Pulmonary Disease," (pp. 411–434), by R. M. Kaplan, E. G. Eakin, A. L. Ries, M. T. Toshima, and C. J. Atkins, in *Handbook of Health Behavior Change*, 2nd edition, by S. A. Shumaker, E. B. Schron, J. K. Ockene, and W. L. McBee (Eds.), 1998, New York: Springer Publishing "Adherence in the Patient With Pulmonary Disease," (pp. 347–361), by R. M. Kaplan and A. L. Ries, in *Pulmonary Rehabilitation: Guidelines to Success*, 2nd edition, by J. Hodgkin, G. L. Connors, & C. W. Bell (Eds.), 2000, Philadelphia: Lippincott.

lung gradually loses its elasticity. This loss of lung elasticity means that the airways are not held open during expiration and tend to collapse. Air gets trapped in these damaged areas, and the lungs become inflated and enlarged ("Patient information series. Chronic obstructive pulmonary disease (COPD)," 2005). Chronic bronchitis is defined as the presence of chronic productive cough for 3 months in each of 2 successive years in a patient in whom other causes of chronic cough have been excluded. It is the result of chronic inflammation of the cells lining the breathing passages (bronchi). The inflammation causes the cells to swell and to produce excess quantities of mucus. The swelling and excess mucus result in a narrowing of the bronchi, which, in turn, obstructs the airflow and produces chronic cough ("Patient information series. Chronic obstructive pulmonary disease (COPD)," 2005).

Symptoms of COPD result from restrictions of airflow into and out of the lungs. It has been estimated that 80% to 90% of all cases of COPD result from long-term tobacco use (Buist, 2006). COPD is the fourth leading cause of death in the United States, and is on the increase in most countries (Buist, 2006; Lopez et al., 2006). It is projected that by 2020,COPD will rank 5th in the world as a cause of disease burden (Rabe et al., 2007). In addition to its effect on life expectancy, COPD results in significant loss in daily function and increases in health care costs (Mannino, 2002), including high rates of hospitalization (Strassels, Smith, & Mahajan, 2001). Following hospitalization, COPD patients remain vulnerable to rehospitalization and death. One-year post-hospitalization mortality rates range from 22% (Almagro et al., 2002) to 36% (Yohannes, Baldwin, & Connolly, 2005).

Patients with COPD experience significant limitations in daily activities. COPD has a profound effect upon functioning and everyday life. The increase in tobacco use among women in the later part of the 20th century (Han et al., 2007; "The rise in chronic obstructive disease mortality," 1989) resulted in increased rates of COPD among women. Current estimates suggest that COPD is diagnosed in approximately 11% of the adult population, and the incidence is increasing. The epidemic of COPD is expanding worldwide (Rabe et al., 2007). The human lung has a large reserve, and patients can have relatively advanced disease before they come to clinical attention. The disease can be present without symptoms for many years, and most patients are first diagnosed late in the course of disease.

Treatment Options

Despite major advances in diagnosis and medical therapeutics, many patients do not receive optimal benefit from standard medical care. While some aspects of COPD are treatable, the medical regimen is extremely complex. Medical management of COPD requires multiple medications. George and colleagues, using self-report measures, noted that only about 37% of patients with chronic lung diseases are fully adherent with their medical treatments (George, Kong, Thoman, & Stewart, 2005). However, treatment may also include respiratory chest physiotherapy techniques, exercise, and advice to quit smoking. Most patients are confronted with complex combinations of antibiotics, bronchodilators, anti-inflammatory drugs, and, in some cases, supplemental oxygen. Pulmonary rehabilitation is one of the most important interventions for COPD (Ries et al., 2007). Surgical interventions, such as lung volume reduction surgery (LVRS) or lung transplantation, may also be appropriate in selected patients (Fishman et al., 2003). However, it is widely recognized that these measures cannot cure COPD.

Some evidence suggests that nonadherence is common among patients with serious illnesses who are in poor health (DiMatteo, Haskard, & Williams, 2007). This is often the case with COPD patients. A variety of behavioral intervention programs that emphasize behavior change and adherence have been shown to improve outcomes for patients with chronic obstructive pulmonary disease (COPD), interstitial lung disease, and other lung diseases that cause activity limitations (Ries, 2007; Ries et al., 2007*).

Adherence

Medical encounters typically end with advice and recommendations. Patients are advised to fill a prescription, take a medication, stay on a prescribed diet, or give up cigarettes (DiMatteo, 2004). Often, medical advice is given by managed care organizations or nonprofit agencies such as the American Lung Association. Chronic disease management modules provide instructions for self-care, and physician records are used as evidence that certain services have been completed by the patient (Dunbar-Jacob, 2005). Several groups offer guidelines. For example, the American Lung Association recommends that people with chronic bronchitis get vaccinated against influenza and pneumococcal pneumonia (see www.lungusa.org). Patients are asked to adhere to many different instructions. Nonadherence is defined as the failure to follow such advice.

Adherence to Pharmacological Interventions

We have reviewed published papers on adherence with the COPD regimen published after 1980. In addition, we examined literature reviews published prior to 1980. Overall, the search revealed few studies that have directly addressed adherence, especially regarding traditional medical regimens for COPD. The studies considered different treatments in diverse samples and employed various definitions of, and measurements for, adherence. Unfortunately, few conclusions, if any, can be drawn from the current literature.

Published studies have considered adherence with regard to a variety of different regimens. Adherence to oxygen therapy in Scotland was reported by Morrison, Skwarski, and MacNee (1995). Among patients with COPD prescribed 24-hour oxygen, only 14% were fully adherent. The average use was 14.9 hours per day, and 44% used their oxygen less than 15 hours per day. These patients also had poor adherence to other aspects of the regimen. Although all patients were requested to have acute arterial blood gas measurements within 12 months, only about half obtained the tests. In another study from the United Kingdom, it was shown that patients who are prescribed oxygen for less than 24 hours (in this case, 15 hours/day) obtained high levels of adherence to the prescription (Restrick et al., 1993). In Denmark, about 66% of patients appear to have appropriate medical follow-up when on oxygen therapy, but adherence with therapy was often low (Ringbaek, 2005). Neri and colleagues studied more than 1,500 patients in Italy. They found that 84% of their sample had a mobile oxygen delivery device but that only 40% of these patients used the device daily (Neri et al., 2006). Some of the more recent studies that measure adherence by examining medication refills are difficult to interpret because they lump asthma and COPD into a single category (Krigsman, Nilsson, & Ring, 2007). Many people with asthma have reversible airways disorders.

Long-term adherence with inhaled medications was evaluated in the Lung Health Study (Rand, Nides, Cowles, Wise, & Connett, 1995). This was one of the first trials to evaluate inhaled bronchodilator medication used regularly over of time. The Lung Health Study was a large clinical trial (N = 3,923) of smoking intervention and the use of bronchodilator therapy in the early stages of COPD. Early in the trial, self-report data suggested that nearly 70% of the patients adhered to the regimen. This rate dropped off only slightly over the next 18 months. In addition to self-reports, the investigators weighed the canisters containing the medications. Self-reports confirmed by canister weights showed that 48% of the patients had good adherence at 1 year. Some nonadherence involved overuse of medication. Further analysis demonstrated that those who overused medication were also likely to incorrectly report their true smoking status.

Personality measures tend not to be good predictors of adherence. A scale designed to assess medication adherence in COPD has been developed and reported by Powell (1994), but it is not clear if it has clinical value because it does a poor job of predicting adherence. A variety of studies have investigated demographic characteristics associated with COPD self-care behaviors. For example, the Lung Health Study suggested that adherence was associated with being married, older, White, and having more severe disease. More adherent patients also had less shortness of breath and were hospitalized or confined to bed less often (Rand et al., 1995). Studies of adherence with nebulizer therapy from the intermittent positive-pressure breathing study showed that about half of the patients were adherent and half were nonadherent. Predictors of adherence included being White, being married, abstaining from alcohol and cigarette use, and having more severe shortness of breath. Further, those patients with more severe disease were also more likely to adhere to the therapy (Turner, Wright, Mendella, & Anthonisen, 1995). There have been very few trials that evaluate interventions to improve adherence. Solomon et al (1998) failed to demonstrate that having instructions given by clinical pharmacy residents significantly improved adherence over usual care.

Some variables thought to predict adherence often fail to do so. For example, it is commonly assumed that heavy drinkers will be less likely to follow the regimen than those who drink less. In the Lung Health Study, alcohol consumption was tested as a predictor of the ability to quit smoking. The results revealed that heavy alcohol use (more than 25 drinks per week) was not a significant predictor of relapse in smoking cessation. However, binge drinking defined as having eight or more drinks per occasion once a month or more was associated with greater relapse (Murray, Istvan, Voelker, Rigdon, & Wallace, 1995).

Estimated or measured adherence values do not appear to converge on a specific rate or even a specific pattern of nonadherence. James and colleagues (1985) reported that only half of their patients took their medicine regularly. Corden and colleagues also found that about half (56%) of their patients failed to comply with home nebulized therapy (Corden & Rees, 1998). The Intermittent Positive Pressure Breathing (IPPB) clinical trial, which used objective assessments of actual time on IPPB therapy, found that only half of the patients used the nebulizer at least 25 minutes per day ("Intermittent positive pressure breathing therapy of chronic obstructive pulmonary disease. A clinical trial," 1983). Adherence does appear to be related to health quality of life. Patients with higher scores on the St. George's Respiratory Questionnaire have been shown to be more likely to comply with nebulized therapy (Corden & Rees, 1998).

Electronic medication monitors may be valuable methods for improving adherence among patients with COPD. Evidence suggests that measures of oxygen expenditure may not be the most accurate estimates of adherence. New methods that allow direct assessment of oxygen inhalation may be more reliable (Lin, Kuna, & Bogen, 2006). One study evaluated 251 COPD patients who participated in a multisite clinical trial of meter dose inhaler therapy. The patients were divided into an intervention and a control group. Using an electronic medication monitor known as the nebulizer chronolog, the intervention group was given feedback on the accuracy of their medication use. Patients who received feedback were significantly more likely to adhere to the regimen and to use medications correctly than those in the control group (Nides et al., 1993).

To date, few studies have systematically evaluated adherence with regard to the COPD regimen, and in these few cases, the focus has been on drug and oxygen therapy. Further, only a few studies evaluating interventions to improve COPD patients' ability to manage their disease have been reported. Several commentaries have offered strategies for enhancing adherence; however, none have been systematically studied. Some individuals with asthma mistakenly stop steroid inhalers but continue bronchodilator inhalers because they do not notice any acute effect from the steroid inhaler (Williams et al., 2007).

Overadherence

Most of the literature on adherence behaviors focuses on the extent to which patients underuse medications. A less common but perhaps equally important problem involves the overuse of medication. Overadherence is a more common problem when medications provide prompt symptomatic relief. Chryssidis and colleagues (1981), for example, studied the use of high doses of aerosol therapy, doses that often exceeded prescription rates. The mean percentage of prescribed dose actually used was 98.5% at 1 month follow-up and 110.8% at 2 month follow-up. Since there was variability for each of these estimates, it appears that some percentage of the patients took considerably more medication than was prescribed (Chryssidis et al., 1981). It is not surprising that patients suffering from COPD, a highly symptomatic disorder, would overuse a medication that provides rapid symptomatic relief. Since the 1980s, surprisingly little attention has been given to medication overuse.

Adherence With Exercise

An important component of most pulmonary rehabilitation programs has been the establishment of a regular exercise regimen. Specific physical conditioning exercises, such as walking, can be undertaken by the patient to help maintain lung function and improve the remainder of the oxygen delivery system (Ries, 1994). Specifically, appropriate physical conditioning exercises can improve maximum oxygen consumption and endurance, reduce heart rate, improve ventilator efficiency, and increase tolerance for exercise. Lacasse and colleagues (2006) reviewed 23 RCTs on pulmonary rehabilitation and found significant improvements on all measured aspects of quality of life, including functional or maximal exercise capacity and dyspnea. Some evidence suggests that community-based programs can significantly improve adherence to exercise in COPD patients (Cockram, Cecins, & Jenkins, 2006). However, Beswick and colleagues (2005) considered 3,261 studies on cardiac rehabilitation and found only a dozen that considered methods for improving adherence.

Few studies have evaluated factors associated with long-term exercise maintenance among COPD patients. However, a rich literature in cardiac rehabilitation may provide useful suggestions. For example, Gupta and colleagues (2007) have shown good maintenance of cardiac rehabilitation benefits. One literature review analyzed 24 studies that had reported 12 or more months of follow-up (Simons-Morton, Calfas, Oldenburg, & Burton, 1998). Long-term maintenance of exercise was associated with supervision of the exercise, availability of equipment, frequent contact with program staff, the inclusion of a behavioral component, involvement in moderate rather than high-intensity activity, and specific interventions to maintain the behavior. Some success has been shown for difficult-to-reach patients. For example, Friedman and colleagues (1997) offered a rehabilitation program to the medically indigent. By individualizing instructions and providing guidance for specific community activities such as mall walking, stair climbing, and use of neighborhood facilities, they were able to obtain a self-reported adherence rate of 90%.

Exercise as a Component of Rehabilitation

A few controlled trials documented the benefits of exercise programs for patients with COPD (Resnikoff & Ries, 1998). Cockcroft, Saunders, and Berry (1981) randomly assigned 39 patients to a 6-week exercise program or to a no-treatment control group. Patients in the exercise group experienced more subjective benefits and a greater increase in the amount of distance they could walk in 12 minutes than did those who received no intervention. However, the length of follow-up was only 2 months. McGavin and coworkers randomly allocated 24 COPD patients to a 3-month unsupervised stair-climbing home exercise program or to a non-exercise control group. The 12 patients in the exercise group noted subjective improvements and an increased sense of well-being and decreased breathlessness. They also reported an objective increase in the 12-minute walk distance and in their maximal level of exercise on a cycle ergometer. These changes did not occur in the control group. However, the length of follow-up was limited to 3 months (McGavin, Gupta, Lloyd, & McHardy, 1977). Ambrosino and coworkers (1981) randomly assigned 23 patients to a 1-month medical and rehabilitative therapy group and 28 patients to medical therapy alone without exercise training. The experimental group improved in exercise tolerance and respiratory pattern, as evidenced by a decrease in respiratory rate and an increase in tidal volume. Again, these changes were not present in the control group.

One argument for the importance of exercise is that programs that do not have an exercise component are less effective. Sassi-Dambron et al. (1995) conducted a randomized clinical trial to evaluate a modified pulmonary rehabilitation program focused on supporting coping strategies for shortness of breath but without exercise training. Eighty-nine patients with COPD were randomly assigned to the 6-week treatment or to a 6-week general health-education control group.

The treatment consisted of instruction and practice in techniques of progressive muscle relaxation, breathing retraining, pacing, self-talk, and panic control. Outcomes included the 6-minute walk test, quality of well-being, depression and anxiety scales, and six commonly used dyspnea shortness of breath measures. There were no significant differences between the treatment and the control groups at the end of treatment or at 6-month follow-ups. The authors conclude that, while dyspnea management strategies are an important component of COPD management, they should be taught in combination with other aspects of comprehensive pulmonary rehabilitation, namely structured exercise training.

We have conducted several studies designed to improve adherence to exercise for patients with COPD. One of these experiments randomly assigned 119 COPD patients to either comprehensive rehabilitation or to an education control group. Pulmonary rehabilitation consisted of 12 4-hour sessions distributed over an 8-week period. The sessions focused on education, physical and respiratory care, psychosocial support, and supervised exercise. The education control group attended four 2-hour sessions that were scheduled twice per month. These education sessions did not include any individual instruction or exercise training. Topics included medical aspects of COPD, pharmacy use, breathing techniques, and a variety of interviews about smoking, life events, and social support. Lectures covered pulmonary medicine, pharmacology, respiratory therapy, and nutrition. Outcome measures included lung function; maximum and endurance exercise tolerance; symptoms such as perceived breathlessness, and perceived fatigue; self-efficacy for walking; and the Centers for Epidemiologic Studies Depression (CES-D) and the Quality of Well-Being scales. The patients were evaluated at the baseline and then again after 2, 6, 12, 24, 36, 48, and 60 months.

Figure 30.1 shows the differences between those in pulmonary rehabilitation and those in the education control groups over the first year of the study. The top portion of the figure shows changes in exercise endurance. Those randomly assigned to rehabilitation had significantly higher endurance at 2, 6, and 12 months. This was complemented by differences in breathlessness; those in the rehabilitation program were less breathless at the end of the treadmill exercise after 2, 6, and 12 months than those in the control group. Similarly, patients in the rehabilitation group were significantly lower in perceived muscle fatigue at each follow-up period (lower section of Figure 30.1) (Ries, Kaplan, Limberg, & Prewitt, 1995). There were no differences between the groups on measures of lung function, depression, or general quality of life. However, both groups experienced reductions in quality of life. Among the exercise variables, benefits tended to relapse toward baseline after 18 months of follow-up.

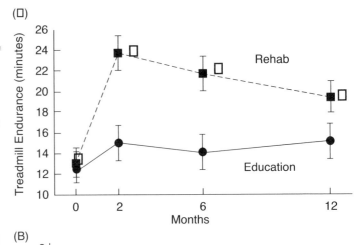

30.1

Results of treadmill endurance exercise tests for patients in the rehabilitation (Rehab) and education groups at baseline and for 12 months of follow-up. A. Exercise endurance time. B. Perceived breathlessness rating at the end of exercise. C. Perceived muscle-fatigue rating at the end of exercise. Asterisks indicate *P* < 0.05 for within-group change from baseline; values and error bars represent the mean (±SD).

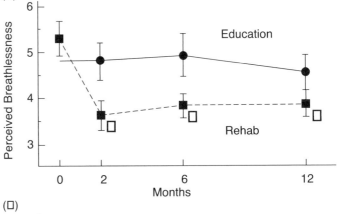

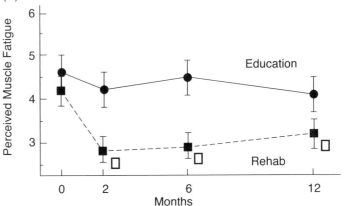

Note. From "Effects of Pulmonary Rehabilitation on Physiologic and Psychosocial Outcomes in Patients with Chronic Obstuctive Pulmonary Disease," by A. L. Ries, R. M. Kaplan, T. M. Lindberg, and L. M. Prewitt, 1995, *Annals of Internal Medicine, 122* (11), pp. 823–832. Copyright 1995 by the American College of Physicians. Reprinted with permission.

We have reason to believe that there is a systematic relationship between adherence to physical activity and a variety of outcomes. In an earlier study, we demonstrated a linear relationship between quartile of adherence with physical activity and exercise endurance measured in minutes. The study involved 57 moderate to severe COPD patients who were participating in a rehabilitation program. All participants were advised to exercise up to 60 minutes per day. Each patient kept a log of physical activity, making it possible to determine self-reported adherence to the exercise component of the program. Each 3 minutes of physical activity per day translated into an estimated 1-minute of improvement on treadmill exercise endurance (Eakin, Kaplan, & Ries, 1993).

In a more recent study, 160 patients with chronic lung disease participated in a comprehensive rehabilitation program. At the end of the rehabilitation program, the patients were randomly assigned to a program designed to improve adherence and maintenance of the rehabilitation lessons or to routine follow-up. Outcome measures included quality of life, symptoms, health care utilization, measures of pulmonary function, measures of psychological function, and survival. All patients were evaluated prior to the pulmonary rehabilitation and then again after the 8-week program had been completed. Following the second evaluation, patients were evaluated at 6 months, 12 months, and 24 months (Ries, Kaplan, Myers, & Prewitt, 2003). The effect of the postrehabilitation intervention was not significant in relation to the control group. Across both groups, the patients were classified according to their adherence to exercise during the follow-up period. Two groups were created—those who were regular walkers and those who walked irregularly. Regular walking was defined as walking most days or every single day, whereas irregular walking was defined as walking some days, rarely, or never. The core psychosocial measures included a generic quality of life measure known as the Quality of Well-Being (QWB) scale. Other measures included the UCSD Shortness of Breath questionnaire and a measure of self-efficacy for walking. Quality-of-life results are summarized in Figure 30.2. Regular walkers maintained better quality of life scores than irregular walkers. Similarly, those who walked on an irregular basis had more shortness of breath than those who walked on a regular basis (Heppner, Morgan, Kaplan, & Ries, 2006).

Our group has produced other evidence that walking adherence is related to better health outcomes. In one of our earlier studies, COPD patients were randomly assigned to one of five groups. One group was designed to increase adherence to physical activity using cognitive-behavior modification. Cognitive-behavior modification combines traditional behavior modification with cognitive therapy and is believed to be superior to either the behavior modification alone or the cognitive component alone. The study also involved a behavioral and a cognitive group. The fourth group got attention, while the fifth group received no treatment. All patients were evaluated at baseline and followed over the course of 12 weeks. Cumulative time spent walking was measured through patient reports in a diary. Those in the cognitive-behavior modification group accumulated significantly more walking time than those in control groups (Figure 30.3). Adherence to physical activity was associated with changes in endurance as evaluated on a treadmill after 12 weeks. Further, these changes in endurance were associated with changes on the QWB scale (Figure 30.4). All three groups experiencing a cognitive or behavioral intervention showed improvements on the QWB, while those in the two control groups declined on the QWB (Atkins, Kaplan, Timms, Reinsch, & Lofback, 1984).

There are several potential explanations for the failure to demonstrate long-term benefits from comprehensive pulmonary rehabilitation. One explanation is that behavioral interventions, without long-term follow-up or maintenance sessions, such as rehabilitation, are inadequate to produce long-term change. Long-term maintenance of behavior change has also been difficult to demonstrate in research on smoking cessation (Ockene et al., 1994b), weight-loss

30.2

Changes in the Quality of Well-Being Scale (QWB)—excluding deaths for regular and irregular walkers at post rehabilitation and 6-, 12-, and 24-month follow-ups. Higher scores indicate better overall health-related quality life.

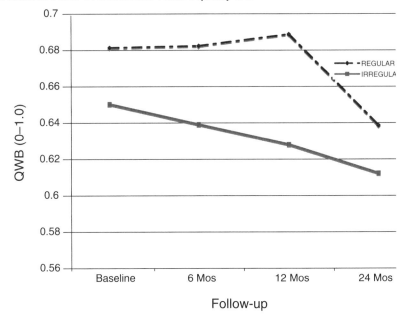

Note. From "Regular Walking and Long-Term Maintenance of Outcomes After Pulmonary Rehabilitation," by P. S. Heppner, C. Morgan, R. M. Kaplan, & A. L. Ries, 2006, *Journal of Cardiopulmonary Rehabilitation 26*(1), pp. 44–53. Copyright 2006 by Lippincott Williams & Wilkins. Reprinted with permission of Lippincott Williams & Wilkins.

(Mann et al., 2007), and exercise adherence (Dubbert, 1992). The finding that patients experience behavior change during treatment that is not maintained after treatment is consistent across a variety of different behavioral interventions (Mann et al., 2007). Discovering ways to maintain behavior change over extended periods of time remains a high priority for research.

In summary, patient adherence to exercise is perhaps the most difficult and least studied component of pulmonary rehabilitation. Exercise requires alteration in lifestyle, coping with uncomfortable sensations, and changes in daily schedules.

Adherence in Smoking Cessation Programs

Because of the well-documented association between smoking and COPD, successful smoking prevention programs are expected to reduce the incidence of these diseases. Smoking cessation programs are also valuable. There is considerable interest in the effects of smoking cessation for smokers with mild airway obstruction who may be at risk for COPD. In addition to the role of smoking as a cause of COPD, active cigarette smoking also affects the course of the illness. For example, cigarette smoking is associated with mucous hypersecretion, acute

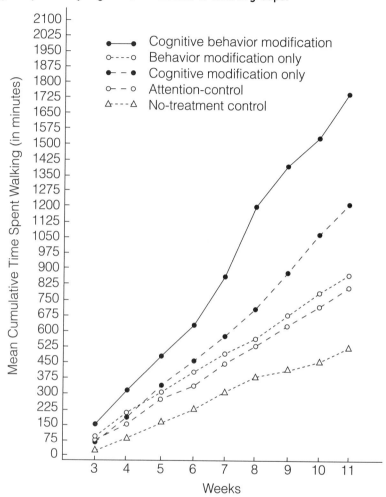

30.3

Walking compliance by cognitive, behavioral, or control groups.

Mean Cumulative Time Spent Walking (in minutes)

- ●——● Cognitive behavior modification
- ○----○ Behavior modification only
- ●- -● Cognitive modification only
- ○- -○ Attention-control
- △---△ No-treatment control

Weeks

Note. From "Behavioral Exercise Programs in the Management of Chronic Obstructive Pulmonary Disease," by C. J. Atkins, R. M. Kaplan, R. M. Timms, S. Reinsch, & K. Lofback, 1984, *Journal of Consulting Clinical Psychology, 52*(4), p. 599. Copyright 1984 by the American Psychological Association. Reprinted with permission of the American Psychological Association.

respiratory illnesses, altered airway reactivity, and increased risk of mortality from other causes, including coronary heart disease. Some of the relations between smoking and problems in the airways have been reviewed elsewhere (Lopez et al., 2006). A variety of studies have suggested that loss in lung function is associated with total duration of cigarette use (Dockery et al., 1988). Longitudinal studies indicate that there is a progressive loss of pulmonary function with continued cigarette smoking. However, there is at least some evidence that there is partial recovery of lung function for those who cease cigarette smoking, particularly for those who do so early in life (Buist, 2006).

30.4

Mean change in QWB (multiplied by 100) by group.

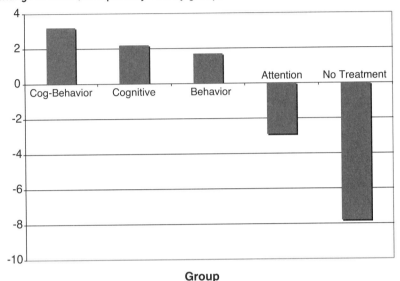

Group

Note: From "Behavioral Exercise Programs in the Management of Chronic Obstructive Pulmonary Disease," by C. J. Atkins, R. M. Kaplan, R. M. Timms, S. Reinsch, & K. Lofback, 1984, *Journal of Consulting Clinical Psychology, 52*(4), p. 599. Copyright 1984 by the American Psychological Association. Reprinted with permission of the American Psychological Association.

Because of the potential benefits of smoking cessation, efforts to improve adherence to smoking cessation programs are of great importance. Evidence has accumulated suggesting that the physician may play a critical role in helping patients to stop smoking and to maintain this behavioral change (Ockene & Zapka, 1997). Several experimental trials have trained physicians to deliver a smoking cessation intervention. The components of the intervention include approaches for taking a smoking history, personalizing the health risks, setting a quit date, prescribing nicotine chewing gum, and counseling techniques for follow-up. In one study, Ockene and associates (1994a) assigned physicians to receive training in behaviorally oriented counseling techniques or to a control group in which patients were provided with only brief advice to stop smoking. Some of the interventions involved the use of nicotine gum, whereas others did not. The results suggested that the behavioral intervention, with or without the use of nicotine gum, resulted in greater reductions in cigarette use among patients. Further, differences between these groups remained at 6-month follow-up. The Agency for Health Care Policy and Research offered guidelines for smoking cessation in primary care medicine (Fiore, 1998). Despite the well-established health consequences of tobacco use, early studies suggested that fewer than one half of physicians commonly advise their patients to give up cigarettes (Ockene, Aney, Goldberg, Klar, & Williams, 1988). By 2006, rates of referral for smoking cessation remained low, although three-quarters of primary-care physicians reported that they advised their smoking patients to quit (Schnoll, Rukstalis, Wileyto, & Shields, 2006). Among those who discuss smoking with their patients, few go much further. For example, only about one in four physicians makes any effort beyond simply stating that the patient should quit smoking (Ockene et al., 1988). One of the biggest challenges in getting patients to quit smoking is the recognition that relapse is common. Most smokers who stop will begin using cigarettes again within 3 months. Among smokers who have abstained for 48 hours, nearly 20% relapse within the first week and an additional 13% relapse during the second week (Gulliver, Hughes, Solomon, & Dey, 1995). About 23% remain smoke free for 6 months. Relapse rates among those who participate in formal programs are somewhat better than those for self-quitters (Brandon, Tiffany, Obremski, & Baker, 1990). Recent studies suggest that those smokers who slip are most likely to relapse. For example, a smoker who takes an occasional cigarette is significantly more likely to relapse than one who does not slip (Baer, Kamarck, Lichtenstein, & Ransom, 1989; Brandon et al., 1990). Readiness to change should also be assessed. Many smokers may be in a "precomtemplation" phase in which they are nonreceptive to messages about quitting. Those who are already contemplating a quit might be better targets for a quitting message (Boudreaux, Carmack, Searinci, & Brantley, 1998; Boudreaux, Hunter, Bos, Clark, & Camargo, 2006).

Perhaps the best predictor of relapse is low personal expectations for remaining smoke free. Using electronic daily diaries, Shiffman and colleagues (Shiffman, 2006; Shiffman et al., 2006) have been able to determine what factors precipitate relapse. These studies suggest that lapses associated with self-reported stress or good mood were more likely to progress to relapses than those associated with eating or drinking.

A large literature on smoking cessation techniques has developed and is best summarized in the AHCPR Smoking Guideline (Fiore, 1998). Overall, self-help groups tend not to achieve better outcomes than control groups (Ranney, Melvin, & Rohweder, 2005). We urge the use of self-help materials in combination with some counseling intervention. Telephone counseling appears to offer significant benefits. In addition, several free 800 numbers are now available. Many of these are summarized at www.helpguide.org/mental/quit_smoking_cessation.htm. Evidence does suggest that physicians and other health care providers can offer brief smoking cessation counseling in combination with pharmacological intervention (Ranney et al., 2005) and that these simple interventions enhance abstinence rates at 6 and 12 months (Morgan et al., 1996). The addition of Nicotine Replacement Therapy has also been shown to increase long-term maintenance. Pharmacotherapy may be more effective for men than for women, particularly when it is used with combination with smoking cessation counseling (Perkins, Grobe, Caggiula, Wilson, & Stiller, 1997).

Summary

The typical regimen for patients with COPD requires many different behaviors. These may include the use of several different medications, exercise, oxygen, respiratory and physiotherapy techniques, and other aspects of self-care. Adherence to this regimen can be challenging. In contrast to nearly every other medical condition, there are relatively few published studies evaluating the benefits of interventions to improve adherence among patients with COPD. Further, we do not know the extent to which overuse of medication is associated with poor outcomes for patients with COPD. Behavioral intervention may enhance adherence with medicine taking, smoking cessation, and exercise. However, considerably more research is necessary to evaluate the long-term benefits of these interventions.

References

Almagro, P., Calbo, E., Ochoa de Echaguen, A., Barreiro, B., Quintana, S., Heredia, J. L., et al. (2002). Mortality after hospitalization for COPD. *Chest, 121*(5), 1441–1448.

Ambrosino, N., Paggiaro, P. L., Macchi, M., Filieri, M., Toma, G., Lombardi, F. A., et al. (1981). A study of short-term effect of rehabilitative therapy in chronic obstructive pulmonary disease. *Respiration, 41*(1), 40–44.

Atkins, C. J., Kaplan, R. M., Timms, R. M., Reinsch, S., & Lofback, K. (1984). Behavioral exercise programs in the management of chronic obstructive pulmonary disease. *Journal of Consulting and Clinical Psychology, 52*(4), 591–603.

Baer, J. S., Kamarck, T., Lichtenstein, E., & Ransom, C. C., Jr. (1989). Prediction of smoking relapse: Analyses of temptations and transgressions after initial cessation. *Journal of Consulting and Clinical Psychology, 57*(5), 623–627.

Beswick, A. D., Rees, K., West, R. R., Taylor, F. C., Burke, M., Griebsch, I., et al. (2005). Improving uptake and adherence in cardiac rehabilitation: Literature review. *Journal of Advanced Nursing, 49*(5), 538–555.

Boudreaux, E., Carmack, C. L., Searinci, I. C., & Brantley, P. J. (1998). Predicting smoking stage of change among a sample of low socioeconomic status, primary care outpatients: Replication and extension using decisional balance and self-efficacy theories. *International Journal of Behavioral Medicine, 5*(2), 148–165.

Boudreaux, E. D., Hunter, G. C., Bos, K., Clark, S., & Camargo, C. A., Jr. (2006). Predicting smoking stage of change among emergency department patients and visitors. *Academic Emergency Medicine, 13*(1), 39–47.

Brandon, T. H., Tiffany, S. T., Obremski, K. M., & Baker, T. B. (1990). Postcessation cigarette use: The process of relapse. *Addictive Behaviors, 15*(2), 105–114.

Buist, S. (2006). COPD: A common disease that is preventable and treatable. *Primary Care Respiratory Journal, 15*(1), 7–9.

Chryssidis, E., Frewin, D. B., Frith, P. A., & Dawes, E. R. (1981). Compliance with aerosol therapy in chronic obstructive lung disease. *New Zealand Medical Journal, 94*(696), 375–377.

Cockcroft, A. E., Saunders, M. J., & Berry, G. (1981). Randomised controlled trial of rehabilitation in chronic respiratory disability. *Thorax, 36*(3), 200–203.

Cockram, J., Cecins, N., & Jenkins, S. (2006). Maintaining exercise capacity and quality of life following pulmonary rehabilitation. *Respirology, 11*(1), 98–104.

Corden, Z., & Rees, P. J. (1998). The effect of oral corticosteroids on bronchodilator responses in COPD. *Respiratory Medicine, 92*(2), 279–282.

DiMatteo, M. R. (2004). Variations in patients' adherence to medical recommendations: A quantitative review of 50 years of research. *Medical Care, 42*(3), 200–209.

DiMatteo, M. R., Haskard, K. B., & Williams, S. L. (2007). Health beliefs, disease severity, and patient adherence: A meta-analysis. *Medical Care, 45*(6), 521–528.

Dockery, D. W., Speizer, F. E., Ferris, B. G., Jr., Ware, J. H., Louis, T. A., & Spiro, A., III. (1988). Cumulative and reversible effects of lifetime smoking on simple tests of lung function in adults. *American Review Respiratory Disease, 137*(2), 286–292.

Dubbert, P. M. (1992). Exercise in behavioral medicine. *Journal of Consulting and Clinical Psychology, 60*(4), 613–618.

Dunbar-Jacob, J. (2005). Chronic disease: A patient-focused view. *Journal of Professional Nursing, 21*(1), 3–4.

Eakin, E. G., Kaplan, R. M., & Ries, A. L. (1993). Measurement of dyspnoea in chronic obstructive pulmonary disease. *Quality of Life Research, 2*(3), 181–191.

Fiore, M. C. (1998). Overview of the agency for health care policy and research guideline. *Tobacco Control, 7*(Suppl.), S14–S16; discussion, S24–S15.

Fishman, A., Martinez, F., Naunheim, K., Piantadosi, S., Wise, R., Ries, A., et al. (2003). A randomized trial comparing lung-volume-reduction surgery with medical therapy for severe emphysema. *New England Journal of Medicine, 348*(21), 2059–2073.

Friedman, D. B., Williams, A. N., & Levine, B. D. (1997). Compliance and efficacy of cardiac rehabilitation and risk factor modification in the medically indigent. *American Journal of Cardiology, 79*(3), 281–285.

George, J., Kong, D. C., Thoman, R., & Stewart, K. (2005). Factors associated with medication nonadherence in patients with COPD. *Chest, 128*(5), 3198–3204.

Gulliver, S. B., Hughes, J. R., Solomon, L. J., & Dey, A. N. (1995). An investigation of self-efficacy, partner support and daily stresses as predictors of relapse to smoking in self-quitters. *Addiction, 90*(6), 767–772.

Gupta, R., Sanderson, B. K., & Bittner, V. (2007). Outcomes at one-year follow-up of women and men with coronary artery disease discharged from cardiac rehabilitation: What benefits are maintained? *Journal of Cardiopulmonary Rehabilitation and Prevention, 27*(1), 11–18, quiz, 19–20.

Han, M. K., Postma, D., Mannino, D., Giardino, N. D., Buist, S., Curtis, J. L., et al. (2007). Gender and COPD: Why it matters. *American Journal of Respiratory and Critical Care Medicine 176*(12), 1179–1184.

Heppner, P. S., Morgan, C., Kaplan, R. M., & Ries, A. L. (2006). Regular walking and long-term maintenance of outcomes after pulmonary rehabilitation. *Journal of Cardiopulmonary Rehabilitation, 26*(1), 44–53.

Intermittent positive pressure breathing therapy of chronic obstructive pulmonary disease. A clinical trial. (1983). *Annals of Internal Medicine, 99*(5), 612–620.

James, P. N., Anderson, J. B., Prior, J. G., White, J. P., Henry, J. A., & Cochrane, G. M. (1985). Patterns of drug taking in patients with chronic airflow obstruction. *Postgraduate Medical Journal, 61*(711), 7–10.

Krigsman, K., Nilsson, J. L., & Ring, L. (2007). Refill adherence for patients with asthma and COPD: Comparison of a pharmacy record database with manually collected repeat prescriptions. *Pharmacoepidemiology and Drug Safety, 16*(4), 441–448.

Lacasse, Y., Goldstein, R., Lasserson, T. J., & Martin, S. (2006). Pulmonary rehabilitation for chronic obstructive pulmonary disease. *Cochrane Database Systemic Reviews,* (4), CD003793.

Lin, S. K., Kuna, S. T., & Bogen, D. K. (2006). A novel device for measuring long-term oxygen therapy adherence: A preliminary validation. *Respiratory Care, 51*(3), 266–271.

Lopez, A. D., Shibuya, K., Rao, C., Mathers, C. D., Hansell, A. L., Held, L. S., et al. (2006). Chronic obstructive pulmonary disease: Current burden and future projections. *European Respiratory Journal, 27*(2), 397–412.

Mann, T., Tomiyama, A. J., Westling, E., Lew, A. M., Samuels, B., & Chatman, J. (2007). Medicare's search for effective obesity treatments: Diets are not the answer. *American Psychologist, 62*(3), 220–233.

Mannino, D. M. (2002). Epidemiology, prevalence, morbidity and mortality, and disease heterogeneity. *Chest, 121*(5), 121S-126S.

McGavin, C. R., Gupta, S. P., Lloyd, E. L., & McHardy, G. J. (1977). Physical rehabilitation for the chronic bronchitic: Results of a controlled trial of exercises in the home. *Thorax, 32*(3), 307–311.

Morgan, G. D., Noll, E. L., Orleans, C. T., Rimer, B. K., Amfoh, K., & Bonney, G. (1996). Reaching midlife and older smokers: Tailored interventions for routine medical care. *Preventative Medicine, 25*(3), 346–354.

Morrison, D., Skwarski, K., & MacNee, W. (1995). Review of the prescription of domiciliary long term oxygen therapy in Scotland. *Thorax, 50*(10), 1103–1105.

Murray, R. P., Istvan, J. A., Voelker, H. T., Rigdon, M. A., & Wallace, M. D. (1995). Level of involvement with alcohol and success at smoking cessation in the lung health study. *Journal of Studies on Alcohol, 56*(1), 74–82.

Neri, M., Melani, A. S., Miorelli, A. M., Zanchetta, D., Bertocco, E., Cinti, C., et al. (2006). Long-term oxygen therapy in chronic respiratory failure: A multicenter Italian study on oxygen therapy adherence (misota). *Respiratory Medicine, 100*(5), 795–806.

Nides, M. A., Tashkin, D. P., Simmons, M. S., Wise, R. A., Li, V. C., & Rand, C. S. (1993). Improving inhaler adherence in a clinical trial through the use of the nebulizer chronolog. *Chest, 104*(2), 501–507.

Ockene, J. K., Adams, A., Pbert, L., Luippold, R., Hebert, J. R., Quirk, M., et al. (1994a). The physician-delivered smoking intervention project: Factors that determine how much the physician intervenes with smokers. *Journal of General Internal Medicine, 9*(7), 379–384.

Ockene, J. K., Aney, J., Goldberg, R. J., Klar, J. M., & Williams, J. W. (1988). A survey of Massachusetts physicians' smoking intervention practices. *American Journal of Preventive Medicine, 4*(1), 14–20.

Ockene, J. K., Kristeller, J., Pbert, L., Hebert, J. R., Luippold, R., Goldberg, R. J., et al. (1994b). The physician-delivered smoking intervention project: Can short-term interventions produce long-term effects for a general outpatient population? *Health Psychology, 13*(3), 278–281.

Ockene, J. K., & Zapka, J. G. (1997). Physician-based smoking intervention: A rededication to a five-step strategy to smoking research. *Addictive Behavior, 22*(6), 835–848.

Patient information series. Chronic obstructive pulmonary disease (COPD). (2005). *American Journal of Respiratory and Critical Care Medicine, 171*(6), P3–P4.

Perkins, K. A., Grobe, J. E., Caggiula, A., Wilson, A. S., & Stiller, R. L. (1997). Acute reinforcing effects of low-dose nicotine nasal spray in humans. *Pharmacology Biochemistry and Behavior, 56*(2), 235–241.

Powell, S. G. (1994). Medication compliance of patients with COPD. *Home Healthcare Nurse, 12*(3), 44–50.

Rabe, K. F., Hurd, S., Anzueto, A., Barnes, P. J., Buist, S. A., Calverley, P., et al. (2007). Global strategy for the diagnosis, management, and prevention of chronic obstructive pulmonary disease: Gold executive summary. *American Journal of Respiratory and Critical Care Medicine, 176*(6), 532–555.

Rand, C. S., Nides, M., Cowles, M. K., Wise, R. A., & Connett, J. (1995). Long-term metered-dose inhaler adherence in a clinical trial. The lung health study research group. *American Journal of Respiratory and Critical Care Medicine, 152*(2), 580–588.

Ranney, L. M., Melvin, C. L., & Rohweder, C. L. (2005). From guidelines to practice: A process evaluation of the national partnership to help pregnant smokers quit. *AHIP Coverage, 46*(4), 50–52.

Resnikoff, P. M., & Ries, A. L. (1998). Maximizing functional capacity. Pulmonary rehabilitation and adjunctive measures. *Respiratory Care Clinics of North America, 4*(3), 475–492.

Restrick, L. J., Paul, E. A., Braid, G. M., Cullinan, P., Moore-Gillon, J., & Wedzicha, J. A. (1993). Assessment and follow up of patients prescribed long term oxygen treatment. *Thorax, 48*(7), 708–713.

Ries, A. L. (1994). The importance of exercise in pulmonary rehabilitation. *Clinics in Chest Medicine, 15*(2), 327–337.

Ries, A. L. (2007). AACP/AACCPR evidence-based guidelines for pulmonary rehabilitation. Round 3: Another step forward. *Journal of Cardiopulmonary Rehabilitation and Prevention, 27*(4), 233–236.

Ries, A. L., Bauldoff, G. S., Carlin, B. W., Casaburi, R., Emery, C. F., Mahler, D. A., et al. (2007). Pulmonary rehabilitation: Joint AACP/AACVPR evidence-based clinical practice guidelines. *Chest, 131*(5 Suppl), S4–S42.

Ries, A. L., Kaplan, R. M., Limberg, T. M., & Prewitt, L. M. (1995). Effects of pulmonary rehabilitation on physiologic and psychosocial outcomes in patients with chronic obstructive pulmonary disease. *Annals of Internal Medicine, 122*(11), 823–832.

Ries, A. L., Kaplan, R. M., Myers, R., & Prewitt, L. M. (2003). Maintenance after pulmonary rehabilitation in chronic lung disease: A randomized trial. *American Journal of Respiratory and Critical Care Medicine, 167*(6), 880–888.

Ringbaek, T. J. (2005). Continuous oxygen therapy for hypoxic pulmonary disease: Guidelines, compliance and effects. *Treatments in Respiratory Medicine, 4*(6), 397–408.

The rise in chronic obstructive disease mortality. (1989). *American Review of Respiratory Disease, 140*(3 Pt. 2), S1–S107.

Sassi-Dambron, D. E., Eakin, E. G., Ries, A. L., & Kaplan, R. M. (1995). Treatment of dyspnea in COPD. A controlled clinical trial of dyspnea management strategies. *Chest, 107*(3), 724–729.

Schnoll, R. A., Rukstalis, M., Wileyto, E. P., & Shields, A. E. (2006). Smoking cessation treatment by primary care physicians: An update and call for training. *American Journal of Preventive Medicine, 31*(3), 233–239.

Shiffman, S. (2006). Reflections on smoking relapse research. *Drug and Alcohol Review, 25*(1), 15–20.

Shiffman, S., Scharf, D. M., Shadel, W. G., Gwaltney, C. J., Dang, Q., Paton, S. M., et al. (2006). Analyzing milestones in smoking cessation: Illustration in a nicotine patch trial in adult smokers. *Journal of Consulting and Clinical Psychology, 74*(2), 276–285.

Simons-Morton, D. G., Calfas, K. J., Oldenburg, B., & Burton, N. W. (1998). Effects of interventions in health care settings on physical activity or cardiorespiratory fitness. *American Journal of Preventive Medicine, 15*(4), 413–430.

Solomon, D. K., Portner, T. S., Bass, G. E., Gourley, D. R., Gourley, G. A., Holt, J. M., et al. (1998). Clinical and economic outcomes in the hypertension and COPD arms of a multicenter outcomes study. *Journal of the American Pharmaceutical Association, 38*(5), 574–585.

Strassels, S. A., Smith, D. H., Sullivan, S. D., & Mahajan, P. S. (2001). The costs of treating COPD in the united states. *Chest, 119,* 344–352.

Turner, J., Wright, E., Mendella, L., & Anthonisen, N. (1995). Predictors of patient adherence to long-term home nebulizer therapy for COPD. The IPPB study group. Intermittent positive pressure breathing. *Chest, 108*(2), 394–400.

Williams, L. K., Joseph, C. L., Peterson, E. L., Wells, K., Wang, M., Chowdhry, V. K., et al. (2007). Patients with asthma who do not fill their inhaled corticosteroids: A study of primary nonadherence. *Journal of Allergy and Clinical Immunology, 120*(5), 1153–1159.

Yohannes, A. M., Baldwin, R. C., & Connolly, M. J. (2005). Predictors of 1-year mortality in patients discharged from hospital following exacerbation of chronic obstructive pulmonary disease. *Age and Aging, 34,* 491–496.

Aging, Cognition, and Diabetes: The Transition From Self-Care to a Caregiver for Diabetes Self-Management

31

Laura H. Coker

Cognitive declines across a broad spectrum, from "normal" age-related declines to dementia, and type 2 diabetes are common among people aged 65 years and older (see chapter 35 for the epidemiology of cognition and diabetes). Briefly, some longitudinal epidemiologic studies have established an association between diabetes mellitus and both Alzheimer's (Leibson et al., 1997; Ott et al., 1996; Yoshitake et al., 1995) and vascular dementias (Ott et al., 1996; Yoshitake et al., 1995) in older adults, while others support the link between diabetes and vascular dementia only (Curb et al., 1999). The relationship between diabetes and dementia is suggestive but does not confirm that type 2 diabetes causes cognitive dysfunction independent of dementia (Coker & Shumaker, 2003). These relationships are under study in the ongoing National Heart, Lung, and Blood Institute (NHLBI) funded Action to Control Cardiovascular Risk in Diabetes—Memory in

Diabetes (ACCORD-MIND) clinical trial, which addresses the effect of diabetes and cardiovascular risk factors on age-associated cognitive declines in men and women age 55 years and over (Williamson et al., 2007).

The gerontologic literature suggests that declining cognitive abilities are important predictors of decrements in self-care behaviors and lifestyle choices that support health maintenance in general. Cognitive declines are also associated with decreased ability to self-manage medical regimens for secondary prevention and treatment of chronic disease. Self-care regimens for diabetes are complex and difficult to manage for people with normal cognitive abilities, and they pose a real challenge to those with impaired thinking, remembering, and planning skills. The transition from self-care to care provided by an "informal" family caregiver provides a way for the cognitively impaired person to maintain diabetic self-management. Ideally, this transition takes place gradually, with both the caregiver and the care recipient negotiating their roles. Regardless, when a caregiver enters the equation, a number of variables are introduced to the ultimate goal of improving management of the care recipient's treatment regimen. These include, but are not limited to, the caregiver's knowledge of the disease process, the complexity of the care required, the physical "work" of providing care, and the caregiver's health. Important interpersonal factors involve the relationship between the care recipient and caregiver, acceptance of the care recipient and caregiver roles, and the combined resources of the care recipient and caregiver. Informal caregivers perform an enormous role in the day-to-day care of dependent elderly with chronic disease in the United States, and this trend will increase with the current demographic of an aging population.

This chapter classifies types of cognitive declines commonly seen in older adults and describes typical functional abilities associated with each type. It also explores the transition from diabetes self-care to care provided by an informal family caregiver. Description of this transition includes a discussion on recognizing the need for a caregiver, followed by a section on emergence of the caregiver. Finally, findings from the literature describe the experiences of the caregiver and the structural and policy issues that suggest that supporting the caregiver is the ultimate strategy for promoting self-management of the cognitively impaired person with diabetes. This exploration uses a biopsychosocial framework by Glasgow & Eakin (1998), which includes six levels of influence that affect diabetes self-management. Finally, we discuss factors that are supportive and those that act as barriers to the well-being of the cognitively impaired diabetes patient, the caregiver, and the dyad they compose.

Types of Cognitive Decline and Effect on Self-Care Behaviors

Cognitive declines are common as one ages, hence the terms *normal cognitive aging* and *age-associated cognitive decline*, which frequently appear in the gerontologic and neuropsychologic literature (Arenberg, 1978; Resnick, Trotman, Kawas, & Zonderman, 1995). Both terms refer to a range of mild to marked declines in cognitive abilities that occurs due to aging rather than to specific disease processes. Age-associated cognitive decline affects memory and the ability to plan, organize, and shift from one task to another while sparing other cognitive abilities such as well-learned verbal skills and vocabulary (La Rue, 1992) (see chapter 35 for an explanation of domain-specific cognitive issues and diabetes). Although cognitive declines due to aging are a source of great concern and social anxiety among older adults (Resnick et al., 2004), the declines do not necessarily predict a downward course to dementia—and generally do not interfere with the ability to conduct daily activities and manage one's own affairs, including one's health.

Mild cognitive impairment (MCI) is a newer classification that continues to be refined and portends further declines in a small subset of people who bear this classification. For example, people with MCI generally exhibit poor cognitive performance (10th percentile or lower) in at least one area in the Modified Consortium to Establish a Registry for Alzheimer's Disease (CERAD) cognitive battery (Morris et al., 1989), a report of some functional impairment that is not severe enough to interfere with basic activities of daily living (ADLs), such as eating, bathing, dressing, and grooming, and absence of a psychiatric disorder or medical condition that could account for the decline in cognition and the absence of dementia. (Petersen et al., 2001). Sources suggest that approximately 15% of people with MCI convert to the classification of dementia every year; however, this figure may be higher in cohorts that include amnestic MCI, which is viewed by most as part of the continuum to dementia, whereas the conversion to dementia is lower in cohorts with nonamnestic MCI. Also, the number of people who convert to dementia also varies depending on whether functional impairment is required for the definition of dementia (Fisk, Merry, & Rockwood, 2003; Lopez et al., 2003). Although the majority of people with MCI are able to manage their own basic ADLs, they may have difficulty with specific instrumental activities of daily living (IADLs) such as cooking, driving, gardening, balancing a checkbook, or using public transportation. People with MCI do have a measurable decline in cognitive functioning, and progression to dementia is higher in this group than in same-age cohorts without MCI. Therefore, the classification of MCI alone suggests that close attention be paid to the patient's ability to adequately manage self-care.

The diagnosis of *all-cause dementia* is reserved for people who meet the criteria set forth in the American Psychiatric Association Diagnostic Manual of Mental Disorders (American Psychiatric Association, 1994). These criteria require that individuals who suffer from cognitive declines score poorly on two or more tests in the CERAD battery (or similar standardized neurological tests); demonstrate a degree of functional decline that makes them dependent on others; not have psychiatric or physical illness that could account for the cognitive decline; and not be abusing alcohol or drugs that could explain the cognitive symptoms.

Significant declines in cognitive functioning associated with dementia have been shown to increase the risk of difficulty performing basic ADLs and IADLs, including self-care behaviors (Kelly-Hayes, Jette, Wolf, D'Agostino, & Odell, 1992; Stuck et al., 1999). Declines in self-care behaviors affect routine health maintenance and preventive health practices, as well as specific daily care regimens that are required for diabetes self-management. The clinical diagnosis of dementia suggests a level of dependency on others that may be met by an informal family caregiver, formal paid assistance, or formal supportive living arrangements such as assisted living or nursing home care.

Aging, Cognition, and Diabetes Self-Management

When cognitive declines result in poor adherence to the medical treatment regimen, the severity of diabetes increases (Sinclair, Girling, & Bayer, 2000). Ideally, precipitous declines in health status can be prevented by early recognition of the need for a caregiver and early identification of an able and enthusiastic person to accept the role. Glasgow & Eakin's (1998) "pyramid of influences" provides a biopsychosocial framework to systematically examine supportive factors, as well as barriers to diabetes self-management. The factors include six levels, arranged from micro- to macro-levels: 1. personal, 2. family and significant other, 3. health care system, 4. worksite or organization, 5. neighborhood and community, 6. media, policy, and culture. This framework may also be useful to evaluate whether these factors differ or are magnified when the patient with diabetes has concomitant cognitive declines and has an informal family caregiver.

In *Level 1: Personal Factors* of Glasgow & Eakin's (1998) framework, the concepts of empowerment, high self-efficacy, and good problem-solving skills are identified as supportive for diabetes self-management, while lack of knowledge and low self-efficacy are named as barriers. When one adds the concept of *aging* as a personal factor, viewed from a biopsychosocial perspective, the effect on self-management can be mixed, depending on health status and developmental stage. For example, aging is often linked to negative health outcomes but holds positive connotations for life-span developmental stages. Erikson (1959) discussed the developmental milestones of old age and the stage of *personal integrity*—described as the ultimate stage of personality development. Older adults operating in this stage have a strong preference to remain independent, to reflect on the mark they are leaving on the world, to be an example to others, and to contribute to the well-being of others, especially their own families. For many older adults, becoming a burden on one's own spouse and children is to be avoided at all costs. However, when faced with significant problems (health, financial, safety), these same older adults can reach out to their spouses and other family members and take an active part in decision making about their own care. Theoretically, being able to recognize the need for and help plan for one's own care facilitates the process of adapting to the role of becoming a care recipient, but this process has not been well studied.

On the other hand, older adults with waning cognitive abilities may lack the judgment or problem-solving skills to assess their need for assistance from others. It may be that empowerment and high self-efficacy, which are supportive factors to older adults with *normal* cognitive functioning, are not as important as "insight" into their abilities in people with impaired cognitive functioning. There is evidence that some cognitively impaired older adults lack insight with respect to their limitations and overestimate their abilities. Cotrell, Wild, & Bader (2006) studied the relationship among cognitive status, deficit awareness, medication management skills, and actual adherence among individuals 65 years and older with mild AD and compared this group to age-matched cognitively normal participants. They found those with AD were seemingly unaware of their cognitive limitations and significantly overpredicted their ability to adhere to timing and dosing requirements.

Also, the literature suggests that *awareness* of one's own cognitive abilities may be more important than cognitive status per se in achieving good adherence. Branin (2001) reported that older adults who expressed greater concern about their memory were more likely to rely on "external props" to prompt flagging skills in memory and organization. Life-span adherence studies report that despite strong evidence for age-related cognitive decline, adults in the "young-old" category adhered adequately and had fewer errors than busy middle-aged adults, whereas the oldest-old had more difficulty adhering (Morrell, Park, Kidder, & Martin, 1997; Park, Hong, Lee, Ha, & Sung, 2004). Individuals who retain a certain level of insight with respect to their cognitive abilities may be able to effectively use scheduling and contextual cues to compensate for their waning cognitive skills. For example, individuals who experience psychomotor slowness, a common sign of age-related cognitive decline, may adjust by simplifying their schedules to provide more time to attend to medication adherence and other self-care activities. Those who are aware of memory problems may adopt any number of behaviors, such as making lists, filling pill dispensers for the week (with or without help), or using a diary to record self-care requirements such as checks on blood pressure, weight, and medication time, dosing, and side effects. Those who retain the ability to plan, coordinate, and set priorities may be able to link contextual cues such as bath time or preparation for bed with self-care activities such as checking feet and taking evening medications (Branin, 2001; Brown & Park, 2003; Gould, McDonald-Miszczak, & King, 1996).

Recognizing the Need for a Caregiver for Diabetes Self-Management

Consistent with Glasgow & Eakin's (1998) diabetes self-management framework, at *Level 2: Family and Significant Other,* family and friends among the diabetic patient's close social network are most likely to recognize when the diabetic person needs help. This is especially important when the patient is cognitively impaired or lacks the insight to ask for help. Elderly people with diabetes display excess cognitive dysfunction that is associated with decrements in self-care and increased dependency needs (Sinclair et al., 2000). The literature records a number of signs of worsening disease or events that may indicate that the patient with diabetes is having difficulty with cognition and/or self-care and needs assistance. These include poorer glycemic control as measured by Hgb A1c (Perlmuter et al., 1984); declines in cognitive screening scores (Sinclair et al., 2000); lower ADL scores or functional declines (Langa et al., 2002; Sinclair et al., 2000); development of neuropathy (Perlmuter et al., 1984); hospitalization for diabetes symptoms (Sinclair et al., 2000); diagnosis of comorbidity such as stroke or heart disease (Langa et al., 2002); complicated medication regimen, including the addition of insulin therapy (Hendra & Taylor, 2004; Silliman, Bhatti, Khan, Dukes, & Sullivan, 1996); declines in vision (Langa et al., 2002); and infection and/or delayed wound healing (Nabuurs-Franssen, Huijberts, Nieuwenhuijzen Kruseman, Willems, & Schaper, 2005). This list of events or signs and symptoms associated with diabetes is not exhaustive, but any one of them may indicate the need for some degree of assistance from someone in monitoring the day-to-day needs of the person with diabetes.

Emergence of a Caregiver for Diabetes Self-Management

Glasgow & Eakin (1998) identify the diabetes patient's family and friends as the source of social support when the patient is dealing with diabetes self-management issues. It follows, therefore, that the older, cognitively impaired patient would also look to his close social network for care. Supportive factors include an environment that is conducive to responding to the patient's specific needs (e.g., glucose monitoring, therapeutic diet, medication regimen), while also actively encouraging the patient to remain independent, active, and as productive as possible. Lack of expected support from one's close network serves as a barrier to the patient's well-being. Ideally, emergence of a capable and dedicated caregiver takes place gradually, so the caregiver has ample opportunity to acquire needed information and to understand which of the patient's needs require caregiver assistance. It is often the case that some of the care activities are maintained by the patient, while others are transferred to the caregiver. Ideally, the caregiver and the care recipient work together, each negotiating roles that are dynamic over time. But how is the caregiver chosen, and who is he or she?

Family systems theory provides a way to think about how the need for care is recognized and how the caregiver role emerges. The theory holds that behaviors within the family system are more intimate and enduring than those outside the system. Within the system, dependency needs are shared and interdependence is accepted as a norm. Therefore, when one person has increased needs for care, a member of the family is likely to recognize and meet that need. As the person in need adapts to the role of the care recipient, another person emerges as the caregiver. When the care recipient is married, the caregiver is most often the spouse (Whitchurch & Constantine, 1993). Also, when the care needs involve intimate physical care, these needs are usually managed by the spousal caregiver. Unmarried care recipients look to other family members for care, and the role is most likely assumed by a close female member—mother, sister, sister-in-law. Male caregivers tend to manage specific tasks, such as heavy physical work like lifting or transferring patients or transporting the patient to medical appointments. Men may also assist by performing typical gender role tasks, such as financial management and home, yard, and automobile maintenance for care recipients who have lost the ability to perform these instrumental activities. Numerous clinical studies have borne out these theoretical underpinnings of the care recipient and caregiver roles (Nabuurs-Franssen et al., 2005; Silliman et al., 1996; Stone, Cafferata, & Sangl, 1987).

Little is known about the process of how the patient and the caregiver negotiate which self-care tasks are to be retained by the patient and which are to be transferred to the caregiver. Ideally, the patient should remain as independent as possible, asking for assistance with only those tasks that are especially complex or physically difficult. But how do the patient and the caregiver sort this out? There is a lack of pertinent psychosocial research in the area of caregiving and role adjustment associated with diabetes self management (Anderson, 1996). The literature on cardiac disease and spousal caregiving suggests that changes in lifestyle (dietary requirements; physical activity), encounters with health professionals, and each spouse's reaction to illness are important sources of stress. Primary coping strategies include seeking "informational support" and "protective buffering" and are used by both the caregiver and care recipient. Care recipients complain of "miscarried helping" referring to perceived loss of independence resulting from the overprotective caregiver (Coyne & Smith, 1991; Coyne, Wortman, & Lehman, 1988; Stewart, Davidson, Meade, Hirth, & Makrides, 2000).

There is some evidence that when cognition is normal or only mildly affected, patients are able to recognize subtle needs and may take the lead in asking for help. Hendra & Taylor (2004) studied adult diabetics with only mild age-associated cognitive decline (Mini Mental State Exam mean score = 26; Folstein, Folstein, & McHugh, 1975) and good functional status (Barthel Index mean score = 19; Collins, Wade, Davies, & Horne, 1988). Although the patients said they provided self-care, they also recognized the need for periodic caregiver assistance when there were changes in the diabetes medication regimen. Cognitively impaired patients often lack insight and fail to recognize when they need help from others. Therefore, they are at high risk for declines in diabetes self-management and development of complications of diabetes and comorbidities.

Caregiving to Promote Diabetes Self-Management

Soon after the caregiver emerges, she will need information about diabetes in general and about the care recipient's needs specifically. Although there is an extensive literature on caregiving to dependent elderly and cognitively impaired persons, surprisingly few studies have addressed specific caregiving tasks performed by informal caregivers to older adults with diabetes. Some of these tasks may be learned through patient education activities (e.g., instructions for checking blood glucose, correct dosage and timing of medications, diet planning) that are provided by the physician and health care team directing the patient's medical regimen. At *Level 3: The Health System* in Glasgow & Eakin's (1998) framework of diabetes self-management, states that advice from one's physician highly influences self-care behaviors. However, in busy medical practices today, time with the physician is brief and the physician's advice is often supplemented by counsel from others who provide education and support to the patient. These professionals (nurses, nutritionists, social workers, psychologists), some of whom hold the credential Certified Diabetes Educator, use innovative teaching methods and scientific and experiential evidence in their practice (Funnell et al., 2006).

The health care setting has provided the scientific expertise, facilities, and personnel for numerous studies of interventions that support self-management for diabetes. These interventions include goal setting and shared decision making between medical personnel and the patient (Heisler et al., 2003; Warsi, Wang, LaValley, Avorn, & Solomon, 2004; Williams, McGregor, Zeldman, Freedman, & Deci, 2004); small-group interventions for self-care skill development (Anderson et al., 1995; Litzelman et al., 1993; Parchman, Arambula-Soloman, Noel, Larme, & Pugh, 2003); and use of technology for patient education (Glasgow, Toobert, & Hamson, 1996). There is also good evidence that the health care system recognizes the value of an ecological approach to self-care, with the patient integrating self-management skills with support from the environment, including family and friends (Fisher, Brownson, O'Toole, Anwuri, & Shetty, 2007; Fisher et al., 2005). The literature is not clear, however, on how the health care system recognizes the need for a family caregiver to assist the patient or how the health care system assists the caregiver in coping with the burden of providing patient care. A medical system that is supportive to diabetes self-management provides a patient-family education component that the caregiver and the care recipient can attend singly or as a dyad, both interacting with the health care team for collaborative goal setting and planned follow-up. Opportunities for the caregiver to schedule sessions alone are ideal, because the caregiver may need to ask questions or express feelings in private. A health care system that does not actively involve the diabetic patient's caregiver creates barriers to diabetes self-management.

Recognizing and Understanding Caregiver Burden

Caregiver burden, the most commonly measured outcome of informal (usually family) caregiving, is thought to emerge from a subjective belief that current and future resources are insufficient to meet the demands imposed by the role (Zarit, Reever, & Bach-Peterson, 1980; Zarit, Todd, & Zarit, 1986). As a result, burden is believed to be a predictor of negative physical and psychological outcomes, such as depression. Caregivers for patients with diabetes are at risk for mild to severe burden because of the chronicity of the disease, the range and complexity of diabetes self-management activities, and comorbidities such as heart disease, visual problems, renal insufficiency, microvascular disease associated with wound healing and amputations, and cognitive decline. Although the range of expected outcomes among those who care for persons with diabetes is broad, surprisingly few studies have addressed these diverse outcomes. If the decline in cognition is mild and occurs in the absence of physical complications of diabetes, the caregiving needs may be limited to monitoring and/or assisting the patient in checking blood sugar, taking medications, maintaining a therapeutic diet, and continuing regular health maintenance and preventive care. Hendra & Taylor (2004) reported that caregivers of diabetic patients randomized to one of three medication regimens—two of which included insulin therapy—reported low stress as measured by the General Health Questionnaire (Goldberg, 1986), a widely used instrument for screening psychological distress. In this case, the diabetes patients were only mildly impaired and could ask for help with new insulin dosages during the course of this short-term study. Another study looked at the effect of a foot ulcer on health-related quality of life (HRQL) for patients with diabetes and their caregivers. Patients' mean age was 60 years, 72% were male, and the duration of diabetes averaged 17 years. At intake, the ulcer was examined and HRQL was measured independently in the patient and the caregiver; these tests were repeated at 20 months. Caregivers and patients whose ulcers healed during the 20 months had a significantly higher HRQL than caregivers and patients whose ulcers had not healed. This study is interesting in that patients and caregivers who had dealt with diabetes for a number of years showed significant declines in HRQL in less than 1 year because of the additional burden posed by a commonly occurring complication of diabetes—a nonhealing foot ulcer (Nabuurs-Franssen et al., 2005).

Many factors related to the caregiver and the care recipient merge or overlap to compound the caregiver's sense of burden, but the chronic nature of diabetes and the likelihood that the physical work of caregiving will increase over time suggest that diabetes caregivers are at high risk. For example, informal care has been shown to increase from 10.1 hours per day when oral medication alone is sufficient to 14.4 hours per day ($p < 0.01$) when insulin therapy is required (Langa et al., 2002). Similarly diabetic care recipients with macrovascular (heart disease and stroke) and microvascular (visual) complications have significantly higher need for informal care (Langa et al., 2002). Silliman et al. (1996) examined family caregiving among a community-based sample of 357 caregivers of patients with type 2 diabetes. Family caregivers, who had a mean age of 65 years, were primarily female (76%) and spouses (71%). Up to 50% of caregivers provided assistance in some type of diabetes-specific care, and more than one-third were present and played a role in the patient's medical appointments. Caregiver involvement increased in association with the patient's functional disability. Caregivers' perceived unmet needs included education about diabetes and diabetes-related care to support them in their diabetes management roles.

While caregivers provide a major contribution to the day-to-day support of patients with diabetes and other chronic illnesses, the burden takes its toll and frequently leads to negative outcomes such as isolation and financial constraint (Gahagan, Loppie, Rehman, Maclellan, & Side, 2007) and declines in emotional and physical health (Schulz et al., 1997). Vulnerable caregivers are at particular risk for undergoing significant health declines and giving up the caregiver role. A recent nationally representative study of 1002 informal caregivers found that 36% were vulnerable and suffering from fair to poor health or experiencing serious health conditions. This group was older (≥65 years), married and had fewer than 12 years of education (Navaie-Waliser et al., 2002). Models of caregiver stress suggest that coping skills and social support may ameliorate stressful outcomes for the caregiver. However, it is also the case that chronic illness may drain supportive resources and lead caregivers to become isolated, overwhelmed, and ill (Stewart et al., 2000). Vulnerable caregivers are an understudied group and are particularly important because they represent the last opportunity for at-home informal care for a large number of care recipients who, without such care, will enter the formal institutional care system, at great cost to both private and public funding sources.

The caregiving literature has focused much attention on the negative or stressful outcomes of caregiving, with the construct of "burden" being the most often studied. However, Pearlin, Mullen, Semple, & Skaff's (1990) model of caregiver stress demonstrates that caregivers bring personal attributes to the caring process, including intrapersonal coping mechanisms and social and/or material resources, that lead them to find personal meaning and a sense of accomplishment or well-being in caregiving, rather than consistently negative outcomes. Gaugler, Kane, & Newcomer (2007) studied caregiver resilience—"the ability of certain caregivers to persevere in at-home caregiving roles while remaining stable or reporting decreasing levels of burden or depressive symptoms." Over a period of 3 years, high caregiver resilience (low perceived burden in the face of frequent care demands) was associated with less frequent institutionalization of the care recipient and loss to follow-up, as well as more frequent care recipient mortality. The interpretation was that the resilient caregiver was able to remain in a caring role throughout the life of the dependent care recipient. More research is needed on the ways in which caregiver resiliency can be supported.

Level 4: Worksite and Organization of Glasgow & Eakin's (1998) diabetes self-management framework is important to the extent that macro-level organizations, such as the workplace and its policies, may ameliorate caregiver burden by supporting the needs of both the caregiver and the care recipient. Many caregivers continue to work outside the home while coping with the additional responsibilities of providing care for another. Working outside the home provides regular social contacts and prevents caregiver isolation, which is an important source of caregiver burden (Rochette, Desrosiers, Bravo, St-Cyr Tribble, & Bourget, 2007). In addition, some workplaces offer flexible schedules and telecommuting, which increases the caregiver's options for work schedules. Other workplaces provide on-site exercise programs, food service with a range of healthy choices, health clinics for minor illnesses and preventive health maintenance, and referral for psychological services. The array of work-related benefits also includes health, dental, and disability insurance, health- and dependent-care spending accounts, and financial counseling services that directly benefit the caregiver. Some larger employers provide support groups for caregivers and elder care programs at or near the workplace, but these are the least frequently offered among the work-related benefits (Walston, 1995). When the care recipient is cognitively impaired or dependent on the caregiver, workplace policies and services that benefit the caregiver also benefit the care recipient. The care recipient who is no longer employed may continue to benefit from group health insurance obtained earlier through the workplace. In this sense, the workplace is very important to the caregiver and to the care recipient with diabetes, and absence of workplace benefits present barriers to diabetes self-management.

Similar to the macro-level benefits from the workplace, according to Glasgow & Eakin's (1998) framework, *Level 5: Neighborhood and Community,* are the supports for and the barriers to diabetes self-management provided by community-based organizations and services. The cognitively impaired patient with diabetes may benefit directly from community-based (senior services, social service, church-sponsored) adult day care programs, which provide a safe and caring environment that also promotes social interaction. Some adult day care programs go beyond these basic offerings and provide rehabilitative and educational activities, entertainment, and outings (Baumgarten, Lebel, Laprise, Leclerc, & Quinn, 2002; Zarit et al., 1998). The patient's caregiver may benefit from the support groups and respite services associated with adult day care services (Baumgarten et al., 2002; Hedrick et al., 1993). A quasi-experimental U.S. study reported that caregivers who used adult day care services for at least 2 days a week for 3 months were less depressed and had less burden than did caregivers who did not use day care services (Zarit et al., 1998). Other innovative models for community-based respite services and their cost-effectiveness are under study (Mason et al., 2007). Safe neighborhoods with shopping, libraries, meeting places, and easy access to parks or "green areas" encourage social and physical activity. There is evidence that adverse neighborhood environment interacts with caregiver status to modify (increase) health-related outcomes (Brummet et al., 2005). Environments that provide little or no sense of community or support for the patient or caregiver place excess burdens on both and serve as barriers to diabetes self-management.

Supporting Caregivers: The Ultimate Diabetes Self-Management Strategy

Level 6: Media, Policy, and Culture of Glasgow & Eakin's (1998) diabetes self-care framework suggests that societal-level influences have not been consistently supportive of diabetes self-management, due in part to the lack of a health policy that promotes healthy living and in part to advertisements and media endorsements that are aimed more at a youth culture than at the maintenance of good health. Patients with diabetes and their caregivers have much to gain from a societal interest in healthy living. There is some evidence that the sheer economics of care provided at home may boost a national discourse on reasons to support caregivers of people with chronic illness. The American Association of Retried Persons (AARP) Public Policy Institute has prepared an issue brief that directly addresses the economic value of unpaid informal care provided at home (Gibson & Houser, 2007). Moreover, the report was made available to the public at large. A conservative estimate of the annual economic value of unpaid informal caregiving activities in 2006 was reported at $354 billion, which is more than the total spending for Medicaid, including both federal and state contributions and both medical and long-term care (Burwell, Sredl, & Eiken, 2006). The brief discusses out-of-pocket cost to caregivers, lost wages and retirement income, and the effects of the long-term-care and health care systems.

Another current work with policy implications comes from social scientists who have spent long careers studying the structure, function, and effects of one person providing informal care for another. New constructs of "patient suffering" and "caregiver compassion" are discussed from a theoretical, hypothesis-generating perspective. The history, definitions, and cultural meanings of suffering and compassion are discussed and a conceptual model of perceived suffering and caregiver compassion and their relation to caregiving and health are provided. This thoughtful work places the discussion of suffering and compassion in the context of family caregiving and aims to promote an empirical approach that will enrich researchers' understanding and lead to strategies that will improve the human condition (Schulz et al., 2007).

Summary

Declining cognitive abilities associated with aging and chronic disease, including diabetes, are important predictors of decrements in self-care behaviors. Self-care regimens for diabetes are complex and difficult to manage in people who have normal cognitive abilities, and they pose a real challenge to those with impaired thinking, remembering, and planning skills. The transition from self-care to care provided by an "informal" family caregiver provides a way for the cognitively impaired older adult to maintain diabetes self-management.

Diabetes self-management skills and behaviors and the resources to encourage or barriers that impede these are described from biopsychosocial (Glasgow & Eakin, 1998) and social ecological (Stokols, 1996) frameworks. The diabetes patient's behaviors are influenced by an environment stratified by a close personal social group composed of family and friends, a larger system-level environment, which includes worksites and the health care system, and the macro-level influences of the community and policy. The patient whose environment holds key resources from which to choose (e.g., social support, accessible health care, healthy diet) is likely to fare better than one who lacks a supportive social group and has limited access to care. This line of thinking suggests that older diabetes patients with cognitive decline are not only more likely to have difficulty with self-management regimens but also are more likely to have difficulty choosing valuable resources from their environment. The informal family caregiver provides a means by which the cognitively impaired patient can receive the type and amount of assistance required through a process of transitioning from total self-care to care provided by a caregiver. Ideally, this transition takes place gradually, with both the caregiver and the care recipient negotiating their roles. Despite a large literature on caregiver burden, few studies report how the caregiver assumes the role and how the patient and the caregiver negotiate how they will work together. Studies are also needed on how the health care system recognizes the need for a caregiver and interacts with the caregiver to maximize patient care and/or to deal with caregiver burden. Although there are some complex studies (Langa et al., 2002; Silliman, 1996), research on diabetes and caregiving is largely at the exploratory and descriptive stages and does not yet address interventions to improve caregiver stress or caregiver outcomes. For example, there is a study of the perceptions and experiences of family members of diabetes patients (Rosa, Sunvisson, & Ahlstrom, 2007); focus groups that address the needs of family caregivers who provide complex care at home (wound care, dialysis) (Hennessy, John, & Anderson, 1999) and culturally competent self-management for Latinos (Vincent, Clark, Zimmer, & Sanchez, 2006); small, subjective quality-of-life studies of caregivers and patients (Awadalla, Ohaeri, Al-Awad, & Tawfig, 2006; Brod, 1998; Li, Lee, Lin, & Amidon, 2004); a small study of children as caregivers to adult patients with diabetes (Jacobson & Wood, 2003); and small clinical treatment trials that incorporate the impact on the caregiver as an outcome (Hendra & Talyor, 2004; Shelmet et al., 2004).

Supporting the family caregiver may be the ultimate diabetes self-management strategy for older, cognitively impaired and/or dependent adults. Research on the economic value of unpaid informal care provided at home has laid some ground to understanding the contribution of family caregivers (Gibson & Houser, 2007; Langa et al., 2002). Research of this kind and research on how to support family caregivers could provide critical information to inform policy that would provide assistance for care in the home, a preference of many and an alternative to costly institutional care.

References

American Psychiatric Association. (1994). *Diagnostic and statistical manual of mental disorders* (4th ed.). Washington, DC: American Psychiatric Association.

Anderson, B. J. (1996). Involving family members in diabetes treatment. In B. J. Anderson & R. R. Rubin (Eds.), *Practical psychology for diabetes clinicians* (pp. 43–50). Alexandria, VA: American Diabetes Association.

Anderson, R. M., Funnel, M. M., Butler, P. M., Arnold, M. S., Fitzgerald, J. T., & Feste, C. C. (1995). Patient empowerment: Results of a randomized controlled trial. *Diabetes Care, 18,* 943–949.

Arenberg, D. (1978). Differences and changes in age in the Benton Visual Retention Test. *Journal of Gerontology, 33,* 534–540.

Awadalla, A. W., Ohaeri, J. U., Al-Awad, S. A., & Tawfig, A. M. (2006). Diabetes mellitus patients family caregivers' subjective quality of life. *Journal of the National Medical Association, 98,* 727–736.

Baumgarten, M., Lebel, P., Laprise, H., Leclerc, C., & Quinn, C. (2002). Adult day care for the frail elderly: Outcomes, satisfaction, and cost. *Journal of Aging and Health, 14,* 237–259.

Branin, J. (2001). The role of memory strategies in medication adherence among the elderly. *Home Health Care Services Quarterly, 20,* 1–16.

Brod, M. (1998). Quality of life issues with diabetes and lower extremity ulcers: Patients and caregivers. *Quality of Life Research, 7,* 365–372.

Brown, S. C., & Park, D. C. (2003). Theoretical models for cognitive aging and implications for translational research in medicine. *Gerontologist, 43*(Special Issue 1), 57–67.

Brummet, B. H., Siegler, I. L., Rohe, W. M., Barefoot, J. C., Vitaliano, P., Surwit, R. S., Feinglos, M. N., & Williams, R. B. (2005). Neighborhood characteristics moderate effects of caregiving on glucose functioning. *Psychosomatic Medicine, 67,* 752–758.

Burwell, B., Sredl, K., & Eiken, S. (2006). *Medicaid long-term care expenditures FY 2005.* Cambridge, MA: The MEDSTAT Group.

Coker, L. H., & Shumaker, S. A. (2003). Type 2 diabetes mellitus and cognition. An understudied issue in women's health. *Journal of Psychosomatic Research, 54,* 129–139.

Collins, C., Wade, D. T., Davies, S., & Horne, V. (1988). The Barthel Index: A reliability study. *International Disability Studies, 10,* 61–63.

Cotrell, V., Wild, K., & Bader, T. (2006). Medication management and adherence among cognitively impaired older adults. *Journal of Gerontological Social Work, 47,* 31–46.

Coyne, J., & Smith, D. (1991). Couples coping with a myocardial infarction: A contextual perspective on wives distress. *Journal of Perspectives on Social Psychology, 61,* 404–412.

Coyne, J., Wortman, C., & Lehman, D. (1988). The other side of support: Emotional overinvolvement and miscarried helping. In B. H. Gottlieb (Ed.), *Marshalling social support: Formats, process, and effects* (pp. 305–330), Newbury Park, CA: Sage.

Curb, J. D., Rodriguez, B. L., Abbott, R. D., Petrovitch, H., Ross, G. W., Masaki, K. H., et al. (1999). Longitudinal association of vascular and Alzheimer's dementias, diabetes, and glucose tolerance. *Neurology, 52,* 971–975.

Erikson, E. H. (1959). *Identity and the life cycle.* New York: International Universities Press.

Fisher, E. B., Brownson, C. A., O'Toole, M. L., Anwuri, V. V., & Shetty, G. (2007). Perspectives on self-management from the Diabetes Initiative of the Robert Wood Johnson Foundation. *Diabetes Educator, 33*(Suppl. 6), 216S–224S.

Fisher, E. B., Brownson, C. A., O'Toole, M. L., Shetty, G., Anwuri, V. V., & Glasgow, R E. (2005). Ecological approaches to self-management: The case of diabetes. *American Journal of Public Health, 95,* 1523–1535.

Fisk, J. D., Merry, H. R., & Rockwood, K. (2003). Variations in case definition affect prevalence but not outcomes of MCI. *Neurology, 61,* 1179–1184.

Folstein, M. F., Folstein, F. E., & McHugh, P. R. (1975). A practical method for grading the cognitive state of patients for the clinician. *Journal of Psychiatric Research, 12,* 189–198.

Funnell, M. M., Anderson, R. M., Nwankwo, R., Gillard, M. L., Butler, P.M., Fitzgerald, J. T., & Two Feathers, J. (2006). A study of certified diabetes educators. *Diabetes Educator, 32,* 359–372.

Gahagan, J., Loppie, C., Rehman, L., Maclellan, M., & Side, K. (2007). Far as I get is the clothesline: The impact leisure on women's health and unpaid caregiving experiences in Nova Scotia, Canada. *Health Care for Women, 28,* 47–68.

Gaugler, J. E., Kane, R. L., & Newcomer, R. (2007). Resilience and transitions from dementia caregiving. *Journal of Gerontology, 62B,* P38–P44.

Gaugler, J. E., & Zarit, S. H. (2001). The effectiveness of adult day services for disabled older people. *Journal of Aging and Social Policy, 12,* 23–27.

Gibson, M. J., & Houser, A. (2007). Valuing the invaluable: A new look at the economic value of family caregiving. Issue Brief: Public Policy Institute. *American Association of Retired Persons,* IB82, 1–12.

Glasgow, R. E., & Eakin, E. G. (1998). Diabetes self-management. In S. Shumaker, E. B. Schron, J. K. Ockene, & W. McBee (Eds.), *Handbook of health behavior change* (2nd ed., pp. 435–461). New York: Springer Publishing.

Glasgow, R. E., Toobert, D. J., & Hampson, S. E. (1996). Effects of a brief office-based intervention to facilitate diabetes dietary self-management. *Diabetes Care, 19,* 835–842.

Goldberg, D. (1986). Use of the general health questionnaire in clinical work. *British Medical Journal, 293,* 1188–1189.

Gould, O., Mcdonald-Miszczak, L., & King, B. (1996). Metacognition and medication adherence: How do older adults remember? *Experimental and Aging Research, 23,* 315–342.

Hedrick, S. C., Rothman, M. L., Chapko, M., Ehreth, J., Diehr, P., Inui, T. S., et al. (1993). Summary and discussion of methods and results of the Adult Day Health Care Evaluation Study. *Medical Care, 31,* SS94–103.

Heisler, M., Vijan, S., Anderson, R. M, Ubel, P. A., Bernstein, S. J., & Hofer, T. P. (2003). When do patients and their physicians agree on diabetes treatment goals and strategies and what difference does it make? *Journal of General Internal Medicine, 18,* 893–902.

Hendra, T. J., & Taylor, C. D. (2004). A randomised trial of insulin on well-being and carer strain in elderly type 2 diabetic subjects. *Journal of Diabetes and Its Complications, 18,* 148–154.

Hennessy, C. H., John, R., & Anderson, L. A. (1999). Diabetes education needs of family members caring for American Indian elders. *Diabetes Educator, 25,* 747–754.

Jacobson, S., & Wood, R. G. (2003). Contributions of children to the care of adults with diabetes. *Diabetes Educator, 30,* 820–826.

Kelly-Hayes, M., Jette, A. M., Wolf, P. A., D'Agostino, R. B., & Odell, P. M. (1992). Functional limitations and disability among elders in the Framingham Study. *American Journal of Public Health, 82,* 841–845.

Langa, K. M., Vijan, S., Hayward, R. A., Chernew, M. E., Blaum, C. S., Kabeto, M. U., et al. (2002). Informal caregiving for diabetes and diabetic complications among elderly Americans. *Journal of Gerontology, 57B,* S177–S186.

La Rue, A. (1992). *Aging and neuropsychological assessment.* New York: Plenum Press.

Leibson, C. L., Rocca, W. A., Hanson, V. A., Cha, R., Kokmen, E., Obrien, P. C., et al. (1997). Risk of dementia among persons with diabetes mellitus: A population-based cohort study. *American Journal of Epidemiology, 145,* 301–308.

Li, T. C., Lee, Y. D., Lin, C. C., & Amidon, R. L. (2004). Quality of life of primary caregivers of elderly with cerebrovascular disease or diabetes hospitalized for acute care and assessment of well-being and functioning using the SF-36 health questionnaire. *Quality of Life Research, 13,* 1081–1088.

Lin, E. H., Katon, W., Rutter, C., Simon, G. E., Ludman, E. J., Von Korff, M., et al. (2006). Effects of enhanced depression treatment on diabetes self-care. *Annals of Family Medicine, 4,* 46–53.

Litzelman, D. K., Slemenda, C. W., Langefeld, C. D., Hayes, M., Welch, M. A., Bild, D. E., et al. (1993). Reduction of lower extremity clinical abnormalities in patients with non-insulin-dependent diabetes mellitus: A randomized, controlled trial. *Annals of Internal Medicine, 119,* 36–41.

Lopez, O. L., Jagust, W. J., Dulberg, C., Becker, J. T., DeKosky, S. T., Fitzpatrick, A., et al. (2003). Risk factors for mild cognitive impairment in the Cardiovascular Health Study Cognition Study: Part 2. *Archives of Neurology, 60,* 1394–1399.

Mason, A., Weatherly, H., Spilsbury, K., Golder, S., Arksey, H., Adamson, J., et al. (2007). The effectiveness and cost-effectiveness of respite for caregivers of frail older people. *Journal of American Geriatric Society, 55,* 290–299.

Morrell, R. W., Park, D. C., Kidder, D. P., & Martin, M. (1997). Adherence to antihypertensive medications across the life span. *Gerontologist, 37,* 609–619.

Morris, J. C., Heyman, A., Mohs, R. C., Hughes J. P., van Belle, G., Fillenbaum, G., et al. (1989). The Consortium to Establish a Registry for Alzheimer's disease (CERAD), Part I: Clinical and neuropsychological assessment of AD. *Neurology, 39,* 1159–1165.

Nabuurs-Franssen, M. H., Huijberts, M. S., Nieuwenhuijzen Kruseman, A. C., Willems, J., & Schaper, N. C. (2005). Health-related quality of life of diabetic foot ulcer patients and their caregivers. *Diabetologia, 48,* 1906–1910.

Navaie-Waliser, M., Feldman, P. H., Gould, D. A., Levine, C., Kuerbis, A. N., & Donelan, K. (2002). When the caregiver needs care: The plight of vulnerable caregivers. *American Journal of Public Health, 92,* 409–413.

Ott, A., Stolk, R. P., Hofman, A., van Harskamp, F., Grobbee, D. E., & Breteler, M. M. (1996). Association of diabetes mellitus and dementia: The Rotterdam Study. *Diabetologia, 39,* 1392–1397.

Parchman, M. L., Arambula-Soloman, T. G., Noel, P. H., Larme, A. C., & Pugh, J. A. (2003). Stage of change advancement for diabetes self-management behaviors and glucose control. *Diabetes Educator, 29,* 128–134.

Park, H. S., Hong, Y. S., Lee, H. J., Ha, E. H., & Sung, Y. A. (2004). Individuals with type 2 diabetes and depressive symptoms exhibited lower adherence with self-care. *Journal of Clinical Epidemiology, 57,* 978–984.

Pearlin, L., Mullan, J., Semple, S., & Skaff, M. (1990). Caregiving and the stress process: An overview of concept and their measures. *Gerontologist, 30,* 583–594.

Perlmuter, L. C., Hakami, M. K., Hodgson-Harrington, C., Ginsberg, J., Katz, J., Singer, D. E., et al. (1984). Decreased cognitive function in aging non-insulin dependent diabetic patients. *American Journal of Medicine, 77,* 1043–1048.

Petersen, R. C., Doody, R., Kurz, A., Mohs, R. C., Morris, J. C., Rabins, R. V., et al. (2001). Current concepts in mild cognitive impairment. *Archives of Neurology, 58,* 1985–1992.

Resnick, S. M., Coker, L. H., Maki, P. M., Rapp, S. R., Espeland, M. A., & Shumaker, S. A. (2004). The Women's Health Initiative Study of Cognitive Aging (WHISCA): A randomized clinical trial of the effects of hormone therapy on age-associated cognitive decline. *Clinical Trials, 1,* 440–450.

Resnick, S. M., Trotman, K. M., Kawas, C., & Zonderman, A. B. (1995). Age-associated changes in specific errors on the Benton Visual Retention Test. *Journals of Gerontology Psychological Sciences and Social Sciences, 50B,* P171–P178.

Rochette, A., Desrosiers, J., Bravo, G., St Cyr Tribble, D., & Bourget, A. (2007). Changes in participation level after spouses first stroke and relationship to burden and depressive symptoms. *Cerebrovascular Disease, 24,* 255–260.

Rosa, S., Sunvisson, H., & Ahlstrom, G. (2007). Lived experiences of significant others of persons with diabetes. *Journal of Clinical Nursing, 16,* 215–222.

Schulz, R., Hebert, R. S., Dew, M. A., Brown, S. L., Scheier, M. F., Veach, S. R., et al. (2007). Patient suffering and caregiver compassion: New opportunities for research, practice, and policy. *Gerontologist, 47,* 4–13.

Schulz, R., Newsom, J., Mittelmark, M., Burton, L., Hirsch, C., & Jackson, S. (1997). Health effects of caregiving: The Caregiver Health Effects Study: An ancillary study of the Cardiovascular Health Study. *Annals of Behavioral Medicine, 19,* 110–116.

Shelmet, J., Schwartz, S., Coppleman, J., Peterson, G., Skovlund, S., Lytzen, L., et al. (2004). Preference and resource utilization in elderly patients. Innolet version vial/syringe. *Diabetes Research and Clinical Practice, 63,* 27–35.

Silliman, R. A., Bhatti, S., Khan, A., Dukes, K. A., & Sullivan, L. M. (1996). The care of older persons with diabetes mellitus: Families and primary care physicians. *Journal of the American Geriatrics Society, 44,* 1314–1321.

Sinclair, A. J., Girling, A. J., & Bayer, A. J. (2000). Cognitive function in older subjects with diabetes mellitus: Impact on diabetes self-management and use of care services. *Diabetes Research and Clinical Practice, 50,* 203–212.

Stewart, M., Davidson, K., Meade, D., Hirth, A., & Makrides, L. (2000). Myocardial infarction: Survivors and spouses' stress, coping, and support. *Journal of Advanced Nursing, 31,* 1351–1360.

Stokols, D. (1996). Translating social ecological theory into guidelines for community health promotion. *American Journal of Health Promotion, 10,* 282–298.

Stone, R., Cafferata, G. L., & Sangl, J. (1987). Caregivers of the frail elderly: A national profile. *Gerontologist, 27,* 616–626.

Stuck, A. E., Walthert, J. M., Nikolaus, T., Bula, C. J., Hohman, C., & Beck, J. C. (1999). Risk factors for functional status decline in community-living elderly people: A systematic literature review. *Social Science and Medicine, 48,* 445–469.

Vincent, D., Clark, L., Zimmer, L. M., Sanchez, J. (2006). Culturally competent diabetes self-management for Latinos. *Diabetes Educator, 32,* 89–97.

Walston, M. R. (1995). Eldercare benefits offered by the best companies to work for in America. *Health Mark Quarterly, 13,* 37–50.

Warsi, A., Wang, P. S., LaValley, M. P., Avorn, J., & Solomon, D. H. (2004). Self-management education programs in chronic disease: A systematic review and methodological critique of the literature. *Archives of Internal Medicine, 164,* 1641–1649.

Whitchurch, G. C., & Constantine, L. L. (1993). Systems theory. In P. G. Boss, W. J. Doherty, R. LaRossa, W. R. Shumm, & S. K. Steinmetz (Eds.), *Sourcebook of family theory and methods* (pp. 325–352). New York: Plenum Press.

Williams, G. C., McGregor, H. A., Zeldman, A., Freedman, Z. R., & Deci, E. L. (2004). Testing a self-determination theory process model for promoting glycemic control through diabetes self-management. *Health Psychology, 23*(1), 58–66.

Williamson, J. D., Miller, M. E., Bryan, R. N., Lazar, R. M., Coker, L. H., Johnson. J., et al. (2007). The Action to Control Cardiovascular Risk in Diabetes, Memory in Diabetes Study (ACCORD-MIND): Rationale, design, and methods. *American Journal of Cardiology, 99*(Suppl.), 112i–122i.

Yoshitake, T., Kiyohara, Y., Kato, I., Ohmura, T., Iwamoto, H., Nakayama, K., et al. (1995). Incidence and risk factors of vascular dementia and Alzheimer's disease in a defined elderly Japanese population: The Hisayama Study. *Neurology, 45,* 1161–1168.

Zarit, S. H., Reever, K. G., & Bach-Peterson, J. (1980). Relatives of the impaired elderly: Correlates of feelings of burden. *Gerontologist, 20,* 649–653.

Zarit, S. H., Stephens, M. A., Townsend, A., & Greene, R. (1998). Stress reduction for family caregivers: Effects of adult day care use. *Journals of Gerontology Psychological Sciences and Social Sciences, 53B,* S267–S277.

Zarit, S. H., Todd, P. P., & Zarit, J. M. (1986). Subjective burden of husbands and wives as caregivers: A longitudinal study. *Gerontologist, 26,* 260–266.

Adherence to Treatment and Lifestyle Changes Among People With Cancer

32

Amy H. Peterman,
David Victorson, and
David Cella

Research on treatment adherence and health behavior change among people with cancer continues to lag behind that for patients with other serious illnesses or the general population. A large portion of the existing literature related to cancer patients is focused simply on documenting rates of adherence to treatment. Significantly less attention has been paid to variables associated with adherence or to interventions designed to improve adherence. One potential reason for the relative lack of attention to adherence in this population is the widely held assumption that patients facing a possibly terminal illness like cancer should adhere without question to whatever recommendations are made. That is, health professionals have assumed that patients will adhere if they believe that the likely alternative is death. However, comparisons of adherence rates among patients with diseases of varying severity do not confirm this assumption (DiMatteo, 2004).

Another factor that may contribute to a limited focus on cancer-related adherence is that, until fairly recently, most cancer treatment was administered intravenously (IV) in a hospital or outpatient clinic setting. Specialized skills are required for IV administration, and there was a pressing need for close patient observation to prevent life-threatening side effects or complications. There were simply fewer opportunities for the kind of self-management that characterizes treatment for other conditions. However, improved supportive care (e.g., antinausea medications, white and red blood cell growth factors), reduced insurance coverage for inpatient stays, and the development of numerous oral cancer therapies have changed the cancer treatment landscape considerably.

Treatment advances, in conjunction with improved early detection methods, have significantly improved survival rates for most types of cancers. Even people diagnosed with more advanced disease, such as metastatic breast cancer, are being told that their cancer can be managed as a chronic condition, similar to diabetes. However, cancer is still a serious, often life-threatening, illness. Despite that, DiMatteo's (2004) authoritative review of 50 years of medical adherence research estimated that about one-fifth of cancer patients don't adhere to some part of their prescribed treatment. Such failure can carry high personal costs, such as higher mortality rates, shorter disease-free survival, greater likelihood of cancer recurrence, and the delayed identification of possible complications of treatment (e.g., osteoporosis) (Adsay et al., 2004; Ballantyne, 2003; De Csepel, Tartter, & Gajdos, 2002; Hershman & Narayanan, 2004; McCready et al., 2000; Van Gerpen & Mast, 2004). On the societal level, cancer-related nonadherence can result in the waste of vast amounts of health care resources and can also create misleading or incorrect results from clinical research (Dunbar-Jacob & Mortimer-Stephens, 2001; Farmer, 1999).

This chapter presents an overview of the literature on adherence among people who have been diagnosed with cancer. It is organized as follow. First, we discuss the potential significance of adherence for treatment success. Second, we cover methods for measuring adherence to cancer treatment. Third, we review investigations that have estimated adherence rates for different treatment-related behaviors in an effort to establish the magnitude of the problem of adherence. Fourth, research investigating various determinants of adherence and interventions to improve adherence are examined. We do not address adherence to cancer prevention and screening behaviors among the general population here, as these topics are well covered elsewhere in this book. The chapter concludes with a discussion of future directions for research.

Relationship of Adherence to Treatment Outcomes: Why Study Adherence in Cancer?

Cancer Treatment

The bottom-line significance of adherence to cancer treatment regimens is assumed to be increased likelihood of treatment success, which should translate into improved physical health and longer survival of the patient. One frequently cited early investigation documented that treatment success was significantly better among patients who received at least 85% of their planned dosages of adjuvant chemotherapy, while disease-free survival was significantly shorter among people who received less than 65% of their planned treatment (Bonadonna & Valagussa, 1981). More recently, a major clinical trial demonstrated a significant survival advantage for people who took tamoxifen for 5 years rather than two or three (Early Breast Cancer Trialists' Collaborative Group, 2005). Although patient adherence was not specifically evaluated, the findings of this and similar dose studies have been generalized to support a role for adherence in treatment outcome. Indeed, a great deal of cancer research is directed toward identifying treatment schedules (e.g., weekly doses rather than every-three-week dosing) and supportive medications (e.g., growth factors G-CSF) that will allow more intense and dense treatment regimens to be administered without intolerable side effects (e.g., Desai et al. 2007; Gridelli et al., 2007). In addition, the dosing schedule is a crucial component of the effectiveness of some medications. Thus, if nonadherence contributes to a patient's receiving less than optimal treatment, such nonadherence may lead to a poorer outcome.

Adherence to recommended follow-up appointments and tests after the conclusion of cancer treatment might be expected to also affect long-term outcome. However, recent research findings are equivocal. Several investigations into the utility of intensive follow-up after cancer treatment have failed to show a benefit to more frequent check-ups (Secco et al., 2000) or the use of state-of-the-art imaging MRI technology in areas where recurrence is most likely (Titu, Nicholson, Hartley, Breen & Monson, 2006). A recent Cochrane systematic review evaluated survival and disease-free survival as they related to the intensity of the follow-up schedule after primary treatment for Stage I–III breast cancer (Rojas et al., 2005). No difference was found for these outcomes in the more than 3,000 women enrolled in these trials.

It is quite difficult to judge the significance of nonadherence, as there are multiple factors that affect outcome, only one of which is adherence. Frequently, the current state of scientific knowledge does not allow an accurate assessment of the impact of treatment. Adjuvant chemotherapy, for example, is given in the absence of any visible evidence of disease. As such, there is no way to reliably monitor the success of treatment, unless the treatment fails and there is a recurrence. Additionally, it is very difficult to specify what a particular patient must do to ensure a response from a treatment: dosage recommendations are made on the basis of group data, and thus any particular individual may need more or less treatment for the cure or control of disease (Barofsky, 1984). Thus, while adherence is likely to play an important role, it is but one of many factors that affect treatment outcomes.

Behavioral and Lifestyle Factors

For many people, a cancer diagnosis is a "wake-up call," motivating them to make long-delayed lifestyle changes. Health care providers are generally in favor of this strategy, making recommendations to stop smoking, eat a balanced diet, increase the consumption of fruit and vegetables, and get regular exercise. Although it's not known whether these behaviors increase the likelihood of treatment success, they are increasingly recognized for their positive impact on quality of life during cancer treatment. For example, several randomized intervention trials (e.g., Mock et al., 2005) have documented that regular exercise minimizes cancer-related fatigue, a common and debilitating side effect of cancer treatment.

In summary, adherence to cancer follow-up care, medication regimens, and health behaviors has the potential to significantly increase survival time and improve quality of life. The actual size of this effect can be debated, and the applicability to any given individual is unknown. Still, the high stakes of cancer care make it incumbent on researchers to continue to focus on this area.

Methods for Measuring Adherence

There are three general categories of measurement available for assessing adherence (Hays & DiMatteo, 1987). These include self-reports, collateral reports, and objective measures. Each of these has particular advantages and disadvantages when applied to the wide variety of treatment-related behaviors required of cancer patients.

That self-reported treatment adherence is frequently inaccurate has been well documented within a general medical population (Cannell, Oksenberg, & Converse, 1977; Dunbar-Jacob et al., 2000). The few investigations that attempted to validate the self-report of cancer patients by comparing self-report data with data from objective measures have shown equivocal results. A comparison of self-report data and adherence rates obtained from blood levels of a drug treatment suggested that adherence rates derived from blood levels were half the self-reported adherence rates (Levine et al., 1987). However, two measures of smoking cessation, cotinine levels and self-reports, among head and neck cancer patients were in agreement 89.6% of the time (Gritz et al., 1993). One hundred percent agreement between self-report and serum drug levels was reported in a study of children and adolescents (Tebbi et al., 1986).

It is, therefore, possible for patients to be relatively accurate reporters of their own behavior. Nonetheless, the variability in these concordance rates suggests that it is necessary to approach self-reports with some skepticism and to consider the context of the treatment. Sources of inaccuracy in self-report by other medical populations are multiple, including fear of embarrassment or rejection by the health care provider, desire for support and approval, and misunderstandings about treatment recommendations (Hays & DiMatteo, 1987). In addition, self-report does not allow for an assessment of unintentional nonadherence due to forgetfulness or neglect: by definition, people can't self-report about nonadherence of which they are unaware. Although these variables have not been investigated with cancer patients, there is no reason to expect that they would not also operate in this population.

Collateral reports of adherence can be obtained from family, friends, and health care providers. These sources have apparently been little used in the cancer population. In apparently the only study to utilize this kind of data, Dolgin, Katz, Doctors, and Siegel (1986) asked physicians to rate their adolescent cancer patients' treatment adherence and to estimate the threat that nonadherence posed to treatment outcome. However, they did not obtain self-reports of adherence, so it was not possible to judge the accuracy of the physicians' report. In early work, physicians' estimates of patients' adherence were found to be quite inaccurate (Caron & Roth, 1968, 1971; Davis, 1966).

Chart reviews have been used extensively as a source of objective information on cancer patient adherence to appointments for IV chemotherapy and follow-ups. Another method that is gaining in popularity and feasibility is the use of pharmacy and insurance records to evaluate the adherence of larger patient populations. For example, Silliman et al. (2002) examined the concordance between prescription refills and self-reported adherence to tamoxifen, finding roughly 90% agreement in this cohort of women older than 65 years.

Pill counts, electronic bottles, and urine or blood levels of medication in the patient's body also provide more objective measures, particularly cancer patients' adherence to oral chemotherapy and supportive medications. For example, the presence of 17-ketogenic steroids in urine has been shown to be a reliable indicator of adherence to oral prednisone in pediatric cancer patients (Festa, Tamaroff, Chasalow, & Lanzkowsky, 1992). However, others have questioned whether drug metabolites are really accurate adherence measures in patients for whom a particular treatment is not effective (i.e., biologically active) (Partridge, Avorn, Wang, & Winer, 2002).

Other investigators have also utilized blood serum levels of drugs and their metabolites to measure adherence (Lebovits et al., 1990; Richardson et al., 1987). Differing adherence rates have been found depending on whether the blood level of the parent drug or the metabolite was used. For example, Richardson et al. found that 77% of a sample of cancer patients were nonadherent to allopurinol as measured by the detection of the drug itself in the blood but that only 43.3% of patients would be classified as nonadherent on the basis of detection of oxipurinol, a metabolite of allopurinol. These authors suggest that such different levels might indicate poor or inconsistent medication ingestion. This interpretation has not been tested empirically, and other authors have questioned the value of this method due to individual variability in drug distribution and metabolism (Lee, Nicholson, Souhami, & Deshmukh, 1992).

Another alternative for measuring adherence to oral medication is the use of an electronic pill bottle that can record the times of day that the bottle is opened. This method is a particularly powerful objective measurement tool because it picks up both intentional and unintentional sources of nonadherence: it can also pick up both underadherence and "overadherence," which has been argued to be of potential concern with cancer patients who may think "more is better" when it comes to drugs that are supposed to kill off their cancerous cells (Partridge et al., 2002). Lee et al. (1992) reported the use of such a container with patients receiving oral chemotherapy. They documented almost perfect adherence to the regimen by comparing the number of bottle openings with the number of openings expected if adherence was perfect. In addition, they were able to reveal the pattern of pill taking by noting discrepancies between the time the bottle was opened and the time it was supposed to be opened. Pill bottles were opened the correct number of times on 80.9% of days.

Given the "fallibility" of individual methods, Hays & DiMatteo (1987) advocated the use of a multitrait, multimethod approach to the assessment of treatment adherence. Thus, patients might be defined as nonadherent if their self-report, the report of their physician or their spouse, or serum drug levels indicated nonadherence to the recommended treatment. The reader is referred to Section III of this book for a more thorough discussion of adherence measurement issues.

Adherence Rates for Cancer Management Behaviors

As with other serious illnesses, the behaviors required for good management of cancer risk and diagnosis are many and varied. For the general population, professional organizations and cancer advocacy groups publish guidelines for screening and early detection tests (Bach, Silvestri, Hanger, & Jett, 2007; Saslow et al. 2007). Although cancer screening and prevention behavior are not covered in this chapter, which is focused on people already diagnosed with cancer, they are a crucial component of the fight against this disease. (See Section II of this book for chapters on health behaviors linked to cancer risk reduction.)

Once a cancer has been diagnosed, additional diagnostic tests may be required to determine if the cancer has spread and, if so, the location of the metastasis. Treatment recommendations will then be presented, and a patient will be asked to adhere to a course that could include surgery, chemotherapy, other anticancer drugs or supportive medications, and radiation therapy. The care regimen may require the patient to attend multiple appointments for treatment and checkups, to take oral or IV medications, to make lifestyle changes, and, finally, to attend specified follow-up visits after treatment completion. In the upcoming sections, we consider various aspects of adherence and self-management in these three categories of cancer-related behavior: cancer treatment, lifestyle changes, and follow-up surveillance to detect possible recurrence or late complications of cancer therapy.

Treatment Refusal

At the far end of the continuum of patient nonadherence is outright treatment refusal. This can be active, with patients informing their physicians that they will not accept treatment, or it may be passive, as when patients simply don't show up for their treatment appointments.

The available data on the prevalence of treatment refusal are fairly limited. Two recent studies retrospectively examined the medical records of women who refused surgical treatment for breast cancer. In one review of 5,339 women in the Geneva Cancer Registry diagnosed with nonmetastatic breast cancer between 1975 and 2000, only 70 (1.3%) women refused the recommended surgery (Verkooijen et al., 2005). Forty-seven percent of those patients opted to receive a different type of therapy, such as hormonal treatment. Surgery is, however, considered to be the mainstay of treatment for early-stage breast cancer. Even controlling for other prognostic factors, those who refused surgery had 2.1 times the chance of dying from breast cancer within 5 years of those on whom operations were performed. Similarly poor outcomes were recorded in a smaller, retrospective chart review study of women who chose to utilize a form of alternative medicine rather than undergo recommended surgery as treatment for their breast cancer (Chang, Glissmeyer, Tonnes, Hudson, & Johnson, 2006).

Treatment refusal is probably more common among people with more advanced cancer. Physicians are also far more likely to support that choice, or at
least to voice understanding of it, when a patient appears to have a limited life
span. Three recently published studies investigated patient and/or physician
perceptions of patients' refusal of cancer treatment. In one study in the Netherlands, interviews were conducted with 30 patients who had refused either a
curative or a noncurative treatment, and 16 physicians with experience in this
area (Van Kleffens, van Baarsen, & van Leeuwen, 2004). As might be expected,
noncurative treatments were more likely to be refused than curative ones. Interestingly, physicians believed that medical information about the disease,
treatment, and prognosis was the critical factor in patients' decisions: patients
reported that their own, or close other's, experience of cancer and treatment
was the single most influential factor in their decision. Taking responsibility for
their own bodies and feeling free to make a choice were also critical aspects for
patients.

The refusal of treatment for non-small-cell lung cancer was investigated
in a sample of nine patients identified through a U.S. Veteran's Administration
(VA) hospital (Sharf, Stelljes, & Gordon, 2005). Analysis of the qualitative data
suggested that four themes accounted for a large portion of these patients' decision making: self-efficacy, threat minimization, fatalism and faith, and distrust
of the medical system. A lack of adequate information, desire to maximize quality of life, and a wish to avoid definitive unpleasant information were additional
themes identified in this study. Contrary to the previously discussed study, a
great deal of dissatisfaction and distrust with physician and the larger health
care system were reported as reasons for avoiding or refusing recommended
treatment.

Partial Adherence to Chemotherapy and
Other Medical Interventions

The treatment context and demands differ greatly for chemotherapy administered intravenously in an oncology clinic and oral antineoplastic therapies that
the patient is responsible for taking on a daily basis. The former is still more
common and evokes a traditional image, popular in the medical literature, of a
passive patient compliantly receiving treatment. In fact, relatively high rates of
adherence have been demonstrated for this form of cancer treatment. This is
particularly true for people being treated for early stage cancer. For example,
a recent report of a four-arm treatment trial for Stage II and III colon cancer
reported that 88.4% of randomized subjects received the treatment as it was
specified by the trial (Haller et al., 2005). Importantly, no compliance differences were noted between treatment arms. Differential compliance for different treatments is an important issue, however. For example, Von Minckwitz et al
(2006) reported on a trial for early-stage breast cancer. In it, 97.7% of subjects
completed the three cycles of a combination chemotherapy, but only 75.4% of
subjects completed the other proscribed regimen.

Investigations of adherence to chemotherapy for more advanced cancers
have reported significantly higher nonadherence rates. For example, Feld et al.
(Feld, Rubinstein, & Thomas, 1994; Feld, Rubinstein, Thomas, & the Lung Cancer

Study Group, 1993) reported on a trial of adjuvant chemotherapy for operable non-small-cell lung cancer. Only 80% of patients enrolled in the trial actually received their first treatment dose, 66% of patients received at least two of the four planned courses of treatment, and only 54% of patients completed all four courses. Another recently reported clinical trial was specifically designed to answer the question of whether the continuation of chemotherapy longer than 12 weeks for late-stage lung cancer resulted in better outcomes (i.e., longer survival, better quality of life) than 12 weeks of chemo followed by monitoring only until relapse (Socinski et al., 2002). There was no difference in survival or health-related quality of life for the two treatment arms, demonstrating that more treatment is not necessarily better in this particularly setting. However, this trial also spoke to the difficulty of adherence to a treatment protocol for patients with advanced cancer: approximately equal numbers of patients on each arm of the trial stopped receiving chemotherapy before 12 weeks. Only 42% of patients actually received more than four cycles of chemotherapy, even though this was the main difference between the two treatment arms. The reasons were varied and included serious treatment toxicity such that the physician deemed the treatment not in the patients' best interests, death, transition to hospice care, and patient choice not to continue the trial often because of worsening illness or significant treatment side effects.

Oral antineoplastic therapies are changing expectations among cancer patients, making them even more responsible for their own care and health than ever before. Nilsson et al. (2006) reported on the use of clinical pharmacy records to obtain the rates at which people with cancer refilled their prescriptions. The majority of these prescriptions were for hormonal antagonist treatments (86%), with the remainder for oral chemotherapies (8.5%) and hormones (5.5%). Of their sample of 141 cancer-related prescriptions, about 14% were filled less than 80% of the recommended times: the authors calculated that those 14% had a median treatment gap of 39 days. Fifty-six percent of prescriptions were filled appropriately, and 30% were actually filled more often than recommended. Contrary to the authors' expectations, these rates didn't differ significantly from refill adherence rates for all other (noncancer) medications.

There is also a growing literature on adherence to tamoxifen and the aromatase inhibitors, which are oral medications usually taken for a period of years to prevent the recurrence of breast cancer. As noted, taking tamoxifen for 5 years provides a significantly greater reduction in risk of recurrence and mortality than does taking it for 1 or 2 years (Early Breast Cancer Trialists' Collaborative Group, 2005). Despite these known benefits, several studies have reported suboptimal adherence rates over a 5 year period. Partridge, Wang, Winer, and Avorn (2003) examined adherence to tamoxifen among 2,378 women beginning tamoxifen for primary breast cancer. Although the percentage of prescriptions filled was relatively high during the first year (87%), the percentage filled decreased to less than 50% of the time by year 4. Another study investigated patterns of tamoxifen use among 516 women with estrogen-receptor-positive breast cancer (Fink, Gurwitz, Rakowski, Guadagnoli, & Silliman, 2004). They found that 17% stopped taking the medication by the second year and that the majority of those who stopped took it less than 1 year. Similarly, Lash, Fox, Westrup, Fink, and Silliman (2006) reported that 31% of their sample of older women diagnosed with stage I–IIIA breast cancer

(N = 462) stopped taking tamoxifen by year 5. A recent study examined tamoxifen use among a cohort of 881 women with stage I or II disease (Kahn, Schneider, Malin, Adams, & Epstein, 2007). Findings indicated that roughly 21% stopped taking tamoxifen by year 4, while 54% of those who stopped did so between the first and third years. Atkins and Fallowfield (2006) interviewed women taking tamoxifen or an aromatase inhibitor in an attempt to distinguish between "intentional" and "unintentional" nonadherence. Of 131 interviewees, 72 (55%) reported occasional nonadherence. Of these, 12 (16.7%) reported that they "chose not to take" their medication on occasion (intentional), while 60 (83.3%) "forgot" to take it (unintentional). These estimates of adherence to oral cancer medication from a number of different samples again suggest rates that are quite similar to those for other serious or chronic conditions. Similar conclusions were reached in a more detailed examination of adherence to oral cancer regimens by Partridge, Avorn, Wang, and Winer (2002).

Adherence to Behavioral Recommendations and Follow-Up

Rates of adherence to behavioral recommendations made during treatment have also been investigated. These recommendations are thought to improve the effectiveness of cancer treatment, decrease the likelihood of relapse, or inhibit the development of other serious health conditions that share common risk factors (Demark-Wahnefried, Peterson, McBride, Lipkus, & Clipp, 2000). Indeed, Denmark-Wahnefried et al. demonstrated strong interest in health promotion programs among a large sample of people who had been recently treated for early-stage breast or prostate cancer. In addition, there was significant variability in the subjects' report of their current level of engagement in healthy behaviors, from a low of 45% who were eating the recommended daily servings of fruit and vegetables to a high of 92% who reported that they did not smoke.

Much higher rates of smoking have been reported among head and neck and lung cancer patients, with estimates of continuing smoking after diagnosis ranging from 23%–35% for the former and from 13%–20% of the latter (Schnoll et al., 2004). In a study that examined rates of participation in a smoking cessation program offered specifically for these patients, 53% of 231 eligible patients declined to participate (Schnoll et al., 2005). Most stated that they intended to quit on their own and did not need additional help to do so. Further work is needed to determine the extent to which this is possible in the midst of intensive treatment.

Behavioral interventions that focus on physical activity and nutrition are far more popular and effective among cancer patients and survivors and are typically well supported by physicians (Brown et al., 2003). Exercise can positively affect psychological, physical, and biological outcomes (Vallance, Courneya, Jones, & Reiman, 2006) that are related to cancer. As with similar programs in healthy populations, adherence to an exercise regimen is moderately difficult for people with cancer. In Mock et al.'s (2005) trial of home-based walking exercise for women with Stage 0–III breast cancer, only 72% of the women were adherent to the prescribed exercise program.

As with other types of treatment-related behaviors, adherence to follow-up visits varies widely. From 77% to 93% of testicular cancer patients kept all of their scheduled follow-up appointments. The actual percentage varied depending upon the type of previous treatment received (Young, Bultz, Russell, & Trew, 1991). Using a different type of follow-up measure, 84% of colon cancer patients who had been treated with surgery adhered to a fairly intensive follow-up procedure, including three hemoccult tests, a clinical examination, and sigmoidoscopy every 3 months (Crowson, Jewkes, Acheson, & Fielding, 1991). Only 22% of breast cancer patients studied by Tomlin and Donegan (1987) completed all recommended follow-up visits for 5 years or more. However, 100% of a medically indigent population with breast cancer completed 5 years of follow-up after treatment (Smith et al., 1995). Finally, 80% of patients diagnosed with colon cancer returned for at least one follow-up colonoscopy after treatment, although this percentage later dropped, then rose steadily over the 7-year period of the investigation (Eckardt, Fuchs, Kanzler, Remmele, & Stienen, 1988).

In summary, rates of adherence to IV chemotherapy, oral chemotherapy and supportive medications, treatment appointments, behavioral changes, and follow-up visits vary widely. In some cases, such as treatment for early-stage cancer, nonadherence rates are quite low. However, for most others important behaviors, nonadherence rates seem to be comparable to those found in the general medical population. This challenges the widely held notion that people will always be adherent to treatment for life-threatening illness. It also affirms the necessity of investigating sources of nonadherence and potential interventions to improve adherence.

Predictors of Adherence

The primary explanation that is consistently advanced for nonadherence to cancer treatments has been their toxic side effects. Although side effect profiles vary widely, many of these medications produce unpleasant reactions such nausea, vomiting, pain, anemia, diarrhea, alopecia, anorexia, cachexia, loss of taste, and fatigue. In an early investigation, toxicity was cited as the major reason for breast cancer patients' not receiving at least 85% of their planned treatment (Lee, 1983). Similarly, the recent studies of endocrine therapy discussed earlier highlight that side effects that impair quality of life (e.g., hot flashes, night sweats) were the primary reason for temporary or permanent treatment discontinuation (Atkins & Fallowfield, 2006; Grunfeld, Hunter, Sikka, & Mittal, 2005; Lash et al., 2006). Several other cancer treatment variables have been associated with adherence. Treatment length was related to poorer adherence, with fewer patients continuing with longer treatments (e.g., Early Breast Cancer Trialists Group, 2005). The anticipation of longer treatment may be enough, in some cases, to decrease adherence. Rivkin et al. (1993) found that patients assigned to a 2 year treatment were less likely to complete even 6 months of treatment than were those assigned to a 1 year treatment arm. The patient's lack of symptoms, the length and type of treatment, and the complexity of the regimen are additional treatment-related variables known to decrease cancer-related adherence (Dunbar-Jacob & Mortimer-Stephens, 2001; McDonald, Amit, & Haynes, 2002).

The relationship of demographic variables to adherence has also been explored. Younger age has been related to lower likelihood of treatment refusal after a new cancer diagnosis (Huchcroft & Snodgrass, 1993), greater likelihood of smoking cessation after treatment for head and neck cancer (Gritz et al., 1993), greater tendency to practice breast self-examinations after breast cancer (Taylor et al., 1984) and better appointment attendance (Berger, Braverman, Sohn, & Morrow, 1988). However, younger women may be less likely to adhere to adjuvant endocrine treatment (Atkins & Fallowfield, 2006). Others have found that age does not affect the likelihood of refusing treatment (Moul, Paulson, & Walther, 1990) or completing treatment (Berger et al., 1988; Jehn, 1994). Older patients still tend to receive lower doses of chemotherapy, probably due to fears about tolerance of toxicity or interactions with other medical conditions. However, these concerns are generally thought to be unfounded, as tolerability of chemotherapy seems to be unrelated to age (Cress, O'Malley, Leiserowitz, & Campleman, 2003; Sargent et al., 2001).

Patients' beliefs about their disease and their treatment regimen also appear to play a role in cancer-related adherence. Several recent studies have demonstrated that adherence can be partially predicted by beliefs about the necessity of the medication and influenced also by beliefs about the short- and long-term costs of taking it. Horne & Weinman (1999) assessed subjects with one of four chronic conditions: asthma, renal disease, cardiac conditions, or cancer. Nineteen percent of the variance in patients' self-reported adherence with prescribed medication was predicted by the balance between beliefs about the necessity of taking the medication to control the illness and concerns about the potential negatives about doing so. Patients reported being concerned about potential long-term adverse events and the potential for dependence on their medication. Negative beliefs about the efficacy of tamoxifen (e.g., nothing would be gained by taking it) and increases in negative beliefs over time predicted lower adherence (Grunfeld et al., 2005; Lash et al., 2006). Similarly, adherence to analgesic regimens is influenced by negative beliefs about the potential for addiction to narcotics (Kirsch, Whitcomb, Donaghy, & Passik, 2002) and the likelihood that medication will provide better relief than other pain control methods (Lai et al., 2002). Another cognitive variable, self-efficacy, was associated with a greater chance of quitting smoking (Schnoll et al., 2002) and of regularly attending hospital appointments (Lev, 1997). Adherence to exercise promotion interventions is also predicted by participants' stage of change and level of perceived control (Courneya et al., 2004).

Interventions to Improve Adherence Among Cancer Patients

Although the past 10 years have brought an increase in knowledge about factors associated with greater adherence to cancer treatment, this knowledge has yet to be translated into testable interventions. In a recent chapter, we presented a case-based description of an adherence-promoting intervention on patient, provider, and health care system variables (Victorson, Peterman, & Cella, 2006). This focus on individually tailored changes exemplifies an approach that could be generalized to all patients where appropriate adherence is a concern. In fact, a recent review of interventions to increase adherence to medication regimens across diseases emphasized the complexity of the successful interventions (McDonald et al., 2002). The authors noted the difficulty of disentangling the necessary from the "nice" components when interventions include multiple appointment reminders, pill counters, and problem solving with trained personnel about barriers to taking medication as prescribed, among others. Although cancer was not one of the diseases for which a randomized intervention trial was described, it is reasonable to assume that these results from other chronic illnesses are generalizable.

Patient navigation is a comprehensive type of intervention that attempts to increase adherence by reducing or removing barriers to quality cancer care (Dohan & Schrag, 2005). Flexibility is a key feature, as the type of provided service differs depending on the barriers identified. Dohan and Schrag's overview of patient navigation programs described a variety of services that are provided in existing programs: improving access to care, including clinical trials, through education and outreach to underserved communities; providing translation services by bilingual, bicultural navigators to minimize communication problems between patients and providers; remedying logistical barriers such as lack of child care during appointments, limited transportation, lack of or insufficient insurance; and addressing systemic barriers such as historical mistrust of health care institutions or the existence of complex, fragmented medical services. The National Cancer Institute recently funded a number of research projects to rigorously examine the impact of patient navigation services in cancer care. To date, reports indicate that the programs are well received and that they increase patient satisfaction (e.g., Steinberg et al., 2006). Data on "harder" outcomes, such as percentage of treatment received or morbidity and mortality rates, are not yet available.

Conclusions and Suggestions for Future Research

Over the past several years, there has been incredible progress in the field of cancer treatment. Improved screening techniques and expanded access to them has allowed the diagnosis of many cancers while still in early, more curable stages. Novel therapies have improved effectiveness while reducing toxic side effects. There is real hope that many cancers can become true "chronic illnesses," rather than imminently life-threatening ones.

The true promise of such scientific discoveries can be enhanced significantly by provider and patient behaviors that support adherence. Clinicians and researchers can look for inspiration in the literature on adherence promotion in other serious illnesses, as well as to the basic cancer research demonstrating the impact of personality, treatment regimen, and patients' beliefs. Thoughtfully designed research will evaluate the utility of patient navigation interventions for improved patient outcomes. If successful, we can begin to untangle the critical components for enhancing adherence and maximizing quality of life and survival.

References

Adsay, N. V., Andea, A., Basturk, O., Kilinc, N., Nassar, H., & Cheng, J. D. (2004). Secondary tumors of the pancreas: An analysis of a surgical and autopsy database and review of the literature. Virchows Archive: *An International Journal of Pathology, 444,* 527–535.

Atkins, L., & Fallowfield, L. (2006). Intentional and non-intentional 835 nonadherence to medication amongst breast cancer patients. *European Journal of Cancer, 42,* 2271–2276.

Bach, P. B., Silvestri, G. A., Hanger, M., Jett, J. R., & American College of Chest Physicians. (2007). Screening for lung cancer: ACCP evidence-based clinical practice guidelines (2nd ed). *Chest, 132*(3 Suppl.), 69S–77S.

Ballantyne, J. C. (2003). Chronic pain following treatment for cancer: The role of opioids. *Oncologist, 8,* 567–575.

Barofsky, I. (1984). Therapeutic compliance and the cancer patient. *Health Education Quarterly, 10,* 43–56.

Berger, D., Braverman, A., Sohn, C. K., & Morrow, M. (1988). Patient compliance with aggressive multimodal therapy for locally advanced breast cancer. *Cancer, 61,* 1453–1455.

Bonadonna, G., & Valagussa, P. (1981). Dose-response effect of adjuvant chemotherapy in breast cancer. *New England Journal of Medicine, 304,* 10–15.

Brown, J. K., Byers, T., Doyle, C., Courneya, K. S., Demark-Wahnefried, W., Kushi, L. H., et al. (2003). Nutrition and physical activity during and after cancer treatment: An American Cancer Society guide for informed choices. *CA—A Cancer Journal for Clinicians, 53,* 268–291.

Cannell, C. E., Oksenberg, L., & Converse, J. M. (Eds.). (1977). *Experiments in interviewing techniques: Field experiments in health reporting, 1971–1977.* Ann Arbor, MI: Survey Research Center, Institute for Social Research.

Caron, H. S., & Roth, H. P. (1968). Patients' cooperation with a medical regimen. *Journal of the American Medical Association, 203,* 922–926.

Caron, H. S., & Roth, H. P. (1971). Objective assessment of cooperation with an ulcer diet: Relation to antacid intake and to assigned physician. *American Journal of Medical Science, 261,* 61–66.

Chang, E. Y., Glissmeyer, M., Tonnes, S., Hudson, T., & Johnson, N. (2006). Outcomes of breast cancer in patients who use alternative therapies as primary treatment. *American Journal of Surgery, 192,* 471–473.

Courneya, K. S., Friedenreich, C. M., Quinney, H. A., Fields, A. L. A., Jones, L. W., & Fairey, A. S. (2004). Predictors of adherence and contamination in a randomized trial of exercise in colorectal cancer survivors. *Psycho-Oncology, 13,* 857–866.

Cress, R. D., O'Malley, C. D., Leiserowitz, G. S., & Campleman, S. L. (2003). Patterns of chemotherapy use for women with ovarian cancer: A population-based study. *Journal of Clinical Oncology, 21*(8), 1530–1535.

Crowson, M. C., Jewkes, A. J., Acheson, N., & Fielding, J. (1991). Haemoccult testing as an indicator of recurrent colorectal cancer: A 5-year prospective study. *European Journal of Surgical Oncology, 17,* 281–284.

Davis, M. S. (1966). Variations in patients' compliance with doctors' orders: Analysis of congruence between survey responses and results of empirical investigations. *Journal of Medical Education, 41,* 1037–1048.

De Csepel, J., Tartter, P. I., & Gajdos, C. (2002). When not to give radiation therapy after breast conservation surgery for breast cancer. *Journal of Surgical Oncology, 74,* 273–277.

Demark-Wahnefried, W., Peterson, B., McBride, C., Lipkus, I., & Clipp, E. (2000). Current health behaviors and readiness to pursue life-style changes among men and women diagnosed with early stage prostate and breast carcinomas. *Cancer, 88,* 674–684.

Desai, S. P., Ben-Josef, E., Normolle, D. P., Francis, I. R., Greenson, J. K., Simeone, D. M., et al. (2007). Phase I study of oxaliplatin, full-dose gemcitabine, and concurrent radiation therapy in pancreatic cancer. *Journal of Clinical Oncology: Official Journal of the American Society of Clinical Oncology, 25,* 4587–4592.

DiMatteo, M. R. (2004). Variations in patients' adherence to medical recommendations: A quantitative review of 30 years of research. *Medical Care, 42,* 200–209.

Dohan, D., & Schrag, D. (2005). Using navigators to improve care of underserved patients. Current practices and approaches. *Cancer, 104,* 848–855.

Dolgin, M. J., Katz, E. R., Doctors, S. R., & Siegel, S. E. (1986). Caregivers' perceptions of medical compliance in adolescents with cancer. *Journal of Adolescent Health Care, 7,* 22–27.

Dunbar-Jacob, J., Erlen, J. A., Schlenk, E. A., Ryan, C. M., Sereika, S. M., & Doswell, W. M. (2000). Adherence in chronic disease. *Annual Review of Nursing Research, 18,* 48–90.

Dunbar-Jacob, J., & Mortimer-Stephens, M. K. (2001). Treatment adherence in chronic disease. *Journal of Clinical Epidemiology, 54,* S57–S60.

Early Breast Cancer Trialists' Collaborative Group. (2005). Effects of chemotherapy and hormonal therapy for early breast cancer on recurrence and 15-year survival: An overview of the randomized trials. *Lancet, 365,* 1687–1717.

Eckardt, V. F., Fuchs, M., Kanzler, G., Remmele, W., & Stienen, U. (1988). Follow-up of pa-
    tients with colonic polyps containing severe atypia and invasive carcinoma. *Cancer, 61,*
    2552–2557.
Fallowfield, L., Atkins, L., Catt, S., Cox, A., Coxon, C., Langridge, C., et al. (2006). Patients' pref-
    erence for administration of endocrine treatments by injection or tablets: Results from a
    study of women with breast cancer. *Annals of Oncology: Official Journal of the European
    Society for Medical Oncology, 17,* 205–210.
Farmer, K. C. (1999). Methods for measuring and monitoring medication regimen adherence in
    clinical trials and clinical practice. *Clinical Therapeutics, 21,* 1074–1090.
Feld, R., Rubinstein, L., & Thomas, P. A. (1994). Adjuvant chemotherapy with cyclophospha-
    mide, doxorubicin, and cisplatin in patients with completely resected Stage I non-small-
    cell lung cancer. *Chest, 106*(6 Suppl.), 307S–309S.
Feld, R., Rubinstein, L., Thomas, P. A., & the Lung Cancer Study Group. (1993). Adjuvant che-
    motherapy with cyclophosphamide, doxorubicin, and cisplatin in patients with completely
    resected Stage I non-small-cell lung cancer. *Journal of the National Cancer Institute, 85,*
    299–306.
Festa, R. S., Tamaroff, M. H., Chasalow, F., & Lanzkowsky, P. (1992). Therapeutic adherence to
    oral medication regimens by adolescents with cancer: I. Laboratory assessments. *Journal
    of Pediatrics, 120,* 807–811.
Fink, A. K., Gurwitz, J., Rakowski, W., Guadagnoli, E., & Silliman, R. A. (2004). Patient beliefs and
    tamoxifen discontinuance in older women with estrogen receptor-positive breast cancer.
    Journal of Clinical Oncology, 22(16), 3309–3315.
Gridelli, C., Maione, P., Illiano, A., Piantedosi, F. V., Favaretto, A., Bearz, A., et al. (2007). Cisplatin
    plus gemcitabine or vinorelbine for elderly patients with advanced non-small-cell lung
    cancer: The MILES-2P studies. *Journal of Clinical Oncology, 25,* 4663–4669.
Gritz, E. R., Carr, C. R., Rapkin, D., Abemayor, E., Chang, L. J. C., Won, W. K., et al. (1993). Predic-
    tors of long-term smoking cessation in head and neck cancer patients. *Cancer Epidemiol-
    ogy, Biomarkers & Prevention, 2,* 261–270.
Grunfeld, E. A., Hunter, M. S., Sikka, P., & Mittal, S. (2005). Adherence beliefs among breast
    cancer patients taking tamoxifen. *Patient Education and Counseling, 59,* 97–102.
Haller, D. G., Catalano, P. J., Macdonald, J. S., O'Rourke, M. A., Frontiera, M. S., Jackson, D. V.,
    et al. (2005). Phase III study of fluorouracil, leucovorin, and levamisole in high-risk Stage
    II and III colon cancer: Final report of Intergroup 0089. *Journal of Clinical Oncology, 23,*
    8671–8678.
Hays, R. D., & DiMatteo, M. R. (1987). Key issues and suggestions for patient compliance assess-
    ment: Sources of information, focus of measures, and nature of response options. *Journal
    of Compliance in Health Care, 2,* 37–53.
Hershman, D., & Narayanan, R. (2004). Patients' beliefs about prescribed medicines and their
    role in adherence to treatment in chronic physical illnesses. *Current Oncology Reports, 6,*
    277–284.
Horne, R., & Weinman, J. (1999). Patients' beliefs about prescribed medicines and their role in
    adherence to treatment in chronic physical illness. *Journal of Psychosomatic Research, 47,*
    555–567.
Huchcroft, S. A., & Snodgrass, T. (1993). Cancer patients who refuse treatment. *Cancer Causes
    and Control, 4,* 179–185.
Jehn, U. (1994). Long-term outcome of postremission chemotherapy for adults with acute my-
    eloid leukemia using different dose intensities. *Leukemia and Lymphoma, 15,* 99–112.
Kahn, K. L., Schneider, E. C., Malin, J. L., Adams, J. L., & Epstein, A. M. (2007). Patient centered
    experiences in breast cancer: Predicting long-term adherence to tamoxifen use. *Medical
    Care, 45,* 431–439.
Kirsh, K. L., Whitcomb, L. A., Donaghy, K., & Passik, S. D. (2002). Abuse and addiction issues
    in medically ill patients with pain: Attempts at clarification of terms and empirical study.
    Clinical Journal of Pain, 18, S52–S60.
Lai, Y. H., Keefe, F. J., Sun, W. Z., Tsai, L. Y., Cheng, P. L., Chiou, J. F., et al. (2002). Relationship
    between pain-specific beliefs and adherence to analgesic regimens in Taiwanese cancer
    patients: A preliminary study. *Journal of Pain and Symptom Management, 24,* 415–423.
Lash, T. L., Fox, M. P., Westrup, J. L., Fink, A. K., & Silliman, R. A. (2006). Adherence to tamoxifen
    over the five-year course. *Breast Cancer Research and Treatment, 99,* 215–220.
Lebovits, A. H., Strain, J. J., Schleifer, S. J., Tanaka, J. S., Bhardwaj, S., & Messe, M. R. (1990). Pa-
    tient noncompliance with self-administered chemotherapy. *Cancer, 65,* 17–22.

Lee, C. R., Nicholson, P. W., Souhami, R. L., & Deshmukh, A. A. (1992). Patient compliance with oral chemotherapy as assessed by a novel electronic technique. *Journal of Clinical Oncology, 10,* 1007–1013.

Lee, Y. N. (1983). Adjuvant chemotherapy (CMF) for breast carcinoma. *American Journal of Clinical Oncology, 6,* 25–30.

Lev, E. L. (1997). Bandura's theory of self-efficacy: Applications to oncology. *Scholarly Inquiry for Nursing Practice, 11,* 21–37.

Levine, A. M., Richardson, J. L., Marks, G., Chan, K., Graham, J., Selser, J. N., et al. (1987). Compliance with oral drug therapy in patients with hematologic malignancy. *Journal of Clinical Oncology, 5,* 1469–1476.

McCready, D. R., Chapman, J. A., Hanna, W. M., Kahn, H. J., Yap, K., Fish, E. B., et al. (2000). Factors associated with local breast cancer recurrence after lumpectomy alone: Postmenopausal patients. *Annals of Surgical Oncology, 7,* 562–567.

McDonald, H. P., Amit, G. X., & Haynes, R. B. (2002). Interventions to enhance patient adherence to medication prescriptions. *Journal of the American Medical Association, 288*(22), 2868–2879.

Mock, V., Frangakis, C., Davidson, N. E., Ropka, M. E., Pickett, M., Poniatowski, B., et al. (2005). Exercise manages fatigue during breast cancer treatment: A randomized controlled trial. *Psycho-Oncology, 14,* 464–477.

Moul, J. W., Paulson, D. F., & Walther, P. J. (1990). Refusal of cancer therapy in testicular cancer: Recognizing and preventing a significant problem. *World Journal of Urology, 8,* 58–62.

Nilsson, J. L. G., Andersson, K., Bergkvist, A., Bjorkman, I., Brismar, A., & Moen, J. (2006). Refill adherence to repeat prescriptions of cancer drugs to ambulatory patients. *European Journal of Cancer Care, 15,* 235–237.

Partridge, A. H., Avorn, J., Wang, P. S., & Winer, E. P. (2002). Adherence to therapy with oral antineoplastic agents. *Journal of the National Cancer Institute, 94,* 652–661.

Partridge, A. H., Wang, P. S., Winer, E. P., & Avorn, J. (2003). Nonadherence to adjuvant tamoxifen therapy in women with primary breast cancer. *Journal of Clinical Oncology, 21,* 602–606.

Richardson, J. L., Marks, G., Johnson, C., Graham, J. W., Chan, K. K., Selser, J., et al. (1987). Path model of multidimensional compliance with cancer therapy. *Health Psychology, 6,* 183–207.

Rivkin, S. E., Green, S., Metch, B., Jewell, W. R., Costanzi, J. J., Altman, S. J., et al. (1993). One versus 2 years of CMFVP adjuvant chemotherapy in axillary node positive and estrogen receptor negative patients: A Southwest Oncology Group Study. *Journal of Clinical Oncology, 11,* 1710–1716.

Rojas, M. P., Telaro, E., Russo, A., Moschetti, I., Coe, L., Fossati, R., et al. (2005). Follow-up strategies for women treated for early breast cancer. *Cochrane Database of Systematic Reviews, 1,* CD001768.

Sargent, D. J., Goldberg, R. M., Jacobson, S. D., Macdonald, J. S., Labianca, R., Haller, D. G., et al. (2001). A pooled analysis of adjuvant chemotherapy for resected colon cancer in elderly patients. *New England Journal of Medicine, 345,* 1091–1097.

Saslow, D., Boetes, C., Burke, W., Harms, S., Leach, M. O., Lehman, C. D., et al. for the American Cancer Society Breast Cancer Advisory Group. (2007). American Cancer Society guidelines for breast screening with MRI as an adjunct to mammography. *CA—A Cancer Journal for Clinicians, 57,* 75–89.

Schnoll, R. A., Malstrom, M., James, C., Rothman, R. L., Miller, S. M., Ridge, J. A., et al. (2002). Correlates of tobacco use among smokers and recent quitters diagnosed with cancer. *Patient Education and Counseling, 46,* 137–145.

Schnoll, R. A., Rothman, R. L., Lerman, C., Miller, S. M., Newman, H., Movsas, B., et al. (2004). Comparing cancer patients who enroll in a smoking cessation program at a comprehensive cancer center with those who decline enrollment. *Head and Neck, 26,* 276–284.

Secco, G. B., Fardelli, R., Rovida, S., Gianquinto, D., Baldi, E., Bonfante, P., et al. (2000). Is intensive follow-up really able to improve prognosis of patients with local recurrence after curative surgery for rectal cancer? *Annals of Surgical Oncology: The Official Journal of the Society of Surgical Oncology, 7*(1), 32–37.

Sharf, B. F., Stelljes, L. A., & Gordon, H. W. (2005). "A little bitty spot and I'm a big man": Patients' perspectives on refusing diagnosis or treatment for lung cancer. *Psycho-Oncology, 14,* 636–646.

Silliman, R. A., Guadagnoli, E., Rakowski, R., Landrum, M. B., Lash, T. L., Wolf, R., et al. (2002). Adjuvant tamoxifen prescription in women 65 years and older with early stage breast cancer. *Journal of Clinical Oncology, 20,* 2660–2662.

Smith, R. G., Landry, J. C., Hughes, L. L., Moore, M. R., Lynn, M. J., Davis, L. W., et al. (1995). Conservative treatment of early-stage breast cancer in a medically indigent population. *Journal of the National Medical Association, 87,* 500–504.

Socinski, M. A., Schell, M. J., Bakri, K., Peterman, A., Lee, J., Unger, P., et al. (2002). Second-line, low-dose, weekly paclitaxel in patients with stage IIIB/IV nonsmall cell lung carcinoma who fail first-line chemotherapy with carboplatin plus paclitaxel. *Cancer, 95,* 1265–1273.

Steinberg, M. L., Fremont, A., Khan, D. C., Huang, D., Knapp, H., Karaman, D., et al. (2006). Lay patient navigator program implementation for equal access to cancer care and clinical trials. Essential steps and initial challenges. *Cancer, 107,* 2669–2677.

Taylor, S. E., Lichtman, R. R., Wood, J. V., Bluming, A. Z., Dosik, G. M., & Leibowitz, R. L. (1984). Breast self-examinations among diagnosed breast cancer patients, *Cancer, 54,* 2528–2532.

Tebbi, C. K., Cummings, K. M., Zevon, J. M. A., Smith, L., Richards, M., & Mallon, J. (1986). Compliance of pediatric and adolescent cancer patients. *Cancer, 58,* 1179–1184.

Titu, L. V., Nicholson, A. A., Hartley, J. E., Breen, D. J., & Monson, J. R. T. (2006). Routine follow-up by magnetic resonance imaging does not improve detection of resectable local recurrences from colorectal cancer. *Annals of Surgery, 243*(3), 348–352.

Tomlin, R., & Donegan, W. L. (1987). Screening for recurrent breast cancer: Its effectiveness and prognostic value. *Journal of Clinical Oncology, 5,* 62–67.

Vallance, J. K. H., Courneya, K. S., Jones, L. W., & Reiman, T. (2006). Exercise preferences among a population-based sample of non-Hodgkin's lymphoma survivors. *European Journal of Cancer Care, 15,* 34–43.

Van Gerpen, R., & Mast, M. E. (2004). Thromboembolic disorders in cancer. *Clinical Journal of Oncology Nursing, 8,* 289–299.

Van Kleffens, T., van Baarsen, B., & van Leeuwen, E. (2004). The medical practice of patient autonomy and cancer treatment refusals: A patients' and physicians' perspective. *Social Science & Medicine, 58,* 2325–2336.

Verkooijen, H. M., Fioretta, G. M., Rapiti, E., Bonnefoi, H., Vlastos, G., et al. (2005). Patients' refusal of surgery strongly impairs breast cancer survival. *Annals of Surgery, 242,* 276–280.

Victorson, D., Peterman, A. H., & Cella, D. (2006). Cancer-related adherence: Background, clinical issues, and promotion strategies. In W. T. O'Donohue & E. R. Levensky (Eds.), *Promoting treatment adherence* (pp. 267–281). Thousand Oaks, CA: Sage.

Von Minckwitz, G., Graf, E., Geberth, M., Eiermann, W., Jonat, W., Conrad, B., et al. (2006). CMF versus goserelin as adjuvant therapy for node-negative, hormone-receptor-positive breast cancer in premenopausal patients: A randomised trial (GABG trial IV-A-93). *European Journal of Cancer, 42,* 1780–1788.

Young, B. J., Bultz, B. D., Russell, J. A., & Trew, M. S. (1991). Compliance with follow-up of patients treated for non-seminomatous testicular cancer. *British Journal of Cancer, 64,* 606.

Adherence and HIV: A Lifetime Commitment

33

Scott D. Rhodes,
Kenneth C.
Hergenrather,
Aimee M. Wilkin, and
Richard Wooldredge

Since the isolation and identification of HIV in 1983, the number of people living with HIV/AIDS (PLWHA) continues to increase. Fortunately, advances in medical treatments have changed the outcomes for PLWHA for the better. Dramatic improvements in HIV treatment came in 1996 when protease inhibitors (PI) and non-nucleoside reverse transcriptase inhibitors (NNRTI) became widely available and were used as part of highly active antiretroviral therapy (HAART) to suppress HIV viral replication and improve immune function.

The profound impact of HAART was illustrated in the late summer of 1998, when the *Bay Area Reporter* published its now-famous headline "No Obits," commemorating the first time since the beginning of the epidemic that the newspaper received no death notices for a week. These initial reports of the decline in mortality coinciding with the use of HAART were striking. In one large cohort, the mortality rate fell from 29.4 deaths/100 person years in 1995 to 8.8 deaths/100 person years by mid-1997 (Palella et al., 1998). Since that time, the number of inpatient hospital beds dedicated to patients with HIV/AIDS in the United States has declined, and PLWHA are leading more productive lives for longer periods of time (Crum et al., 2006; Hergenrather, Rhodes, & Clark, 2004, 2006; Schackman et al., 2006).

However, despite advances in treatment, maintaining patient adherence to HIV medications (defined as the extent to which a therapeutic regimen is correctly taken) is challenging, in part because of the complexity of the treatment regimes and side effects. Other challenges to adherence for PLWHA include the need to take other medications, such as opportunistic infection (OI) prophylaxis.

This chapter explores adherence to HIV medications by examining what is currently known about adherence and HIV disease progression; exploring the facilitators of and barriers to adherence among various subgroups of PLWHA, including men who have sex with men (MSM), adolescents, homeless populations, pregnant women, those with comorbidities such as mental illness and substance use and abuse histories, and populations in developing countries; defining and measuring adherence; reviewing the state of interventions developed to improve adherence; and proposing future directions and research needs.

Adherence and Disease Progression and Outcomes

Strict adherence to HAART has been shown to suppress HIV viral loads, increase CD4+ lymphocyte counts and immune system function, improve clinical health, and decrease AIDS-related mortality. However, to maximize its benefit, HAART requires unusually high levels of adherence when compared to other regimens (Paterson et al., 2000). PLWHA taking protease inhibitor-based regimens must adhere to their schedule 95% of the time to achieve an 80% likelihood of having a viral load below the limit of detection. Put another way, they can miss no more than three doses a month of a twice-a-day regimen (Paterson et al., 2000).

With less than 95% adherence, the probability of viral suppression falls dramatically (Paterson et al., 2000; Altice, Mostashari, & Friedland, 2001). Adherence rates between 50% and 80% may promote drug resistance due to ongoing viral replication in the presence of suboptimal drug levels. If adherence falls below 50%, HAART drug levels tend to be too low to affect viral replication.

Suboptimal adherence to prescribed medication is not unique to HAART. Adherence rates ranging from 36% to 70% among various populations of PLWHA have been reported (Arnsten et al., 2002; Heckman, Catz, Heckman, Miller, & Kalichman, 2004). One study of 3,788 young men and women on HAART reported a mean annual adherence rate of 36%, and only 26% of individuals had adherence of 80% or better (Becker, Dezii, Burtcel, Kawabata, & Hodder, 2002).

The success of HAART relies on adherence to potentially complicated medical regimens for extremely long periods of time. Given recent findings that stopping or interrupting HAART can be harmful (El-Sadr et al., 2006), the commitment to staying on HIV medications after starting is likely a lifetime one. Interruptions in medication adherence permit HIV to resume its typical rapid replication of as many as 10^{10} viral particles produced per day (Perelson et al., 1997) and promote the development of drug-resistant variants of HIV, with potential cross-resistance across entire classes of medications (Hecht et al., 1998). This scenario limits future treatment options for the individual and poses a potential public health risk through the transmission of these strains to others (Friedland & Williams, 1999; McNabb et al., 2001).

Adherence to HAART

Factors associated favorably or adversely with medication adherence in PLWHA can be organized into six domains, as presented in Figure 33.1. Although many of these may provide insight into populations that may benefit from tailored interventions or into potentially modifiable factors for an individual, they are not completely predictive of response to HAART.

Demographic factors associated with decreased adherence in different settings include younger age, African American race, low level of educational attainment, homelessness or unstable housing, and decreased income (Altice et al., 2001; Golin et al., 2002; Kleeberger et al. 2001).

Cognitive and psychological factors that have been found to be associated with decreased HIV medication adherence include having relatively little knowledge about how to take prescribed medications and about the importance of adherence and doubting the efficacy of the medications (Altice et al., 2001; Catz, Kelly, Bogart, Benotsch, & McAuliffe, 2000). Compromised cognitive functioning, forgetfulness, and depression are other key factors that adversely affect adherence (Ammassari et al., 2004; Chesney et al., 2000; Golin et al., 2002). An interesting construct that has been identified as a barrier is "seeing positive results" from treatment that in turn leads to the feeling that one no longer needs medication (Adam, Maticka-Tyndale, & Cohen, 2003).

Behavioral factors that have been found to predict decreased adherence include alcohol and substance use and abuse (Ammassari et al., 2004; Hinkin

33.1

Domains affecting adherence to HAART and viral load among persons living with HIV/AIDS.

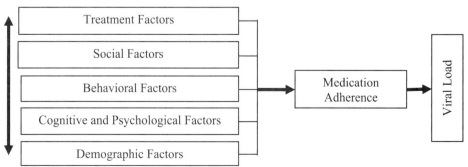

et al., 2007). The use of adherence aids such as pill boxes and timers has been associated with improved adherence to HAART (Andrade et al., 2005; Fogarty et al., 2002).

Provider characteristics have long been associated with health behaviors (Rhodes & Benfield, 2006) and clearly affect adherence to HAART. Reduced adherence among PLWHA is associated with lack of trust in the provider in terms of their skill and their real or perceived abilities to be nonjudgmental and maintain confidentiality (Beach, Keruly, & Moore, 2006; Schneider, Kaplan, Greenfield, Li, & Wilson, 2004).

Social factors also have an influence on adherence. PLWHA who report having less social support and being more socially isolated have lower adherence than those who have increased social support and report not being socially isolated (Catz et al., 2000). Some PLWHA may perceive that taking medications may serve to reveal their serostatus to others, such as coworkers (Meystre-Agustoni, Dubois-Arber, Cochand, & Telenti, 2000).

Finally, the type of treatment regimen is associated with adherence. Complexity and timing of dosing, side effects, food requirements, and how well adherence fits within one's lifestyle can influence adherence rates (Catz et al., 2000; Nieuwkerk, Gisolf, Sprangers, & Danner, 2001). The presence of side effects from medications can be challenging, especially when the benefits of treatment such as delaying disease progression may not have an immediately tangible result.

HAART Adherence Among Subgroups

Certain subgroups of PLWHA have even further challenges to HAART adherence. Economic and social strain and developmental processes experienced by some vulnerable and marginalized populations likely exacerbate adherence issues, since even among affluent and educated populations adherence rates as low as 67% are reported (Deloria-Knoll et al., 2004). Perceptions and beliefs related to efficacy of HAART, the stigma associated with an HIV/AIDS diagnosis, and attitudes toward illness vary by subgroup and can profoundly affect adherence (Parker & Aggleton, 2003).

Men Who Have Sex With Men

Men who have sex with men (MSM) make up a large percentage of the individuals living with HIV/AIDS in the United States and in Europe. Some MSM may not adhere to their treatment regimen because of internalized homophobia, which may lead them to deny their own same-sex behavior. Their infection may present a conflict, since to acknowledge their HIV-positive serostatus may imply that they must acknowledge this behavior. Internalized homophobia also may affect relationships with providers (Klitzman & Greenberg, 2002; Rhodes & Hergenrather, 2002). By not sharing the challenges they face with their providers or other supportive individuals, some MSM may impair their own ability to explore solutions to these challenges. Other complications may include feelings of guilt regarding their HIV-positive status (Madru, 2003).

Just as racism has been identified as a cause for compromised heath outcomes among racial and ethnic minorities (Institute of Medicine, 2003), homophobia and heterosexism also exist within a broad historical and contemporary context (Rhodes, McCoy, Hergenrather, Omli, & DuRant, 2007; Rhodes & Yee, 2006). MSM may have reduced access to high-quality health services, care, and programs that meet their particular needs (Willging, Salvador, & Kano, 2006). Many providers are uncomfortable discussing HIV or the sexual health of MSM in general, which in turn may discourage disclosures necessary for appropriate care and services (Rhodes & Hergenrather, 2002; Rhodes & Yee, 2006). For example, the provider may fail to engage a same-sex partner in efforts to increase adherence, despite evidence that partner support is beneficial (Power et al., 2003).

To increase HAART adherence among MSM living with HIV/AIDS, providers must: maintain nonhomophobic assumptions and attitudes; distinguish sexual behavior from identity; communicate clearly and sensitively; use gender-neutral terms; and, perhaps most important, recognize how personal provider attitudes affect clinical judgments (Rhodes & Hergenrather, 2002; Rhodes, Yee, & Hergenrather, 2006; Rhodes et al., 2007).

Most of what is currently known about the challenges faced by MSM living with HIV/AIDS came from the early epicenters of the U.S. epidemic, which are large urban areas with long histories of service provision, including treatment, care, and prevention (McKinney, 2002). These epicenters do not fully reflect the unique characteristics of the current epidemic (Rhodes et al., 2007). Those living outside large urban areas are more likely to have providers with less experience dealing with HIV and less opportunity to participate in clinical trials for AIDS treatments (Ellerbrock et al., 2004; Rhodes, Hergenrather, Wilkin, Alegria-Ortega, & Montaño, 2006).

Adolescents

While adhering to HAART is challenging enough for adults, adolescents living with HIV/AIDS face some unique challenges that may make adherence even more difficult. The reasons for these challenges are numerous and overlap to some degree with those already identified. Developmentally, adolescents often feel invincible or immortal. They are prone to live in the moment and may not realize the long-term consequences of their actions (DeWit, Offord, & Wong, 1997). While this way of thinking is beneficial as adolescents try new roles and activities and take healthy risks, adolescents living with HIV/AIDS may not have immediate incentives for maintaining adherence to HAART. Taking the medications often does not make them feel better and can, in fact, make them feel worse. Moreover, they may not feel any worse if they inconsistently take or stop taking their medications, and this lack of immediate negative consequences can reinforce feelings of invincibility. Helping adolescents focus on the long-term health consequences of their adherence choices is a significant but necessary challenge in promoting HAART adherence (Koenig & Bachanas, 2006; Parsons et al., 2006).

Peer acceptance and support during adolescence are important developmentally (Resnick, Harris, & Blum, 1993). Adolescents living with HIV fear rejection, abandonment, and stigma and may not tell their family, friends, and sexual partners of their HIV status. Many adolescents avoid treatment and care, fearing that seeking care will reveal their HIV status (Rao, Kekwaletswe, Hosek, Martinez, & Rodriguez, 2007; Steele, Nelson, & Cole, 2007). Their fears are not without reason, as some adolescents with HIV are alienated from their families as a result of their HIV status or sexual orientation. Thus, their housing situation is often unstable, increasing the difficulty of making and keeping appointments, refilling prescriptions before they run out, and adhering to HAART. Furthermore, follow-up efforts by clinics (e.g., reminder calls, letters) are problematic when contact information changes or when adolescents have not told family members of their HIV status. Adolescents trying to conceal their HIV status find it difficult to keep medications handy and thus may not remember to take them regularly (Koenig & Bachanas, 2006; Rao et al., 2007).

Psychosocial, mental health, and substance-use problems, common among adolescents with HIV, also make adherence challenging for adolescents. Comparing demographically and socially similar adolescents with and without HIV infection, researchers found that adolescents living with HIV were significantly more likely to have been sexually abused, to have engaged in unprotected sex with causal partners, to have had sex under the influence of drugs, to have engaged in sex for money, to have had another sexually transmitted disease, to have used several types of illicit drugs, to have been incarcerated, to have dropped out of school, to have a history of psychiatric hospitalization, and to not be living at home (Steele et al., 2007). Thus, adherence to HAART is seriously challenged.

Over a quarter of a century into the pandemic, a subgroup of adolescents who are living with HIV/AIDS is emerging: adolescents who were infected through vertical transmission as infants 10–20 years ago. These adolescents may have similar challenges to those infected, but further research is needed to understand their unique adherence needs.

There are few efficacious interventions designed to increase adherence among adolescents living with HIV/AIDS. Promising findings, however, suggest that peer group-level interventions focused on the dynamics of HIV may improve adherence, as may having an understanding of the reasons for adhering to therapies and effective management of side effects, and improved communication with providers (Koenig & Bachanas, 2006).

Homeless Populations

Ensuring proper treatment of HIV/AIDS and adhering to HAART can be extremely difficult for PLWHA without stable housing. Meeting food and shelter priorities often leaves little time for medical appointments. The lack of privacy, risk of physical or verbal abuse, theft of medications, and lack of a secure place to store medications or to lie down during the day compound the discomforts associated with HIV and HAART. Ideally, homeless PLWHA need a stable residence and routine to properly adhere to HAART. Although some transitional housing for HIV-infected individuals exists in larger metropolitan areas, in many communities such individuals face a lack of available housing, long waiting lists, and policies that exclude active substance users or former inmates. Most housing, rehabilitation, or transitional programs available to homeless persons with HIV infection require sobriety for admission or continued residence. Thus, such supports become attainable only when homeless individuals with co-occurring addiction disorders become extremely ill, and typically when HIV disease is advanced (Smith, DeWeaver, & Reece, 2006; Tommasello, Gillis, Lawler, & Bujak, 2006).

Homeless populations also are at risk for discontinuity of care. They often have limited access to health care services, and their utilization of these services may be infrequent (i.e., only when they require urgent care). Homeless persons tend to have increased rates of arrest and incarceration due to loitering, sleeping, or drinking in public places. These periods of detention or incarceration can interrupt their health care.

A variety of steps can be taken to increase adherence to HAART among homeless PLWHA. For example, written instructions that include simple graphics (for those with low literacy) and color coding have been associated with increased HAART adherence among homeless PLWHA (Conanan et al., 2003). Furthermore, providers who rehearse with homeless PLWHA which drugs to take and when to take them have been successful in increasing adherence (Conanan et al., 2003). Consumer advocates, specifically formerly homeless persons, have increased adherence by navigating the treatment process and overcoming the communication barriers that homeless people sometimes experience in their encounters with health care providers. These advocates know the reality of "living on the street" and may have creative solutions that providers and other caregivers cannot imagine, given their very different frames of reference.

Adherence among homeless populations also has been improved through the implementation of directly observed therapy (DOT; Mitty, Macalino, Taylor, Harwell, & Flanigan, 2003). DOT requires homeless PLWHA to come to a clinic or other location to take their medications. This may be burdensome for clinic staff; however, adherence for indigent PLWHA who use DOT is higher than among those who do not (Santos, Adeyemi, & Tenorio, 2006; Wohl et al., 2004).

Pregnant Women

Worldwide, the number of women infected with HIV/AIDS has grown exponentially, and most women living with HIV are of reproductive age. Without treatment, 15% to 30% of babies born to HIV-positive mothers will be HIV infected (Centers for Disease Control and Prevention, 1994); however, preventive treatment of women during pregnancy combined with short-term treatment of newborns with AZT can significantly decrease perinatal HIV transmission (Centers for Disease Control and Prevention, 1994; Connor et al., 1994). With the progress in HAART and other management strategies, the rate of perinatal transmission of HIV has plummeted in the United States to less than 2% (Centers for Disease Control and Prevention, 2006). Unfortunately, even among those with access to care and treatment, not all pregnant PLWHA adhere to the recommended regimens. Poor treatment of women and racial minorities in the health care system, clients' lack of trust in health care providers, and a lack of accurate information about the treatment and prevention of HIV are barriers to adherence among pregnant women (Sowell, Phillips, Seals, Misener, & Rush, 2001). Furthermore, increased adherence among pregnant women has been associated with women's perception of how strongly their health care providers believe in AZT; social support from family, friends, and peers; and accurate knowledge about HIV, pregnancy, and AZT (Desai & Mathur, 2003; Siegel, Lekas, Schrimshaw, & Johnson, 2001; Sowell, Murdaugh, Addy, Moneyham, & Tavokoli, 2002). Providers' attitudes about pregnancy in women living with HIV/AIDS may greatly impact treatment uptake and clients' adherence to prevent vertical transmission. For example, some providers' attitudes may preclude women who get pregnant or want to get pregnant from having the information they need to make informed decisions and to improve pregnancy outcomes (Sowell et al., 2001).

Finally, despite the fact that AZT is safe for fetuses (Perinatal HIV Guidelines Working Group, 2002; Siu, Yeung, Pang, Chiu, & Lau, 2005), some pregnant PLWHA choose not to adhere to AZT to reduce vertical transmission because they fear that the medication will have unintended and harmful effects on their unborn children (Siegel & Gorey, 1997; Siegel et al., 2001; Sowell et al., 2001).

PLWHA and Comorbidities: Substance Use and Mental Health

It is estimated that nearly 50% of PLWHA receiving care for HIV in the United States have or have had a comorbidity of substance abuse or mental illness within the past 12 months—five to seven times higher than in the general U.S. population (Bing et al., 2001). Substance use negatively impacts adherence to HAART by impairing cognition, judgment, and short-term memory. Factors associated with decreased adherence among PLWHA who use illicit drugs include worries about the possible side effects of illicit drug use in conjunction with HAART. In one study, for example, PLWHA who were using cocaine or heroin and were eligible to take HAART believed that taking HAART while actively using cocaine would harm their bodies; thus, they had very low rates of adherence (Sharpe, Lee, Nakashima, Elam-Evans, & Fleming, 2004).

Nonadherence to HAART has been associated with depression and psychological stress (Elliott, Russo, & Roy-Byrne, 2002; Markowitz et al., 1998; Singh et al., 1996). PLWHA diagnosed with depression are likely to exhibit a general pessimism about the future and have poorer adherence to treatment regimens than do nondepressed PLWHA.

PLWHA with comorbidity of substance abuse and mental illness are likely to face greater morbidity and decreased quality of life and to participate in unsafe sexual and needle-sharing behaviors, leading to HIV transmission and further re-infection. Enabling HIV-infected substance abusers to reduce or end their substance use through treatment programs may produce the best results for medication adherence to HAART (Avants, Warburton, Hawkins, & Margolin, 2000; Boyer & Indyk, 2006; Chander, Himelhoch, & Moore, 2006; Colfax & Guzman, 2006; Kelly et al., 1993; Shapiro et al., 1999; Sherbourne et al., 2000; Willenbring, 2005). PLWHA who are in substance abuse treatment programs are significantly more likely to adhere to HAART (Battaglioli-Denero, 2007).

Interventions designed to increase adherence among PLWHA with a comorbidity of substance abuse and mental illness may include the application of cognitive-behavioral therapy and structured interviewing. These approaches may focus on changing deficiencies in clients' knowledge of HIV diagnosis and of the importance of adhering to the medical protocol and the ramifications of nonadherence; increasing prescribed medication self-efficacy; promoting the management of side effects; using social supports; decreasing perceptions that HAART regimens are too complex; and improving attitudes toward medication and diagnosis. However, these strategies require that public and private options be available for the treatment of mental illness and substance abuse.

Populations in Developing Countries

For PLWHA in developing countries, the fundamental barriers to adherence include limited access to counseling and testing services to determine serostatus and limited access to HAART. Only 10% of people who need HIV testing in low- and middle-income countries have access to counseling and testing services; thus, most are unaware of their serostatus (Furber, Hodgson, Desclaux, & Mukasa, 2004). Furthermore, the predominant approach to health care and the provision of health care services in developing countries is modeled on acute care—but, for HIV treatment, a chronic disease model is more appropriate. Such a model encompasses regular and ongoing follow-up, data management, and the use of communication tools that are efficient and that protect confidentiality. Access and adherence to HAART are also limited by cost—for PLWHA living in developing countries, paying even modest prices for drugs can be impossible. Criteria for access to subsidized HAART differ profoundly around the world and can be based on social characteristics, level of income, profession, and number of dependents (Desclaux, 2003).

Despite more than 25 years of awareness of HIV/AIDS, the stigmatization of PLWHA and those related to, caring for, and otherwise connected to PLWHA and HIV/AIDS prevention remains strong. Access to antiretroviral drugs may reduce stigma because, as HIV/AIDS is perceived as a chronic but manageable condition, one of the factors that amplify stigma—fear of contagion and inevitable death—is lessened (Hawkins, 2006). However, stigma is also a tool used by cultures to exclude those felt to have broken its rules, and the dominant stereotype of people living with HIV casts them as immoral (Stanley, 1999).

Taking HAART also may be stigmatizing. PLWHA often hide their medicines because relatives and other community members might reject them if they were aware of the PLWHA's medical status (Furber et al., 2004).

Thus, PLWHA in developing countries face fundamental barriers to adherence. First, they must have access to resources for counseling and testing to learn their serostatus. Second, infrastructures must exist to deliver HAART. Currently, more than 95% of PLWHA live in developing countries, and very few within this population have access to HAART. Finally, PLWHA in developing countries face similar but often greater challenges to pay for HAART and have worries about confidentiality and stigma.

Summary

This review of the identified facilitators of and barriers to adherence, while not exhaustive, offers an overview and highlights important considerations in adherence to HAART among populations for whom adherence may pose extraordinary challenges. Of course, these challenges may overlap or be shared by other populations. For example, stigma associated with HIV exists within most populations and is not unique to the challenges of living with HIV within developing countries.

Defining and Measuring Adherence

Valid measures of adherence are key to identifying PLWHA who are not adhering to regimens and to developing and evaluating meaningful interventions designed to increase adherence. However, operationalizing adherence through measurement is problematic. Common methods for measuring adherence to

HAART include drug concentrations in blood and urine, direct observation, pill count, physician ratings, and self-report. Monitoring of pharmacy refills of antiretroviral medications may also be a useful tool for assessing adherence (Gross et al., 2006). Use of medication-event monitoring system (MEMS) caps on drug bottles is the current state-of-the-art method for measuring adherence. MEMS caps have computer chips embedded in them that record the date and time whenever the cap of a medication bottle is opened; however, they are expensive and thus their use is limited (Bova et al., 2005).

Self-report measures are most commonly used because of their relatively low cost, ease of administration, minimal participant burden, flexibility in administration and timing, and potential to yield specific information regarding dosing behavior, such as timing with food (Simoni, Pearson, Pantalone, Marks, & Crepaz, 2006). On the other hand, self-report remains a coarse measure of adherence and is subject to threats such as recall bias and social desirability effects. Self-report of adherence to HAART tends to overestimate adherence and generally does not distinguish individuals by levels of adherence.

Another consideration is that adherence requirements may differ by potency. More potent and more recently developed medications, including nonnucleoside reverse transcriptase therapy (NNRTI) and ritonavir-boosted protease inhibitor therapy, seem to be capable of reliably suppressing viral load in patients at more moderate levels of adherence (King, Brun, & Kempf, 2005; Maggiolo et al., 2005). Moreover, the ability of medication-resistant virus to replicate differs by medication. For example, for single protease inhibitors, drug resistance may occur at adherence levels ranging from 80% to 95%, while for NNRTI, drug resistance may not occur even at adherence levels as low as 2% (Bangsberg et al., 2006). Thus, patterns of adherence may be more critical than overall adherence. Discontinuation of HAART for more than 48 hours is an independent risk factor for NNRTI resistance, even controlling for average adherence over time (Bangsberg et al., 2006; Spacek et al., 2006). As a result, rapid changes in HAART lead to changes in adherence goals. Thus, adherence measurement must include and identify specific levels and specific patterns of adherence that put the health of PLWHA at risk and particular regimens at risk for resistance.

Interventions Designed to Improve Adherence

Studies and intervention strategies have approached improving adherence to HAART from multiple frameworks. These frameworks reflect the array of complex factors that affect adherence, as presented in Figure 33.1. Unfortunately, a lack of consistent predictors of adherence remains (Hill, Kendall, & Fernandez, 2003), and many different measures that may not be directly comparable have been used in adherence studies. Studies differ in design, sample composition, types of adherence measurements, and outcome measures. A quantitative meta-analysis of 19 randomized controlled trials of various adherence interventions using the outcome measures of 95% adherence to HAART or undetectable HIV viral load found that intervention participants were more likely (odds ratio = 1.5; 95% confidence interval: 1.16–1.94) to achieve 95% adherence than those randomized to control groups. Viral load also was positively affected by adherence interventions, although the results were not statistically significant

(Simoni et al., 2006). Interventions studied included counseling (one-on-one or group) provided by health care providers such as physicians, nurses, or mental health counselors. More than half the studies used study staff to deliver interventions, and both the length of time per counseling visit and the number of visits varied considerably. Overall, 62% of those in the intervention groups and 50% of those in the control groups achieved optimal adherence. Although some interventions targeted PLWHA who were at high risk for nonadherence, many were provided to all persons on HAART, conceivably diluting the ability to detect differences in groups (Gordon, 2006). In a similar meta-analysis that included randomized and nonrandomized studies, interventions that targeted PLWHA with known poor adherence had stronger effects than those that had broader enrollment (Amico, Harman, & Johnson, 2006).

A recent trial examined the use of a cognitive behavioral adherence intervention for PLWHA starting or changing HAART regimens. Participants in the intervention groups received five sessions of cognitive behavioral and motivational components (with or without a 2 week trial of placebo medications), while those in the comparison group received usual care (Wagner et al., 2006). Adherence rates in all groups were high with modest treatment effects at week 24 (mean percentage of pills taken 89% in the intervention group and 81% in the control group). Unfortunately, these treatment effects were extinguished by week 48. There were no differences between groups in virologic control. The researchers speculated that a new approach in adherence interventions tailored to the needs of individuals may be necessary.

Another potential strategy for improving adherence among PLWHA is to use a case-management approach. Case management is a client-centered approach that coordinates the provisions of service. It includes intensive, ongoing, individualized counseling, support, and service brokerage by a trained case-management professional. Areas addressed include the relationship between HIV risk (both treatment nonadherence and re-infection) and issues such as substance abuse, treatment for STDs, mental health, and social and cultural factors. A recent study (Kushel et al., 2006), using a nonrandomized prospective observational cohort, reported an association between receiving case management and self-reported adherence in homeless and marginally housed PLWHA. Groups that accessed case management at higher rates had larger increases in CD4+ lymphocyte counts than the groups that did not receive case management. However, no relationship was found between case management and viral load suppression. Case management may be a promising approach for increasing adherence to HAART among PLWHA.

The use of directly administered antiretroviral therapy (DAART) has engendered interest as a strategy to improve adherence. A setting that may be particularly suited for DAART is a structured environment where clients make regular contact with the health care system, such as a methadone clinic. In a recent report, DAART was examined among 82 PLWHA on methadone treatment for injecting-drug use. Clients received a dose of HAART on each morning they received methadone and took prepackaged doses with them for "off" days or evening use. At 1 year, 56% of DAART participants had an undetectable viral load, whereas only 32% in the methadone and non-DAART arms ($p = .009$) and 33% in the no-methadone arm ($p = .001$; Lucas et al., 2006) had such results. A randomized trial that compared (1) daily delivery of prepackaged medications with

extra doses for nondelivery times, (2) intensive adherence case management (weekly individual sessions for 6 months to overcome adherence barriers and self-administered HAART), and (3) standard of care (including quarterly case management visits) found no statistically significant differences in viral suppression or self-reported adherence at 6-month follow-up (Wohl et al., 2006).

Other potentially useful strategies to improve adherence are medication reminder devices such as beepers, pill boxes, and telephone calls. Supportive telephone calls to improve adherence rates in participants were tested in one study; although the intervention did not improve virologic outcomes, an increase in self-reported adherence was found (Collier et al., 2005). The use of a population already enrolled in a clinical trial may have blunted the intervention's potential effectiveness, since participants in clinical trials may be more likely to be adherent than others. Medication reminder devices need to be tailored to individuals and may be most helpful in people with memory impairment (Andrade et al., 2005).

Machtinger and Bangsberg (2007) have proposed a seven-step framework to support adherence, which includes (1) developing patient-centered relationships, (2) using motivational interviewing techniques, (3) addressing the known impediments to adherence, (4) screening regularly for poor adherence, (5) utilizing adherence aids, (6) expanding pharmacy services or directly observed therapy, and (7) creating an adherence program to formalize attention to this issue. Because it is clear that a single approach will not suit each PLWHA, strategies to match adherence interventions to the populations or individuals most likely to benefit from them are needed.

Conclusions and Future Directions

Maintaining health while living with HIV includes adhering to pharmacological treatment regimens, clinical and treatment appointments, and recommendations for safer sex and safer drug use practices. In this chapter, we focused on adherence to pharmacological treatment regimens, specifically HAART. Further research is needed to understand adherence among PLWHA, including adherence to pharmacological treatment regimens, clinical and treatment appointments, and recommendations for safer sex and safer drug use behaviors. Future research also must address a variety of important issues facing adherence, including (1) how to help patients decide when to initiate therapy (e.g., identifying when the patient is psychologically ready to commit to strictly adhering to a potentially lifelong regimen); (2) the rapidly advancing treatment options available to PLWHA and their providers; (3) the evolving technology that can be harnessed via monitoring devices or reminders; (4) the potential benefit of continual or ongoing adherence intervention over the traditional approach of a short-term or limited intervention for the promotion of long-term adherence; and (5) the changing face of HIV/AIDS. In the United States, the epidemic has become more rural and disproportionately affects those of lower social-economic status. Approaches must be developed, implemented, and tested to appropriately meet the needs of these populations. As the HIV/AIDS epidemic continues to evolve and change, adherence research has much to do in order to understand the challenges facing PLWHA, to develop accurate and meaningful measures of adherence, and to increase long-term adherence among PLWHA.

References

Adam, B. D., Maticka-Tyndale, E., & Cohen, J. J. (2003). Adherence practices among people living with HIV. *AIDS Care, 15*(2), 263–274.

Altice, F. L., Mostashari, F., & Friedland, G. H. (2001). Trust and the acceptance of and adherence to antiretroviral therapy. *Journal of Acquired Immune Deficiency Syndromes, 28*(1), 47–58.

Amico, K. R., Harman, J. J., & Johnson, B. T. (2006). Efficacy of antiretroviral therapy adherence interventions: A research synthesis of trials, 1996 to 2004. *Journal of Acquired Immune Deficiency Syndromes, 41*(3), 285–297.

Ammassari, A., Antinori, A., Aloisi, M. S., Trotta, M. P., Murri, R., Bartoli, L., et al. (2004). Depressive symptoms, neurocognitive impairment, and adherence to highly active antiretroviral therapy among HIV-infected persons. *Psychosomatics, 45*(5), 394–402.

Andrade, A. S., McGruder, H. F., Wu, A. W., Celano, S. A., Skolasky, R. L., Jr., Selnes, O. A., et al. (2005). A programmable prompting device improves adherence to highly active antiretroviral therapy in HIV-infected subjects with memory impairment. *Clinical Infectious Diseases, 41*(6), 875–882.

Arnsten, J. H., Demas, P. A., Grant, R. W., Gourevitch, M. N., Farzadegan, H., Howard, A. A., et al. (2002). Impact of active drug use on antiretroviral therapy adherence and viral suppression in HIV-infected drug users. *Journal of General Internal Medicine, 17*(5), 377–381.

Avants, S. K., Warburton, L. A., Hawkins, K. A., & Margolin, A. (2000). Continuation of high-risk behavior by HIV-positive drug users. Treatment implications. *Journal of Substance Abuse Treatment, 19*(1), 15–22.

Bangsberg, D. R., Acosta, E. P., Gupta, R., Guzman, D., Riley, E. D., Harrigan, P. R., et al. (2006). Adherence-resistance relationships for protease and non-nucleoside reverse transcriptase inhibitors explained by virological fitness. *AIDS, 20*(2), 223–231.

Battaglioli-Denero, A. M. (2007). Strategies for improving patient adherence to therapy and long-term patient outcomes. *Journal of the Association of Nurses in AIDS Care, 18*(1 Suppl.), S17–S22.

Beach, M. C., Keruly, J., & Moore, R. D. (2006). Is the quality of the patient-provider relationship associated with better adherence and health outcomes for patients with HIV? *Journal of General Internal Medicine, 21*(6), 661–665.

Becker, S. L., Dezii, C. M., Burtcel, B., Kawabata, H., & Hodder, S. (2002). Young HIV-infected adults are at greater risk for medication nonadherence. *Medscape General Medicine, 4*(3), 21.

Bing, E. G., Burnam, M. A., Longshore, D., Fleishman, J. A., Sherbourne, C. D., London, A. S., et al. (2001). Psychiatric disorders and drug use among human immunodeficiency virus-infected adults in the United States. *Archives of General Psychiatry, 58*(8), 721–728.

Bova, C. A., Fennie, K. P., Knafl, G. J., Dieckhaus, K. D., Watrous, E., & Williams, A. B. (2005). Use of electronic monitoring devices to measure antiretroviral adherence: Practical considerations. *AIDS and Behavior, 9*(1), 103–110.

Boyer, A., & Indyk, D. (2006). Shaping garments of care: Tools for maximizing adherence potential. *Social Work in Health Care, 42*(3–4), 151–166.

Catz, S. L., Kelly, J. A., Bogart, L. M., Benotsch, E. G., & McAuliffe, T. L. (2000). Patterns, correlates, and barriers to medication adherence among persons prescribed new treatments for HIV disease. *Health Psychology, 19*(2), 124–133.

Centers for Disease Control and Prevention. (1994). Birth outcomes following zidovudine therapy in pregnant women. *Journal of the American Medical Association, 272*(1), 17.

Centers for Disease Control and Prevention. (2006). Achievements in public health. Reduction in perinatal transmission of HIV infection—United States, 1985–2005. *Morbidity and Mortality Weekly Report, 55*(21), 592–597.

Chander, G., Himelhoch, S., & Moore, R. D. (2006). Substance abuse and psychiatric disorders in HIV-positive patients: Epidemiology and impact on antiretroviral therapy. *Drugs, 66*(6), 769–789.

Chesney, M. A., Ickovics, J. R., Chambers, D. B., Gifford, A. L., Neidig, J., Zwickl, B., et al. (2000). *Self-reported adherence to antiretroviral medications among participants in HIV clinical trials: The AACTG adherence instruments.* Patient Care Committee & Adherence Working Group of the Outcomes Committee of the Adult AIDS Clinical Trials Group (AACTG). *AIDS Care, 12*(3), 255–266.

Colfax, G., & Guzman, R. (2006). Club drugs and HIV infection: A review. *Clinical Infectious Diseases, 42*(10), 1463–1469.

Collier, A. C., Ribaudo, H., Mukherjee, A. L., Feinberg, J., Fischl, M. A., & Chesney, M. (2005). A randomized study of serial telephone call support to increase adherence and thereby improve virologic outcome in persons initiating antiretroviral therapy. *Journal of Infectious Diseases, 192*(8), 1398–1406.

Conanan, B., London, K., Martinez, L., Modersbach, D., O'Connell, J., O'Sullivan, M., et al. (2003). *Adapting your practice: Treatment and recommendations for homeless patients with HIV/AIDS*. Nashville, TN: Health Care for the Homeless Clinicians' Network, National Health Care for the Homeless Council.

Connor, E. M., Sperling, R. S., Gelber, R., Kiselev, P., Scott, G., O'Sullivan, M. J., et al. (1994). Reduction of maternal-infant transmission of human immunodeficiency virus type 1 with zidovudine treatment. Pediatric AIDS Clinical Trials Group Protocol 076 Study Group. *New England Journal of Medicine, 331*(18), 1173–1180.

Crum, N. F., Riffenburgh, R. H., Wegner, S., Agan, B. K., Tasker, S. A., Spooner, K. M., et al. (2006). Comparisons of causes of death and mortality rates among HIV-infected persons: Analysis of the pre-, early, and late HAART (highly active antiretroviral therapy) eras. *Journal of Acquired Immune Deficiency Syndromes, 41*(2), 194–200.

Deloria-Knoll, M., Chmiel, J. S., Moorman, A. C., Wood, K. C., Holmberg, S. D., & Palella, F. J. (2004). Factors related to and consequences of adherence to antiretroviral therapy in an ambulatory HIV-infected patient cohort. *AIDS Patient Care and STDs, 18*(12), 721–727.

Desai, N., & Mathur, M. (2003). Selective transmission of multidrug resistant HIV to a newborn related to poor maternal adherence. *Sexually Transmitted Infections, 79*(5), 419–421.

Desclaux, A. (2003). Equity in access to aids treatment in Africa: Pitfalls in achievements. In A. Castro & M. Singer (Eds.), *Unhealthy health policy: A critical anthropological examination*. Walnut Creek, CA: AltaMira.

DeWit, D. J., Offord, D. R., & Wong, M. (1997). Patterns of onset and cessation of drug use over the early part of the life course. *Health Education and Behavior, 24*(6), 746–758.

Ellerbrock, T. V., Chamblee, S., Bush, T. J., Johnson, J. W., Marsh, B. J., Lowell, P., et al. (2004). Human immunodeficiency virus infection in a rural community in the United States. *American Journal of Epidemiology, 160*(6), 582–588.

Elliott, A. J., Russo, J., & Roy-Byrne, P. P. (2002). The effect of changes in depression on health related quality of life (HRQOL) in HIV infection. *General Hospital Psychiatry, 24*(1), 43–47.

El-Sadr, W. M., Lundgren, J. D., Neaton, J. D., Gordin, F., Abrams, D., Arduino, R. C., et al. (2006). Cd4+ count-guided interruption of antiretroviral treatment. *New England Journal of Medicine, 355*(22), 2283–2296.

Fogarty, L., Roter, D., Larson, S., Burke, J., Gillespie, J., & Levy, R. (2002). Patient adherence to HIV medication regimens: A review of published and abstract reports. *Patient Education and Counseling, 46*(2), 93–108.

Friedland, G. H., & Williams, A. (1999). Attaining higher goals in HIV treatment: The central importance of adherence. *AIDS, 13*(Suppl.1), S61–S72.

Furber, A. S., Hodgson, I. J., Desclaux, A., & Mukasa, D. S. (2004). Barriers to better care for people with AIDS in developing countries. *British Medical Journal, 329*(7477), 1281–1283.

Golin, C. E., Liu, H., Hays, R. D., Miller, L. G., Beck, C. K., Ickovics, J., et al. (2002). A prospective study of predictors of adherence to combination antiretroviral medication. *Journal of General Internal Medicine, 17*(10), 756–765.

Gordon, C. M. (2006). Commentary on meta-analysis of randomized controlled trials for HIV treatment adherence interventions. Research directions and implications for practice. *Journal of Acquired Immune Deficiency Syndromes, 43*(Suppl.1), S36–S40.

Gross, R., Yip, B., Re, V. L., III, Wood, E., Alexander, C. S., Harrigan, P. R., et al. (2006). A simple, dynamic measure of antiretroviral therapy adherence predicts failure to maintain HIV-1 suppression. *Journal of Infectious Diseases, 194*(8), 1108–1114.

Hawkins, T. (2006). Appearance-related side effects of HIV-1 treatment. *AIDS Patient Care and STDs, 20*(1), 6–18.

Hecht, F. M., Grant, R. M., Petropoulos, C. J., Dillon, B., Chesney, M. A., Tian, H., et al. (1998). Sexual transmission of an HIV-1 variant resistant to multiple reverse-transcriptase and protease inhibitors. *New England Journal of Medicine, 339*(5), 307–311.

Heckman, B. D., Catz, S. L., Heckman, T. G., Miller, J. G., & Kalichman, S. C. (2004). Adherence to antiretroviral therapy in rural persons living with HIV disease in the United States. *AIDS Care, 16*(2), 219–230.

Hergenrather, K. C., Rhodes, S. D., & Clark, G. (2004). Employment-seeking behavior of persons with HIV/AIDS: A theory-based approach. *Journal of Rehabilitation, 70*(4), 21–30.

Hergenrather, K. C., Rhodes, S. D., & Clark, G. (2006). Windows to work: Exploring employment-seeking behaviors of persons with HIV/AIDS through photovoice. *AIDS Education and Prevention, 18*(3), 243–258.

Hill, Z., Kendall, C., & Fernandez, M. (2003). Patterns of adherence to antiretrovirals: Why adherence has no simple measure. *AIDS Patient Care and STDs, 17*(10), 519–525.

Hinkin, C. H., Barclay, T. R., Castellon, S. A., Levine, A. J., Durvasula, R. S., Marion, S. D., et al. (2007). Drug use and medication adherence among HIV-1 infected individuals. *AIDS and Behavior, 11*(2), 185–194.

Institute of Medicine. (2003). *Unequal treatment: Confronting racial and ethnic disparities in health care.* Washington, DC: National Academy Press.

Kelly, J. A., Murphy, D. A., Bahr, G. R., Koob, J. J., Morgan, M. G., Kalichman, S. C., et al. (1993). Factors associated with severity of depression and high-risk sexual behavior among persons diagnosed with human immunodeficiency virus (HIV) infection. *Health Psychology, 12*(3), 215–219.

King, M. S., Brun, S. C., & Kempf, D. J. (2005). Relationship between adherence and the development of resistance in antiretroviral-naive, HIV-1-infected patients receiving lopinavir/ritonavir or nelfinavir. *Journal of Infectious Diseases, 191*(12), 2046–2052.

Kleeberger, C. A., Phair, J. P., Strathdee, S. A., Detels, R., Kingsley, L., & Jacobson, L. P. (2001). Determinants of heterogeneous adherence to HIV-antiretroviral therapies in the multicenter AIDS cohort study. *Journal of Acquired Immune Deficiency Syndromes, 26*(1), 82–92.

Klitzman, R. L., & Greenberg, J. D. (2002). Patterns of communication between gay and lesbian patients and their health care providers. *Journal of Homosexuality, 42*(4), 65–75.

Koenig, L. J., & Bachanas, P. J. (2006). Adherence to medications for HIV: Teens say, "too many, too big, too often." In M. E. Lyon & L. J. D'Angelo (Eds.), *Teenagers, HIV, and AIDS: Insights from youths living with the virus* (pp. 45–65). Westport, CT: Praeger.

Kushel, M. B., Colfax, G., Ragland, K., Heineman, A., Palacio, H., & Bangsberg, D. R. (2006). Case management is associated with improved antiretroviral adherence and cd4+ cell counts in homeless and marginally housed individuals with HIV infection. *Clinical Infectious Diseases, 43*(2), 234–242.

Lucas, G. M., Mullen, B. A., Weidle, P. J., Hader, S., McCaul, M. E., & Moore, R. D. (2006). Directly administered antiretroviral therapy in methadone clinics is associated with improved HIV treatment outcomes, compared with outcomes among concurrent comparison groups. *Clinical Infectious Diseases, 42*(11), 1628–1635.

Machtinger, E. L., & Bangsberg, D. R. (2007). Seven steps to better adherence: A practical approach to promoting adherence to antiretroviral therapy. *AIDS Reader, 17*(1), 43–51.

Madru, N. (2003). Stigma and HIV: Does the social response affect the natural course of the epidemic? *Journal of the Association of Nurses in AIDS Care, 14*(5), 39–48.

Maggiolo, F., Ravasio, L., Ripamonti, D., Gregis, G., Quinzan, G., Arici, C., et al. (2005). Similar adherence rates favor different virologic outcomes for patients treated with nonnucleoside analogues or protease inhibitors. *Clinical Infectious Diseases, 40*(1), 158–163.

Markowitz, J. C., Kocsis, J. H., Fishman, B., Spielman, L. A., Jacobsberg, L. B., Frances, A. J., et al. (1998). Treatment of depressive symptoms in human immunodeficiency virus-positive patients. *Archives of General Psychiatry, 55*(5), 452–457.

McKinney, M. M. (2002). Variations in rural aids epidemiology and service delivery models in the United States. *Journal of Rural Health, 18*(3), 455–466.

McNabb, J., Ross, J. W., Abriola, K., Turley, C., Nightingale, C. H., & Nicolau, D. P. (2001). Adherence to highly active antiretroviral therapy predicts virologic outcome at an inner-city human immunodeficiency virus clinic. *Clinical Infectious Diseases, 33,* 700–705.

Meystre-Agustoni, G., Dubois-Arber, F., Cochand, P., & Telenti, A. (2000). Antiretroviral therapies from the patient's perspective. *AIDS Care, 12*(6), 717–721.

Mitty, J. A., Macalino, G., Taylor, L., Harwell, J. I., & Flanigan, T. P. (2003). Directly observed therapy (DOT) for individuals with HIV: Successes and challenges. *Medscape General Medicine, 5*(1), 30.

Nieuwkerk, P., Gisolf, E., Sprangers, M., & Danner, S. (2001). Adherence over 48 weeks in an antiretroviral clinical trial: Variable within patients, affected by toxicities and independently predictive of virological response. *Antiviral Therapy, 6*(2), 97–103.

Palella, F. J., Jr., Delaney, K. M., Moorman, A. C., Loveless, M. O., Fuhrer, J., Satten, G. A., et al. (1998). Declining morbidity and mortality among patients with advanced human immunodeficiency virus infection. HIV outpatient study investigators. *New England Journal of Medicine, 338*(13), 853–860.

Parker, R., & Aggleton, P. (2003). HIV and AIDS-related stigma and discrimination: A conceptual framework and implications for action. *Social Science and Medicine, 57*(1), 13–24.

Parsons, G. N., Siberry, G. K., Parsons, J. K., Christensen, J. R., Joyner, M. L., Lee, S. L., et al. (2006). Multidisciplinary, inpatient directly observed therapy for hiv-1-infected children and adolescents failing HAART: A retrospective study. *AIDS Patient Care STDs, 20*(4), 275–284.

Paterson, D. L., Swindells, S., Mohr, J., Brester, M., Vergis, E. N., Squier, C., et al. (2000). Adherence to protease inhibitor therapy and outcomes in patients with HIV infection. *Annals of Internal Medicine, 133*(1), 21–30.

Perelson, A. S., Essunger, P., Cao, Y., Vesanen, M., Hurley, A., Saksela, K., et al. (1997). Decay characteristics of HIV-1-infected compartments during combination therapy rapid turnover of plasma virions and cd4 lymphocytes in hiv-1 infection. *Nature, 387*(6629), 188–191.

Perinatal HIV Guidelines Working Group. (2002). Public health service task force recommendations for use of antiretroviral drugs in pregnant hiv-1 infected women for maternal health and interventions to reduce perinatal HIV-1 transmission in the United States. *MMWR, 51*(18), 1–38.

Power, R., Koopman, C., Volk, J., Israelski, D. M., Stone, L., Chesney, M. A., et al. (2003). Social support, substance use, and denial in relationship to antiretroviral treatment adherence among HIV-infected persons. *AIDS Patient Care and STDs, 17*(5), 245–252.

Rao, D., Kekwaletswe, T. C., Hosek, S., Martinez, J., & Rodriguez, F. (2007). Stigma and social barriers to medication adherence with urban youth living with HIV. *AIDS Care, 19*(1), 28–33.

Resnick, M. D., Harris, L. J., & Blum, R. W. (1993). The impact of caring and connectedness on adolescent health and well-being. *Journal of Paediatric and Child Health, 29*(Suppl. 1), S3–9.

Rhodes, S. D., & Benfield, D. (2006). Community-based participatory research: An introduction for the clinician researcher. In J. D. Blessing (Ed.), *Physician assistant's guide to research and medical literature* (2nd ed., pp. 105–118). Philadelphia: F. A. Davis.

Rhodes, S. D., & Hergenrather, K. C. (2002). Exploring hepatitis b vaccination acceptance among young men who have sex with men: Facilitators and barriers. *Preventive Medicine, 35*(2), 128–134.

Rhodes, S. D., Hergenrather, K. C., Wilkin, A., Alegria-Ortega, J., & Montaño, J. (2006). Preventing HIV infection among young immigrant Latino men: Results from focus groups using community-based participatory research. *Journal of the National Medical Association, 98*(4), 564–573.

Rhodes, S. D., McCoy, T., Hergenrather, K. C., Omli, M. R., & DuRant, R. H. (2007). Exploring the health behavior disparities of gay men in the United States: Comparing gay male university students to their heterosexual peers. *Journal of LGBT Health Research, 3*(1), 15–23.

Rhodes, S. D., & Yee, L. J. (2006). Public health and gay and bisexual men: A primer for practitioners, clinicians, and researchers. In M. Shankle (Ed.), *The handbook of lesbian, gay, bisexual, and transgender public health: A practitioner's guide to service* (pp. 119–143). Binghamton, NY: Haworth.

Rhodes, S. D., & Yee, L. J. (2007). Using hepatitis A and B vaccination as a paradigm for effective HIV vaccine delivery. *Sexual Health, 4*(2), 121–127.

Rhodes, S. D., Yee, L. J., & Hergenrather, K. C. (2006). A community-based rapid assessment of HIV behavioural risk disparities within a large sample of gay men in southeastern USA: A comparison of African American, Latino and white men. *AIDS Care, 18*(8), 1018–1024.

Santos, C. Q., Adeyemi, O., & Tenorio, A. R. (2006). Attitudes toward directly administered antiretroviral therapy (DAART) among HIV-positive inpatients in an inner city public hospital. *AIDS Care, 18*(7), 808–811.

Schackman, B. R., Gebo, K. A., Walensky, R. P., Losina, E., Muccio, T., Sax, P. E., et al. (2006). The lifetime cost of current human immunodeficiency virus care in the United States. *Medical Care, 44*(11), 990–997.

Schneider, J., Kaplan, S. H., Greenfield, S., Li, W., & Wilson, I. B. (2004). Better physician-patient relationships are associated with higher reported adherence to antiretroviral therapy in patients with HIV infection. *Journal of General Internal Medicine, 19*(11), 1096–1103.

Shapiro, M. F., Morton, S. C., McCaffrey, D. F., Senterfitt, J. W., Fleishman, J. A., Perlman, J. F., et al. (1999). Variations in the care of HIV-infected adults in the United States: Results from the HIV cost and services utilization study. *Journal of the American Medical Association, 281*(24), 2305–2315.

Sharpe, T. T., Lee, L. M., Nakashima, A. K., Elam-Evans, L. D., & Fleming, P. L. (2004). Crack cocaine use and adherence to antiretroviral treatment among HIV-infected Black women. *Journal of Community Health, 29*(2), 117–127.

Sherbourne, C. D., Hays, R. D., Fleishman, J. A., Vitiello, B., Magruder, K. M., Bing, E. G., et al. (2000). Impact of psychiatric conditions on health-related quality of life in persons with HIV infection. *American Journal of Psychiatry, 157*(2), 248–254.

Siegel, K., & Gorey, E. (1997). HIV-infected women: Barriers to AZT use. *Social Science and Medicine, 45*(1), 15–22.

Siegel, K., Lekas, H. M., Schrimshaw, E. W., & Johnson, J. K. (2001). Factors associated with HIV-infected women's use or intention to use AZT during pregnancy. *AIDS Education and Prevention, 13*(3), 189–206.

Simoni, J. M., Pearson, C. R., Pantalone, D. W., Marks, G., & Crepaz, N. (2006). Efficacy of interventions in improving highly active antiretroviral therapy adherence and HIV-1 RNA viral load: A meta-analytic review of randomized controlled trials. *Journal of Acquired Immune Deficiency Syndrome, 43*(Suppl.1), S23–S35.

Singh, N., Squier, C., Sivek, C., Wagener, M., Nguyen, M. H., & Yu, V. L. (1996). Determinants of compliance with antiretroviral therapy in patients with human immunodeficiency virus: Prospective assessment with implications for enhancing compliance. *AIDS Care, 8*(3), 261–269.

Siu, S. S., Yeung, J. H., Pang, M. W., Chiu, P. Y., & Lau, T. K. (2005). Placental transfer of zidovudine in first trimester of pregnancy. *Obstetrics and Gynecology, 106*(4), 824–827.

Smith, B. D., DeWeaver, K. L., & Reece, M. (2006). A comparison study of homeless and non-homeless HIV-positive persons enrolled in mental health care. *Journal of HIV/AIDS & Social Services, 5*(1), 5–20.

Sowell, R. L., Murdaugh, C. L., Addy, C. L., Moneyham, L., & Tavokoli, A. (2002). Factors influencing intent to get pregnant in HIV-infected women living in the southern USA. *AIDS Care, 14*(2), 181–191.

Sowell, R. L., Phillips, K. D., Seals, B. F., Misener, T. R., & Rush, C. (2001). HIV-infected women's experiences and beliefs related to AZT therapy during pregnancy. *AIDS Patient Care and STDs, 15*(4), 201–209.

Spacek, L. A., Shihab, H. M., Kamya, M. R., Mwesigire, D., Ronald, A., Mayanja, H., et al. (2006). Response to antiretroviral therapy in HIV-infected patients attending a public, urban clinic in Kampala, Uganda. *Clinical Infectious Diseases, 42*(2), 252–259.

Stanley, L. D. (1999). Transforming AIDS: The moral management of stigmatized identity. *Anthropology & Medicine, 6*, 103–120.

Steele, R. G., Nelson, T. D., & Cole, B. P. (2007). Psychosocial functioning of children with AIDS and HIV infection: Review of the literature from a socioecological framework. *Journal of Developmental and Behavioral Pediatrics, 28*(1), 58–69.

Tommasello, A. C., Gillis, L. M., Lawler, J. T., & Bujak, G. J. (2006). Characteristics of homeless HIV-positive outreach responders in urban U.S. and their success in primary care treatment. *AIDS Care, 18*(8), 911–917.

Wagner, G. J., Kanouse, D. E., Golinelli, D., Miller, L. G., Daar, E. S., Witt, M. D., et al. (2006). Cognitive-behavioral intervention to enhance adherence to antiretroviral therapy: A randomized controlled trial (CCTG 578). *AIDS, 20*(9), 1295–1302.

Willenbring, M. L. (2005). Integrating care for patients with infectious, psychiatric, and substance use disorders: Concepts and approaches. *AIDS, 19*(Suppl. 3), S227–S237.

Willging, C. E., Salvador, M., & Kano, M. (2006). Brief reports: Unequal treatment: Mental health care for sexual and gender minority groups in a rural state. *Psychiatric Services, 57*(6), 867–870.

Wohl, A. R., Garland, W. H., Squires, K., Witt, M., Larsen, R., Kovacs, A., et al. (2004). The feasibility of a community-based directly administered antiretroviral therapy program. *Clinical Infectious Diseases, 38* (Suppl 5), S388–S392.

Wohl, A. R., Garland, W. H., Valencia, R., Squires, K., Witt, M. D., Kovacs, A., et al. (2006). A randomized trial of directly administered antiretroviral therapy and adherence case management intervention. *Clinical Infectious Diseases, 42*(11), 1619–1627.

Lifestyle Change and Adherence Issues Among Patients With Heart Disease

34

Laura L. Hayman

Atherosclerotic cardiovascular disease (CVD) is a major cause of morbidity and premature mortality in women and men in the United States, as well as most of the rest of the developed world, and many developing countries (Rosamond et al., 2007). Accumulated data indicate that atherosclerotic-CVD processes begin early in life and are influenced over time by the interaction of genetic and behavioral factors and environmental exposures. Within the multidisciplinary community of cardiovascular health care professionals, these data have placed emphasis on a life course approach to prevention of CVD with individual and public health efforts beginning early in life (Hayman & Hughes, 2006; Hayman et al., 2007). Similarly, extensive evidence amassed over the past four decades points to established, potentially modifiable risk factors and unhealthy lifestyle behaviors as important determinants of cardiovascular morbidity and mortality. Central to both prevention and management of CVD are healthy lifestyle behaviors and adherence to therapeutic regimens that emphasize lifestyle change.

This chapter provides an overview of evidence supporting the need for prevention and management of CVD, presents key elements of science-based guidelines and recommendations for lifestyle change for individuals with documented atherosclerotic CVD, and includes strategies to promote adherence that are applicable across health care and community settings. Implications for clinical and public health practice and future research are integrated throughout the chapter and included in the summary.

The Need for Prevention and Management of CVD

In the United States and globally, atherosclerotic cardiovascular conditions, particularly coronary heart disease (CHD) and cerebrovascular disease (i.e., stroke), are leading causes of disability and premature death (Rosamond et al., 2007). In every year since 1900 (except 1918), CVD accounted for more deaths than any other single cause or group of causes of death in the United States. If all forms of CVD were eliminated, life expectancy would increase by approximately 7 years (Rosamond et al., 2007). CVD risk reduction and evidence-based medical therapies play a critically important role in reducing the age-adjusted mortality due to CHD (Ford et al., 2007). Specifically, Ford and colleagues (2007) applied an updated version of the IMPACT mortality model to data for the years 1980–2000 on the use and effectiveness of specific cardiac treatments and changes in risk factors among U.S. adults 25 to 84 years of age. The IMPACT model incorporates major potentially modifiable risk factors for CHD, including smoking, high blood pressure, elevated total cholesterol, obesity, diabetes, and physical inactivity, as well as standard medical and surgical treatments for CHD. Results indicated that approximately half the decline in U.S. deaths from CHD in the period studied may be attributable to reductions in major risk factors, and approximately half is due to evidence-based medical therapies. These results are consistent with earlier U.S. and international studies and underscore the importance of potentially modifiable risk factors and behaviors in preventing mortality from CHD.

The results of the INTERHEART study, a case-control study conducted in 52 countries and designed to examine the effect of CVD risk factors and unhealthy lifestyle behaviors on incident CHD, indicated that nine potentially modifiable risk factors accounted for 90% of the population-attributable risk for incident CHD in men and 94% in women (Yusuf et al., 2004). In part on the basis of these findings, the World Heart Foundation (WHF), the American Heart Association (AHA), and the World Health Organization (WHO) issued a collaborative statement advocating that each country develop and implement plans for prevention and management of CVD, including primary prevention beginning early in life (Smith et al., 2004). In addition to targeting behavioral and lifestyle risk factors for intervention, the recommendations also emphasized the importance of addressing specific cultural, social, and environmental determinants of CVD (Smith et al., 2004).

Disparities in Prevention and Management of CVD

While substantial progress has been made in reducing CHD mortality in the United States over the past three decades, disparities remain pervasive (Bonow, Grant, & Jacobs, 2005; Davis, Vinci, Okwuosa, Chase, & Huang, 2007; Jones, 2007; Mensah, Mokdad, Ford, Greenlund, & Croft, 2005). Many population subgroups defined by race, ethnicity, gender, socioeconomic status, educational level, and/ or geography demonstrate an excess burden of CHD and its attendant risk factors (Bonow et al., 2005; Davis et al., 2007; Mensah, 2005). Several national population-based surveys indicate that substantial disparities exist in risk factor prevalence, indices of mortality, and overall quality of life among U.S. adults 18 years of age and older (Mensah, 2005). Specifically, in men, the highest prevalence of obesity (29.2%) was observed in Mexican Americans who had completed a high school education. Independent of educational status, Black women had a high prevalence of obesity (47.3%). Hypertension prevalence was highest among Blacks (39.8%), regardless of gender or educational status. A major independent risk factor for CVD, hypertension has earlier onset, is more difficult to control, and is associated with more end-organ damage among Blacks than among other racial and ethnic groups (Davis et al., 2007).

Consistent with earlier studies, Mensah (2005) and colleagues also documented inverse associations among education, income and poverty status, and ischemic heart disease (CHD) and stroke. Among Medicare enrollees, rates of hospitalization for congestive heart failure hospitalization were higher among Blacks, Hispanics, and American Indian/Alaska Natives than among Whites; stroke hospitalization was highest in Blacks. Hospitalizations for Chronic Heart Failure (CHF) and stroke were highest in the southeastern United States. Finally, Blacks had higher death rates for diseases of the heart at all ages than did Whites (Mensah, 2005).

Intra-individual clustering of CVD risk factors and adverse health behaviors is well documented and known to accelerate atherogenic processes (Grundy et al., 2005; Gustat, Srinivasan, Elkasabany, & Berenson, 2002; Park, Zhu, Palaniappan, Heshka, Carnethon, & Heymsfield, 2003). More recently, attention has focused on racial, ethnic, gender, and geographic differences in multiple-risk-factor clustering (Davis, 2007; Jones, 2007; Mensah, 2005). Similarly, social-ecological determinants of disparities in multiple-risk-factor clustering and comorbid behaviors have emerged as important areas of transdisciplinary inquiry. While more research is needed to guide and inform evidence-based guidelines for prevention and management of CVD, accumulated results support the need for both clinical and public health efforts that target multiple risk factors and comorbid behaviors and that tailor strategies to individuals and families from minority populations.

Evidence-Based Guidelines for Prevention and Management of CVD: Emphasis on Lifestyle Modification

Numerous clinical trials have prompted and informed practice guidelines for primary and secondary prevention of CVD. In this chapter we emphasize recent recommendations for lifestyle change for individuals with documented athero-sclerotic–CVD, also referred to as secondary prevention. It is noteworthy, how-ever, that heart-healthy behaviors, including patterns of dietary intake, physical activity and smoke-free lifestyles and environments and therapeutic lifestyle change (TLC), are the cornerstone of evidence-based primary and secondary-prevention guidelines, respectively (Kavey et al., 2003; Mosca et al., 2007; Pearson, Blair, Daniels, et al., 2002; Smith et al., 2006).

During the past two decades, practice guidelines for secondary preven-tion of CVD have been issued and updated periodically with recommenda-tions based on evidence generated primarily from clinical trials and systematic meta-analyses. The AHA, in collaboration with the American College of Cardi-ology (ACC) and with the endorsement of the National Heart, Lung, and Blood Institute (NHLBI), recently revised secondary-prevention guidelines classify intervention recommendations on the basis of level of evidence (Smith et al., 2006). Targets for intervention include smoking, blood pressure control, lipid management, physical activity, and weight and diabetes management (Smith et al., 2006). The recent AHA/ACC guidelines (Smith et al., 2006) support and broaden aggressive risk-reduction therapies for individuals with established coronary, and other atherosclerotic vascular disease, including peripheral arte-rial disease, carotid artery disease, and atherosclerotic aortic disease. Indeed, a growing body of evidence confirms that aggressive comprehensive risk-factor management improves survival, reduces recurrent events and the need for in-terventional procedures, and improves quality of life for individuals with estab-lished heart disease (Smith et al., 2006).

The specific pharmacotherapeutic recommendations for secondary pre-vention of CVD are beyond the purpose and scope of this chapter and have been published elsewhere (Braun & Hughes, 2007; Artinian, Yucha, & Dungan, 2007). Lifestyle modification, however, remains a central component of second-ary prevention and is viewed as essential for achieving treatment goals and preventing recurrent events. Importantly, these lifestyle change recommen-dations are consistent with those of the AHA/American Association of Car-diovascular and Pulmonary Rehabilitation (AACVPR), which emphasize that all cardiac rehabilitation and secondary-prevention programs consist of core components that aim to optimize cardiovascular risk reduction, foster healthy behaviors and compliance with these behaviors, reduce disability, and promote an active lifestyle for patients with cardiovascular disease (Balady et al., 2007). They also emphasize theory-based principles of behavior change and patient counseling and encourage clinicians to evaluate and manage psychological fac-tors (i.e., depression, anxiety, anger and hostility, social isolation, marital and family distress, sexual dysfunction and adjustment, and substance use) as part of CVD risk-factor management for individuals with documented CVD. Strate-gies suggested for increasing adherence to lifestyle change are discussed in this chapter and included in Table 34.1.

Adherence Issues Among Patients With CVD

The central and essential role of adherence to lifestyle modification and medication recommendations in preventing recurrent events in patients

34.1 Actions to Increase Adherence to Treatment Recommendations

Actions by patients	Specific strategies
Patients must engage in essential treatment behaviors	
▪ Decide to control risk factors and modify adverse health behaviors ▪ Negotiate goals with provider ▪ Develop skills for adopting and maintaining recommended behaviors ▪ Monitor progress toward goals ▪ Resolve problems that block achievement of goals	▪ Understand rationale, importance of commitment ▪ Develop communication skills ▪ Use reminder systems ▪ Use self-monitoring skills ▪ Develop problem solving skills, use social support networks
Patients must communicate with providers about treatment services	
	▪ Define own needs and preferences on basis of experience ▪ Validate rationale for continuing to follow recommendations

Actions by providers	Specific strategies
Providers must foster effective communication with patients	
▪ Provide clear, direct messages about importance of behavioral change and/or pharmacotherapy ▪ Include patterns in decisions about treatment goals and related strategies ▪ Incorporate evidence-based behavioral strategies into counseling	▪ Assess patient's health literacy; tailor communication accordingly ▪ Provide instruction in multiple modes including verbal and written rationale for treatments ▪ Develop skills in communicating/counseling ▪ Use tailoring and contracting strategies ▪ Negotiate goals and plan for treatment ▪ Anticipate barriers to adherence and discuss solutions ▪ Use active listening ▪ Develop multicomponent strategies (i.e., cognitive and behavioral) ▪ Determine methods of evaluating outcomes ▪ Use self-report or electronic data ▪ Use telephone and other forms of follow-up including e-health technologies
Providers must document and respond to patients' progress towards goals ▪ Create and maintain an evidence-based practice ▪ Assess patient's adherence at each visit and in telephone follow-up ▪ Develop reminder systems to ensure identification and follow-up of patient status	

34.1 Actions to Increase Adherence to Treatment Recommendations *(Continued)*	
Actions by health care organizations	**Specific strategies**
Health care organizations must ▪ Develop an environment that supports both prevention and treatment interventions with integrated systems of care ▪ Provide tracking and reporting systems ▪ Provide training and education for providers ▪ Provide adequate reimbursement for allocation of time for all health care professionals Health care organizations must develop and implement integrated systems of care including core components of the Chronic Care Model to improve adherence and health outcomes in patients with CVD	▪ Develop and implement training in behavioral science and multidisciplinary models of health care delivery ▪ Use preappointment reminders ▪ Use telephone follow-up ▪ Schedule flexible office hours ▪ Provide group/individual counseling for patients and families ▪ Develop computer-based programs (electronic medical records) ▪ Require continuing education courses in communication and behavioral counseling ▪ Develop and implement incentives tied to desired patient and provider outcomes ▪ Incorporate multidisciplinary models of care including nursing case management ▪ Implement pharmacy patient profile and recall review systems ▪ Use electronic transmission storage of patient's self-monitored data ▪ Obtain patient data on lifestyle behavior before visit ▪ Provide continuous quality improvement training

Adapted from Miller, Hill, Kottke, and Ockene (1997) and Ockene, Hayman, Pasternak, Shron, E., & Dunbar-Jacob (2002).

with documented CVD is well established. Consistent with social-ecological models of health, optimal strategies for increasing adherence to preventive and therapeutic regimens consider individual (patient-level), provider, and health care system factors (Miller, Hill, Kottke, & Ockene, 1997; Ockene, Hayman, Pasternak, Schron, & Dunbar-Jacob, 2002).

Individual Factors That Affect Adherence in Patients With CVD

Substantial research attention has focused on individual, patient-level factors and adherence behaviors in both the prevention and the management of

CVD. Systematic reviews of the literature (Burke, Dunbar-Jacob, & Hill, 1997; Dunbar-Jacob, Schlenk, Burke, & Matthews, 1998; Ockene et al., 2002) and evidence-based statements (Miller et al., 1997) point to the importance of considering psychological, cognitive, motivational, somatic, and behavioral factors as individual-level targets for increasing adherence. Research on these patient-level factors, however, has not yielded consistent results across studies.

Depression and depressive symptoms are common in patients recovering from cardiac events (such as acute myocardial infarction) and following interventional procedures such as coronary artery bypass surgery (Ariyo, Haan, & Tangen, 2000; Burg, Benedetto, & Soufer, 2003). Major depression has been observed to develop in 20% of post myocardial infarction patients; approximately 33% of patients have clinically significant symptoms of depression (Ziegelstein, 2001). While some earlier studies did not observe associations between negative affective states and adherence behaviors (Emery, Hauck, & Blumenthal, 1992; Graveley & Oseasohn, 1991; Nelson, Stason, Neutra, Solomon, & McArdle, 1978), others and more recent studies (DiMatteo, Lepper, & Croghn, 2000; Ziegelstein, 2001) suggest that depression and depressive symptoms have a detrimental effect on adherence to recommendations for post-myocardial infarction therapy, including completion rates, and clinical outcomes in cardiac rehabilitation (Caulin-Glaser, Maciejewski, Snow, LaLonde, & Mazure, 2007). In addition, depression has been associated with self-report of medication nonadherence in an outpatient population of patients with documented CHD (Gehi, Haas, Pipkin & Whooley, 2005). Depressive symptoms have also been observed to predict medication nonadherence in heart failure patients (Morgan et al., 2006) and other documented cardiovascular conditions (Bane, Hughes, & McElnay, 2006). The relationship of depression to health outcomes in patients with established CVD, particularly CHD, has been investigated extensively. Recent meta-analyses indicate that there are positive associations between depression and/or depressive symptoms and adverse health outcomes in post-myocardial infarction patients (Barth, Schumacher, & Herrmann-Lingen, 2004; vanMelle, de Jonge, & Spijkerman, 2004) and implicate biobehavioral and biological mechanisms as possible links. As noted earlier, because of the evidence base in this area, depression is included in current practice guidelines as an important target for assessment and management in patients with CVD.

Cognitive variables, including attitudes regarding therapeutic regimens (Fitzgerald & Phillipov, 2000; Frank, 1997) and self-efficacy (the extent to which an individual believes he can change a behavior), have been associated with adherence to a number of CVD-related health behaviors (Burke et al., 1997; Burns & Evon, 2007; Cheng & Boey, 2002; Ewart, Taylor, Reese, & DeBusk, 1983; King, 2001). Because of the extensive database linking self-efficacy and adherence behaviors relevant to CVD, self-efficacy is emphasized in current guidelines as an important target for assessment and intervention.

More recently, attention has focused on health literacy, the knowledge and fundamental ability to manage illness as well as to navigate the health care system (Baker, Wolf, Feinglass, & Thompson, 2008). A study of 3,260 Medicare managed-care enrollees followed for an average of 67.8 months indicated that poor health literacy in elder adults (≥65 years of age) predicts all-cause and cardiovascular mortality (Baker et al., 2008). Specifically, hazard ratios (adjusted for demographic factors, socioeconomic status, and baseline health) for all-cause mortality were 1.52 (95% CI: 1.26–1.83) for participants with inadequate health literacy and 1.13 (95% CI: 0.90–1.41) for participants with marginal health literacy (Baker, 2007). In addition, risk-adjusted rates of cardiovascular death were higher in participants with inadequate health literacy.

The authors suggest several plausible mechanisms to explain the higher mortality in patients with inadequate health literacy, including less knowledge regarding CVD and poor self-management skills for hypertension, diabetes, and heart failure. While this prospective cohort study did not directly measure adherence behaviors and had some methodological limitations, including a failure to measure confounding variables (i.e., cognitive function), the results point to the need for attention to health literacy in teaching, counseling, and managing chronic disease in patients with CVD.

Health literacy is just emerging as a major patient-level determinant of adherence behaviors, with some research demonstrating an association between inadequate health literacy and low medication-refill adherence in CVD patients (Gazmararian et al., 2006). Considering the complexity of therapeutic regimens for patients with multiple risk factors and CVD, health literacy is an important area of inquiry. Data are lacking, however, on effective interventions for improving adherence to recommendations regarding lifestyle and medication in CVD patients with low health literacy.

Provider Factors That Affect Adherence in Patients With CVD

Substantial evidence indicates that provider interventions have a significant effect on patients' adherence to lifestyle changes in CVD-related health behaviors, including patterns of smoking behavior, alcohol use, and dietary intake (Burke et al., 2001; Fiore, Bailey, & Cohen, 1996; Ockene, Adams, Turley, Wheeler, & Herbert, 1999). Research has demonstrated that brief provider interventions positively influence both initiation and maintenance of such behavior change (Ockene et al., 1999). Unfortunately, as documented in several studies, physician/provider adherence to evidence-based recommendations, including screening for CVD risk factors and behaviors and counseling regarding behavioral change strategies, is much less than optimal (Kim, Hofer, & Kerr, 2003; Pearson et al., 2000; Sueta et al., 1999). A recent online study of 500 randomly selected physicians, including 300 primary-care physicians, 100 obstetricians/gynecologists, and 100 cardiologists, supports the need for educational interventions designed to increase awareness and adoption of CVD prevention guidelines among health care providers (Mosca et al., 2005). Specifically, this experimental case study tested physician accuracy in assessing CVD risk level of high-, intermediate-, and low-risk patients according to evidence-based guidelines. As assessed by the Framingham risk score, all physician groups were likely to assign intermediate-risk women to a low-risk category. It is noteworthy that assignment of risk level significantly predicted recommendations for lifestyle interventions and pharmacotherapy. Importantly, and consistent with results of other studies, physicians did not rate themselves as very effective in their ability to help patients make the therapeutic lifestyle changes necessary for preventing and managing CVD (Mosca et al., 2005). Methodological limitations, including restricting the study to three categories of physicians and low survey response rate, were acknowledged by the authors; however, the results are consistent with earlier research in this area of provider behavior.

These results suggest the need for interventions designed to increase providers' knowledge and awareness of and adherence to evidence-based guidelines for CVD prevention and management, as well as improvements in physician competencies in behavior-change counseling. As discussed later, they also suggest the need for integrated systems of care that emphasize multidisciplinary team approaches to risk-factor management and encouraging behavioral change in patients with CVD.

System-Level Factors That Affect Adherence in Patients With CVD

In this context, system-level factors refer to both the settings or environments in which patients with established CVD are managed and the processes that influence delivery of care. Substantial research has focused on the influence of such factors on patient adherence to therapeutic regimens, as well as provider adherence to evidence-based guidelines for management of CVD. Institutional or system-level policies establish expectations for care and can facilitate or impede adherence-related activities. For example, as discussed later, systems of care that value, encourage, and reward providers' adherence to evidence-based guidelines normally have mechanisms in place that enable physicians to track patients' risk-factor levels (i.e., lipids, blood pressure, body weight) and monitoring and to follow up until treatment goals are achieved. Robust information technology and integrated systems of care, generally lacking within the current U.S. health system structure, are necessary for effective preventive interventions (including both primary and secondary prevention of CVD) and are likely to enhance patient and provider adherence behaviors. An important additional characteristic of adherence-enhancing health care systems is a multidisciplinary collaborative team approach that optimizes the contributions of professionals from the many disciplines involved in the management of patients with CVD.

Strategies for Increasing Adherence and Improving Outcomes in Patients With CVD

Substantial evidence, including a recent meta-analysis, indicates that multidisciplinary, multicomponent secondary-prevention programs are effective in reducing recurrent acute cardiovascular events and all-cause mortality, and improving health-related quality of life and functional status in individuals with CVD (Clark, Hartling, Vandermeer, & McAlister, 2005). It is noteworthy that almost half (45%) of the 63 randomized trials included in this meta-analysis were identified as nurse-led or nurse-managed programs. As illustrated in landmark and recent clinical and community-based trials, improving adherence and health outcomes in CVD patients from diverse racial, ethnic, and sociodemographic backgrounds is achievable but will require major reforms in current systems of care (Ades et al., 2000; Becker et al., 2005; DeBusk et al., 1994; Fonarow, Gawlinski, Moughrabi, & Tillisch, 2001; Gordon et al., 2002; Haskell et al., 2006;

Vale, Jelinek, & Best, 2003). The key elements of successful secondary CVD-prevention programs identified in this research are consistent with the core components or pillars of the Chronic Care Model as defined by Wagner, Austin, and vonKorff (1996) and Bodenheimer and colleagues (2002), including self-management support, decision support (i.e., evidence-based clinical practice guidelines), computerized clinical information systems, community resources and policies (i.e., linkages between provider organizations and community-based resources), delivery system design (i.e., case-managed, multidisciplinary team approach), and health care organization (i.e., structure, goals, and values of provider organization that prioritize provision of chronic care). More specifically, as operationalized in secondary CVD-prevention programs, essential elements of effective programs include systems for coordination of services with multiple providers (case-managed, multidisciplinary teams); comprehensive lifestyle management programs that incorporate evidence-based principles of behavior change, including self-management support and enhanced social support; clinical information systems (computerized participant management, tracking, reporting, and outcomes analysis systems); and efficient mechanisms for patient follow-up to monitor adherence, safety, and effectiveness of interventions. An essential additional component of effective nurse-led, case-managed programs is the use of evidence-based protocols and algorithms for management of patients with single- and multiple-risk factors (Allen & Scott, 2003; Berra, Miller, & Fair, 2006).

The Stanford Coronary Risk Intervention Project (SCRIP), a landmark clinical trial that included a nurse case-managed, multidisciplinary team approach (and several features of the chronic care model) illustrates the potential of secondary-prevention programs and their core elements to reduce morbidity and mortality in patients with CVD (Haskell et al., 1994). Specifically, SCRIP tested the hypothesis that intensive multiple-risk-factor reduction over a period of 4 years would significantly reduce the rate of progression of coronary artery atherosclerosis in men (n = 259) and women (n = 41) (mean age, 56+/− 7.4 years) with documented coronary artery disease. Participants were randomly assigned to the multicomponent, multiple-risk-reduction intervention that was coordinated by advanced-practice nurses in collaboration with a multidisciplinary team or to physician-delivered usual care (UC). Components included baseline assessment conducted by nurses and dietitians, evidence-based individualized risk-reduction goals, protocol-driven medication algorithms for lipid management, bimonthly clinic visits, and individual follow-up by telephone and/or mail by nurses to monitor participants' progress toward achieving their goals. Strategies for risk- reduction and behavioral change were evidence based, theoretically derived, and individualized, with emphasis placed on helping each participant (in the intervention arm) to reach the best possible outcome (as defined by evidence-based practice guidelines). Intermediate and minimal goals were used selectively to enhance motivation and program adherence. As part of the individualized, risk-reduction behavioral change interventions, participants met with the SCRIP nurse (immediately postrandomization) to develop goals and to design a program that targeted dietary intake, physical activity, weight status, and smoking behavior. Referral and follow-up with members of the multidisciplinary SCRIP team was initiated by the nurse case manager and based on the participant's baseline risk assessment. For example, all participants in the risk-reduction program (intervention arm) were instructed by a dietitian on how to implement a heart-healthy pattern of dietary intake, with goals set for total fat, saturated fat, cholesterol, carbohydrate, and protein intake. Consideration of the participant's food preferences and resources was an important part of the plan. In compliance with guidelines developed by the SCRIP team for home-based exercise training of cardiac patients, each participant had an individualized physical activity program. Current smokers and those who had recently quit were provided an individualized smoking-cessation or relapse-prevention program by a staff psychologist. Each participant in the risk-reduction intervention arm was provided verbal and written instructions for an individualized risk-reduction, behavioral-change plan; progress toward achieving the goals outlined in those plans was monitored through bimonthly clinic visits and telephone follow-up that also provided opportunity for continued education and counseling.

SCRIP results indicated that an intensive physician-directed, nurse case-managed multidisciplinary, multicomponent, individualized program conducted over a period of 4 years can significantly improve the risk profile in individuals with documented CVD and can favorably alter progression of coronary atherosclerosis (Haskell et al., 1994). Small changes were observed in the UC group, whereas participants in the intervention arm had a 22% reduction in atherogenic low-density lipoprotein cholesterol (LDL-C), a 20% reduction in triglycerides, a 4% reduction in body weight, and a 24% reduction in intake of dietary fat; cardioprotective high-density lipoprotein cholesterol (HDL-C) increased by 12%, and exercise capacity increased by 20%. In addition, the risk-reduction group demonstrated a rate of narrowing of diseased coronary artery segments that was 47% lower than the rate for participants in the UC group, and the intervention group had significantly fewer hospitalizations for clinical events (25 vs. 44) than the UC group.

Building on the SCRIP approach and including other core elements of the Chronic Care Model (described earlier), subsequent clinical and community-based trials were designed to reduce risk factors, adverse health behaviors, and recurrent events in individuals with CVD (Ades et al., 2000; DeBusk et al., 1994; Fonarow et al., 2001; Gordon et al., 2002; Vale et al., 2003). More recently, the effectiveness of multifactor risk-reduction programs has been examined in medically underserved individuals at high risk for CVD (Becker et al., 2005; Haskell et al., 2006). The Heart Disease on the Mend (HDOM) project, for example, was designed to evaluate the effectiveness of a team-based disease-management approach to multifactor CVD risk reduction in patients with limited or no health insurance and low family income. Participants (n = 148; 57% women; 57% Hispanic; 64% uninsured) were recruited from free clinics and hospitals and randomized to UC or UC plus team management. All participants had at least one risk factor for CVD, and 25% self-reported personal history of CVD. The program was physician directed, delivered by nurses and dietitians, and guided by the SCRIP model and included comprehensive lifestyle modifications and pharmacotherapy. Program features included patient counseling, point-of-care lipid and glucose testing, use of existing resources in the community, telephone and mail follow-up, and theory-based strategies for patient self-management. Primary outcomes, LDL-C and systolic blood pressure (SBP), were measured at 12 months; 91% of participants assessed at baseline were retained through the 12-month data point. Participants in the HDOM disease management program (intervention arm) demonstrated significantly larger decreases in selected risk factors, including the primary outcomes, SBP and LDL-C, than the group receiving UC. In addition, more patients in the disease-management program moved from high-risk to lower-risk categories (as defined by recent guidelines) for selected risk factors, including physical activity and nutrition. While this study was limited to one geographic region and included a small sample, the results indicate the potential of a team-based, multidisciplinary disease-management approach in reducing risk and long-term disease burden in underserved populations.

Taken together, results of clinical and community-based studies demonstrate the promise and potential of innovative multidisciplinary models and integrated systems of care for reducing morbidity and mortality and improving quality of life in diverse populations of patients with CVD. They also underscore the feasibility and effectiveness of the Chronic Care Model and its core components in improving outcomes for individuals with CVD. However, a limitation of most research in this area and a fertile area for future research is assessment and examination of adherence as an outcome. Specifically, a clearer delineation of the relationship between patient adherence to therapeutic regimens and cardiovascular health outcomes, as well as adherence-enhancing multilevel strategies and specific factors that improve adherence behaviors on the individual patient and provider levels, is needed. As presented in Table 34.1 and placed in the context of the evidence accumulated to date, results also reaffirm the need for a multilevel, ecological approach to increasing adherence to lifestyle modifications and pharmacological regimens through efforts that extend beyond the individual patient and include providers, systems of care, and broader sociocontextual factors.

Summary

While substantial progress has been made in reducing CHD mortality in the United States over the past 30 years, cardiovascular diseases remain a major cause of death and disability in men and women. As discussed in this chapter, many population subgroups, defined by race, ethnicity, gender, socioeconomic status, educational level, and geography, demonstrate an excess burden of CVD and its attendant risk factors (Bonow et al., 2005; Davis et al., 2007; Mensah, 2005). Research is needed to inform and guide clinical and public health efforts, as well as multilevel policies designed to reduce the documented disparities in the prevention and treatment of CVD.

Evidence-based guidelines for secondary prevention of CVD (Balady et al., 2007; Mosca et al., 2007; Smith et al., 2006) emphasize therapeutic behavioral- lifestyle change and assessment and management of psychosocial risk factors as part of comprehensive risk-reduction strategies for individuals with established CVD. Indeed, a growing body of evidence confirms that aggressive, comprehensive risk-factor management improves survival, reduces recurrent events and the need for interventional procedures, and improves the quality of life for individuals with established heart disease (Smith et al., 2006). Adherence to lifestyle modification and medication recommendations is essential to achieving treatment goals and preventing recurrent events. Consistent with social-ecological models of health and behavior, accumulated evidence supports the need and potential for multilevel strategies for increasing adherence to therapeutic regimens. While numerous studies have shown that multicomponent, multilevel interventions result in improved outcomes for individuals with CVD, most studies have neglected to assess either the impact of the intervention on adherence behaviors or the added value of behavioral counseling beyond maximizing the medical management of CVD. In addition, while more research is needed to inform and guide effective strategies at the individual patient, provider, and health care system level, the need to disseminate and apply in practice existing evidence-based, adherence-enhancing strategies is equally as important.

As discussed in this chapter, substantial evidence indicates that multidisciplinary, multicomponent secondary-prevention programs are effective in reducing recurrent acute cardiovascular events and improving quality of life in individuals with CVD. The key elements of successful programs identified in seminal and recent research are consistent with the core components of the Chronic Care Model (Bodenheimer et al., 2002; Wagner et al., 1996) and underscore the promise and potential of innovative models and integrated systems of care for reducing morbidity and mortality and improving quality of life in diverse populations of patients with CVD.

References

Ades, P. A., Pashkow, F. J., Fletcher, G., Pina, I. L., Zohman, L. R., & Nestor, J. R. (2000). A controlled trial of cardiac rehabilitation in the home setting using electrocardiographic and voice transtelephonic monitoring. *American Heart Journal, 139,* 543–548.

Allen, J. K., & Scott, L. B. (2003). Alternative models in the delivery of primary and secondary prevention programs. *Journal of Cardiovascular Nursing, 18,* 150–156.

Ariyo, A. A., Haan, M., & Tangen, C. M. (2000). Depressive symptoms and risks of coronary heart disease mortality in elderly Americans. *Circulation, 102,* 1773–1779.

Artinian, N. T., Yuccha, C. B., & Dungan, J. (2007). Management of hypertension. In D. Moser & B. Riegel (Eds.), *Cardiac nursing: A companion to Braunwald's heart disease* (pp. 1205–1219). St Louis, MO: Saunders/Elsevier.

Baker, D. W., Wolf, M. S., Feinglass, J., & Thompson, J. A. (2008). Health literacy, cognitive abilities, and mortality among elderly persons. *Journal of General Internal Medicine, 23,* 723–726.

Balady, G. J., Williams, M. A., Ades, P. A., Bittner, V., Cosmos, P., Foody, J. M., et al. (2007). Core components of cardiac rehabilitation/secondary prevention programs: 2007 update. *Circulation, 115,* 2675–2682.

Bane, C., Hughes, C. M., & McElnay, J. C. (2006). The impact of depressive symptoms and psychosocial factors on medication adherence in cardiovascular disease. *Patient Education and Counseling, 80,*187–193.

Barth, J., Schumacher, M., & Herrmann-Lingen, C. (2004). Depression as a risk factor for mortality in patients with coronary heart disease: A meta-analysis. *Psychosomatic Medicine, 66,* 802–813.

Becker, D. M., Yanek, L. R., Johnson, W. R., Garrett, D., Moy, T. F., Reynolds, S. S., et al. (2005). Impact of a community-based multiple risk factor intervention on cardiovascular risk in black families with a history of premature coronary disease. *Circulation, 111,* 1298–1304.

Berra, K., Miller, N. H., & Fair, J. M. (2006). Cardiovascular disease prevention and disease management: A critical role for nursing. *Journal of Cardiopulmonary Rehabilitation, 26,* 197–206.

Bodenheimer, T., Wagner, E. H., & Grumbach, K. (2002). Improving primary care for patients with chronic illness. *Journal of the American Medical Association, 288,* 1775–1779.

Bonow, R. O., Grant, A. O., & Jacobs, A. K. (2005). The cardiovascular state of the union: Confronting healthcare disparities. *Circulation, 111,* 1205–1207.

Braun, L. T., & Hughes, S. (2007). Management of dyslipidemia. In D. Moser & B. Riegel (Eds.), *Cardiac nursing: A companion to Braunwald's heart disease* (pp. 1189–1204). St Louis, MO: Saunders/Elsevier.

Burg, M., Benedetto, C., & Soufer, R. (2003). Depressive symptoms and mortality after coronary artery bypass graft surgery (CABG) in men. *Psychosomatic Medicine, 65,* 508–510.

Burke, L. E., Dunbar-Jacob, J. M., & Hill, M. N. (1997). Compliance with cardiovascular disease prevention strategies: A review of the research. *Annals of Behavioral Medicine, 19,* 239–263.

Burns, J. W., & Evon, D. (2007). Common and specific process factors in cardiac rehabilitation: independent and interactive effects of the working alliance and self-efficacy. *Health Psychology, 26,* 684–692.

Caulin-Glaser, T., Maciejewski, P. K., Snow, R., LaLonde, M., & Mazure, C. (2007). Depressive symptoms and sex affect completion rates and clinical outcomes in cardiac rehabilitation. *Preventive Cardiology, 10,* 15–21.

Cheng, T. Y. L., & Boey, K. W. (2002). The effectiveness of a cardiac rehabilitation program on self-efficacy and exercise tolerance. *Clinical Nursing Research, 11,* 10–21.

Clark, A. M., Hartling, L., Vandermeer, B., & McAlister, F. A. (2005). Meta-analysis: Secondary prevention programs for patients with coronary artery disease. *Annals of Internal Medicine, 143,* 659–672.

Davis, A. M., Vinci, L. M., Okwuosa, T. M., Chase, A. R., & Huang, E. S. (2007). Cardiovascular health disparities: A systematic review of health care interventions. *Medical Care Research and Review, 64,* 29–69.

DeBusk, R. F., Miller, N. H., Superko, H. R., Dennis, C. A., Thomas, R. J., Lew, H. T., et al. (1994). A case-management system for coronary risk factor modification after acute myocardial infarction. *Annals of Internal Medicine, 120,* 721–729.

DiMatteo, M. R., Lepper, H. S., & Croghn, T. W. (2000). Depression is a risk factor for noncompliance with medical treatment: Meta-analysis of the effects of anxiety and depression on patient adherence. *Archives of Internal Medicine, 160,* 2101–2107.

Dunbar-Jacob, J., Schlenk, E. A., Burke, L. E., & Matthews, J. T. (1998). Predictors of patient adherence: Patient characteristics. In S. A. Shumaker, E. Schron, J. Ockene, & W. L. McBee (eds.), *Handbook of health behavior change* (2nd ed., pp. 491–514). New York: Springer Publishing.

Emery, C., Hauck, E. R., & Blumenthal, J. A. (1992). Exercise adherence or maintenance among older adults: 1-year follow-up study. *Psychology of Aging, 7,* 466–470.

Evangelista, L. S., & Pike, N. A. (2007). Promoting adherence to treatment. In D. Moser & B. Riegel (Eds.), *Cardiac nursing: A companion to Braunwald's heart disease* (pp. 1283–1296). St Louis, MO: Saunders/Elsevier.

Ewart, C. K., Taylor, C. B., Reese, L. B., & DeBusk, R. F. (1983). Effects of early post-myocardial infarction exercise testing on self-perception and subsequent physical activity. *American Journal of Cardiology, 51,* 1076–1080.

Fiore, M. D., Bailey, W. C., & Cohen, S. J. (1996). *Smoking cessation: Clinical practice guideline.* No. 18 (96-06592). Rockville, MD: U.S. Department of Health and Human Services, Agency for Health Care Policy and Research and Centers for Disease Control and Prevention.

Fitzgerald, S. P., & Phillipov, G. (2000). Patient attitudes to commonly promoted medical interventions. *Medical Journal of Australia, 172,* 9–12.

Fletcher, B., Berra, K., Ades, P., Braun, L. T., Burke, L. E., Durstine, J. L., et al. (2005). Managing abnormal blood lipids: A collaborative approach. *Circulation, 112,* 3184–3209.

Fonarow, G. C., Gawlinski, A., Moughrabi, S., & Tillisch, J. H. (2001). Improved treatment of coronary heart disease by implementation of a Cardiac Hospitalization Atherosclerosis Management Program (CHAMP). *American Journal of Cardiology, 87,* 819–822.

Ford, E. S., Ajani, U. A., Croft, J. B., Critchley, J. A., Labarthe, D. R., Kittke, T. E., et al. (2007). Explaining the decrease in U.S. deaths from coronary disease, 1980–2000. *New England Journal of Medicine, 356,* 2388–2398.

Frank, E. (1997). Enhancing patient outcomes: Treatment adherence. *Journal of Clinical Psychiatry, 58*(Suppl. 1), 11–14.

Gazmararian, J. A., Kripalani, S., Miller, M. J., Echt, K. V., Ren, J., & Rask, K. (2006). Factors associated with medication refill adherence in cardiovascular-related diseases: A focus on health literacy. *Journal of General Internal Medicine, 21,* 1215–1221.

Gehi, A., Haas, D., Pipkin, S., & Whooley, M. A. (2005). Depression and medication adherence in outpatients with coronary heart disease: Findings from the Heart and Soul Study. *Archives of Internal Medicine, 165,* 2508–2513.

Gordon, N. F., English, C. D., Contactor, A. S., Salmon, R. D., Leighton, R. F., Franklin, B. A., et al. (2002). Effectiveness of three models for comprehensive cardiovascular disease risk reduction. *American Journal of Cardiology, 89,* 1263–1268.

Gordon, N. F., Salmon, R. D., Mitchell, B. S., Faircloth, G. C., Levinrad, L. I., Salmon, S., et al. (2001). Innovative approaches to comprehensive cardiovascular disease risk reduction in clinical and community-based settings. *Currents in Atherosclerosis, 3,* 498–506.

Graveley, E. A., & Oseasohn, C. S. (1991). Multiple drug regimens: Medication compliance among veterans 65 years and older. *Research in Nursing and Health, 14,* 51–58.

Grundy, S. M., Cleeman, J. I., Daniels, S. R., Donato, K. A., Eckel, R. H., Franklin, B. A., et al. (2005). Diagnosis and management of the metabolic syndrome. *Circulation, 112,* 2735–2752.

Gustat, J., Srinivasan, S. R., Elkasabany, A., & Berenson, G. (2002). Relation of self-rated measures of physical activity to multiple risk factors of insulin resistance syndrome in young adults: The Bogalusa Heart Study. *Journal of Clinical Epidemiology, 55,* 997–1006.

Haskell, W. L., Alderman, E. L., Fair, J. M., Maron, D. J., Mackey, S. F., Superko, R., et al. (1994). Effects of multiple risk factor reduction on coronary atherosclerosis and clinical cardiac events in men and women with coronary artery disease: The Stanford Coronary Risk Intervention project (SCRIP). *Circulation, 89,* 975–990.

Haskell, W. L., Berra, K., Arias, E., Christopherson, D., Clark, A., George, J., et al. (2006). Multifactor cardiovascular disease risk reduction in medically underserved high-risk patients. *American Journal of Cardiology, 98,* 1472–1479.

Hayman, L. L., Meininger, J. C., Daniels, S. R., McCrindle, B. W., Helden, L., Ross, J., et al. (2007). Primary prevention of cardiovascular disease in nursing practice: Focus on children and youth. *Circulation, 116,* 344–357.

Hayman, L. L., & Hughes, S. (2006 November 4). Prevention of cardiovascular disease: A life course ecological perspective. *Journal of Cardiovascular Nursing, 21,* 500–501.

Jones, D. W. (2007, November 4). *Delivering the promise: Progress, challenges and opportunities.* Presidential address. American Heart Association Scientific Sessions, Orlando, FL.

Kavey, R. E., Daniels, S. R., Lauer, R. M., Atkins, D. L., Hayman, L. L., & Taubert, K. (2003). American Heart Association guidelines for primary prevention of atherosclerotic cardiovascular disease beginning in childhood. *Circulation, 107,* 1562–1566.

Kim, C., Hofer, T. P., & Kerr, E. A. (2003). Review of evidence and explanations for suboptimal screening and treatment of dyslipidemia in women: A conceptual model. *Journal of General Internal Medicine, 18,* 854–863.

Mensah, G. A., Mokdad, A. H., Ford, E. S., Greenlund, K. J., & Croft, J. B. (2005). State of disparities in cardiovascular health in the United States. *Circulation, 111,* 1233–1241.

Miller, N. H., Hill, M., Kottke, T., & Ockene, I. S. (1997). The multilevel compliance challenge: A call to action. A statement for healthcare professionals. *Circulation, 95,* 1085–1090.

Miller, R. R., Sales, A. E., Kopjar, B., Fin, S. D., & Bryson, C. L. (2005). Adherence to heart-healthy behaviors in a sample of the U.S. population. *Preventing chronic disease: public health research practice and policy* [serial online]. Retrieved July 23, 2007, from http://www.cdc.gov/pcd/issues/2005/apr/04_0115.htm

Morgan, A. L., Masoudi, F. A., Havranek, E. P., Jones, P. G., Peterson, P. N., Krumholtz, H. M., et al. for the Cardiovascular Outcomes Research Consortium (CORC). (2006). Difficulty taking medications, depression, and health status in heart failure patients. *Journal of Cardiology, 1,* 54–60.

Mosca, L., Banka, C. L., Benjamin, E. J., Berra, K., Bushnell, C., Dolor, R. J., et al. (2007). Evidence-based guidelines for cardiovascular disease prevention in women: 2007 update. *Circulation, 115,* 1481–1501.

Mosca, L., Linfante, A. H., Benjamin, E. J., Berra, K., Hayes, S. N., Walsh, B. W., et al. (2005). National study of physician awareness and adherence to cardiovascular disease prevention guidelines. *Circulation, 111,* 499–510.

Nelson, E. C., Stason, W. B., Neutra, R. R., Solomon, H. S., & McArdle, P. J. (1978). Impact of patient perceptions on compliance with treatment for hypertension. *Medical Care, 16,* 893–906.

Ockene, J. K. (2001). Strategies to increase adherence to treatment. In L. E. Burke & I. S. Ockene (Ed.), *Compliance in healthcare and research* (pp. 43–55). Armonk, NY: Futura Publishing.

Ockene, J. K., Adams, A., Turley, T. G., Wheeler, E. V., & Herbert, J. R. (1999). Brief physician- and nurse practitioner-delivered counseling for high-risk drinkers: Does it work? *Archives of Internal Medicine, 159,* 2198–2205.

Ockene, I. S., Hayman, L. L., Pasternak, R. C., Shron, E., & Dunbar-Jacob, F. (2002). Task Force #4-Adherence issues and behavior changes: achieving a long-term solution. *Journal of the American College of Cardiology, 40,* 630–640.

Ockene, I. S., Herbert, J. R., Ockene, J. K., Merriam, P. A., Hurley, T. G., & Saperia, G. M. (1996). Effect of training and a structured office practice on physician-delivered nutrition counseling: The Worcester-Area Trial for Counseling in Hyperlipidemia (WATCH). *American Journal of Preventive Medicine, 12,* 252–258.

O'Malley, P. G., & Greenland, P. (2007). The promise of preventive interventions depends on robust health care delivery. *Archives of Internal Medicine, 167,* 532.

Park, Y. W., Zhu, S., Palaniappan, L., Heshka, S., Carnethon, M. R., & Heymsfield, S. B. (2003). The metabolic syndrome: Prevalence and associated risk factor findings in the U.S. population from the Third National Health and Nutrition Examination Survey, 1988–1994. *Archives of Internal Medicine, 163,* 427–436.

Pearson, T. A., Blair, S. N., Daniels, S. R., Eckel, R. H., Fair, J. M., Fortmann, S. P. et al. (2002). AHA guidelines for primary prevention of cardiovascular disease and stroke: 2002 Update. *Circulation, 106,* 388–391.

Pearson, T. A., Laurora, I., Chu, H., & Kafonek, S. (2000). The Lipid Treatment Assessment Project (L-TAP): A multicenter survey to evaluate the percentages of dyslipidemic patients receiving lipid-lowering therapy and achieving low-density lipoprotein cholesterol goals. *Archives of Internal Medicine, 160,* 459–467.

Rosamond, W., Flegal, K., Friday, G., Furie, K., Go, A., Greenlund, K., et al. (2007). Heart disease and stroke statistics—2007 update. *Circulation, 115,* e69–e171.

Smith, S. C., Allen, J., Blair, S. N., Bonow, R. O., Brass, L. M., Fonarow, G. C., et al. (2006). AHA/ACC guidelines for secondary prevention for patients with coronary and other atherosclerotic vascular disease: 2006 update. *Circulation, 113,* 2363–2372.

Smith, S. C., Jackson, R., Pearson, T. A., Fuster, V., Yusuf, S., Faergeman, O., et al. (2004). Principles for national and regional guidelines on cardiovascular disease prevention. *Circulation, 109,* 3112–3121.

Sueta, C. A., Chowdhury, M., Boccuzzi, S. J., Smith, S. C., Alexander, C. M., Londhe, A., et al. (1999). Analysis of the degree of undertreatment of hyperlipidemia and congestive heart failure secondary to coronary artery disease. *American Journal of Cardiology, 84,* 1303–1307.

Vale, M. J., Jelinek, M. V., & Best, J. D. (2003). Coaching patients on achieving cardiovascular health (COACH): A multicenter randomized trial in patients with coronary heart disease. *Archives of Internal Medicine, 163,* 2775–2783.

vanMelle, J. P., de Jonge, P., & Spijkerman, T. A. (2004). Prognostic association of depression following myocardial infarction with mortality and cardiovascular events: A meta-analysis. *Psychosomatic Medicine, 66,* 814–822.

Wagner, E. H., Austin, B. T., & vonKorff, M. (1996). Organizing care for patients with chronic illness. *The Millbank Quarterly, 73,* 511–544.

Yusuf, S., Hawken, S., Ounpuu, S., Dans, T., Avezum, A., Lanas, F., et al. (2004). Effect of potentially modifiable risk factors associated with myocardial infarction in 52 countries (the INTERHEART study): Case-control study. *Lancet, 364,* 937–952.

Ziegelstein, R. C. (2001). Depression in patients recovering from a myocardial infarction. *Journal of the American Medical Association, 286,* 1621–1627.

Does Cognition Influence Type 2 Diabetes-Related Adherence?

35

David L. Mount

Clinical Case Example 1

The patient is a 56-year-old male with a high school education who reports occasional difficulty with mental organization that is most pronounced when he has to listen to multiple conversations. He reports accumulating mild to moderate problems with forgetfulness, concentration, word finding, and irritability. He believes his job is in jeopardy because he is experiencing increased episodic problems with completing work assignments. The patient is concerned that he cannot proficiently comply with medical instructions. He notes forgetting to schedule medical appointments, and his diabetes-related self-care monitoring is highly inconsistent. While he is frustrated with his fluctuating medical status, he denies any significant depression or anxiety. When questioned about his past history of self-managing health related changes, he states that he is overly compliant with all medical treatments. In fact, the patient notes that he has typically monitored his health and wellness with good vigilance since his family history is significant for diabetes and cardiovascular disease.

The patient reports being diagnosed with Type 2 diabetes approximately 8 years ago. For the past 2 years, he has reported inconsistent adherence to diet, exercise, and other health-protective behavior relevant to achieving glycemic control. The patient reports multiple episodes of errors in medication management, with two related hospitalizations. His mediation regimen for the past 3 years has included oral hypoglycemic and insulin medications, with mixed dosage between lunch and dinner. His medical records indicated that his A1c levels have averaged from 7.8 to 9.2 for the past year. His medical history is remarkable for hypertension for approximately 3 years, and his body mass index is 36. There is no evidence of diabetes-related neuropathy, retinopathy, or nephropathy. His medical history is unremarkable for neuroimaging evaluation, substantiated via medical record review.

The patient denies any prior history of neurocognitive assessment, which is confirmed via his medical record. On a self-report measure of psychological distress, the patient does not endorse symptoms suggestive of psychological distress. On the basis of the patient's age, education level, occupation, and reported history of academic performance, his performance on neurocognitive testing suggests evidence of generally low-average to below-normal abilities in most domains assessed, including memory, speed of information processing, attention and concentration, visual-spatial skills, verbal fluency, and manual dexterity. There is evidence of reduced mental efficiency on tasks requiring complex problem solving and/or multitasking.

From the standpoint of this patient's potential for adhering to a complex medical regimen, his current neurocognitive liabilities warrant concern regarding his ability to effectively self-manage his diabetes-related activities of daily living. It is anticipated that unless cognitive compensatory devices are put in place, his current cognitive resources will adversely limit his potential to adhere to a demanding medical management regimen. This neurocognitive testing provides an objective psychometric understanding of the patient's current cognitive strengths and weaknesses that can inform the tailoring of his medical regimen. It behooves his health care providers to monitor the patient for additional changes in cognitive functioning, particularly given his history of hypertension, which is independently predictive of deterioration in brain functioning, neurocognitive resources, and risk for cerebrovascular event.

Does Cognition Influence Type 2 Diabetes–Related Adherence?

Introduction

The World Health Organization is forecasting that diabetes will afflict 300 million persons by 2025 (King, Aubert, & Herman, 1998). Type 2 diabetes has no cure and is disproportionately prevalent among persons who have family history of diabetes, who are overweight, who are members of a racial or ethnic minority, who are of lower socioeconomic status, and who are middle aged or older (Bell & Polonsky, 2001).

Efforts to prevent type 2 diabetes have met with multiple challenges that represent a combination of biological and environmental factors. In efforts to achieve successful management of this chronic disease state, a premium is placed on patients' adhering to medical regimen(s) that work to maintain adequate blood sugar control. Both cross-sectional and well-known longitudinal studies, including the United Kingdom Prospective Diabetes Study, the Diabetes Control and Complications Trial, and the Kumomoto Trial, show evidence that successful glycemic control translates into reduced and/or delayed medical complications, fewer hospitalizations, and decreased medical costs (American Diabetes Association, 2003a; Aring, Jones, & Falko, 2005; Poncelet, 2003; Ratner, 2001; Stearne et al., 1998). It is estimated that the cost for financing chronic disease can increase substantially depending on age, sex, and chronic condition profile (Fishman, Von Korff, Lozano, & Hecht, 1997). Three-year costs for treating adults with type 2 diabetes who also had coronary heart disease and hypertension were more than three times those for treating adults with type 2 diabetes only, that is, $46,879 instead of $14,233 (Gilmer et al., 2005). Past, current, and forecast health care spending suggest a trend toward escalating direct and indirect costs linked to type 2 diabetes (Zimmet, Alberti, & Shaw, 2001).

This existing body of research speaks very little to the intersection of cognitive functioning on adherence to type 2 diabetes regimens. As both human and financial cost projections are being used to understand the impact of diabetes, the ramifications of cognitive dysfunction within this population on adherence to medical regimens has been slowly emerging. Epidemiological studies underscore a connection between diabetes and dementia (Biessels et al., 2006; Boyle, Wilson, Aggarwal, Tang, & Bennett, 2006; Luchsinger et al., 2007; Ott et al., 1996). This chapter seeks to underscore how and to what extent the evidence base supports a diabetes-cognition interaction. The chapter also discusses how acquired cognitive impairments in the type 2 diabetes population might influence adherence. The foundation of this discussion is a review of findings from cross-sectional, meta-analysis, and longitudinal research studies.

Metabolic Control and Adhering to Medical Regimen Components

Type 2 diabetes is a blood sugar dysregulation disorder and is associated with insulin resistance, insulin deficiency, or both. Type 2 diabetes generally has an insidious onset and progresses relatively slowly, and it is estimated that persons can remain undiagnosed for as long as 7 years (Harris, Klein, Welborn, & Knuiman, 1992). When it comes to specifying metabolic control in diabetes, a key benchmark is the hemoglobin A1c value. This value is most clearly associated with likelihood of developing additional medical complications.

A hemoglobin A1c 7% is at present a consensus reference marker for adequate blood sugar control (American Diabetes Association, 2003b; Centers for Disease Control and Prevention Primary Prevention Working Group, 2004). In an effort to achieve metabolic control, physicians may recommend changes in diet, weight loss, medications, or some combination of the three. For people who are unable to achieve metabolic control using prescribed lifestyle interventions, the next treatment strategy is likely to involve treatment with oral agents (e.g., sulfonylureas, repaglinide, metformin, thiazolidinediones) and/or insulin. More than 50% of persons diagnosed with type 2 diabetes are prescribed exogenous insulin and/or some type of diabetes-related medicine (Harris, Klein, Welborn, & Knuiman, 1992), and this trend is increasing (Austin, 2006; Fan, Koro, Fedder, & Bowlin, 2006; Koro, Bowlin, Bourgeois, & Fedder, 2004; Morris, 2001).

Taking diabetes-related medications as prescribed maximizes clinical benefit; however, the fluctuations in adhering to medical regimen components are an enduring challenge (Dunbar-Jacob & Mortimer-Stephens, 2001; Paterson et al., 2000). Rates of noncompliance for medications range from 20% to as high as 80% (Boccuzzi et al., 2001; Cramer, 2004; Shenolikar, Balkrishnan, Camacho, Whitmire, & Anderson, 2006). Although some components of the medical regimen plan are more difficult to achieve compliance with than others, adherence to prescribed medication protocol is a major deficit area.

Poor medication adherence in diabetes care is associated with increased all-cause mortality (hazard ratio = 1.43; 95% CI 1.13–1.82; P = 0.003) and diabetes-related deaths (1.66; 1.20–2.30; P = 0.002) over a 7-year period after adjusting for relevant confounders (Kuo et al., 2003). When poor medication adherence is a patient-care factor, there is a greater likelihood that such patients will also demonstrate excessive health utilization, ranging from preventable hospitalization to premature mortality due to disease-related complications (Fillenbaum et al., 2004; Ho et al., 2006; Vik et al., 2006). Inadequate metabolic control due to medication nonadherence has an estimated price tag of $100 billion a year (O'Connor, 2006).

Cognitive Functioning and Medical Adherence

Knowledge of a person's cognitive abilities can be useful across a broad range of related activities of daily living. Cognitive functioning represents the capacity for information processing, learning, remembering, analyzing, making reasonable decisions, and executing a plan of action (Baltes, Staudinger, & Lindenberger, 1999; Hultsch, Hammer, & Small, 1993). Our cognitive abilities promote our potential for functional independence and safety in carrying out activities germane to daily living. When cognitive abilities fail, there is increased potential for self-care errors. As shown in Figure 35.1, multiple neurocognitive markers can affect the mental reasoning abilities necessary for tracking details intertwined in the daily disease-management process.

Although the research is primarily correlational in nature, the study of cognitive functioning and components of patient-oriented medical adherence is emerging as a promising and prudent area of scientific inquiry (Cavanagh, Van Beck, Muir, & Blackwood, 2002; Hinkin et al., 2002; Insel, Morrow, Brewer, & Figueredo, 2006; McDonald, Garg, & Haynes, 2002; Okuno, Yanagi, & Tomura, 2001). While health status is a key factor in well-being and cognitive functioning (Morrow-Howell, Hinterlong, Rozario, & Tang, 2003; Small et al., 2006), the relationship between medication adherence and cognitive functioning suggests that cognitive resources are a factor in medication noncompliance (Kalichman et al., 2005). Research shows that lower performance on psychometric tests

Chapter 35 Does Cognition Influence Type 2 Diabetes-Related Adherence?

697

35.1

Neurocognitive markers of everyday functioning.

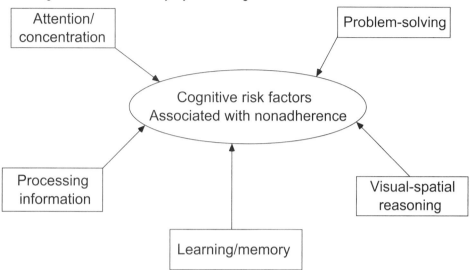

of cognitive abilities, as well as low literacy, is inversely related to medication adherence (Hutchison, Jones, West, & Wei, 2006; Kripalani et al., 2006; Maddigan, Farris, Keating, Wiens, & Johnson, 2003). In 2001, Salas and associates published data from the Rotterdam Study in which the researchers related impaired cognitive function to adherence to antihypertensive drugs in older adults. After adjustment for age, sex, education, income, living situation, and smoking, the findings indicated that persons who were cognitively impaired were twice as likely to have adherence problems with antihypertensive medicine as were persons without cognitive impairment. In addition, persons living alone were approximately three times as likely to be medication nonadherent.

For persons suffering from diseases of the immune system (i.e., HIV-infected persons), a trend toward lower medication adherence increases as patients are expected to cope with complex medication regimens (e.g., taking multiple medications and adhering to food requirements). Persons at higher risk for medication nonadherence have been shown to demonstrate cognitive deficits including problematic information processing sequencing, slowed problem solving related to how to self-management variability in medical symptoms, and fluctuation in memory functions (Hinkin et al., 2002).

Other factors such as psychiatric illness (Jeste et al., 2003; Piette, Heisler, Ganoczy, McCarthy, & Valenstein, 2007), environmental demands (Martin & Park, 2003), and age-associated cognitive changes (Insel, Morrow, Brewer, & Figueredo, 2006) are shown to increase medication-taking errors and risk for failure to take medicines as prescribed. These risks are also elevated in persons who have undergone changes in higher-order thinking skills, particularly memory. Although the literature regarding type 2 diabetes populations is not well developed or understood, it is nevertheless possible to speculate, on the basis of findings on adherence among those with other chronic diseases, findings that are traditionally understood to have neurocognitive connections.

Risk for Cognitive Decline in Type 2 Diabetes

Although study findings are not complete or always consistent, there is growing speculation that individuals diagnosed with type 2 diabetes can carry an elevated risk for cognitive decline. Some of the earlier reports noted that memory problems seemed to emerge in persons experiencing type 2 diabetes-related complications of peripheral neuropathy and/or elevated A1c levels (Perlmuter et al., 1984). Just over a decade later, Strachan and colleagues (1997) published findings that validated the observations of Perlmuter and associates. In their meta-analysis approach, and on the basis of research published between 1980 and 1995, Strachan and colleagues found that, indeed, there was a connection between a vulnerability in verbal memory and type 2 diabetes.

Supplementing these findings, multisite longitudinal studies, including the Rotterdam Study (Ott et al., 1996), the Honolulu-Asia Aging Study (Peila, Rodriguez, & Launer, 2002), and the Epidemiology of Vascular Aging Study (Fontbonne, Berr, Ducimetiere, & Alperovitch, 2001) have also found that risk to cognitive functions are increased in type 2 diabetes. Verbal memory is one particular cognitive asset that is at risk in type 2 diabetes. This memory process refers to the ability to remember words, narrative passages, and verbal items. This ability can be evaluated by asking the patient to recall information from a short story or a set of items from a word list.

Older cohorts have been the focus of choice when investigating the risk for non-age-related cognitive changes in type 2 diabetes. When studying younger type 2 diabetes cohorts, non-age-related changes in information processing speed are observed. The work of Ryan and Geckle (2000), for example, employed a cross-sectional methodology investigating differences in cognitive functions in 50 persons ranging in age from 34 to 65 years old with type 2 diabetes. This study highlighted cognitive deficits in psychometrically estimated information-processing reaction time. Information-processing speed is a cognitive asset thought to be correlated with global cognitive capacity. This cognitive skill can be stratified into several tasks: simple reaction time tasks (all stimuli require a response), recognition reaction time tasks (patients must discriminate using what was learned), and choice reaction time task (patients are required to respond to only one of the two possible stimuli). Whereas speed of information processing is a strong neurocognitive asset in younger years, the ability to handle situational tasks requiring quick acquisition of information, multitasking, or efficiency in the mental manipulation of multiple pieces of information declines with advancing age (Alloway, Gathercole, & Pickering, 2006; Miyake, Friedman, Rettinger, Shah, & Hegarty, 2001; Park et al., 2002).

In a middle-aged cohort from the Whitehall II study, Kumari and Marmot (2005) compared cognitive performance among three groups: those with diagnosed Type 2 diabetes, those with diagnosed impaired glucose tolerance, and persons with euglycemia. They found that persons with diabetes performed poorer on cognitive measures (men: OR, 2.45; 95% CI, 1.77 to 3.38; women: OR, 1.83; 95% CI, 1.09 to 3.08). In an earlier case-control study focused on persons younger than age 55 years with type 2 diabetes, Dey and colleagues (1997) found that those with diabetes had suboptimal performance on neuropsychological tests measuring attention, repetition, and memory. However, no differences between those with diabetes and controls were observed for other measures of neurocognitive functioning (e.g., tasks of comprehension, visual naming, visual-spatial ability, or math skills).

As noted in their published findings on the Atherosclerosis Risk in Communities cohort, a large biracial, multisite, longitudinal investigation of middle-aged individuals, Knopman et al. (2001) observed that persons with type 2 diabetes demonstrated problems with language-skills tasks, specifically word fluency, which measures the speed and flexibility of verbal thought processes, as well as assessing an individual's ability to generate as many words as possible within a fixed time limit.

The type 2 diabetes population is not a homogenous population. When persons with well-controlled type 2 diabetes are compared with relatively healthy individuals without diabetes, there are practically no discernable differences between them on behavioral tasks that measure verbal memory, except when duration of diabetes is considered (Cosway, Strachan, Dougall, Frier, & Deary, 2001). Duration of diabetes as a brain-cognition threshold marker is reported in the literature (Stewart & Liolitsa, 1999). Similar findings were reported from a sample of 16,596 women ages 70–81, with and without type 2 diabetes. In this study, the odds that a study participant would have poor cognition were approximately twice as great for those persons with longer duration of type 2 diabetes (Logroscino, Kang, & Grodstein, 2004).

Physiological Markers and Brain Functioning

Some biomarkers are reported to drive the relationship between diabetes and brain function more than others. Type 2 diabetes is largely a disease of the aging process; however, one must keep in mind that there are various types of aging, including chronological aging, physiological aging, and mental aging. It is generally accepted that chronic stress and chronic physical diseases accelerate physiological changes in multiple organ systems independent of age (Roth et al., 2004; Sieck, 2003). As some brain functions are more sensitive to the effects of aging than others, neurobiological and contextual factors such as environmental demands and cultural experiences independently and simultaneously influence underlying neural circuits that activate and deactivate cognitive processes (Baltes, Staudinger, & Lindenberger, 1999; Park & Gutchess, 2006; Salthouse, 1996; Von Dras & Blumenthal, 2000).

The poor supply of glucose to the brain can also cause neurological symptoms such as drowsiness, confusion, loss of consciousness, seizures, and permanent brain damage. Elevated blood glucose levels can damage small blood vessels (microvascular disease) that in turn affect the eyes (diabetic retinopathy), kidneys (nephropathy), and nerves (neuropathy). Elevated blood sugar or hyperglycemia is a significant complication experienced in type 2 diabetes. Elevated blood sugar is shown to decrease acetylcholine synthesis in rat brain (Welsh & Wecker, 1991). Acetylcholine is a neurotransmitter that appears to be involved in learning and memory and is severely diminished in the brains of persons with Alzheimer's disease.

As diabetes is a constellation of signs and symptoms, a salient feature of poor glycemic control is increased risk for atherosclerosis. Atherosclerosis, a disease of vessel wall thickness and plaques of the carotid arteries, is a risk factor for non-age-related changes in brain functioning (Hofman et al., 1997) and a consequence of several lifestyle factors (e.g., cigarette smoking, sedentary lifestyle, obesity). Reporting on their findings from the Rotterdam Study, Hofman and associates found that atherosclerosis is associated with dementia, and the odds ratio for Alzheimer's disease in those with severe atherosclerosis compared with those without atherosclerosis was 3.0 (95%, CI 1.5–6.0; $p = 0.001$).

Similar to atherosclerosis, hypertension is shown to alter brain functions (den Heijer et al., 2005; Kilander, Nyman, Boberg, Hansson, & Lithell, 1998). Variables that may alter (i.e., moderate) the relationship of hypertension to brain functioning include age, education, several characteristics of elevated blood pressure or hypertension, and the presence of concurrent diseases (Waldstein, 2003). The data suggest that while hypertension is a risk for cerebrovascular health independent of type 2 diabetes, the joint contributions of both diseases elevate stroke mortality (Hu et al., 2005).

Cognitive Functioning and Patient Care Planning

Verbal Fluency

Changes in any of these cognitive domains can have adverse consequences for following a diabetes regimen. Mild word generation problems can affect social processes. Verbal fluency deficits in diabetes can affect spontaneous speech. This issue is most problematic when the primary-care team has a short window to collect information from patients during follow-up visits. Some patients become relatively skilled at masking this problem. A consequence of verbal fluency deficits is that patients will likely have problems generating accurate representations of their diabetes self-management. If health care providers are unaware that such problems exist, the patient-provider interface will have multiple challenges, including the belief that the patient is unmotivated and not interested in talking with members of the health care team.

Verbal fluency problems may also cause the patient to be perceived as depressed. This misjudgment will unfortunately cause a strain in the relationship between primary-care providers and the patients they care for. As patients are likely to feel misunderstood, there is the potential that the diabetes care recipient will become uninterested in his own care and will resist complying with medical recommendations. When patients are unsuccessful in achieving stable diabetes control, consultation with a health care professional specializing in diabetes and neurocognitive functioning can provide an opportunity to rethink the existing diabetes care regimen. Such professionals should be knowledgeable about psychometric measures that are sensitive to changes in neuropsychological functioning within this chronic disease population.

Information Processing Speed

Cognitive reaction to information can alter a patient's ability to understand information presented through either an auditory or a visual medium. The primary care environment generally makes an assumption that patients have relatively equivalent information-processing efficiency. This belief represents a ubiquitous process operating throughout health service delivery. In the event that information is presented at a rate faster than the patient's neurocognitive processing can encode and organize it, it is highly likely that the patient will not remember what has been discussed. The primary care team will want to intervene around this issue by attending to the accuracy of each patient's understanding of the information presented. It is estimated that 50%–80% of persons with type 2 diabetes have knowledge and skill deficits in self-care-related activities and experience a significant relapse in self-management adherence 6 months after receiving initial treatment instructions (Norris, Engelgau, & Narayan, 2001).

While skill deficits in diabetes care may be unrelated to challenges in cognitive processing, investigating the influence of such a process on the acquisition of care skills is in many cases warranted. A key to assisting patients with below-average information processing speed is allowing them an adequate amount of time to process information. An additional strategy is to repeat information and verify that the patient has correctly understood the instructions.

Cognitive impairment in type 2 diabetes is not commonly understood or recognized and is likely to be missed during primary care clinic visits. With the proportion of adults with type 2 growing and the rates of nonadherence to diabetes medical regimen rapidly increasing in the United States, the number of persons living with both type 2 diabetes and cognitive impairment is expected to present a massive public health problem. The demand for translational science has pushed basic science, epidemiological, and clinical trial researchers to think more broadly about the bidirectional pathways of diabetes on body, brain, and society. A type 2 diabetes body-mind paradigm on adherence has the potential to provide a platform that models and investigates the underlying differences in patient outcomes, particularly given the body of research emerging in the study of neurobiology and cognitive function, with particular attention to brain plasticity, cognitive health, culture, and successful mental aging (Chua, Chen, & Park, 2006; Gutchess et al., 2006; Park & Gutchess, 2006).

Implications From the Clinical Case

The case presented at the beginning of this chapter has multiple implications that might shed light on the cognitive mechanisms potentially connected to an individual's ability to develop and maintain self-care skills, to benefit from diabetes-related education, and to follow a prescribed treatment regimen. When cognitive functions become unstable or specific neurocognitive abilities start to diminish, it is important that health care providers tailor the medication regimen to patients' cognitive strengths and weaknesses, taking into account the complexity of the medication regimen.

Diabetes care is heavily language driven. When persons present for a medical visit, the majority of the interface is verbally driven, and patients' ability to understand the information discussed with the provider has implications for their ability to execute self-care skills after the medical visit. Since face-to-face contact time with health care providers is limited, problems with verbal fluency may hinder individuals' ability to effectively communicate issues that might place them at further safety risk with regard to self-management of their diabetes. Patients with diabetes can experience deficits in new learning and memory functioning that can affect diabetes education as well as their ability to remember what is discussed during a clinic visit. Peoples with diabetes can also experience deficits in higher-order cognitive functions. Such patients may evidence weaknesses in their ability to process and respond to verbal instructions of increasing complexity. Deficits in higher-order cognitive functioning are hallmarks of problems in planning, self-monitoring, self-regulating, flexibility in mental processing, and problem solving. As with other chronic diseases that have a neurological connection, the signs and symptoms of type 2 diabetes-related neuropsychological disturbance vary in the rate at which they progress and can range from deficits in concentration, declarative memory, visual understanding, acquisition of new information, and word finding to deficits in ability to remember vital information, mental agility, and emotional stability.

The development of strategies to improve how patients learn health information are of particular interest in the management of chronic disease (Rogers, Wallace, & Weiss, 2006; Safeer, Cooke, & Keenan, 2006; Schillinger et al., 2002). This suggests that benefits from health education are generally influenced by a combination of cognitive factors, including risk perception, motivation, self-efficacy, reasoning, knowledge, and general intellectual functioning (Bandura, 1998; Whitehead, 2001). However, health care providers need to be aware that the potential for completing tasks of relatively moderate to high complexity is reduced when cognitive agility or cognitive efficiency is compromised (Perneczky et al., 2006; Tabert et al., 2002). As noted by Lezak (1995), brain-behavior relationships have implications for proficiency in activities of daily living. Self-managing a diabetes regimen involves performance of a complex variety of functions related to filtering, selecting, focusing, shifting, and tracking information. Since there is typically a huge amount of available information to attend to, a person must be able to filter this potential information and attend to only the most relevant sources.

Discussion

Diabetes control is a unifying goal of care, but many elements weigh in on the achievability of diabetes control, including who is receiving the care and who is delivering the care. Poor diabetes management increases risk for secondary medical complications ranging from heart disease, erectile dysfunction in men, and polycystic ovary disease in women to blindness, stroke, end-stage renal disease, and lower-extremity amputations, polypharmacy, and premature death. The rate of complications associated with type 2 diabetes nonadherence places increasing demands on health care providers at all levels.

Diabetes Adherence and Cognitive Functioning

Type 2 diabetes is a regimen-intensive disease that requires an assortment of complex mental skills. Cognitive problems in diabetes may affect the patient's ability to correctly identify appropriate medications, awareness of physiological responses to self-care behaviors, ability to remember to take medications at scheduled times, and ability to fill prescriptions in a timely manner. The evidence base for type 2 diabetes-related cognitive dysfunction and adherence capacity is relatively sparse at this time, and future research will be needed to fill this gap while simultaneously educating providers of direct-service care about the patient self-management challenges associated with alterations in cognition. Effectively matching a patient's cognitive strengthens and weaknesses with patient care regimen planning is a promising and innovative strategy for reducing problematic nonadherence.

Conclusions and Future Implications

The risk for dementia appears to be significantly greater for persons diagnosed with type 2 diabetes than in the general population. However, correlation does not warrant a conclusion of causation. While the literature does not fully support the proposition that all persons diagnosed with type 2 diabetes experience cognitive impairment, or that all cognitive abilities are affected equally, it is worth reiterating that diabetes self-management can place demands on a variety of cognitive resources.

Persons treated for diabetes require care from primary-care physicians and various allied health professionals, including diabetes educators, nurses, pharmacists, and physical activity specialists. The patient-oriented diabetes regimen is a full-time job that requires, among other activities, keeping vaccinations up to date; checking feet every day; taking daily aspirin and other prescribed medications; monitoring blood pressure; managing stress; and planning ahead for health care visits.

In summary, adherence to diabetes-related therapies is a major issue in diabetes care, and strategies for improving adherence are desperately needed. Cognitive functioning in diabetes has an impact on medical regimen planning, tailored intervention programs, lifestyle management, and health behavior practices. It seems highly important for science to determine whether differences in diabetes care outcomes are influenced by a set of cognitive skills such as attention to details, multitasking, complex problem solving, and remembering information and how these affect self-care behaviors, particularly checking blood sugar, taking medicines, and following up on medical appointments. Elucidating the mechanisms by which cognitive dysfunction is a barrier for diabetes-related adherence would provide insight as to what cognitive remediation strategies are needed and how technological innovations might be employed to strengthen adherence behavior.

Given the cost of diabetes care, shifts in philosophy from a focus on intervention to one on prevention, and the burgeoning interest in pay-for-performance, it is imperative that a fuller picture be developed of diabetes-related medical adherence. It is anticipated that, as the body of evidence grows in type 2 diabetes adherence research, brain-behavior research will add to the process of tailored intervention planning to reduce risk for nonadherence to medical regimens. A potential barrier in coordinating diabetes and neurocognitive care will involve restructuring the traditional primary-care team. Health service providers will find that holistic management of patients with type 2 diabetes supports a realistic chance to effectively close gaps in disparate adherence to diabetes regimens.

References

Alloway, T. P., Gathercole, S. E., & Pickering, S. J. (2006). Verbal and visuospatial short-term and working memory in children: Are they separable? *Child Development, 77*(6), 1698–1716.

American Diabetes Association. (2003a). Economic costs of diabetes in the U.S. in 2002. *Diabetes Care, 26*(3), 917–932.

American Diabetes Association. (2003b). Screening for Type 2 Diabetes. *Diabetes Care, 26*(Suppl. 1), S21–S24.

Aring, A. M., Jones, D. E., & Falko, J. M. (2005). Evaluation and prevention of diabetic neuropathy. *American Family Physician, 71*(11), 2123–2128.

Austin, R. P. (2006). Polypharmacy as a risk factor in the treatment of type 2 diabetes. *Diabetes Spectrum, 19*(1), 13–16.

Baltes, P. B., Staudinger, U. M., & Lindenberger, U. (1999). Lifespan psychology: Theory and application to intellectual functioning. *Annual Review Psychology, 50,* 471–507.

Bandura, A. (1998). Health promotion from the perspective of social cognitive theory. *Psychology & Health, 13,* 623–649.

Bell, G. I., & Polonsky, K. S. (2001). Diabetes mellitus and genetically programmed defects in [beta]-cell function. *Nature, 414*(6865), 788–791.

Biessels, G. J., De Leeuw, F. E., Lindeboom, J., Barkhof, F., & Scheltens, P. (2006). Increased cortical atrophy in patients with Alzheimer's Disease and type 2 diabetes mellitus. *Journal of Neurology, Neurosurgery & Psychiatry, 77*(3), 304–307.

Boccuzzi, S. J., Wogen, J., Fox, J., Sung, J. C., Shah, A. B., & Kim, J. (2001). Utilization of oral hypoglycemic agents in a drug-insured U.S. population. *Diabetes Care, 24*(8), 1411–1415.

Boyle, P. A., Wilson, R. S., Aggarwal, N. T., Tang, Y., & Bennett, D. A. (2006). Mild cognitive impairment: Risk of Alzheimer Disease and rate of cognitive decline. *Neurology, 67*(3), 441–445.

Cavanagh, J. T., Van Beck, M., Muir, W., & Blackwood, D. H. (2002). Case-control study of neuro-cognitive function in euthymic patients with bipolar disorder: An association with mania. *British Journal of Psychiatry, 180,* 320–326.

Centers for Disease Control and Primary Prevention Working Group. (2004). Primary prevention of type 2 diabetes mellitus by lifestyle intervention: Implications for health policy. *Annals of Internal Medicine, 140*(11), 951–957.

Chua, H. F., Chen, W., & Park, D. C. (2006). Source memory, aging and culture. *Gerontology, 52*(5), 306–313.

Cosway, R., Strachan, M. W., Dougall, A., Frier, B. M., & Deary, I. J. (2001). Cognitive function and information processing in type 2 diabetes. *Diabetic Medicine, 18*(10), 803–810.

Cramer, J. A. (2004). A systematic review of adherence with medications for diabetes. *Diabetes Care, 27*(5), 1218–1224.

Den Heijer, T., Launer, L. J., Prins, N. D., van Dijk, E. J., Vermeer, S. E., Hofman, A., et al. (2005). Association between blood pressure, white matter lesions, and atrophy of the medial temporal lobe. *Neurology, 64*(2), 263–267.

Dey, J., Misra, A., Desai, N. G., Mahapatra, A. K., & Padma, M. V. (1997). Cognitive function in younger type II diabetes. *Diabetes Care, 20*(1), 32–35.

Dunbar-Jacob, J., & Mortimer-Stephens, M. K. (2001). Treatment adherence in chronic disease. *Journal of Clinical Epidemiology, 54*(12, Suppl. 1), S57–S60.

Fan, T., Koro, C. E., Fedder, D. O., & Bowlin, S. J. (2006). Ethnic disparities and trends in glycemic control among adults with type 2 diabetes in the U.S. from 1988 to 2002. *Diabetes Care, 29*(8), 1924–1925.

Fillenbaum, G. G., Hanlon, J. T., Landerman, L. R., Artz, M. B., O'Connor, H., Dowd, B., et al. (2004). Impact of inappropriate drug use on health services utilization among representative older community-dwelling residents. *American Journal of Geriatric Pharmacotherapy, 2*(2), 92–101.

Fishman, P., Von Korff, M., Lozano, P., & Hecht, J. (1997). Chronic care costs in managed care. *Health Affairs, 16*(3), 239–247.

Fontbonne, A., Berr, C., Ducimetiere, P., & Alperovitch, A. (2001). Changes in cognitive abilities over a 4-year period are unfavorably affected in elderly diabetic subjects: Results of the Epidemiology of Vascular Aging Study. *Diabetes Care, 24*(2), 366–370.

Gilmer, T. P., O'Connor, P. J., Rush, W. A., Crain, A. L., Whitebird, R. R., Hanson, A. M., et al. (2005). Predictors of health care costs in adults with diabetes. *Diabetes Care, 28*(1), 59–64.

Gispen, W. H., & Biessels, G. J. (2000). Cognition and synaptic plasticity in diabetes mellitus. *Trends Neurosciences, 23*(11), 542–549.

Gutchess, A. H., Yoon, C., Luo, T., Feinberg, F., Hedden, T., Jing, Q., et al. (2006). Categorical organization in free recall across culture and age. *Gerontology, 52*(5), 314–323.

Harris, M. I., Klein, R., Welborn, T. A., & Knuiman, M. W. (1992). Onset of NIDDM occurs at least 4–7 yr before clinical diagnosis. *Diabetes Care, 15*(7), 815–819.

Hinkin, C. H., Castellon, S. A., Durvasula, R. S., Hardy, D. J., Lam, M. N., Mason, K. I., et al. (2002). Medication adherence among HIV+ adults: Effects of cognitive dysfunction and regimen complexity. *Neurology, 59*(12), 1944–1950.

Ho, P. M., Rumsfeld, J. S., Masoudi, F. A., McClure, D. L., Plomondon, M. E., Steiner, J. F., et al. (2006). Effect of medication nonadherence on hospitalization and mortality among patients with diabetes mellitus. *Archives of Internal Medicine, 166*(17), 1836–1841.

Hofman, A., Ott, A., Breteler, M. M., Bots, M. L., Slooter, A. J., van Harskamp, F., et al. (1997). Atherosclerosis, apolipoprotein E, and prevalence of dementia and Alzheimer's Disease in the Rotterdam Study. *Lancet, 349*(9046), 151–154.

Hu, G., Sarti, C., Jousilahti, P., Peltonen, M., Qiao, Q., Antikainen, R., et al. (2005). The impact of history of hypertension and type 2 diabetes at baseline on the incidence of stroke and stroke mortality. *Stroke, 36*(12), 2538–2543.

Hultsch, D. F., Hammer, M., & Small, B. J. (1993). Age differences in cognitive performance in later life: Relationships to self-reported health and activity life style. *Journal of Gerontology, 48,* 1–11.

Hutchison, L. C., Jones, S. K., West, D. S., & Wei, J. Y. (2006). Assessment of medication management by community-living elderly persons with two standardized assessment tools: A cross-sectional study. *American Journal of Geriatric Pharmacotherapy, 4*(2), 144–153.

Insel, K., Morrow, D., Brewer, B., & Figueredo, A. (2006). Executive function, working memory, and medication adherence among older adults. *Journal of Gerontology: Psychological Sciences and Social Sciences, 61*(2), P102–P107.

Jeste, S. D., Patterson, T. L., Palmer, B. W., Dolder, C. R., Goldman, S., & Jeste, D. V. (2003). Cognitive predictors of medication adherence among middle-aged and older outpatients with schizophrenia. *Schizophrenia Research, 63*(1–2), 49–58.

Kalichman, S. C., Cain, D., Fuhrel, A., Eaton, L., Di Fonzo, K., & Ertl, T. (2005). Assessing medication adherence self-efficacy among low-literacy patients: Development of a pictographic visual analogue scale. *Health Education Research, 20*(1), 224–235.

Kilander, L., Nyman, H., Boberg, M., Hansson, L., & Lithell, H. (1998). Hypertension is related to cognitive impairment: A 20-year follow-up of 999 men. *Hypertension, 31*(3), 780–786.

King, H., Aubert, R. E., & Herman, W. H. (1998). Global burden of diabetes, 1995–2025: Prevalence, numerical estimates, and projections. *Diabetes Care, 21*(9), 1414–1431.

Knopman, D., Boland, L. L., Mosley, T., Howard, G., Liao, D., Szklo, M., et al. (2001). Cardiovascular risk factors and cognitive decline in middle-aged adults. *Neurology, 56*(1), 42–48.

Koro, C. E., Bowlin, S. J., Bourgeois, N., & Fedder, D. O. (2004). Glycemic control from 1988 to 2000 among U.S. adults diagnosed with type 2 diabetes: A preliminary report. *Diabetes Care, 27*(1), 17–20.

Kripalani, S., Henderson, L. E., Chiu, E. Y., Robertson, R., Kolm, P., & Jacobson, T. A. (2006). Predictors of medication self-management skill in a low-literacy population. *Journal of General Internal Medicine, 21*(8), 852–856.

Kumari, M., & Marmot, M. (2005). Diabetes and cognitive function in a middle-aged cohort: Findings from the Whitehall II study. *Neurology, 65*(10), 1597–1603.

Kuo, Y. F., Raji, M. A., Markides, K. S., Ray, L. A., Espino, D. V., & Goodwin, J. S. (2003). Inconsistent use of diabetes medications, diabetes complications, and mortality in older Mexican Americans over a 7-year period: Data from the Hispanic established population for the epidemiologic study of the elderly. *Diabetes Care, 26*(11), 3054–3060.

Lezak, M. D. (1995). *Neuropsychological assessment* (3rd ed.). New York: Oxford University Press.

Logroscino, G., Kang, J. H., & Grodstein, F. (2004). Prospective study of type 2 diabetes and cognitive decline in women aged 70–81 years. *British Medical Journal, 328*(7439), 548.

Luchsinger, J. A., Reitz, C., Patel, B., Tang, M.-X., Manly, J. J., & Mayeux, R. (2007). Relation of diabetes to mild cognitive impairment. *Archives of Neurology, 64*(4), 570–575.

Maddigan, S. L., Farris, K. B., Keating, N., Wiens, C. A., & Johnson, J. A. (2003). Predictors of older adults' capacity for medication management in a self-medication program: A retrospective chart review. *Journal of Aging and Health, 15*(2), 332–352.

McDonald, H. P., Garg, A. X., & Haynes, R. B. (2002). Interventions to enhance patient adherence to medication prescriptions: Scientific review. *JAMA, 288*(22), 2868–2879.

Miyake, A., Friedman, N. P., Rettinger, D. A., Shah, P., & Hegarty, M. (2001). How are visuospatial working memory, executive functioning, and spatial abilities related? A latent-variable analysis. *Journal of Experimental Psychology: General, 130*(4), 621–640.

Morris, A. D. (2001). The reality of type 2 diabetes treatment today. *International Journal of Clinical Practice, 1,* 32–35.

Morrow-Howell, N., Hinterlong, J., Rozario, P. A., & Tang, F. (2003). Effects of volunteering on the well-being of older adults. *Journal of Gerontology: Psychological Sciences and Social Sciences, 58*(3), S137–S145.

Norris, S. L., Engelgau, M. M., & Narayan, K. M. (2001). Effectiveness of self-management training in type 2 diabetes: A systematic review of randomized controlled trials. *Diabetes Care, 24*(3), 561–587.

O'Connor, P. J. (2006). Improving medication adherence: Challenges for physicians, payers, and policy makers. *Archives of Internal Medicine, 166*(17), 1802–1804.

Okuno, J., Yanagi, H., & Tomura, S. (2001). Is cognitive impairment a risk factor for poor compliance among Japanese elderly in the community? *European Journal of Clinical Pharmacology, 57*(8), 589–594.

Ott, A., Stolk, R. P., Hofman, A., van Harskamp, F., Grobbee, D. E., & Breteler, M. M. (1996). Association of diabetes mellitus and dementia: the Rotterdam Study. *Diabetologia, 39*(11), 1392–1397.

Ott, A., Stolk, R. P., van Harskamp, F., Pols, H. A., Hofman, A., & Breteler, M. M. (1999). Diabetes mellitus and the risk of dementia: The Rotterdam Study. *Neurology, 53*(9), 1937–1942.

Park, D., & Gutchess, A. (2002). Aging, cognition, and culture: A neuroscientific perspective. *Neuroscience & Biobehavioral Reviews, 26*(7), 859–867.

Park, D., & Gutchess, A. (2006). The cognitive neuroscience of aging and culture. *Current Directions in Psychological Science, 15*(3), 105–108.

Park, D. C., Lautenschlager, G., Hedden, T., Davidson, N. S., Smith, A. D., & Smith, P. K. (2002). Models of visuospatial and verbal memory across the adult life span. *Psychology and Aging, 17*(2), 299–320.

Paterson, D. L., Swindells, S., Mohr, J., Brester, M., Vergis, E. N., Squier, C., et al. (2000). Adherence to protease inhibitor therapy and outcomes in patients with HIV infection. *Annals of Internal Medicine, 133*(1), 21–30.

Peila, R., Rodriguez, B. L., & Launer, L. J. (2002). Type 2 diabetes, APOE gene, and the risk for dementia and related pathologies: The Honolulu-Asia Aging Study. *Diabetes, 51*(4), 1256–1262.

Perlmuter, L. C., Hakami, M. K., Hodgson-Harrington, C., Ginsberg, J., Katz, J., Singer, D. E., et al. (1984). Decreased cognitive function in aging non-insulin-dependent diabetic patients. *American Journal of Medicine, 77*(6), 1043–1048.

Perneczky, R., Pohl, C., Sorg, C., Hartmann, J., Komossa, K., Alexopoulos, P., et al. (2006). Complex activities of daily living in mild cognitive impairment: Conceptual and diagnostic issues. *Age and Ageing, 35*(3), 240–245.

Piette, J. D., Heisler, M., Ganoczy, D., McCarthy, J. F., & Valenstein, M. (2007). Differential medication adherence among patients with schizophrenia and comorbid diabetes and hypertension. *Psychiatric Services, 58*(2), 207–212.

Poncelet, A. N. (2003). Diabetic polyneuropathy. Risk factors, patterns of presentation, diagnosis, and treatment. *Geriatrics, 58*(6), 16–18, 24–15, 30.

Ratner, R. E. (2001). Glycemic control in the prevention of diabetic complications. *Clinical Cornerstone, 4*(2), 24–37.

Rogers, E. S., Wallace, L. S., & Weiss, B. D. (2006). Misperceptions of medical understanding in low-literacy patients: Implications for cancer prevention. *Cancer Control, 13*(3), 225–229.

Roth, G. S., Mattison, J. A., Ottinger, M. A., Chachich, M. E., Lane, M. A., & Ingram, D. K. (2004). Aging in rhesus monkeys: Relevance to human health interventions. *Science, 305*(5689), 1423–1426.

Ryan, C. M., & Geckle, M. O. (2000). Circumscribed cognitive dysfunction in middle-aged adults with type 2 diabetes. *Diabetes Care, 23*(10), 1486–1493.

Safeer, R. S., Cooke, C. E., & Keenan, J. (2006). The impact of health literacy on cardiovascular disease. *Vascular Health and Risk Management, 2*(4), 457–464.

Salas, M., In't Veld, B. A., van der Linden, P. D., Hofman, A., Breteler, M., & Stricker, B. H. (2001). Impaired cognitive function and compliance with antihypertensive drugs in elderly: The Rotterdam Study. *Clinical Pharmacology & Therapeutics, 70*(6), 561–566.

Salthouse, T. A. (1996). The processing-speed theory of adult age differences in cognition. *Psychology Review, 103*(3), 403–428.

Schillinger, D., Grumbach, K., Piette, J., Wang, F., Osmond, D., Daher, C., et al. (2002). Association of health literacy with diabetes outcomes. *Journal of the American Medical Association, 288*(4), 475–482.

Shenolikar, R. A., Balkrishnan, R., Camacho, F. T., Whitmire, J. T., & Anderson, R. T. (2006). Race and medication adherence in Medicaid enrollees with type-2 diabetes. *Journal of the National Medical Association, 98*(7), 1071–1077.

Sieck, G. C. (2003). Physiology of aging. *Journal of Applied Physiology, 95*(4), 1333–1334.

Small, G. W., Silverman, D. H., Siddarth, P., Ercoli, L. M., Miller, K. J., Lavretsky, H., et al. (2006). Effects of a 14-day healthy longevity lifestyle program on cognition and brain function. *American Journal of Geriatric Psychiatry, 14*(6), 538–545.

Stearne, M., Palmer, S., Hammersley, M., Franklin, S., Spivey, R., & Levy, J., et al. (1998). Tight blood pressure control and risk of macrovascular and microvascular complications in type 2 diabetes: UKPDS 38. UK Prospective Diabetes Study Group. *British Medical Journal, 317*(7160), 703–713.

Stewart, R., & Liolitsa, D. (1999). Type 2 diabetes mellitus, cognitive impairment and dementia. *Diabetic Medicine, 16*(2), 93–112.

Strachan, M. W., Deary, I. J., Ewing, F. M., & Frier, B. M. (1997). Is type II diabetes associated with an increased risk of cognitive dysfunction? A critical review of published studies. *Diabetes Care, 20*(3), 438–445.

Tabert, M. H., Albert, S. M., Borukhova-Milov, L., Camacho, Y., Pelton, G., & Liu, X. (2002). Functional deficits in patients with mild cognitive impairment: Prediction of AD. *Neurology, 58*(5), 758–764.

Vik, S. A., Hogan, D. B., Patten, S. B., Johnson, J. A., Romonko-Slack, L., & Maxwell, C. J. (2006). Medication nonadherence and subsequent risk of hospitalisation and mortality among older adults. *Drugs and Aging, 23*(4), 345–356.

Von Dras, D. D., & Blumenthal, H. T. (2000). Biological, social-environmental, and psychological dialecticism: An integrated model of aging. *Basic and Applied Social Psychology, 22*(3), 199–212.

Waldstein, S. R. (2003). The relation of hypertension to cognitive function. *Current Directions in Psychological Science, 12*(1), 9–13.

Welsh, B., & Wecker, L. (1991). Effects of streptozotocin-induced diabetes on acetylcholine metabolism in rat brain. *Neurochemistry Research, 16*(4), 453–460.

Whitehead, D. (2001). A social cognitive model for health education/health promotion practice. *Journal of Advanced Nursing, 36*(3), 417–425.

Winograd, C. H. (1984). Mental status tests and the capacity for self-care. *Journal of the American Geriatric Society, 32*(1), 49–55.

Zimmet, P., Alberti, K. G., & Shaw, J. (2001). Global and societal implications of the diabetes epidemic. *Nature, 414*(6865), 782–787.

Lifestyle Change and Adherence: The Broader Context

Section 7

Sally A. Shumaker
Editor

As discussed throughout this volume, obstacles to adherence may arise from a number of factors, including individual differences; the complexity of a particular regimen; behavioral or biological disincentives to changing behaviors; poor communication between individuals and their health providers; public policies and social contexts that reinforce negative health behaviors; and the complex needs of specific populations. Furthermore, though improving, there is a persistent inadequacy in the theoretical models used to help investigators frame questions and to assist them in better understanding adherence and behavior change. Also, defining, measuring, and interpreting information about adherence continues to be a formidable challenge for both researchers and health providers. In spite of these problems, however, there is an implicit assumption throughout this book that better adherence is almost always worth pursuing and will usually result in improved health outcomes for most individuals. Thus, our focus to this point has been on identifying and pursuing methods to enhance adherence and the adoption and maintenance of healthy behaviors.

In this final section—expanded from the earlier edition—the authors step back from the assumption that adherence is prima facie good and should be relentlessly pursued by both consumers and health care providers. They consider the possible unintended consequences of good adherence, who in society is ultimately responsible for health behavior changes, the underlying ethical issues inherent in the contracts between health providers and their patients, how much adherence is actually enough, and, after several years now of investigating interventions to enhance adherence, what we have actually learned.

Updating their chapter from the earlier edition, Czajkowski, Chesney, and Smith discuss the potential consequences of adherence in experimental studies that include placebo and treatment groups in the chapter "Adherence and the Placebo Effect." They consider how various factors, including one's belief in the efficacy of treatment, can produce treatment-like effects in the placebo condition. Further, this placebo effect is strengthened by adherence. These authors suggest that as long as the placebo effect is treated as a nuisance variable rather than as a real phenomenon worthy of study in its own right, differences in adherence rates between treatment and placebo groups may lead to incorrect interpretations of data and, ultimately, inaccurate recommendations for clinical care. Health care providers may be underutilizing the strength of personal commitment embodied in the placebo effect to improve health. Czajkowski, Chesney, and Smith describe several models to explain the placebo effect and discuss its implications for clinical research and for assumptions regarding treatment efficacy.

In "Collaboration Between Professionals and Mediating Structures in the Community: Social Determinants of Health and Community-Based Participatory Research," Cashman and Forlano provide an updated and expanded perspective from the chapter in the earlier edition by Ribisl and Humphreys. In the earlier chapter, Ribisl and Humphrey described a "third path" between individual and social responsibility for health status in which collaboration with organizations and institutions is critical. Cashman and Forlano build on this framework and consider the powerful means for effecting change embodied in taking into account the social determinants of health (SDOH), coupled with the methods available within community-based participatory research (CBPR). The authors argue that SDOH provides a philosophical underpinning for action that is directed toward transforming power relations from ones that permit inequity and injustice to ones that promote equity. In the section on SDOH Cashman and Forlano provide a definition of the concept and supporting evidence of its impact on health behaviors. In addition, they consider how SDOH can influence inequalities in health care, and they update the reader on current research, barriers to investigating and impacting SDOH, and actions that can be taken within this area. Complementing SDOH, the authors describe CBPR as a method that can be used to build productive partnerships. They provide a current definition of this concept and the methods implied in conducting research from a CBPR perspective. In addition, they consider the relative strengths of CBPR, the limits and challenges to applying it to health related research, and how CBPR can be used to enhance sustained health behavior changes. The authors provide a compelling and innovative approach to the complex systems in which health behaviors exist—a natural addition to the several chapters within the volume that approach adherence and health behavior change and maintenance from a systems or social ecological model.

In her chapter on "Ethical Issues in Lifestyle Change and Adherence," King expands on and updates the chapter by Faden in the earlier editions of this book. Providing an in-depth and critical analysis of the degree to which ethics help frame the factors that underlie adherence and health behavior change, King examines issues in lifestyle change and adherence from the perspective of normative ethics—the moral theory addressing the way individuals, institutions, or societies ought to act. She discusses the key moral issues related to lifestyle change and adherence in each of four relationships, and describes the emerging relevant principles and rules as each relationship is discussed. These relationships include the ethics of the health professional-patient relationship; the ethics of the researcher-subject relationship; the ethics of the government-citizenry relationship; and the ethics of the payer-client relationship. Finally, King cautions the reader about the critical distinction between adherence in the clinical setting versus lifestyle changes for the general public, and the blurring of these two heretofore clearly distinct domains as the tendency to medicalize nondisease states (e.g., prediabetic, estrogen deficient) is becoming a more common strategy used to persuade healthy individuals to change behaviors or take preventive medications. This chapter underscores the complex ethical aspects that are critical to our consideration of how and when we attempt to alter human behavior, and what defines good for the individual and the society at large.

In a new chapter to this third edition of the book, Haskard, DiMatteo, and Williams ask the provocative question "Adherence and Health Outcomes—How Much Does Adherence Matter?" In addressing this question, the authors consider what they define as the ultimate issue regarding the efficacy of adherence—does it improve health outcomes? They then provide a critical review of the evidence linking adherence rates to health improvements across a number of diseases and conditions including CVD, cancer, HIV, diabetes, transplant patients, and depression. Further, they explore differences in the link between adherence and health status among adults and pediatric populations. Haskard et al. review the methodological issues, mediating factors, and various interventions to enhance adherence as they explore the fundamental issue of whether or not adherence enhances health. In general, they provide convincing data on the basic premise that people do better when they adhere to pharmacological and behavioral treatments. However, as noted by the authors, optimum rates of adherence with specific conditions are less clear, thus leading to ambiguity regarding ideal treatment protocols and clinical care recommendations. This chapter provides an excellent grounding in the key meaning of adherence and brings the reader back to some fundamental questions in this area of research.

Since the previous edition of our book, a number of efforts have been undertaken to enhance treatment adherence and health behavior change, with varying degrees of success. In this final and new chapter, Bowen and Boehmer consider the "Lessons Learned: What We Know Doesn't Work and What We

Shouldn't Repeat." They divide their chapter into two sets of "don'ts." The first set relates to what has been learned within specific lines of research. Through specific examples from research, they consider issues such as focusing too much on the individual and not enough on the environment, overgeneralizing from one group to another, making assumptions about mechanisms without the support of science, and the critical differences between changing and maintaining behavior. In the second set of "don'ts," Bowen and Boehmer consider issues related to the process of doing research. Here they provide provocative evidence of the consequences that occur in terms of compromised science when health behavior researchers enter a study as an afterthought. In addition, they provide several vivid examples of the contradictions that occur between public policy and evidence-based health care practices—a fitting cautionary end note to the complex arena embodied in this text on health behavior change and maintenance.

Adherence and the Placebo Effect

36

Susan M. Czajkowski,
Margaret A. Chesney,
and Ashley W. Smith

Traditionally, adherence has been viewed as a critical element in the success of a treatment or health regimen, for without it patients may not receive the full benefits of treatment. Given the importance of adherence to treatment success, other chapters in this volume focus on factors that *predict* or influence adherence to a specific treatment and on strategies for increasing adherence. In contrast, in this chapter we consider adherence from another perspective: the potential *effects* of adherence on treatment effectiveness and health outcomes.

A series of studies has found that, across a range of diseases and treatments, patients who demonstrate better adherence to *either* an active treatment *or* to a placebo have better health outcomes and, in particular, lower mortality, than those who have poorer adherence. The mortality benefits associated with adherence to placebo have been explained in two ways: first, as resulting from biases inherent in performing analyses based on patient responses (such as adherence) in randomized clinical trials, and, second, as reflecting a "healthy adherer" effect in which the act of adherence is a marker for a set of healthy behaviors, such as healthy diet, physical activity, and adherence to other medications and regimens, that are themselves responsible for the lower mortality risk. While acknowledging the merit of these explanations, we propose an additional explanation for the consistent finding of an placebo adherence-mortality relationship: that, in addition to its role in maximizing the *active, specific* effects of the treatment, adherence may also increase treatment effectiveness by activating nonspecific or *placebo* effects that influence treatment success. Thus, the mere act of adhering to a treatment regimen may in itself produce positive health outcomes, regardless of the actual efficacy of the intervention, because of a placebo effect.

We begin with a brief review of studies documenting an association between adherence to treatment and health outcomes. We then outline a hypothetical model of the role adherence may play in enhancing the nonspecific, or placebo, effects of an intervention and thus in affecting treatment outcome. A brief overview of placebo effects is presented, including a discussion of possible mechanisms through which placebos exert their influence. Applying the model, we then suggest an explanation for why adherence to a treatment may enhance a placebo response and, finally, discuss implications of the model for both clinical applications and research.

The Relationship of Adherence to Treatment Outcome

A number of studies have now documented an association between adherence, to either active treatment or placebo, and health outcomes. Good adherence to either treatment or placebo has been associated with benefit, and poor adherence with negative effects, in studies of treatments for myocardial infarction (Coronary Drug Project Research Group, 1980; Verter & Friedman, 1984; Horwitz et al., 1990); congestive heart failure (Granger et al., 2005); arrhythmias (Irvine et al., 1999); cancer (Dolin et al., 1982; Pizzo et al., 1983); and schizophrenia (Pledger, 1992), as well as in studies of preventive therapies for cardiovascular disease and cancer (e.g., the Physicians Health Study, a primary prevention trial of aspirin alternating with beta carotene; Glynn, Buring, Manson, LaMotte, & Hennekens, 1994). A recent meta-analysis of 21 studies (46,847 participants) that included eight clinical trials with placebo arms (19,633 participants) showed that good adherence to placebo was associated with lower mortality (odds ratio 0.56, 95% confidence interval 0.43 to 0.74) than poor adherence to placebo, as was good adherence to beneficial drug therapy (0.55, 0.49 to 0.62; Simpson et al., 2006).

In one of the earliest studies to document this effect, the Coronary Drug Project (CDP) (Coronary Drug Project Research Group, 1980), male patients who had experienced a myocardial infarction within 3 months of study entry were randomly assigned to either a condition in which they received clofibrate or to a placebo control group. The results showed no significant difference in 5-year mortality between the two groups: for the 1,103 men treated with clofibrate,

36.1 The Influence of Adherence on 5-Year Mortality Rates in the Coronary Drug Project		
Treatment group		
Adherence	Clofibrate	Placebo
Good adherers (> 80% adherence)	15.0% (15.7)[a]	15.1% (16.4)
Poor adherers (< 80% adherence)	24.6% (22.5)	28.2% (25.8)

Note. From "Influence of Adherence to Treatment and Response of Cholesterol on Mortality in the Coronary Drug Project," by The Coronary Drug Project Research Group, 1980, *The New England Journal of Medicine, 8,* pp. 1038–1041. Copyright 1980 by The Massachusetts Medical Society. Reprinted with permission of The Massachusetts Medical Society.
[a]The figures in parentheses are adjusted for 40 baseline characteristics.

5-year mortality was 20%; for the 2,789 men given placebo, it was 20.9%. Further analyses performed to determine whether adherence to clofibrate influenced 5-year mortality showed that good adherers (defined as patients who took 80% or more of the drug during the 5-year follow-up period) had a significantly lower 5-year mortality (15%) than did poor adherers (24.6%). However, this was true for those receiving the placebo as well; good adherers to placebo had significantly lower mortality than poor adherers to placebo (15.1% for good adherers and 28.2% for poor adherers). Furthermore, this effect held even when multivariate statistical methods were used to adjust for baseline differences between the two groups on 40 variables that were related to 5-year mortality (e.g., indices of disease severity, use of hypertensive medication; see Table 36.1).

In the CDP, flaws in the way adherence was measured may account for the relationship found between adherence and mortality. Adherence was determined by physician estimates of the number of pills taken by patients each day. These estimates were based not only on the number of pills returned by patients at their clinic visits but also on physicians' interviews in which patients were questioned about problems with the medication, including side effects, that may have affected adherence to the regimen. Because of the subjective nature of the latter measure of adherence, assessments of patients' adherence may have been influenced by physicians' assessments of the health of individual patients. Thus, the healthier patients may have been assigned to the high-adherence group, and their lower mortality rate may have simply reflected this bias in assignment to the adherence "condition."

However, similar results have been found in other studies using more objective measures of adherence. For example, in the Aspirin Myocardial Infarction Study (AMIS), in which adherence was assessed using three different measures (pill count, urine salicylate, and platelet aggregation), lower mortality rates were found for good adherers to the aspirin treatment (6.1%) and to placebo (5.1%) than for poor adherers to either aspirin (21.9%) or placebo (22%). An analysis of the relationship of adherence to mortality in the Beta-Blocker Heart Attack Trial (BHAT) also found good adherers to have better health outcomes than poor adherers: patients who demonstrated poor adherence, whether assigned to treatment or placebo, were twice as likely to die within 1 year of follow-up as patients with good adherence (Horwitz et al., 1990). Other studies demonstrating this effect include trials of antibiotic prophylaxis to reduce fever or infection in cancer patients (Dolin et al., 1982; Pizzo et al., 1983) and a trial of chlorpromazine versus placebo in schizophrenic patients (Pledger, 1992).

These results have most often been used to demonstrate the problems associated with analyzing clinical trial data on adherence using subgroups on the basis of patient responses, since individuals who demonstrate good adherence may differ from poor adherers on any number of variables that may also cause differences in mortality (Coronary Drug Project Research Group, 1980; Friedman, Furberg, & DeMets, 1996). Perhaps the healthier patients in these studies were better able to tolerate the medication and so adhered better to it, while the sicker patients were less able to tolerate it and so discontinued using it. Alternatively, the results of these studies have been explained as reflecting a "healthy adherer" effect, in which good adherence is considered a marker for an overall healthy lifestyle and poor adherence may reflect adverse health behaviors, habits, or characteristics (Simpson et al., 2006). For example, the poor adherers in studies such as the CDP may have been individuals who exhibited some unmeasured (and therefore unadjusted for) adverse behavior or characteristic (e.g., psychiatric conditions, drug or alcohol abuse) that caused them to be negligent about taking their medication. If these individuals were also less healthy than adherers, which might be expected, their survival rates over the 5-year follow-up period would be lower than those in the "high-adherence" group. In this case, both adherence and mortality would result from a third, unmeasured variable—such as psychiatric condition or alcohol/drug abuse—and would actually be unrelated to each other when that third variable was controlled.

Many of the studies cited here used multivariate analyses to control for sociodemographic, medical, psychosocial, lifestyle, and other health-related factors that might account for the adherence-mortality relationship in an attempt to determine the variable or variables that underlie this relationship (Coronary Drug Project Research Group, 1980; Glynn et al., 1994; Granger et al., 2005; Horwitz et al., 1990; Irvine et al., 1999). Adjustment for these variables, including medical history, various indices of disease severity, psychosocial factors such as stress, and unhealthy behaviors such as smoking and alcohol use did not appreciably weaken the adherence-mortality association. Nevertheless, it is possible that some key explanatory variable was not measured and therefore not able to be used in the adjusted analyses. For example, Kellet (1990) suggests that depression, which has been independently associated with mortality in coronary artery disease and myocardial infarction patients (Barth, Schumacher, & Herrmann-Lingen, 2004; Carney & Freedland, 2003; Frasure-Smith, Lesperance, & Talajic, 1993; Glassman & Shapiro, 1998; van Melle et al., 2004) and with adherence to cardiovascular treatment regimens, cardiac risk factor modification, and cardiac rehabilitation (Blumenthal, Williams, Wallace, Williams, & Needles, 1982; Guiry, Conroy, Hickey, & Mulcahy, 1987; Kronish et al., 2006; Rieckmann et al., 2006), may have contributed to both low levels of adherence and higher mortality in the heart disease treatment trials (AMIS, CDP, and BHAT).

A recent study calls into question the extent to which a "healthy adherer" effect is responsible for the relationship between adherence (whether to active drug treatment or placebo) and positive health outcomes, including survival (Rasmussen, Chong, & Alter, 2007). In this longitudinal study of a large (N = 31,455) cohort of elderly patients with acute myocardial infarction (MI), adherence to evidence-based therapies for MI (based on pharmacy refill records) was associated in dose-response fashion to mortality, with high adherers to beta-blockers and statins at lowest risk for mortality, moderate adherers to these drugs at higher risk, and low adherers at greatest risk. However, this graded relationship was not found for calcium channel blockers, which have not been shown to improve post-MI survival. One might expect that, if a placebo-adherence relationship exists, adherence to a non-evidence-based (and therefore, presumably, noneffective, at least in terms of mortality) therapy would show the same kind of graded, dose-response relationship with mortality as would adherence to a biologically active therapy. However, there are several differences between the Rasmussen et al. (2007) study and the placebo-controlled trials finding placebo-adherence effects. The main difference is that the Rasmussen et al. (2007) study is a longitudinal cohort study of a group of elderly patients seen in clinical practice settings, rather than a placebo-controlled trial. There are many differences between patients who volunteer to participate in a clinical trial and those being seen in clinical practice that may account for the discrepant findings, including health status, health-related behaviors, and even expectations about treatment effectiveness. Other differences include the use of pharmacy refill data in the Rasmussen et al. (2007) study (rather than pill counts, which are the primary adherence measures used in the clinical trials) and analyses using survival curves in the Rasmussen et al. (2007) study (rather than simple percentages of patients who survived in the active treatment and placebo groups in the studies that showed a placebo-adherence effect). Thus, while the Rasmussen et al. (2007) findings raise questions about healthy adherer effects and placebo-based adherence, too many methodological and analytic differences exist between their study and the clinical trials that find such placebo-adherence effects to rule out the existence of either of these phenomena.

Of clinical trials, however, at least two studies have failed to find a relationship between adherence to placebo and health outcomes. In the Lipid Research Clinics-Coronary Primary Prevention Trial (LRC-CPPT), a primary prevention trial of cholesterol lowering as a way to reduce coronary heart disease risk, no evidence of a relationship between adherence to placebo and fatal or nonfatal MI (the primary outcome) was found after adjustment for baseline measures of risk, including serum lipid levels (Lipid Research Clinics Program, 1984). And no relationship between placebo adherence and arrhythmic mortality was found in the Cardiac Arrhythmia Suppression Trial (CAST), a three-arm, double-blind, placebo-controlled randomized clinical trial of two anti-arrhythmic agents in patients with ventricular arrhythmias following MI. The trial was stopped early due to increased mortality in the active-treatment arms (encainide and flecainide), and, as expected, adherence to treatment was associated with increased arrhythmic mortality in the active treatment arms, but no association was found for the placebo group (Oblas-Manno et al., 1996). Questions have been raised about the CAST placebo adherence findings, due to problems such as low power (analyses were based on only nine arrhythmic deaths) and the limited nature of the adherence data used (only pill counts from the first follow-up visit were used; Avins, personal communication). In addition, it is interesting to note that of the seven clinical trials that have investigated the association between adherence to placebo and health outcome, the two that did not find an effect were the only trials that did not use total mortality as the primary outcome and the only two to analyze adherence as a continuous variable (Avins, personal communication). Secondary analyses of data are currently under way to examine these and other differences between studies that found the effect and those that have not and to better understand the basis for the relationship between placebo adherence and mortality found in most of the studies.

Apart from their value in justifying intent-to-treat approaches to data analysis in clinical trials, some have argued that the finding of a relationship between placebo adherence and mortality reflects an interesting phenomenon that deserves study in its own right—that the act of adherence itself may enhance psychosocial characteristics or qualities that generate positive health outcomes (Epstein, 1984; Horwitz & Horwitz, 1993). Epstein (1984) raises the possibility that patient expectations about the efficacy of treatment may play a role in the relationship between adherence and health outcomes found in these studies. Horwitz and colleagues (Horwitz & Horwitz, 1993; Horwitz et al., 1990) suggest that adherence may be a marker not only for a healthy lifestyle but also for a variety of psychological, social, and behavioral variables that may affect the outcomes of treatment (e.g., a patient's ability to control aspects of life that affect disease progression; optimism or resilience in the face of adversity) and recommend further research using more extensive and refined measures of psychosocial and behavioral factors.

We agree that the relationship between adherence and placebo found in these studies may be attributable to bias or to adherence acting as a surrogate for healthy lifestyle behaviors. However, in this chapter we explore the possibility that the act of adherence may affect health outcomes by activating the nonspecific or placebo effects of an intervention. In the next section, we propose a hypothetical model that demonstrates the ways in which adherence might influence treatment outcome via nonspecific effects.

Model: The Nonspecific Effects of Adherence

The model proposed here is one in which adherence to an intervention is seen as enhancing not only the effects of active treatment components but also the effects of nonspecific components of that intervention. Specifically, the model suggests that adherence enhances the following nonspecific components that can influence intervention outcomes: (1) patient and provider *expectancies* of the intervention's success, and (2) the *social support* available to the patient from the provider and others in the patient's environment.

In several chapters in this volume, expectancies and social support have been described as predictors of adherence. The model presented here suggests that these factors may also be "effects" of adherence. Adherence influences the expectancy of treatment success to the extent that patients who follow an intervention develop the expectation that they will experience positive health outcomes. Conversely, patients who do not adhere should have a diminished expectancy of positive outcomes from the intervention. Patient adherence also impacts provider expectancies regarding the outcome of the intervention. For example, a physician is more likely to expect lower serum cholesterol levels in a patient who is adhering to a prescribed low-fat diet than a patient who continues to eat a high-fat diet. Patient adherence may also influence the amount of social support extended to patients by providers and others in the patient's social network, since adhering to a prescribed medical regimen is likely to be rewarded by positive responses from family, friends, and caretakers.

As portrayed in the model, the relationship between adherence and the nonspecific components of treatment is a reciprocal one. Expectancies and social support are affected by adherence and, in turn, influence subsequent adherence. For example, the patient who adheres to the low-fat diet and meets with a physician who expresses a positive expectancy for lower cholesterol levels and praises the patient for adhering is more likely to continue adhering to the prescribed diet.

In the model, expectancy and social support are considered not only in terms of their relationship to adherence but also in terms of their roles as nonspecific factors influencing treatment outcomes. This aspect of the model is based on evidence that these two variables are important in influencing health outcomes (Agras, Horne, & Taylor, 1982; Berkman, Leo-Summers, & Horwitz, 1992; Hovell et al., 1986; Williams et al., 1992). Thus, the perspective added by this model is that the expectancies and social support fostered by adherence may have an affect on health that is independent of any active treatment the patient may receive.

Finally, the literature indicates that nonspecific effects are influenced by some of the same factors known to influence adherence. These factors include patient characteristics (e.g., attitudes toward the provider, self-efficacy, and positive expectancies) and intervention characteristics (e.g., therapeutic setting, provider characteristics, treatment cost, and method of treatment delivery). Figure 36.1 shows these characteristics as having effects on adherence and on nonspecific treatment components; in addition, patient characteristics can directly influence specific treatment effects (e.g., due to individual differences in sensitivity to the therapeutic agent).

Overview of the Placebo Effect

Shapiro and Shapiro (1984, p. 372) define a placebo as "any therapy or component of therapy that is deliberately used for its nonspecific, psychological, or psychophysiological effect, or that is used for its presumed specific effect but is without specific activity for the condition being treated." A placebo effect is defined as "the psychological or psychophysiological effect produced by placebos" (Shapiro & Shapiro, 1984, p. 372). This definition implies that active treatments may have placebo components and that the effects of specific therapies (i.e., nonplacebos) are often due to both placebo and nonplacebo effects (Shapiro & Shapiro, 1984).

Historically, the term "placebo" has referred to inactive pills or tablets given to control subjects in drug trials. Over time, however, the term "placebo effect" has come to refer to a variety of nonspecific effects on health outcomes that are integrally related to the delivery and monitoring of treatment but that are not attributable to the specific therapeutic agent under study. In this chapter, the terms "placebo" and "nonspecific" are used interchangeably.

36.1

The effects of adherence on health outcomes.

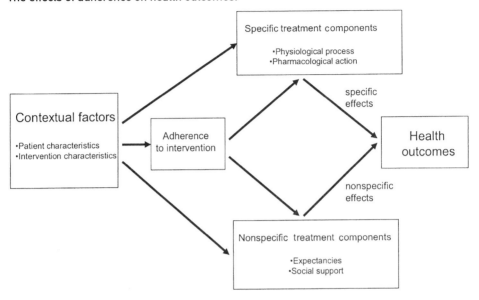

The nonspecific effects of treatments are well documented in the literature on medical and behavioral interventions. Placebo effects have been studied in medical conditions as diverse as pain (Peck & Coleman, 1991); ulcerative colitis (Meyers & Janowitz, 1989) and irritable bowel syndrome (Dobrilla, Imbimbo, Piazzi, & Benzi, 1990); and congestive heart failure (Archer & Leier, 1992; Packer, 1990). Beecher (1955), in his classic review of placebo responses in patients suffering a wide variety of illnesses, found that in 35% of patients (averaged across the studies), symptoms were "satisfactorily relieved" by the placebo.

Placebo effects have received increased attention in clinical trials that have found greater than expected improvements in the health of participants in placebo control groups, in some cases equivalent to or greater than those observed in participants receiving active treatment. In the area of hypertension control, for instance, a number of studies, including the Multiple Risk Factor Intervention Trial (Multiple Risk Factor Intervention Trial Research Group, 1982), the Hypertension Detection and Follow-up Program (Hypertension Detection and Follow-up Program Cooperative Group, 1979), and the Australian National Blood Pressure Study (Management Committee, 1980), found significant and persistent reductions in blood pressure in usual care or placebo control groups. Similar results have been reported in several other studies that compared the effects of behavioral treatments for hypertension (e.g., relaxation training, biofeedback, cognitive restructuring) with the effects of placebo treatment (e.g., flexibility training) or blood pressure monitoring alone (Agras, Taylor, Kraemer, Southam, & Schneider, 1987; Chesney, Black, Swan, & Ward, 1987; Jacob et al., 1986; Ward, Swan, & Chesney, 1987). The results of these studies stimulated inquiry into possible explanations for the significant improvements or changes found for control groups and focused attention on the impact of nonspecific and behavioral factors on control groups in clinical trial research (Kramer & Shapiro, 1984).

It is important to note that in the clinical trials mentioned here, as well as in other studies, nonspecific effects have been demonstrated to involve not only improvements in subjective symptoms but also objectively measured cardio-vascular risk factor and end organ changes (Gould, Davies, Mann, Altman, & Raftery, 1981). Indeed, the physiological effects of placebos are acknowledged as being very powerful: placebos can induce addiction and have been reported to be more effective than, or even to reverse the effects of, some pharmacologic agents (Shapiro & Shapiro, 1984). In addition, the range of physiological processes that have been shown to exhibit placebo effects are very broad and include inhibited gastric acid secretion, reduced adrenocortical activity, and decreased serum lipoproteins (Bush, 1974).

Mechanisms of the Placebo Effect

The recognition that nonspecific treatment components may influence health outcomes raises questions regarding the mechanisms underlying these effects. Placebos are thought to exert their effects through both *psychological* and *biological* mechanisms (Wilkins, 1985).

Psychological Mechanisms

Models that focus on the psychological mechanisms underlying the placebo effect fall into two categories: (1) *learning theory* models, which explain placebo effects as classical conditioning phenomena, and (2) *cognitively oriented* models, which emphasize the role of mental processes, such as expectancy.

Learning Theory Models

Models based on a learning theory approach focus on the placebo effect as a *conditioned response*. According to this explanation, the complex of stimuli surrounding the administration of a drug (e.g., taking a pill) become conditioned stimuli because of their repeated association with drug administration and relief from suffering during the person's developmental history (Wickramasekera, 1985). For example, a patient who derives pain relief from aspirin may eventually respond in a similar fashion to medications with similar characteristics (e.g., small, white pills). Support for the learning theory model involves mostly animal research, which has confirmed the conditioning of physiologic and pharmacologic responses as an important element in placebo phenomena (Ader, 1985). This model is useful in explaining placebo effects associated with the administration of drugs; however, it is less applicable to situations involving nonpharmacologic treatments, such as behavioral or lifestyle interventions.

Cognitive Models

Currently, the most widely accepted cognitively based explanation for the placebo effect is that it is based on people's expectations of therapeutic benefit or success. The expectancy model of placebo effects is similar to an early cognitively based hypothesis that postulated a relationship between people's response to placebo and their suggestibility. However, although it is commonly believed that individuals who score high on measures of suggestibility are more prone to the placebo response, no consistent relationship has been found between this response and either suggestibility or hypnotizability (Evans, 1985).

Another early cognitive model of placebo effects involved anxiety reduction, resulting from an individual's belief in the pain reducing effects of a treatment. According to this model, placebo effects are attributable to decreased perceptions of pain and distress associated with anxiety reduction. This hypothesis was supported by studies showing that for chronically anxious individuals, feelings of reduced anxiety following placebo ingestion lead to a significant increase in pain tolerance (Evans, 1985). While the anxiety-reduction hypothesis addresses the effects of placebos on pain, it does not generalize easily to the many other physiological processes affected by placebos.

More recently, studies have shown that individuals' expectations regarding the effects of a drug or treatment influence their responses to placebo treatments. For example, study participants who received a caffeine placebo and were led to expect improved performance on a psychomotor task showed improved performance relative to participants who received the caffeine placebo and were told they could expect impairment (Fillmore, Mulvihill, & Vogel-Sprott, 1994). Similarly, the belief that alcohol has been consumed and expectations about the effects of alcohol have been shown to influence a variety of responses to consumption of nonalcoholic beverages, including pain reduction (Cutter, Maloof, Kurtz, & Jones, 1976) and alcohol craving (Ludwig, Wikler, & Stark, 1974). Study participants given placebos that were described as analgesics have also reported less pain than no-treatment controls (Liberman, 1964; Gelfand, Ullman, & Krasner, 1963), and the content of placebo instructions has been found to be a powerful influence on study participants' responses to dental pain (Gryll & Katahn, 1978). Other studies have demonstrated changes in physiological responses such as blood pressure and pulse rate based on participants' expectancies about the effects of the placebo being administered (Kirsch & Weixel, 1988). Ross and Olson (1981), in an examination of double-blind drug outcome studies, conclude that participants' expectancies are key determinants of placebo responses and that participants provided placebos will respond in ways that are congruent with expected symptoms or physical responses.

Studies in clinical settings have also shown that responses to treatment are mediated by patient expectancies generated within the therapeutic relationship. In one study, students who expected a relaxation procedure to produce an immediate lowering of blood pressure had significantly lower systolic blood pressures immediately following the procedure than did a group of participants who were led to believe that the relaxation training would produce a delayed effect (Agras et al., 1982). In contrast, Wadden (1984) found no differences in blood pressure reduction between participants assigned to a cognitive therapy condition, which involved a positive expectancy of blood pressure change, and those assigned to relaxation therapy. Results from several other studies, however, suggest that the effects of relaxation therapy may be primarily due to nonspecific factors, such as positive expectancy or social support (Brauer, Horlick, Nelson, Farquhar, & Agras, 1979; Luborsky et al., 1982).

Evidence suggests that the placebo effect is influenced not only by patient expectancies but also by doctor or experimenter expectations. For example, when the physician believes a powerful drug is being used in a double-blind study, the placebo effect is stronger than if he or she believes the medication is less effective (Evans, 1985). Thus, the physician's belief about a drug's efficacy may be communicated to the patient and appears to mediate treatment effectiveness.

An individual's expectations about treatment success may be influenced by a variety of factors. For example, the social support received from family, friends, and health providers may enhance patients' beliefs or expectations about the efficacy of therapy. When a spouse is supportive of the patient's receiving a specific form of therapy, the patient may come to believe that such therapy will be beneficial. The effect of social support from members of a patient's network can be especially powerful when those others are seen as credible sources of information and when the patient has a great deal of faith in them. Plotkin (1985) emphasizes the impact of the patients' faith in the therapist as an important condition for behavioral change to occur in therapy.

The powerful influence of social support on health outcomes, including morbidity and mortality, is now well documented (Berkman et al., 1992; Williams et al., 1992). Given these effects, one might expect that supportive interactions with health care personnel might influence response to treatment. One study demonstrated a positive effect for personalized care, operationalized as greater personal attention and warmth shown to the patient, on blood pressure reduction in hypertensives (Hovell et al., 1986). In this study, patients receiving personalized care differed significantly in the magnitude of their blood pressure reductions from those receiving usual care. Several other studies have documented similar differences in the effects of personalized and usual care, although the mechanisms for such effects remain unknown (Dunbar, Marshall, & Hovell, 1979; Finnerty, Mattie, & Finnerty, 1973). Hovell et al. (1986) have speculated that personalized care may evoke a generalized relaxation response and suggest that future research is needed to determine the mechanisms underlying the effects of social support on blood pressure reduction. One mechanism through which social support may affect cardiovascular health, including the development of hypertension, is through effects on biological processes, such as neuroendocrine or hemodynamic functioning. This hypothesis has received support from a series of studies that have shown that interpersonal support, characterized by the presence of a friend or supportive other during a challenging experimental task, reduces blood pressure reactivity to stress (Christenfeld et al., 1997; Edens, Larkin, & Abel, 1992; Fontana, Diegnan, Villeneuve, & Lepore, 1999; Gerin et al., 1992; Kamarck, Manuck, & Jennings, 1990; Lepore, Allen, & Evans, 1993).

Neurobiological Models

Developments in recent years, particularly in neuroscience and biochemistry, including new tools such as functional magnetic resonance imaging (fMRI) and positron emission tomography (PET), have provided new insights into pathways by which placebos may exert effects. A detailed review of the full range of potential neurobiological mechanisms of the placebo effect that are currently being proposed is beyond the scope of this chapter. Among those most relevant to the issue of adherence and the placebo effect is the evidence that the placebo may activate the endogenous opioid system and the neural circuitry underlying reward mechanisms (Benedetti et al., 2005; Benedetti et al., 2008).

In their original research on placebo analgesia, Levine, Gordon, and Fields (1978) hypothesized that placebo effects resulting in pain reduction are based on expectancies that activate the endorphin system. There is substantial evidence from studies of both clinical and experimentally induced pain that administration of placebo with the expectation of analgesia is associated with reduction in reports of pain that are reversed by either hidden or open administration of naloxone (see Amanzio and Benedetti, 1999; Benedetti, 1996).

The endogenous opioid system and its activation of μ-opioid receptors is thought to be important in animal and human responses to novel and potentially threatening environmental stimuli (Filliol et al., 2000; Zubieta et al., 2003). This neurotransmitter system is implicated in the regulation of neuroendocrine functions, stress responses, emotional states, and pain. (Akil et al., 1984; Sora et al., 1997; Zubieta et al., 2001, 2003).

Using fMRI, researchers found that placebo administered under the condition of expectancy (for pain relief) was associated with reductions in activity of regions of the brain known to be pain-responsive (the rostral anterior cingulate, the insular cortex, and the thalamus) (Wager et al., 2004). Using PET and molecular imaging techniques, Zubieta and his colleagues examined the effects of administration of placebo with expectancy on the activity of the endogenous opioid system on μ-opioid receptors in healthy human volunteers who were exposed to deep sustained muscle pain (Zubieta et al., 2005). To circumvent the activation of antinociceptive (pain-inhibiting) responses to sustained pain, which could interfere with the placebo responses, this team of investigators used an adaptive system that maintained the pain over time by increasing the pain stimulus as volunteer ratings of the pain declined. With this experimental procedure, Zubieta and his research team observed, for the first time, significant placebo-induced neurotransmission in both higher and subcortical brain regions that was mediated by the μ-opioid receptors. This work "takes the investigation of placebo effects directly into the realm of human brain neurotransmission, addressing the function of a single neurotransmitter system" (Zubieta et al., 2005, p. 7759). As noted earlier, the μ-opioid receptor-mediated neurotransmission system is implicated not only in the modulation of pain but also in emotional responses (Zubieta et al., 2003) and stress responses, including those on the cardiovascular system (Akil et al., 1984).

Among the brain regions involved in the μ-opioid receptor-mediated neurotransmission are the pregenual and subgenual rostal anterior cigulate, the dorsolateral prefrontal cortex, the insular cortex, and the nucleus accumbens. This latter region, the nucleus accumbens, responds to anticipated rewards in studies conducted in nonhuman primates and in rodents. It is also a region potentially implicated in the placebo effect in Parkinson's disease, which is thought to be related to placebo-activated dopamine release (de la Fuente-Fernandez et al., 2002, 2004).

On the basis of observations in Parkinson's Disease, de la Fuente-Fernandez and his colleagues proposed the hypothesis that the placebo effect is mediated by activation of the brain circuitry underlying reward mechanisms and linked to the expectation of therapeutic benefit (de la Fuente-Fernandez et al., 2001). Confirmation of this hypothesis is provided by Scott, Zubieta, and their colleagues who, using functional molecular imaging, demonstrated that not only is activation of dopamine release in the nucleus accumbens observed in response to placebo administration but there are individual differences in neurochemical responses (e.g., dopamine release) and psychophysiological responses (pain ratings) that are associated with individual differences in reward expectation processing (Scott et al., 2007).

Returning to the issue of adherence and the placebo effect, participants in trials or patients in clinical practice who adhere to placebos may be more likely to develop greater "reward expectancies" than those who are aware of their own nonadherence. These patients would therefore have greater placebo responses. The earlier discussion suggests that the placebo effect is mediated by neural reward mechanisms and the μ-opioid receptor-mediated neurotransmission system. This neurotransmission system is involved in behavioral and physiological responses to the environment, including the modulation of pain, emotional responses to events, and both psychological and physiological responses to stress. Thus, this proposed mechanism may at least in part explain some of the health-related changes associated with adherence to placebos discussed in this chapter.

Adherence and the Placebo Effect

Returning to the thesis outlined earlier that adherence may activate or enhance placebo effects, how might adherence influence these effects? There are two leading explanations: (1) adherence per se activates nonspecific components of treatment, and (2) certain characteristics of individuals who adhere to a treatment enhance the nonspecific components of treatment.

With the first explanation, given the hypothesis discussed in the previous section that expectancies of therapeutic benefit or success activate placebo effects, then any factor in a therapeutic situation that enhances such expectancies would indirectly influence placebo effects, as well. Adherence to treatment may be one such factor, since adherence is integrally related to patient expectancies in a therapeutic situation.

Patient adherence to treatment is influenced by the expectation that the treatment will produce the desired effect (e.g., lower cholesterol, reduced weight). For example, individuals will be more likely to adhere to a low-calorie diet if they believe that doing so will be effective in producing weight loss *and* if they see themselves as capable of adhering to the diet. Bandura (1977) refers to the former belief as an outcome expectancy (the belief that a given behavior will lead to a particular outcome) and the latter as an efficacy expectation (the belief that "one can successfully execute the behavior required to produce outcomes"). According to Bandura (1977), success in a therapeutic situation is based on the acquisition of expectancies of increased personal effectiveness, or efficacy expectancies. High-efficacy expectancies are related to perseverance at a task (e.g., adherence) and thus to maintenance of therapeutic improvement.

Expectations about treatment effectiveness and one's ability to comply with a treatment are thus important determinants of actual adherence to treatment.

However, as noted earlier, the relationship is reciprocal, since expectancies of success can also be a consequence of complying with treatment: the more one adheres to the treatment regimen, the more likely one is to expect treatment success. By complying with treatment, the patient enhances the expectation that the treatment will work. Adherence may also affect patients' generalized feelings of well-being and increase their expectations that they can control other aspects of their lives, such as health-related behaviors (Epstein, 1984), ultimately leading to changes in these behaviors (e.g., quitting smoking, adhering to other medications, and adopting healthy dietary and exercise regimens). While there are cognitive and social reasons for expecting health behaviors to cluster, few studies have found significant associations among health behaviors, with the exception of the documented link between smoking and alcohol consumption. National and health-plan level data suggest that a very small percentage of the population meets multiple recommended levels of positive health behaviors at once (e.g., Pronk et al., 2004; Berrigan, Dodd, Troiano, Krebs-Smith, & Barbash, 2003). However, there is some evidence that changing one behavior has implications for other behaviors. For example, intervention research has shown that having a more fit lifestyle is associated with improvements in diet (O'Halloran et al., 2001). Similarly, research by King and colleagues (1996) showed that reduced smoking behavior is associated with increased physical activity and that self-efficacy for smoking cessation was significantly associated with self-efficacy for increasing physical activity. It is possible that perceptions of control and more generalized self-efficacy are important mediators of positive health behavior adoption (i.e., change). Expectancies of change and improvement may therefore be important as both antecedents and consequences of adherence.

If this is true, then efforts to increase adherence (especially by enhancing expectancies of treatment success) may increase treatment effectiveness not only because they maximize the extent to which the patient receives active treatment but also because these adherence-induced expectancies activate placebo responses to treatment. In the same way, social support may influence patients' beliefs or expectations about the efficacy of treatment and thus influence nonspecific treatment responses.

The second explanation of how adherence influences placebo effects, that there are certain characteristics of adherers that activate nonspecific components of treatment, may also be based on an expectancy effect. For example, if adherers are more likely to have an enhanced sense of control over events in their lives and are therefore more likely to believe that they can affect their health positively by complying with treatment recommendations, then treatment effectiveness may result primarily from the greater expectancies for treatment success held by these individuals, rather than from the treatment itself. This may be true of behavioral treatments, as well as medical treatments. For example, one recent randomized study showed that the perception of adherence to healthy exercise levels (in the absence of increased workloads) predicted weight loss and other health benefits (Crum & Langer, 2007). In this study, female hotel workers were given information about the benefits of exercise on their health and were then randomized to one of two conditions: one group was told that their housekeeping work satisfied the CDC's recommendations for physical activity, while the other group was not told that their work was good exercise. Those who were told that their work satisfied recommended physical activity levels had improved outcomes (greater weight loss, improved body composition, and re-duced blood pressure) after 4 weeks than did the women who were not told this information. The study authors attributed this change to a placebo effect—that increasing the *perceived* level of exercise alone resulted in health benefits.

While the results of this study are intriguing and merit further investiga-tion, the authors fail to control for or measure differences in the *actual* levels of physical activity of the two groups, which could be the source of the differ-ences found in health benefits between the groups. The authors state that hotel managers reported no alterations in housekeepers' workloads over the 4-week study, but it is possible that the information provided to the "informed" work-ers, that housekeeping is good exercise, stimulated them to alter the *intensity* of their physical activity while working; perhaps applying the label "exercise" to the work they were performing caused them to more vigorously perform that work, resulting in the health benefits that were found. To explore this possibil-ity, the use of accelerometers or other devices to monitor the intensity of work-ers' physical activity, as well as measurement of fitness level before and after the study period for both "informed" and "control" groups, would be required.

Other characteristics that differentiate adherers from nonadherers (e.g., "hardiness" or greater resiliency under stress, optimism) may also be impor-tant determinants of treatment success to the extent that they influence pa-tient expectations regarding treatment outcomes. More adherent individuals may also be more likely to engage in a variety of health-related behaviors, such as adopting healthier diets and exercise regimens and avoiding stressors, than nonadherers. Adoption of these behaviors, which may increase expectations of better health, may also contribute to better medical outcomes in these individu-als. These may have implications for mental health, as well as physical health. For example, one recent intervention among breast cancer survivors found that both a nutrition intervention and a psycho-educational intervention resulted in better physical functioning and fewer depressive symptoms than were found in a group that received standard care (Scheier et al., 2005). The effects of the nutrition intervention were mediated in part by self-efficacy expectations.

Finally, Horwitz and Horwitz (1993) suggest that in individuals with chronic disease, adherence may reflect better adaptation to the stress of illness and an enhanced capability to respond to such stress. This enhanced adaptive response may itself generate both positive health-related behaviors and increased ex-pectancies for treatment success, both of which may result in improvements in health.

Implications and Research Directions

There has been no research to date that adequately tests the model proposed in this chapter concerning the role that adherence may play in enhancing non-specific treatment effects. This may be partly because of the lack of attention paid to nonspecific treatment components in health research. Although placebo effects are acknowledged as being of sufficient importance to necessitate the inclusion of placebo controls in most studies of medical or behavioral interven-tions, biomedical researchers have not made use of the placebo condition as an opportunity to examine and better understand the nonspecific effects of treatment. Instead, placebos have traditionally been viewed as nuisance variables to be controlled for, rather than as variables that are important for study in their own right or as important adjuncts to active treatment (Evans, 1985). This is in contrast to the emphasis on nonspecific factors in psychotherapy outcome studies (Frank, 1971; Garfield, 1980, 1982; Smith, Glass, & Miller, 1980; Stone, Imber, & Frank, 1966). In this literature, psychotherapy researchers have identified a number of nonspecific factors, or "common ingredients," as being important contributors to positive therapy outcomes, regardless of the particular mode of therapy used (Garfield, 1982). The nonspecific factor thought to be most central to therapeutic outcome is the patient's expectation of benefit (Frank, 1961, 1983; Garfield, 1982; Goldstein, 1962), which has also been implicated as an important mechanism underlying placebo effects.

The model presented in this chapter suggests that adherence to treatment may affect health outcomes by enhancing or activating nonspecific effects of treatment (e.g., expectancies, social support). This has important implications for clinical trials and other research studies involving interventions, since there are several situations in which such adherence-induced placebo effects could lead to inaccurate conclusions about treatment efficacy.

As stated earlier, secondary analyses of data by Avins et al. (personal communication) are being conducted to confirm the placebo-adherence effect, to determine conditions under which this effect is likely to occur, and to better understand the basis for the relationship between placebo adherence and mortality that has been found. The results of these analyses should provide important information concerning the existence and nature of this effect.

While placebo control conditions are commonly used in studies involving the evaluation of drug therapies, studies evaluating other types of interventions (especially behavioral or lifestyle interventions) often do not use placebo conditions or use inadequate placebo controls. This is a result of the difficulty of designing a placebo control condition when the treatment is behavioral in nature. When the treatment is pharmacological, it is possible to manufacture a pill that is identical in every respect (e.g., in appearance) to the pharmacological agent being used. But it is often difficult to devise a placebo for a behavioral treatment that is identical to the treatment itself in every way except that it has no active component (Buck & Donner, 1982). Clearly, given the possibility that adherence to an intervention may affect the evaluation of a treatment's effectiveness, the design of placebo conditions for all studies involving patient adherence to some intervention, whether behavioral or pharmacological in nature, should be given serious consideration.

Problems may arise even when adequate placebo controls are used if adherence rates differ between the treatment and the control groups. One reason for different adherence rates that could influence patient expectations regarding treatment success (and therefore affect treatment effectiveness through those expectations) is that some patients receiving treatment who are particularly sensitive to physiological cues and sensations might interpret the presence or absence of such sensations as indicating whether or not they are receiving the active treatment (Wilkins, 1985). Because patients in the active treatment group would be more likely to become "unblinded" in this way, and therefore more likely to adhere to treatment and to expect a successful outcome, it would be difficult to pull apart the actual treatment effect from an expectancy-induced effect. In this case, a more positive outcome for the treatment group could be inaccurately attributed to treatment efficacy when it was actually due to increased expectations of treatment success. This suggests that adherence rates in the treatment and the placebo conditions should always be assessed to rule out the possibility that adherence-induced placebo effects are responsible for any effects found.

The model presented in this chapter has implications not only for the internal validity of studies that involve adherence to interventions but also for the generalizability of such studies. For example, one disadvantage of prerandomization screening (also known as the "run-in" phase of a clinical trial) is that by screening out nonadherers, any effects found for a particular treatment can be generalized only to those individuals who are likely to adhere to a treatment regimen. Since these individuals may have certain psychosocial characteristics that affect their adherence behavior (e.g., high self-efficacy) and that may also affect treatment success, the finding of a treatment effect would be applicable only to a narrow subgroup of patients, those who adhere to treatment. More studies are needed of the characteristics of nonadherers and the ways in which they are similar to or differ from good adherers to determine whether the results of studies using "run-ins" can be generalized to those individuals who are typically less adherent.

Future research should attempt to (1) determine whether adherence-induced expectations do in fact activate placebo effects, and (2) identify and evaluate aspects of the act of adherence or characteristics of those who comply that may enhance placebo effects. Furthermore, clinical trials and other studies that evaluate the effects of interventions should use designs that allow researchers to distinguish between or control for these effects. Rosenthal (1985) and Ross and Buckalew (1985) suggest experimental designs that can be used to better understand how nonspecific effects may impact evaluations of treatment effectiveness. A method that may help clarify whether or not patient expectancies are mediating the effects of adherence on mortality and morbidity is a causal modeling approach that tests the effect of adherence on health outcomes directly and indirectly (via expectancy as a mediating variable). Aspects of the model presented in this chapter can also be tested experimentally. Examples of this approach include laboratory studies in which participants' expectations about the effects of a particular treatment are manipulated (see Agras et al., 1982; Fillmore et al., 1994; Kirsch & Weixel, 1988). A classic design in this regard is the balanced placebo design proposed by Marlatt and Rohsenow (1980), which allows independent evaluation of drug effects, expectancy effects, and their interaction. Design of studies to include a placebo and nonplacebo control group may also clarify expectancy effects.

Some behavioral and biomedical researchers have called for increased attempts to understand and harness the power of the placebo effect to benefit patients in clinical practice settings (Benson & Friedman, 1996; Chaput de Saintonge & Herxheimer, 1994; Connelly, 1991). Clearly, more attention should be focused on the role of nonspecific factors in health-related research, similar to the prominent role given to such factors in psychotherapy outcome research (Garfield, 1982). Perhaps certain components of health care interventions, such as enhanced expectations of benefit or perceived social support available from the health care provider, are "common ingredients" that enhance health-related outcomes regardless of the treatment or disease process involved. Future research should focus on identifying such common ingredients and using them to increase the effectiveness of health-related interventions.

References

Ader, R. (1985). Conditioned immunopharmacological effects in animals: Implications for a conditioning model of pharmacotherapy. In L. White, B. Tursky, & G. E. Schwartz (Eds.), *Placebo: Theory, research and mechanisms* (pp. 306–331). New York: Guilford Press.

Agras, W. S., Horne, M., & Taylor, C. B. (1982). Expectation and blood pressure lowering effects of relaxation. *Psychosomatic Medicine, 44,* 389–395.

Agras, W. S., Taylor, C. B., Kraemer, H. C., Southam, M. A., & Schneider, O. A. (1987). Relaxation training for essential hypertension at the worksite: II. The poorly controlled hypertensive. *Psychosomatic Medicine, 49,* 264–273.

Akil, H., Watson, S. J., Young, E., Lewis, M. E., Khachaturian, H., & Walker, J. M. (1984). Endogenous opioids: Biology and function. *Annual Review of Neuroscience, 7,* 223–255.

Amanzio, M., & Benedetti, F. (1999). Neuropharmacological dissection of placebo analgesia: Expectation-activated opioid systems versus conditioning-activated specific subsystems. *Journal of Neuroscience, 19,* 484–494.

Archer, T. P., & Leier, C. V. (1992). Placebo treatment in congestive heart failure. *Cardiology, 81,* 125–133.

Bandura, A. (1977). Self-efficacy: Toward a unifying theory of behavior change. *Psychological Review, 84,* 191–215.

Barth, J., Schumacher, M., & Herrmann-Lingen, H. (2004). Depression as a risk factor for mortality in patients with coronary heart disease: A meta-analysis. *Psychosomatic Medicine, 66,* 802–813.

Beecher, H. K. (1955). The powerful placebo. *Journal of the American Medical Association, 159,* 1602–1606.

Benedetti, F. (1996). The opposite effects of the opiate antagonist naloxone and the cholecystokinin antagonist proglumide on placebo analgesia. *Pain, 64,* 535–543.

Benedetti, F., Mayberg, H. S., Wager, T. D., Stohler, C. S., & Zubieta, J. K. (2005). Neurobiological mechanisms of the placebo effect. *Journal of Neuroscience, 25,* 10390–10402.

Benson, H., & Friedman, R. (1996). Harnessing the power of the placebo effect and renaming it "remembered wellness." *Annual Review of Medicine, 47,* 193–199.

Berkman, L. F., Leo-Summers, L., & Horwitz, R. I. (1992). Emotional support and survival after myocardial infarction. *Annals of Internal Medicine, 117,* 1003–1009.

Berrigan, D., Dodd, K., Troiano, R. P., Krebs-Smith, S. M., & Barbash, R. B. (2003). Patterns of health behavior in U.S. adults. *Preventive Medicine, 36,* 615–623.

Blumenthal, J. A., Williams, R. S., Wallace, A. G., Williams, R. B., & Needles, T. L. (1982). Physiological and psychological variables predict compliance to prescribed exercise therapy in patients recovering from myocardial infarction. *Psychosomatic Medicine, 44,* 519–527.

Brauer, A. P., Horlick, L., Nelson, E., Farquhar, J. W., & Agras, W. S. (1979). Relaxation therapy for essential hypertension. *Journal of Behavioral Medicine, 2,* 21–29.

Buck, C., & Donner, A. (1982). The design of controlled experiments in the evaluation of nontherapeutic interventions. *Journal of Chronic Diseases, 35,* 531–538.

Bush, P. J. (1974). The placebo effect. *Journal of the American Pharmaceutical Association, 14,* 671–672.

Carney, R. M., & Freedland, K. E. (2003). Depression, mortality, and medical morbidity in patients with coronary heart disease. *Biological Psychiatry, 54,* 241–247.

Chaput de Saintonge, D. M., & Herxheimer, A. (1994). Harnessing placebo effects in health care. *Lancet, 344,* 995–998.

Chesney, M. A., Black, G. W., Swan, G. E., & Ward, M. M. (1987). Relaxation training for essential hypertension at the worksite: 1. The untreated mild hypertensive. *Psychosomatic Medicine, 49,* 250–263.

Christenfeld, N., Gerin, W., Linden, W., Sanders, M., Mathur, J., Deich, J. D., et al. (1997). Social support effects on cardiovascular reactivity: Is a stranger as effective as a friend? *Psychosomatic Medicine, 59,* 388–398.

Colloca, L., Tinazzi, M., Recchia, S., Le Pera, D., Fiaschi, A., Benedetti, F., et al. (2008). Learning potentiates neurophysiological and behavioral placebo analgesic responses. *Pain,* June 5 [epub ahead of print].

Connelly, R. J. (1991). Nursing responsibility for the placebo effect. *Journal of Medicine and Philosophy, 16,* 325–341.

Coronary Drug Project Research Group. (1980). Influence of adherence to treatment and response of cholesterol on mortality in the Coronary Drug Project. *New England Journal of Medicine, 18,* 1038–1041.

Crum, A. J., & Langer, E. J. (2007). Mind-set matters: Exercise and the placebo effect. *Psychological Science, 18*(2), 165–171.

Cutter, H. S., Maloof, B., Kurtz, N. R., & Jones, W. C. (1976). "Feeling no pain": Differential responses to pain by alcoholics and non-alcoholics before and after drinking. *Journal of Studies on Alcohol, 37,* 273–277.

De la Fuente-Fernandez, R., Schulzer, R., & Stoessl, A. J. (2002). The placebo effect in neurological disorders. *Lancet Neurology, 1,* 85–91.

De la Fuente-Fernandez, R., Schulzer, R., & Stoessl, A. J. (2004). Placebo mechanisms and reward circuitry: Clues from Parkinson's disease. *Biological Psychiatry, 56,* 67–71.

Dobrilla, G., Imbimbo, B. P., Piazzi, L., & Benzi, G. (1990). Long-term treatment of irritable bowel syndrome with cimetropium bromide: A double-blind placebo controlled clinical trial. *Gut, 31,* 355–358.

Dolin, R., Reichman, R., Madore, H. P., Maynard, R., Linton, P. N., & Webber-Jones, J. (1982). A controlled trial of amantadine and rimantadine in the prophylaxis of influenza A infection. *New England Journal of Medicine, 307,* 580–583.

Dunbar, J., Marshall, G., & Hovell, M. (1979). Behavioral interventions in compliance. In R. B. Haynes, D. W. Taylor, & D. L. Sackett (Eds.), *Compliance with therapeutic and preventive regimens* (pp. 174–190). Baltimore: Johns Hopkins University Press.

Edens, J. L., Larkin, K. T., & Abel, J. L. (1992). The effect of social support and physical touch on cardiovascular reactions to mental stress. *Journal of Psychosomatic Research, 36*(4), 371–381.

Epstein, L. (1984). The direct effects of compliance on health outcome. *Health Psychology, 3,* 385–393.

Evans, F. J. (1985). Expectancy, therapeutic instructions and the placebo response. In L. White, B. Tursky, & G. E. Schwartz (Eds.), *Placebo: Theory, research and mechanisms* (pp. 215–278). New York: Guilford Press.

Filliol, D., Ghozland, S., Chluba, J., Martin, M., Matthes, H.W., Simonin, F., et al. (2000). Mice deficient for delta- and mu-opioid receptors exhibit opposing alterations of emotional responses. *Nature Genetics, 25,* 195–200.

Fillmore, M. T., Mulvihill, L. E., & Vogel-Sprott, M. (1994). *Psychopharmacology, 115,* 383–388.

Finnerty, F. A., Jr., Mattie, E. C., & Finnery, E. A., III. (1973). Hypertension in the inner city I: Analysis of clinic dropouts. *Circulation, 47,* 73–75.

Fontana, A. M., Diegnan, T., Villeneuve, A., & Lepore, S. J. (1999). Nonevaluative social support reduces cardiovascular reactivity in young women during acutely stressful performance situations. *Journal of Behavioral Medicine, 22,* 75–91.

Frank, J. D. (1961). *Persuasion and healing: A comparative study of psychotherapy.* Baltimore: Johns Hopkins University Press.

Frank, J. D. (1971). Therapeutic factors in psychotherapy. *American Journal of Psychotherapy, 25,* 350–361.

Frank, J. D. (1983). The placebo is psychotherapy. *Behavioral and Brain Sciences, 6,* 291–292.

Frasure-Smith, N., Lesperance, F., & Talajic, M. (1993). Depression following myocardial infarction: Impact on 6-month survival. *Journal of the American Medical Association, 270,* 1819–1825.

Friedman, L., Furberg, C., & DeMets, D. (1996). *Fundamentals of clinical trials.* St. Louis, MO: Mosby Year Book.

Garfield, S. L. (1980). *Psychotherapy: An eclectic approach.* New York: Wiley.

Garfield, S. L. (1982). Eclecticism and integration in psychotherapy. *Behavior Therapy, 13,* 610–623.

Gelfand, S., Ullman, L. P., & Krasner, L. (1963). The placebo response: An experimental approach. *Journal of Nervous and Mental Disorders, 136,* 379–387.

Gerin, W., Pieper, C., Levy, R., & Pickering, T. G. (1992). Social support in social interaction: A moderator of cardiovascular reactivity. *Psychosomatic Medicine, 54,* 324–336.

Glassman, A. H., & Shapiro, P. A. (1998). Depression and the course of coronary artery disease. *American Journal of Psychiatry, 155,* 4–11.

Glynn, R. J., Buring, J. E., Manson, J. E., LaMotte, F., & Hennekens, C. H. (1994). Adherence to aspirin in the prevention of myocardial infarction: The Physicians' Health Study. *Archives of Internal Medicine, 154,* 2649–2657.

Goldstein, A. P. (1962). *Therapist-patient expectancies in psychotherapy.* New York: Macmillan.

Gould, B. A., Davies, A. B., Mann, S., Altman, D. G., & Raftery, E. B. (1981). Does placebo lower blood pressure? *Lancet, 2,* 1377–1381.

Granger, B. B., Swedberg, K., Ekman, I., Granger, C. B., Olofsson B., McMurray, J. J. V., et al. (2005). Adherence to candesartan and placebo and outcomes in chronic heart failure in the CHARM programme: Double-blind, randomised, controlled clinical trial. *Lancet, 366,* 2005–2011.

Grevert, P., & Goldstein, A. (1977). Effects of naloxone on experimentally produced ischemic pain and on mood in human subjects. *Proceedings of the National Academy of Sciences USA, 74,* 1291–1294.

Grevert, P., & Goldstein, A. (1978). Endorphins: Naloxone fails to alter experimental pain or mood in humans. *Science, 199,* 1093–1095.

Gryll, S. L., & Katahn, M. (1978). Situational factors contributing to the placebo effect. *Psychopharmacology, 57,* 253–261.

Guiry, E., Conroy, R. M., Hickey, N., & Mulcahy, R. (1987). Psychological response to an acute coronary event and its effect on subsequent rehabilitation and lifestyle change. *Clinical Cardiology, 10,* 256–260.

Horwitz, R. I., Viscoli, C. M., Berkman, L., Donaldson, R. M., Horwitz, S. M., Murray, C. J., et al. (1990). Treatment adherence and risk of death after a myocardial infarction. *Lancet, 336,* 542–545.

Hovell, M. E., Black, D. R., Mewborn, C. R., Geary, D., Agras, W. S., Kamachi, K., et al. (1986). Personalized versus usual care of previously uncontrolled hypertensive patients: An exploratory analysis. *Preventive Medicine, 15,* 673–684.

Howritz, R. I., & Horwitz, S. M. (1993). Adherence to treatment and health outcomes. *Archives of Internal Medicine, 153,* 1863–1868.

Hypertension Detection and Follow-up Program Cooperative Group. (1979). 5-year findings of the Hypertension Detection and Follow-up Program: I. Reduction in mortality of persons with high blood pressure, including mild hypertension. *Journal of the American Medical Association, 242,* 2562–2571.

Irvine, J., Baker, B., Smith, J., Jandciu, S., Paquette, M., Cairns, J., et al. (1999). Poor adherence to placebo or amiodarone therapy predicts mortality: Results from the CAMIAT study. *Psychosomatic Medicine, 61,* 566–575.

Jacob, R. G., Shapiro, A. P., Reeves, R. A., Johnsen, A. M., McDonald, R. H., & Coburn, P. C. (1986). Relaxation therapy for hypertension: Comparison of effects with concomitant placebo, diuretic and beta blocker. *Archives of Internal Medicine, 146,* 2335–2340.

Kamarck, T. W., Manuck, S. B., & Jennings, J. R. (1990). Social support reduces cardiovascular reactivity to psychological challenge: A laboratory model. *Psychosomatic Medicine, 52,* 42–58.

Kellet, J. M. (1990). Compliance and clinical trials in heart disease. *Lancet, 336,* 1003.

King, T. K., Marcus, B. H., Pinto, B. M., Emmons, K. M., & Abrams, D. B. (1996). Cognitive-behavioral mediators of changing multiple behaviors: Smoking and a sedentary lifestyle. *Preventive Medicine, 25*(6), 684–691.

Kirsch, I., & Weixel, L. J. (1988). Double-blind versus deceptive administration of a placebo. *Behavioral Neuroscience, 102,* 319–323.

Kramer, M. S., & Shapiro, S. H. (1984). Scientific challenges in the application of randomized trials. *Journal of the American Medical Association, 252,* 2739–2745.

Kronish, I. M., Rieckmann, N., Halm, E. A., Shimbo, D., Vorchheimer, D., Haas, D. C., et al. (2006). Persistent depression affects adherence to secondary prevention behaviors after acute coronary syndromes. *Journal of General Internal Medicine, 21,* 1178–1183.

Lepore, S. J., Allen, K. A., & Evans, G. W. (1993). Social support lowers cardiovascular reactivity to an acute stressor. *Psychosomatic Medicine, 55,* 518–524.

Levine, J. D., Gordon, M. C., & Fields, H. L. (1978). The mechanism of placebo analgesia. *Lancet, 2,* 654–657.

Levine, J. D., Gordon, N. C., Jones, R. T., & Fields, H. L. (1978). The narcotic antagonist naloxone enhances clinical pain. *Nature, 272,* 826–827.

Levine, J. D., Gordon, N. C., & Melds, H. L. (1979). Naloxone dose dependently produces analgesia and hyperalgesia in postoperative pain. *Nature, 278,* 740–741.

Liberman, R. (1964). An experimental study of the placebo phenomenon under three different situations of pain. *Journal of Psychiatric Research, 2,* 233–246.

Lipid Research Clinics Program. (1984). The Lipid Research Clinics Coronary Primary Prevention Trial results II: The relationship of reduction in incidence of coronary heart disease to cholesterol lowering. *Journal of the American Medical Association, 251,* 365–374.

Luborsky, L., Crits-Christoph, P., Brady, J. P., Kron, R. E., Weiss, T., Cohen, M., et al. (1982). Behavioral versus pharmacological treatments for essential hypertension—A needed comparison. *Psychosomatic Medicine, 44,* 203–213.

Ludwig, A. M., Wikler, A., & Stark, L. H. (1974). The first drink: Psychological aspects of craving. *Archives of General Psychiatry, 30,* 539–547.

Management Committee. (1980). The Australian therapeutic trial in mild hypertension. *Lancet, 1*(8181), 1261–1267.

Marlatt, G. A., & Rohsenow, D. J. (1980). Cognitive processes in alcohol use: Expectancy and the balanced placebo design. In N. K. Mello (Ed.), *Advances in substance abuse: Behavioral and biological research* (pp. 159–199). Greenwich, CT: JAI Press.

Meyers, S., & Janowitz, H. D. (1989). The "natural history" of ulcerative colitis: An analysis of the placebo response. *Journal of Clinical Gastroenterology, 11,* 33–37.

Mihic, D., & Binkert, E. (1978). *Is placebo analgesia mediated by endorphine?* Paper presented at the Second World Congress on Pain, Montreal, Quebec, Canada.

Multiple Risk Factor Intervention Trial Research Group. (1982). Multiple Risk Factor Intervention Trial: Risk factor changes and mortality results. *Journal of the American Medical Association, 248,* 1465–1477.

Oblas-Manno, D., Friedmann, E., Brooks, M. M., Thomas, S. A., Haakenson, C., Morris, M., et al. Adherence and arrhythmic mortality in the Cardiac Arrhythmia Suppression Trial (CAST). (1996). *Annals of Epidemiology, 6,* 93–101.

O'Halloran, P., Lazovich, D., Patterson, R. E., Harnack, L., French, S., Curry, S. J., et al. (2001) Effect of health lifestyle pattern on dietary change. *American Journal of Health Promotion, 16*(1), 27–33.

Packer, M. (1990). The placebo effect in heart failure. *American Heart Journal,* 120, 1579–1582.

Peck, C., & Coleman, G. (1991). Implications of placebo therapy for clinical research and practice in pain management. *Theoretical Medicine, 12,* 247–270.

Pizzo, P. A., Robichaud, K. J., Edwards, B. K., Schumaker, C., Kramer, B. S., & Johnson, A. (1983). Oral antibiotic prophylaxis in patients with cancer: A double-blind randomized placebo-controlled trial. *Journal of Pediatrics, 102,* 125–133.

Pledger, G. W. (1992). Basic statistics: Importance of adherence. *Journal of Clinical Research in Pharmacoepidemiology, 6,* 77–81.

Plotkin, E. B. (1985). A psychological approach to placebo: The role of faith in therapy and treatment. In L. White, B. Tursky, & G. E. Schwartz (Eds.), *Placebo: Theory, research and mechanisms* (pp. 237–254). New York: Guilford Press.

Pronk, N. P., Anderson, L. H., Crain, A. L., Martinson, B. C., O'Connor, P. J., Sherwood, N. E., et al. (2004). Meeting recommendations for multiple healthy lifestyle factors: Prevalence, clustering, and predictors among adolescent, adult, and senior health plan members. *American Journal of Preventive Medicine, 27*(Suppl.), 25–33.

Rasmussen, J. N., Chong, A., & Alter, D. A. (2007). Relationship between adherence to evidence-based pharmacotherapy and long-term mortality after acute myocardial infarction. *Journal of the American Medical Association, 297,* 177–186.

Rieckmann, N., Gerin, W., Kronish, I. M., Burg, M. M., Chaplin, W. F., Kong, G., et al. (2006). Course of depressive symptoms and medication adherence after acute coronary syndromes: An electronic medication monitoring study. *Journal of the American College of Cardiology, 48,* 2215–2222.

Rosenthal, R. (1985). Designing, analyzing, interpreting and summarizing placebo studies. In L. White, B. Tursky, & G. E. Schwartz (Eds.), *Placebo: Theory, research and mechanisms* (pp. 110–136). New York: Guilford Press.

Ross, M., & Olson, J. M. (1981). An expectancy-attribution model of the effects of placebos. *Psychological Review, 88,* 408–437.

Ross, S., & Buckalew, L. W. (1985). Placebo agentry: Assessment of drug and placebo effects. In L. White, B. Tursky, & G. E. Schwartz (Eds.), *Placebo: Theory, research and mechanisms* (pp. 67–82). New York: Guilford Press.

Scheier, M. F., Helgeson, V. S., Schulz, R., Colvin, S., Berga, S., Bridges, M. W., et al. (2005). Interventions to enhance physical and psychological functioning among younger women who are ending nonhormonal adjuvant treatment for early-stage breast cancer. *Journal of Clinical Oncology, 23,* 4298–4311.

Shapiro, A. K., & Shapiro, E. (1984). Patient-provider relationships and the placebo effect. In J. D. Matarazzo, S. M. Weiss, J. A Herd, N. E. Miller, & S. M. Weiss (Eds.), *Behavioral health: A handbook of health enhancement and disease prevention* (pp. 371–383). New York: Wiley.

Simpson, S. H., Eurich, D. T., Majumdar, S. R., Padwal, R. S., Tsuyuki, R. T., Varney, J., et al. (2006). A meta-analysis of the association between adherence to drug therapy and mortality. *British Medical Journal, 333,* 15.

Smith, M. L., Glass, E. V., & Miller, T. I. (1980). *The benefits of psychotherapy.* Baltimore, MD: Johns Hopkins University Press.

Sora, I., Takahashi, N., Funada, M., Ujike, H., Revay, R. S., Donovan, D. M., et al. (1997). Opiate receptor knockout mice define mu receptor roles in endogenous nociceptive responses and morphine-induced analgesia. *Proceedings of the National Academies of Science USA, 94,* 1544–1549.

Stone, A. R., Imber, S. D., & Frank, J. D. (1966). The role of non-specific factors in short-term psychotherapy. *Australian Journal of Psychology, 18,* 210–217.

Van Melle, J. P., de Jonge, P., Spijkerman, T. A., Tijssen, J. G., Ormel, J., van Veldhuisen, D. J., et al. (2004). Prognostic association of depression following myocardial infarction with mortality and cardiovascular events: A meta-analysis. *Psychosomatic Medicine, 66,* 814–822.

Verter, J., & Friedman, L. (1984). Adherence measures in the Aspirin Myocardial Infarction Study (AMIS). *Controlled Clinical Trials* (abstract), *5,* 306.

Wadden, T. (1984). Relaxation therapy for essential hypertension: Specific or nonspecific effects? *Journal of Psychosomatic Research, 28,* 53–61.

Wager, T. D., Rilling, J. K., Smith, E. E., Sokolik, A., Casey, K. L., Davidson, R. J., et al. (2004). Placebo-induced changes in fMRI in the anticipation and experience of pain. *Science, 303,* 1162–1167.

Ward, M. M., Swan, G. E., & Chesney, M. A. (1987). Arousal reduction treatments for mild hypertension: A meta-analysis of recent studies. In S. Julius (Ed.), *Handbook of hypertension. Vol. 10: Behavioral factors in hypertension* (pp. 285–302). New York: Elsevier.

Wickramasekera, I. (1985). A conditioned response model of the placebo effect: Predictions from the model. In L. White, B. Tursky, & G. E. Schwartz (Eds.), *Placebo: Theory, research and mechanisms* (pp. 255–287). New York: Guilford Press.

Wilkins, W. (1985). Placebo controls and concepts in chemotherapy and psychotherapy research. In L. White, B. Tursky, & G. E. Schwartz (Eds.), *Placebo: Theory, research and mechanisms* (pp. 83–109). New York: Guilford Press.

Williams, R. B., Barefoot, J. C., Califf, R. M., Haney, T. L., Saunders, W. B., Pryor, D. B., et al. (1992). *Journal of the American Medical Association, 267,* 520–524.

Zubieta, J. K., Ketter, T. A., Bueller, J. A., Xu, Y., Kilbourn, M. R., Young, E. A., et al. (2003). Regulation of human affective responses by anterior cingulate and limbic mu-opioid neurotransmission. *Archives of General Psychiatry, 60,* 1145–1113.

Zubieta, J. K., Smith, Y. R., Bueller, J. A., Xu, Y., Kilbourn, M. R., Jewett, D. M., et al. (2001). Regional mu opioid receptor regulation of sensory and affective dimensions of pain. *Science, 292,* 311–315.

Collaboration Between Professionals and Mediating Structures in the Community: Social Determinants of Health and Community-Based Participatory Research

37

Suzanne B. Cashman
and Laurie G. Forlano

With a focus on identifying ways in which providers and colleagues can help individuals develop healthier lifestyle practices, many chapters in this book emphasize micro-level analyses and provide rich information about effective interventions for behavior change. This micro focus represents a necessary but not sufficient approach to the goal of improving health. In this chapter, we consider social determinants of health (SDOH) and community-based participatory research (CBPR). Both are powerful means for effecting change. SDOH provides a philosophical underpinning for action aimed at transforming power relations from ones that permit inequity and injustice to ones that promote equity. CBPR offers a method for building and capitalizing on productive partnerships that result in empowered communities acting to improve health.

Together, these two approaches help frame a language of health behavior that more clearly articulates the values of equity, social justice, and the common good. (See also chapter 38, "Ethical Issues in Lifestyle Change and Adherence," for a further discussion of equity framing in adherence research.)

When the second edition of this volume was published a decade ago, this chapter addressed "whether health is primarily a personal responsibility or a societal obligation" (Ribisl & Humphreys, 1998, p. 535). In laying out their thesis, the chapter's authors presented strengths and weaknesses of the individual as well as the paternalistic approaches to health and suggested a "third way" that would highlight the advantages while reducing the disadvantages of each approach. This "third path" consisted of collaboration with mediating structures, defined as organizations and institutions (e.g., churches, families, voluntary associations, and neighborhoods) that "stand between individuals' private lives and the larger public domains" (Ribisl & Humphreys, 1998, p. 539). In suggesting that collective approaches are based on "doing with" rather than "doing for" or "doing to," the authors concluded that health promotion and behavior change initiatives could be most effective if they adopted a collaborative or partnership model and took advantage of the best elements that community control and decision making offer. In this chapter, we build on these ideas and advance the need to address social determinants of health and consider community-based participatory research.

Increasingly, models of health use ecological approaches that recognize the interconnectedness of individuals and the context of the communities in which they live (Wilcox, 2007). Yet, despite the development of these models and the knowledge that many advances in the conquest of diseases have come from structural approaches and macro interventions such as environmental and policy changes that alter the norms in which we live, a preponderance of health promotion activities continues to be directed toward encouraging individuals to adopt healthier approaches to living. In focusing the majority of our efforts on the individual, we risk failing to attain our full potential for improved health (McKinlay, 1998). We must use our understanding of SDOH and the potential of CBPR if we are to make meaningful, lasting changes (Navarro et al., 2006).

The Ecological Approach

The choice of language and how we elect to frame issues are powerful influencers of action (Hofrichter, 2003; Leichter, 2003). For example, it is widely stated that the factors affecting an individual's health status include genetic makeup, environment, and medical care, as well as lifestyle and health behaviors (McGinnis, Williams-Russo, & Knickman, 2002; O'Hara, 2005). With lifestyle and behavioral factors accounting for approximately 50% of an individual's health status (Regan & Brookins-Fisher, 1997), policymakers suggest that we need to pay more attention to *individuals'* lifestyle "choices" and behaviors (McGinnis et al., 2002). Placing the majority of our efforts at this level, however, ignores the power of context in which individuals live and work. The decrease in tobacco use provides a good example of context, as behavioral change did not reach significant levels until laws, regulations, social norms, taxes, and other societal factors were implemented in conjunction with individually focused aids for quitting and for avoiding initiating tobacco use (Schneider, 2006).

Almost 30 years ago, in an essay about health care in America, Crawford (1979) challenged what he saw as the then prevailing victim-blaming approach to health promotion. He asserted that this focus substituted an ideology of individual responsibility for an understanding of the complexities of social causation of disease and disability and suggested that the individual approach "ignored what is known about human behavior" and minimized "the importance of evidence about the environmental assault on health." Crawford lamented the fact that individuals were being held responsible for achieving a level of health that was influenced by environmental factors beyond their control and castigated those who asserted that, while environmental factors might be relevant, there was little that could be done to effect change at this level (Crawford, 1979).

Writing at about the same time, Brofenbrenner (1977, 1979) proposed an ecological perspective on health in which behavior was viewed as simultaneously being affected by and affecting multiple levels of influence. In dividing environmental influences on behavior into micro-, meso-, exo-, and macro-systems, he reinforced the importance of addressing the SDOH as a means of achieving meaningful change and noted that ecological models view behavior and the social environment as inextricably intertwined. Consequently, to improve health, SDOH need to be addressed, with actions and interventions complementing one another and occurring simultaneously on all levels.

In 1988, McLeroy and colleagues (1988) proposed an ecological model for health promotion that specified patterned behavior as the outcome of interest, with behavior determined by intrapersonal factors; interpersonal processes and primary groups; institutional factors; community factors; and public policy. This model extends Brofenbrenner's by dividing the macro-system into community factors and public policy. Both are relevant to health promotion and behavior change. McLeroy et al.'s ecological model offers a comprehensive approach that captures a wide range of strategies available for health promotion interventions and programs and, again, reminds us of the importance of focusing on SDOH and on working at multiple levels simultaneously.

While applying the ecological model has been shown to be effective in identifying environmental causes of behavior and suitable environmental interventions, using this model can result in charges of coercion, paternalism, and invasion of privacy (McLeroy, Bibeau, Steckler, & Glanz, 1988). To avoid these charges and to maximize the model's effectiveness, the active involvement of communities in defining issues and selecting foci of change with accompanying appropriate interventions, implementation, and evaluation is needed. While not a panacea, the process of engaging in community consensus building around health concerns and issues initiates needed consciousness raising regarding causes and responsibilities for health and illness (Wallerstein & Bernstein, 1988).

Social Determinants of Health (SDOH)

Definition and Background

The social determinants of health (SDOH) are defined similarly but with nuanced differences by various theorists and researchers. Synthesizing these definitions, Raphael (2007) concluded that SDOH represent the "economic and social conditions that influence the health of individuals, communities, and jurisdictions as a whole." These determinants influence an individual's health directly, as well as indirectly, through the extent to which a person has access to the physical, social, and personal resources to identify and achieve personal aspirations, satisfy needs, and cope with the environment. Thus, SDOH is about the "quantity and quality of a variety of resources that a society makes available to its members" (Raphael, 2007). In short, SDOH captures elements related to the social gradient, stress, early life, social exclusion, work, unemployment, social support, addiction, food, and transport (Wilkinson & Marmot, 1998).

Engels (1845/1987), and Virchow (1848/1985), two prominent figures in health and medicine, reported that factors related to a society's structure, such as political, economic, and social forces, exerted important influences on health. After investigating a typhus epidemic in Upper Silesia, Virchow did not recommend that the region adopt a behavioral model of health. Rather, he risked his career by asserting that unfair social structures that included tax policies and feudalism were responsible for residents' unsanitary conditions and poor diet and that it was these factors that had been a catalyst for the epidemic. He challenged the power structure by asking, "Do we not always find diseases of the populace traceable to defects in society?" and encouraged physicians to become advocates for the poor, working for change at the level of social structures.

The World Health Organization's (WHO) constitution states that health is "a state of complete physical, mental and social well-being" (World Health Organization, 1948). Premising its view of health on this definition, 40 years later, in 1986, the First International Conference on Health Promotion drafted what has become known as the Ottawa Charter. Based on strong principles of equity, the Charter identified the prerequisites of health as peace, shelter, education, food, income, a stable ecosystem, sustainable resources, social justice, and equity. Despite that Charter's principles having been reaffirmed at subsequent international meetings, in the United States, however, the major focus of health promotion has been on lifestyle approaches associated with behavioral change, rather than on society's larger structural elements (Baum, 2007; Raphael & Farrell, 2002). Nevertheless, local efforts that engage community voices have identified governmental and other institutional decisions as appropriate areas of activity for improving health (Minkler, 1997; Minkler & Wallerstein, 2003). Moreover, the U.S. blueprint for improving population health states that "communities, states, and national organizations will need to take a multi-disciplinary approach to achieving health equity—an approach that involves improving health, education, housing, labor, justice, transportation, agriculture, and the environment" (U.S. Department of Health and Human Services, 2000, p. 16; Metzler, 2007).

In the United Kingdom, two reports, the Black Report (1980) and the Health Divide (1992), have energized the SDOH approach by keeping the influence of social structures in the purview of policy makers. These reports described how members of the lowest employment-level groups were more likely than those at higher levels of employment to experience a wide range of diseases and premature death from illness and injury throughout the life cycle (Townsend, Davidson, & Whitehead, 1992). The authors reported health differences in a step-wise progression across the socioeconomic range, with professionals having the best and manual laborers the worst health. The researchers concluded that material conditions such as income, working conditions, and quality of food and housing were the primary determinants of outcomes and noted that health inequalities were socioeconomically driven. The significance of these two reports cannot be understated—they mark the first time that the government of a Western industrialized nation acknowledged that a wide range of social policies influenced levels of health and that these policies were deemed appropriate for government action (Benzeval, 2002).

Evidence Supporting SDOH

In the past century, industrialized nations witnessed significant improvements in health status on a wide range of measures. While access to medical care and changes in individual behaviors are responsible for part of these improvements, the main contributors to increased longevity and decreases in morbidity are improvements in material conditions, including more widespread education, safe food, improved housing, and better sanitation. In a recent seminal study of the macro-economic determinants of health, researchers concluded that the "empirical evidence is overwhelming that poverty, measured at the levels of societies as well as individuals, is causally related to poor health of societies and individuals, respectively" (Subramanian, Belli, & Kawachi, 2002, p. 287). There are multiple ways in which poverty can affect health. Income provides the ability to purchase shelter, food, and warmth and, in many instances, the ability to participate in society. Poverty is stressful and frequently results in heightened levels of anxiety that can damage health. Additionally, a low income limits a person's choices and represents a major barrier to healthful behavior changes (Benzeval, Judge, & Whitehead, 1995). It is estimated that the cumulative effect of income-related exposures may mean that the highest 5% of income earners live approximately 25% longer than the bottom 5% (Rogot, 1992) and that an individual 18 years of age or older who lives below the poverty threshold can expect 8.5 fewer health-adjusted life years than a person of the same age who lives above that threshold (Muennig, Franks, Jia, Lubetkin, & Gold, 2005).

Writing in 2002 under the auspices of the Center for Social Justice Foundation for Research and Education and focusing on social exclusion, Raphael concluded that while "an unhealthy material environment and unhealthy behaviors have direct harmful effects, . . . the worries and insecurities of daily life and the lack of supportive environment also have an influence" (Raphael, 2002, p. xi). The concept of social exclusion helps us understand the interrelationships among three important and influential aspects of low-income people's lives: material disadvantage, excessive psychosocial stress, and unhealthy behaviors (Raphael, 2002). "Social exclusion is defined as a multi-dimensional process, in which various forms of exclusion are combined: participation in decision-making and political processes, access to employment and material resources, and integration into common cultural processes. When combined, they create acute forms of exclusion that find a spatial representation in particular neighborhoods" (Raphael, 2002, p. 30).

Examining cardiovascular disease and noting that only a small proportion of the variation in incidence of heart disease is explained by medical and lifestyle risk factors, animal researchers have identified the biological and psychological mechanisms by which chronic stress and hierarchy create illness (Sapolsky & Share, 1994; Shively, Laird, & Anton, 1997). These stress models reflect the experience of life lived on a low income and help explain the relationship between low income and cardiovascular as well as other diseases. "Chronic anxiety, insecurity, low self-esteem, social isolation, and lack of control over work appear to undermine mental and physical health" (Brunner & Marmot, 1999, p. 41). It has been posited that, by disturbing the usual homeostatic equilibrium by repeated activation of the related "fight or flight" response, social differences affect neuroendocrine, physiological, and metabolic variables—the precursors of ill health and disease (Brunner & Marmot, 1999; Kunst, Groenhof, & Mackenbach, 1998; Stansfield & Marmot, 2002). Additionally, stress has been shown to be associated with changes in allostatic load, resulting in bodily wear and tear (McEwen, 2003), as well as higher levels of cortisol excretion, leading in time to excess weight gain (McEwen, 1998a, 1998b). Furthermore, adding to this toll on the body is the positive association between the psychosocial stress of living in poverty and the likelihood of adopting behaviors such as tobacco use and lack of physical activity that are related to poor health (Wardle & Gibson, 2002). Individuals who have adequate coping mechanisms, coupled with opportunities to control their environments, are better able to return rapidly to a resting level and thus resist stress-related conditions (Marmot & Wilkinson, 1999).

Ten years ago, researchers concluded that there was a body of evidence that demonstrated the accumulating effect of a lifetime of poor socioeconomic conditions on adult health outcomes. It is now understood that an early life spent in adverse socioeconomic conditions can result in lasting increases in the risk of cardiovascular disease, respiratory disease, diabetes, and some cancers (Smith, Hart, Blane, Gillis, & Hawthorne, 1997). Without structural changes that address the social determinants of health, encouraging the adoption of healthy lifestyles and behavior change to reduce risk may simply be too little, too late. Moreover, focusing exclusively on individual behavior change may set people up to fall short of their goals and possibly even exacerbate the ill effects of a life characterized by high stress levels. In contrast, behavior change developed through using approaches focused on SDOH and associated with community-based participatory research (CBPR) engages people at the level of their primary concerns and marshals the community's energy and creativity to develop structures and systems that encourage the desired changes. Ultimately, understanding the SDOH is essential "because the health gradient [cannot] be attributed, in the main, to differences in diet, smoking or other aspects of 'lifestyle'" (Marmot, 2004, p. 241; see also Dovell, 2006). To improve health status through effecting behavior change, a community-engaged SDOH approach that incorporates multiple strategies and interventions and includes cross sector collaborations is needed.

Inequalities in Health Contributing to Evidence of SDOH

While empirical evidence related to the effect of a society's income distribution on population health suggests that income inequality is related to health levels (Kawachi, Kennedy, & Wilkinson, 1999; Ram, 2005), studies of economic inequality and health have found the effects of income inequality to be inconsistent or relatively small. As a consequence, researchers continue to debate the degree to which income inequality per se affects population health (Abbott, 2007). One hypothesis drawn from this body of research is that the relationship between income inequality and poor health is not universal. Rather, it may depend on a government's social policies and the effect of those policies on reducing the impact of economic inequalities (Kawachi et al., 1999), as well as on the specific mechanisms by which income inequality is hypothesized to affect health (Subramanian et al., 2002). This hypothesis is consistent with evidence offered by SDOH researchers who have concluded that the most important social determinant of health is income inequality (the actual income gap between people), rather than absolute income. Indeed, evidence of differences in health status across an entire socioeconomic gradient, not just between rich and poor, demonstrates that the larger the gap, the lower the health status of the overall population (Marmot & Wilkinson, 1999).

Inequality is affected by government policies that focus on tax structure; education and job training; investment in children, particularly their education and their early developmental years; transfer payments; minimum wages and benefits; and availability of capital. An inverse relationship characterizes the degree of inequality within a geographic area and the amount of resources invested in social infrastructure and social safety net organizations. Ramifications of this inverse relationship are not reserved for the less well off exclusively; the well off in economically unequal communities have greater rates of health problems than their counterparts in communities characterized by relative economic equality (Lynch et al., 1998).

Current Activity Related to SDOH

Recognizing that in the later decades of the 20th century the world had largely moved away from action on the social determinants, early in the 21st century, the WHO committed to returning to its original concerns. To refocus activity on the social roots of ill health and health inequality, in 2005, the WHO constituted a global Commission on the Social Determinants of Health (CSDH). The Commission's charge is to catalyze policy and institutional change that addresses social determinants of health within countries, among institutions working in global health, and within WHO itself (Irwin et al., 2006). Knowledge Networks comprised of scientists and practitioners have been established and charged with compiling evidence related to policies and interventions to eliminate social barriers to health. In a recent report to the Commission, authors concluded that to effect change, "political will combined with the evidence offers the most powerful response to the negative effects of social determinants" (Kelly, Morgan, Bonnefoy, Butt, & Bergman, 2007, p. 7).

In the United States, the National Association of County and City Health Officials (NACCHO) has taken a strong SDOH approach to recommendations for future public health activity. In a book entitled *Health and Social Justice* (Hofrichter, 2003), the editor quotes Beauchamp (1988, p. 14) as stating that, to reclaim its historical focus on "collective control over conditions affecting the common health," public health must return to a focus on broad-based social reform. Several premises, including the belief that health is a "collective public good, actively produced by institutions and social policies," that "population health outcomes are primarily the result of social and political forces, not lifestyles or behavior," and that "an accumulation of negative social conditions and lack of fundamental resources contribute to health inequalities," frame NACCHO's recommendations for how local health departments might tackle health inequities. Thus, rather than simply asking why an individual uses tobacco products, the question should be more broadly framed so that it asks, "What social conditions and economic policies, along with systematic practices of tobacco companies, predispose people to the stress that encourages smoking?" In order to effect change, public health is being encouraged to move away from accepting social conditions without exploring how they have developed and to question how behavior is linked to and affected by the socioeconomic context and conditions in which it occurs.

Barriers to Employing the SDOH Approach

Despite accumulating evidence and extensive discussion in the literature regarding the social determinants of health and their influence on health status and rising medical care costs, little attention has been paid in the policy arena to effecting change in these determinants. While public health has long been noted for its efforts to focus activity and change upstream rather than downstream, even public health as a profession and as a movement has been noticeably absent from identifying effective policy levers related to making change at the level of the SDOH. Why is that?

Several barriers to working at the level of the SDOH pose significant challenges to public health. They include (1) ideological issues related to an ongoing debate about the relative contribution of medical, lifestyle, and societal explanations for health; (2) political issues that are raised when health workers are employed by the very governments whose policies may compromise health; (3) institutional issues that result in workers electing the course of least resistance, thus choosing to focus activity at the level of lifestyle change, rather than at the level of social conditions and institutional policies; (4) personal issues of knowledge and competence that result in workers remaining in the domains of medical treatment and lifestyle change, rather than those of community organizing and development; and (5) attitudinal and motivational issues that render issues of poverty too overwhelming to tackle, thus keeping health workers in arenas that seem to offer more control, even though they may not be particularly effective (Raphael, 2004). Together, these challenges represent significant barriers to improving health through an SDOH approach.

Recommendations for Action

The strong associations between people's material circumstances and their health, coupled with the importance of one's relative position in the social hierarchy, suggest a need to focus on the fundamental structural determinants of the social environment (Marmot, 2007; Wilkinson, 1999). Moreover, correcting social inequalities has been shown to improve the health of whole populations (Navarro, et al., 2006). Unlike policies related to modifying individually oriented risk factors that lie between distal causes and disease, approaches based in population health focus on developing healthy public policies that call for governmental, institutional, and organizational action (McKinlay, 1998). They require intersector cooperation (Murphy, 2004) and focus on reducing the burden of disadvantage, particularly related to employment, income, and education (Wilkinson, 1999). In a recent discussion on promoting population health and reducing disparities, policy researchers recommended approaches that (1) benefit individuals regardless of their own resources and actions; (2) target special needs of resource-poor groups that may face barriers to implementing recommended interventions; and (3) promote policies that increase socioeconomic resources that are available to resource-poor groups (Link & Phelan, 2005).

At the global level, the slow uptake of activity aimed at policy change has led the WHO European Regional Office (The International Centre for Health and Society at the University College of London) to compile evidence on the social determinants of health in a way that policy makers can find helpful. The resulting document, *The Solid Facts,* summarizes SDOH in 10 messages and is being used to formulate health policy (Wilkinson & Marmot, 2003). In addition, WHO leaders have called for the development and implementation of pro-equity health policies that go beyond a focus on income by addressing "systematic disparities in health between more and less advantaged social groups" (Braveman, Starfield, & Geiger, 2001, p. 679) and by intervening in the social factors that influence health (Baum, 2007; Vega & Irwin, 2004). At the municipal level, this approach has been captured in the Healthy Cities movement, which promotes initiatives aimed at improving health by changing local social structures and environments. Incorporating elements of the community-based participatory research approach, Healthy Cities calls for including community members' voices in identifying community issues (Blackwell & Colmenar, 2000; Norris & Pittman, 2000; Raphael, 2003). This pro-equity approach requires intersectoral cooperation—even in the face of administrative and budgeting structures in the public sector that make such collaborative action difficult. Addressing health and health inequities at this level will likely remove the veil that has shielded health from the political arena and presented it as an apolitical entity. The need to develop a "politics of health" and to acknowledge the profoundly political nature of health was posited recently by a team of academics from the United Kingdom (Bambra, Fox, & Scott-Samuel, 2005). They suggest that failing to see the political nature of health policy results in a lack of understanding of the degree to which the political context affects how health policy is formulated. Furthermore, individuals and groups with the greatest power have a vested interest in maintaining this failure of understanding.

Building a more inclusive society (Schulz & Sankaran, 2006) is suggested as a way to address the social determinants of health and thus improve health status. The need to rethink health policy at the macro as well as the micro level has also been recommended. In the United States, the Department of Health and Human Services (DHHS) recommended that a Federal Leadership Council be created under its auspices. This Council would leverage government-wide resources to improve health and reduce inequities (Hofrichter, 2006). Coordination among departments, including labor, education, defense, justice, energy, and transportation, would occur at the regional and local levels; strategies have been identified at the political, professional, and organizational levels to address the multiple barriers to such intersectoral collaboration (Syme, Lefkowitz, & Krimgold, 2002). In Canada, a resource for health professionals, lay workers, volunteers, and activists provides a primer for action on SDOH (Ontario Prevention Clearinghouse, 2007).

A further initiative that could increase the likelihood that the SDOH would be incorporated into policy changes focuses on educating the polity about the consequences for all of increasing inequality and poverty on health. One example in the United States is the *Guide to Community Preventive Services,* an evidence-based review of interventions that have been shown to be effective at a community level (Zaza, Briss, & Harris, 2005). For example, the Task Force "highly recommended" an increase in housing vouchers and center-based child care for low-income children from birth to age 3. Educating the public using the vehicle of a Surgeon General's report on the SDOH could also have a powerful effect on policies that would improve health. The high profile that these initiatives have garnered indicates that such a report would feature the important role that SDOH plays, thereby stimulating action (Lurie, 2002).

Complementing the idea of a Surgeon General's report on the SDOH is the *Index of Social Health* that the Fordham Institute for Innovation in Social Policy has published since 1990 (Miringoff & Miringoff, 1999). Consisting of 16 health and well-being indicators, the Index captures elements of SDOH that include availability of affordable housing, rates of unemployment, average weekly wages, inequality, child poverty, and violent crime. Additionally, Health Impact Assessments (HIA), defined as "a combination of procedures, methods and tools by which a policy program or project may be judged as to its potential effects on the health of a population and the distribution of those effects within the population" (European World Health Organization, 1999, p. 4), are suggested as a mechanism for developing healthy public policies. A goal of HIA is the integration of diverse assessment methods that use health promotion as a unifying lens (Bhatia, 2003). With an emphasis on the social, economic, and environmental conditions that influence health (Kemm, 2001), health equity is frequently an underlying value of HIAs (Parry & Stevens, 2001). As demonstrated by one recent example of a community participatory research approach in developing a health impact assessment, the significance of the HIA is in its joining diverse disciplinary interests and practices that value experiential and intuitive knowledge. Moreover, as a mechanism for promoting political accountability and community capacity development, the HIA process can result in the development of political analysis tools that reflect community values and needs, thus supporting the participation of lay people in ensuring institutional accountability (Bhatia, 2003).

Progress on building the science base for interventions in the SDOH has been made. Nevertheless, we continue to know too little about the mechanisms through which nonmedical determinants affect health. This is particularly true in the case of socioeconomic status and a range of social conditions. Research into causal mechanisms is needed to ensure that our policy interventions are evidence based (Lurie, 2002) and that they derive from the perspective of a "critical social science" (Fay, 1987). Examples of areas where such research could be particularly effective are in the health consequences of tax and income transfer policies, labor market policies, and social service policies. Concomitantly, we must change our language to embrace SDOH and social justice. In the interim, using the CBPR approach—which by definition engages communities and works with them to effect needed structural changes—can result in modifications in community structures that not only permit but also encourage healthier behaviors.

Community-Based Participatory Research (CBPR)

Given the complexities related to individual behavior change and the social determinants of health, it is reasonable to question how one might integrate the two approaches. Furthermore, the important question regarding how to most efficiently and effectively investigate health behavior change within an ecologic context remains. While traditional research methodology serves a valued and important purpose, when researching multifaceted issues such as the nuances of human behavior, health disparities, and how the complexities of the communities in which people live might affect behavior, a different research approach is warranted. More important, traditional research approaches that focus only on individual-level behaviors risk preventing recognition of the broader context of health and disease and ignoring the roles of social and environmental factors (Israel, Schulz, Parker, & Becker, 1998). In contrast, participatory research "ensures that research results may in fact address real needs and will actually be used" (Green and Mercer, 2001, p. 1926).

Definition of CBPR

"CBPR is a collaborative research approach that is designed to ensure and establish structures for participation by communities affected by the issue being studied, representatives of organizations, and researchers in all aspects of the research process to improve health and well-being through taking action, including social change" (Viswanathan et al., 2004, p. 77). CBPR encompasses the concepts of co-learning, shared decision making, and mutual ownership of the research and its products (Viswanathan et al., 2004). It is intended to intimately involve communities in the research process so that the resulting knowledge reflects their needs. This approach is particularly well suited to the area of health behavior change, as it allows for the design of interventions that consider the unique qualities of the community in which the interventions are to be implemented. Consequently, CBPR is intended to foster sustained health behavior change by focusing on an ecological approach that includes political change.

Israel and her colleagues shed light on CBPR by describing it as "a partnership approach to research that equitably involves, for example, community members, organizational representatives, and researchers in all aspects of the research process" (Israel, Engels, Schulz, & Parker, 2005, p. 5). In identifying key elements of participatory research, the importance of participation, influence, and control of nonacademic researchers in the process of creating knowledge and change is emphasized. Israel also calls upon health behavior researchers to recognize the community as a social and cultural entity by actively engaging the community in the research process.

Cornwall and Jewkes (1995) elaborate on the definition of participatory research when they describe the CBPR process as a series of reflections and actions, carried out "*with* local people rather than *on* them" (p. 1667, italics added). Traditional research studies rarely include the participants in most aspects of the research design, analysis, and implementation. Some traditional researchers may believe that a participatory approach is incompatible with "real" or "rigorous" research. This attitude accompanies the intention of removing bias from the study. Nevertheless, there is growing acceptance of inclusive participatory methods that render a study's results more applicable and pertinent to the targeted participants. Rather than serving the needs of academic researchers, participatory research reminds us of the goal of research: to serve and improve the health and well-being of the people and communities being studied. As research in the field of behavior change explores the motivations and challenges inherent in behavior, it must also address the ecological context discussed earlier in this chapter by including the broader aspects of the community environment and social factors that inevitably affect behavior. For behavior change promotions and interventions to be successful, the workings and structures that currently (or could in the future) influence behavior change in individuals within the community must be considered.

The CBPR Approach

CBPR is an approach that draws upon the full range of research designs and can include qualitative and quantitative data collection and analysis. It is used in developing health promotion interventions (Lantz, Israel, Schulz, & Reyes, 2006) and has been shown to be beneficial in developing policy processes and environmental change (Vasquez, Minkler, & Shepard, 2006). The CBPR approach is strongly linked to individual behavior change through the context of community-based interventions that address the SDOH. Thus, CBPR considers address the broader context of health, environment, culture, and community, thereby making behavior change more approachable and feasible for individuals. CBPR enhances research relevance by involving the knowledge and experience of people with relevant lived experience, rather than relying on outside researcher input alone (Altman, 1995). Developing partnerships and community assessments are initial elements of CBPR. The community context is used to define research questions and, eventually, interventions such as health promotion campaigns or behavior change strategies. Research products are shared equally and focus on effective program and policy changes that will produce lasting health behavior change and sustainable positive health outcomes (Israel et al., 1998).

The development of partnerships is a key component of CBPR and serves a significant purpose in relation to health behavior change and health promotion. In its attempt to reach the heart of the community and to benefit from community knowledge and expertise, CBPR is unique in its emphasis on relationships with nontraditional public health partners and reaches past barriers to partners and relationships that were previously out of reach. Adhering to the principles of good participatory research means that "activities critical in partnership development include sharing decision-making, defining principles of collaboration, establishing research priorities, and securing funding" (Metzler et al., 2003, p. 804).

Partnership building in and of itself can lead to positive actions related to health behavior change. Partnerships created via participatory research strategies often result in relationships that facilitate significant collective action. Developing partnerships constitutes an integral step in the process toward social action and community empowerment through the development of networks of organizations and individuals.

In its partnership-building process, investigators associated with The Healthy Neighborhoods Project in West Contra County, California, discovered that the community had much to offer to the health promotion and research projects targeting its residents. The project used a community-organizing approach and created an authentic partnership between residents, community-based organizations, the health department, and often others, such as the housing, crime and safety, business, and transportation sectors (Minkler, 2000). Through the participatory research processes of this project, among other results, transportation services were improved and security measures for high-risk neighborhoods increased. The community-wide changes that took place through the Healthy Neighborhoods Project demonstrated how CBPR engages communities to address the social determinants of health, thereby improving the likelihood that health behavior change will result. Without community engagement, it is possible that these key factors could be missed and change would be impossible, regardless of the theoretical efficacy of any given health promotion intervention.

One of the most critical junctions of the research process is the development of the research question. Traditionally, in health promotion and behavior change, the question is developed by hypothesizing the reasons for a specific disease state in a certain population. Researchers then work from this hypothesis to develop an intervention that they theorize will encourage and inspire change in a certain health behavior, such as physical activity, sexual practices, or tobacco use. While this is obviously a well-tested approach to research, CBPR adds an additional component to crafting the research question, or the definition of the problem to be addressed: community members are involved in the discussions. "With the community playing a key role, epidemiologists may have to put aside their topic of interest and predetermined methods so that the community can help determine the issue and how it is to be investigated, as well as toward what ends" (Leung, Yen, & Minkler, 2004, p. 501). Leung argues that involving community members in the development of the research question strengthens researchers' ability to learn about community networks and therefore their ability to write informed hypotheses and collect data.

Strengths of CBPR

While the benefits of using the CBPR approach must be balanced by the challenges that accompany its use, CBPR is gaining acceptance as a valid research approach. The strengths of CBPR lie in its ability to address a broad context, value local resources, develop collaborative and trusting relationships with communities, build capacity, and effect policy change.

Broad Context

Working with community members to define the research question or issue can be a means to the end of addressing the broader context of health promotion and disease prevention. In East Harlem, New York, a community coalition that included care providers, community-based organizations, and community members was created in order to conduct a survey research study in a population with an exceptionally high prevalence of diabetes (Horowitz, Williams, &

Bickell, 2003). Before health behavior change researchers could design interventions to encourage individual-level behavior change, they acknowledged that gaining a broad community-level picture was an important part of the initiative. This study found that most residents of this community had the knowledge they needed regarding their medicines but that underlying conditions were preventing them from attending to their personal diabetes care. Factors such as transportation and financial challenges ranked high on their lists of concerns (Horowitz et al., 2003). Without the use of participatory community-based research, these underlying social and economic factors might not have been identified and incorporated into the overall intervention design and solution.

Without community participation, health promotion interventions can sometimes miss the mark. An example is seen in the Community Intervention Trial for Smoking Cessation (COMMIT). This large project had modest success in changing the behavior of light to moderate smokers but had no marked effect on the higher risk heavy-smoker group. A community-based intervention in several matched communities, COMMIT did not permit flexibility in intervention design between and among communities. While this consistency across settings serves the purpose of testing the same intervention, it necessarily ignores the unique underlying social factors in each community. At the study's conclusion, the authors agreed that "the standardized protocol may have constrained some communities from undertaking activities that might have had greater impact" (COMMIT Research Group, 1995, p. 190). In addition, they "felt that the protocol did not permit emphasis on some kind of policy or environmental changes that might have been quite powerful" (COMMIT Research Group, 1995, p. 190). While it is challenging to attain the rigor of traditional scientific design with community-based approaches, the strategies proposed in CBPR can combine the two and, in the end, strengthen the results.

Valuing Local Resources and Community Collaboration

A reward of partnerships built through CBPR is the multitude of skills and knowledge gained from the involvement of individuals and community organizations. Participatory research emphasizes the role of communities as collaborators in research. It involves communities and aims to support the structures of those communities in order to improve their health (Israel et al., 1998). Minkler (2005) discusses the strengths of this approach and notes that "by deeply valuing lay knowledge, CBPR can uncover hidden contributors to health and social problems" (p. 6).

The Kahnawake schools diabetes prevention project is a good example of utilizing local resources and community collaboration in a health promotion project (Macaulay et al., 1997). It also demonstrates the importance of this component in a population not traditionally involved in research. This project was implemented in a Canadian Mohawk community, one with a long-term goal of primary prevention of type 2 diabetes. Kahnawake is represented through a community advisory board of 25 volunteers from the health, educational, political, recreational, social, spiritual, economic, and private sectors and the full-time project staff (Macaulay et al., 1997). Researchers noted that the community members' "collective wisdom adds a perspective that broadens interpretations, increases the project's effectiveness, helps to decrease harm and improves the credibility of oral and written results, which saves the community from potential stigmatization" (Macaulay et al., 1997, p. 779). The community members involved in the project's design and implementation were able to give researchers their perspectives on critical aspects of the project, such as the population to be targeted, advocating for respect for community acceptance of interventions and reminding the research team of relevant local customs and practices. These were integral parts of the overall research plan and led to a successful outcome. Although not all the targeted health outcomes were reached, community collaboration and empowerment were certainly increased. These are welcome secondary outcomes of participatory research and are often the precursors of behavior change.

Establishing Trust

Participatory research has been said to be more inclusive of communities that are more often marginalized in traditional research, partly because of the ability of the CBPR approach to foster trust through collaboration. Populations that have previously been taken advantage of in research studies are historically skeptical of researchers, questioning their motives and approaches. This historical lack of trust can make it difficult to recruit and retain participants from these populations for research studies. Attributing the culture of distrust to such grievous violations such as the Tuskegee syphilis study, researchers have found that, for example, African Americans have a marked distrust of the medical community and that this is a prominent barrier to participation in research (Corbie-Smith, Thomas, Williams, & Moody-Ayers, 1999).

Practiced ethically and with adherence to CBPR principles, community-based research can involve community members and their representatives in all phases of the research project—from defining the research question to owning and implementing the results (Cashman, et al., 2008). Participatory research, with its more inclusive and transparent methodology, may well alleviate some of the trust issues previously seen in traditional research methods. In their review of three urban health promotion projects, Metzler et al. (2003) determined that the "challenge of community-based research partnerships is to overcome historical breaches of trust and discrepancies in power to build relationships across boundaries of race and class" (p. 809). The projects reviewed in this study did indeed have some success in combating these challenges.

Research to Action—Relevance

A common criticism of public health research is its limited ability to translate into realistic, effective action. The CBPR approach challenges some of this criticism through its goal of effecting social action and environmental change. By the very nature of its participatory paradigm, CBPR increases the relevance of resulting recommended interventions and therefore translates more easily into realistic practice.

Limitations and Challenges of CBPR

Criticisms of CBPR focus on the extent to which the CBPR approach embodies scientific rigor. Additionally, some researchers question the ability of CBPR to identify causes and determine the effect of an intervention. Even those who advocate for CBPR as a research approach and who value its contributions to health promotion and disease prevention recognize that it is challenging to implement. Challenges arise in three areas (1) Institutional Review Board human subjects protocol approval (Malone, Yerger, McGruder, & Froelicher, 2006); (2) obtaining funding (Minkler, Blackwell, Thompson, & Tamir, 2003); and (3) balancing pressures from both academic researchers and community members in adhering to CBPR principles and practices (Green & Mercer, 2001).

Logistical obstacles also arise when trying to maintain full community participatory status, as often the community members are contributing as volunteers. Additionally, given the time needed to focus on process, it can be challenging to maintain community members' interest, and community champions may move on. Furthermore, priorities may change in a community during the time that the research project is being carried out, and motivation to remain involved may wax and wane. Expectations for community-based projects may be set too high, with timelines that are unrealistic given the need to change long-standing social and environmental contexts and practices. Yet, the results of community-based research often lay the groundwork and develop the supporting structures needed to facilitate change.

When addressing specific health outcomes as results of behavior change, community-based programs may not show immediate results. Outcomes such as changes in body mass index for physical activity promotions or glycated hemoglobin levels for diabetes prevention programs, for example, may not occur within the time frame of the research project, as these particular outcomes require longer timelines for measurable change (Daniel et al., 1999).

Relating CBPR to Behavior Change

Through the CBPR approach, research on behavior change within the community context can flourish. Because CBPR allows for more inclusive approaches that often result in addressing social determinants of health and environmental factors that affect community and individual health, it ultimately leads to more effective programs and interventions to support behavior change. The collaborative, community-engaged approach serves as a conduit, linking individual and population-based approaches to health promotion. The development of partnerships and collaborative structures in communities is a fundamental building block of CBPR; relationships that develop through these partnerships assist in health behavior change efforts by focusing on underlying causes and striving for social justice.

Schulz and her colleagues (Schulz et al., 2002) investigated these principles through their work in the East Side Village Health Worker Partnership. They found that interventions that consider the local perspective can serve a dual purpose of meeting local community priorities for change (more police presence, adequate street lighting) and addressing fundamental, structural issues that shape behavior (e.g., housing, poverty) and that may be of more immediate concern to the academic partners. This dual purpose of CBPR can in turn affect the likelihood that healthy behavior changes will occur. While behavior change takes place at an individual level, individuals are part of a larger community; they influence community norms and customs while in turn being influenced by them.

Laverack and Labonte (2000) offer a description of the differences between initiatives that work within communities and those that work on communities. The former describes an approach that engages communities in the very early stages of disease prevention, in defining the issues and priorities that are most important to the people actually living in the community itself. This approach, which characterizes the CBPR strategy, can result in increases in community capacity and power; these increases in capacity are themselves a desired outcome of the intervention. It follows, therefore, that from this increased capacity is born an environment that is more amenable to behavior change outcomes. The second approach refers to health promotion programs designed primarily by outside agencies, with little regard for community interests or priorities. This approach more often targets particular health behaviors as the desired health outcome. One approach is not necessarily always more successful than the other. However, interventions that begin within and engage communities create a sense of ownership in the problem and the solution. This approach often results in more sustainable positive healthful changes, while simultaneously creating a stronger community network.

The work of the Chicago Southeast Diabetes Community Action Coalition is a good example of this concept of community capacity building (Giachello et al., 2003). While traditional health promotion activities to combat diabetes usually rely on health education to change individual lifestyle practices, the CBPR approach will often address components that contribute to problems such as diabetes in struggling communities. The researchers in the Chicago project utilized CBPR to engage the community in identifying the root causes and social determinants of their priority health issues. As part of their research process, local community members interested in diabetes were offered training sessions that provided information about the disease, approaches to community building, and methods of research. This reduced the "gap" between outside researchers and community lay persons, while affording the community an opportunity to build upon its own strengths and to utilize those strengths for future projects.

Communities can also use skills fostered through those developing CBPR partnerships to advocate for policy and environmental changes that support health promotion efforts. In the Chicago diabetes project, the collaborative team recognized that "health education and increased surveillance in a system without reform will only serve to further frustrate a population that has few options in general" (Giachello et al., 2003). While healthy lifestyles are indeed worthwhile goals, many residents of high-risk communities cannot adopt these healthier practices. In many cases, they have no healthy options. Using CBPR as a basis for health behavior change, researchers found that the primary vehicles for health promotion and health behavior change resided in building community control, resources, and capacities toward economic, social, and political change (Laverack & Labonte, 2000).

Summary

Community-based participatory research is becoming an increasingly valued approach to behavior change and health promotion research. This methodology contributes to the field of health behavior change by providing a means of examining the larger, contextual setting of human behavior that exists beyond the individual. The social determinants of health and the ecological perspective are vital aspects of health promotion activities. Without considering these perspectives and building on the insight they provide, interventions from health promotion initiatives can miss key elements contributing to the health issue addressed. CBPR gives us a way to investigate these crucial elements, while still maintaining scientific quality and relevance. This participatory approach increases the value of health promotion research, while simultaneously helping a community build its own capacity to address public health challenges that stem from any of the array of social determinants of health. It also allows us to consider the broader context of health and disease, place value on local resources, increase community capacity, and enhance the relevance of the research. Remarkably, studies that incorporate a community's view of its health needs frequently find that community-driven concerns are consistent with the view that societal factors are the primary driving forces affecting health (Raphael, 2001).

The strength of the CBPR approach, combined with efforts to trace the causes of poor health encompassed in SDOH, allows communities and researchers alike to aim for a more effective translation of research into public health practice that includes social and political change. With the power of research, communities can feel more confident in advancing their struggle to meet basic needs, such as transportation, housing, job security, access to healthy foods, and physical safety. The use of CBPR allows us to consider behavior change at the community and population level, set within the context of social determinants of health. Combining strategies that encompass individuals and the communities in which they live and work results in health promotion efforts that bring about measurable improvement.

References

Abbott, S. (2007). The psychosocial effects on the health of socioeconomic inequalities. *Critical Public Health, 17*(2), 151–158.

Altman, D. G. (1995). Sustaining interventions in community systems: On the relationship between researchers and communities. *Health Psychology, 14*(6), 526–536.

Bambra, C., Fox, D., & Scott-Samuel, A. (2005). Towards a politics of health. *Health Promotion International, 20*(2), 187–193.

Baum, F. (2007). Cracking the nut of health equity: Top down and bottom up pressure for action on the social determinants of health. *Promotion and Education, 14*(2), 90–95.

Beauchamp, D. (1988). *Health of the republic epidemics, medicine and moralism as challenges to democracy.* Philadelphia: Temple University Press.

Benzeval, M. (2002). *Reducing inequalities in health: A European perspective.* London: Routledge.

Benzeval, M., Judge, K., & Whitehead, M. (Eds.). (1995). *Tackling inequalities in health: An agenda for action.* London: King's Fund.

Bhatia, R. (2003). Swimming upstream in a swift current: Public health institutions and inequality. In R. Hofrichter (Ed.), *Health social justice: Politics, ideology, and inequity in the distribution of disease* (pp. 557–578). San Francisco: Jossey-Bass.

Blackwell, A. G., & Colmenar, R. (2000). Community-building: From local wisdom to public policy. *Public Health Reports, 115,* 161–166.

Braveman, P., Starfield, B., & Geiger, H. J. (2001). World health report 2000: How it removes equity from the agenda for public health monitoring and policy. *British Medical Journal, 323*(7314), 678–681.

Brofenbrenner, U. (1977). Toward an experimental ecology of human development. *American Psychologist, 32,* 513–531.

Brofenbrenner, U. (1979). *The ecology of human development.* Cambridge, MA: Harvard University Press.

Brunner, E., & Marmot, M. (1999). Social organization, stress, and health. In M. Marmot & R. G. Wilkinson (Eds.), *Social determinants of health* (pp. 17–43). New York: Oxford University Press Inc.

Cashman, S. B., Adeky, S., Allen, A. J., Corburn, J., Israel, B. A., Montano, J., et al. (2008). The power and the promise: Working with communities to analyze data, interpret findings, and get to outcomes. *American Journal of Public Health, 98*(8), 1407–1417.

COMMIT Research Group. (1995). Community Intervention Trial for Smoking Cessation (COMMIT). *American Journal of Public Health, 85*(2), 183–192.

Corbie-Smith, G., Thomas, S. B., Williams, M. V., & Moody-Ayers, S. (1999). Attitudes and beliefs of African Americans toward participation in medical research. *Journal of General Internal Medicine, 14*(9), 537–546.

Cornwall, A., & Jewkes, R. (1995). What is participatory research? *Social Science and Medicine, 41,* 1667–1676.

Crawford, R. (1979). Individual responsibility and health politics in the 1970's. In S. Reverby & D. Rosner (Eds.), *Health care in America: Essays in social history.* Philadelphia: Temple University Press.

Daniel, M., Green, L. W., Marion, S. A., Gamble, D., Herbert, C. P., Hertzman, C., et al. (1999). Effectiveness of community-directed diabetes prevention and control in a rural aboriginal population in British Columbia, Canada. *Social Science and Medicine, 48*(6), 815–832.

Dovell, R. (2006). *Beyond health services and lifestyle. A social determinants approach to reporting on the health status of the interior health population.* Ottawa: Interior Health Authority.

Engels, F. (1845/1987). *The condition of the working class in England.* New York: Penguin Classics.

European World Health Organization. (1999). *Centre for health policy. Health impact assessment: Main concepts and suggested approach* (Gothenburg consensus paper). Brussels: Author.

Fay, B. (1987). *Critical social science: Liberation and its limits.* Ithaca, NY: Cornell University Press.

Giachello, A. L., Arrom, J. O., Davis, M., Sayad, J. V., Ramirez, D., Nandi, C., et al. (2003). Reducing diabetes health disparities through community-based participatory action research: The Chicago southeast diabetes community action coalition. *Public Health Reports, 118*(4), 309–323.

Green, L. W., & Mercer, S. L. (2001). Can public health researchers and agencies reconcile the push from funding bodies and the pull from communities? *American Journal of Public Health, 91*(12), 1926–1929.

Hofrichter, R. (2003). The politics of health inequities: Contested terrain. In R. Hofrichter (Ed.), *Health and social justice: Politics, ideology, and inequity in the distribution of disease* (pp. 1–56). San Francisco: Jossey-Bass.

Hofrichter, R. (Ed.). (2006). *Tackling health inequities through public health practice: A handbook for action.* Washington, DC: National Association of County and City Health Officials.

Horowitz, C. R., Williams, L., & Bickell, N. A. (2003). A community-centered approach to diabetes in East Harlem. *Journal of General Internal Medicine, 18*(7), 542–548.

Irwin, A., Valentine, N., Brown, C., Loewenson, R., Solar, O., Brown, H., et al. (2006). The commission on social determinants of health: Tackling the social roots of health inequities. *PLoS Medicine, 3*(6), e106.

Israel, B. A., Engels, F., Schulz, A. J., & Parker, E. A. (Eds.). (2005). *Methods in community-based participatory research for health.* San Francisco: Jossey-Bass.

Israel, B. A., Schulz, A. J., Parker, E. A., & Becker, A. B. (1998). Review of community-based research: Assessing partnership approaches to improve public health. *Annual Review of Public Health, 19,* 173–202.

Kawachi, I., Kennedy, B. P., & Wilkinson, R. G. (Eds.). (1999). *The society and population health reader, Vol. 1: Income inequality and health.* New York: Oxford: University Press.

Kelly, M., Morgan, A., Bonnefoy, J., Butt, J., & Bergman, V. (2007). *The social determinants of health: Development of an evidence base for political action.* Geneva: World Health Organization.

Kemm, J. (2001). Health impact assessment: A tool for healthy public policy. *Health Promotion International, 16*(1), 79–85.

Kunst, A., Groenhof, F., & Mackenbach, J. (1998). Occupational class and cause specific mortality in middle aged men in 11 European countries: Comparison of population based studies. *British Medical Journal, 316,* 1636–1642.

Lantz, P., Israel, B., Schulz, A., & Reyes, A. (2006). Community-based participatory research: Rationale and relevance for social epidemiology. In J. Oakes & J. Kaufman (Eds.), *Methods in social epidemiology* (pp. 239–266). San Francisco: Jossey-Bass.

Laverack, G., & Labonte, R. (2000). A planning framework for community empowerment goals within health promotion. *Health Policy Planning, 15*(3), 255–262.

Leichter, H. M. (2003). "Evil habits" and "personal choices": Assigning responsibility for health in the 20th century. *Milbank Quarterly, 81*(4), 603–626.

Leung, M. W., Yen, I. H., & Minkler, M. (2004). Community based participatory research: A promising approach for increasing epidemiology's relevance in the 21st century. *International Journal of Epidemiology, 33*(3), 499–506.

Link, B., & Phelan, J. (2005). Fundamental sources of health inequalities. In D. Mechanic, L. Rogut, & D. Colby (Eds.), *Policy challenges in modern health care.* New Brunswick, NJ: Rutgers University Press.

Lurie, N. (2002). What the federal government can do about the nonmedical determinants of health. *Health Affairs (Millwood), 21*(2), 94–106.

Lynch, J. W., Kaplan, G. A., Pamuk, E. R., Cohen, R. D., Heck, K. E., Balfour, J. L., et al. (1998). Income inequality and mortality in metropolitan areas of the United States. *American Journal of Public Health, 88*(7), 1074–1080.

Macaulay, A. C., Paradis, G., Potvin, L., Cross, E. J., Saad-Haddad, C., McComber, A., et al. (1997). The Kahnawake schools diabetes prevention project: Intervention, evaluation, and baseline results of a diabetes primary prevention program with a native community in Canada. *Preventive Medicine, 26*(6), 779–790.

Malone, R. E., Yerger, V. B., McGruder, C., & Froelicher, E. (2006). "It's like Tuskegee in reverse": A case study of ethical tensions in institutional review board review of community-based participatory research. *American Journal of Public Health, 96*(11), 1914–1919.

Marmot, M. (2004). *The status syndrome: How social standing affects our health and longevity.* New York: Holt.

Marmot, M. (2007). Achieving health equity: From root causes to fair outcomes. *Lancet, 370*(9593), 1153–1163.

Marmot, M., & Wilkinson, R. (Eds.). (1999). *Social determinants of health.* New York: Oxford University Press.

McEwen, B. S. (1998a). Protective and damaging effects of stress mediators. *New England Journal of Medicine, 338*(3), 171–179.

McEwen, B. S. (1998b). Stress, adaptation, and disease. Allostasis and allostatic load. *Annals of the New York Academy of Sciences, 840,* 33–44.

McEwen, B. S. (2003). Interacting mediators of allostasis and allostatic load: Towards an understanding of resilience in aging. *Metabolism: Clinical and Experimental, 52*(10 Suppl. 2), 10–16.

McGinnis, J. M., Williams-Russo, P., & Knickman, J. R. (2002). The case for more active policy attention to health promotion. *Health Affairs (Millwood), 21*(2), 78–93.

McKinlay, J. B. (1998). Paradigmatic obstacles to improving the health of populations—implications for health policy. *Salud Publica de Mexico, 40*(4), 369–379.

McLeroy, K. R., Bibeau, D., Steckler, A., & Glanz, K. (1988). An ecological perspective on health promotion programs. *Health Education Quarterly, 15*(4), 351–377.

Metzler, M. (2007). Social determinants of health: What, how, why, and now. *Preventing Chronic Disease, 4*(4), A85.

Metzler, M. M., Higgins, D. L., Beeker, C. G., Freudenberg, N., Lantz, P. M., Senturia, K. D., et al. (2003). Addressing urban health in Detroit, New York City, and Seattle through community-based participatory research partnerships. *American Journal of Public Health, 93*(5), 803–811.

Minkler, M. (2000). Using participatory action research to build healthy communities. *Public Health Reports, 115*(2–3), 191–197.

Minkler, M. (2005). Community-based research partnerships: Challenges and opportunities. *Journal of Urban Health, 82*(2 Suppl. 2), ii3–12.

Minkler, M. (Ed.). (1997). *Community organizing and community building for health.* New Brunswick, NJ: Rutgers University Press.

Minkler, M., Blackwell, A. G., Thompson, M., & Tamir, H. (2003). Community-based participatory research: Implications for public health funding. *American Journal of Public Health, 93*(8), 1210–1213.

Minkler, M., & Wallerstein, N. (2003). *Community based participatory research for health.* San Francisco: Jossey-Bass.

Miringoff, M. L., & Miringoff, L. (1999). *The social health of the nation: How America is really doing.* New York: Oxford University Press.

Muennig, P., Franks, P., Jia, H., Lubetkin, E., & Gold, M. R. (2005). The income-associated burden of disease in the United States. *Social Science and Medicine, 61*(9), 2018–2026.

Murphy, B. (2004). In search of the fourth dimension of health promotion: Guiding principles for action. In H. Keleher & B. Murphy (Eds.), *Understanding health: A determinants approach* (pp. 152–169). Melbourne, Australia: Oxford University Press.

Navarro, V., Muntaner, C., Borrell, C., Benach, J., Quiroga, A., Rodriguez-Sanz, M., et al. (2006). Politics and health outcomes. *Lancet, 368*(9540), 1033–1037.

Norris, T., & Pittman, M. (2000). The healthy communities movement and the coalition for healthier cities and communities. *Public Health Reports, 115,* 118–124.

O'Hara, P. (2005). *Creating social and health equity: Adopting an Alberta social determinants of health framework.* Edmonton, Canada: Edmonton Social Planning Council.

Ontario Prevention Clearinghouse. (2007). *Primer to action: Social determinants of health.* Toronto: Ontario Chronic Disease Prevention Alliance and the Canadian Cancer Society—Ontario Division.

Parry, J., & Stevens, A. (2001). Prospective health impact assessment: Pitfalls, problems, and possible ways forward. *British Medical Journal, 323*(7322), 1177–1182.

Ram, R. (2005). Income inequality, poverty, and population health: Evidence from recent data for the United States. *Social Science and Medicine, 61*(12), 2568–2576.

Raphael, D. (2001). Evaluation of quality of life initiatives in health promotion. In I. Rootman, D. McQueen, & M. Goodstadt (Eds.), *Evaluating health promotion initiatives: Principles and practice* (pp. 123–147). Geneva: World Health Organization.

Raphael, D. (2002). *Social justice is good for our hearts: Why societal factors—not lifestyles—are major causes of heart disease in Canada and elsewhere.* Unpublished manuscript, Toronto.

Raphael, D. (2003). Toward the future: Policy and community actions to promote population health. In R. Hofrichter (Ed.), *Health social justice: Politics, ideology, and inequity in the distribution of disease* (pp. 453–468). San Francisco: Jossey-Bass.

Raphael, D. (2004). Introduction to the social determinants of health. In D. Raphael (Ed.), *Social determinants of health: Canadian perspectives* (pp. 1–18). Toronto: Canadian Scholars' Press.

Raphael, D. (2007). *Social determinants of health listserv.* Retrieved November 13, 2006, from http://quarts.atkinson.yorku.ca/QuickPlace/draphael/main.nsf/

Raphael, D., & Farrell, E. (2002). Beyond medicine and lifestyle: Addressing the societal determinants of cardiovascular disease in North America. *Leadership in Health Services, 15,* 1–5.

Regan, P., & Brookins-Fisher, J. (1997). *Community health in the 21st century.* Needham Heights, MA: Allyn & Bacon.

Ribisl, K. M., & Humphreys, K. (1998). Collaboration between Professionals and Mediating Structures in the Community: Toward a "Third Way" in Health Promotion. In S. A. Shumaker, E. B. Schron, J. K. Ockene, W. L. McBee (Eds.), *The Handbook of Health Behavior Change* (2nd ed., pp. 535–554). New York: Springer Publishing.

Rogot, E. (1992). *A mortality study of 1.3 million persons by demographic, social, and economic factors: 1979–85 follow-up.* Bethesda, MD: National Institutes of Health.

Sapolsky, R. M., & Share, L. J. (1994). Rank-related differences in cardiovascular function among wild baboons: Role of sensitivity to glucocorticoids. *American Journal of Primatology, 32,* 261–275.

Schneider, M. J. (2006). *Introduction to public health.* Boston: Jones & Bartlett.

Schulz, A. J., Parker, E. A., Israel, B. A., Allen, A., Decarlo, M., & Lockett, M. (2002). Addressing social determinants of health through community-based participatory research: The East Side Village Health worker Partnership. *Health Education and Behavior, 29*(3), 326–341.

Schulz, P., & Sankaran, S. (2006). *Inclusion: Societies that foster belonging improve health.* Toronto: Ontario Clearinghouse.

Shively, C. A., Laird, K. L., & Anton, R. F. (1997). The behavior and physiology of social stress and depression in female cynomolgus monkeys. *Biological Psychiatry, 41,* 871–872.

Shumaker, S. A., Ockene, J. K., Schron, E. B., & McBee, W. L. (Eds.). (1998). *The handbook of health behavior change.* New York: Springer Publishing Company.

Smith, G. D., Hart, C., Blane, D., Gillis, C., & Hawthorne, V. (1997). Lifetime socioeconomic position and mortality: Prospective observational study. *British Medical Journal, 314*(7080), 547–552.

Stansfield, S., & Marmot, M. (Eds.). (2002). *Stress and the heart: Psychosocial pathways to coronary heart disease.* London: BMJ Books.

Subramanian, S. V., Belli, P., & Kawachi, I. (2002). The macroeconomic determinants of health. *Annual Review of Public Health, 23,* 287–302.

Syme, S. L., Lefkowitz, B., & Krimgold, B. K. (2002). Incorporating socioeconomic factors into U.S. health policy: Addressing the barriers. *Health Affairs (Millwood), 21*(2), 113–118.

Townsend, P., Davidson, N., & Whitehead, M. (Eds.). (1992). *Inequalities in health: The Black Report and the health divide.* New York: Penguin.

U.S. Department of Health and Human Services. (2000). *Healthy People 2010.* Retrieved May 22, 2008, from www.healthypeople.gov/about/goals.htm

Vasquez, V. B., Minkler, M., & Shepard, P. (2006). Promoting environmental health policy through community based participatory research: A case study from Harlem, New York. *Journal of Urban Health, 83*(1), 101–110.

Vega, J., & Irwin, A. (2004). Tackling health inequalities: New approaches in public policy. *Bulletin of the World Health Organization, 82*(7), 482–483.

Virchow, R. (1848/1985). *Collected essays on public health and epidemiology.* Cambridge: Science History Publications.

Viswanathan, M., Ammerman, A. E., Eng, E., Gartlehner, G., Lohr, K. N., Griffith, D., et al. (2004). *Community-based participatory research: Assessing the evidence. Evidence report/technology assessment no. 99.* No. AHRQ Publication 04-E022-2. Rockville, MD: Agency for Healthcare Research and Quality.

Wallerstein, N., & Bernstein, E. (1988). Empowerment education: Freire's ideas adapted to health education. *Health Education Quarterly, 15*(4), 379–394.

Wardle, J., & Gibson, E. L. (2002). Impact of stress on diet: Processes and implications. In S. Stansfeld & M. G. Marmot (Eds.), *Stress and the heart: Psychosocial pathways to coronary heart disease* (pp. 124–149). London: BMJ Books.

Wilcox, L. S. (2007). Onions and bubbles: Models of the social determinants of health. *Preventing Chronic Disease, 4,* A83.

Wilkinson, R., & Marmot, M. (Eds.). (2003). *Social determinants of health: The solid facts* (2nd ed.). Copenhagen: World Health Organization.

Wilkinson, R. G. (1999). Putting the picture together: Prosperity, redistribution, health, and welfare. In M. Marmot & R. G. Wilkinson (Eds.), *Social determinants of health* (pp. 256–274). New York: Oxford University Press.

Wilkinson, R. G., & Marmot, M. G. (1998). *Social determinants of health: The solid facts.* Copenhagen: World Health Organization.

World Health Organization. (1948). *Constitution of the World Health Organization.* Retrieved May 22, 2008, from http://policy.who.int/cgi-bin/om_isapi.dll?hitsperheading=on&infobase=basicdoc&record={9D5}&softpage=Document42

Zaza, S., Briss, P. A., & Harris, K. W. (Eds.). (2005). *The guide to community preventive services. What works to promote health?* New York: Oxford University Press.

Ethical Issues in Lifestyle Change and Adherence

38

Nancy M. P. King

In this chapter, I examine issues in lifestyle change and adherence from the perspective of normative ethics—that is, moral theory that addresses the way individuals, institutions, or societies ought to act. Moral deliberation and justification in normative ethics ordinarily rest on action guides. These action guides are often expressed as rules or principles; in addition, however, ethical analysis may be based on rights theory, which requires an examination of reciprocal rights and duties within a relationship, or on virtue theory, which employs considerations of moral character.

These action guides serve as the centerpiece of modern ethical theory. They do not stand alone, however. Moral analysis requires choosing which action guides to employ, as well as considering the relationships among those chosen,

I am greatly indebted to Ruth R. Faden for her contribution to previous editions of the *Handbook*.

in addition to applying them to particular circumstances. Each of these analytical steps is subject to controversy and disagreement (Beauchamp & Childress, 2008). Perhaps most important, human moral agency may only rarely fit neatly into a single model of moral reasoning. It is likely that people think through moral choices more by using "moral eclecticism"—that is, the propensity to mix and match different kinds of moral considerations and analyses—than by applying a single philosophical model (Churchill, King, & Schenck, 2005). The universe of available moral action guides among which to choose has also been expanded by inclusion of models reflecting a diversity of cultural and religious perspectives (Guinn, 2006; Prograis & Pellegrino, 2007).

Structures of principles and rules, rights, and virtues can be used to analyze questions of morality in particular concrete situations and arenas of social life. Often, such analysis is referred to as "applied ethics." Numerous areas of applied ethics have been identified, such as business ethics, journalism ethics, and health care ethics.

Four areas of applied ethics with particular relevance to the themes of this volume are the ethics of the health professional-patient relationship; the ethics of the researcher-study participant relationship; the ethics of the government-citizenry relationship; and the ethics of the payer-client relationship. This chapter considers the key moral issues related to lifestyle change and adherence in each of these relationships. Relevant principles and rules emerge as each relationship is discussed.

Two distinct but related questions of adherence are considered in this volume: adherence in a clinical context and questions of lifestyle change for the general public. The ethical issues raised by adherence to prescribed medical regimens for the clinically ill may often be substantively different from the issues raised by adoption of recommendations of the Surgeon General or the American Heart Association regarding healthy lifestyles. And, although such differences seem stark, the distance between the "well" and the "ill" can be minimized rhetorically by the process, increasingly common in health care, of "medicalization." Medicalization is the tendency to label nondisease states, including risk factors for the development of common disorders, as medical conditions. For example, it has become commonplace to use labels like "prediabetic" to persuade asymptomatic individuals to adopt lifestyle changes and sometimes even to penalize physicians who fail to so counsel such patients. Increased knowledge about genetic contributions to common multifactorial disorders can also "medicalize" a healthy individual's genetic heritage, as a result of identifying in that person an increased likelihood of developing a disorder. Sometimes medicalization increases recognition of the risks to health posed by some nondisease states; the metabolic syndrome might be one example. Other instances of medicalization may be premature or counterproductive. It is important to consider possible differences in lifestyle change and adherence for different populations in the discussion that follows and to note how these differences can become blurred, although a full exploration is beyond the scope of this chapter.

The Clinician-Patient Relationship

Much of the emphasis in this volume is on adherence and lifestyle issues in health care services and the clinical encounter. Chapter 6, for example, considers how different models of the provider-patient relationship affect adherence. Medical ethics also considers different models of the doctor-patient relationship. One such approach argues that the doctor-patient relationship in particular, and all health professional-patient relationships generally, are dominated by two competing models of moral responsibility—the beneficence model and the autonomy model (Beauchamp & McCullough, 1984). Discussion of the conflict between beneficence and autonomy dominated early thinking in bioethics. Since then, analysis and application of these two models has become far more nuanced, and both their interdependence and their complementarity with other models are more fully recognized (Beauchamp & Childress, 2008). For the purposes of this chapter, however, it is useful to begin with a rather broad description of each.

According to the beneficence model, the primary obligation of clinicians is to seek the best balance of good over harm for their patients. Goods and harms are understood in medical terms: the chief goods are health, the prevention or elimination of disease and injury, relief from pain and suffering, the amelioration of disabilities, and the prolongation of life. The principal harms at issue are death, disease, disability, pain, and suffering. In the autonomy model, the values and beliefs of the patient and the patient's own assessment of what is in his or her best interests become the primary moral considerations. If the patient's values conflict with the values of medicine, the clinician's primary moral obligation is to respect and facilitate the patient's preferences. Both models speak to important moral truths about the health professional-patient relationship. However, when starkly drawn, their requirements can conflict, and it becomes necessary to bring them into balance by identifying the limits of each in a particular context.

The perspective of the beneficence model can provide strong moral support for adherence interventions in clinical settings. Under this model, clinicians have a moral obligation, an affirmative duty, to take actions that will preserve the health of their patients and protect them from disease and injury. Thus, clinicians who do not take seriously their obligations to secure the adherence of their patients to medically indicated regimens are morally blameworthy. This moral obligation was given legal force in a California case in which a physician was held liable for not adequately informing his patient of the risks of failing to have a Pap test (*Truman v. Thomas,* 1980). Nonetheless, there are legal, moral, and practical limits to the clinician's obligation to act to secure patient adherence. Even in the court decision just mentioned, the physician's responsibility was limited to adequately informing the patient so that she would be equipped to decide for herself whether to take his advice.

If it is not reasonably possible for clinicians to implement adherence interventions or otherwise secure adherence, they have no obligation to do so. As discussion throughout this volume demonstrates, clinicians' abilities to secure adherence depend on a host of factors, including the amount of time and the kinds of skills needed to be successful in promoting adherence in clinical contexts. Similarly, assessing the clinician's obligation to secure adherence also requires considering the relative moral priority of competing clinical duties in a context of limited resources. When the amount of time and dollars to be spent on clinical encounters is limited, what priority is to be placed on activities that can cure disease and allay suffering, rather than those that can prevent deterioration or promote health? Although clinicians may have a prima facie obligation to seek adherence to medical regimens and lifestyle recommendations, these obligations may be less weighty than other duties that compete for the clinician's attention. The strength of the clinician's obligation further depends on the strength of the evidence that, in given circumstances, adherence improves health outcomes; this requires not only knowledge of the epidemiologic literature but some application of that evidence to the individual patient. Thus, determining what steps clinicians should reasonably be expected to take to promote lifestyle change and adherence in patients is an important inquiry that depends both on particular circumstances and on continued developments in the rapidly changing health care environment.

The most important limit on the clinician's duty to "secure" adherence is the role of the individual whose adherence is sought. The autonomy model does not provide clinicians with a direct moral warrant for securing adherence to medical recommendations. According to the autonomy model, if the patient's values do not include improving his health prospects by altering lifestyle or adhering to medications, then the clinician is obligated to respect that value preference. This is not to say, however, that the autonomy model releases clinicians from any obligation in relation to adherence and lifestyle change. At minimum, respect for the patient's autonomy requires the clinician to ascertain the basis for the patient's position and, in particular, to establish whether the patient's rejection of the clinician's recommendation is based on an adequate understanding of what is at stake. The *Truman v. Thomas* decision can thus be interpreted as a reflection of the autonomy model, as well as the beneficence model. The physician in the case admitted that, although he repeatedly recommended a Pap smear and his patient repeatedly refused, he never probed beyond her refusal to determine whether she understood its consequences.

It cannot be assumed that laypersons' understandings of disease conform to medical understandings; therefore, laypersons and clinicians will not necessarily agree about the importance of medical recommendations for disease prevention. Moreover, even when their understanding is similar, it cannot be assumed that laypersons and clinicians place similar weight on what the clinician identifies as in a patient's medical best interests in relation to that person's other life priorities. Indeed, it is now widely recognized that informed decision making is best understood as a process of mutual learning in the clinician-patient relationship, whereby both clinician and layperson come to appreciate the other's reasoning and perspective and seek the best course of action for the patient under the circumstances. Discussions throughout this volume of the health beliefs model, including its dimensions, strengths, and limitations (e.g., chapters 2, 3, & 28), parallel this ethical analysis of autonomy by recognizing that decision making about adherence is a complex calculus of preferences, perceptions, priorities, and circumstances. The contribution of ethics to this increasingly nuanced understanding of health behavior change is simply the recognition that the physician's duty to support and enhance the patient's autonomy (Faden & Beauchamp, 1986) may require addressing these differences in viewpoint as part of the decision-making relationship.

What if the clinician ascertains that the patient has a correct understanding of what is at stake in refusing to adhere to medical recommendations and still wishes to ignore them? Both beneficence and autonomy suggest that the clinician is required to attempt to persuade the patient to change her position.

The obligation to promote the patient's good requires the clinician to attempt to persuade the patient that she will benefit from adherence. Persuasive interventions, properly constrained, do not violate obligations to respect patient autonomy (Faden & Beauchamp, 1986)—to the contrary, they often promote autonomous decision making by providing necessary information. However, if, after reasonable attempts at persuasion, the patient's decision remains unchanged, it must be respected.

It is essential to distinguish persuasion—defined as using reason to convince the patient to adopt the clinician's viewpoint as her own—from manipulation and coercion, which can appear similar (Faden & Beauchamp, 1986). Manipulation can be defined as using means other than reasoning, such as emotional appeals (for example, to fear), to bring the patient to a particular decision. Manipulation may or may not be morally permissible; that determination depends on the circumstances. Advertising campaigns often make use of manipulation, and the techniques of advertising (for example, music, imagery, and the addition of emotion to information) are often used to promote lifestyle changes such as exercise, smoking cessation, and diet modification. In such contexts, manipulation can be morally acceptable. In contrast, a classic example of manipulation that may be morally unacceptable is a physician's informing a smoker that something suspicious has been seen on a lung X-ray, intentionally misreading a benign finding in order to frighten the patient into quitting smoking (Smith & Churchill, 1986). Coercion—that is, seeking to achieve a given outcome by force or threat—is always and by definition morally illicit. An example might be a clinician's refusal to continue providing health care to a patient who does not give up smoking.

While it is morally necessary to distinguish among persuasion, manipulation, and coercion, it is not always easy to do so. Clean distinctions—especially between manipulation and persuasion and between acceptable and unacceptable manipulation—depend on the totality of circumstances and can be elusive. To help determine whether a given action is ethically permissible, the clinician should consider whether its goal is to ensure the patient's adherence or to ensure that the patient is well equipped to assess his own benefit and make his own choices, assisted by the clinician's education, advice, and support.

Increased recognition of the need to promote and support individuals' autonomy has been reflected in the adherence literature over time. What was once referred to as the problem of "compliance with doctor's orders" has become the problem of "adherence to the recommendations of professionals." Yet, even this second adherence formulation is not wholly satisfactory. A more desirable formulation would be something like "helping individuals make informed and reflective choices about whether to adopt or reject professional recommendations." Progress has also been made in expanding clinicians' views of what can be in the patient's best interests beyond a strictly medical perspective. Finally, both beneficence and autonomy find common cause in the recognition that neither can be adequately promoted by examining the clinician-patient relationship in isolation. Bioethics has moved beyond an exclusive focus on decision-making dyads to examine the roles and responsibilities of institutional actors (Henderson et al., 2005; Institute of Medicine, 2002). As is discussed extensively in this volume (e.g., chapters 2, 3, & 37), it is now also necessary to consider how the wider web of social structures, networks, and relationships supports or impedes individual lifestyle change.

As noted, although contrasting the beneficence model of professional-patient relationships with the autonomy model helps highlight the central moral issues raised by adherence and lifestyle interventions in clinical settings, this approach draws too stark a contrast between competing moral principles and fails to capture much of the contextual richness of the clinician-patient relationship. An alternative approach in moral theory, frequently referred to as the care perspective, draws attention to issues of responsiveness and compassion in the moral life, including the need to respond to that which is unique and particular about the other in a moral relationship (Areen, 1988; Hanen & Nielsen, 1987; Noddings, 2002). The care perspective reminds us to refrain from being formulaic in our approach to moral issues. In clinical encounters, each patient brings a unique history and life experience. From the care perspective, helping individuals make informed and reflective choices about medical regimens or lifestyle changes requires compassionate attention to the needs of the patient as a unique individual.

Uncertainty also plays a critical role in the ethics of adherence in the physician-patient relationship. The recent explosion in empirical data relating to health behavior and lifestyle has also led to greatly increased awareness of the gaps, ambiguities, and uncertainties inherent in those data, their interpretation, and their application. In providing decision-making assistance, professionals should recognize that there is genuine epistemic uncertainty about the value of many medical recommendations for lifestyle change. Challenges to the validity of medical knowledge, opinions, and recommendations almost always have a legitimate basis and should be taken seriously. As many recent examples have shown, and as other chapters in this volume describe in more detail, the medical community has a notable history of being wrong in its predictions and recommendations regarding both health risks and protective behavior (see, e.g., chapter 40). Patients of the past who refused to increase their consumption of eggs and who refused to take swine flu shots were at the time considered to be "noncompliers" who held "false beliefs" by contemporary medical standards. And medical recommendations about a variety of preventive regimens, such as postmenopausal hormone therapy for women, the best diet for weight control, and the type of exercise regimen best calculated to maintain physical function, have undergone recent and repeated revisions, leading to understandable public confusion and even disillusion.

To a significant extent, this sort of disagreement between patient and physician is an epistemic problem about the nature of medical knowledge and its evidentiary base, in a context of ever-evolving scientific theories of disease and illness. At stake is whether physicians can offer anything stronger than medical opinions, a far cry from traditional "doctor's orders." In addition, these disagreements reflect the changing social context of medical science and are resolved not only by the acquisition of better data but also by the recognition that successful lifestyle change depends on much more than convincing data: not only on medical opinion but on a supportive relationship that places adherence in the context of the life and needs of each individual.

The Researcher–Study Participant Relationship

The ethics of the researcher-study participant relationship has a different tradition and a different social imperative from that of the physician-patient relationship. In the clinical context, ethics is guided, at least in part, by the assumption that both clinician and patient share the goal of seeking to improve the patient's welfare. By contrast, in research the primary goal is not to benefit the study participant but to produce generalizable scientific knowledge. Because the welfare of the study participant is not central to the research enterprise, there is no beneficence model in research ethics corresponding to that in clinical ethics. As a result, overriding the obligation to respect the autonomy of study participants is extremely difficult to justify, even by appeal to arguments grounded in beneficence or conceptions of the public good.

The implications of this understanding for considering adherence issues in research are fairly straightforward. In general, it is morally impermissible for researchers to fail to fulfill their obligations to (1) seek valid informed consent from study participants, and (2) respect potential participants' decisions to refuse to participate or to drop out of studies—even when honoring these obligations compromises the scientific integrity of their research. When tensions arise between respecting the refusals of study participants and promoting their cooperation, the interventions of researchers should be restricted to persuasion and to inducements that do not substantially undermine the voluntariness of study participants' decisions.

Although researchers are not generally viewed as having an obligation to promote study participants' good, they are nonetheless increasingly viewed as having a related but distinguishable obligation to minimize harms to study participants arising from their research participation. This "nonmaleficence" obligation has been seen as underpinning the researcher-study participant relationship since the beginning of research ethics in the United States (National Commission, 1979) but has recently taken on special force in instances where research participation has the potential to disadvantage study participants.

Two examples are relevant to prevention research. First, in the Kennedy-Krieger Institute decision, researchers who were testing different lead abatement strategies in Baltimore low-income housing were held to have a responsibility to the welfare of resident children whose blood lead concentrations, measured for study purposes, exceeded safe levels (*Grimes v. Kennedy Krieger Institute, Inc.*, 2001). The court's reasoning is controversial and the decision's applicability is limited, but the case has reawakened vigorous discussion of the researcher-study participant relationship.

Second, since, as noted, the evidentiary support for many preventive regimens can be flawed or lacking, randomized controlled trials can provide a useful way to assess the effectiveness of preventive health care. Comparisons between the long-term health of study participants who practice preventive regimens and that of those who do not is usually more accurate if participants are randomly assigned, and even more accurate if the assignment can be blinded—which can be easy to do with some preventive drug regimens but impossible with other behavior-based regimens, like diet and exercise.

For a potential participant, the challenge is to understand and agree to take the chance that a prophylactic regimen in which he believes strongly may be safely forgone for what may be a long period of time. For researchers and oversight bodies, the challenge is to ensure clarity about the nature of the evidence that exists and that is needed to justify research to determine the efficacy of what may have come to be common practice. Even research that poses few risks of harm to well-informed participants can be unethical if the trial design cannot answer the question asked or if the study data cannot be meaningfully analyzed—that is to say, it is not fair to subject study participants even to inconvenience if there is little or no chance that their inconvenience will benefit science (Emanuel, Wendler, & Grady, 2000). Large-scale epidemiologic studies of preventive interventions may be more likely than other randomized trials to pose these kinds of ethical challenges because of their design complexities.

Imagine translating the recent controversy over the short- and long-term effects of the Atkins diet into a randomized trial of different Atkins-type diets and trying to monitor weight, serum cholesterol, body fat percentage, disease outcomes, and other measures over time. How should the risks of harm and potential benefits of such a study be described for potential participants? How can the conduct of the study be adequately monitored? How should it take account of changing information about the safety and effectiveness of the Atkins diet? Randomized controlled trials that involve behavior-based interventions and seek to measure disease-related outcomes can require following the cohort for a very long time, as the expected effect sizes may be quite small and event rates are often low. Replacing a clinical outcome with a surrogate measure can shorten the duration of a trial but may also weaken the significance of the data. Moreover, there is considerable evidence that adherence to the placebo arm in a trial can sometimes improve health outcomes significantly, which signals the existence of considerable uncertainty about the relationship between adherence and health outcomes generally: is it causal, only an association (see chapter 40)? This combination of complexities in prevention research helps to explain why large studies are not undertaken more often. The result, of course, is continued uncertainty, smaller studies, persisting gaps in the evidence base, and decision making based on limited evidence. This example is just one illustration of how complex the ethical and social context of prevention and prevention research can be.

The Government-Citizenry Relationship

That government has both the obligation and the right to protect the public health is clear. What is less clear is the scope of this government obligation. What kinds of threats to health are covered under this government obligation? What means should the government use to control these threats?

The answers to these questions turn on a complex of principles and values, including, most prominently, respect for autonomy, justice, public welfare, and utility. How the demands of these principles are to be balanced or blended depends critically on one's theory of the state—in this instance, on one's theory of the liberal state in a democratic society.

In the government-citizenry relationship, the counterparts of the benefi-cence and autonomy models have been described as the paternalism model and the "rugged individual" model (Ribisl & Humphreys, 1998) or the "public inter-est viewpoint" and the "libertarian viewpoint" (Callahan, 2000). Paternalism is defined as the overriding of autonomous choice for beneficent reasons, that is, the determination that someone other than the affected individual—in this case, the government—knows what is best for the individual. Bioethics scholars have expressed concerns about paternalism in health education efforts, while at the same time advocating for restrictive government regulatory action where appropriate (Faden, 1987). Bioethics scholars have likewise expressed concern about the increasing focus on personal responsibility for health, while at the same time seeking to protect decisional autonomy (Minkler, 2000). What may at first appear to be contradictory in such arguments is rather an acknowledgment of different decision-making contexts, as well as the articulation of a model in-termediate to the extremes of paternalism and individual self-sufficiency.

Strong state action is most clearly morally demanded when the health of innocent parties is placed at risk by the actions of others and there is a feasible way to remove the risk through regulation or environmental control. Classic examples include asbestos and lead exposures in the workplace or the home, unsafe appliances, and carcinogenic food additives. Many expressions of the type of state action discussed here are, by nature, coercive—that is, designed to change behavior by threat of legal sanction. In the government-citizenry rela-tionship, legal coercion is morally acceptable when it reflects the appropriate workings of the democratic process.

State action is demanded in these cases by a complex of principles, includ-ing justice and utility. It should be noted that these cases do not raise relevant autonomy issues: that is, there is no substantive conflict, in these examples, between the demands of justice and obligations to respect autonomy. (To be facetious, one rarely asserts a liberty right to be exposed to lead or asbestos.)

It is also significant that lead and asbestos exposure represent classic examples of the victim-blaming scenarios that appear frequently in the health behavior change literature. Interventions designed to change indi-vidual behavior, rather than the use of state action to change the root causes of exposure, often focus attention on the wrong end of the equation. Health education interventions to promote the wearing of respiratory protective gear among workers in inadequately ventilated plants, to encourage more vigilant behavior among tenants in lead-contaminated apartments, or to train migrant workers to wear gloves while using pesticides in the fields are morally sus-pect, if not unconscionable, when governmental action is possible, more ap-propriate under the circumstances, and likely to be more effective. In these examples, government is in a position to improve ventilation in the workplace, to require lead abatement in rental housing, and to ban highly toxic pesticides and to mandate the availability of protective gear and shower facilities for farmworkers, making it unjust to rely on individual action alone (chapter 37; Steinbrook, 2006).

The moral issues are somewhat more complicated when we move to cases where there are plausibly some autonomy interests at issue, but no weighty liberty values. Classic examples are the controversy over seat belts and air bags in automobiles and the freedom of motorcyclists to forgo wearing helmets. To put the argument somewhat simplistically, those opposed to compulsory seat belt or helmet legislation claim, among other things, a liberty right to drive unharnessed. Those opposed to mandatory air bags claim, among other things, a liberty right to decide whether they wish to pay the additional costs of air bag installation, which are passed on to consumers.

The position one takes in relation to these controversies depends to a significant extent on the value one places on these particular liberty interests in comparison to the value placed on other principles. (In the case of helmets and seat belts, for example, it is reasonable to consider whether society should share the increased costs of medical treatment when those not wearing seat belts or motorcycle helmets are injured.) Whether media campaigns or other forms of behavioral interventions are morally preferable or morally questionable alternatives to regulation turns on a complex balancing of these competing values and principles.

Of course, all health issues do not entail strong arguments for coercive state action. Individual autonomy may outweigh other considerations; effective technological or regulatory solutions may not exist, or, if they do, they may be inadequate to the problem. In such instances, behavioral interventions directed at individuals by governmental entities are appropriate. Examples include governmental promotion of oral hygiene, breast self-exam, safer sexual practices, and exercise.

As in the clinician-patient relationship, in the government-citizen relationship when autonomy interests are strong it is important to evaluate behavioral interventions in terms of their effects on autonomous choice. However, it is not always possible to reach consensus about which health issues entail strong autonomy interests, in part because of fundamental disagreements about the role of social and cultural influences on individual choices and actions (chapter 2; Steinbrook, 2006). The classic lifestyle issues of diet and exercise may fall into this area of disagreement. Consider, for example, the difference between a governmental requirement that the amount of trans fats be listed on all food packaging and a ban on trans fats in prepared and packaged foods. The former requirement provides the citizenry with the information needed to make healthier food choices but does not in itself ensure that healthier choices are available. The latter requirement ensures the availability of trans fat-free food choices, but at the expense of individual autonomy.

Finally, any evaluation of the ethics of government lifestyle change and adherence interventions must recognize that there are instances in which regulatory or environmental intervention is morally preferable but politically inadvisable or impossible. How government officials and researchers ought to proceed under such circumstances is difficult to stipulate in the abstract. As other chapters in this volume make clear, circumstances are likely to arise in which interventions directed at individuals are morally permissible as the only available strategy for dealing with a health problem. Increasingly, however, health promotion and disease prevention has taken on an ecological perspective (chapter 37), acknowledging the connections between individual actions and their social context and recognizing that institutional and society-wide changes, including regulatory changes, may be imperative.

The Payer-Client Relationship

In addition to the aforementioned relationships, the relationship between health insurers (or other payers) and their clients is increasingly important in the arena of health behavior change, for two reasons. First, discussions about whether and when to pay for prevention and health maintenance are becoming more common. In addition to familiar preventive services such as Pap tests and mammograms, many insurers pay for other services, as well, both for healthy clients and for clients with chronic diseases such as diabetes. Second, as health insurance moves further away from community rating and experience rating becomes ever more elaborate, insurers and other payers are more likely to increase health insurance premiums for individuals identified as being at increased genetic or behavioral risk (Stone 1990) and to lower premium costs only upon demonstration of successful behavior change, such as smoking cessation, weight loss, or blood pressure control (Mello & Rosenthal, 2008; Morreim, 2000; Steinbrook, 2006). The relationship between payers and clinicians may similarly be affected by patients' success, or lack thereof, through payer-imposed reporting requirements (Bishop & Brodkey, 2006) and "pay-for-performance" programs (AMA Council on Ethical and Judicial Affairs, 2005), detailed discussion of which is beyond the scope of this chapter.

The payer-client relationship implicates the same tensions between beneficence and autonomy that arise in the relationships already discussed, with several important differences. First, this relationship may be clearly contractual, or individuals may be the direct beneficiaries of a contractual relationship between the payer and their employer. Second, individuals may or may not have the ability to choose other health insurance plans. Thus, the responsibilities of the payer may depend on the freedom of the client. When the payer is governmental—as is the case for Medicare and Medicaid—individuals' choices may be especially constrained by their circumstances, but the stakes for payers grow higher as the costs of chronic disease-related health care increase.

For these reasons, another important difference lies in the way that payers make use of information. Whether the payer's goal is to benefit patients by offering incentives for behavior change or to benefit stockholders by saving money and increasing profitability is often an open question. Positive incentives, such as insurer coverage for preventive services, are more likely to have beneficent intent than are negative incentives, such as increased premiums for failure to change behavior (or for failure to demonstrate the effectiveness of behavior change). Even so, it is not clear how the information payers might use to assess premiums should be interpreted. Whether prevention is effective and whether various payer incentives to practice prevention are fair and reasonable are empirical questions that merit careful investigation, especially in the rapidly changing health insurance market.

Finally, as Morreim has noted, the task of determining how to apply these kinds of incentives is morally problematic in yet another way. Meaningfully measuring adherence is potentially very intrusive upon individuals' privacy, while refraining from intrusion is likely to reward deception (Morreim, 2000). Indeed, the very ability to ascertain whether adherence improves health or saves money requires a significant privacy tradeoff—one that is largely familiar and accepted in prevention research but that is far more sensitive outside the research context.

Common Issues Across Relationships

Discussion of these four relationships—physician and patient, investigator and study subject, individual and government, payer and client—reveals some important common issues. First, the process of assessing the respective responsibilities of the parties to each relationship necessitates the same comparison and balancing of principles, though in each case the context and conclusions will differ. Second, in each relationship, several considerations are key, most notably the empirical question of uncertainty regarding the evidence available to prove or disprove the effectiveness of lifestyle change in improving health and the concomitant normative question about what counts as effectiveness in health behavior change. Is it improved health—measured by fewer illness episodes, or decreased need for treatment interventions, or in some other way? Is it longer life? Is it lower health care costs over a person's lifetime? Is it better quality of life, by self-report or by some other measure? Third, each relationship embodies a tension—albeit a productive and necessary tension—between autonomy and beneficence.

An emerging issue held in common across each of these relationships is the significance of the genetic contribution to health. As has been extensively debated in the literature, the current trend toward the "geneticization" of health behavior and the concomitant search for genetic predispositions, gene-environment interactions, and the genetic contributions to common multifactorial disorders and conditions has important implications for how society views individual autonomy in health behavior change.

If individuals are considered able to effect change, then persuasion will take on a more significant role. If, however, individuals' health is viewed as determined by genetic risk factors, then interventions that place less emphasis on individual choice—such as regulation and coercive sanctions—could become more common. The geneticization of health behavior could reduce the tendency toward victim blaming, but at considerable expense, by unduly downplaying the capacity of individuals to effect behavior change and thereby improve their health. Moreover, this trend could exaggerate the role of the genetic contribution to health and deemphasize inherent uncertainty about the significance of genetic information for individuals (Koenig & Stockdale, 2000). If lifestyle change is achieved by prematurely labeling people with new diagnoses solely on the basis of their genetic heritage, then that achievement may come at some moral cost. The possible costs include issues discussed throughout this volume: stigmatization, guilt, the inappropriate manipulation of information necessary for informed decision making, and a focus on individual behavior to the exclusion of attention to the social and cultural determinants of health behavior change.

Finally, perhaps there is yet another common tension, at the policy level, between the costs of prevention and its goals. Effective promotion of health behavior change—efforts that address the social, cultural, economic, and political context in which individuals act and live—may not only be expensive but also may involve sometimes-profound changes in the communities in which we live and work (chapters 2 & 37) and invoke important social values. Some deep changes may be welcome; others will certainly not be; all are likely to foster public debate and discussion.

The Social Context of Ethics in Health Behavior Change

This chapter focuses on traditional moral principles, most notably beneficence, justice, and autonomy, as they relate to lifestyle change and adherence. One variant of the justice and autonomy themes not yet discussed is the morality of devoting significant attention to promoting healthier lifestyles while at the same time millions of Americans lack access to basic health services. Any thorough examination of the ethics of lifestyle change and adherence must address not only whether the characteristics of specific interventions conform to our moral obligations, narrowly construed, but also whether the resources needed to mount these interventions have been fairly allocated in a broader sense.

A rich understanding of autonomy includes recognition that decision-making relationships in health care should support and facilitate autonomous decision making by individuals. Thus, addressing the social and structural determinants of health is both a way to avoid the victim blaming of individually focused responsibility for health behavior change and a means of identifying additional levels of responsibility for making more choices available and fostering more fully informed decision making. Understood in this way, the ethics of health behavior change must not fail to take account of the system of health care delivery, of which prevention and lifestyle change form one part.

The ethics of lifestyle change and adherence must also consider the goals of an intervention and how the intervention's success is measured. If the objective is to encourage people to make informed and voluntary decisions regarding their health, then the primary evaluation criterion should be the quality of the choices made by those at which interventions are aimed, more than the choices themselves. The correct evaluation criterion, then, is not how many subjects stayed in the trial but how well they understood what was involved in participating in the trial, regardless of whether they consented or refused, stayed in or dropped out. The issue becomes not how many individuals with hypertension took their medications according to directions but how many made an informed, reflective decision about whether they wanted to take the medication as recommended.

In other words, morally sound evaluation of the success of health behavior change should include mutual, ongoing education about what constitutes good decision making about health and about how health behavior is integrated into the lives of individuals, cultures, and communities. Patients, the public, and health care professionals must learn from one another what works and does not work and why, so that progress in the field is built on using sound data to develop interventions that are both effective for and respectful of all concerned.

References

AMA Council on Ethical and Judicial Affairs. (2005). *Physician pay-for-performance programs.* CEJA Report 3-I-05. Retrieved April 17, 2008, from http://www.ama-assn.org/go/cejareports

Areen, J. (1998). A need for caring. *Michigan Law Review, 86,* 967–1082.

Beauchamp, T. L., & Childress, J. (2008) *Principles of biomedical ethics* (6th ed.). New York: Oxford University Press.

Beauchamp, T. L., & McCullough, L. B. (1984). *Medical ethics.* Englewood Cliffs, NJ: Prentice-Hall.

Bishop, G., & Brodkey, A. M. (2006). Personal responsibility and physician responsibility—West Virginia's Medicaid plan. *New England Journal of Medicine, 355,* 756–758.

Callahan, D. (2000). Freedom, healthism, and health promotion: Finding the right balance. In D. Callahan (Ed.), *Promoting healthy behavior: How much freedom? Whose responsibility?* (pp. 138–152). Washington, DC: Georgetown University Press.

Churchill, L. R., King, N. M. P., & Schenck, D. (2005). Ethics in medicine: An introduction to moral tools and traditions. In N. M. P. King, R. P. Strauss, L. R. Churchill, S. E. Estroff, G. E. Henderson, & J. Oberlande (Eds.), *The social medicine reader* (2nd ed.), Vol. 1, *Patients, doctors, and illness* (pp. 169–185). 2005. Durham, NC: Duke University Press.

Emanuel, E. J., Wendler, D., & Grady, C. (2000). What makes clinical research ethical? *Journal of the American Medical Association, 283,* 2701–2711.

Faden, R. R. (1987). Ethical issues in government sponsored public health campaigns. *Health Education Quarterly, 14*(1), 27–37.

Faden, R. R., & Beauchamp, T. L., with King, N. M. P. (1986). *A history and theory of informed consent.* New York: Oxford University Press.

Grimes v. Kennedy Krieger Institute, Inc., 366 Md. 29, 782 A.2d 807 (Md. 2001).

Guinn, D. E. (Ed.). (2006). *Handbook of bioethics and religion.* New York: Oxford University Press.

Hanen, M., & Nielsen, K. (Eds.). (1987). Science, morality and feminist theory. *Canadian Journal of Philosophy, 13*(Suppl.).

Henderson, G. E., Estroff, S. E., Churchill, L. R., King, N. M. P., Oberlander, J., & Strauss, R. P. (Eds.). (2005). *The social medicine reader* (2nd ed.), Vol. II, *Social and cultural contributions to health, difference, and inequality.* Durham, NC: Duke University Press.

Institute of Medicine. (2002). *Unequal treatment: Confronting racial and ethnic disparities in health care.* Washington, DC: National Academy of Sciences.

Koenig, B. A., & Stockdale, A. (2000). The promise of molecular medicine in preventing disease: Examining the burden of genetic risk. In D. Callahan (Ed.), *Promoting healthy behavior: How much freedom? Whose responsibility?* (pp. 116–137). Washington, DC: Georgetown University Press.

Mello, M. M., & Rosenthal, M. B. (2008). Wellness programs and lifestyle discrimination–The legal limits. *New England Journal of Medicine, 359,* 192–199.

Minkler, M. (2000). Personal responsibility for health: Contexts and controversies. In D. Callahan (Ed.), *Promoting healthy behavior: How much freedom? Whose responsibility?* (pp. 1–22). Washington, DC: Georgetown University Press.

Morreim, E. H. (2000). Sticks and carrots and baseball bats: Economic and other incentives to modify health behavior. In D. Callahan (Ed.), *Promoting health behavior: How much freedom? Whose responsibility?* (pp. 56–75). Washington, DC: Georgetown University Press.

National Commission for the Protection of Human Subjects of Biomedical and Behavioral Research. (1979). *The Belmont Report: Ethical principles and guidelines for the protection of human subjects of research.* Retrieved April 17, 2008, from http://ohsr.od.nih.gov/guidelines/belmont.html

Noddings, N. (2002). *Starting at home: Caring and social policy.* Berkeley: University of California Press.

Prograis, L. J., & Pellegrino, E. D. (2007). *African-American bioethics: Culture, race, and identity.* Washington, DC: Georgetown University Press.

Ribisl, K. M., & Humphreys, K. (1998). Collaboration between professionals and mediating structures in the community: Toward a "third way" in health promotion. In S. A. Shumaker, E. B. Schron, J. B. Ockene, & W. L. McBee (Eds.), *Handbook of health behavior change* (2nd ed., pp. 535–554). New York: Springer Publishing Company.

Smith, H. L., & Churchill, L. R. (1986). *Professional ethics and primary care medicine: Beyond dilemmas and decorum.* Durham, NC: Duke University Press.

Steinbrook, R. (2006). Imposing personal responsibility for health. *New England Journal of Medicine, 355,* 753–756.

Stone, D. (1990). Preventing chronic disease: The dark side of a bright idea. In *Chronic disease and disability: Beyond the acute medical model.* Papers commissioned for the Pew Health Policy Program. Washington, DC: National Academies Press.

Truman v. Thomas, 165 Cal. Rptr. 308, 611 P.2d 902 (Cal 1980).

Adherence and Health Outcomes: How Much Does Adherence Matter?

39

Kelly B. Haskard,
M. Robin DiMatteo,
and Summer L.
Williams

Patient adherence (also known as patient compliance) involves the degree to which patients follow their medical provider's recommendations for varied health regimens, including taking medications, making changes to diet, exercising, attending follow-up appointments, completing screenings, and attending to a host of lifestyle changes and treatment activities. Rates of nonadherence vary widely across disease conditions and treatment requirements, but, on average, at least a quarter of patients are nonadherent (DiMatteo, 2004a). Average rates of

This work was supported by a Robert Wood Johnson Foundation Investigator Award in Health Policy Research, by a grant from the National Institute on Aging 5R03AG27552–02, and by the Committee on Research of the U.C. Riverside Academic Senate. The views expressed in this chapter are those of the authors alone and do not imply endorsement by the funding sources.

nonadherence in the treatment of various common conditions include 20.9% for cancer, 32.5% for diabetes, 30% for end-stage renal disease, and 34.5% for sleep disorders (DiMatteo, 2004b).

Patients may have numerous reasons for their nonadherence. Ickovics and Meisler (1997) described patient, regimen, clinical setting, disease characteristics, and the provider-patient relationship as broad categories of factors that affect adherence. Nonadherence has economic outcomes, such as unnecessary hospitalizations, wasted medical visits, and unused prescriptions, to name a few. Nonadherence also diminishes the quality of the physician-patient relationship, as trust deteriorates and physician and patient frustration intensifies.

Ultimately, outcomes of health and disease management serve as the most important endpoints in determining the value of adherence. For example, the efficacy of medication adherence can be determined by several outcomes, including reduction of symptoms, alteration of disease course, decrease in pain, improvement in functioning, and even increase in life expectancy. Answering the important question of whether patient adherence "matters" is the purpose of the current chapter. This chapter addresses disease-specific evidence from studies describing the relationship between treatment adherence and relevant outcomes and presents broader evidence from qualitative and quantitative reviews that address this issue. The role of adherence in the outcomes of placebo treatment is also considered, as the beneficial effects of adhering to a placebo introduce consideration of possible psychosocial and biological mechanisms in the adherence-outcomes relationship. Finally, we examine the role of interventions to improve adherence in terms of their potential to improve patients' health outcomes.

Adherence-Outcome Relationship Across Diseases

The relationship between patient adherence and treatment outcomes is critically important to examine in a range of disease realms, where the requirements of adherence and the potential for its benefit vary widely. Studies of heart disease and myocardial infarction (MI), for example, point to a strong relationship between adherence and mortality risk. Specifically, patients whose adherence to the medication clofibrate was at least 80% had a lower risk of death over the ensuing 5 years. In this study, as is examined in more detail later, patients who were adherent to a placebo also had a lower risk of death than did those who were nonadherent to a placebo (Coronary Drug Project Research Group, 1980). The Beta-blocker Heart Attack Trial demonstrated that men whose medication adherence was less than 75% had two and a half times the likelihood of dying in the year after experiencing an MI of those with better adherence. This result occurred even when psychosocial factors, including social support and stress, which may independently affect mortality, were controlled for (Horwitz et al., 1990). In other research, women with heart disease who were poorly adherent to propranolol had three times the risk of dying over a 25-month follow-up period than did those with good adherence (Gallagher, Viscoli, & Horwitz, 1993). Hypertension patients have better control of their blood pressure when they are more adherent. Comparisons of hypertensives with low (<50%), medium (50%–79%), and high (≥80%) adherence revealed significantly greater blood pressure control in the highly adherent patients. Even after controlling for demographic factors, effective management of blood pressure was 45% better in highly adherent patients (Bramley, Gerbino, Nightengale, & Frech-Tamas, 2006). Poor blood pressure control can result in stroke or MI, among other life-threatening conditions; thus, serious, long-term negative outcomes can result from lower patient adherence.

Adherence to HIV medication can be particularly important; adherence is linked to various short-term and long-term disease outcomes, including viral load, CD4 cell count, and, ultimately, survival (Wainberg & Friedland, 1998). HIV medication management can involve significant challenges, of course, because of the complexity of the regimens, which often require taking multiple medications that have dosing schedules that challenge the conduct of daily life and that cause disturbing (and sometimes debilitating) side effects. Ideal outcomes in HIV include "undetectable" viral load, a high CD4 immune cell count, and prevention of drug resistance; these conditions may be achievable only with perfect, or near-perfect, adherence to treatment. HIV may be one of the conditions where the link between adherence and outcomes has been strongest and the level of adherence needed has been given the most research attention.

For HIV-positive patients taking protease inhibitors, one study showed that 21.7% of patients with adherence greater than 95% sustained virologic failure, whereas about 82% of patients who were less than 70% adherent did so (Paterson et al., 2000). In this study, higher CD4 counts and less frequent hospitalizations were also associated with better adherence. In other research that focused on behavior rather than medication, failure to achieve "undetectable" viral loads was associated with failure to keep appointments among HIV-positive patients following a protease inhibitor regimen (Lucas, Chaisson, & Moore, 1999). Recent treatment regimens for HIV/AIDS involving antiretroviral therapy have shown that less than 95% adherence was associated with greater likelihood of virologic failure (one definition of which was viral load at or greater than 200 HIV RNA copies/ml at week 24 of follow-up) (Collier et al., 2005). In a study that modeled both clinical and economic outcomes of HAART (highly active antiretroviral therapy), the authors differentiated between typical and ideal adherence, finding that 16.9 additional years of life were associated with typical adherence, whereas 19.2 additional years were associated with "ideal" adherence. Typical adherence also meant a loss of 12% in quality-adjusted life years (Munakata et al., 2006). Factors leading to better adherence may include positive provider-patient interactions and communication and greater confidence in one's ability to adhere. Although the effect on outcomes was not directly tested in this study, one could predict that effective and positive provider-patient communication is associated with better adherence and ultimately with improved treatment outcomes (Johnson et al., 2006).

Adherence to cancer treatment is associated with longer survival times and a reduced probability of cancer recurrence. Nonadherence can lead to the failure to contain localized disease. For example, irregular attendance at radiation therapy or chemotherapy appointments and premature discontinuation of treatment may increase the risk of metastasis and can increase the chances of metastasis and of disease recurrence (cf. Andersen, Kiecolt-Glaser, & Glaser, 1994). In one study, rural breast cancer patients of minority ethnicity who underwent breast conservation therapy and radiation had reduced rates of survival when they did not adhere to their radiation protocols (Li et al., 2000). Conversely, in other work, individuals with colon cancer who completed adjuvant chemotherapy had a significantly higher rate of survival (Dobie et al., 2006).

Medication nonadherence among heart transplant patients has been found to predict adverse outcomes. This serious medical procedure requires complex follow-up care that can mean the difference between transplant success and failure. In one study of heart transplant patients taking immunosuppressive medication, nonadherent patients experienced significantly more transplant coronary artery disease over a 5-year follow-up period than did those who were adherent. Earlier and more frequent adverse clinical events were associated with poorer adherence (Dobbels, De Geest, Van Cleemput, Droogne, & Vanhaecke, 2004). In another study of adherence following heart transplant, failure to adhere to the prescribed medication regimen was significantly related to rejection of the transplant and development of coronary artery disease (Dew et al., 1999).

Adherence to diabetes regimens is also associated with more positive health outcomes, including better glycemic control. Diabetes is a chronic condition requiring multifaceted regimens involving medications, dietary restrictions, and insulin injections, among other therapeutic approaches. One study of glycemic control among 20 type 1 diabetes patients indicated that better control was associated with higher self-reported adherence to dietary restrictions (approaching traditional significance levels; $p < .10$) (Strychar et al., 1998). In an intervention in which "high-risk" diabetes patients received a blood glucose monitoring guide to self-management, a significantly greater number of patients in the intervention group experienced improved glycemic control (i.e., improved hemoglobin levels) (Moreland et al., 2006).

Recurrence or relapse of depression has been associated with discontinued antidepressant treatment. The probability of relapse or recurrence of depressive episodes increases when medication to control the symptoms of this mood disorder is not taken consistently. Early discontinuation of antidepressant treatment (defined as fewer than 4 prescriptions filled in a 6-month period) has been found to be associated with greater likelihood of recurring or relapsing (risk ratio = 1.77) (Melfi et al., 1998). An adherence intervention that involved greater involvement by health care providers in patients' care through visits, phone calls, and symptom monitoring resulted in greater improvement in the symptoms of depression, although not a significant reduction in the likelihood of relapse (Katon et al., 2001).

Among patients with hepatitis, adherence to medications is associated with better virologic response. In one study, patients who were more than 80% adherent had higher rates of virologic response (i.e., absence of HCV RNA) than did those who were less than 80% adherent to combination therapy with interferon (McHutchison et al., 2002).

Pharmacological treatments are not the only regimens for which adherence can affect patient outcomes. Considerable evidence indicates that adherence to behavioral treatments is associated with better outcomes. For example, better adherence by elderly hospitalized patients to a set of protocols, including orientation, mobility, and therapeutic activities, significantly reduced rates of patient delirium (Inouye, Bogardus, Williams, Leo-Summers, & Agostini, 2003).

There are some studies, of course, that have not shown a connection between adherence and better health outcomes. In the Medical Outcomes Study, for example, patients with hypertension, diabetes, MI, and congestive heart disease self-reported their levels of adherence, and the relationship between adherence and various health outcomes from the SF-36 was examined, and no consistent relationship of adherence to health outcomes was found (Hays et al., 1994). These results may be interpreted in a variety of ways, including the possibility that there were difficulties in adherence measurement, the fact that some medications and regimens may not have a strong effect on outcomes regardless of level of adherence, and the possibility that other factors, such as genetics, may play a greater role than adherence in determining disease progression.

Review Evidence Supporting the Relationship Between Adherence and Outcomes

Many quantitative reviews have been conducted to assess the relationship between adherence and health outcomes. One of the earliest reviews of this relationship included six studies and demonstrated that adherence was related to positive health outcomes in five out of the six investigations (Epstein, 1984). A meta-analysis of the relationship between adherence and outcomes across diseases indicated that the odds of a good health outcome are 2.88 times higher if a person is adherent and that there is a 26% greater risk of poor health outcomes in the context of nonadherence (DiMatteo, Giordani, Lepper, & Croghan, 2002). This effect is moderated by a number of factors; the relationship between adherence and outcomes was strongest in intestinal disease, hypertension, hypercholesterolemia, and sleep apnea (all p < .01). Analyses of moderators demonstrated a stronger relationship between adherence and outcomes for chronic illnesses than for acute illnesses and, among less severe illnesses, in nonmedication regimens and in pediatric populations. Further, studies that measured more subjective outcomes, such as pain, showed stronger effects than did those with more objective outcomes, such as blood pressure (DiMatteo et al., 2002). Additional quantitative review has shown a relationship between adherence and what may be considered the ultimate outcome, lower mortality risk. A meta-analysis of 21 studies of adherence to drug therapy showed significantly lower probability of death among "good" adherers than among those who were "poor" adherers (Simpson et al., 2006).

Research and Methodological Issues in the Adherence–Outcomes Relationship

Research studies of specific diseases and reviews of multiple disease conditions overwhelmingly demonstrate a positive, although not large, correlation between higher levels of adherence and better health outcomes. Several conceptual and methodological issues regarding this relationship are relevant to consider. First, the level of adherence necessary to achieve a positive health outcome may vary considerably from one disease to another. In HIV, for example, it has been clinically proposed that 95% adherence to some medications is essential so that drug resistance does not occur. Some of the newer classes of medications may require only 80% adherence, although the efficacy of reduced levels of medication adherence and the implications for a variety of health outcomes are yet to be empirically determined (Johnson & Chesney, 2006).

Second, every medical condition may have a different definition of appropriate adherence, making comparison of the adherence-outcome relationship across conditions quite difficult. For example, studies suggest that for the treatment of sinusitis, similar outcomes resulted from 3 days and 10 days of antibiotic treatment (Kravitz & Melnikow, 2004). On the other hand, evidence is robust that a level of 80% adherence is essential for effective antihypertensive medication treatment, as well as for some orally administered cancer therapies (Paterson et al., 2000).

Third, the form of the relationship between adherence and outcomes may not be completely clear. Whereas most general linear model statistics test linear trends, it is possible that relationships between adherence and outcomes could be curvilinear or could follow a more complex trend, such as an initial reduction in effectiveness followed by a rapid and robust improvement in health outcomes. Or, a lower slope relating adherence to health outcomes may occur below a certain adherence threshold, whereas higher levels of adherence may produce a stronger correlation with health outcomes. Another possibility is that, above a certain threshold of adherence, there may be marginal improvements or even no added benefits to health outcomes (Kravitz & Melnikow, 2004).

Fourth, the relationship between adherence and treatment outcomes is likely to depend upon the circumstances surrounding care. Adherence achieved by closely monitored patients in clinical trials may be considerably higher than that exhibited by patients in the general population, influencing evidence for the effectiveness of treatment and for the relationship between adherence and efficacy (Horwitz & Horwitz, 1993). Further, the "intention to treat" and the actual receipt of treatment (as a result of adhering properly) may be quite different and may strongly influence evidence about outcomes. In clinical trials, there may be a wide range of adherence levels that "confound" the relationship between treatments and outcomes (Simpson et al., 2006).

Fifth, studies of the adherence-outcome relationship are correlational, and causal inferences must be made with caution. Certainly, if adherence is assessed well before health outcomes are determined, it may be possible to use temporal evidence for the likelihood that adherence causes outcomes, and not the reverse. It is always possible, however, that a "third variable" causes both adherence and outcomes, bringing about their correlation with each other. Examples might be patient poverty or ethnic minority status, which limits access to resources needed for adherence and also accounts for significant disparities in health outcomes (Betancourt, Carrillo, & Green, 1999).

Sixth, there is evidence that, in some cases, better patient adherence leads to worse health outcomes, most notably when treatment is the result of a medical error or is inappropriate for a particular patient. A meta-analysis of the relationship between adherence to drug therapy and patient mortality included two studies in which medication therapy was actually harmful to patients and those with better adherence had a greater mortality risk (Simpson et al., 2006).

It is also possible that patients may recognize the risk of inappropriate therapy and the possibility that adherence makes their health worse; in response, they may make a deliberate choice to be nonadherent.

The Relationship of Adherence to Placebo and Outcomes

Findings from numerous studies suggest that adherence to placebo may result in better outcomes than nonadherence to placebo. (See Czajkowski, Chesney, and Smith, 1990, for a more detailed discussion of the relationship between placebo and adherence.) The result of a meta-analytic study demonstrated that good adherence to a drug placebo was also associated with lower risk of mortality (Simpson et al., 2006). This finding, replicating the early work of Epstein (1984), suggests that there may be more to the positive outcome effects of adherence than simply the physiological and pharmacological aspects of treatment. Specifically, when the effect on health or disease outcomes does not depend on whether the treatment is an active drug or a placebo, a "main effect" of adherence occurs.

One of the first confirmations of this "main effect" was Epstein's finding that in five of six studies, adherence improved health outcomes regardless of the "active" nature of treatment (Epstein, 1984). This study suggested that the actions of a medication and the ensuing outcomes result not only from the specific, pharmacological properties of the medication but also from beneficial "nonspecific" therapeutic effects. A review conducted almost a decade later offered further evidence that patients who expect their treatment to be effective may, in turn, practice healthier lifestyle habits that facilitate achievement of the desired outcome (Horwitz & Horwitz, 1993).

Individual empirical studies have had similar findings. A study of cancer patients' adherence to oral antibiotics to reduce the chance of infection found that those patients with the highest levels of adherence were least likely to develop fever or infections, regardless of whether they received the active therapy or a placebo (Pizzo et al., 1983). Similarly, a study of patients undergoing alcohol withdrawal and taking beta-blockers to combat symptoms found a relationship between nonadherence and greater likelihood of alcohol relapse; the placebo condition findings mirrored those of the nonplacebo condition (Gottlieb, Horwitz, Kraus, Segal, & Viscoli, 1994).

A number of plausible explanations for these findings are possible. First, patients' expectations of the effectiveness of treatment could work to create a "self-fulfilling prophecy." Second, health habits such as eating a healthy diet, exercising, getting adequate sleep, and cutting back or eradicating harmful health habits (such as alcohol use or tobacco use) can complement medication in facilitating health outcomes (Horwitz & Horwitz, 1993). Third, the act of adherence may enhance adaptation and/or active coping behaviors that help to reduce or alleviate the stresses of serious illness (Horwitz & Horwitz, 1993). For example, a hypertensive patient who expects that medication will reduce the risk of stroke and heart attack may concurrently relax more, eat a healthier diet, begin walking for exercise, and even quit smoking.

Fourth, adherent patients may have stronger feelings of internal health-related locus of control and feel more positive about their health. Their optimistic thought processes and sense of well-being may have direct, and positive, physiological and immunological effects, although of course it is also possible that those who feel better are thus more optimistic (Epstein, 1984). Optimistic thought processes are also associated with changes in immune functioning, as has been demonstrated in studies of HIV-positive individuals (Taylor, Kemeny, Reed, Bower, & Gruenewald, 2000). Specifically, optimism has been associated with greater numbers of helper T cells and greater natural killer cell activity (Segerstrom, Taylor, Kemeny, & Fahey, 1998). Optimism is also related to disease management in that patients who engage in positive thinking may cope better and subsequently experience more positive health outcomes (Fournier, De Ridder, & Bensing, 2002).

Not every study shows positive effects of adherence to placebos, however. A study of prevention of type 2 diabetes involved administration of metformin or a placebo; those who were adherent to metformin had a 24.8% reduction in risk over nonadherent patients. For placebo patients, however, adherers had a nonsignificant reduction in risk over nonadherers (Walker et al., 2006). It is possible that in this research, adherence may have been less important in the preventive regimens than in the regimens for a diagnosed condition. Findings that adherence to a placebo can have beneficial effects on health outcomes, however, leads us to further explore the nonbiological mechanisms through which adherence can be effective.

Mechanisms for the Relationship Between Adherence and Health Outcomes

Most medications have some pharmacological effects, and for many patients those effects are directly related to preventing or managing their disease or to achieving improvement in their symptoms. Evidence for the efficacy and safety of medication likely argue in favor of patients' adhering to all aspects of their prescribed regimen, including the dosage, timing of, and circumstances surrounding treatment. These circumstances may both affect and be affected by the medication regimen. For example, adherence may increase with and/or be increased by the availability of social support, which itself may affect and even be affected by the patients' health outcomes. Specifically, a more adherent patient might encourage family members to offer social support, and that social support might translate directly into more beneficial health outcomes (DiMatteo, 2004a).

There may be personal characteristics, such as conscientiousness, that provide advantage to the adherent patient (Gallagher et al., 1993). More conscientious people have been found to have better health behaviors than those who are less conscientious (Friedman et al., 1993).

Personality traits or psychological makeup might provide another explanation as to how adherence to placebo results in better outcomes. Adherent individuals may be more optimistic that their health will improve and their symptoms will abate, whereas pessimistic individuals may fail to adhere because they have little hope that their treatment will work. In addition, individuals who are more adherent might have greater resilience to stress and/or more active coping strategies. Those who do not adhere may not cope well, on the other hand, or may use emotion-focused coping strategies, rather than the active strategy of choosing to be adherent. Furthermore, patient expectations and confidence that treatment is likely to work for them may affect both their likelihood of being adherent and their health outcomes (Horwitz & Horwitz, 1993). Patients are more likely to adhere if they believe treatment will work, and such patients are motivated and capable of following the regimen. A physician's confidence that treatment will help the patient to achieve the desired outcome may motivate patient adherence and contribute to more positive health outcomes for the patient (Czajkowski, Chesney, & Smith, 1990).

The lifestyle of individuals who are more adherent might provide another clue to better understanding the adherence-outcome relationship. Individuals who adhere might already have healthier habits, such as eating a low-fat diet, exercising more frequently, sleeping enough, following better hygiene practices, engaging in stress-reduction strategies, and exhibiting fewer risky or health-compromising behaviors than nonadherent individuals. Some researchers have described this as the "Healthy Adherer Effect" (Gallagher et al., 1993; Pizzo et al., 1983; Simpson et al., 2006). In addition, adherent patients may expect to have better health outcomes, making adherence to healthy lifestyle regimens easier for them because they are more motivated and confident about the expected end result of improved health (Andersen et al., 1994). On the other hand, nonadherent patients may not receive necessary information about how to improve their health habits because of limitations in communication and lack of rapport with their health care providers (Andersen et al., 1994).

Adherent patients might simply be initially healthier and have fewer complex regimens and treatments to which they must adhere (Gallagher et al., 1993; Pizzo et al., 1983). Patients who have difficulty with adherence may face more treatment challenges, more difficulties with medication side effects, and worse disease parameters than those for whom adherence is easier (Horwitz & Horwitz, 1993).

Some negative factors might mediate the relationship between adherence and outcomes, as well. Specifically, nonadherence may be a result of depression and mediate the relationship between depression and poor health outcomes (DiMatteo, Lepper, & Croghan, 2000). In one study of patients who were prescribed aspirin after Acute Coronary Syndrome, depressed, nondepressed, and intermittently depressed patients were compared over a 3-month period (Kronish et al., 2006). The persistently depressed patients took the least number of correct doses of aspirin across the entire measurement period, and, although mortality was not assessed, the findings indicated that nonadherence might represent the link to higher mortality risk in these patients. Findings also indicated that continuously depressed patients had poorer health behaviors; they were less likely to quit smoking, undergo cardiac rehabilitation, exercise, and modify their diet (Kronish et al., 2006).

Additional evidence demonstrating a link among depression, adherence, and outcomes can be found in the case of asthmatic patients. In a study of economically vulnerable patients who had recently been hospitalized for asthma-related emergencies and who were electronically monitored for adherence, patients with a greater number of depressive symptoms were

5.5 times more likely to be nonadherent to their prescribed regimen than those with fewer symptoms (Smith et al., 2006). Adherence, outcomes, and depression may be linked because pessimism, low energy, and poor motivation can create a situation in which adherence becomes difficult to achieve. Such research suggests the need for further studies of the adherence-outcome relationship to control for personal, psychological, and regimen factors that may affect this association.

Interventions, Adherence, and Outcomes

Addressing patient challenges to adherence has involved intervention research designed to alleviate some of the problems that stand in the way of patient adherence. Several studies suggest that health outcomes can be improved by enhancing patient adherence, and that barriers to adherence such as ineffective physician-patient communication, poor understanding of the treatment, the severity of the patient's condition, and emotional and mental health challenges can be improved to enhance adherence. Roter and colleagues (1998) conducted a meta-analysis of educational, behavioral, and affective intervention programs to improve patient adherence. These studies measured both subjective and objective health outcomes such as blood pressure, hospitalizations, survival, disability, pain, and gains in knowledge. Results indicated that interventions to improve patient adherence helped to lower the blood pressure levels of hypertensive patients. Cancer patients had improved survival times and lower recurrence rates as a result of interventions to improve their adherence. And adherence-enhancing interventions for patients on mental health regimens were associated with fewer hospitalizations (Roter et al., 1998).

In another meta-analysis of 95 independent samples of behavior-focused, educational, and combined interventions to improve adherence, 31 studies included a measure of health outcomes for a particular disease. The authors did not evaluate the relationship between adherence and outcomes (instead focusing on the effect of the interventions on adherence) but noted that there is an unknown relationship between adherence and health outcomes and that this relationship may depend on the disease and outcome in question (Peterson, Takiya, & Finley, 2003). Randomized controlled trials of interventions to improve adherence are extremely important because, with randomized experiments, it is possible to assess the causal effects of adherence on health outcomes. Further, studies of interventions to improve health and treatment outcomes that include an adherence or medication-taking intervention component would allow the assessment of both main effects and interactions of the adherence intervention on a variety of health and survival outcomes.

Conclusion and Implications

The role of patient adherence in determining patients' health outcomes is broad, particularly in light of the multiplicity of potential regimens for numerous conditions, as well as the myriad outcomes that are possible for any given condition. There are both conceptual and methodological issues of importance in terms of what is known about the relationship between adherence and outcomes and what areas require further study.

Several conceptual questions remain important to consider. Convincing evidence exists for the adherence-outcome relationship in several chronic and severe illnesses, including heart disease, HIV/AIDS, and cancer. There are fewer studies of the adherence-outcomes relationship in pediatric conditions, however, than there are for adult conditions; meta-analytic evidence suggests, however, that the adherence-outcome relationship may be even stronger in pediatric than in adult populations (DiMatteo, 2004b). Next, low levels of adherence challenge health outcomes in important ways for many illness conditions, but the optimal level of adherence necessary for the treatment of many medical conditions has not yet been determined. In conditions where 80% adherence is acceptable, should patients be told what they will gain in striving for 90%? If for some conditions (e.g., sinusitis) taking antibiotics for 3 of 10 days is enough for a good outcome, should patients be told not to worry if they miss 7 days of medication? Or, better still, should they be prescribed only 3 days' supply? If the process of adhering itself does something good for patients, shouldn't they know what constitutes appropriate adherence for their condition so that they can reap the benefits of achieving it? Also, the mediators and moderators of the adherence-outcomes relationship are challenging to untangle. Such factors as patients' disease severity and physical and mental health status are issues that require further examination. An important next step for future research is to clearly elucidate these pathways.

It is important to compare adherent and nonadherent individuals to determine how they differ on psychosocial factors such as optimism or coping strategies and to assess the effect of these on outcomes (Horwitz & Horwitz, 1993). It is evident that being adherent can involve health behaviors well beyond simply taking medication. Systematic study is needed of the broader self-efficacy over health and lifestyle behaviors that may be an important link to a patient's achieved health outcomes to add to our understanding of this area (Gottlieb et al., 1994).

Several important methodological questions require study. First, it is clear that robust measurement of both adherence behavior and outcomes, as well as their potential mediating or moderating factors, is critical. Electronic assessments of adherence may be the most accurate, but they are also expensive and are not feasible in standard clinical practice. Good measurement may involve the use of multiple approaches to adherence assessment (DiMatteo, 2004b; Garber, Nau, Erickson, Aikens, & Lawrence, 2004). Next, there is a need for more research into aspects of the physician-patient relationship that may influence both adherence and outcomes. It is important to determine, for example, the extent to which physicians discuss the benefits of certain medications with their patients and options to deal with side effects or other barriers to adherence and thereby fully involve their patients in decision making. These areas of communication about adherence are crucial but remain relatively understudied (Ballard-Reisch, 1990; Kaplan, Gandek, Greenfield, Rogers, & Ware, 1995). Third, many of the studies described here involve medication adherence. It is important to explore nonmedication regimens, such as dietary changes or exercise programs. For example, how does adherence to a dietary or exercise regimen

affect outcomes for obese patients and for those with chronic diseases that require lifelong behavioral management?

There remain conceptual and methodological issues in understanding the
adherence-outcomes relationship. Patient adherence may sometimes be critical,
but it is also clear that positive health outcomes rely on more than the pharmacological effects of a drug. Patients' psychological mind-set, behaviors, and beliefs and expectations, as well as the communication they have with their doctor,
play a significant role in adherence and the enhancement of health outcomes.

References

Andersen, B. L., Kiecolt-Glaser, J. K., & Glaser, R. (1994). A biobehavioral model of cancer stress
    and disease course. *American Psychologist, 49,* 389–404.
Ballard-Reisch, D. (1990). A model of participative decision making for physician-patient
    interaction. *Health Communication, 2,* 91–104.
Betancourt, J. R., Carrillo, J. E., & Green, A. R. (1999). Hypertension in multicultural and minor-
    ity populations: Linking communication to compliance. *Current Hypertension Reports, 1,*
    482–488.
Bramley, T. J., Gerbino, P. P., Nightengale, B. S., & Frech-Tamas, F. (2006). Relationship of blood
    pressure control to adherence with antihypertensive monotherapy in 13 managed care
    organizations. *Journal of Managed Care Pharmacy, 12*(3), 239–245.
Collier, A. C., Ribaudo, H., Mukherjee, A. L., Feinberg, J., Fischl, M. A., & Chesney, M. (2005). A
    randomized study of serial telephone call support to increase adherence and thereby im-
    prove virologic outcome in persons initiating antiretroviral therapy. *Journal of Infectious
    Diseases, 192,* 1398–1406.
Coronary Drug Project Research Group. (1980). Influence of adherence to treatment and re-
    sponse of cholesterol on mortality in the Coronary Drug Project. *New England Journal of
    Medicine, 303,* 1038–1041.
Czajkowski, S. M., Chesney, M. A., & Smith, A. W. (1990). Adherence and the placebo effect. In
    S. A. Shumaker, E. B. Schron, & J. K. Ockene (Eds.), *The handbook of health behavior change*
    (1st ed., pp. 515–534). New York: Springer Publishing Company.
Dew, M. A., Kormos, R. L., Roth, L. H., Murali, S., DiMartini, A., & Griffith, B. P. (1999). Early
    post-transplant medical compliance and mental health predict physical morbidity and
    mortality one to three years after heart transplantation. *Journal of Heart and Lung Trans-
    plantation, 18,* 549–562.
DiMatteo, M. R. (2004a). Social support and patient adherence to medical treatment: A meta-
    analysis. *Health Psychology, 23,* 207–218.
DiMatteo, M. R. (2004b). Variations in patients' adherence to medical recommendations: A
    quantitative review of 50 years of research. *Medical Care, 42,* 200–209.
DiMatteo, M. R., Giordani, P. J., Lepper, H. S., & Croghan, T. W. (2002). Patient adherence and
    medical treatment outcomes: A meta-analysis. *Medical Care, 40,* 794–811.
DiMatteo, M. R., Lepper, H. S., & Croghan, T. W. (2000). Depression is a risk factor for noncom-
    pliance with medical treatment: Meta-analysis of the effects of anxiety and depression on
    patient adherence. *Archives of Internal Medicine, 160,* 2101–2107.
Dobbels, F., De Geest, S., van Cleemput, J., Droogne, W., & Vanhaecke, J. (2004). Effect of late
    medication non-compliance on outcome after heart transplantation: A 5-year follow-up.
    The Journal of Heart and Lung Transplantation, 23, 1245–1251.
Dobie, S. A., Baldwin, L. M., Dominitz, J. A., Matthews, B., Billingsley, K., & Barlow, W. (2006).
    Completion of therapy by Medicare patients with stage III colon cancer. *Journal of the
    National Cancer Institute, 98,* 610–619.
Epstein, L. H. (1984). The direct effects of compliance on health outcome. *Health Psychology,
    3,* 385–393.
Fournier, M., De Ridder, D., & Bensing, J. (2002). Optimism and adaptation to chronic disease:
    The role of optimism in relation to self-care options of type 1 diabetes mellitus, rheuma-
    toid arthritis and multiple sclerosis. *British Journal of Health Psychology, 7,* 409–432.

Friedman, H. S., Tucker, J. S., Tomlinson-Keasey, C., Schwartz, J. E., Wingard, D. L., & Criqui, M. H. (1993). Does childhood personality predict longevity? *Journal of Personality and Social Psychology, 65,* 176–185.

Gallagher, E. J., Viscoli, C. M., & Horwitz, R. I. (1993). The relationship of treatment adherence to the risk of death after myocardial infarction in women. *Journal of the American Medical Association, 270,* 742–744.

Garber, M. C., Nau, D. P., Erickson, S. R., Aikens, J. E., & Lawrence, J. B. (2004). The concordance of self-report with other measures of medication adherence: A summary of the literature. *Medical Care, 42,* 649–652.

Gottlieb, L. D., Horwitz, R. I., Kraus, M. L., Segal, S. R., & Viscoli, C. M. (1994). Randomized controlled trial in alcohol relapse prevention: Role of atenolol, alcohol craving, and treatment adherence. *Journal of Substance Abuse Treatment, 11,* 253–258.

Hays, R. D., Kravitz, R. L., Mazel, R. M., Sherbourne, C. D., DiMatteo, M. R., Rogers, W. H., et al. (1994). The impact of patient adherence on health outcomes for patients with chronic disease in the Medical Outcomes Study. *Journal of Behavioral Medicine, 17,* 347–360.

Horwitz, R. I., & Horwitz, S. M. (1993). Adherence to treatment and health outcomes. *Archives of Internal Medicine, 153,* 1863–1868.

Horwitz, R. I., Viscoli, C. M., Berkman, L., Donaldson, R. M., Horwitz, S. M., Murray, C. J., et al. (1990). Treatment adherence and risk of death after a myocardial infarction. *Lancet, 336,* 542–545.

Ickovics, J. R., & Meisler, A. W. (1997). Adherence in AIDS clinical trials: A framework for clinical research and clinical care. *Journal of Clinical Epidemiology, 50,* 385–391.

Inouye, S. K., Bogardus, S. T., Jr., Williams, C. S., Leo-Summers, L., & Agostini, J. V. (2003). The role of adherence on the effectiveness of nonpharmacologic interventions: Evidence from the delirium prevention trial. *Archives of Internal Medicine, 163,* 958–964.

Johnson, M. O., & Chesney, M. A. (2006). The value and challenges of improving adherence to antiretroviral therapy for human immunodeficiency virus. *Medical Care, 44,* 891–892.

Johnson, M. O., Chesney, M. A., Goldstein, R. B., Remien, R. H., Catz, S., Gore-Felton, C., et al. (2006). Positive provider interactions, adherence self-efficacy, and adherence to antiretroviral medications among HIV-infected adults: A mediation model. *AIDS Patient Care and STDS, 20,* 258–268.

Kaplan, S. H., Gandek, B., Greenfield, S., Rogers, W., & Ware, J. E. (1995). Patient and visit characteristics related to physicians' participatory decision-making style. Results from the Medical Outcomes Study. *Medical Care, 33,* 1176–1187.

Katon, W., Rutter, C., Ludman, E. J., Von Korff, M., Lin, E., Simon, G., et al. (2001). A randomized trial of relapse prevention of depression in primary care. *Archives of General Psychiatry, 58,* 241–247.

Kravitz, R. L., & Melnikow, J. (2004). Medical adherence research: time for a change in direction? *Medical Care, 42,* 197–199.

Kronish, I. M., Rieckmann, N., Halm, E. A., Shimbo, D., Vorchheimer, D., Haas, D. C., et al. (2006). Persistent depression affects adherence to secondary prevention behaviors after acute coronary syndromes. *Journal of General Internal Medicine, 21,* 1178–1183.

Li, B. D., Brown, W. A., Ampil, F. L., Burton, G. V., Yu, H., & McDonald, J. C. (2000). Patient compliance is critical for equivalent clinical outcomes for breast cancer treated by breast-conservation therapy. *Annals of Surgery, 231,* 883–889.

Lucas, G. M., Chaisson, R. E., & Moore, R. D. (1999). Highly active antiretroviral therapy in a large urban clinic: Risk factors for virologic failure and adverse drug reactions. *Annals of Internal Medicine, 131,* 81–87.

McHutchison, J. G., Manns, M., Patel, K., Poynard, T., Lindsay, K. L., Trepo, C., et al. (2002). Adherence to combination therapy enhances sustained response in genotype-1-infected patients with chronic hepatitis C. *Gastroenterology, 123,* 1061–1069.

Melfi, C. A., Chawla, A. J., Croghan, T. W., Hanna, M. P., Kennedy, S., & Sredl, K. (1998). The effects of adherence to antidepressant treatment guidelines on relapse and recurrence of depression. *Archives of General Psychiatry, 55,* 1128–1132.

Moreland, E. C., Volkening, L. K., Lawlor, M. T., Chalmers, K. A., Anderson, B. J., & Laffel, L. M. (2006). Use of a blood glucose monitoring manual to enhance monitoring adherence in adults with diabetes: A randomized controlled trial. *Archives of Internal Medicine, 166,* 689–695.

Munakata, J., Benner, J. S., Becker, S., Dezii, C. M., Hazard, E. H., & Tierce, J. C. (2006). Clinical and economic outcomes of nonadherence to highly active antiretroviral therapy in patients with human immunodeficiency virus. *Medical Care, 44,* 893–899.

Paterson, D. L., Swindells, S., Mohr, J., Brester, M., Vergis, E. N., Squier, C., et al. (2000). Adherence to protease inhibitor therapy and outcomes in patients with HIV infection. *Annals of Internal Medicine, 133,* 21–30.

Peterson, A. M., Takiya, L., & Finley, R. (2003). Meta-analysis of trials of interventions to improve medication adherence. *American Journal of Health Systems and Pharmacy, 60,* 657–665.

Pizzo, P. A., Robichaud, K. J., Edwards, B. K., Schumaker, C., Kramer, B. S., & Johnson, A. (1983). Oral antibiotic prophylaxis in patients with cancer: A double-blind randomized placebo-controlled trial. *Journal of Pediatrics, 102*(1), 125–133.

Roter, D. L., Hall, J. A., Merisca, R., Nordstrom, B., Cretin, D., & Svarstad, B. (1998). Effectiveness of interventions to improve patient compliance: A meta-analysis. *Medical Care, 36,* 1138–1161.

Segerstrom, S. C., Taylor, S. E., Kemeny, M. E., & Fahey, J. L. (1998). Optimism is associated with mood, coping, and immune change in response to stress. *Journal of Personality and Social Psychology, 74,* 1646–1655.

Simpson, S. H., Eurich, D. T., Majumdar, S. R., Padwal, R. S., Tsuyuki, R. T., Varney, J., et al. (2006). A meta-analysis of the association between adherence to drug therapy and mortality. *British Medical Journal, 333,* 15–20.

Smith, A., Krishnan, J. A., Bilderback, A., Riekert, K. A., Rand, C. S., & Bartlett, S. J. (2006). Depressive symptoms and adherence to asthma therapy after hospital discharge. *Chest, 130,* 1034–1038.

Strychar, I. M., Blain, E., Rivard, M., Gelinas, M. D., Radwan, F., & Crawhall, J. C. (1998). Association between dietary adherence measures and glycemic control in outpatients with type 1 diabetes mellitus and normal serum lipid levels. *Journal of the American Dietetic Association, 98,* 76–79.

Taylor, S. E., Kemeny, M. E., Reed, G. M., Bower, J. E., & Gruenewald, T. L. (2000). Psychological resources, positive illusions, and health. *American Psychologist, 55,* 99–109.

Wainberg, M. A., & Friedland, G. (1998). Public health implications of antiretroviral therapy and HIV drug resistance. *Journal of the American Medical Association, 279,* 1977–1983.

Walker, E. A., Molitch, M., Kramer, M. K., Kahn, S., Ma, Y., Edelstein, S., et al. (2006). Adherence to preventive medications: Predictors and outcomes in the Diabetes Prevention Program. *Diabetes Care, 29,* 1997–2002.

Lessons Learned: What We Know Doesn't Work and What We Shouldn't Repeat

40

Deborah J. Bowen
and Uli Boehmer

The importance and central role of health behavior in improving human's health cannot be disputed. This book contains analyses and summaries of specific research questions on the study of health behavior. However, there are some issues or themes that cut across health behavior areas in the form of lessons learned, sometimes through painful experience. These lessons do not usually fit neatly into the standard format of a research report. Here we list several of these issues for consideration. They are in the form of "don'ts," or directions that we recommend you not repeat. We divide them into the "don'ts" that stem from a specific line of research and the "don'ts" that come from the process of doing research.

Research Don'ts

Don't Focus on Individual-Level Issues Without Considering the Environment

Any new strategy for disease control and prevention must recognize that human behavior is a major determinant of health outcomes (Hiatt & Rimer, 1999). A recent Institute of Medicine (IOM) report (Board on Population Health and Public Health Practice, 2005) estimates that lifestyle changes could prevent a significant number of deaths, and a recent position paper by the Centers for Disease Control and Prevention (CDC) (Gerberding, 2005) called for actions to reduce the burden of chronic disease through lifestyle changes. However, much of what we have considered to date rests with individual level variables—behaviors initiated and reported by participants in studies (Bowen et al., 2008). There is a growing interest and increasing research focus on the larger causes of human choices as a way to develop clearer and more lasting explanations for patterns of behavior. We must place more emphasis on the social, structural, and environmental causes of these lifestyle choices than has currently been done. Social and behavioral science research is critical to cancer prevention and control because translating knowledge into practice at the population level requires new methods for promoting social and behavioral change (including identifying cultural barriers to change), improved cancer communications, and continuous evaluation of the outcomes of cancer interventions. The recent focus on the social and structural causes of chronic disease also calls for increased research and training on societal interventions to reduce health disparities (Bowen et al., 2008).

One issue that illustrates this point is obesity reduction. The United States has spent a long time and billions of dollars figuring out that it is really impossible to lose weight and maintain the loss with traditional weight-loss programs. While we have been doing this, the epidemic of obesity in the United States and in western Europe has become a critical and frightening public health issue, arguably the most pressing health issue today. We virtually ignored the larger social and environmental foci that helped shape our obesity problem, separately and in conjunction with the focus on individual skills training. Given the lack of these behavioral and individual approaches to obesity reduction and prevention, the field is looking to the social, cultural, and environmental causes of this health issue. Does this mean that understanding the individual causes of human behavior is no longer necessary? Not at all. It simply means that humans are social creatures and that they are influenced by their social systems. Therefore, if we want to change behavioral patterns that lead to a negative health outcome, we need to consider the larger forces at play in shaping and influencing our individual choices and, ultimately, our health.

Don't Assume That the Cause of a Health Problem Is Solely Biological or Psychological/Social in Nature Until You Have Examined the Evidence

The assumption of a biological cause when social factors are also important is implicit in some of the new emphasis on genetic causes of health differences.

The National Institutes of Health's (NIH) definition of a disparity focuses on the difference between two subgroups. There is no inherent cause of disparity to be found in this definition, and no assumption is made about the role of biology in the definition. However, recent published definitions of disparity (Baquet & Carter-Pokras, 2002) focus on the social causes of disparities and on the social construction of conditions that lead to disparities, like racism. The word "disparities" is becoming increasingly associated with social or behavioral causes and less with biological differences. This shift in definition means that more emphasis should then be placed on research that identifies the social causes of disparities and the potential interventions that can reverse or eliminate them.

One current area of research that is drawing much attention from researchers, both positive and negative, is the area of genetic research as applied to health disparities. Whether a genetic difference can be considered a disparity hits at the heart of the controversy over the definition of a disparity. Do all biological differences fit into a disparity definition? Given that generally women are born with a uterus and men are not, are rates of uterine cancer to be classified as disparities? The field of health disparities would benefit from clarity of definition as we move forward in the identification of methods to reduce disparities in health.

Don't Assume That Lessons From One Group Automatically Fit Another

For years, while the biomedical model prevailed with little challenge, most research was conducted on men. The findings were later applied to women, with the implicit operating assumption that women are "little men" and that differences between men and women were not relevant (Haynes, 2000). For example, testing of drug treatments was historically conducted in men, but women later were prescribed these drugs. Pharmaceutical industries argued for the exclusion of women, citing safety concerns for women and their potential fetuses. Multiple examples indicate that this approach was incorrect and even shortsighted, since the drugs were prescribed to women as soon as they were approved by the U.S. Food and Drug Administration (FDA). Thus, the effectiveness and the safety of the medication for women were established only after the drugs were on the market and actively used by consumers. An FDA analysis of the labels of approved drugs indicated that 22% of labels report gender-related difference in the effects of medications (Evelyn et al., 2001). Some FDA-approved drugs had to be taken off the market when the dangers they posed for women became apparent (e.g., terfenadine [Seldane] in 1998) (U.S. Government Accountability Office, 2001).

This lesson does not apply only to drug safety and effectiveness. It applies just as much to behaviors. Safe-sex behaviors aimed at HIV prevention cannot be implemented by the promotion of similar interventions for women and men. An intervention that teaches safe-sex behaviors only to women without taking into account that some women's negotiation of safe-sex behaviors may be compromised by their unequal status in power is likely to be ineffective (Tinker, Finn, & Epp, 2000). Other research demonstrates that there are gender differences in the ability to change behaviors related to chronic diseases: smoking, physical inactivity, and high fat intake (O'Hea, Wood, & Brantley, 2003). Men and women do not view these behaviors from the same perspectives, and therefore, changing some of these risk behaviors requires gender-specific interventions (O'Hea et al., 2003).

We must acknowledge an end to a "one size fits all" era and acknowledge the need for different tools for different groups. Sexually transmitted diseases (STDs) and HIV/AIDS provide good examples of the importance of this issue. Racial differences in STDs and HIV/AIDS rates have been documented, and research confirms that Blacks have higher rates of HIV infection and other STDs (Celentano et al., 2005; Hallfors, Iritani, Miller, & Bauer, 2007; Halpern et al., 2004). The prevailing assumption is that the best intervention for STDs is to reduce individuals' risk behaviors. The applicability of this premise to Blacks has been called into question by studies that demonstrate that STDs and HIV infection rates are higher in Blacks regardless of individual risk behaviors (Hallfors et al., 2007; Halpern et al., 2004). One likely explanation is same-race partner choice among Blacks and a greater tendency among Blacks than Whites to choose discordant coupling (the pairing of a high-risk individual with a low-risk-behavior partner). This discordance in risk behaviors in couples increases the likelihood of STD and HIV transmission among Blacks, regardless of individual risk behaviors (Hallfors et al., 2007). Different and targeted interventions targeted at Blacks are therefore necessary to reduce the documented differences.

Don't Make Assumptions About the Mechanism of Behavior Change Without Supporting Evidence

The field of youth smoking prevention in the United States is an excellent example of the need to be clear about what is behind behavior change. The original smoking prevention programs for youth were school based and focused on imparting knowledge about the harmful health effects of tobacco use. The idea was that youth did not fully understand or appreciate these long-term chronic disease effects, and therefore the best way to keep youth from smoking was to fully inform them of these harmful health effects. These early programs had no effect on the onset of smoking in young people (Thomas & Perera, 2006). Therefore, investigators focused on the social influences model of smoking prevention intervention, which is based on the finding that many youth who smoked also had friends who smoked. The "Just say no" programs, which taught youth skills to use in social interactions about tobacco use, were a result of this wave of research. These programs had no lasting effects on tobacco use, either (Peterson, Kealey, Mann, Marek, & Sarason, 2000). The current, perhaps more informed approach to reducing smoking among youth focuses on the mass media and reduction of exposure to tobacco in purchasing situations through advertising and via promotion of tobacco products by tobacco companies. These approaches carry promise for greater and longer-lasting effectiveness on use of tobacco among youth. Smoking cessation researchers spent approximately 40 years trying ineffective interventions because, in part, they did not stop to fully understand the mechanism of smoking behavior in youth. Identifying the mechanisms of behavioral choices—in this case, the influence of mass media advertising on youth smoking behavior—before trying various interventions is likely to promote more effective interventions.

Don't Assume That Maintenance of Initial Change Is Easy

Health behavior change is a critical and essential piece of behavioral approaches to disease prevention. However, the initial change in risk-related behaviors (e.g., a reduction in smoking) must be maintained over long periods of time to influence individual risk for developing disease. Countless studies have described short-term gains in behavior change but limited maintenance of the changed behavior. Sustained change needs to be studied separately, with interventions designed to *target* the maintenance of the newly achieved behavior. One example of this phenomenon was studied in research that focused on school-based youth behavioral change programs. Investigators identified significant initial changes in the targeted behaviors, including tobacco use, physical activity, and eating behaviors. However, only when individual classroom efforts were combined with community change was youth behavior change maintained over years (Ranney et al., 2006; Sowden, Arblaster, & Stead, 2003). The intervention that produced the initial change was not an efficacious means of maintaining behaviors, and it therefore had to be coupled with other types of intervention plans (e.g., changes in environmental cues and supports) if the changes were to be maintained.

Process Don'ts

Don't Settle for Second Place in Large Collaborative Disease Endpoint Studies

The shift over the past 30 years from a focus on the treatment of acute illnesses and chronic diseases to chronic disease prevention has led to a role for health behavior change that is central to improving disease rates. The data to support this shift come from large national or international studies in which the behaviors of interest are measured and disease outcomes are tracked. Most of these studies used a medical model approach to behavior change, where individuals were randomized to treatment or observed over time for specific disease outcomes. However, the focus on behavior change has provided opportunities to learn more about the role of behavior and its determinants in large populations samples. For example, the Women's Health Initiative (WHI) serves as a model for how to include social and behavioral scientists both as drivers of procedures for behavior change (e.g., diet change) and as experts in selecting the appropriate measures of a large-scale disease endpoint study, thereby allowing for several key behavioral hypotheses to be tested (Matthews et al., 1997). The WHI measures of interest included multiple psychosocial assessments, including quality of life, depression, sleep disturbance, sexual functioning, and anger and hostility, and the behavioral outcomes of the three major randomized trials were improved health behavior (dietary fat reduction, hormone therapy (HT) adherence, and calcium/vitamin D adherence). Access to these data was shared by behavioral and biomedical scientists, allowing for multiple papers and abstracts to be created through the Behavioral Committee and by psychosocial and behavioral colleagues across the country. Analyses of the WHI data are ongoing, and these data stand as the most integrated source of information on the behavioral and psychosocial aspects of women's health in the world. These resources came about because of the determination of the initial group of social scientists to be included in the process of decision making about what to measure and because of the vision of the WHI Steering Committee members, who recognized that behavior was essentially a key aspect of the study in that all of the key interventions required expertise in behavior change and methods to enhance adherence.

Don't Assume That Policies Are Driven by Good Science

In 1983, the Drug Abuse Resistance Education curriculum (D.A.R.E.) was introduced nationally (U.S. Government Accountability Office, 2003), and it became the most widely used school-based substance abuse prevention program, operating in about 80% of all school districts in the United States (U.S. Government Accountability Office, 2003). There is no centralized accounting of the funds for D.A.R.E., which are provided by a variety of sources, including federal, state, local, and private sources (Shepard, 2001). Estimates of the total funds used for this program vary. D.A.R.E. itself estimates its costs at $215 million annually, which includes more than $41 million in federal funding, according to the Office of National Drug Control Policy (ONDCP) (Shepard, 2001). The main goal of D.A.R.E. is to provide children with information about drug abuse and to teach them the skills to live drug-free lives. In the 1990s, a number of studies were published that concluded that D.A.R.E. is not effective in preventing youth from using drugs and alcohol (U.S. Government Accountability Office, 2003). In 2003, the Government Accounting Office (GAO) published a report that concluded there were no significant differences in illicit drug use between students who had gone through the D.A.R.E. program in the fifth or sixth grade and students in a control group who had not attended D.A.R.E. (U.S. Government Accountability Office, 2003). Further, the D.A.R.E. program had no significant long-term impact on whether youth used illicit drugs, and those who had attended D.A.R.E. and those who had not did not differ significantly in their attitudes toward drug use and in their ability to resist peer pressure. Yet the D.A.R.E. programs continue to receive funding, perhaps because of the influence of law enforcement on funding and policy.

Abstinence-only education in sexual and reproductive health programs is another example of an education program designed to alter risky behaviors that was never tested for efficacy prior to implementation. The funding for abstinence-until-marriage programs comes from federal sources established through the 1996 Welfare Reform Act. The funding comes from the U.S. Department of Health and Human Services and increased steadily, from about $73 million in 2001 to about $158 million in 2005 (U.S. Government Accountability Office, 2006). The program's goal is to reduce the incidence of sexually transmitted diseases and unintended pregnancies. The intervention involves delivering to youth a curriculum that promotes abstaining from sexual intercourse until marriage. The Choosing the Best program (http://www.choosingthebest.org/), which focuses on abstinence, has eight defining characteristics: (1) it teaches the social, psychological, and health gains from abstinence, (2) it promotes abstinence from sexual activity as the standard for all school-age children, (3) it stresses that abstinence is the only certain way to avoid pregnancy, sexually transmitted diseases, and other health problems, (4) it holds out the premise that a mutually faithful monogamous marriage is the standard of human sexual activity, (5) it asserts that sexual activity outside marriage is likely to have harmful effects, (6) it teaches that bearing children out of wedlock is likely to have harmful consequences for the child, the child's parents, and society, (7) it teaches young people how to reject sexual advances and how alcohol and drug use increases vulnerability to sexual advances; and (8) it stresses the importance of attaining self-sufficiency before engaging in sexual activity.

Recently, the GAO reported on the scientific accuracy of materials used in abstinence-until-marriage education programs and their effectiveness (U.S. Government Accountability Office, 2006). The review concluded that some of the materials included in the program were inaccurate about the effectiveness of contraception in preventing sexually transmitted diseases and HIV. The report did not directly address the effectiveness of abstinence programs and noted that the determination of effectiveness was hampered by the lack of scientifically valid evaluations. There is a lack of rigorously conducted research using experimental designs (e.g., intervention and control groups) and of follow-up assessments collected over a long enough time period to allow effects to be assessed reliably (U.S. Government Accountability Office, 2006). Data from a more recent and scientifically rigorous study concluded that abstinence programs are not effective (Trenholm et al., 2007). Young people who had gone through abstinence-only education did not differ in rates of abstinence from sex, number of sexual partners, age of initiation of sexual activities, and rates of unprotected sex from those who had not (Trenholm et al., 2007). Abstinence education program did not reduce the targeted behaviors, and it is unlikely that they reduced the incidence of sexually transmitted diseases and unwanted pregnancies, though these outcomes were not directly assessed as part of the study. Yet, the abstinence program remains the intervention of choice nationally for controlling these critical health issues for youth as expressed in the federal budget for fiscal year 2008, which allocated $204 million to abstinence-only education (White House, 2007).

Don't Assume That Companies Have Public Health Priorities

The phrase "follow the money" as advice for identifying the underlying rationale for an event indicates the power of money as a motivator. Financial motives are often key in explaining the actions of individuals or groups that seek to influence health-related policy. One recent example is the tobacco industry's opposition to the Occupation and Safety Administration Air Indoor Quality Rule (Bryan-Jones & Bero, 2003). This rule was implemented to provide protection through ventilation from secondhand smoke, yet it was withdrawn in 2001 after multiple hearings and efforts by the tobacco industry stalled or derailed the policy process. Using strategies such as continuing to debate and dispute the negative health effects of smoking (which have been publicly and scientifically proven for years) and promoting media coverage of the tobacco industry position, the industry group effectively blocked the rule from taking effect. States, rather than the federal government, now create rules to regulate indoor air policies, though these too have been actively opposed by tobacco industry-affiliated consultants and scientists (Bryan-Jones & Bero, 2003). Though progress on this issue at the state level is promising, ultimately the demise of a national-level policy on this issue makes it more difficult to fight on a coherent and integrated level, thereby weakening the ability of antitobacco advocates to realize health-promoting policies.

This type of influence—for-profit corporations acting in their own best interests and against the best health interests of the public at large—occurs at a global level. For example, Germany's tobacco reduction advocacy system is tangled in a web of tobacco company advocacy groups, resulting in the highest prevalence of tobacco use in Europe (Gruning, Gilmore, & McKee, 2006). Documented relationships between national trade and humanitarian aid policies in developing countries by the tobacco companies effectively blocks tobacco control in developing countries where tobacco use rates are growing (Lawrence & Collin, 2004; Warner, 2005). These international issues highlight the clash between economic gain for some and efforts designed to protect and promote the health of the general population (see chapter 38 for further consideration of this point from an ethical perspective).

Even when the policy is a scientific recommendation for more policy, large corporate organizations may attempt to influence the outcome. For example, two internationally known scientists reported on the U.S. government's efforts, backed and influenced by the major food companies, to influence the United Nation's position on healthy eating and, specifically, to add sugar to both sweet and nonsweet foods (Brownell & Nestle, 2004). The UN report recommended straightforward changes to behavior—eat more fruit and vegetable foods, reduce sugar consumption—to prevent or slow the rising international epidemic of obesity. The U.S. Department of Health and Human Services issued a detailed critique of the UN's report, charging the UN with inaccurate science (Brownell & Nestle, 2004). These food company tactics did not ultimately work, and the policies were carried forward by the UN report and recommended for worldwide acceptance.

Conclusions

We have identified issues that come up in our work and that represent lessons learned from conducting research in health-behavior change and adherence. The research lessons are very different from the process lessons, with the primary distinguishing factor being the level of control individual researchers have over the issues. As researchers exert more control over the issues, we have the opportunity to use science to inform public policy and practice, which can be rewarding for scientists and have positive effects on health outcomes. If we ignore these research lessons, we run the risk of conducting scientific studies that do not take into account all of the evidence and that therefore are not of the highest quality possible. Ignoring environmental influences, for example, will lead us to only partially understand the causes of obesity or tobacco use. This partial understanding may delay our responses to the real and complex issues in public health.

The same level of control, however, is not always possible with regard to some of the process lessons. The last two examples provided suggest that public policies are outside the individual researcher's control. One process lesson deals with allowing special interest groups to set policies (e.g., the focus on DARE and on abstinence). The second lesson deals with the influence of corporate interests on policies. Though individual researchers do not control these types of influences, they can share information and band together to advocate for the use of evidence in setting health policy, and they can conduct research in a way that is directly relevant and accessible to policy makers. These types of lessons are not often taught in scientific or graduate settings and must usually be learned through experience, though some professional societies provide technical assistance on how to link research to policy agendas. For example, learning to anticipate political opposition to specific scientific positions as the science is being published or considered for policy decisions might help scientists to create presentations that are more convincing. Understanding and anticipating the impact of corporations on the public health choices that we wish to influence through our own scientific findings will help us as scientists prepare to counter such opposition.

References

Baquet, C., & Carter-Pokras, O. (2002). What is a "health disparity"? *Public Health Reports, 117,* 426–434.

Board on Population Health and Public Health Practice. (2005). *Estimating the contributions of lifestyle-related factors to preventable death: A workshop summary.* Washington, DC: Institute of Medicine.

Bowen, D. J., Moinpour, C., Thompson, B., Andersen, M. R., Meischke, H., & Cochrane, B. (2008). Creation of a framework for public health intervention design. In S. Miller, D. Bowen, R. Croyle, & J. Rowland (Eds.), *Handbook of behavior and cancer.* Washington, DC: American Psychological Association.

Brownell, K. D., & Nestle, M. (2004, January 23). The sweet and lowdown on sugar. *The New York Times,* p. 23.

Bryan-Jones, K., & Bero, L. A. (2003). Tobacco industry efforts to defeat the occupational safety and health administration indoor air quality rule. *American Journal of Public Health, 93*(4), 585–592.

Celentano, D. D., Sifakis, F., Hylton, J., Torian, L. V., Guillin, V., & Koblin, B. A. (2005). Race/ethnic differences in HIV prevalence and risks among adolescent and young adult men who have sex with men. *Journal of Urban Health, 82*(4), 610–621.

Evelyn, B., Toigo, T., Banks, D., Pohl, D., Gray, K., Robins, B., et al. (2001). *Women's participation in clinical trials and gender-related labeling: A review of new molecular entities approved 1995–1999.* Rockville, MD: Office of Special Health Issues, Office of International and Constituent Relations, Office of the Commissioner, U.S. Food and Drug Administration.

Gerberding, J. L. (2005). Protecting health—the new research imperative. *Journal of the American Medical Association, 294*(11), 1403–1406.

Gruning, T., Gilmore, A. B., & McKee, M. (2006). Tobacco industry influence on science and scientists in Germany. *American Journal of Public Health, 96*(1), 20–32.

Hallfors, D. D., Iritani, B. J., Miller, W. C., & Bauer, D. J. (2007). Sexual and drug behavior patterns and HIV and STD racial disparities: The need for new directions. *American Journal of Public Health, 97*(1), 125–132.

Halpern, C. T., Hallfors, D., Bauer, D. J., Iritani, B., Waller, M. W., & Cho, H. (2004). Implications of racial and gender differences in patterns of adolescent risk behavior for HIV and other sexually transmitted diseases. *Perspectives on Sexual and Reproductive Health, 36*(6), 239–247.

Haynes, S. G. (2000). The role of women in health care and research. In M. B. Goldman & M. C. Hatch (Eds.), *Women and health* (pp. 25–26). San Diego: Academic Press.

Hiatt, R. A., & Rimer, B. K. (1999). A new strategy for cancer control research. *Cancer Epidemiology Biomarkers and Prevention, 8*(11), 957–964.

Lawrence, S., & Collin, J. (2004). Competing with kreteks: Transnational tobacco companies, globalisation, and Indonesia. *Tobacco Control, 13*(Suppl. 2), ii96–ii103.

Matthews, K. A., Shumaker, S. A., Bowen, D. J., Langer, R. D., Hunt, J. R., Kaplan, R. M., et al. (1997). Women's health initiative. Why now? What is it? What's new? *American Psychologist, 52*(2), 101–116.

O'Hea, E. L., Wood, K. B., & Brantley, P. J. (2003). The transtheoretical model: Gender differences across 3 health behaviors. *American Journal of Health Behavior, 27*(6), 645–656.

Peterson, A. V., Jr., Kealey, K. A., Mann, S. L., Marek, P. M., & Sarason, I. G. (2000). Hutchinson Smoking Prevention Project: Long-term randomized trial in school-based tobacco use prevention—results on smoking. *Journal of the National Cancer Institute, 92*(24), 1979–1991.

Ranney, L., Melvin, C., Lux, L., McClain, E., Morgan, L., & Lohr, K. N. (2006). Tobacco use: Prevention, cessation, and control. *Evidence Report Technology Assessment (Full Report)* 140, 1–120.

Shepard, I. E. M. (2001). *The economic costs of D.A.R.E.* Research Paper Number 22. Syracuse, NY: Le Moyne College, Institute of Industrial Relations.

Sowden, A., Arblaster, L., & Stead, L. (2003). Community interventions for preventing smoking in young people. *Cochrane Database of Systematic Reviews, 1,* CD001291.

Thomas, R., & Perera, R. (2006). School-based programmes for preventing smoking. *Cochrane Database of Systematic Reviews, 3,* CD001293.

Tinker, A., Finn, K., & Epp, J. (2000). *Improving women's health: Issues & interventions.* Washington, DC.: World Bank.

Trenholm, C., Devaney, B., Fortson, K., Quay, L., Wheeler, J., & Clark, M. (2007). *Impacts of four Title V, Section 510 abstinence education programs.* Princeton, NJ: Mathematica Policy Research.

U.S. Government Accountability Office. (2001). *Drug safety: Most drugs withdrawn in recent years had greater health risks for women.* Retrieved from http://www.gao.gov/new.items/ d01754.pdf

U.S. Government Accountability Office. (2003). *Youth illicit drug use prevention: DARE long-term evaluations and federal efforts to identify effective programs.* Retrieved from http:// www.gao.gov/new.items/d03172r.pdf

U.S. Government Accountability Office. (2006). *Abstinence education: Efforts to assess the accuracy and effectiveness of federally funded programs.* Retrieved from http://www.gao.gov/ new.items/d0787.pdf

Warner, K. E. (2005). The role of research in international tobacco control. *American Journal of Public Health, 95*(6), 976–984.

White House. (2007). *2008 budget fact sheets.* Retrieved September 29, 2007, from http://www. whitehouse.gov/infocus/budget/BudgetFY2008.pdf

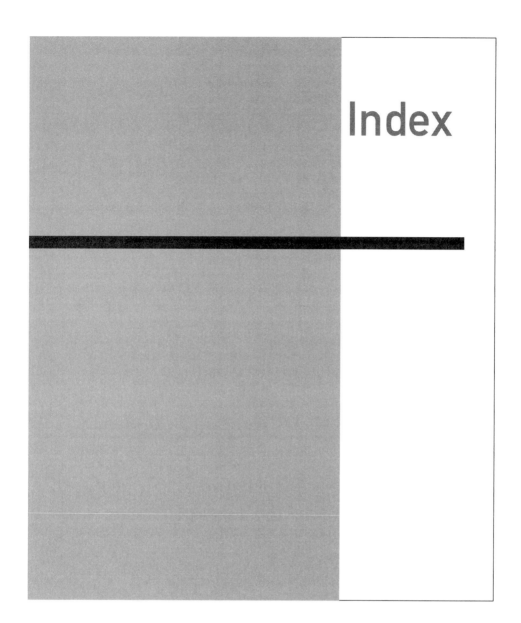

Index

SPRINGER PUBLISHING COMPANY

An Introduction to the US Health Care System

Sixth Edition

Steven Jonas, MD, MPH, FACPM
Raymond L. Goldsteen, DrPH
Karen Goldsteen, PhD, MPH

Completely expanded and updated to account for the latest changes in the U.S. health care system, this bestselling text remains the most concise and balanced introduction to the domestic health care system. Like its predecessors, it provides an accessible overview of the basic components of the system: health care personnel, hospitals and other institutions, the federal government, financing and payment mechanisms, and managed care. Finally, it provides an insightful look at the prospects for health care reform.

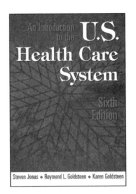

Steven Jonas, a revered expert in public health, has enlisted his colleagues, Drs. Raymond and Karen Goldsteen, to add their expertise in public health, health policy, and management to this outstanding volume. All students of health care administration and policy, as well as practicing health professionals who simply want a relatively brief overview of the system, will find it useful.

Partial Table of Contents

Health Care Systems • U.S. Health Care System • Future of the U.S. Health Care System • Health Care Workforce • Physicians • Nursing • Physicians' Assistants • Health Care Workforce Outside the Hospital and Physician Office

Hospitals and Other Health Care Institutions • Hospital Structure • Public General Hospitals • The Hospital in the Present Era • Long-Term Care: The Example of Nursing Homes • Primary and Ambulatory Care • Primary Care • Ambulatory Care

Government and the Health Care System • The Constitutional Basis of Government Authority in Health Care • The Health Care Functions of Government • The Federal Government and the Provision of Health Services • State Governments' Role in Health Services • Local Governments' Role in Health Services • Problems in Public Health

Financing and Payment of Health Care • How Much Is Spent • Where the Money Comes From, Within the System • Where the Money Goes • How the Money Is Paid Out: Providers, Payers, and Payments • Equity of Health Care • Efficiency of Health Care • A National Scorecard

2007 · 328pp · Softcover · 978-0-8261-0214-0

11 West 42nd Street, New York, NY 10036-8002 • **Fax: 212-941-7842**
Order Toll-Free: 877-687-7476 • **Order Online: www.springerpub.com**

SPRINGER PUBLISHING COMPANY

Toward Equity in Health

A New Global Approach to Health Disparities

Barbara C. Wallace, PhD, Editor

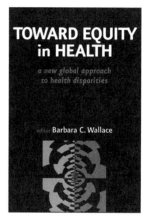

"This is quite possibly the most comprehensive examination of health disparities written in the last two decades. Wallace and her colleagues have contributed a body of work that will engage scholars, advocates, policy makers, and educators. More importantly, however, it will challenge conventional thinking about disparities and offer a body of work rich in the material from which a new paradigm for health, equity, and human rights will be constructed."

—**Robert E. Fullilove,** EdD, Professor of Clinical Sociomedical Sciences
Associate Dean for Community and Minority Affairs ,
Mailman School of Public Health, Columbia University

"Dr. Wallace's edited collection provides a comprehensive and compelling overview of the new interdisciplinary scholarship on health equity. It's recommended for students, researchers, and practitioners in public health, social science and other health-related disciplines."

—**Nicholas Freudenberg,** DrPH , Distinguished Professor of Public Health
Hunter College and Graduate Center, City University of New York

Partial Contents:

PART 1: New Theory, Paradigms, and Perspectives • **PART 2:** New Procedures and Policies—Implications for Funders, Researcheers, and Policy Makers • **PART 3:** The Legacy and Role of Racism—Implications and Recommendations for Research and Practice

PART 4: Collaborations, Partnerships, and Community-Based Participatory Research • **PART 5:** New Internet Technology—Achieving Wide Dissemination and Global Rearch • **PART 6:** Training Community Health Workers and Peer Educators

PART 7: Closing Gaps in Health for Special Populations • **PART 8:** Closing the Education and Health Gaps—Addressing Dual Inter-Related Disparities Through Effective Engagement

2007 · 592 pp · Hardcover · 978-0-8261-0313-0

11 West 42nd Street, New York, NY 10036-8002 • Fax: 212-941-7842
Order Toll-Free: 877-687-7476 • Order Online: www.springerpub.com

SPRINGER PUBLISHING COMPANY

Solving Life's Problems
A 5-Step Guide to Enhanced Well-Being

Arthur M. Nezu, PhD, ABPP
Christine Maguth Nezu, PhD, ABPP
Thomas D'Zurilla, PhD

Yes, You Can! Learn How to:
- Cope Better with Stressful Life Problems and Circumstances
- Increase Your Ability to Stick with a Diet or Lifestyle Change
- Decrease Emotional Stress
- Improve Your Personal Relationships.

Guided by an easy, new 5-step program called ADAPT, these life changes ARE possible!

ADAPT is based on a proven-effective method of behavioral intervention called Problem-Solving Therapy (PST), and is simple enough to apply to even the busiest schedules.

The ADAPT Method 5 Little Steps To Solving Life's Big Problems
1. Attitude: Enhancing Your Problem-Solving Capacity
2. Defining Your Problem and Setting Realistic Goals
3. Being Creative in Problem Solving
4. Predicting the Consequences and Developing a Solution Plan
5. Trying Out Your Solution and Determining if It Works

If you are searching for enhanced well-being, the ADAPT method will quickly steer you in the right direction, and provide the lifelong skills you need to better define the problems you may be facing, choose effective solutions, and improve the quality of your life.

2006 · 124pp · Softcover · 978-0-8261-1489-1

11 West 42nd Street, New York, NY 10036-8002 • **Fax: 212-941-7842**
Order Toll-Free: 877-687-7476 • **Order Online: www.springerpub.com**